With more than 2.5 million copies of their bestselling *Counter* books in print, Annette Natow and Jo-Ann Heslin have provided American consumers with the very best references for informed eating, food shopping and restaurant dining. Now these nutrition experts present the ultimate encyclopedia of food values—in a one-volume, easy-to-use reference that answers every question about eating.

THE MOST COMPLETE FOOD COUNTER

- MORE nutrient values than any other counter book available

- MORE thorough, up-to-date nutritional values listed

- MORE reliable for anyone seeking sound nutrition information

- MORE restaurant chains represented

- MORE take-out items

- MORE important folic acid values

- MORE than just nutritional counts—including an extensive A to Z dictionary of easy-to-understand nutrition terms, to help you make sense of the news.

Books by Annette B. Natow and Jo-Ann Heslin

The Antioxidant Vitamin Counter
The Calorie Counter
The Cholesterol Counter (Fifth Edition)
The Diabetes Carbohydrate and Calorie Counter
Eating Out Food Counter
The Fat Attack Plan
The Fat Counter (Fourth Edition)
The Food Shopping Counter
Megadoses
No-Nonsense Nutrition for Kids
The Pocket Encyclopedia of Nutrition
The Pocket Fat Counter (Second Edition)
The Pocket Protein Counter
The Pregnancy Nutrition Counter
The Protein Counter
The Sodium Counter
The Supermarket Nutrition Counter (Second Edition)

Published by POCKET BOOKS

For orders other than by individual consumers, Pocket Books grants a discount on the purchase of **10 or more** copies of single titles for special markets or premium use. For further details, please write to the Vice President of Special Markets, Pocket Books, 1230 Avenue of the Americas, 9th Floor, New York, NY 10020-1586.

For information on how individual consumers can place orders, please write to Mail Order Department, Simon & Schuster Inc., 100 Front Street, Riverside, NJ 08075.

THE MOST COMPLETE FOOD COUNTER

ANNETTE B. NATOW, PH.D., R.D.
JO-ANN HESLIN, M.A., R.D.

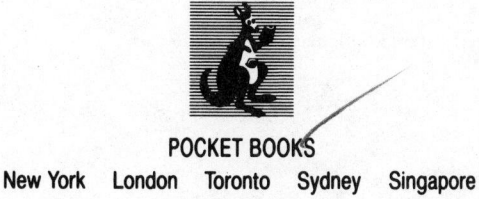

POCKET BOOKS
New York   London   Toronto   Sydney   Singapore

The authors and publisher of this book are not physicians and are not licensed to give medical advice. The information in this book has been collected for the convenience of the reader. The nutrient values for prepared foods are subject to change and might currently vary from listings herein, which are based on research conducted in 1998. Such information does not constitute a recommendation or endorsement of any individual, institution, or product, nor is it intended as a substitute for personalized consultation with your physician. The authors and publisher disclaim any liability arising directly or indirectly from the use of this book.

Information from food labels, manufacturers, and processors. The values are based on research conducted through the first half of 1998. Manufacturers' ingredients are subject to change and may vary in different regions, so current values may differ from those listed in this book.

An *Original* Publication of POCKET BOOKS

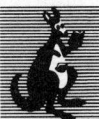

POCKET BOOKS, a division of Simon & Schuster Inc.
1230 Avenue of the Americas, New York, NY 10020

Copyright © 1999 by Annette Natow and Jo-Ann Heslin

Library of Congress Cataloging-in-Publication Data

Natow, Annette B.
    The most complete food counter / Annette B. Natow, Jo-Ann Heslin.
        p.   cm.
    ISBN 0–671–02561–9
    1. Food—Composition—Tables.   I. Heslin, Jo-Ann.   II. Title
TX551.N3964   1999
613.2′8—dc21   99-17169
                                                   CIP

ISBN: 0-671-02561-9

First Pocket Books trade paperback printing March 1999

10 9 8 7 6 5 4 3 2

Cover photo by FoodPix

Text design by C. Linda Dingler

Printed in the U.S.A.

To our families
who support us through every project:
Harry, Allen, Irene, Sarah, Meryl, Marty, Laura,
George, Emily, Steven, Joseph, Kristen and Karen.

". . . foods, though so numerous and so varied in form,
can be reduced to rather simple terms."

MARY SWARTZ ROSE, PH.D.
Feeding the Family
The Macmillan Company, 1919

ACKNOWLEDGMENTS

Without the tireless cooperation of Steven Natow, M.D. and Stephen Llano, *The Most Complete Food Counter* would never have been completed. A special thanks to our insightful and supportive agent, Nancy Trichter, and our wonderfully perceptive editor, Jane Cavolina.

Our thanks also to all the food manufacturers who graciously shared their data.

DO YOU KNOW...

Which fruit has more vitamin C than an orange?

Which foods enhance your sexual drive?

Which herb has been shown to help depression?

Which vitamin protects against birth defects?

Why your eyes tear when you peel an onion?

Which spice relieves motion sickness?

Which vitamin can reduce cholesterol?

Which beans may help prevent breast cancer?

What substances in wine reduce the risk of heart disease?

Which form of vitamin E is best for you?

Which common drink, other than milk, makes your teeth stronger?

That taking medication with grapefruit juice can be dangerous?

CONTENTS

INTRODUCTION

Calories, fat, protein, carbohydrate, fiber, calcium, sodium, potassium, vitamins A, C and folic acid—the list of these nutrients is long. Because your body is working all the time (even when you are sleeping), you need a source of calories and other nutrients to keep you going. It's reassuring to know that you can get all of them in the foods you enjoy. Different foods have different assortments of nutrients; some foods, like meat and cheese, are high in protein; others, like milk and yogurt, have lots of calcium. Fruits and vegetables are good sources of vitamins and fiber. When you eat a variety of foods, you get all the nutrients you need. *The Most Complete Food Counter* will help you make sure that you do. It is the most comprehensive nutrition resource, listing nutrition values for over 21,000 foods along with a dictionary that explains nutrition terms in simple language.

Calories

You get calories from the fat, protein, and carbohydrate in foods. Fat has the most calories of the three, more than twice as many as protein and carbohydrate. One teaspoon of olive oil (fat) has 40 calories, while a teaspoon of either sugar (carbohydrate) or unsweetened gelatin (protein) has only 16 calories.

Most men need about 2,400 calories a day, while most women need as few as 1,800. If a person is very active, calorie intake can go as high as 3,900 for men and 3,000 for women. Very few people need this many calories. (See also page 819).

Fat

Eating too much fat is not healthy. But some fat is needed by the body. How do you figure out how much to eat? A government recommendation, the Daily Value (DV) for a 2,000-calorie diet, is 65 grams or less of fat a day. As a rule of thumb, if you are an average-weight, moderately active adult, and you want a benchmark for your total fat grams each day, simply divide your weight in half.

It's not always easy to tell if a food is high in fat by looking at it. Some visible fat can be seen on slices of roast beef or bacon or in foods like butter, margarine, and oil. But in many foods—like milk, eggs, cheese, avocados, pastries, and nuts—the fat is not so obvious. That's when *The Most Complete Food Counter* comes in handy. (See also page 823).

Saturated Fat (Sat fat)

Saturated fats are solid fats found in meat, butter, ice cream, and margarine. Most saturated fats raise the body's cholesterol level; others, like some of the saturated fat in chocolate and beef, do not. People with high cholesterol levels are at greater risk for a heart attack. Research suggests that saturated fat may also increase the risk for ovarian cancer in women. The government recommendation, the Daily Value (DV) for a 2,000-calorie diet, is 20 grams or less of saturated fat a day. (See also page 835).

Cholesterol (Chol)

Although the body needs cholesterol to function normally, when the blood level gets too high it's not healthy. Some of the cholesterol can be deposited in the arteries, narrowing them and interfering with normal blood flow. Cholesterol can be made in the body. Strict vegetarians, who eat no animal foods, make all the cholesterol they need. Most experts suggest that people limit their cholesterol intake to 300 milligrams or less a day. (See also page 820)

Protein

Protein is in every cell and substance in the body except for urine and bile (a digestive juice). It is used for growth, repair, and replacement of cells worn out in daily living. Most experts recommend a protein intake of 51 to 64 grams a day for a woman weighing 140 pounds and 62 to 77 grams for a man weighing 170 pounds. As high protein foods are popular, many people eat much more than that amount. (See also page 834).

Carbohydrate (Carbo)

Carbohydrates include sugars, starches, and fiber. A healthy intake is between 50 and 60 percent of the calories eaten. In a 2,000-calorie diet that would be 250 to 300 grams of carbohydrate. But only a small portion of that, 50 to 60 grams, should come from sugar in sweets. (See also page 819).

Fiber

Fiber is the part of plants that is not digested. Adequate fiber helps you avoid constipation, control weight, lower cholesterol, and protects against some cancers. The average fiber intake of Americans is about 15 grams a day, which is only one-half of the 25 to 30 grams recommended by experts. (See also page 824).

Calcium

There is more calcium in the body than any other mineral, about two pounds in the average person. Adequate calcium through the growing years is needed to build strong bones to help protect against fractures later in life. The government recommended Adequate Intake (AI) for calcium is 1,000 milligrams a day for adults aged 19 to 50 and 1,200 milligrams for those 51 and over. The average daily intake of calcium is only about one-half of this amount. (See also page 819).

Sodium (Sod)

Sodium is an important mineral in the body, but there is slight danger of getting too little of it. Almost all foods contain sodium, either naturally or as added salt. Table salt is a mixture of sodium and chloride, another mineral. Americans, on average, eat two to three teaspoons of salt a day. That's equal to 4,000 to 6,000 milligrams of sodium. This is about twice the recommended Daily Value (DV) of less than 2,400 milligrams. (See also page 836)

Potassium (Potas)

Potassium is a mineral with important roles in the body. Adequate potassium may lower blood pressure. Some medicines (diuretics or "water pills") used to treat high blood pressure may cause potassium to be lost from the body. Laxative use over a long time can do this also. Foods high in potassium may be suggested to compensate for the loss, sometimes along with a supplement. The recommended Daily Value (DV) for potassium is 3,500 milligrams. Americans average about 3,000 milligrams a day. (See also page 834)

Vitamin C (Vit C)

The Recommended Daily Allowance (RDA) for vitamin C is 60 milligrams a day. Americans average an intake of over 100 milligrams. An intake of 200 milligrams of the vitamin saturates the body so that any extra vitamin C is passed out of the body in urine. Doses of over 2 grams may cause diarrhea. Smoking increases the need for vitamin C, and it is recommended that smokers have 100 milligrams of the vitamin each day. (See also page 839).

Folic Acid (Folic)

One of the B vitamins, folic acid protects against some birth defects. It also reduces blood levels of a protein, homocysteine, that is believed to be a risk factor for heart disease. The Recommended Dietary Allowance (RDA) for folic acid is 400 micrograms for those aged 14 and older, with higher levels during pregnancy and breastfeeding. Americans' average intake of folic acid is about 300 micrograms. (See also page 824).

Vitamin A (Vit A)

The active form of vitamin A is found only in animal foods like eggs, milk, cheese, and fish liver oils (cod, halibut) that are taken as supplements. Beta-carotene in dark, leafy vegetables and yellow fruits and vegetables can be converted to active vitamin A in the body. Vitamin A is needed for healthy eyes and skin, for normal bone growth and reproduction, and aids immune function. The Recommended Dietary Allowance (RDA) for vitamin A is 5,000 International Units (IU) a day for males 11 and older and 4,000 IUs a day for females 11 and older. The RDA for children is lower, ranging from 1,875 IU for infants to 3,500 for those 7 to 10. (See also page 838).

USING YOUR MOST COMPLETE FOOD COUNTER

The Most Complete Food Counter lists the calories, fat, saturated fat, cholesterol, protein, carbohydrate, fiber, calcium, sodium, potassium, vitamins A, C, and folic acid in more than 21,000 foods. These are key nutrients for you to consider when you are choosing foods. Fat, saturated fat, cholesterol, and sodium are nutrients you may want to limit. You can be more liberal with the others, aiming for moderate amounts of protein and higher amounts of the rest. Recommended intake for all nutrients counted is described in the introduction. There are still other nutrients needed for good health, but when you eat a variety of foods containing the nutrients listed in this counter, you will automatically get the other necessary nutrients along with them.

Now you will be able to compare your usual food selections with others that are available so you can make the best choices. With this information at your fingertips, you'll find it easy to have a healthier diet. For example, when you want to select pizza, look up the pizza category on page 459. You will see over 155 listed so you can find one that is best for you. Please note that a dash (—) appears in many entries. A dash simply means that analysis was not done for that nutrient. It is not the same as a "0," which indicates that there is none of the nutrient in that food.

The Most Complete Food Counter has foods listed alphabetically. For each category, you will find nonbranded (generic) foods are listed first in alphabetical order, followed by an alphabetical listing of brand-name foods. The nonbranded listing will help you determine values for foods when you do not find your favorite brand listed. They also help you to evaluate generic and store brands. Large categories are divided into subcategories such as canned, fresh, frozen, and refrigerated to make it easier to find what you are looking for. Many categories have take-out and home recipe subcategories. Look there for foods you take-out or order in a store or restaurant because these foods are not nutrition labeled.

The Most Complete Food Counter is divided into three sections. Part One, Brand Name, Nonbranded (Generic) and Take-Out Foods; Part Two, Restaurant Chains; and Part Three, All the Facts A to Z, a nutrition dictionary to help you understand all the terms you read and hear about.

Most foods are listed alphabetically. But, in some cases, foods are grouped by category. For example, a tuna salad sandwich and tuna salad are found under the category TUNA DISHES. Other group categories include:

DEFINITIONS

as prep (as prepared): refers to food that has been prepared according to package directions

home recipe: describes homemade dishes; those included can be used as a guide to similar products you may prepare or take-out food you buy ready-to-eat

lean and fat: describes meat with some fat on its edges that is not cut away before cooking, or poultry prepared with skin and fat as purchased

lean only: lean portion, trimmed of all visible fat

shelf stable: refers to prepared products found on the supermarket shelf that are ready-to-eat or to be heated and do not require refrigeration

take-out: describes prepared dishes that you purchase ready-to-eat; those included serve as a guide to similar products you may purchase

ABBREVIATIONS AND MEASURES

avg = average
diam = diameter
fl = fluid
frzn = frozen
g = gram
in = inch
lb = pound
lg = large
med = medium
mg = milligram
oz = ounce
pkg = package
pt = pint
prep = prepared
qt = quart
reg = regular
sec = second
serv = serving
sm = small
sq = square
tbsp = tablespoon
tr = trace
tsp = teaspoon
w/ = with
w/o = without
< = less than

EQUIVALENT MEASURES

1 tablespoon	=	3 teaspoons
4 tablespoons	=	¼ cup
8 tablespoons	=	½ cup
12 tablespoons	=	¾ cup
16 tablespoons	=	1 cup
1000 milligrams	=	1 gram
28 grams	=	1 ounce

LIQUID MEASURE

2 tablespoons	=	1 ounce
¼ cup	=	2 ounces
½ cup	=	4 ounces
¾ cup	=	6 ounces
1 cup	=	8 ounces
2 cups	=	1 pint
4 cups	=	1 quart

DRY MEASURE

4 ounces	=	¼ pound
8 ounces	=	½ pound
12 ounces	=	¾ pound
16 ounces	=	1 pound

NOTES

Discrepancies in figures are due to rounding, product reformulation, and reevaluation. Labeling law allows rounding of values. Because most of the data is analysis data, obtained directly from manufacturers and not from labels, in some cases our values may not be exactly the same as label information because they have not been rounded.

All FAT values of foods are given in grams (g).

All saturated fat (SAT FAT) values are given in grams (g).

All cholesterol (CHOL) values are given in milligrams (mg).

All PROTEIN values are given in grams (g).

All carbohydrate (CARBO) values are given in grams (g).

All FIBER values are given in grams (g).

All CALCIUM values are given in milligrams (mg).

All sodium (SOD) values are given in milligrams (mg).

All potassium (POTAS) values are given in milligrams (mg).

All vitamin C (VIT C) values are given in milligrams (mg).

All folic acid (FOLIC) values are given in micrograms (mcg).

All vitamin A (VIT A) values are given in International Units (IUs).

tr (trace) is the value used when a food contains less than one calorie, less than one gram of fat, saturated fat, protein, carbohydrate or fiber, less than one milligram of cholesterol, calcium, sodium, potassium or vitamin C, less than one microgram of folic acid, or less than one International Unit of vitamin A.

A dash (—) indicates data was not available.

0 (zero) indicates that there is none of the nutrient in that food.

PART ONE

BRAND NAME, NONBRANDED (GENERIC) AND TAKE-OUT FOODS

FOOD	PORTION	CALORIES	FAT	SAT FAT	CHOL	PROTEIN	CARBO	FIBER	CALCIUM	SOD	POTAS	VIT C	FOLIC	VIT A
ABALONE														
fresh fried	3 oz	161	6	1	80	17	9	—	32	502	—	—	5	—
raw	3 oz	89	1	tr	72	15	5	—	27	255	—	—	4	—
ACEROLA														
fresh	1	2	tr	—	0	tr	tr	—	1	0	7	81	—	37
ACEROLA JUICE														
juice	1 cup	51	1	—	0	1	12	—	24	7	235	3872	—	1232
ADZUKI BEANS														
canned sweetened	1 cup	702	tr	—	0	11	163	—	66	646	353	—	—	—
dried cooked	1 cup	294	tr	—	0	17	57	—	63	18	1224	0	—	13
yokan sliced	3¼ in slices	112	tr	—	0	1	26	—	12	36	19	—	—	—
EDEN														
Organic	½ cup (4.6 oz)	110	0	0	0	7	19	5	40	10	250	—	—	—
ALE														
(*see* BEER AND ALE, and MALT)														
ALFALFA														
sprouts	1 cup	40	tr	tr	0	1	1	—	10	2	26	3	12	51
sprouts	1 tbsp	1	tr	tr	0	tr	tr	—	1	0	2	tr	1	5
ALLSPICE														
ground	1 tsp	5	tr	tr	0	tr	1	—	13	1	20	1	—	10
ALMONDS														
almond butter honey & cinnamon	1 tbsp	96	8	1	0	3	4	—	43	2	120	tr	10	0
almond butter w/ salt	1 tbsp	101	9	1	0	2	3	—	43	75	121	tr	10	0
almond butter w/o salt	1 tbsp	101	10	1	0	2	3	—	43	2	121	tr	10	0
almond meal	1 oz	116	5	tr	0	11	8	—	120	2	390	—	—	0
almond paste	1 oz	127	8	1	0	3	12	—	65	3	184	tr	16	0
dried blanched	1 oz	166	15	1	0	6	5	—	70	3	213	tr	11	0
dried unblanched	1 oz	167	15	1	0	6	6	—	75	3	208	tr	16	0
dry roasted unblanched	1 oz	167	15	1	0	5	7	—	80	3	219	tr	18	0
dry roasted unblanched salted	1 oz	167	15	1	0	5	7	—	80	260	219	tr	18	0
oil roasted blanched salted	1 oz	174	16	2	0	5	5	—	55	3	197	tr	18	0
oil roasted unblanched	1 oz	176	16	2	0	6	5	—	66	3	194	tr	18	0
BEER NUTS														
Almonds	1 pkg (1 oz)	180	14	—	0	5	7	—	8	51	—	—	—	—
DOLE														
Blanched Slivered	1 oz	170	14	—	0	6	5	—	—	4	—	—	—	—
Blanched Whole	1 oz	170	14	—	0	6	5	—	—	4	—	—	—	—

FOOD	PORTION	CALORIES	FAT	SAT FAT	CHOL	PROTEIN	CARBO	FIBER	CALCIUM	SOD	POTAS	VIT C	FOLIC	VIT A
DOLE (CONT.)														
Chopped Natural	1 oz	170	14	—	0	6	5	—	—	4	—	—	—	—
Sliced Natural	1 oz	170	14	—	0	6	5	—	—	4	—	—	—	—
Whole Natural	1 oz	170	14	—	0	6	5	—	—	4	—	—	—	—
HAIN														
Almond Butter Natural Raw	2 tbsp	190	18	2	0	8	3	—	80	120	—	0	—	0
Almond Butter Toasted	2 tbsp	220	19	2	0	8	3	—	80	210	—	0	—	0
LANCE														
Smoked	1 pkg (0.7 oz)	120	11	1	0	6	3	—	20	130	75	—	—	—
NUTELLA														
Spread	1 tbsp (0.5 oz)	85	5	—	0	1	9	—	20	5	—	—	—	—
PLANTERS														
Almonds	1 oz	170	15	1	0	6	5	3	60	0	190	—	—	—
Gold Measure Slivered	1 pkg (2 oz)	340	31	3	0	12	11	4	150	0	390	—	—	—
Honey Roasted	1 oz	160	14	1	0	5	7	2	60	190	165	—	—	—
AMARANTH														
(see also CEREAL, COOKIES)														
uncooked	1 cup (6.8 oz)	729	13	3	0	28	129	30	298	41	714	8	96	0
ARROWHEAD														
Seeds	¼ cup (1.6 oz)	170	2	1	0	7	29	3	80	0	170	0	—	0
HEALTH VALLEY														
Fast Menu Amaranth With Garden Vegetables	7½ oz	140	3	—	0	8	16	8	43	140	100	5	10	5010
ANASAZI BEANS														
ARROWHEAD														
Dried	¼ cup (1.5 oz)	150	1	0	0	10	27	9	60	0	460	0	—	0
BEAN CUISINE														
Dried	½ cup	115	1	—	0	8	—	5	—	5	310	—	62	—
ANCHOVY														
CANNED														
in oil	1 can (1.6 oz)	95	4	1	—	13	0	—	104	1651	245	—	—	—
in oil	5	42	2	tr	—	6	0	—	46	734	109	—	—	—
FRESH														
fillets	3 (0.4 oz)	21	1	—	—	2	tr	—	20	—	—	0	—	0
raw	3 oz	62	4	1	—	17	0	—	125	88	325	—	—	—
ANISE														
seed	1 tsp	7	tr	—	0	tr	1	—	14	tr	30	—	—	—
ANTELOPE														
roasted	3 oz	127	2	1	107	25	0	—	4	46	316	—	—	—

APPLE

FOOD	PORTION	CALORIES	FAT	SAT FAT	CHOL	PROTEIN	CARBO	FIBER	CALCIUM	SOD	POTAS	VIT C	FOLIC	VIT A
CANNED														
sliced sweetened	1 cup	136	1	tr	0	tr	34	—	4	7	138	1	1	103
DRIED														
cooked w/ sugar	½ cup	116	tr	tr	0	tr	29	—	4	27	137	1	—	22
cooked w/o sugar	½ cup	172	tr	tr	0	tr	20	—	4	26	134	1	0	22
rings	10	155	tr	tr	0	1	42	—	9	56	288	3	—	0
DEL MONTE														
Sliced	⅓ cup (1.4 oz)	80	0	0	0	0	23	5	0	310	—	1	—	0
SONOMA														
Pieces	10-12 pieces (1.4 oz)	110	0	0	0	0	29	4	0	0	—	2	—	0
FRESH														
w/o skin sliced & cooked	1 cup	91	tr	tr	0	tr	23	—	8	1	150	tr	1	75
w/o skin sliced & microwaved	1 cup	96	tr	tr	0	tr	25	—	8	1	159	tr	1	68
DOLE														
Apple	1	80	1	—	0	0	18	5	—	0	170	—	—	—
TASTEE														
Candy Apple	1 (3 oz)	160	5	2	0	3	26	4	—	20	—	4	—	0
Caramel Apple	1 (3 oz)	160	5	2	0	3	26	4	—	20	—	4	—	0
FROZEN														
sliced w/o sugar	½ cup	41	tr	tr	0	tr	11	—	4	3	67	tr	1	29
MRS. PAUL'S														
Apple Fritters	2	270	9	—	5	4	35	—	20	500	—	9	—	—
STOUFFER'S														
Escalloped	1 cup (6 oz)	180	3	0	0	0	37	3	0	70	130	48	—	0

APPLE JUICE

FOOD	PORTION	CALORIES	FAT	SAT FAT	CHOL	PROTEIN	CARBO	FIBER	CALCIUM	SOD	POTAS	VIT C	FOLIC	VIT A
frzn as prep	1 cup	111	tr	tr	0	tr	28	—	14	17	301	1	1	—
frzn not prep	6 oz	349	1	tr	0	1	87	—	43	54	945	4	2	—
AFTER THE FALL														
Organic	1 bottle (10 oz)	110	0	0	0	0	28	—	0	25	300	0	—	0
Vermont Apple	1 bottle (10 oz)	110	0	0	0	1	27	—	0	24	300	1	—	0
Vermont Apple	1 bottle (8 oz)	90	0	0	0	0	22	—	0	20	240	0	—	0
Vermont Harvest Moon Sparkling Apple Cider	8 fl oz	110	0	0	0	1	27	—	0	5	—	9	—	0
APPLE & EVE														
Cider	6 fl oz	80	0	0	0	0	16	—	9	0	188	0	—	76
Juice	6 fl oz	80	0	0	0	0	16	—	9	0	188	0	—	76
Nothin' But Juice	6 fl oz	78	0	0	0	0	18	—	7	0	154	1	—	161
BRUCE														
Lite	½ cup	88	0	0	0	tr	20	—	—	25	—	9	—	6000

FOOD	PORTION	CALORIES	FAT	SAT FAT	CHOL	PROTEIN	CARBO	FIBER	CALCIUM	SOD	POTAS	VIT C	FOLIC	VIT A
EVERFRESH														
Apple Juice	1 can (8 oz)	110	0	0	0	0	29	0	—	10	—	—	—	—
HI-C														
Jammin' Apple	8 fl oz	130	0	0	0	0	31	—	—	30	—	60	—	—
HOOD														
Select Cider	1 cup (8 oz)	120	0	0	0	0	30	—	—	2	—	—	—	—
MINUTE MAID														
Box	8.45 fl oz	120	0	0	0	0	29	—	—	30	—	—	—	—
Juices To Go	1 can (11.5 fl oz)	160	0	0	0	0	40	—	—	40	—	—	—	—
Juices To Go	1 bottle (10 fl oz)	140	0	0	0	0	35	—	—	35	—	—	—	—
Juices To Go	1 bottle (16 fl oz)	110	0	0	0	0	28	—	—	30	—	—	—	—
Naturals	8 fl oz	110	0	0	0	0	28	—	—	30	—	—	—	—
MOTT'S														
From Concentrate as prep	8 fl oz	120	0	0	0	0	29	0	0	20	250	2	—	0
Fruit Basket Cocktail as prep	8 fl oz	120	0	0	0	0	29	0	20	5	300	15	—	0
Natural	8 fl oz	120	0	0	0	0	29	0	0	20	250	2	—	0
OCEAN SPRAY														
100% Juice	8 fl oz	110	0	0	0	0	28	0	—	35	240	0	—	0
ODWALLA														
Live Apple	8 fl oz	140	0	0	0	0	34	0	0	25	—	1	—	0
RED CHEEK														
From Concentrate	8 fl oz	120	0	0	0	0	29	0	0	20	250	2	—	0
Natural	8 fl oz	120	0	0	0	0	29	0	0	20	250	2	—	0
SENECA														
Clarifed frzn, as prep	8 fl oz	120	0	0	0	0	30	0	0	24	245	60	—	0
Granny Smith frzn as prep	8 fl oz	120	0	0	0	0	30	0	0	24	315	60	—	0
Natural frzn as prep	8 fl oz	120	0	0	0	0	30	0	0	24	245	60	—	0
SIPPIN' PAK														
100% Pure	8.45 fl oz	110	0	0	0	0	28	—	—	25	240	—	—	—
SNAPPLE														
Apple Crisp	10 fl oz	140	0	0	0	0	36	—	0	30	—	0	—	0
TREE OF LIFE														
East Coast Apple	8 fl oz	120	0	0	0	tr	30	—	—	25	—	4	—	—
TROPICANA														
Season's Best	8 fl oz	110	0	0	0	0	28	—	—	10	200	—	—	—
Season's Best	1 container (6 fl oz)	80	0	0	0	0	21	—	—	5	150	—	—	—
Season's Best	1 container (8 fl oz)	110	0	0	0	0	28	—	—	10	200	—	—	—

FOOD	PORTION	CALORIES	FAT	SAT FAT	CHOL	PROTEIN	CARBO	FIBER	CALCIUM	SOD	POTAS	VIT C	FOLIC	VIT A
TROPICANA (CONT.)														
Season's Best	1 container (10 fl oz)	140	0	0	0	0	35	—	—	15	250	—	—	—
Season's Best	1 can (11.5 fl oz)	160	0	0	0	0	40	—	—	25	280	—	—	—
Season's Best	1 bottle (10 fl oz)	140	0	0	0	0	35	—	—	15	250	—	—	—
Season's Best	1 bottle (7 fl oz)	100	0	0	0	0	24	—	—	10	175	—	—	—
VERYFINE														
100% Juice	1 bottle (10 oz)	150	0	0	0	0	38	0	0	20	—	2	—	0
Juice-Ups	8 fl oz	120	0	0	0	0	30	0	0	35	—	60	—	0
APPLESAUCE														
MOTT'S														
Chunky	5 oz	110	0	0	0	0	26	2	0	0	90	1	—	0
Cinnamon	5 oz	120	0	0	0	0	29	1	0	0	85	2	—	0
Fruit Snacks Apple Spice	4 oz	70	0	0	0	0	18	1	0	0	95	2	—	0
Fruit Snacks Cinnamon	4 oz	90	0	0	0	0	23	1	0	0	70	1	—	0
Fruit Snacks Sweetened	4 oz	90	0	0	0	0	22	1	0	0	70	1	—	0
Sweetened	5 oz	110	0	0	0	0	28	1	0	0	85	2	—	0
SENECA														
Cinnamon	½ cup	100	0	0	0	0	24	3	0	0	105	60	—	0
Golden Delicious	½ cup	100	0	0	0	0	24	3	0	0	105	60	—	0
McIntosh	½ cup	100	0	0	0	0	24	3	0	0	105	60	—	0
Natural	½ cup	60	0	0	0	0	15	3	0	0	105	2	—	0
Regular	½ cup	100	0	0	0	0	24	3	0	0	105	60	—	0
TREE OF LIFE														
Applesauce	½ cup (4.3 oz)	50	0	0	0	0	15	2	—	15	—	—	—	—
WHITE HOUSE														
Chunky	4 oz	80	0	0	0	0	22	1	—	5	—	—	—	—
APRICOT JUICE														
DEL MONTE														
Nectar	8 fl oz	140	0	0	0	1	35	1	0	15	—	30	—	2500
KERN'S														
Nectar	6 fl oz	110	0	0	0	1	27	—	—	0	200	27	—	2500
LIBBY														
Nectar	1 can (11.5 fl oz)	220	0	0	0	1	52	—	40	10	370	60	—	3500
APRICOTS														
CANNED														
halves heavy syrup pack w/ skin	1 cup (9.1 oz)	214	tr	tr	0	1	55	—	22	10	361	8	4	3174

FOOD	PORTION	CALORIES	FAT	SAT FAT	CHOL	PROTEIN	CARBO	FIBER	CALCIUM	SOD	POTAS	VIT C	FOLIC	VIT A
halves water pack w/ skin	1 cup (8.5 oz)	65	tr	tr	0	2	16	—	19	7	465	8	4	3142
halves water pack w/o skin	1 cup (8 oz)	51	tr	tr	0	2	12	—	19	25	350	4	4	4109
heavy syrup w/ skin	3 halves	70	tr	tr	0	tr	18	—	7	3	119	3	1	1046
juice pack w/ skin	3 halves	40	tr	tr	0	1	10	—	10	3	139	4	—	1421
light syrup w/ skin	3 halves	54	tr	tr	0	tr	14	—	10	3	117	2	1	1124
puree from heavy syrup pack w/ skin	¾ cup (9.1 oz)	214	tr	tr	0	1	55	—	22	10	361	8	4	3174
puree from light pack w/ skin	¾ cup (8.9 oz)	160	tr	tr	0	1	42	—	28	10	349	7	4	3344
puree from water pack w/ skin	¾ cup (8.5 oz)	65	tr	tr	0	2	16	—	19	7	465	8	4	3142
puree juice pack w/ skin	1 cup (8.7 oz)	119	tr	tr	0	2	31	—	30	9	409	12	—	4195
water pack w/ skin	3 halves	22	tr	tr	0	1	5	—	7	2	161	3	2	1086
water pack w/o skin	4 halves	20	tr	tr	0	1	5	—	8	10	139	2	2	1629
DEL MONTE														
Halves Unpeeled In Heavy Syrup	½ cup (4.5 oz)	100	0	0	0	0	26	1	0	10	—	5	—	2000
Halves Unpeeled Lite	½ cup (4.3 oz)	60	0	0	0	0	16	1	0	10	—	5	—	2000
LIBBY														
Halves Unpeeled Lite	½ cup (4.4 oz)	60	0	0	0	1	13	1	0	10	105	1	—	400
DRIED														
halves cooked w/o sugar	½ cup	106	tr	tr	0	2	27	—	20	4	611	2	0	2954
DEL MONTE														
Sun Dried	⅓ cup (1.4 oz)	80	0	0	0	2	25	6	20	5	—	5	—	4500
SONOMA														
Dried	10 pieces (1.4 oz)	120	0	0	0	2	31	1	20	0	—	0	—	400
FRESH														
apricots	3	51	tr	tr	0	1	12	—	15	1	313	11	9	2769
FROZEN														
sweetened	½ cup	119	tr	tr	0	1	30	—	12	5	277	11	—	2033
ARROWHEAD														
fresh boiled	1 med (⅓ oz)	9	tr	—	0	1	2	—	1	2	106	—	—	0
ARROWROOT														
flour	1 cup (4.5 oz)	457	tr	tr	0	tr	113	4	51	3	14	0	9	0
ARTICHOKE														
CANNED														
PROGRESSO														
Hearts	2 pieces (2.9 oz)	35	0	0	0	2	6	1	0	240	—	1	—	0

FOOD	PORTION	CALORIES	FAT	SAT FAT	CHOL	PROTEIN	CARBO	FIBER	CALCIUM	SOD	POTAS	VIT C	FOLIC	VIT A
PROGRESSO (CONT.)														
Hearts Marinated	⅓ cup (3 oz)	160	14	2	0	1	6	1	20	290	—	9	—	100
FRESH														
DOLE														
Large Whole	1	23	tr	—	0	2	5	3	—	65	241	7	—	0
FROZEN														
cooked	1 pkg (9 oz)	108	1	tr	0	7	22	—	50	127	634	12	285	394

ASIAN FOOD

(*see also* DINNER, EGG ROLLS, PASTA, SUSHI)

FOOD	PORTION	CALORIES	FAT	SAT FAT	CHOL	PROTEIN	CARBO	FIBER	CALCIUM	SOD	POTAS	VIT C	FOLIC	VIT A
CANNED														
chow mein chicken	1 cup	95	tr	tr	8	7	18	—	45	725	418	tr	—	150
LA CHOY														
Bi-Pack Beef Pepper	¾ cup	80	2	1	17	7	10	2	20	950	170	21	—	350
Bi-Pack Chow Mein Chicken	¾ cup	80	3	1	18	7	8	1	10	970	225	15	—	100
Bi-Pack Chow Mein Pork	¾ cup	80	4	tr	14	5	7	2	20	950	275	12	—	150
Bi-Pack Chow Mein Shrimp	¾ cup	70	1	tr	19	7	6	1	40	860	210	15	—	100
Bi-Pack Sweet & Sour Chicken	¾ cup	120	2	tr	13	7	18	2	20	440	400	15	—	400
Bi-Pack Teriyaki Chicken	¾ cup	85	2	1	20	8	8	1	20	850	230	12	—	200
Dinner Chow Mein Chicken	¾ pkg	300	17	8	16	12	29	2	89	1800	240	3	—	150
Entree Beef Pepper Oriental	¾ cup	100	4	2	36	7	12	2	20	1340	170	9	—	450
Entree Chow Mein Beef	¾ cup	40	2	1	16	5	5	2	80	960	150	2	—	150
Entree Chow Mein Chicken	¾ cup	70	4	1	16	5	2	4	80	850	165	3	—	150
Entree Chow Mein Meatless	¾ cup	25	tr	tr	0	1	5	2	60	860	175	5	—	100
Entree Chow Mein Shrimp	¾ cup	35	1	tr	50	4	4	2	80	940	280	6	—	100
Entree Sweet & Sour Chicken	¾ cup	240	2	1	19	8	47	1	20	1420	235	4	—	350
Entree Sweet & Sour Pork	¾ cup	250	4	1	18	6	48	1	20	1540	215	4	—	125
FRESH														
wonton wrappers	1	23	tr	tr	1	1	5	—	4	46	7	0	1	1
AZUMAYA														
Won Ton Wraps	1 (8 g)	23	tr	—	—	1	5	—	1	50	—	tr	—	—
FROZEN														
BANQUET														
Chow Mein Chicken	1 pkg (9 oz)	400	7	2	30	9	28	3	20	850	—	9	—	500

FOOD	PORTION	CALORIES	FAT	SAT FAT	CHOL	PROTEIN	CARBO	FIBER	CALCIUM	SOD	POTAS	VIT C	FOLIC	VIT A
BIRDS EYE														
Easy Recipe Meal Starter Oriental Stir Fry as prep	1 serv	280	8	2	69	8	30	2	40	336	—	27	—	1000
Easy Recipe Meal Starter Spicy Asian	1 serv	280	8	2	69	8	30	2	40	336	—	27	—	1000
Easy Recipe Meal Starter Teriyaki Stir Fry as prep	1 serv	280	8	2	69	8	30	2	40	336	—	27	—	1000
CHUN KING														
Beef Pepper Steak	1 pkg (13 oz)	300	4	1	10	15	50	5	20	1670	—	36	—	750
Chow Mein Chicken	1 pkg (13 oz)	370	14	5	45	16	45	4	40	2010	—	9	—	500
Imperial Chicken	1 pkg (13 oz)	460	10	3	25	17	59	5	40	1670	—	0	—	1000
Sweet & Sour Pork	1 pkg (13 oz)	450	6	3	20	12	66	4	20	1180	—	5	—	1000
Walnut Chicken	1 pkg (13 oz)	460	19	5	35	19	56	5	60	1820	—	0	—	0
GREEN GIANT														
Create A Meal LoMein Stir Fry as prep	1¼ cups (10 oz)	320	70	2	60	30	35	4	60	980	—	18	—	1500
Create A Meal Sweet & Sour Stir Fry as prep	1¼ cups (10 oz)	290	7	1	60	27	29	5	80	460	—	18	—	4500
Create A Meal Szechuan Stir Fry as prep	1¼ cups (10 oz)	340	15	4	60	28	22	5	60	1280	—	36	—	4000
Create A Meal Teriyaki Stir Fry as prep	1¼ cups (10 oz)	240	6	1	55	27	18	4	60	940	—	42	—	750
LEAN CUISINE														
Chicken Chow Mein With Rice	1 pkg (9 oz)	220	5	1	35	12	33	3	20	560	300	0	—	1500
Chicken Oriental w/ Vegetables & Vermicelli	1 pkg (9 oz)	250	6	2	35	19	30	4	20	530	350	12	—	300
Oriental Style Dumplings	1 pkg (9 oz)	300	6	2	20	10	51	2	40	520	500	15	—	1500
Teriyaki Stir Fry	1 pkg (10 oz)	290	4	1	25	17	48	4	40	590	430	9	—	1750
LUIGINO'S														
Chicken & Almonds With Rice	1 pkg (8 oz)	250	8	2	20	12	33	3	60	770	—	0	—	100
Chop Suey Pork With Rice	1 pkg (8.5 oz)	210	4	1	15	10	34	2	60	980	—	0	—	0
Lo Mein Chicken	1 pkg (8 oz)	320	5	2	15	13	35	3	60	950	—	0	—	200
Lo Mein Shrimp	1 pkg (8 oz)	190	3	1	15	8	31	4	60	980	—	0	—	0

FOOD	PORTION	CALORIES	FAT	SAT FAT	CHOL	PROTEIN	CARBO	FIBER	CALCIUM	SOD	POTAS	VIT C	FOLIC	VIT A
LUIGINO'S (CONT.)														
Oriental Beef & Peppers With Rice	1 pkg (8 oz)	230	5	2	10	8	38	2	60	820	—	0	—	0
PASTA FAVORITES														
Chicken Lo Mein	1 pkg (10.5 oz)	270	6	1	20	11	43	5	40	1060	—	9	—	3500
RICE GOURMET														
Chicken Teriyaki Rice Bowl	1 bowl (10.9 oz)	430	6	1	25	19	77	1	60	1210	—	12	—	2000
STOUFFER'S														
Chicken Chow Mein w/ Rice	1 pkg (10.6 oz)	260	5	1	25	13	40	3	40	1090	280	6	—	1750
TYSON														
Stir Fry Kit With Yoshida Oriental Sauce	10.6 oz	330	10	—	80	24	37	—	—	1740	—	—	—	—
Sweet & Sour Kit With Sweet & Sour Sauce	14.85 oz	440	9	—	—	20	71	—	—	1300	—	—	—	—
WEIGHT WATCHERS														
Smart Ones Chicken Chow Mein	1 pkg (9 oz)	200	2	1	25	12	34	3	20	570	—	5	—	1500
Smart Ones Hunan Style Rice & Vegetables	1 pkg (10.34 oz)	250	7	2	5	7	39	8	60	630	—	9	—	750
Smart Ones King Pao Noodles & Vegetables	1 pkg (10 oz)	260	10	2	5	8	35	5	60	690	—	6	—	750
Smart Ones Spicy Szechaun Style Vegetables & Chicken	1 pkg (9 oz)	220	2	1	10	11	39	3	150	730	—	2	—	750
MIX														
LA CHOY														
Dinner Classics Egg Foo Young	2 patties + 3 oz sauce	170	7	2	275	8	20	1	60	1390	270	—	—	150
Dinner Classics Pepper Steak	¾ cup	180	9	3	60	17	9	1	20	760	490	—	—	300
Dinner Classics Sweet & Sour	¾ cup	310	6	1	50	32	30	tr	40	860	360	3	—	600
TAKE-OUT														
cha siu bao steamed buns w/ chicken filling	1 (2.3 oz)	160	3	1	15	5	26	tr	0	300	—	0	—	0
chicken teriyaki w/ rice	1 serv (11 oz)	430	6	1	25	19	77	1	60	1210	—	12	—	2000

FOOD	PORTION	CALORIES	FAT	SAT FAT	CHOL	PROTEIN	CARBO	FIBER	CALCIUM	SOD	POTAS	VIT C	FOLIC	VIT A
chop suey w/ beef & pork	1 cup	300	17	4	68	26	13	—	81	1053	425	33	—	600
chow mein chicken	1 cup	255	10	4	75	31	10	—	58	718	473	10	—	280
chow mein vegetable	1 serv (8 oz)	90	3	0	0	3	15	4	40	1010	—	9	—	1250
spring roll deep fried	3.5 oz	202	9	—	—	6	24	—	—	—	—	—	—	—
sweet & sour pork	1 serv (8 oz)	250	8	3	30	6	37	2	20	1500	—	9	—	200
szechuan chicken w/ lo mein	1 cup (5.3 oz)	190	1	0	5	10	35	0	20	560	—	1	—	200

ASPARAGUS

CANNED

FOOD	PORTION	CALORIES	FAT	SAT FAT	CHOL	PROTEIN	CARBO	FIBER	CALCIUM	SOD	POTAS	VIT C	FOLIC	VIT A
spears	½ cup	24	1	tr	0	3	3	—	—	—	—	—	116	—

DEL MONTE

FOOD	PORTION	CALORIES	FAT	SAT FAT	CHOL	PROTEIN	CARBO	FIBER	CALCIUM	SOD	POTAS	VIT C	FOLIC	VIT A
Salad Tips Tender Green	½ cup (4.4 oz)	20	0	0	0	2	3	1	0	420	—	18	—	400
Spears Cut Tender Green	½ cup (4.4 oz)	20	0	0	0	2	3	1	0	420	—	18	—	400
Spears Extra Long Tender Green	½ cup (4.4 oz)	20	0	0	0	2	3	1	0	420	—	18	—	400
Spears Tender Green	½ cup (4.4 oz)	20	0	0	0	2	3	1	0	420	—	18	—	400
Tips Tender Green	½ cup (4.4 oz)	20	0	0	0	2	3	1	0	420	—	18	—	400

GREEN GIANT

FOOD	PORTION	CALORIES	FAT	SAT FAT	CHOL	PROTEIN	CARBO	FIBER	CALCIUM	SOD	POTAS	VIT C	FOLIC	VIT A
Cut Spears	½ cup (4.2 oz)	20	0	0	0	2	3	1	0	420	—	9	—	400
Cut Spears 50% Less Sodium	½ cup (4.2 oz)	20	0	0	0	2	3	1	0	210	—	9	—	400
Extra Long Spears	4.5 oz	20	0	0	0	2	3	1	0	400	—	12	—	400
Spears	4.5 oz	20	0	0	0	2	3	1	0	450	—	12	—	400

LESUEUR

FOOD	PORTION	CALORIES	FAT	SAT FAT	CHOL	PROTEIN	CARBO	FIBER	CALCIUM	SOD	POTAS	VIT C	FOLIC	VIT A
Spears Extra Large	4.5 oz	20	0	0	0	2	3	1	0	440	—	12	—	400

SENECA

FOOD	PORTION	CALORIES	FAT	SAT FAT	CHOL	PROTEIN	CARBO	FIBER	CALCIUM	SOD	POTAS	VIT C	FOLIC	VIT A
Asparagus	½ cup	20	0	0	0	2	3	2	20	264	175	20	—	200

FRESH

DOLE

FOOD	PORTION	CALORIES	FAT	SAT FAT	CHOL	PROTEIN	CARBO	FIBER	CALCIUM	SOD	POTAS	VIT C	FOLIC	VIT A
Spears	5	18	0	—	0	2	2	2	—	0	264	9	—	604

FROZEN

FOOD	PORTION	CALORIES	FAT	SAT FAT	CHOL	PROTEIN	CARBO	FIBER	CALCIUM	SOD	POTAS	VIT C	FOLIC	VIT A
cooked	4 spears	17	tr	tr	0	2	3	—	14	2	131	15	81	491
cooked	1 pkg (10 oz)	82	1	tr	0	9	14	—	68	12	640	72	395	2397

BIG VALLEY

FOOD	PORTION	CALORIES	FAT	SAT FAT	CHOL	PROTEIN	CARBO	FIBER	CALCIUM	SOD	POTAS	VIT C	FOLIC	VIT A
Spears	5-6 (3 oz)	20	0	0	0	2	3	1	20	0	—	24	—	600

GREEN GIANT

FOOD	PORTION	CALORIES	FAT	SAT FAT	CHOL	PROTEIN	CARBO	FIBER	CALCIUM	SOD	POTAS	VIT C	FOLIC	VIT A
Harvest Fresh Cuts	⅔ cup (3 oz)	25	0	0	0	2	4	1	0	85	—	12	—	400

ATEMOYA

FOOD	PORTION	CALORIES	FAT	SAT FAT	CHOL	PROTEIN	CARBO	FIBER	CALCIUM	SOD	POTAS	VIT C	FOLIC	VIT A
fresh	½ cup	94	1	—	—	1	24	—	—	2	314	9	—	10

FOOD	PORTION	CALORIES	FAT	SAT FAT	CHOL	PROTEIN	CARBO	FIBER	CALCIUM	SOD	POTAS	VIT C	FOLIC	VIT A
AVOCADO														
FRESH														
avocado	1	324	31	5	0	4	15	—	22	21	1204	16	124	1230
mashed	1 cup	370	35	6	0	5	17	—	25	24	1378	18	142	1407
BACON														
(*see also* BACON SUBSTITUTES)														
breakfast strips cooked	3 strips	156	12	4	36	10	tr	0	5	714	—	0	1	0
pan fried	3 strips	109	9	3	16	6	tr	0	2	303	—	0	1	0
BLACK LABEL														
Center Cut cooked	3 slices (0.5 oz)	70	6	2	15	5	0	0	0	260	—	0	—	0
Cooked	2 slices (0.5 oz)	80	7	3	15	5	0	0	0	330	—	0	—	0
Low Salt cooked	2 slices (0.5 oz)	80	7	3	15	5	0	0	0	230	—	0	—	0
HILLSHIRE														
Bacon	1 slice	120	12	—	—	2	tr	—	—	150	—	—	—	—
HORMEL														
Bacon Bits	1 tbsp (7 g)	30	2	1	5	3	0	0	0	250	—	0	—	0
Bacon Pieces	1 tbsp (7 g)	25	2	1	10	3	0	0	0	180	—	0	—	0
Microwave cooked	2 slices (0.5 oz)	70	5	2	15	5	0	0	0	230	—	0	—	0
JONES														
Sliced	1 slice	130	13	—	25	2	tr	—	—	150	—	—	—	—
OLD SMOKEHOUSE														
Cooked	2 slices (0.5 oz)	80	7	3	15	5	0	0	0	280	—	0	—	0
OSCAR MAYER														
Bacon Bits	1 tbsp (0.2 oz)	25	2	1	5	3	0	0	0	220	—	0	—	0
Bacon Pieces	1 tbsp (0.2 oz)	25	2	1	5	2	0	0	0	170	—	0	—	0
Center Cut cooked	2 slices (0.4 oz)	70	5	2	15	4	0	0	0	270	—	0	—	0
Cooked	2 slices (0.5 oz)	70	6	2	15	4	0	0	0	290	—	0	—	0
Lower Sodium cooked	2 slices (0.5 oz)	70	5	2	15	5	1	0	0	200	—	0	—	0
Thick Cut cooked	1 slice (0.4 oz)	60	5	2	10	4	0	0	0	250	—	0	—	0
RANGE BRAND														
Cooked	2 slices (0.7 oz)	100	9	4	20	7	0	0	0	460	—	0	—	0
RED LABEL														
Cooked	2 slices (0.5 oz)	80	7	3	15	5	0	0	0	330	—	0	—	0
SHANNON														
Irish	1 oz	70	5	2	—	6	0	—	—	—	—	1	—	—

FOOD	PORTION	CALORIES	FAT	SAT FAT	CHOL	PROTEIN	CARBO	FIBER	CALCIUM	SOD	POTAS	VIT C	FOLIC	VIT A
BACON SUBSTITUTES														
bacon substitute	1 strip	25	2	tr	0	1	1	—	2	117	14	0	3	7
BAC-OS														
Pieces	1½ tbsp	30	1	0	0	3	2	0	—	130	130	—	—	—
HARVEST DIRECT														
Bacon Bits	3.5 oz	320	15	2	0	40	24	17	—	2000	1750	—	—	—
LIGHTLIFE														
Fakin' Bacon	3 strips (2 oz)	79	3	tr	0	9	6	—	—	233	—	—	—	—
LOUIS RICH														
Turkey Bacon	1 slice (0.5 oz)	35	3	1	15	2	0	0	0	180	—	0	—	0
MCCORMICK														
Bac'n Pieces	2 tsp	20	tr	—	0	2	1	—	—	140	—	—	—	—
MORNINGSTAR FARMS														
Breakfast Strips	2 (0.5 oz)	60	5	1	0	2	2	tr	0	220	15	0	—	0
MR. TURKEY														
Slice	1	25	2	—	10	3	0	—	—	170	—	—	—	—
WORTHINGTON														
Stripples	2 strips (0.5 oz)	60	5	1	0	2	2	tr	0	220	15	0	—	0
BAGEL														
FRESH														
cinnamon raisin	1 (3½ in)	194	1	tr	0	7	39	—	13	229	—	1	—	52
cinnamon raisin toasted	1 (3½ in)	194	1	tr	0	7	39	—	13	229	—	tr	—	47
egg	1 (3½ in)	197	2	tr	17	8	38	—	9	359	48	tr	16	77
egg toasted	1 (3½ in)	197	2	tr	17	8	38	—	9	358	48	tr	11	70
oat bran	1 (3½ in)	181	1	tr	0	8	38	—	9	360	—	tr	—	3
oat bran toasted	1 (3½ in)	181	1	tr	0	8	38	—	9	360	—	tr	—	3
onion	1 (3½ in)	195	1	tr	0	8	38	2	53	379	72	0	16	0
plain	1 (3½ in)	195	1	tr	0	8	38	2	53	379	72	0	16	0
plain toasted	1 (3½ in)	195	1	tr	0	8	38	2	53	379	72	0	11	0
poppy seed	1 (3½ in)	195	1	tr	0	8	38	2	53	379	72	0	16	0
ALVARADO ST. BAKERY														
Sprouted Wheat	1 (3.3 oz)	260	1	0	0	9	54	2	—	400	—	—	—	—
Sprouted Wheat Cinnamon/Raisin	1 (3.3 oz)	280	1	0	0	9	59	3	—	270	—	—	—	—
Sprouted Wheat Onion/Poppyseed	1 (3.3 oz)	320	2	0	0	11	66	2	—	410	—	—	—	—
Sprouted Wheat Sesame	1 (3.3 oz)	320	4	1	0	11	64	2	—	410	—	—	—	—
FROZEN														
AMY'S ORGANIC														
Cinnamon Raisin	1 (3.5 oz)	240	2	0	0	8	52	3	—	480	—	—	—	—
Plain	1 (3.5 oz)	230	2	0	0	8	48	2	—	490	—	—	—	—
Poppy Seed	1 (3.5 oz)	230	2	0	0	8	48	2	—	480	—	—	—	—
Sesame	1 (3.5 oz)	240	2	0	0	8	48	2	—	480	—	—	—	—

FOOD	PORTION	CALORIES	FAT	SAT FAT	CHOL	PROTEIN	CARBO	FIBER	CALCIUM	SOD	POTAS	VIT C	FOLIC	VIT A
GREAT STARTS														
Ham & Cheese On A Bagel	3 oz	240	8	—	—	12	28	—	100	600	—	4	—	300
SARA LEE														
Blueberry	1 (2.8 oz)	210	1	1	0	7	43	3	—	230	—	—	—	—
Cinnamon Raisin	1 (2.8 oz)	220	1	0	0	8	45	3	—	320	—	—	—	—
Egg	1 (2.8 oz)	210	1	1	0	7	44	2	—	460	—	—	—	—
Oat Bran	1 (2.8 oz)	210	1	0	0	8	42	3	—	570	—	—	—	—
Onion	1 (2.8 oz)	210	0	0	0	7	44	2	—	540	—	—	—	—
Plain	1 (2.8 oz)	210	1	0	0	8	43	2	—	500	—	—	—	—
Poppy Seed	1 (2.8 oz)	210	1	0	0	8	41	2	—	570	—	—	—	—
Sesame Seed	1 (2.8 oz)	210	2	1	0	8	42	2	—	530	—	—	—	—
TREE OF LIFE														
Onion	1 (3 oz)	210	0	0	0	8	44	0	20	115	—	0	—	0
Plain	1 (3 oz)	210	0	0	0	8	44	0	20	115	—	0	—	0
Poppy	1 (3 oz)	210	0	0	0	8	44	0	20	115	—	0	—	0
Raisin	1 (3 oz)	210	0	0	0	8	45	tr	20	115	—	0	—	0
Sesame	1 (3 oz)	210	0	0	0	8	44	0	20	115	—	0	—	0
BAKING POWDER														
baking powder	1 tsp	2	0	0	0	0	1	—	270	488	1	0	0	0
low sodium	1 tsp	5	0	0	0	0	2	—	217	4	505	0	0	0
CALUMET														
Baking Powder	¼ tsp (1 g)	0	0	0	0	0	0	0	60	100	0	0	—	0
CLABBER GIRL														
Baking Powder	1 tsp	0	0	0	0	tr	1	—	84	435	tr	—	—	—
DAVIS														
Baking Powder	1 tsp	6	0	0	0	0	2	—	—	450	0	—	—	—
WATKINS														
Baking Powder	¼ tsp (1 g)	0	0	0	0	0	0	0	0	150	—	0	—	0
BAKING SODA														
baking soda	1 tsp	0	0	0	0	0	0	—	0	1259	0	0	0	0
ARM & HAMMER														
Baking Soda	1 tsp	0	0	0	0	0	0	—	tr	1368	tr	—	—	—
BALSAM PEAR														
leafy tips cooked	½ cup	10	tr	—	0	1	2	—	12	4	174	16	25	503
leafy tips raw	½ cup	7	tr	—	0	1	1	—	20	3	145	21	—	416
pods cooked	½ cup	12	tr	—	0	1	3	—	6	4	198	21	—	70
BAMBOO SHOOTS														
CANNED														
sliced	1 cup	25	1	tr	0	2	4	—	10	9	104	1	—	11
KA-ME														
Sliced	½ cup (4.5 oz)	15	0	0	0	1	3	1	—	10	—	—	—	—
LA CHOY														
Sliced	¼ cup	6	tr	tr	0	tr	1	tr	3	2	25	—	—	tr

FOOD	PORTION	CALORIES	FAT	SAT FAT	CHOL	PROTEIN	CARBO	FIBER	CALCIUM	SOD	POTAS	VIT C	FOLIC	VIT A
FRESH														
cooked	½ cup	15	tr	tr	0	2	2	—	14	5	640	0	—	0
raw	½ cup	21	tr	tr	0	2	1	—	10	3	405	3	—	15

BANANA

FOOD	PORTION	CALORIES	FAT	SAT FAT	CHOL	PROTEIN	CARBO	FIBER	CALCIUM	SOD	POTAS	VIT C	FOLIC	VIT A
banana chips	1 oz	147	10	8	0	1	17	2	5	2	152	2	4	—
powder	1 tbsp	21	tr	tr	0	tr	5	—	1	0	92	tr	—	19
DOLE														
Fresh	1	120	1	—	0	1	28	3	—	0	380	11	—	70
RAINFOREST FARMS														
Slices Dried	5 slices (1.3 oz)	60	0	0	0	1	12	—	—	10	—	15	—	—

BANANA JUICE

FOOD	PORTION	CALORIES	FAT	SAT FAT	CHOL	PROTEIN	CARBO	FIBER	CALCIUM	SOD	POTAS	VIT C	FOLIC	VIT A
LIBBY														
Nectar	1 can (11.5 fl oz)	190	0	0	0	0	47	—	—	35	190	60	—	—

BARBECUE SAUCE

(*see also* SAUCE)

FOOD	PORTION	CALORIES	FAT	SAT FAT	CHOL	PROTEIN	CARBO	FIBER	CALCIUM	SOD	POTAS	VIT C	FOLIC	VIT A
barbecue	1 cup	188	5	1	0	5	32	—	48	2038	436	18	—	2170
HAIN														
Honey	1 tbsp	14	1	—	0	0	1	—	—	120	—	—	—	—
HEALTHY CHOICE														
Hickory	2 tbsp (1.1 oz)	26	0	0	0	tr	6	tr	1	229	—	4	—	9
Hot & Spicy	2 tbsp (1.1 oz)	25	0	0	0	tr	6	tr	1	229	—	2	—	8
Original	2 tbsp (1.1 oz)	25	0	0	0	tr	6	tr	1	229	—	2	—	8
HEINZ														
Select	1 oz	40	0	0	0	0	9	—	—	275	115	1	—	—
Select Hickory	1 oz	35	0	0	0	0	8	—	—	260	105	1	—	—
Thick & Rich Cajun Style	1 oz	35	0	0	0	0	8	—	—	360	100	—	—	—
Thick & Rich Chunky	1 oz	30	0	0	0	1	6	—	—	380	100	1	—	400
Thick & Rich Hawaiian Style	1 oz	40	0	0	0	0	10	—	—	210	65	—	—	—
Thick & Rich Hickory Smoke	1 oz	35	0	0	0	0	8	—	—	380	90	1	—	200
Thick & Rich Mesquite Smoke	1 oz	30	0	0	0	0	7	—	—	380	90	1	—	300
Thick & Rich Mushroom	1 oz	30	0	0	0	1	6	—	—	460	100	—	—	400
Thick & Rich Old Fashioned	1 oz	35	0	0	0	0	8	—	—	350	95	—	—	200
Thick & Rich Onion	1 oz	30	0	0	0	0	7	—	—	420	95	—	—	300
Thick & Rich Original	1 oz	35	0	0	0	0	8	—	—	390	90	—	—	500
Thick & Rich Texas Hot	1 oz	30	0	0	0	0	7	—	—	390	85	1	—	200

FOOD	PORTION	CALORIES	FAT	SAT FAT	CHOL	PROTEIN	CARBO	FIBER	CALCIUM	SOD	POTAS	VIT C	FOLIC	VIT A
HOUSE OF TSANG														
Hong Kong	1 tbsp (0.6 oz)	10	0	0	0	0	2	0	0	150	—	0	—	0
HUNT'S														
Barbeque	¼ cup (2.2 oz)	57	tr	tr	0	1	14	1	11	887	—	11	—	38
Bold Hickory	2 tbsp (1.2 oz)	47	tr	0	0	tr	11	1	1	283	—	5	—	10
Bold Original	2 tbsp (1.2 oz)	46	tr	0	0	tr	11	1	1	315	—	3	—	13
Hickory	2 tbsp (1.2 oz)	38	tr	0	0	tr	9	1	1	410	—	2	—	9
Hickory & Brown Sugar	2 tbsp (1.3 oz)	75	tr	0	0	tr	18	1	30	382	—	1	—	11
Honey Hickory	2 tbsp (1.2 oz)	38	tr	0	0	tr	9	1	1	410	—	2	—	9
Honey Mustard	2 tbsp (1.2 oz)	48	tr	0	0	tr	12	1	1	450	—	3	—	10
Hot & Spicy	2 tbsp (1.2 oz)	48	tr	0	0	tr	12	1	1	450	—	3	—	10
Light	2 tbsp (1.2 oz)	23	tr	0	0	tr	6	1	9	169	—	1	—	27
Mesquite Barbecue	2 tbsp (1.2 oz)	40	tr	0	0	1	9	1	1	361	—	1	—	7
Mild	2 tbsp (1.2 oz)	41	tr	0	0	tr	10	1	1	381	—	1	—	9
Mild Dijon	2 tbsp (1.2 oz)	39	tr	0	0	tr	9	tr	1	400	—	2	—	7
Original	2 tbsp (1.2 oz)	39	tr	0	0	tr	9	1	12	399	—	1	—	30
Teriyaki	2 tbsp (1.2 oz)	46	tr	0	0	1	11	1	2	351	—	5	—	5
KRAFT														
Char-Grill	2 tbsp (1.3 oz)	60	0	0	0	0	13	0	0	460	45	0	—	0
Extra Rich Original	2 tbsp (1.2 oz)	50	0	0	0	0	12	0	0	440	45	0	—	0
Hickory Smoke	2 tbsp (1.2 oz)	40	0	0	0	0	9	0	0	420	30	0	—	100
Hickory Smoke Onion Bits	2 tbsp (1.2 oz)	45	0	0	0	0	11	0	0	360	25	0	—	0
Honey	2 tbsp (1.3 oz)	50	0	0	0	0	13	0	0	360	25	0	—	0
Honey Hickory	2 tbsp (1.3 oz)	60	0	0	0	0	14	0	0	370	30	0	—	0
Honey Mustard	2 tbsp (1.3 oz)	60	0	0	0	0	13	0	0	300	30	0	—	0
Hot	2 tbsp (1.2 oz)	40	0	0	0	0	9	0	0	520	25	0	—	0
Hot Hickory Smoke	2 tbsp (1.2 oz)	40	0	0	0	0	9	0	0	380	35	0	—	100
Kansas City Style	2 tbsp (1.2 oz)	50	0	0	0	0	11	0	0	310	100	0	—	0
Mesquite Smoke	2 tbsp (1.2 oz)	40	0	0	0	0	9	0	0	420	30	0	—	100
Molasses	2 tbsp (1.3 oz)	70	0	0	0	0	16	0	20	390	105	0	—	0
Onion Bits	2 tbsp (1.2 oz)	45	0	0	0	0	11	0	0	360	30	0	—	0
Original	2 tbsp (1.2 oz)	40	0	0	0	0	9	0	0	420	30	0	—	100
Roasted Garlic	2 tbsp (1.2 oz)	50	0	0	0	0	12	0	0	360	40	0	—	0
Spicy Honey	2 tbsp (1.3 oz)	60	0	0	0	0	14	0	0	360	25	0	—	0
Teriyaki	2 tbsp (1.3 oz)	60	1	0	0	tr	12	0	0	440	80	0	—	0
Thick 'N Spicy Brown Sugar	2 tbsp (1.2 oz)	60	0	0	0	0	15	0	0	350	60	0	—	0
Thick 'N Spicy Hickory Bacon	2 tbsp (1.2 oz)	60	1	0	0	0	13	0	0	570	45	0	—	100
Thick 'N Spicy Hickory Smoke	2 tbsp (1.2 oz)	50	0	0	0	0	12	0	0	450	40	0	—	100
Thick 'N Spicy Honey	2 tbsp (1.3 oz)	60	0	0	0	0	13	0	0	360	80	0	—	100

FOOD	PORTION	CALORIES	FAT	SAT FAT	CHOL	PROTEIN	CARBO	FIBER	CALCIUM	SOD	POTAS	VIT C	FOLIC	VIT A
KRAFT (CONT.)														
Thick 'N Spicy Honey Mustard	2 tbsp (1.3 oz)	60	0	0	0	0	14	0	0	310	50	0	—	0
Thick 'N Spicy Hickory Smoke	2 tbsp (1.2 oz)	50	0	0	0	0	12	0	0	440	70	0	—	0
Thick 'N Spicy Honey	2 tbsp (1.2 oz)	60	0	0	0	0	13	0	0	350	95	0	—	200
Thick 'N Spicy Kansas City Style	2 tbsp (1.3 oz)	60	0	0	0	0	14	0	0	310	110	0	—	0
Thick 'N Spicy Mesquite Smoke	2 tbsp (1.2 oz)	50	0	0	0	0	12	0	0	440	40	0	—	100
Thick 'N Spicy Original	2 tbsp (1.2 oz)	50	0	0	0	0	12	0	0	440	75	0	—	200
LAWRY'S														
Dijon Honey	¼ cup	203	1	tr	0	5	27	tr	—	1768	340	—	—	—
RED WING														
"K" Sauce	2 tbsp (1.2 oz)	45	0	0	0	0	9	0	0	410	—	0	—	200
WATKINS														
Bold	2 tsp (0.4 oz)	25	0	0	0	0	5	0	0	290	—	0	—	450
Honey	2 tsp (0.4 oz)	25	0	0	0	0	6	0	0	290	—	0	—	100
Mesquite	2 tsp (0.4 oz)	25	0	0	0	0	5	0	0	300	—	0	—	100
Original	2 tsp (0.4 oz)	25	0	0	0	0	5	0	0	300	—	0	—	100
Smokehouse	2 tsp (0.4 oz)	25	0	0	0	0	5	0	0	300	—	0	—	100
BARLEY														
flour	1 cup (5.2 oz)	511	2	tr	0	15	110	15	47	6	457	0	12	0
malt flour	1 cup (5.7 oz)	585	3	1	0	17	127	12	60	18	363	1	62	31
pearled cooked	1 cup (5.5 oz)	193	1	tr	0	4	44	6	17	5	146	0	25	11
pearled uncooked	1 cup (7 oz)	704	2	tr	0	20	155	31	58	18	560	0	46	44
ARROWHEAD														
Barley	¼ cup (1.7 oz)	170	1	0	0	5	37	6	20	0	140	0	—	0
Hulless	¼ cup (1.6 oz)	140	1	0	0	5	35	6	0	0	230	0	—	0
BASIL														
ground	1 tsp	4	tr	—	0	tr	1	—	30	tr	48	1	—	131
WATKINS														
Liquid Spice	1 tbsp (0.5 oz)	120	14	2	0	0	0	0	0	0	—	0	—	0
BASS														
freshwater raw	3 oz	97	3	1	58	16	0	—	68	59	303	—	—	—
sea cooked	3 oz	105	2	1	45	20	0	—	11	74	279	—	—	181
sea raw	3 oz	82	2	tr	35	16	0	—	9	58	218	—	—	157
BAY LEAF														
crumbled	1 tsp	2	tr	tr	0	tr	tr	—	5	tr	3	tr	—	37
WATKINS														
Bay Leaves	¼ tsp (0.5 g)	0	0	0	0	0	0	0	0	0	—	0	—	0
BEAN SPROUTS														
LA CHOY														
Bean Sprouts	⅔ cup	8	tr	tr	0	1	1	tr	—	20	25	15	—	—

BEANS

(see also individual names)

FOOD	PORTION	CALORIES	FAT	SAT FAT	CHOL	PROTEIN	CARBO	FIBER	CALCIUM	SOD	POTAS	VIT C	FOLIC	VIT A
CANNED														
baked beans w/ beef	½ cup	161	5	2	29	8	22	—	60	632	426	2	—	283
refried beans	½ cup	134	1	1	—	8	23	—	59	534	495	8	—	—
ALLEN														
Baked	½ cup (4.5 oz)	150	1	1	0	6	29	8	40	350	—	0	—	0
B&M														
99% Fat Free Baked Beans	½ cup (4.6 oz)	160	1	0	0	8	31	7	60	220	—	0	—	0
Baked With Honey	½ cup (4.7 oz)	170	2	0	0	8	30	8	60	450	—	0	—	0
Barbeque Baked Beans	½ cup (4.7 oz)	170	2	1	<5	7	32	6	80	360	—	0	—	0
Brick Oven Baked	½ cup (4.6 oz)	180	2	1	5	8	32	7	60	390	—	0	—	0
Extra Hearty Baked	½ cup (4.6 oz)	190	2	1	<5	8	36	8	60	450	—	0	—	0
BROWN BEAUTY														
Mexican Beans With Jalapeno	½ cup (4.5 oz)	120	1	0	0	7	21	7	40	370	—	0	—	200
BUSH'S														
Baked	½ cup (4.6 oz)	150	1	tr	<5	7	29	7	60	550	—	0	—	0
Baked With Onions	½ cup (4.6 oz)	150	2	1	5	7	26	6	40	500	—	tr	—	<100
Homestyle Baked	½ cup (4.6 oz)	160	2	1	5	6	28	8	40	480	—	tr	—	800
Vegetarian	½ cup (4.6 oz)	140	1	0	0	6	24	6	40	550	—	tr	—	500
CAMPBELL														
Barbecue Beans	½ can (7⅞ oz)	210	4	—	—	10	43	—	80	900	—	5	—	500
Home Style Beans	½ can (8 oz)	220	4	—	—	11	48	—	100	820	—	5	—	300
Hot Chili Beans	½ can (7¾ oz)	180	4	—	—	10	38	—	100	870	—	6	—	750
Old Fashioned Beans In Molasses & Brown Sugar Sauce	½ can (8 oz)	230	3	—	—	11	49	—	100	730	—	6	—	100
Pork & Beans In Tomato Sauce	½ can (8 oz)	200	3	—	—	10	43	—	100	770	—	2	—	500
Vegetarian	½ can (7¾ oz)	170	1	—	—	11	40	—	100	780	—	—	—	750
CASA FIESTA														
Refried	3.5 oz	110	2	—	—	6	17	—	32	299	—	6	—	131
CHI-CHI'S														
Refried	½ cup (4.2 oz)	100	1	0	0	5	18	4	20	580	—	0	—	200
Refried Beans Fat Free	½ cup (4.2 oz)	120	0	0	0	5	17	4	20	570	—	0	—	200
Refried Beans Vegetarian	½ cup (4.2 oz)	100	1	0	0	5	18	4	20	580	—	0	—	200
CREST TOP														
Pork And Beans	½ cup (4.5 oz)	130	1	1	0	7	21	6	40	330	—	0	—	100

FOOD	PORTION	CALORIES	FAT	SAT FAT	CHOL	PROTEIN	CARBO	FIBER	CALCIUM	SOD	POTAS	VIT C	FOLIC	VIT A
EDEN														
Organic Baked w/ Sweet Sorghum & Orangic Mustard	½ cup (4.6 oz)	150	0	0	0	8	27	7	100	130	460	—	—	—
FRIEND'S														
Maple Baked	8 oz	240	2	1	<5	14	52	11	100	890	910	—	—	—
Original Baked	½ cup (4.6 oz)	170	1	0	<5	8	32	7	60	390	—	0	—	0
GEBHARDT														
Chili	4 oz	115	1	tr	0	7	21	5	45	580	460	4	—	3
Refried	4 oz	100	2	1	2	7	20	7	39	490	420	2	—	—
Refried Jalapeno	4 oz	115	2	—	2	6	19	7	37	270	400	2	—	8
GREEN GIANT														
Pork And Beans w/ Tomato Sauce	½ cup (4.5 oz)	120	1	0	0	5	23	4	60	490	—	0	—	0
Spicy Chili	½ cup (4.5 oz)	110	1	0	0	6	20	5	40	490	—	0	—	200
Three Bean Salad	½ cup (4.2 oz)	90	0	0	0	3	20	4	60	490	—	0	—	400
HEALTH VALLEY														
Boston Baked	7½ oz	190	tr	—	0	8	41	5	80	300	710	15	5	304
Boston Baked No Salt Added	7.5 oz	190	tr	—	0	8	41	5	80	20	710	15	5	304
Fast Menu Honey Baked Organic Beans With Tofu Weiner	7½ oz	150	4	—	0	11	15	16	100	140	260	0	—	5000
Vegetarian With Miso	7½ oz	180	1	—	0	8	38	5	59	60	640	tr	5	2555
HEARTLAND														
Iron Kettle Baked	½ cup (4.6 oz)	150	1	0	<5	5	29	5	40	400	—	0	—	0
HORMEL														
Beans & Wieners	1 can (7.5 oz)	290	12	4	50	11	34	6	60	1310	—	0	—	200
HUNT'S														
Big John's Beans & Fixin's	½ cup (4.7 oz)	127	4	1	3	7	23	6	7	590	—	5	—	16
Pork & Beans	½ cup (4.5 oz)	130	1	tr	tr	6	28	4	5	516	—	3	—	19
KID'S KITCHEN														
Microwave Meals Beans & Weiners	1 cup (7.5 oz)	310	13	5	45	13	37	8	80	760	—	6	—	200
LITTLE PANCHO														
Refried & Green Chili	½ cup	80	0	0	0	6	15	—	20	330	350	—	—	100
MCILHENNY														
Spicy	1 oz	7	tr	tr	0	1	1	1	13	19	—	1	—	41
OLD EL PASO														
Mexe-Beans	½ cup (4.6 oz)	110	1	0	0	7	19	7	40	630	—	0	—	200
Refried	½ cup (4.2 oz)	110	2	1	<5	6	17	5	40	500	—	0	—	0
Refried Fat Free	½ cup (4.4 oz)	110	0	0	0	6	20	6	40	480	—	0	—	0

FOOD	PORTION	CALORIES	FAT	SAT FAT	CHOL	PROTEIN	CARBO	FIBER	CALCIUM	SOD	POTAS	VIT C	FOLIC	VIT A
OLD EL PASO (CONT.)														
Refried Spicy	½ cup (4.3 oz)	140	3	2	<5	6	22	6	40	560	—	0	—	0
Refried Vegetarian	½ cup (4.1 oz)	100	1	0	0	6	16	6	40	490	—	0	—	0
Refried With Cheese	½ cup (4.2 oz)	130	4	2	5	7	18	6	80	500	—	0	—	0
Refried With Green Chilies	½ cup (4.3 oz)	110	1	0	<5	6	19	6	40	720	—	0	—	0
Refried With Sausage	½ cup (4.1 oz)	200	13	5	10	7	14	8	40	360	—	0	—	0
ROSARITA														
Refried	4 oz	100	2	1	0	7	18	6	43	480	420	—	—	tr
Refried Spicy	4 oz	100	2	1	0	7	19	6	45	500	460	—	—	—
Refried Vegetarian	4 oz	100	2	1	0	7	18	6	42	480	430	—	—	0
Refried With Bacon	4 oz	110	2	1	14	7	20	6	45	560	440	1	—	—
Refried With Green Chilies	4 oz	90	2	1	0	7	18	6	42	460	420	5	—	—
Refried With Nacho Cheese	4 oz	110	2	1	2	7	20	6	40	490	470	—	—	—
Refried With Onions	4 oz	110	2	1	0	7	21	6	46	490	460	1	—	—
TACO BELL														
Home Originals Fat Free Refried Beans	½ cup (4.6 oz)	110	0	0	0	7	21	6	40	460	—	0	—	0
Home Originals Fat Free Refried Beans w/ Mild Chilies	½ cup (4.5 oz)	110	0	0	0	7	20	5	40	480	—	0	—	0
Home Originals Refried Beans	½ cup (4.7 oz)	140	3	1	0	5	23	7	40	530	—	0	—	300
TRAPPEY														
Mexi-Beans With Jalapeno	½ cup (4.5 oz)	130	2	1	0	7	22	8	40	460	—	0	—	500
Pork And Beans	½ cup (4.5 oz)	110	1	1	0	5	21	7	40	710	—	0	—	500
Pork And Beans With Jalapeno	½ cup (4.5 oz)	130	2	1	0	5	24	6	60	610	—	0	—	0
VAN CAMP'S														
Baked Beans Fat Free	½ cup (4.6 oz)	130	0	0	0	7	28	5	40	430	350	—	0	0
Baked Beans Premium	½ cup (4.6 oz)	140	1	0	0	7	29	5	40	520	350	—	0	0
Beanee Weenee	1 cup (9 oz)	320	14	4	40	16	35	8	60	1240	700	—	8	500
Beanee Weenee Baked Flavor	1 cup (9 oz)	410	14	4	40	18	58	10	80	1210	730	—	8	300
Beanee Weenee Barbeque	1 cup (9 oz)	340	14	4	40	17	43	8	60	1150	730	—	8	1000
Brown Sugar Beans	½ cup (4.6 oz)	170	3	1	5	72	31	6	40	410	400	—	0	0
Mexican Style Chili Beans	½ cup (4.6 oz)	110	2	1	0	7	21	8	20	430	330	—	120	500

FOOD	PORTION	CALORIES	FAT	SAT FAT	CHOL	PROTEIN	CARBO	FIBER	CALCIUM	SOD	POTAS	VIT C	FOLIC	VIT A
VAN CAMP'S (CONT.)														
Pork And Beans	½ cup (4.6 oz)	110	2	1	0	6	24	6	40	490	330	—	0	0
Vegetarian In Tomato Sauce	½ cup (4.6 oz)	110	1	0	0	6	23	5	40	400	360	—	0	0
WAGON MASTER														
Pork And Beans	½ cup (4.5 oz)	110	1	1	0	5	21	7	40	710	—	0	—	500
FROZEN														
NATURAL TOUCH														
Nine Bean Loaf	1 in slice (3 oz)	160	8	2	<5	8	13	5	40	350	190	1	—	1500
MIX														
BEAN CUISINE														
Florentine Beans With Bow Ties	½ cup	199	7	2	6	9	27	—	—	450	—	—	—	—
Pasta & Beans Country French With Gemelli	½ cup	214	8	1	tr	6	27	—	—	369	—	—	—	—
MELTING POT														
Terrazza Napoli Mixed Beans	1 cup	200	2	0	<5	9	41	2	20	460	—	6	—	200
TAKE-OUT														
baked beans	½ cup	190	6	2	6	7	27	—	77	532	452	1	61	0
barbecue beans	3.5 oz	120	tr	tr	0	4	26	—	40	460	—	2	—	200
four bean salad	3.5 oz	100	tr	tr	0	4	20	—	40	280	—	5	—	500
BEAR														
simmered	3 oz	220	11	—	—	28	0	—	4	—	—	—	—	—
BEAVER														
simmered	3 oz	141	5	—	—	23	0	—	14	39	269	2	—	—
BEECHNUTS														
dried	1 oz	164	14	2	0	2	10	—	0	—	—	—	—	—
BEEF														
(*see also* BEEF DISHES, VEAL)														
CANNED														
corned beef	3 oz	85	5	4	—	10	0	—	17	—	—	—	—	20
corned beef	1 oz	71	4	—	24	—	—	—	—	—	—	—	—	—
ARMOUR														
Chopped Beef	2 oz	170	15	—	49	7	2	—	—	810	—	—	—	—
Corned Beef	2 oz	120	7	—	45	15	1	—	—	490	—	—	—	—
Potted Meat	1 can (3 oz)	120	8	—	80	11	0	—	—	820	—	—	—	—
Potted Meat	¼ cup (2.2 oz)	90	6	—	60	8	0	—	—	600	—	—	—	—
Tripe	3 oz	90	2	—	125	18	0	—	—	100	—	—	—	—
HORMEL														
Corned Beef	2 oz	120	7	3	50	15	0	0	0	490	—	0	—	0
Cubed Beef	½ cup (4.9 oz)	130	3	1	60	25	0	0	0	600	—	0	—	0
Potted Meat	4 tbsp (2 oz)	100	8	4	50	7	0	0	20	610	—	0	—	0

FOOD	PORTION	CALORIES	FAT	SAT FAT	CHOL	PROTEIN	CARBO	FIBER	CALCIUM	SOD	POTAS	VIT C	FOLIC	VIT A
TREET														
50% Less Fat	2 oz	120	8	—	45	6	4	—	—	750	—	—	—	—
Beef	2 oz	150	12	—	50	6	4	—	—	770	—	—	—	—
UNDERWOOD														
Roast Beef	2.08 oz	140	11	5	45	9	tr	—	—	360	140	—	—	—
Roast Beef Mesquite Smoked	2.08 oz	126	11	5	45	9	tr	—	—	300	140	—	—	—
Roast Beef Light	2.08 oz	90	6	2	30	9	2	—	—	210	160	—	—	—
DRIED														
HORMEL														
Pillow Pack	10 slices (1 oz)	45	1	tr	20	8	0	0	0	1010	—	0	—	0
FRESH														
bottom round lean & fat trim 0 in Choice roasted	3 oz	172	8	3	66	24	0	—	4	56	327	0	10	0
bottom round lean & fat trim 0 in Select braised	3 oz	171	6	2	82	27	0	—	4	43	259	0	9	0
bottom round lean & fat trim 0 in Select roasted	3 oz	150	24	2	66	24	0	—	4	56	330	0	11	0
bottom round lean & fat trim 0 in braised	3 oz	193	26	3	82	26	0	—	4	43	257	0	9	0
bottom round lean & fat trim ¼ in Choice braised	3 oz	241	15	6	81	24	0	—	5	42	239	0	8	0
bottom round lean & fat trim ¼ in Choice roasted	3 oz	221	14	5	68	22	0	—	5	53	302	0	10	0
bottom round lean & fat trim ¼ in Select braised	3 oz	220	13	5	81	25	0	—	5	42	241	0	8	0
bottom round lean & fat trim ¼ in Select roasted	3 oz	199	11	4	68	23	0	—	5	54	307	0	10	0
brisket flat half lean & fat trim 0 in braised	3 oz	183	8	3	81	26	0	—	5	53	246	0	7	0
brisket flat half lean & fat trim ¼ in braised	3 oz	309	24	9	81	21	0	—	5	48	206	0	5	0
brisket point half lean & fat trim 0 in braised	3 oz	304	24	10	78	20	0	—	7	57	198	0	6	0
brisket point half lean & fat trim ¼ in braised	3 oz	343	29	12	79	19	0	—	7	55	188	0	5	0

FOOD	PORTION	CALORIES	FAT	SAT FAT	CHOL	PROTEIN	CARBO	FIBER	CALCIUM	SOD	POTAS	VIT C	FOLIC	VIT A
brisket whole lean & fat trim 0 in braised	3 oz	247	17	6	79	23	0	—	6	55	220	0	6	0
brisket whole lean & fat trim ¼ in braised	3 oz	327	27	11	80	27	0	—	7	52	196	0	5	0
chuck arm pot roast lean & fat trim 0 in braised	3 oz	238	14	6	85	25	0	—	8	53	224	0	8	0
chuck arm pot roast lean & fat trim ¼ in braised	3 oz	282	20	8	85	23	0	—	9	51	210	0	8	0
chuck blade roast lean & fat trim 0 in braised	3 oz	284	21	8	88	23	0	—	11	56	200	0	5	0
chuck blade roast lean & fat trim ¼ in braised	3 oz	293	22	9	88	23	0	—	11	55	197	0	5	0
corned beef brisket cooked	3 oz	213	16	5	83	15	tr	—	7	964	123	—	—	—
eye of round lean & fat trim 0 in Choice roasted	3 oz	153	5	8	59	24	0	—	4	53	333	0	6	0
eye of round lean & fat trim 0 in Select roasted	3 oz	137	4	1	59	24	0	—	4	53	333	0	6	0
eye of round lean & fat trim ¼ in Choice roasted	3 oz	205	12	5	62	23	0	—	5	50	305	0	6	0
eye of round lean & fat trime ¼ in Select roasted	3 oz	184	10	4	61	23	0	—	5	51	310	0	6	0
flank lean & fat trim 0 in braised	3 oz	224	14	6	62	23	0	—	6	60	287	0	7	0
flank lean & fat trim 0 in broiled	3 oz	192	11	5	58	22	0	—	6	69	342	0	7	0
ground extra lean broiled medium	3 oz	217	14	5	71	22	0	—	6	59	266	0	8	—
ground extra lean broiled well done	3 oz	225	14	5	84	24	0	—	7	70	314	0	9	—
ground extra lean fried medium	3 oz	216	14	5	69	21	0	—	6	59	265	0	7	—
ground extra lean fried well done	3 oz	224	14	5	79	24	0	—	7	69	306	0	9	—
ground extra lean raw	4 oz	265	19	8	78	21	0	—	7	75	321	0	9	—
ground lean broiled medium	3 oz	231	16	6	74	21	0	—	9	65	256	0	8	—
ground lean broiled well done	3 oz	238	15	6	86	24	0	—	10	76	296	0	9	—

FOOD	PORTION	CALORIES	FAT	SAT FAT	CHOL	PROTEIN	CARBO	FIBER	CALCIUM	SOD	POTAS	VIT C	FOLIC	VIT A
ground regular broiled medium	3 oz	246	18	7	76	20	0	—	9	70	248	0	8	—
ground regular broiled well done	3 oz	248	17	7	86	23	0	—	10	79	278	0	9	—
porterhouse steak lean & fat trim ¼ in Choice broiled	3 oz	260	19	8	70	21	0	—	7	52	299	0	6	0
porterhouse steak lean only trim ¼ in Prime broiled	3 oz	185	9	4	68	24	0	—	6	56	346	0	7	0
rib eye small end lean & fat trim 0 in Choice broiled	3 oz	261	19	8	70	21	0	—	11	54	293	0	6	0
rib large end lean & fat trim 0 in roasted	3 oz	300	24	10	72	20	0	—	8	55	251	0	6	0
rib large end lean & fat trim ¼ in broiled	3 oz	295	24	10	69	18	0	—	9	54	258	0	5	0
rib large end lean & fat trim ¼ in roasted	3 oz	310	25	10	72	19	0	—	8	54	245	0	6	0
rib small end lean & fat trim 0 in broiled	3 oz	252	18	7	70	21	0	—	11	54	293	0	6	0
rib small end lean & fat trim ¼ in broiled	3 oz	285	22	9	71	20	0	—	11	53	276	0	6	0
rib small end lean & fat trim ¼ in roasted	3 oz	295	24	10	71	19	0	—	11	53	272	0	5	0
rib whole lean & fat trim ¼ in Choice broiled	3 oz	306	25	10	70	19	0	—	10	53	262	0	5	0
rib whole lean & fat trim ¼ in Choice roasted	3 oz	320	27	11	72	19	0	—	9	53	252	0	6	0
rib whole lean & fat trim ¼ in Prime roasted	3 oz	348	30	12	72	19	0	—	10	54	254	0	6	0
rib whole lean & fat trim ¼ in Select broiled	3 oz	274	21	9	69	19	0	—	10	54	269	0	5	0
rib whole lean & fat trim ¼ in Select roasted	3 oz	286	23	9	71	19	0	—	9	54	260	0	6	0
shank crosscut lean & fat trim ¼ in Choice simmered	3 oz	224	12	5	68	26	0	—	25	52	344	0	8	0

FOOD	PORTION	CALORIES	FAT	SAT FAT	CHOL	PROTEIN	CARBO	FIBER	CALCIUM	SOD	POTAS	VIT C	FOLIC	VIT A
short loin top loin lean & fat trim 0 in Choice broiled	3 oz	193	10	4	65	23	0	—	7	57	327	0	7	0
short loin top loin lean & fat trim 0 in Choice broiled	1 steak (5.4 oz)	353	19	7	119	43	0	—	13	104	597	0	12	0
short loin top loin lean & fat trim 0 in Select broiled	1 steak (5.4 oz)	309	14	5	119	44	0	—	13	104	601	0	12	0
short loin top loin lean & fat trim ¼ in Choice braised	3 oz	253	18	7	68	22	0	—	8	54	294	0	6	0
short loin top loin lean & fat trim ¼ in Choice broiled	1 steak (6.3 oz)	536	38	15	143	46	0	—	16	114	623	0	13	0
short loin top loin lean & fat trim ¼ in Prime broiled	1 steak (6.3 oz)	582	43	17	143	46	0	—	16	114	623	0	13	0
short loin top loin lean & fat trim ¼ in Select broiled	1 steak (6.3 oz)	473	31	12	140	46	0	—	16	114	631	0	13	0
short loin top loin lean only trim 0 in Choice broiled	1 steak (5.2 oz)	311	14	5	113	43	0	—	12	101	590	0	12	0
short loin top loin lean only trim ¼ in Choice broiled	1 steak (5.2 oz)	314	15	6	112	42	0	—	12	100	582	0	12	0
shortribs lean & fat Choice braised	3 oz	400	36	15	80	18	0	—	10	43	191	—	4	—
t-bone steak lean & fat trim ¼ in Choice broiled	3 oz	253	18	7	70	21	0	—	7	52	302	0	6	0
t-bone steak lean only trim ¼ in Choice broiled	3 oz	182	9	4	68	24	0	—	6	56	346	0	7	0
tenderloin lean & fat trim 0 in Select broiled	3 oz	194	11	4	72	23	0	—	6	52	341	0	6	0
tenderloin lean & fat trim ¼ in Choice broiled	3 oz	259	19	7	73	21	0	—	7	50	310	0	5	0
tenderloin lean & fat trim ¼ in Choice roasted	3 oz	288	22	9	73	20	0	—	8	55	340	0	7	0
tenderloin lean & fat trim ¼ in Choice broiled	3 oz	208	12	5	72	23	0	—	6	52	338	0	6	0
tenderloin lean & fat trim ¼ in Prime broiled	3 oz	270	20	8	73	21	0	—	7	50	308	0	5	0

FOOD	PORTION	CALORIES	FAT	SAT FAT	CHOL	PROTEIN	CARBO	FIBER	CALCIUM	SOD	POTAS	VIT C	FOLIC	VIT A
tenderloin lean & fat trim ¼ in Select roasted	3 oz	275	21	8	73	21	0	—	8	48	277	0	6	0
tenderloin lean only trim 0 in Select broiled	3 oz	170	7	3	71	24	0	—	6	54	356	0	6	0
tenderloin lean only trim ¼ in Choice broiled	3 oz	188	10	4	71	24	0	—	6	54	356	0	6	0
tenderloin lean only trim ¼ in Select broiled	3 oz	169	7	3	71	24	0	—	6	54	356	0	6	0
tip round lean & fat trim 0 in Choice roasted	3 oz	170	8	3	69	24	0	—	5	54	319	0	7	0
tip round lean & fat trim 0 in Select roasted	3 oz	158	6	2	69	24	0	—	4	55	321	0	7	0
tip round lean & fat trim ¼ in Choice roasted	3 oz	210	13	5	70	23	0	—	5	53	301	0	6	0
tip round lean & fat trim ¼ in Prime roasted	3 oz	233	15	6	70	22	0	—	5	53	299	0	6	0
tip round lean & fat trim ¼ in Select roasted	3 oz	191	10	4	70	23	0	—	5	53	308	0	6	0
top round lean & fat trim 0 in Choice braised	3 oz	184	6	2	77	30	0	—	3	38	280	0	8	0
top round lean & fat trim 0 in Select braised	3 oz	170	5	2	77	30	0	—	3	38	280	0	8	0
top round lean & fat trim ¼ in Choice braised	3 oz	221	11	4	77	29	0	—	4	38	266	0	7	0
top round lean & fat trim ¼ in Choice broiled	3 oz	190	9	3	72	26	0	—	6	51	356	0	10	0
top round lean & fat trim ¼ in Choice fried	3 oz	235	13	5	82	28	0	—	5	58	399	0	10	0
top round lean & fat trim ¼ in Prime broiled	3 oz	195	9	3	72	26	0	—	5	51	367	0	10	0
top round lean & fat trim ¼ in Select braised	3 oz	175	7	3	72	26	0	—	6	51	356	0	10	0
top round lean & fat trim ¼ in Select braised	3 oz	199	8	3	77	29	0	—	4	38	269	0	7	0

FOOD	PORTION	CALORIES	FAT	SAT FAT	CHOL	PROTEIN	CARBO	FIBER	CALCIUM	SOD	POTAS	VIT C	FOLIC	VIT A
top sirloin lean & fat trim 0 in Choice broiled	3 oz	194	10	4	76	25	0	—	10	55	328	0	8	0
top sirloin lean & fat trim 0 in Select broiled	3 oz	166	6	3	76	25	0	—	9	55	334	0	6	0
top sirloin lean & fat trim ¼ in Choice broiled	3 oz	228	14	6	76	23	0	—	10	53	309	0	8	0
top sirloin lean & fat trim ¼ in Choice fried	3 oz	277	19	8	83	24	0	—	10	59	336	0	7	0
top sirloin lean & fat trim ¼ in Select broiled	3 oz	208	12	5	76	24	0	—	10	54	314	0	8	0
tripe raw	4 oz	111	4	2	107	16	0	—	—	52	305	4	2	0
HEALTHY CHOICE														
Ground Extra Lean	4 oz	130	4	2	55	22	2	0	0	230	—	0	—	0
LAURA'S LEAN														
Eye Of Round	4 oz	150	5	2	60	26	0	—	—	85	—	—	—	—
Flank Steak	4 oz	160	7	3	65	24	0	—	—	75	—	—	—	—
Ground	4 oz	180	10	6	60	23	0	—	—	75	—	—	—	—
Ground Round	4 oz	160	7	3	65	24	0	—	—	75	—	—	—	—
Ribeye Steak	4 oz	150	5	2	65	26	0	—	—	60	—	—	—	—
Sirloin Tip Round	4 oz	140	5	2	65	25	0	—	—	65	—	—	—	—
Sirloin Top Butt	4 oz	140	5	2	60	25	0	—	—	90	—	—	—	—
Strip Steak	4 oz	150	5	2	50	25	0	—	—	85	—	—	—	—
Tenderloins	4 oz	150	6	3	75	24	0	—	—	75	—	—	—	—
Top Round	4 oz	140	4	2	65	26	0	—	—	80	—	—	—	—
MAVERICK RANCH														
Ground Round Extra Lean	4 oz	130	4	2	60	24	0	—	—	65	—	—	—	—
FROZEN														
patties broiled medium	3 oz	240	17	7	80	21	0	—	9	66	250	0	8	—
READY-TO-EAT														
HEALTHY CHOICE														
Deli-Thin Roast Beef	6 slices (2 oz)	60	2	1	25	11	1	0	0	520	—	0	—	0
Fresh-Trak Roast Beef	1 slice (1 oz)	30	1	0	10	5	0	0	0	260	—	0	—	0
JORDAN'S														
Healthy Trim 97% Fat Free Roast Beef Medium	1 slice (1 oz)	30	1	1	20	6	0	0	0	130	—	0	—	0
Healthy Trim 97% Fat Free Roast Beef Rare	1 slice (1 oz)	30	1	1	20	6	0	0	0	130	—	0	—	0

FOOD	PORTION	CALORIES	FAT	SAT FAT	CHOL	PROTEIN	CARBO	FIBER	CALCIUM	SOD	POTAS	VIT C	FOLIC	VIT A
WEIGHT WATCHERS														
Deli Thin Oven Roasted Cured	5 slices (⅓ oz)	10	tr	—	5	2	tr	—	—	85	—	—	—	—
TAKE-OUT														
roast beef medium	2 oz	70	2	1	30	12	0	—	—	210	—	—	—	—
roast beef rare	2 oz	70	2	1	30	12	0	—	—	210	—	—	—	—
BEEF DISHES														
CANNED														
corned beef hash	3 oz	155	10	5	—	10	9	—	11	—	—	—	—	—
ARMOUR														
Corned Beef Hash	1 cup (8.3 oz)	440	30	—	100	19	23	—	—	840	—	—	—	—
Roast Beef Hash	1 cup (8.4 oz)	400	25	—	95	20	23	—	—	1460	—	—	—	—
Roast Beef In Gravy	½ cup (4.6 oz)	150	4	—	75	25	3	—	—	640	—	—	—	—
Stew	1 cup (8.6 oz)	220	12	—	30	8	21	—	—	1250	—	—	—	—
DINTY MOORE														
Meatball Stew	1 cup (8.4 oz)	250	15	7	40	13	17	2	20	1120	—	0	—	1250
Sliced Potatoes & Beef	1 can (7.5 oz)	230	9	4	35	10	28	4	40	1080	—	0	—	0
Stew	1 cup (8.3 oz)	230	14	7	40	11	16	2	20	950	—	0	—	2000
Stew	1 cup (8.2 oz)	230	14	7	40	11	16	2	20	950	—	0	—	1000
HORMEL														
Beef Goulash	1 can (7.5 oz)	230	11	5	50	13	19	3	40	1040	—	0	—	300
Roast Beef With Gravy	2 oz	60	2	1	30	11	1	0	0	280	—	0	—	0
MARY KITCHEN														
Corned Beef Hash	1 cup (8.3 oz)	410	27	10	80	21	22	2	20	1020	—	0	—	0
Roast Beef Hash	1 cup (8.3 oz)	390	24	10	70	21	22	2	20	790	—	0	—	0
Roast Turkey Hash	1 can (14.9 oz)	420	11	3	110	39	42	3	40	1800	—	2	—	0
Sausage Hash	1 cup (8.3 oz)	410	27	9	85	20	23	2	20	1020	—	4	—	0
FROZEN														
HOT POCKET														
Stuffed Sandwich Barbecue	1 (4.5 oz)	340	12	5	25	13	45	1	150	850	—	2	—	300
Stuffed Sandwich Beef & Cheddar	1 (4.5 oz)	360	18	9	50	14	36	tr	300	830	—	2	—	300
Stuffed Sandwich Beef Fajita	1 (4.5 oz)	360	17	8	40	14	39	5	60	780	—	1	—	1250
LEAN POCKETS														
Stuffed Sandwich Beef & Broccoli	1 (4.5 oz)	250	7	3	50	9	37	7	40	710	—	5	—	200
LUIGINO'S														
Creamed Sauce Shaved Cured Beef With Croutons	1 pkg (8 oz)	360	20	6	60	15	29	3	200	810	—	0	—	750

FOOD	PORTION	CALORIES	FAT	SAT FAT	CHOL	PROTEIN	CARBO	FIBER	CALCIUM	SOD	POTAS	VIT C	FOLIC	VIT A
LUIGINO'S (CONT.)														
Egg Noodles Rich Gravy Swedish Meatballs	1 pkg (9 oz)	340	15	4	80	16	36	3	40	820	—	0	—	200
Egg Noodles Rich Gravy Swedish Meatballs	1 cup (7.5 oz)	280	12	3	70	13	30	3	40	690	—	0	—	200
MRS. PATERSON'S														
Aussie Pie Philly Steak	1 (5.5 oz)	420	24	8	40	11	39	2	20	860	—	0	—	500
TYSON														
Microwave BBQ Sandwich	1 sandwich	200	3	—	30	15	29	—	—	600	—	—	—	—
MIX														
CASBAH														
Gyro as prep	1 patty (2 oz)	145	5	2	63	2	12	tr	20	456	—	0	—	50
HAMBURGER HELPER														
BBQ Beef as prep	1 cup	320	10	4	55	21	37	1	20	760	460	0	60	500
Beef Pasta as prep	1 cup	270	10	4	50	20	26	tr	40	910	300	0	60	0
Beef Romanoff as prep	1 cup	280	10	4	50	20	27	0	60	920	340	0	60	0
Beef Stew as prep	1 cup	250	10	4	50	18	26	2	20	750	480	0	8	500
Beef Taco as prep	1 cup	310	11	4	50	20	31	1	40	930	370	0	60	500
Beef Teriyaki as prep	1 cup	290	10	4	50	18	34	2	60	990	300	0	40	500
Cheddar 'n Bacon as prep	1 cup	350	16	6	65	24	28	tr	100	890	400	0	60	100
Cheddar Melt as prep	1 cup	310	12	5	55	20	31	tr	80	900	330	0	60	0
Cheddar Spirals Reduced Sodium as prep	1 cup	320	14	5	60	21	27	1	100	650	720	0	60	500
Cheeseburger Macaroni as prep	1 cup	360	16	6	65	23	31	tr	100	1000	440	0	60	0
Cheesy Italian as prep	1 cup	330	14	5	60	22	29	tr	100	920	400	0	60	300
Cheesy Shells as prep	1 cup	340	14	5	60	22	30	tr	100	850	400	0	60	100
Chili Macaroni as prep	1 cup	290	10	4	55	19	30	tr	20	870	400	0	40	1000
Fettuccine Alfredo as prep	1 cup	310	13	5	55	20	26	1	80	850	330	0	60	0
Four Cheese Lasagne as prep	1 cup	330	14	5	55	21	31	0	100	860	410	0	60	200
Italian Herb Reduced Sodium as prep	1 cup	270	10	4	50	19	29	2	20	650	570	0	60	500
Italian Rigatoni as prep	1 cup	280	10	4	50	19	29	1	20	870	340	0	40	300

FOOD	PORTION	CALORIES	FAT	SAT FAT	CHOL	PROTEIN	CARBO	FIBER	CALCIUM	SOD	POTAS	VIT C	FOLIC	VIT A
HAMBURGER HELPER (CONT.)														
Lasagne as prep	1 cup	280	10	4	50	19	30	0	0	990	340	0	60	0
Meat Loaf as prep	⅙ loaf	270	14	6	110	24	11	0	40	580	380	0	16	0
Mushroom & Wild Rice as prep	1 cup	310	12	5	55	20	30	2	100	880	400	0	40	100
Nacho Cheese as prep	1 cup	320	13	5	55	22	30	tr	100	930	420	0	60	0
Pizza Pasta as prep	1 cup	290	10	4	50	19	31	0	60	760	410	0	40	300
Pizzabake as prep	⅙ pie	270	10	4	45	17	28	tr	40	720	320	0	40	200
Potatoes Au Gratin as prep	1 cup	290	14	5	55	18	24	2	60	820	500	0	8	100
Potatoes Stroganoff as prep	1 cup	270	12	5	55	18	25	2	60	870	510	0	8	0
Ravioli as prep	1 cup	280	10	4	50	20	30	1	20	840	410	0	60	400
Rice Oriental as prep	1 cup	310	10	4	55	19	35	0	0	1050	300	0	40	0
Salisbury as prep	1 cup	270	10	4	50	19	26	tr	40	790	290	0	40	300
Southwestern Beef Reduced Sodium as prep	1 cup	300	10	4	50	20	32	2	20	650	610	0	60	500
Spaghetti as prep	1 cup	300	11	4	55	21	29	tr	20	940	430	0	60	500
Stroganoff as prep	1 cup	320	13	5	55	21	30	0	100	830	370	0	60	100
Swedish Meatballs as prep	1 cup	300	14	5	55	19	24	tr	20	780	320	0	40	400
Three Cheeses as prep	1 cup	340	15	5	55	21	32	tr	80	830	350	0	60	100
Zesty Italian as prep	1 cup	320	11	4	55	21	34	tr	20	890	470	0	60	300
Zesty Mexican as prep	1 cup	300	11	4	50	19	32	1	60	730	400	0	40	750
SHELF-STABLE														
DINTY MOORE														
Microwave Cup Corned Beef Hash	1 pkg (7.5 oz)	350	22	9	60	19	19	2	20	850	—	0	—	0
Microwave Cup Hearty Burger Stew	1 pkg (7.5 oz)	240	13	5	40	12	19	3	60	930	—	0	—	1750
Microwave Cup Stew	1 pkg (7.5 oz)	190	10	5	40	11	15	2	20	900	—	0	—	1500
HORMEL														
Microcup Meals Stew	1 cup (7.5 oz)	190	10	4	35	11	15	2	20	900	—	1	—	500
LUNCH BUCKET														
Beef Stew	1 pkg (7.5 oz)	180	11	—	40	8	13	—	—	870	—	—	—	—
TAKE-OUT														
irish stew	1 cup (7 oz)	280	16	9	—	23	10	—	17	—	—	11	—	10
roast beef sandwich plain	1	346	14	4	52	22	33	—	54	792	316	2	40	210

FOOD	PORTION	CALORIES	FAT	SAT FAT	CHOL	PROTEIN	CARBO	FIBER	CALCIUM	SOD	POTAS	VIT C	FOLIC	VIT A
roast beef sandwich w/ cheese	1	402	18	9	77	32	27	—	183	1634	345	0	41	193
roast beef submarine sandwich w/ tomato lettuce & mayonnaise	1	411	13	7	73	29	44	—	41	845	330	6	45	412
steak sandwich w/ tomato lettuce salt & mayonnaise	1	459	14	4	73	30	52	—	91	798	525	6	89	367
stew w/ vegetables	1 cup	220	11	4	71	16	15	—	29	292	613	17	—	5690
BEEFALO														
roasted	3 oz	160	5	2	49	26	0	—	21	70	390	8	15	—
BEER AND ALE														
alcohol free beer	7 fl oz	50	tr	—	—	1	11	—	5	3	40	—	15	—
beer light	12 oz can	100	0	0	0	tr	5	—	18	10	64	0	15	0
beer regular	12 oz can	146	0	0	0	1	13	—	18	19	89	0	21	0
pilsener lager beer	7 fl oz	85	tr	—	—	1	13	—	4	4	55	—	6	—
COORS														
Beer	12 oz	132	0	0	0	tr	30	—	9	10	75	—	—	—
Extra Gold	12 oz	147	0	0	0	tr	32	—	8	10	77	—	—	—
Light	12 oz	101	0	0	0	tr	13	—	11	10	62	—	—	—
KILLIAN'S														
Beer	12 oz	212	0	0	0	tr	29	—	10	10	68	—	—	—
KINGSBURY														
Nonalcoholic	12 fl oz	60	0	0	0	—	—	—	—	—	—	—	—	—
WINTERFEST														
Beer	12 oz	167	0	0	0	1	38	—	7	11	114	—	—	—
BEETS														
CANNED														
harvard	½ cup	89	tr	tr	0	1	22	—	13	199	201	3	—	—
pickled	½ cup	75	tr	tr	0	1	19	—	13	301	169	3	—	7
sliced	½ cup	27	tr	tr	0	1	6	—	—	—	—	—	—	—
DEL MONTE														
Pickled Crinkle Style Sliced	½ cup (4.5 oz)	80	0	0	0	1	19	2	0	380	—	4	—	0
Sliced	½ cup (4.3 oz)	35	0	0	0	1	8	2	0	290	—	2	—	0
Whole	½ cup (4.3 oz)	35	0	0	0	1	8	2	0	290	—	2	—	0
Whole Tiny	½ cup (4.3 oz)	35	0	0	0	1	8	2	0	290	—	2	—	0
GREEN GIANT														
Harvard	⅓ cup (3.1 oz)	60	0	0	0	tr	15	2	0	270	—	0	—	0
Sliced	½ cup (4.2 oz)	35	0	0	0	1	8	2	0	260	—	0	—	0
Sliced No Salt Added	½ cup (4.2 oz)	35	0	0	0	1	8	2	0	60	—	0	—	0
Whole	½ cup (4.2 oz)	35	0	0	0	1	8	2	0	260	—	0	—	0

FOOD	PORTION	CALORIES	FAT	SAT FAT	CHOL	PROTEIN	CARBO	FIBER	CALCIUM	SOD	POTAS	VIT C	FOLIC	VIT A
LESUEUR														
Baby Whole	½ cup (4.3 oz)	35	0	0	0	1	8	2	0	260	—	0	—	0
SENECA														
Cut	½ cup	35	0	0	0	0	9	2	0	264	210	4	—	0
Diced	½ cup	35	0	0	0	0	9	2	0	264	210	4	—	0
Harvard	½ cup	90	0	0	0	1	21	1	20	144	210	6	—	0
Pickled	2 tbsp	20	0	0	0	0	6	0	0	48	70	0	—	0
Pickled With Onions	2 tbsp	20	0	0	0	0	6	0	0	48	70	0	—	0
Sliced	½ cup	35	0	0	0	0	9	2	0	264	210	4	—	0
Whole	½ cup	35	0	0	0	0	9	2	0	264	210	4	—	0
FRESH														
greens cooked	½ cup	20	tr	tr	0	2	4	—	82	173	654	18	—	3672
greens raw	½ cup	4	tr	tr	0	tr	1	—	23	38	104	6	—	1159
greens raw chopped	½ cup	4	tr	tr	0	tr	1	—	23	38	104	6	—	1159
raw sliced	½ cup (2.4 oz)	29	tr	tr	0	1	7	—	11	53	221	3	74	26
sliced cooked	½ cup (3 oz)	38	tr	tr	0	1	9	—	14	65	259	3	68	30
whole cooked	2 (3.5 oz)	44	tr	tr	0	2	10	—	16	77	306	4	80	35
whole raw	2 (5.7 oz)	70	tr	tr	0	3	16	—	27	126	530	8	178	61

BEVERAGES

(*see* BEER AND ALE, CHAMPAGNE, COFFEE, DRINK MIXERS, FRUIT DRINKS, ICED TEA, LIQUOR/LIQUEUR, MALT, MILKSHAKE, MINERAL/BOTTLED WATER, SODA, SPORTS DRINKS, TEA/HERBAL TEA, WINE, WINE COOLER)

BISCUIT

FROZEN

FOOD	PORTION	CALORIES	FAT	SAT FAT	CHOL	PROTEIN	CARBO	FIBER	CALCIUM	SOD	POTAS	VIT C	FOLIC	VIT A
GREAT STARTS														
Egg Canadian Bacon & Cheese	5.2 oz	420	22	—	—	16	37	—	250	1845	—	1	—	—
Sausage	4.7 oz	410	22	—	—	14	36	—	100	1180	—	—	—	—
JIMMY DEAN														
Chicken Twin	2 (3.2 oz)	280	13	4	25	9	32	2	—	870	—	—	—	—
Sausage Twin	2 (3.4 oz)	330	21	7	30	10	25	2	—	900	—	—	—	—
Steak Twin	2 (3.2 oz)	270	13	5	25	10	26	2	—	660	—	—	—	—
RUDY'S FARM														
Ham Twin	2 (3 oz)	160	3	1	20	10	23	1	—	790	—	—	—	—
Sausage & Cheese Twin	2 (3 oz)	290	18	6	30	9	22	1	—	570	—	—	—	—
Sausage Twin	2 (2.7 oz)	296	18	6	30	9	22	1	—	580	—	—	—	—
HOME RECIPE														
buttermilk	1 (2 oz)	212	10	3	2	4	27	—	141	348	73	tr	7	49
plain	1 (2 oz)	212	10	3	2	4	27	—	141	348	73	tr	7	49
MIX														
buttermilk	1 (2 oz)	191	7	2	—	4	28	1	105	544	107	—	3	—
plain	1 (2 oz)	191	7	2	—	4	28	1	105	544	107	—	3	—
ARROWHEAD														
Biscuit Mix	¼ cup (1.2 oz)	120	1	0	0	5	23	3	200	200	180	0	—	0

FOOD	PORTION	CALORIES	FAT	SAT FAT	CHOL	PROTEIN	CARBO	FIBER	CALCIUM	SOD	POTAS	VIT C	FOLIC	VIT A
BISQUICK														
Mix	½ cup (2 oz)	240	8	2	0	4	37	—	80	700	80	—	—	—
Reduced Fat	⅓ cup (1.4 oz)	150	3	1	0	2	28	1	40	460	—	—	40	—
HEALTH VALLEY														
Buttermilk Biscuit Mix not prep	1 oz	100	1	—	0	4	20	3	20	170	250	1	14	3
JIFFY														
As prep	1	150	7	3	3	2	30	2	150	384	—	0	—	0
Biscuit	¼ cup (1.1 oz)	130	5	1	0	2	22	1	100	320	—	0	—	0
Buttermilk as prep	1	170	4	2	5	3	29	tr	60	380	—	0	—	0
READY-TO-EAT														
ARNOLD														
Old Fashioned	1	60	3	—	—	1	8	—	20	100	—	—	—	—
REFRIGERATED														
buttermilk	1 (1 oz)	98	4	1	0	2	14	—	6	341	45	0	—	0
plain	1 (1 oz)	98	4	1	—	2	14	tr	6	341	45	0	—	0
ROMAN MEAL														
Biscuit	2 (2.4 oz)	180	4	1	0	4	34	1	12	456	310	0	—	0
Honey Nut Oat Bran	1 (1.5 oz)	131	5	1	0	2	21	1	9	278	175	0	—	0
TAKE-OUT														
buttermilk	1	127	6	1	—	2	17	—	17	368	78	0	3	—
plain	1 (35 g)	276	34	9	5	4	13	—	90	584	86	0	6	98
tea biscuit	1 (3 oz)	210	3	2	0	5	30	1	150	370	—	0	—	200
w/ egg	1	315	20	6	232	11	24	—	154	655	160	0	29	649
w/ egg & bacon	1	457	31	10	353	17	29	—	189	999	250	3	29	191
w/ egg & sausage	1	582	39	15	302	19	41	—	155	1142	319	tr	40	635
w/ egg & steak	1	474	28	9	272	18	37	—	138	888	306	tr	28	704
w/ egg cheese & bacon	1	477	31	11	261	16	33	—	164	1261	230	2	37	648
w/ ham	1	387	18	11	25	13	44	—	161	1433	197	tr	8	133
w/ sausage	1	485	32	14	34	12	40	—	128	1071	198	tr	9	56
w/ steak	1	456	26	7	26	13	44	—	115	795	233	tr	11	65
BISON														
roasted	3 oz	122	2	1	70	24	0	—	7	48	307	—	—	—
BLACK BEANS														
CANNED														
ALLEN														
Seasoned	½ cup (4.5 oz)	120	2	1	0	7	20	7	40	410	—	0	—	0
EDEN														
Organic	½ cup (4.6 oz)	100	0	0	0	7	18	6	60	15	280	—	—	—
Organic w/ Ginger & Lemon	½ cup (4.6 oz)	120	0	0	0	7	21	7	60	200	300	—	—	—
GREEN GIANT														
Black Beans	½ cup (4.5 oz)	50	0	0	0	6	18	5	40	400	—	0	—	0

FOOD	PORTION	CALORIES	FAT	SAT FAT	CHOL	PROTEIN	CARBO	FIBER	CALCIUM	SOD	POTAS	VIT C	FOLIC	VIT A
HEALTH VALLEY														
Fast Menu Organic Black Beans With Tofu Weiners	7½ oz	150	1	—	0	14	20	15	179	170	280	tr	88	4184
Fast Menu Western Black Beans With Garden Vegetable	7½ oz	160	5	—	0	16	14	14	150	250	260	1	—	5000
OLD EL PASO														
Black Beans	½ cup (4.6 oz)	100	1	0	0	7	17	7	40	400	—	0	—	0
Refried	½ cup (4.2 oz)	120	2	0	0	6	18	6	60	340	—	0	—	0
PROGRESSO														
Black Beans	½ cup (4.6 oz)	100	1	0	0	7	17	7	40	400	—	0	—	0
TRAPPEY														
Seasoned	½ cup (4.5 oz)	120	2	1	0	7	20	7	40	410	—	0	—	0
DRIED														
cooked	1 cup	227	1	tr	0	15	41	—	47	1	611	0	256	10
MIX														
BEAN CUISINE														
Black Turtle	½ cup	115	1	—	0	8	—	5	—	5	310	—	62	—
Pasta & Beans Black Beans With Fusilli	½ cup	174	4	1	tr	6	27	—	—	453	—	—	—	—
MAHATMA														
Black Beans & Rice	1 cup	200	2	0	0	8	39	6	80	850	—	0	—	0
BLACKBERRIES														
canned in heavy syrup	½ cup	118	tr	—	0	2	30	—	27	3	127	4	34	280
unsweetened frzn	1 cup	97	1	—	0	2	24	—	44	2	211	5	51	172
ALLEN-WOLCO														
Canned	½ cup (5.3 oz)	60	1	0	0	2	13	9	40	20	—	0	—	200
BIG VALLEY														
Frozen	⅔ cup (4.9 oz)	70	0	0	0	1	15	4	30	0	—	24	—	0
BLACKBERRY JUICE														
KOOL-AID														
Scary Blackberry Ghoul-Aid Drink as prep w/ sugar	1 serv (8 oz)	100	0	0	0	0	25	0	0	0	0	6	—	0
BLACKEYE PEAS														
CANNED														
w/pork	½ cup	199	4	1	17	7	40	—	21	840	427	1	—	0
ALLEN														
Blackeye Peas	½ cup (4.5 oz)	110	1	1	0	7	18	4	20	340	—	0	—	0
Fresh Shell	½ cup (4.4 oz)	120	1	1	0	7	21	6	40	350	—	0	—	0
With Bacon	½ cup (4.5 oz)	105	2	1	0	7	20	5	40	390	—	0	—	0
With Snaps	½ cup (4.4 oz)	120	1	1	0	8	20	5	40	420	—	0	—	0

FOOD	PORTION	CALORIES	FAT	SAT FAT	CHOL	PROTEIN	CARBO	FIBER	CALCIUM	SOD	POTAS	VIT C	FOLIC	VIT A
DORMAN														
Fresh Shell	½ cup (4.4 oz)	120	1	1	0	7	21	6	40	350	—	0	—	0
EAST TEXAS FAIR														
Blackeye Peas	½ cup (4.5 oz)	110	1	1	0	7	18	4	20	340	—	0	—	0
Fresh Shell	½ cup (4.4 oz)	120	1	1	0	7	21	6	40	350	—	0	—	0
With Snaps	½ cup (4.4 oz)	120	1	1	0	8	20	5	40	420	—	0	—	0
GREEN GIANT														
Blackeye Peas	½ cup (4.4 oz)	90	0	0	0	6	16	3	40	250	—	0	—	0
HOMEFOLKS														
Fresh Shell	½ cup (4.4 oz)	120	1	1	0	7	21	6	40	350	—	0	—	0
With Jalapeno	½ cup (4.4 oz)	120	1	1	0	7	20	5	40	580	—	0	—	0
With Snaps	½ cup (4.4 oz)	120	1	1	0	8	20	5	40	420	—	0	—	0
SUNSHINE														
With Bacon	½ cup (4.5 oz)	105	2	1	0	7	20	5	40	390	—	0	—	0
TRAPPEY														
With Bacon	½ cup (4.5 oz)	120	2	1	0	7	19	5	20	350	—	0	—	0
With Bacon & Jalapeno	½ cup (4.4 oz)	110	2	1	0	6	19	5	20	470	—	0	—	0
DRIED														
HURST														
HamBeens California w/ Ham	1 serv	120	1	0	0	8	22	7	40	73	—	0	—	0
FROZEN														
BIRDS EYE														
Blackeye Peas	½ cup (2.8 oz)	110	1	0	0	7	21	4	20	10	—	1	—	0
FRESH LIKE														
Fresh Like	3.5 oz	138	1	—	—	10	24	1	28	6	440	4	—	81
BLINTZE														
EMPIRE														
Apple	2 (4.4 oz)	220	6	2	<5	6	36	5	0	260	—	5	—	0
Blueberry	2 (4.4 oz)	190	4	1	10	4	36	2	0	260	—	5	—	0
Cheese	2 (4.4 oz)	200	6	2	20	11	29	3	40	310	—	1	—	0
Cherry	2 (4.4 oz)	200	4	1	10	5	38	3	0	280	—	2	—	0
Potato	2 (4.4 oz)	190	6	2	10	6	32	3	20	530	—	1	—	0
GOLDEN														
Apple Raisin	1 (2.25 oz)	80	2	0	10	3	16	—	—	145	55	—	—	—
Blueberry	1 (2.25 oz)	90	1	0	10	2	18	—	—	150	45	—	—	—
Cheese	1 (2.25 oz)	80	2	1	13	6	13	—	—	135	50	—	—	—
Cherry	1 (2.25 oz)	95	1	0	5	3	18	—	—	145	70	—	—	100
Potato	1 (2.25 oz)	90	4	1	5	3	15	—	—	170	135	—	—	—
TAKE-OUT														
cheese	1 (2.7 oz)	160	9	4	65	5	15	tr	300	240	—	0	—	4500
BLUEBERRIES														
canned in heavy syrup	1 cup	225	1	—	0	2	56	—	7	9	102	3	4	164

FOOD	PORTION	CALORIES	FAT	SAT FAT	CHOL	PROTEIN	CARBO	FIBER	CALCIUM	SOD	POTAS	VIT C	FOLIC	VIT A
fresh	1 cup	82	1	—	0	1	20	—	9	9	129	19	9	145
unsweetened frzn	1 cup	78	1	—	0	1	19	—	12	1	83	4	10	126
BIG VALLEY														
Frozen	¾ cup (4.9 oz)	70	0	0	0	0	12	4	0	0	—	11	—	0
SONOMA														
Dried	¼ cup (1.3 oz)	140	0	0	0	1	33	5	0	0	—	0	—	0

BLUEBERRY JUICE
AFTER THE FALL														
Maine Coast	1 cup (8 oz)	90	0	0	0	0	25	0	0	20	—	5	—	0

BOAR
wild roasted	3 oz	136	4	1	—	24	0	—	13	—	—	—	—	—

BOK CHOY
DOLE														
Shredded	½ cup	5	tr	—	0	1	1	—	—	23	88	16	—	1050

BONIATO
fresh	½ cup	90	tr	—	—	1	20	—	—	7	612	11	—	220

BORAGE
fresh chopped cooked	3½ oz	25	1	—	0	2	4	—	102	88	491	33	—	4385
raw chopped	½ cup	9	tr	—	0	1	1	—	41	35	207	15	—	1848

BOYSENBERRIES
in heavy syrup	1 cup	226	tr	—	0	3	57	—	23	9	230	16	88	102
unsweetened frzn	1 cup	66	tr	—	0	1	16	—	36	2	183	4	84	89

BRAINS
beef pan-fried	3 oz	167	13	3	1696	11	0	—	8	134	301	3	5	0
beef simmered	3 oz	136	11	2	1746	9	0	—	8	102	204	1	6	0
lamb braised	3 oz	124	9	2	1737	11	0	—	10	114	175	10	4	0
lamb fried	3 oz	232	19	5	2128	14	0	—	18	133	304	20	6	0
pork braised	3 oz	117	8	2	2169	10	0	0	8	77	—	12	3	0
veal braised	3 oz	115	8	—	2635	10	0	—	13	133	181	11	3	0
veal fried	3 oz	181	14	—	1802	12	0	—	9	150	401	12	5	0
ARMOUR														
Pork Brains In Milk Gravy	⅔ cup (5.5 oz)	150	5	—	3500	16	10	—	—	550	—	—	—	—

BRAN
corn	⅓ cup	56	tr	tr	0	2	21	21	11	2	11	0	1	18
oat cooked	½ cup	44	tr	tr	0	4	13	—	11	1	101	0	7	—
oat dry	½ cup	116	3	tr	0	8	31	7	27	1	266	0	24	—
rice dry	⅓ cup	88	6	1	0	4	14	6	16	1	416	0	18	—
ARROWHEAD														
Oat Bran	⅓ cup (1.4 oz)	150	3	0	0	8	23	7	40	0	280	0	—	0
Wheat Bran	¼ cup (0.6 oz)	30	1	0	0	3	7	6	0	0	180	0	—	0
GOOD SHEPHERD														
Wheat Bran	1 oz	80	1	—	0	4	18	3	—	5	330	—	—	—

FOOD	PORTION	CALORIES	FAT	SAT FAT	CHOL	PROTEIN	CARBO	FIBER	CALCIUM	SOD	POTAS	VIT C	FOLIC	VIT A
H-O														
Super Bran	⅓ cup	110	2	0	0	7	18	3	—	0	90	—	—	—
HEALTH VALLEY														
Fast Menu Oat Bran Pilaf With Garden Vegetables	7½ oz	210	7	—	0	7	30	15	51	330	260	5	45	6174
HODGSON MILL														
Oat	¼ cup (1.3 oz)	120	3	1	0	6	23	6	20	3	—	0	—	0
Wheat	¼ cup (0.5 oz)	30	1	0	0	2	10	7	20	0	139	0	—	0
MOTHER'S														
Oat Bran	½ cup	150	3	1	0	8	24	6	20	0	230	—	8	0
QUAKER														
Oat Bran	½ cup	150	3	1	0	8	24	6	20	0	230	—	8	0
ROMAN MEAL														
Oat	1 oz	94	3	tr	0	5	13	5	19	3	0	0	—	0
STONE-BUHR														
Oat	⅓ cup (1 oz)	90	2	0	0	4	20	4	20	0	—	0	—	0

BRAZIL NUTS

FOOD	PORTION	CALORIES	FAT	SAT FAT	CHOL	PROTEIN	CARBO	FIBER	CALCIUM	SOD	POTAS	VIT C	FOLIC	VIT A
dried unblanched	1 oz	186	19	5	0	4	4	—	50	0	170	tr	1	0

BREAD

(*see also* BAGEL, BISCUIT, BREADSTICK, CROISSANT, ENGLISH MUFFIN, MUFFIN, ROLL, SCONE)

FOOD	PORTION	CALORIES	FAT	SAT FAT	CHOL	PROTEIN	CARBO	FIBER	CALCIUM	SOD	POTAS	VIT C	FOLIC	VIT A
CANNED														
boston brown	1 slice (1.6 oz)	88	1	tr	—	2	20	2	31	284	143	0	3	39
B&M														
Brown Bread	½ in slice (2 oz)	130	1	0	0	3	29	2	40	390	—	0	—	0
Brown Bread Raisins	½ in slice (2 oz)	130	1	0	0	3	29	2	40	360	—	0	—	0
FROZEN														
KINERET														
Challah	⅛ loaf (2 oz)	150	4	1	15	5	25	1	0	220	—	0	—	0
NEW YORK														
Garlic	1 slice (2 oz)	190	8	2	0	3	27	1	0	390	—	0	—	0
Garlic Reduced Fat	1 slice (2 oz)	160	4	1	0	4	29	1	0	340	—	0	—	0
Texas Garlic Toast	1 in slice (1.4 oz)	160	9	2	0	3	17	1	0	260	—	0	—	100
HOME RECIPE														
banana	1 slice (2 oz)	195	6	1	26	3	33	—	13	181	81	1	7	278
cornbread as prep w/ 2% milk	1 piece (2.3 oz)	173	5	1	26	4	28	—	162	428	96	tr	12	180
cornbread as prep w/ whole milk	1 piece (2.3 oz)	176	5	1	28	4	28	—	161	428	95	tr	12	158
datenut	½ in slice	92	3	—	15	2	15	—	17	63	—	—	—	—
irish soda bread	1 slice (2 oz)	174	3	1	11	4	34	—	49	239	160	1	6	116
pita whole wheat	1-6 in	247	1	—	0	—	—	—	12	—	—	—	—	—
pumpkin	1 slice (1 oz)	94	4	1	13	1	15	—	5	89	26	tr	3	1540

FOOD	PORTION	CALORIES	FAT	SAT FAT	CHOL	PROTEIN	CARBO	FIBER	CALCIUM	SOD	POTAS	VIT C	FOLIC	VIT A
white as prep w/ nonfat dry milk	1 slice	78	1	tr	0	2	15	—	9	95	32	0	8	12
white as prep w/ 2% milk	1 slice	81	2	tr	1	2	14	—	16	104	41	tr	12	22
white as prep w/ whole milk	1 slice	82	2	tr	1	2	14	—	16	104	41	tr	2	14
whole wheat	1 slice	79	2	tr	0	2	15	—	9	98	89	0	13	0
MIX														
cornbread	1 piece (2 oz)	189	6	2	37	4	29	1	44	467	77	tr	7	123
AUNT JEMIMA														
Corn Bread Easy Mix	⅓ cup (1.3 oz)	150	4	1	0	2	26	1	0	450	40	—	0	—
DROMEDARY														
Corn Bread	1 piece (2 in x 2 in)	130	3	—	—	3	20	—	60	480	65	—	—	100
NATURAL OVENS														
Cracked Wheat	2 slices (2.4 oz)	140	1	0	0	8	38	4	200	140	—	—	120	—
English Muffin Bread	2 slices (2.4 oz)	140	1	0	0	7	35	2	100	140	—	—	20	—
Executive Fitness Sunny Millet	2 slices (2.6 oz)	160	2	0	0	10	37	4	200	70	—	—	80	—
Garden Bread	1 oz	50	1	0	0	4	14	1	60	100	—	—	80	—
Glorious Cinnamon & Raisin Fat Free	2 slices (2.1 oz)	110	1	0	0	8	30	3	250	140	—	—	80	—
Honey 'N Flax	2 slices (2.5 oz)	140	1	0	0	6	30	4	120	140	—	—	60	—
Hunger Filler Bread	2 slices (2.1 oz)	110	2	0	0	6	28	5	300	140	—	—	120	—
Light Wheat	2 slices (2.2 oz)	84	1	0	0	7	30	5	200	140	—	—	120	—
Nutty Natural Wheat Bread	2 slices (2.5 oz)	140	2	0	0	7	32	6	300	140	—	—	120	—
Seven Grain Herb	2 slices (2.5 oz)	140	1	0	0	8	30	4	200	140	—	—	120	—
Soft Hearth Whole Wheat	2 slices (2 oz)	100	2	0	0	8	30	4	300	140	—	—	80	—
Soft Sandwich Very Low Fat	2 slices (2.3 oz)	110	1	0	0	6	26	2	200	140	—	—	80	—
Stay Slim	2 slices (2 oz)	100	2	0	0	10	20	4	240	140	—	—	60	—
READY-TO-EAT														
baguette whole wheat	2 oz	140	0	0	0	6	29	1	0	360	—	0	—	0
cracked wheat	1 slice	65	1	tr	—	2	12	1	11	135	44	—	10	—
egg	1 slice (1.4 oz)	115	2	1	20	4	19	—	37	197	46	0	28	30
french	1 slice (1 oz)	78	1	tr	0	3	15	1	21	172	32	0	9	0
french	1 loaf (1 lb)	1270	18	4	0	43	230	—	499	2633	409	tr	—	tr

FOOD	PORTION	CALORIES	FAT	SAT FAT	CHOL	PROTEIN	CARBO	FIBER	CALCIUM	SOD	POTAS	VIT C	FOLIC	VIT A
gluten	1 slice	47	tr	tr	0	2	8	—	24	104	—	0	7	—
italian	1 slice (1 oz)	81	1	tr	0	3	15	1	23	175	33	0	9	0
italian	1 loaf (1 lb)	1255	4	1	0	41	256	—	77	2656	336	0	—	0
navajo fry	1 (5 in diam)	296	9	2	0	6	48	—	210	625	67	0	11	0
navajo fry	1 (10.5 in diam)	527	15	3	0	11	85	—	373	1112	118	0	20	0
oat bran	1 slice	71	1	tr	0	3	12	1	19	122	—	—	—	0
oat bran reduced calorie	1 slice	46	1	tr	0	2	10	—	13	81	24	0	—	—
oatmeal	1 slice	73	1	tr	—	2	13	1	18	162	38	—	7	—
oatmeal reduced calorie	1 slice	48	1	tr	0	2	10	—	26	89	—	—	—	—
pita	1 reg (2 oz)	165	1	tr	0	5	33	1	52	322	72	0	14	0
pita	1 sm (1 oz)	78	tr	tr	0	3	16	1	24	152	34	0	7	0
pita whole wheat	1 reg (2 oz)	170	2	tr	0	6	35	5	10	340	108	0	—	0
pita whole wheat	1 sm (1 oz)	76	1	tr	0	3	16	2	4	151	48	0	—	0
protein	1 slice	47	tr	tr	0	2	8	—	24	104	—	0	7	—
pumpernickel	1 slice	80	1	tr	0	3	15	2	22	215	661	0	11	0
raisin	1 slice	71	1	tr	0	2	14	—	17	101	59	—	9	—
rice bran	1 slice	66	1	tr	0	1	12	—	19	119	—	—	—	—
rye	1 slice	83	1	tr	0	3	16	2	23	211	53	—	16	0
rye reduced calorie	1 slice	47	1	tr	0	2	9	—	18	93	23	—	—	—
seven grain	1 slice	65	1	tr	0	3	12	2	24	127	53	tr	12	0
sourdough	1 slice (1 oz)	78	1	tr	0	3	15	1	21	172	32	0	9	0
vienna	1 slice (1 oz)	78	1	tr	0	3	15	1	21	172	32	0	9	0
wheat reduced calorie	1 slice	46	1	tr	—	2	10	3	18	117	—	—	—	—
wheat berry	1 slice	65	1	tr	0	2	12	1	26	132	50	0	—	0
wheat bran	1 slice	89	1	tr	0	3	17	3	27	175	82	—	—	0
wheat germ	1 slice	74	1	tr	—	3	14	—	25	157	72	—	16	—
white	1 slice	67	1	tr	0	2	12	1	27	135	30	0	8	0
white reduced calorie	1 slice	48	1	tr	0	2	10	2	22	104	18	—	—	—
white toasted	1 slice	67	1	tr	0	2	13	—	27	136	30	0	6	0
white cubed	1 cup	80	1	tr	0	2	15	—	38	154	34	tr	—	tr
whole wheat	1 slice	70	1	tr	—	3	13	2	20	149	71	—	14	—
ALVARADO ST. BAKERY														
Barley	1 slice (1.2 oz)	70	1	0	0	3	15	2	—	140	—	—	—	—
California Style	1 slice (1.2 oz)	60	1	0	0	3	10	2	—	150	—	—	—	—
French	1 slice (1.2 oz)	80	1	0	0	3	15	2	—	125	—	—	—	—
Multi-Grain	1 slice (1.2 oz)	60	1	0	0	3	11	2	—	160	—	—	—	—
Multi-Grain No-Salt	1 slice (1.2 oz)	60	1	0	0	3	11	2	—	0	—	—	—	—
Oat Berry	1 slice (1.2 oz)	70	1	0	0	3	13	2	—	150	—	—	—	—
Raisin	1 slice (1.1 oz)	80	1	0	0	3	15	2	—	105	—	—	—	—
Rye Seed	1 slice (1.2 oz)	60	1	0	0	3	11	2	—	150	—	—	—	—

FOOD	PORTION	CALORIES	FAT	SAT FAT	CHOL	PROTEIN	CARBO	FIBER	CALCIUM	SOD	POTAS	VIT C	FOLIC	VIT A
ALVARADO ST. BAKERY (CONT.)														
Sourdough	1 slice (1.2 oz)	80	1	0	0	3	15	2	—	125	—	—	—	—
Wheat	1 slice (1.3 oz)	90	1	0	0	3	18	3	—	170	—	—	—	—
ARNOLD														
12 Grain Natural	1 slice (0.8 oz)	60	0	0	0	2	10	1	—	100	—	—	—	—
Augusto Pan De Aqua	1 oz	80	1	—	0	3	14	1	20	150	—	—	—	—
Bran'nola Country Oat	1 slice (1.3 oz)	90	3	0	0	3	16	3	20	130	—	—	—	—
Bran'nola Dark Wheat	1 slice (1.3 oz)	90	3	0	0	4	15	3	20	150	—	—	—	—
Bran'nola Hearty Wheat	1 slice (1.3 oz)	100	3	0	0	3	15	3	20	160	—	—	—	—
Bran'nola Nutty Grains	1 slice (1.3 oz)	90	2	0	0	3	14	3	20	120	—	—	—	—
Bran'nola Original	1 slice (1.3 oz)	90	2	0	0	3	16	3	20	150	—	—	—	—
Cinnamon Chip	1 slice	80	2	—	0	2	13	tr	—	90	—	—	—	—
Cinnamon Raisin	1 slice (0.9 oz)	70	1	0	0	2	13	1	—	85	—	—	—	—
Country Bran Bakery Light	1 slice (0.8 oz)	40	tr	0	0	2	7	3	—	80	—	—	—	—
Cranberry	1 slice (0.9 oz)	70	1	0	0	2	14	1	0	80	—	0	—	0
French Twin Loaves Francisco	2 slices (2 oz)	150	2	—	—	5	27	—	60	280	—	—	—	—
French Stick Francisco	1 slice (1 oz)	70	2	—	—	3	12	—	20	110	—	—	—	—
French Stick Savoni	1 oz	80	tr	—	0	3	15	1	20	—	—	—	—	—
Italian Bakery Light	1 slice (0.7 oz)	40	tr	0	0	2	7	2	—	90	—	—	—	—
Italian Francisco	1 slice (1 oz)	70	1	—	—	3	12	—	20	110	—	—	—	—
Italian Stick Francisco	1 oz	90	1	—	—	3	17	—	20	110	—	—	—	—
Oatmeal Bakery	1 slice	60	1	0	0	2	12	2	—	95	—	—	—	—
Oatmeal Bakery Light	1 slice	40	tr	0	0	2	8	2	—	100	—	—	—	—
Oatmeal Raisin	1 slice (0.9 oz)	60	tr	0	0	2	12	2	—	90	—	—	—	—
Pita Wheat	½ pocket (1 oz)	71	0	—	—	3	16	—	70	—	—	—	—	—
Pita White	½ pocket (0.5 oz)	71	0	0	—	3	16	—	70	—	—	—	—	—
Pumpernickel	1 slice (1.1 oz)	70	1	0	0	3	15	1	20	200	—	—	—	—
Rye Bakery Soft Light	1 slice (1.1 oz)	40	tr	0	0	2	7	2	—	90	—	—	—	—
Rye Bakery Soft Seeded	1 slice (1.1 oz)	70	1	0	0	2	14	1	20	170	—	—	—	—
Rye Bakery Soft Unseeded	1 slice (1.1 oz)	70	1	0	0	2	14	1	20	170	—	—	—	—
Rye Dill	1 slice (1.1 oz)	60	1	0	0	2	10	1	20	140	—	—	—	—
Rye Real Jewish Dijon	1 slice	70	tr	—	0	3	15	1	20	210	—	—	—	—

FOOD	PORTION	CALORIES	FAT	SAT FAT	CHOL	PROTEIN	CARBO	FIBER	CALCIUM	SOD	POTAS	VIT C	FOLIC	VIT A
ARNOLD (CONT.)														
Rye Real Jewish Melba Thin	1 slice (0.7 oz)	40	tr	0	0	2	9	1	—	95	—	—	—	—
Rye Real Jewish Unseeded	1 slice	80	tr	—	0	3	16	1	20	180	—	—	—	—
Rye Real Jewish With Caraway	1 slice	70	tr	—	0	3	13	1	20	150	—	—	—	—
Rye Real Jewish Without Seeds	1 slice (1.1 oz)	70	tr	0	0	3	15	1	20	150	—	—	—	—
Sourdough Francisco	1 slice	90	1	—	0	3	19	1	20	250	—	—	—	—
Wheat Brick Oven	1 slice (0.8 oz)	60	2	0	0	2	9	2	20	100	—	—	—	—
Wheat Golden Light	1 slice (0.8 oz)	40	tr	0	0	2	7	2	—	90	—	—	—	—
Wheat Natural	1 slice (1.3 oz)	80	1	0	0	3	15	2	—	180	—	—	—	—
Wheat Berry Honey	1 slice (1.1 oz)	80	2	0	0	3	13	2	—	140	—	—	—	—
White Brick Oven	1 slice (0.8 oz)	60	1	0	0	2	11	1	20	130	—	—	—	—
White Country	1 slice (1.3 oz)	100	2	tr	0	3	18	1	—	200	—	—	—	—
White Extra Fiber Brick Oven	1 slice (0.9 oz)	50	tr	0	0	2	10	2	—	90	—	—	—	—
White Light Brick Oven	1 slice (0.8 oz)	40	tr	0	0	2	10	2	60	95	—	—	—	—
White Premium Light	1 slice	40	tr	0	0	2	7	2	—	90	—	—	—	—
White Thin Sliced Brick Oven	1 slice	40	tr	—	0	1	7	tr	—	75	—	—	—	—
Whole Wheat 100% Light Brick Oven	1 slice (0.8 oz)	40	tr	—	0	2	6	3	—	85	—	—	—	—
Whole Wheat 100% Stoneground	1 slice (0.8 oz)	50	1	0	<5	2	8	2	—	100	—	—	—	—
AUGUST BROS.														
Pumpernickel	1 slice	80	1	—	0	3	14	1	20	210	—	—	—	—
Rye Onion	1 slice	80	1	—	0	3	14	1	20	210	—	—	—	—
Rye Thin Unseeded	1 slice	40	—	—	0	2	8	1	—	110	—	—	—	—
Rye With Seeds	1 slice (1 lb loaf)	80	1	—	0	3	14	1	20	210	—	—	—	—
Rye Without Seeds	1 slice	80	1	—	0	3	14	1	20	210	—	—	—	—
Rye N' Pump	1 slice	90	1	—	0	3	18	1	20	220	—	—	—	—
BEEFSTEAK														
Pumpernickel	1 slice (1 oz)	70	1	0	0	3	13	1	—	180	40	—	—	—
Rye Hearty	1 slice (1 oz)	70	1	0	0	3	13	1	—	170	45	—	—	—
Rye Light	2 slices (1.6 oz)	70	1	0	0	5	17	5	150	250	65	—	—	—
Rye Mild	2 slices (1.4 oz)	90	1	0	0	4	18	2	60	240	65	—	—	—
Rye Soft	1 slice (1 oz)	70	1	0	0	3	13	1	—	180	40	—	—	—

FOOD	PORTION	CALORIES	FAT	SAT FAT	CHOL	PROTEIN	CARBO	FIBER	CALCIUM	SOD	POTAS	VIT C	FOLIC	VIT A
BEEFSTEAK (CONT.)														
Wheat Hearty	1 slice (1 oz)	70	1	0	0	3	13	1	60	160	70	—	—	—
Wheat Soft	1 slice (1 oz)	70	1	0	0	3	13	tr	40	150	50	—	—	—
White Robust	1 slice (1 oz)	70	1	0	0	3	13	tr	40	140	35	—	—	—
BREAD DU JOUR														
Austrian Wheat	3 in slice (1 oz)	130	2	0	0	6	26	2	80	280	105	—	—	—
French	3 in slice (1 oz)	130	1	0	0	6	26	1	100	300	65	—	—	—
BROWNBERRY														
Bran'nola Country Oat	1 slice	90	2	—	0	4	18	3	23	166	—	—	—	—
Bran'nola Hearty Wheat	1 slice	88	2	—	0	4	17	3	18	197	—	—	—	—
Bran'nola Nutty Grains	1 slice	85	2	—	0	2	17	3	2	144	—	—	—	—
Bran'nola Original	1 slice	85	1	—	0	4	18	3	11	137	—	—	—	—
Health Nut	1 slice	71	3	—	0	2	12	3	7	158	—	—	—	—
Oatmeal Natural	1 slice	63	1	—	0	2	13	1	13	144	—	—	—	—
Oatmeal Soft	1 slice	48	1	—	0	2	10	2	1	82	—	—	—	—
Raisin Bran	1 slice	61	1	—	0	2	12	2	7	108	—	—	—	—
Raisin Cinnamon	1 slice	66	1	—	0	2	12	1	5	107	—	—	—	—
Raisin Walnut	1 slice	68	3	—	0	2	11	2	5	96	—	—	—	—
Wheat Apple Honey	1 slice	69	2	—	0	2	11	2	5	148	—	—	—	—
Wheat Soft	1 slice	74	2	—	0	2	12	1	27	127	—	—	—	—
CEDAR'S														
Mountain Bread Six Grain	1 piece (2.4 oz)	200	4	0	0	7	35	4	150	380				
DAMASCUS BAKERIES														
Mountain Shepard Lahvash	⅓ loaf (2 oz)	135	0	0	0	5	28	2	40	90	—	0	—	0
DICARLO'S														
Foccaccia	⅛ bread (2 oz)	130	2	0	0	4	25	1	—	260	—	—	—	—
French Parisian	2 slices (1 oz)	70	1	0	0	3	14	tr	40	150	—	—	—	—
FREIHOFER'S														
Country Potato	1 slice (1.3 oz)	100	1	0	0	3	19	1	0	200	—	0	—	0
Country White	1 slice (1.3 oz)	100	1	0	0	3	19	tr	20	220	—	0	—	0
Wheat Light	1 slice (1.6 oz)	80	0	0	0	5	17	4	80	180	—	0	—	0
White Light	2 slices (1.6 oz)	80	1	0	0	4	18	4	60	210	—	0	—	0
Whole Wheat 100%	1 slice (1.3 oz)	90	2	0	0	4	16	2	0	160	—	0	—	0
HOME PRIDE														
Hearty Buttermilk & Biscuit White	1 slice (1.3 oz)	100	2	0	0	3	18	tr	100	280	70	—	—	—

FOOD	PORTION	CALORIES	FAT	SAT FAT	CHOL	PROTEIN	CARBO	FIBER	CALCIUM	SOD	POTAS	VIT C	FOLIC	VIT A
HOME PRIDE (CONT.)														
Hearty Deli Rye	1 slice (2 oz)	140	2	0	0	5	26	3	40	350	85	—	—	—
Hearty Golden Honey Wheat	1 slice (1.3 oz)	90	2	0	0	5	18	2	80	210	80	—	—	—
Hearty Honey Oats & Cracked Wheat	1 slice (1.4 oz)	100	2	0	0	4	19	2	80	210	90	—	—	—
Hearty Seven Grain Multi Grain	1 slice (1.3 oz)	100	2	0	0	4	17	2	60	200	90	—	—	—
Honey Wheat	1 slice (1 oz)	70	1	0	0	3	13	1	40	150	55	—	—	—
Seven Grain	1 slice (0.9 oz)	60	1	0	0	3	12	1	20	130	60	—	—	—
Wheat	1 slice (0.9 oz)	70	1	0	0	3	13	1	40	140	55	—	—	—
Wheat Light	3 slices (2.1 oz)	110	2	0	0	6	25	6	200	300	75	—	—	—
White	1 slice (0.9 oz)	70	1	0	0	2	13	0	40	160	40	—	—	—
White Grain	1 slice (1 oz)	60	1	0	0	3	13	2	40	140	—	—	—	—
White Light	3 slices (0.9 oz)	110	2	0	0	6	25	6	100	320	70	—	—	—
Whole Wheat Hearty 100% Stoneground	1 slice (1.4 oz)	90	2	0	0	5	18	3	60	250	100	—	—	—
MATTHEW'S														
9 Grain & Nut	1 slice	80	3	—	0	3	9	2	20	100	—	—	—	—
Cinnamon	1 slice	70	1	—	0	3	13	2	20	100	—	—	—	—
Golden	1 slice	70	1	—	0	2	14	1	20	125	—	—	—	—
Oat Bran	1 slice	65	0	—	0	3	12	2	60	110	—	—	—	—
Pita Whole Wheat	1	210	2	—	0	10	45	7	100	390	—	—	—	—
Sodium Free	1 slice	70	2	—	0	3	12	2	20	<5	—	—	—	—
Whole Wheat	1 slice	70	1	—	0	3	12	2	20	130	—	—	—	—
MEDITARRANEAN MAGIC														
Focaccia	⅕ loaf (1.8 oz)	140	2	0	0	4	27	tr	0	550	—	0	—	0
MONKS' BREAD														
Hi-Fibre	1 slice	50	1	—	0	3	13	—	20	110	—	—	—	—
Raisin	1 slice	70	2	—	0	3	10	—	20	85	—	—	—	—
Sunflower & Bran	1 slice	70	1	—	0	3	12	2	20	80	—	—	—	—
White	1 slice	60	1	—	0	3	10	—	20	95	—	—	—	—
Whole Wheat 100% Stoneground	1 slice	70	1	—	0	3	13	—	20	110	—	—	—	—
PARISIAN														
French Stick Extra Sour	2 oz	150	1	—	—	8	27	—	25	311	—	—	—	—
French Stick Sweet	2 oz	154	2	—	—	7	27	—	26	331	—	—	—	—
PEPPERIDGE FARM														
7 Grain Hearty Slice	2 slices	180	2	0	0	5	36	2	—	340	—	—	—	—
Cinnamon	1 slice	90	3	—	0	2	15	2	—	110	—	—	—	—

FOOD	PORTION	CALORIES	FAT	SAT FAT	CHOL	PROTEIN	CARBO	FIBER	CALCIUM	SOD	POTAS	VIT C	FOLIC	VIT A
PEPPERIDGE FARM (CONT.)														
Cracked Wheat	1 slice	70	1	—	0	2	13	1	—	140	—	—	—	—
Crunchy Oat 1 ½ lb Loaf	2 slices	190	4	1	0	8	34	3	60	290	—	—	—	—
Date Walnut	1 slice	90	3	—	0	2	14	2	—	110	—	—	—	—
French Fully Baked	2 oz	150	2	—	0	5	28	1	40	320	—	—	—	—
French Twin	1 oz	80	1	—	0	3	15	0	20	160	—	—	—	—
Honey Bran	1 slice	90	1	—	0	3	18	1	—	160	—	—	—	—
Italian Brown & Serve	1 oz	80	1	1	0	2	14	0	20	150	—	—	—	—
Italian Sliced	1 slice	70	1	—	0	2	12	—	—	125	—	—	—	—
Oatmeal	1 slice	70	1	—	0	2	12	1	20	160	—	—	—	—
Oatmeal 1 ½ lb Loaf	1 slice	90	1	—	0	3	17	1	20	200	—	—	—	—
Oatmeal Light	1 slice	45	0	0	0	2	9	1	—	95	—	—	—	—
Oatmeal Very Thin Sliced	1 slice	40	1	—	0	1	8	—	—	80	—	—	—	—
Pumpernickel Family	1 slice	80	1	—	0	3	15	2	20	230	—	—	—	—
Pumpernickel Party	4 slices	60	1	—	0	2	12	1	20	160	—	—	—	—
Raisin With Cinnamon	1 slice	90	2	—	0	2	16	1	20	100	—	—	—	—
Rye Dijon	1 slice	50	1	—	0	2	9	1	20	180	—	—	—	—
Rye Dijon Thick Sliced	1 slice	70	1	—	0	3	15	2	20	260	—	—	—	—
Rye Family	1 slice (32 g)	80	1	—	0	3	16	2	20	220	—	—	—	—
Rye Party	4 slices	60	1	—	0	2	12	1	20	250	—	—	—	—
Rye Seedless Family	1 slice	80	1	—	0	3	16	2	20	210	—	—	—	—
Rye Soft	1 slice	70	1	—	0	2	12	—	—	120	—	—	—	—
Sesame Wheat	2 slices	190	3	1	0	7	36	3	60	340	—	—	—	—
Sprouted Wheat	1 slice	70	2	—	0	3	11	2	—	100	—	—	—	—
Vienna Light	1 slice	45	0	0	0	2	10	1	20	100	—	—	—	—
Vienna Thick Sliced	1 slice	70	1	—	0	2	13	0	20	125	—	—	—	—
Wheat 1 ½ lb Loaf	1 slice	90	2	—	0	3	18	2	20	190	—	—	—	—
Wheat Family	1 slice	70	1	—	0	2	13	2	20	130	—	—	—	—
Wheat Light	1 slice	45	0	0	0	2	9	1	20	90	—	—	—	—
Wheat Very Thin Sliced	1 slice	35	0	0	0	2	7	0	20	75	—	—	—	—
White Country	2 slices	190	2	1	0	7	38	2	60	340	—	—	—	—
White Large Family Thin Slice	1 slice	70	1	—	0	2	13	0	20	150	—	—	—	—
White Sandwich	2 slices	130	2	—	0	4	24	0	40	260	—	—	—	—
White Thin Slice	1 slice	80	2	—	0	2	14	0	20	130	—	—	—	—
White Toasting	1 slice	90	1	—	0	3	17	1	20	200	—	—	—	—
White Very Thin Sliced	1 slice	40	0	0	0	1	8	0	20	80	—	—	—	—

FOOD	PORTION	CALORIES	FAT	SAT FAT	CHOL	PROTEIN	CARBO	FIBER	CALCIUM	SOD	POTAS	VIT C	FOLIC	VIT A
PEPPERIDGE FARM (CONT.)														
Whole Wheat Thin Slice	1 slice	60	1	—	0	2	12	2	20	110	—	—	—	—
ROMAN MEAL														
Brown & Serve Mini Loaf	½ loaf (2 oz)	136	2	tr	0	5	24	1	65	275	69	0	—	0
Cracked Wheat	1 slice (1.4 oz)	92	2	tr	0	4	15	2	24	129	45	0	—	0
Hearty Wheat Light	1 slice (0.8 oz)	42	tr	tr	0	2	7	2	26	102	11	0	—	0
Honey Nut Oat Bran	1 slice (1 oz)	72	2	tr	0	3	11	1	24	129	45	0	—	0
Honey Oat Bran	1 slice (1 oz)	70	1	tr	0	3	12	1	23	132	39	0	—	0
Oat	1 slice (1 oz)	69	1	tr	0	3	12	1	19	100	45	0	—	0
Oat Bran	1 slice (1 oz)	68	1	tr	0	3	12	1	31	136	27	0	—	0
Oat Bran Light	1 slice (0.8 oz)	42	tr	tr	0	2	7	2	25	100	20	0	—	0
Round Top	1 slice (1 oz)	67	1	tr	0	3	12	1	33	142	34	0	—	0
Sandwich	1 slice (0.8 oz)	55	1	tr	0	2	10	1	27	115	28	0	—	0
Seven Grain	1 slice (1 oz)	67	1	tr	0	3	12	1	23	142	35	0	—	0
Seven Grain Light	1 slice (0.8 oz)	42	1	tr	0	2	7	3	27	101	11	0	—	0
Sourdough Light	1 slice (0.8 oz)	41	tr	tr	0	2	7	3	28	115	10	0	—	0
Sourdough Whole Grain Light	1 slice (0.8 oz)	40	tr	tr	0	2	7	3	26	104	18	0	—	0
Sun Grain	1 slice (1 oz)	70	2	tr	0	3	11	1	22	135	45	0	—	1
Twelve Grain	1 slice (1 oz)	70	2	tr	0	3	11	1	23	140	27	0	—	3
Twelve Grain Light	1 slice (0.8 oz)	42	tr	tr	0	2	7	3	28	104	10	0	—	tr
Wheat Light	1 slice (0.8 oz)	41	tr	tr	0	2	7	3	27	102	22	0	—	0
Wheatberry Honey	1 slice (1 oz)	67	1	tr	0	3	12	1	23	139	35	0	—	0
Wheatberry Light	1 slice (0.8 oz)	42	tr	tr	0	2	7	2	26	102	14	0	—	0
White Light	1 slice (0.8 oz)	41	tr	tr	0	2	7	3	28	105	9	0	—	0
Whole Grain 100%	1 slice (1.4 oz)	91	1	tr	0	4	16	2	33	198	80	0	—	0
Whole Grain Sourdough	1 slice (1 oz)	66	1	tr	0	3	12	1	16	141	43	0	—	0
Whole Wheat 100%	1 slice (1 oz)	64	1	tr	0	3	11	2·	24	141	66	0	—	0
Whole Wheat 100% Light	1 slice (0.8 oz)	42	tr	tr	0	3	7	2	30	102	1	0	—	0
SAHARA														
Pita Oat Bran	½ pocket (1 oz)	66	tr	—	0	2	14	2	36	163	—	—	—	—
Pita White	½ pocket	78	1	—	—	3	16	—	39	147	27	0	—	15
STROEHMANN														
White Whole Special Recipe	1 slice	70	1	—	0	3	13	—	80	160	25	—	—	—
White Whole Special Recipe Kids	1 slice	60	tr	—	0	2	12	—	40	150	20	—	—	—

FOOD	PORTION	CALORIES	FAT	SAT FAT	CHOL	PROTEIN	CARBO	FIBER	CALCIUM	SOD	POTAS	VIT C	FOLIC	VIT A
SUNMAID														
Raisin	1 slice	70	tr	tr	0	2	13	1	—	85	—	—	—	—
TREE OF LIFE														
100% Spelt	1 slice (1.8 oz)	130	3	1	10	4	22	3	20	290	—	0	—	0
Millet	1 slice (1.8 oz)	130	2	0	0	3	25	2	20	240	—	0	—	0
Rye Sour Dough	1 slice (1.8 oz)	110	0	0	0	3	24	5	70	30	—	0	—	0
Sprouted Seven Grain	1 slice (1.8 oz)	110	2	0	0	3	20	2	0	140	—	0	—	0
VALLEY LAHVOSH														
Valley Wraps	1 (1 oz)	100	1	0	0	4	19	1	20	125	—	0	—	0
WONDER														
Calcium Enriched	1 slice (1 oz)	70	1	0	0	3	12	tr	300	150	—	0	—	0
Cinnamon Raisin	1 slice (1 oz)	70	1	0	0	3	14	tr	20	100	—	—	—	—
Cracked Wheat	1 slice (1 oz)	70	1	0	0	3	14	1	40	150	45	—	—	—
French	1 slice (1 oz)	80	2	0	0	3	15	tr	40	160	35	—	—	—
French Light	2 slices (1.6 oz)	80	1	0	0	5	18	5	150	210	45	—	—	—
Granola	1 slice (1.5 oz)	100	2	0	0	5	19	2	40	210	90	—	—	—
Honey Bran Light	2 slices (1.6 oz)	80	1	0	0	5	18	6	150	190	70	—	—	—
Italian	1 slice (1.1 oz)	80	1	0	0	3	15	tr	60	190	35	—	—	—
Italian Family	1 slice (1 oz)	70	1	0	0	3	13	tr	40	170	30	—	—	—
Italian Light	2 slices (1.6 oz)	80	1	0	0	5	18	5	150	230	50	—	—	—
Kid	1 slice (0.9 oz)	70	1	0	0	2	13	tr	40	150	35	—	—	—
Light Calcium Enriched	2 slices (1.6 oz)	80	1	0	<5	5	18	5	300	240	—	0	—	0
Nine Grain Light	2 slices (1.6 oz)	80	1	0	0	5	18	6	150	230	60	—	—	—
Oatmeal Light	2 slices (1.6 oz)	90	0	0	0	5	19	4	150	230	60	—	—	—
Rye	1 slice (1 oz)	70	1	0	0	3	13	1	—	170	45	—	—	—
Rye Light	2 slices (1.6 oz)	70	1	0	0	5	17	5	100	220	55	—	—	—
Sourdough	1 slice (1.2 oz)	90	2	0	0	3	17	tr	40	180	40	—	—	—
Sourdough Light	2 slices (1.6 oz)	80	1	0	0	5	18	5	150	250	50	—	—	—
Texas Toast	1 slice (1.4 oz)	100	1	0	0	3	19	1	60	220	50	—	—	—
Vienna	1 slice (1 oz)	70	1	0	0	3	13	tr	40	170	30	—	—	—
Wheat Calcium Light	2 slices (1.6 oz)	80	1	0	0	5	18	6	300	240	65	—	—	—
Wheat Family	1 slice (0.9 oz)	70	1	0	0	3	13	tr	40	150	50	—	—	—
Wheat Golden Country Style	2 slices (1.4 oz)	100	2	0	0	4	19	1	60	220	75	—	—	—
Wheat Light	2 slices (1.6 oz)	80	1	0	0	5	18	6	150	230	50	—	—	—
White	1 slice (0.9 oz)	70	1	0	0	2	13	tr	40	150	35	—	—	—

FOOD	PORTION	CALORIES	FAT	SAT FAT	CHOL	PROTEIN	CARBO	FIBER	CALCIUM	SOD	POTAS	VIT C	FOLIC	VIT A
WONDER (CONT.)														
White Calcium	2 slices (1.6 oz)	100	1	0	0	4	20	1	500	240	50	—	—	—
White Calcium Light	2 slices (1.6 oz)	80	1	0	0	5	18	5	300	260	50	—	—	—
White Light	2 slices (1.6 oz)	80	1	0	0	5	18	5	150	230	50	—	—	—
White With Buttermilk	1 slice (1 oz)	80	1	0	0	3	14	tr	60	180	50	—	—	—
Whole Wheat 100%	1 slice (1 oz)	70	1	0	0	3	12	2	40	180	70	—	—	—
Whole Wheat 100% Soft	2 slices (1.6 oz)	110	2	0	0	4	21	1	60	240	80	—	—	—
Whole Wheat 100% Stoneground	1 slice (1.2 oz)	80	2	0	0	4	14	2	60	190	85	—	—	—
ZA														
Pit-Za Hearty Multi-Grain	1/9 bread (2 oz)	130	2	0	0	5	25	2	0	210	—	4	—	0
Pit-Za Salt-Free Garlic Whole Wheat	1/9 bread (2 oz)	150	1	0	0	7	28	3	0	10	—	4	—	0
REFRIGERATED														
ROMAN MEAL														
Loaf	1 slice (1 oz)	85	3	1	0	2	13	1	6	199	43	0	—	0
STEFANO'S														
Stuffed Bread Broccoli & Cheese	1/2 bread (6 oz)	450	17	6	25	19	54	7	350	830	—	1	—	1500
TAKE-OUT														
chapatis as prep w/ fat	1 bread (1.6 oz)	95	2	1	3	3	18	3	10	180	101	0	11	221
focaccia onion	1 piece (4.6 oz)	282	10	1	0	6	43	2	20	536	114	2	43	5
focaccia rosemary	1 piece (3.5 oz)	251	7	1	0	6	40	2	13	535	68	tr	38	2
focaccia tomato olive	1 piece (4.7 oz)	270	8	1	0	6	42	2	31	683	122	3	39	85
garlic bread	2 slices (2 oz)	190	8	2	0	3	27	1	0	290	—	0	—	0
naan	1 bread (3.5 oz)	286	9	5	46	7	43	2	54	546	107	tr	53	1400
paratha	1 bread (2.1 oz)	201	10	7	27	4	23	2	10	268	78	0	11	1995

BREAD COATING

DON'S CHUCK WAGON

FOOD	PORTION	CALORIES	FAT	SAT FAT	CHOL	PROTEIN	CARBO	FIBER	CALCIUM	SOD	POTAS	VIT C	FOLIC	VIT A
All Purpose Mix	1/4 cup (1 oz)	100	0	0	0	4	20	1	0	580	—	0	—	0
Fish & Chips Mix	1/4 cup (1 oz)	100	0	0	0	3	21	1	0	740	—	0	—	0
Fish Mix	1/4 cup (1 oz)	95	0	0	0	3	21	1	0	940	—	0	—	0
Frying Mix Chicken	1/4 cup (1 oz)	95	0	0	0	3	21	1	0	850	—	0	—	0

FOOD	PORTION	CALORIES	FAT	SAT FAT	CHOL	PROTEIN	CARBO	FIBER	CALCIUM	SOD	POTAS	VIT C	FOLIC	VIT A
DON'S CHUCK WAGON (CONT.)														
Frying Mix Seafood Seasoned	¼ cup (1 oz)	95	1	0	0	2	21	1	0	990	—	0	—	0
Mushroom Mix	¼ cup (1 oz)	95	0	0	0	3	21	1	0	990	—	0	—	0
Onion Ring Mix	¼ cup (1 oz)	100	0	0	0	3	21	1	0	690	—	0	—	0
GOLDEN DIPT														
Breading Frying Mix	1 oz	90	0	0	0	3	20	—	—	630	—	—	—	—
Chicken Frying Mix	1 oz	90	0	0	0	2	20	—	—	1430	—	—	—	—
Onion Ring Mix	1 oz	100	0	0	0	2	22	—	—	570	—	—	—	—
KA-ME														
Tempura Batter Mix	1 oz	100	0	0	0	2	22	0	—	5	—	—	—	—
LITTLE CROW														
Fryin' Magic	0.5 oz	43	tr	—	0	1	8	—	—	542	—	—	—	—
MRS. DASH														
Crispy Coating	2 tbsp (0.6 oz)	65	1	—	0	5	10	—	—	3	229	—	—	—
OVEN FRY														
Extra Crispy For Chicken	⅛ pkg (0.5 oz)	60	1	0	0	2	10	0	0	420	30	0	—	0
Extra Crispy For Pork	⅛ pkg (0.5 oz)	60	2	0	0	2	11	0	0	340	20	0	—	0
SHAKE 'N BAKE														
Buffalo Wings	⅒ pkg (0.4 oz)	40	1	0	0	0	8	0	0	300	15	0	—	100
Classic Italian Chicken or Pork	⅛ pkg (0.4 oz)	40	1	0	0	1	7	0	0	270	30	0	—	0
Country Mild Recipe	⅛ pkg (0.3 oz)	35	2	1	0	0	5	0	0	240	10	0	—	100
Glazes Barbecue Chicken Or Pork	⅛ pkg (0.4 oz)	45	1	0	0	0	9	0	0	410	35	0	—	200
Glazes Honey Mustard Chicken Or Pork	⅛ pkg (0.4 oz)	45	1	0	0	0	9	0	0	300	20	0	—	0
Glazes Tangy Honey Chicken Or Pork	⅛ pkg (0.4 oz)	45	1	0	0	0	9	0	0	300	45	0	—	100
Home Style Flour Recipe For Chicken	⅛ pkg (0.4 oz)	40	1	0	0	tr	7	0	0	470	15	0	—	0
Hot & Spicy Chicken Or Pork	⅛ pkg (0.4 oz)	40	1	0	0	1	7	0	0	170	20	0	—	0
Original For Chicken	⅛ pkg (0.4 oz)	40	1	0	0	1	7	0	0	220	20	0	—	100
Original For Fish	¼ pkg (0.7 oz)	80	2	0	0	2	14	tr	0	350	25	0	—	100
Original For Pork	⅛ pkg (0.4 oz)	45	1	0	0	1	8	0	0	230	20	0	—	0

FOOD	PORTION	CALORIES	FAT	SAT FAT	CHOL	PROTEIN	CARBO	FIBER	CALCIUM	SOD	POTAS	VIT C	FOLIC	VIT A
BREAD MACHINE MIX														
DROMEDARY														
Country White	½ in slice (2 oz)	140	1	1	0	4	28	1	0	230	—	0	—	0
Italian Herb	½ in slice (1.8 oz)	140	3	2	0	4	25	1	40	250	—	0	—	0
Stoneground Wheat	½ in slice (1.8 oz)	140	2	1	0	4	26	2	20	200	—	0	—	0
PILLSBURY														
Cracked Wheat	¹⁄₁₂ pkg (1.3 oz)	130	2	0	0	4	25	2	0	260	—	0	—	0
SASSAFRAS														
Apricot Oatmeal	1 slice (1.4 oz)	140	1	0	0	5	29	2	0	190	—	0	—	100
WANDA'S														
Dried Tomato Cheddar	¼ cup mix per serv (1.2 oz)	140	0	0	0	6	22	3	40	230	—	0	—	100
European White	¼ cup mix per serv (1.2 oz)	130	0	0	0	6	26	1	20	115	—	0	—	0
Oatmeal	¼ cup mix per serv (1.2 oz)	120	0	0	0	5	24	1	20	350	—	0	—	0
Oatmeal Cinnamon	¼ cup mix per serv (1.2 oz)	120	0	0	0	7	19	1	20	280	—	0	—	0
Old World Rye	¼ cup mix per serv (1.9 oz)	90	0	0	0	4	27	3	20	300	—	0	—	0
Onion	¼ cup mix per serv (1.2 oz)	120	0	0	0	4	25	1	0	270	—	0	—	0
Orange Cinnamon	¼ cup mix per serv (1.3 oz)	130	0	0	0	4	28	1	0	90	—	0	—	100
Oregano Garlic	¼ cup mix per serv (1.2 oz)	130	1	0	0	5	25	2	40	270	—	0	—	0
Rosemary Basil	¼ cup mix per serv (1.2 oz)	130	0	0	0	4	26	1	0	250	—	0	—	0
Rye	¼ cup mix per serv (1.2 oz)	120	0	0	0	4	25	1	0	270	—	0	—	0
Rye Caraway	¼ cup mix per serv (1.2 oz)	120	0	0	0	4	25	1	0	270	—	0	—	0
Sourdough	¼ cup mix per serv (1.2 oz)	120	0	0	0	5	25	1	0	160	—	0	—	0
Sunflower Sesame Poppyseed	¼ cup mix per serv (1.2 oz)	120	0	0	0	5	25	2	40	310	—	0	—	0
Ten Grain	¼ cup mix per serv (1.4 oz)	140	0	0	0	6	27	3	0	160	—	2	—	0
Wheat	¼ cup mix per serv (1.2 oz)	130	0	0	0	4	26	2	40	270	—	0	—	0
White	¼ cup mix per serv (1.2 oz)	130	0	0	0	4	26	1	0	250	—	0	—	0
Whole Wheat	¼ cup mix per serv (1.3 oz)	130	0	0	0	6	26	4	40	330	—	0	—	0

FOOD	PORTION	CALORIES	FAT	SAT FAT	CHOL	PROTEIN	CARBO	FIBER	CALCIUM	SOD	POTAS	VIT C	FOLIC	VIT A
BREADCRUMBS														
dry	1 cup	426	6	1	—	14	78	5	245	930	239	—	—	—
dry seasonsed	1 cup (4 oz)	441	3	1	—	17	85	5	119	3180	324	—	—	—
fresh	⅔ cup	76	1	tr	0	4	14	1	31	153	34	0	10	0
4C														
Salt Free	1 tbsp (0.5 oz)	50	1	—	—	2	10	—	20	0	115	—	—	—
Seasoned	1 tbsp (0.5 oz)	50	1	—	—	2	10	—	20	270	20	—	—	—
Toasted	1 tbsp (0.5 oz)	50	1	—	—	2	10	—	20	110	15	—	—	—
Toasted Salt Free	1 tbsp (0.5 oz)	50	1	—	—	2	10	—	20	0	15	—	—	—
ARNOLD														
Italian	½ oz	50	tr	0	0	2	8	tr	—	200	—	—	—	—
Plain	½ oz	50	tr	0	0	2	8	tr	—	80	—	—	—	—
CONTADINA														
Plain	⅓ cup	100	2	—	—	3	19	1	60	700	—	—	—	—
DEVONSHEER														
Italian Style	1 oz	104	1	—	0	4	20	1	23	408	—	—	—	—
Plain	1 oz	108	1	—	0	4	21	1	25	272	—	—	—	—
PROGRESSO														
Italian Style	¼ cup (1 oz)	110	2	0	0	4	20	1	40	430	—	0	—	0
Lemon Herb	¼ cup (0.9 oz)	100	1	0	0	3	20	2	40	480	—	0	—	0
Plain	¼ cup (1 oz)	100	2	0	0	4	19	1	40	210	—	0	—	0
Tomato Basil	¼ cup (1.1 oz)	120	2	0	0	4	22	2	80	750	—	2	—	0
BREADFRUIT														
breadfruit	3.5 oz	109	tr	—	0	—	—	—	tr	—	—	—	—	—
fresh	¼ small	99	tr	—	0	1	26	—	17	2	470	28	—	38
seeds cooked	1 oz	48	1	tr	0	2	9	—	12	—	—	—	—	—
seeds raw	1 oz	54	2	tr	0	2	8	—	10	—	—	2	—	73
seeds roasted	1 oz	59	tr	tr	0	2	11	—	24	—	—	—	—	—
BREADNUTTREE SEEDS														
dried	1 oz	104	tr	tr	0	2	23	—	27	—	—	—	13	61
BREADSTICKS														
plain	1	41	1	tr	0	1	7	—	2	66	12	0	—	—
plain	1 sm	25	1	tr	0	1	4	—	2	66	12	0	—	0
ANGONOA														
Cheese	5 (1 oz)	120	3	1	0	4	20	1	80	270	—	0	—	0
Cheese Mini	16 (1 oz)	120	3	1	0	4	20	1	40	120	—	0	—	0
Garlic	6 (1 oz)	120	2	0	0	4	21	1	0	390	—	0	—	0
Italian Style Plain	5 (1 oz)	120	3	1	0	4	20	1	100	280	—	0	—	0
Low Sodium With Sesame Seed	6 (1 oz)	130	4	1	0	4	19	2	100	65	—	0	—	0
Onion	6 (1 oz)	120	2	1	0	4	21	2	20	200	—	0	—	0
Pizza Mini	26 (1 oz)	120	2	0	0	4	21	1	40	180	—	0	—	0
Sesame Mini	16 (1 oz)	130	4	1	0	4	19	2	60	220	—	0	—	0
Sesame Royale	6 (1 oz)	130	4	1	0	4	18	2	40	210	—	0	—	0

FOOD	PORTION	CALORIES	FAT	SAT FAT	CHOL	PROTEIN	CARBO	FIBER	CALCIUM	SOD	POTAS	VIT C	FOLIC	VIT A
ANGONOA (CONT.)														
Whole Wheat Mini	14 (1 oz)	130	4	1	0	4	19	3	40	220	—	0	—	0
BREAD DU JOUR														
Italian	1 (1.9 oz)	130	2	0	0	5	25	1	150	280	110	—	—	—
Sourdough	1 (1.9 oz)	130	1	0	0	5	25	1	150	280	110	—	—	—
J.J. CASSONE														
Garlic	1 (1.6 oz)	150	3	0	0	5	26	2	20	—	260	0	—	0
KEEBLER														
Garlic	2	30	tr	tr	0	1	6	—		20	15	—	—	—
Onion	2	30	tr	tr	0	1	6	—		25	15	—	—	—
Plain	2	30	tr	tr	0	1	6	—		30	15	—	—	—
Sesame	2	30	1	tr	0	1	5	—	20	30	15	—	—	—
LANCE														
Cheese	2	20	0	0	0	tr	4	—		40	10	—	—	—
Garlic	2	30	0	0	0	tr	5	—		40	10	—	—	—
Plain	2	30	0	0	0	tr	5	—		50	10	—	—	—
Sesame	2	30	0	0	0	1	4	—		50	10	—	—	—
NEW YORK														
Garlic Soft	1 (1.5 oz)	140	4	1	0	3	23	1	0	220	—	0	—	0
ROMAN MEAL														
Brown & Serve Soft	1 (2.7 oz)	181	3	tr	0	7	32	3	65	275	69	0	—	0
Refrigerated	1 (1.4 oz)	117	4	1	0	3	18	1	8	274	58	0	—	0
STELLA D'ORO														
Deli Garlic Fat Free	5	60	0	0	0	2	12	—		120	—	—	—	—
Deli Original Fat Free	5	60	0	0	0	2	12	—		130	—	—	—	—
Garlic	1	35	1	—	0	1	6	—		55	—	—	—	—
Grissini Garlic Fat Free	3	60	0	—	0	2	12	—		120	—	—	—	—
Grissini Original Fat Free	3	60	0	—	0	2	12	—		130	—	—	—	—
Onion	1	40	1	—	0	1	6	—		38	—	—	—	—
Regular	1	40	1	—	0	1	7	—		40	—	—	—	—
Regular Sodium Free	2	80	2	—	0	2	14	—		0	—	—	—	—
Sesame Low Fat	2	70	1	—	0	2	14	—		90	—	—	—	—
Sesame Sodium Free	1	50	3	—	0	1	7	—		0	—	—	—	—
Traditional Garlic Fat Free	2	70	0	0	0	2	15	—		150	—	—	—	—
Traditional Original Fat Free	2	70	0	0	0	2	15	—		150	—	—	—	—
Wheat	1	40	1	—	0	1	6	—		20	—	—	—	—

BREAKFAST BAR

(*see also* BREAKFAST DRINKS, NUTRITIONAL SUPPLEMENTS)

FOOD	PORTION	CALORIES	FAT	SAT FAT	CHOL	PROTEIN	CARBO	FIBER	CALCIUM	SOD	POTAS	VIT C	FOLIC	VIT A
CARNATION														
Chewy Chocolate Chip	1 (1.26 oz)	150	6	3	0	2	22	tr	500	80	—	15	—	1250

FOOD	PORTION	CALORIES	FAT	SAT FAT	CHOL	PROTEIN	CARBO	FIBER	CALCIUM	SOD	POTAS	VIT C	FOLIC	VIT A
CARNATION (CONT.)														
Chewy Peanut Butter Chocolate Chip	1 (1.26 oz)	140	5	2	0	3	21	tr	500	90	—	15	—	1250
GLENNY'S														
Sunrise Bee Pollen	1 (1.5 oz)	190	8	—	—	5	22	—	—	—	—	—	—	—
Sunrise Ginseng	1 (1.5 oz)	160	7	—	—	1	24	—	—	—	—	—	—	—
Sunrise Spirulina	1 (1.5 oz)	140	5	—	—	3	21	—	—	—	—	—	—	—
NUTRI-GRAIN														
Apple Cinnamon	1 (1.3 oz)	140	3	1	0	2	27	1	0	60	—	0	100	750
Blueberry	1 (1.3 oz)	140	3	1	0	2	27	1	0	60	—	0	100	750
Peach	1 (1.3 oz)	140	3	1	0	2	27	1	0	60	—	0	100	750
Raspberry	1 (1.3 oz)	140	3	1	0	2	27	1	0	60	—	0	100	750
Strawberry	1 (1.3 oz)	140	3	1	0	2	27	1	0	60	—	0	100	750

BREAKFAST DRINKS

(*see also* BREAKFAST BAR, NUTRITIONAL SUPPLEMENTS)

FOOD	PORTION	CALORIES	FAT	SAT FAT	CHOL	PROTEIN	CARBO	FIBER	CALCIUM	SOD	POTAS	VIT C	FOLIC	VIT A
orange drink powder	3 rounded tsp	93	0	0	0	0	24	—	46	4	40	98	116	1490
orange drink powder as prep w/ water	6 oz	86	0	0	0	0	22	—	46	9	37	91	107	1376
CARNATION														
Instant Breakfast Cafe Mocha	1 pkg + skim milk (9 fl oz)	220	1	tr	6	12	39	1	500	216	—	30	—	2250
Instant Breakfast Cafe Mocha	1 pkg	130	1	0	<5	4	28	1	350	100	—	27	—	1750
Instant Breakfast Cafe Mocha	1 can (10 fl oz)	220	3	1	5	12	35	0	500	210	—	30	—	2250
Instant Breakfast Classic Chocolate Malt	1 pkg + skim milk (9 fl oz)	220	1	1	6	12	39	1	500	240	—	30	—	2250
Instant Breakfast Classic Chocolate Malt	1 pkg	130	2	1	<5	4	26	1	250	130	—	27	—	1750
Instant Breakfast Creamy Milk Chocolate	1 pkg	130	1	1	<5	4	28	1	300	100	—	27	—	1750
Instant Breakfast Creamy Milk Chocolate	1 pkg + skim milk (9 fl oz)	220	1	1	8	12	39	1	500	240	—	30	—	2250
Instant Breakfast Creamy Milk Chocolate	8 fl oz	220	3	2	10	12	36	1	500	220	—	0	—	1250
Instant Breakfast Creamy Milk Chocolate	1 can (10 fl oz)	220	3	1	5	12	37	1	500	230	—	30	—	2250
Instant Breakfast French Vanilla	1 pkg + skim milk	220	1	tr	6	12	39	0	500	240	—	30	—	2250

FOOD	PORTION	CALORIES	FAT	SAT FAT	CHOL	PROTEIN	CARBO	FIBER	CALCIUM	SOD	POTAS	VIT C	FOLIC	VIT A
CARNATION (CONT.)														
Instant Breakfast French Vanilla	1 pkg	130	0	0	<5	4	27	0	350	110	—	27	—	1750
Instant Breakfast No Sugar Added Classic Chocolate	1 pkg	70	2	1	<5	4	11	1	250	120	—	27	—	1750
Instant Breakfast No Sugar Added Classic Chocolate	1 pkg + skim milk (9 fl oz)	160	2	1	6	12	24	1	500	240	—	30	—	2250
Instant Breakfast No Sugar Added Creamy Milk Chocolate	1 pkg	70	1	1	<5	4	12	1	300	90	—	27	—	1750
Instant Breakfast No Sugar Added Creamy Milk Chocolate	1 pkg + skim milk (9 fl oz)	160	1	1	6	12	24	1	500	216	—	30	—	2250
Instant Breakfast No Sugar Added French Vanilla	1 pkg	70	0	0	<5	4	12	0	350	90	—	27	—	1750
Instant Breakfast No Sugar Added French Vanilla	1 pkg + skim milk (9 fl oz)	150	1	tr	6	12	24	0	500	216	—	30	—	2250
Instant Breakfast No Sugar Added Strawberry Creme	1 pkg + skim milk (9 fl oz)	150	1	tr	6	12	24	0	500	216	—	30	—	2250
Instant Breakfast No Sugar Added Strawberry Creme	1 pkg	70	0	0	<5	4	12	0	350	90	—	27	—	1750
Instant Breakfast Strawberry Creme	1 pkg + skim milk	220	1	tr	6	12	39	0	500	288	—	30	—	2250
Instant Breakfast Strawberry Creme	1 pkg	130	0	0	<5	4	28	0	350	160	—	27	—	1750
BROAD BEANS														
canned	1 cup	183	1	tr	0	14	32	—	67	1161	620	5	84	26
dried cooked	1 cup	186	1	tr	0	13	33	—	62	8	456	1	177	26
fresh cooked	3½ oz	56	tr	tr	0	5	10	—	18	41	193	20	—	270
BROCCOFLOWER														
fresh raw	½ cup (1.8 oz)	16	tr	tr	0	1	3	—	16	12	150	44	29	76
DOLE														
Fresh	⅕ head	35	0	0	0	3	7	—	—	30	280	—	—	—
BROCCOLI														
FRESH														
chinese broccoli (gai lan) cooked	1 cup (3.1 oz)	19	1	tr	0	1	3	2	88	6	230	0	87	1441
DOLE														
Spear	1 med	40	1	—	0	5	4	5	—	75	572	139	—	721

FOOD	PORTION	CALORIES	FAT	SAT FAT	CHOL	PROTEIN	CARBO	FIBER	CALCIUM	SOD	POTAS	VIT C	FOLIC	VIT A
FROZEN														
chopped cooked	½ cup	25	tr	tr	0	3	5	—	47	22	166	37	52	1741
AMY'S ORGANIC														
Pocket Sandwich Broccoli & Cheese	1 (4.5 oz)	270	10	4	15	8	37	3	—	560	—	—	—	—
BIG VALLEY														
Chopped	¾ cup (3 oz)	25	0	0	0	2	4	2	20	20	—	42	—	200
Cuts	¾ cup (3 oz)	25	0	0	0	2	4	2	20	20	—	42	—	200
BIRDS EYE														
Baby Broccoli Blend	1 cup (3.4 oz)	70	2	0	0	4	8	3	20	30	—	18	—	1500
Baby Florets	1 cup (3 oz)	25	0	0	0	2	4	2	20	20	—	36	—	500
In Cheese Sauce	½ cup (3.9 oz)	110	5	2	5	3	7	2	60	500	—	27	—	400
FRESH LIKE														
Spear	3.5 oz	26	tr	—	—	3	5	1	55	32	224	57	—	2084
GREEN GIANT														
Butter Sauce	4 oz	50	2	1	<5	2	7	2	40	330	—	42	—	300
Cheese Sauce	⅔ cup (3.9 oz)	70	3	1	<5	3	9	2	60	520	—	42	—	1000
Chopped	¾ cup (2.8 oz)	25	0	0	0	2	4	2	20	25	—	30	—	400
Cuts	1 cup (2.9 oz)	25	0	0	0	2	4	2	20	25	—	36	—	500
Harvest Fresh Cut	⅔ cup (3.2 oz)	25	0	0	0	2	4	2	20	150	—	42	—	400
Harvest Fresh Spears	3.5 oz	25	0	0	0	2	4	2	40	125	—	36	—	400
Select Florets	1 ⅓ cups (2.9 oz)	25	0	0	0	2	4	2	20	25	—	36	—	500
Select Spears	3 oz	25	0	0	0	2	4	2	20	25	—	30	—	500
PEPPERIDGE FARM														
Broccoli With Cheese In Pastry	1	230	16	—	—	5	18	—	60	380	—	12	—	400
STOUFFER'S														
Au Gratin	1 serv (4 oz)	100	4	2	10	5	10	2	100	450	230	18	—	400
TREE OF LIFE														
Broccoli	1 cup (3.1 oz)	25	0	0	0	2	4	2	20	20	—	36	—	500

BROWNIE

FROZEN

PEPPERIDGE FARM

FOOD	PORTION	CALORIES	FAT	SAT FAT	CHOL	PROTEIN	CARBO	FIBER	CALCIUM	SOD	POTAS	VIT C	FOLIC	VIT A
Monterey Hot Fudge Chocolate Chunk Brownie	1	480	26	14	65	5	56	—	40	200	—	—	—	—
Newport Hot Fudge Brownie	1	400	20	10	80	4	50	—	40	160	—	—	—	—
WEIGHT WATCHERS														
Brownie A La Mode	1 (3.14 oz)	190	4	2	5	5	34	2	100	170	—	0	—	200
Double Fudge Brownie Parfait	1 (5.3 oz)	190	3	2	5	6	39	2	200	170	—	0	—	0

FOOD	PORTION	CALORIES	FAT	SAT FAT	CHOL	PROTEIN	CARBO	FIBER	CALCIUM	SOD	POTAS	VIT C	FOLIC	VIT A
HOME RECIPE														
plain	1 (0.8 oz)	112	7	2	17	2	12	1	14	82	42	tr	4	184
w/nuts	1 (0.8 oz)	95	6	1	18	1	11	—	9	51	35	tr	—	20
MIX														
plain	1 (1.2 oz)	139	7	1	9	1	20	1	6	83	61	—	—	—
plain low calorie	1 (0.8 oz)	84	2	1	0	1	16	1	3	21	69	0	1	0
BETTY CROCKER														
Brownie With Hot Fudge MicroRave Single	1	350	12	3	0	5	55	—	40	260	310	—	—	—
Frosted MicroRave	1	180	7	2	0	1	21	—	—	120	155	—	—	—
Fudge Family Size	1	150	5	1	10	1	22	—	—	100	75	—	—	—
Fudge Light	1	100	1	—	0	1	21	—	—	90	75	—	—	—
Fudge MicroRave	1	150	6	2	0	2	22	—	—	110	150	—	—	—
Fudge Regular Size	1	150	6	1	15	1	23	—	—	105	80	—	—	—
Supreme Caramel	1	120	4	1	10	1	21	—	—	115	60	—	—	—
Supreme Frosted	1	160	6	2	10	1	26	—	—	120	105	—	—	—
Supreme German Chocolate	1	160	7	2	10	1	24	—	—	110	100	—	—	—
Supreme Original	1	140	6	1	10	1	21	—	—	80	65	—	—	—
Supreme Party	1	160	6	2	10	1	26	—	—	110	90	—	—	—
Supreme Walnut	1	140	7	1	10	1	18	—	—	80	80	—	—	—
Walnut MicroRave	1	160	7	2	0	2	21	—	—	95	150	—	—	—
ESTEE														
Lite	2	100	4	2	0	tr	23	1	0	0	140	0	—	0
JIFFY														
Fudge as prep	1	160	4	1	7	1	28	tr	80	150	—	0	—	0
READY-TO-EAT														
plain	1 lg (2 oz)	227	9	2	10	3	36	1	16	175	84	—	—	39
plain	1 sm (1 oz)	115	5	1	5	1	18	1	8	88	42	—	—	20
w/ nuts	1 (1 oz)	100	4	2	14	1	16	—	13	59	50	tr	—	70
w/o nuts	1 (2 oz)	243	10	3	9	3	39	—	25	153	83	3	4	10
FRITO LAY														
Fudge Nut	3 oz	360	14	—	8	3	56	—	—	225	180	2	—	—
GREENFIELD														
Brownie HomeStyle	1 (1.4 oz)	120	0	0	0	2	29	1	20	65	—	0	—	0
HOSTESS														
Brownie Bites	5 (2 oz)	260	14	4	50	4	32	2	—	125	190	—	—	—
Brownie Bites Walnut	5 (2 oz)	270	15	4	50	4	31	2	—	140	190	—	—	—
LANCE														
Brownie	1 pkg (78 g)	320	12	3	5	4	52	—	—	210	25	4	—	—
LITTLE DEBBIE														
Fudge	1 pkg (2.1 oz)	270	13	3	15	2	39	1	20	170	—	0	—	0
Fudge	1 pkg (3.6 oz)	450	21	4	20	4	65	2	20	280	—	0	—	0
Fudge	1 pkg (2.9 oz)	360	17	3	15	3	52	1	20	230	—	0	—	0

FOOD	PORTION	CALORIES	FAT	SAT FAT	CHOL	PROTEIN	CARBO	FIBER	CALCIUM	SOD	POTAS	VIT C	FOLIC	VIT A
LITTLE DEBBIE (CONT.)														
Fudge	1 pkg (2.5 oz)	310	15	3	15	3	44	1	20	190	—	0	—	0
PEPPERIDGE FARM														
Charlotte Fudgey Brownie	1	220	11	4	25	3	28	2	—	105	—	—	—	—
Tahoe Milk Chocolate Pecan	1	210	10	3	25	3	30	1	—	100	—	—	—	—
Westport Fudgey Brownies w/ Walnuts	1	220	11	4	25	3	28	2	—	105	—	—	—	—
SWEET REWARDS														
Double Fudge	1 (1.1 oz)	110	0	0	0	2	25	tr	60	100	—	—	—	—
Fat Free Brownie	1 bar (1 oz)	90	0	0	0	2	21	<1	tr	90	—	—	—	—
TASTYKAKE														
Brownie	1 (85 g)	340	14	3	20	4	53	5	—	220	—	—	—	—

BRUSSELS SPROUTS

FOOD	PORTION	CALORIES	FAT	SAT FAT	CHOL	PROTEIN	CARBO	FIBER	CALCIUM	SOD	POTAS	VIT C	FOLIC	VIT A
FRESH														
cooked	½ cup	30	tr	tr	0	2	7	3	28	17	247	48	47	561
cooked	1 sprout	8	tr	tr	0	1	2	—	7	4	67	13	13	151
raw	½ cup	19	tr	tr	0	1	4	—	18	11	171	37	27	389
DOLE														
Sprouts	½ cup	19	tr	—	0	1	4	2	—	11	171	37	—	389
FROZEN														
cooked	½ cup	33	tr	tr	0	3	6	—	19	18	254	36	79	459
BIG VALLEY														
Whole	5-8 pieces (3 oz)	35	0	0	0	3	6	1	0	9	—	62	—	500
BIRDS EYE														
Burssels Sprouts	6 (3 oz)	35	0	0	0	3	7	3	20	15	—	54	—	500
FRESH LIKE														
Sprouts	3.5 oz	37	tr	—	—	3	7	1	29	21	344	70	—	738
GREEN GIANT														
Butter Sauce	⅔ cup (3.6 oz)	60	2	2	<5	3	9	4	20	270	—	42	—	200

BUCKWHEAT

FOOD	PORTION	CALORIES	FAT	SAT FAT	CHOL	PROTEIN	CARBO	FIBER	CALCIUM	SOD	POTAS	VIT C	FOLIC	VIT A
flour whole groat	1 cup	402	4	tr	0	15	85	—	—	—	—	0	64	—
groats roasted cooked	½ cup	91	tr	tr	0	3	20	—	7	4	88	0	14	—
groats roasted uncooked	½ cup	283	2	tr	0	10	61	—	14	9	263	0	35	—
WOLFF'S														
Brown Groats Roasted	1 cup (8 oz)	900	4	—	—	16	188	—	20	—	—	—	—	—
Flour	1 cup (8 oz)	860	5	—	—	24	170	—	50	—	—	—	—	—
Kasha Coarse cooked	¼ cup (1.6 oz)	170	2	0	0	64	35	2	0	10	220	0	—	0
Kasha Fine cooked	¼ cup (1.6 oz)	170	2	0	0	64	35	2	0	10	220	0	—	0

FOOD	PORTION	CALORIES	FAT	SAT FAT	CHOL	PROTEIN	CARBO	FIBER	CALCIUM	SOD	POTAS	VIT C	FOLIC	VIT A
WOLFF'S (CONT.)														
Kasha Medium cooked	¼ cup (1.6 oz)	170	2	0	0	64	35	2	0	10	220	0	—	0
Kasha Whole cooked	¼ cup (1.6 oz)	170	2	0	0	64	35	2	0	10	220	0	—	0
White Grits	1 cup (8 oz)	840	3	—	—	24	173	—	20	—	—	—	—	—
BUFFALO														
water buffalo roasted	3 oz	111	2	1	52	23	0	—	13	48	266	—	8	—
BULGUR														
cooked	½ cup	76	tr	tr	0	3	17	—	9	5	62	0	17	—
uncooked	½ cup	239	tr	—	0	9	53	—	25	12	287	0	19	—
CASBAH														
Pilaf Mix as prep	1 cup	200	1	0	0	6	42	4	40	450	—	32	—	700
Salad Mix as prep	⅔ cup	90	tr	0	0	3	20	1	50	350	—	22	—	550
GOOD SHEPHERD														
Bulgur	¼ cup (43 g)	150	1	—	0	4	33	1	20	0	165	—	—	—
HODGSON MILL														
Bulgur	¼ cup (1.4 oz)	120	1	0	0	6	24	1	20	0	—	0	—	0
BURDOCK ROOT														
cooked	1 cup	110	tr	—	0	3	26	—	62	5	450	—	—	0
raw	1 cup	85	tr	—	0	2	20	—	48	6	363	4	—	0
BUTTER														
(*see also* BUTTER BLENDS, BUTTER SUBSTITUTES, MARGARINE)														
clarified butter	3½ oz	876	99	62	256	tr	0	—	tr	—	—	0	—	3750
stick	1 stick (4 oz)	813	92	57	248	1	tr	—	27	937	29	0	3	3468
stick	1 pat (5 g)	36	4	3	11	tr	tr	—	1	41	1	0	tr	153
whipped	1 pat (4 g)	27	3	2	8	tr	tr	—	1	31	1	—	tr	116
whipped	4 oz	542	61	38	165	1	tr	—	18	625	20	0	2	2312
CABOT														
Stick	1 tsp	35	4	3	11	0	0	—	1	41	—	—	—	200
Unsalted Stick	1 tsp	35	4	3	11	0	0	—	1	0	—	—	—	200
CRYSTAL														
Salted Stick	1 tbsp (0.5 oz)	102	11	7	43	tr	tr	0	3	89	4	tr	0	422
Unsalted Stick	1 tbsp (0.5 oz)	102	11	7	43	tr	tr	0	3	1	4	tr	0	422
HOTEL BAR														
Stick	1 tsp	35	4	—	—	0	0	—	—	35	—	—	—	200
KELLER'S														
Stick	1 tsp	35	4	—	—	0	0	—	—	35	—	—	—	—
LAND O'LAKES														
Light Stick	1 tbsp	50	6	4	20	0	0	—	—	70	—	—	—	500
Light Unsalted Stick	1 tbsp	50	6	4	15	0	0	—	—	5	—	—	—	500
Stick	1 tbsp (0.5 oz)	100	11	7	30	0	0	—	—	85	—	—	—	400
Unsalted Stick	1 tbsp (0.5 oz)	100	11	7	30	0	0	—	—	0	—	—	—	400

FOOD	PORTION	CALORIES	FAT	SAT FAT	CHOL	PROTEIN	CARBO	FIBER	CALCIUM	SOD	POTAS	VIT C	FOLIC	VIT A
LAND O'LAKES (CONT.)														
Unsalted Tub	1 tbsp	60	7	5	20	0	0	—	—	0	—	—	—	—
Whipped	1 tbsp (0.3 oz)	70	7	5	20	0	0	—	—	55	—	—	—	200

BUTTER BEANS

CANNED

ALLEN

FOOD	PORTION	CALORIES	FAT	SAT FAT	CHOL	PROTEIN	CARBO	FIBER	CALCIUM	SOD	POTAS	VIT C	FOLIC	VIT A
Baby	½ cup (4.5 oz)	120	1	1	0	7	22	6	20	460	—	0	—	0
Large	½ cup (4.5 oz)	120	1	0	0	7	20	7	40	290	—	0	—	0
GREEN GIANT														
Butter Beans	½ cup (4.5 oz)	90	0	0	0	6	16	4	40	450	—	0	—	0
SUNSHINE														
Butter Beans	½ cup (4.5 oz)	120	1	0	0	7	23	8	40	370	—	0	—	0
TRAPPEY														
Baby White With Bacon	½ cup (4.5 oz)	130	2	1	0	8	21	6	0	350	—	0	—	0
Large White With Bacon	½ cup (4.5 oz)	110	1	0	0	6	21	6	0	300	—	0	—	0
VAN CAMP'S														
Butter Beans	½ cup	110	1	0	0	8	22	7	40	430	530	—	0	0
FROZEN														
BIRDS EYE														
Butter Beans	½ cup (2.7 oz)	100	0	0	0	6	20	4	20	130	—	2	—	0
Speckled	½ cup (2.7 oz)	100	0	0	0	6	20	4	20	130	—	2	—	0

BUTTER BLENDS

(*see also* BUTTER, BUTTER SUBSTITUTES, MARGARINE)

BLUE BONNET

FOOD	PORTION	CALORIES	FAT	SAT FAT	CHOL	PROTEIN	CARBO	FIBER	CALCIUM	SOD	POTAS	VIT C	FOLIC	VIT A
Better Blend Stick	1 tbsp	90	11	2	—	0	0	—	—	95	—	—	—	500
Better Blend Tub	1 tbsp	90	11	2	0	0	0	—	—	95	10	—	—	500
Better Blend Unsalted Stick	1 tbsp	90	11	1	5	0	0	—	—	0	0	—	—	500
BRUMMEL & BROWN														
Spread Make With Yogurt	1 tbsp (0.5 oz)	50	5	1	0	0	0	—	—	95	—	—	—	500
COUNTRY MORNING														
Blend Light Stick	1 tbsp (0.5 oz)	50	6	3	10	0	0	—	—	110	—	—	—	750
Blend Light Tub	1 tbsp (0.5 oz)	50	6	3	5	0	0	—	—	90	—	—	—	750
Blend Stick	1 tbsp	100	11	3	0	0	0	—	—	90	—	—	—	400
Blend Tub	1 tbsp	100	11	2	0	0	0	—	—	80	—	—	—	400
Blend Unsalted Stick	1 tbsp	100	11	3	0	0	0	—	—	0	—	—	—	400

BUTTER SUBSTITUTES

(*see also* BUTTER BLENDS, MARGARINE)

BUTTER BUDS

FOOD	PORTION	CALORIES	FAT	SAT FAT	CHOL	PROTEIN	CARBO	FIBER	CALCIUM	SOD	POTAS	VIT C	FOLIC	VIT A
Mix	1 tsp (2 g)	5	0	0	0	0	2	—	—	75	—	—	—	—
Sprinkles	1 tsp (2 g)	5	0	0	0	0	2	—	—	120	—	—	—	—

FOOD	PORTION	CALORIES	FAT	SAT FAT	CHOL	PROTEIN	CARBO	FIBER	CALCIUM	SOD	POTAS	VIT C	FOLIC	VIT A
MOLLY MCBUTTER														
Cheese	1 tsp	5	0	0	0	0	1	—	—	125	0	—	—	—
Light Sodium	1 tsp	5	0	0	0	0	1	—	—	90	0	—	—	—
Natural Butter	1 tsp	5	0	0	0	0	1	—	—	180	0	—	—	—
Roasted Garlic	1 tsp	5	0	0	0	0	1	—	—	125	0	—	—	—
MORNINGSTAR FARMS														
Roasted Soy Butter	2 tbsp (1.1 oz)	170	11	2	0	6	10	1	0	170	150	0	—	0
MRS. BATEMAN'S														
Butterlike Baking Butter	1 tbsp (0.5 oz)	36	1	tr	<5	0	8	0	0	20	—	0	—	0
Butterlike Saute Butter	1 tbsp (0.5 oz)	40	2	1	5	0	8	0	0	60	—	0	—	0
NATURAL TOUCH														
Roasted Soy Butter	2 tbsp (1.1 oz)	170	11	2	0	6	10	1	0	170	150	0	—	0
WATKINS														
Butter Sprinkles	1 tsp (2 g)	5	0	0	0	0	1	0	0	170	—	0	—	0
Imitation Butter Flavored Mist	1 tbsp (0.5 oz)	120	14	2	0	0	0	0	0	0	—	0	—	0
BUTTERBUR														
canned fuki chopped	1 cup	3	tr	—	0	tr	tr	—	42	5	15	15	—	0
fresh fuki raw	1 cup	13	tr	—	0	tr	3	—	97	7	616	30	—	47
BUTTERNUTS														
dried	1 oz	174	16	tr	0	7	3	—	15	0	119	—	—	—
BUTTERSCOTCH														
(*see also* CANDY)														
NESTLE														
Morsels Butterscotch	1 tbsp	80	4	4	—	0	10	—	—	15	—	—	—	—
CABBAGE														
(*see also* COLESLAW)														
FRESH														
chinese pak-choi raw shredded	½ cup	5	tr	tr	0	1	1	—	37	23	88	16	—	1050
chinese pak-choi shredded cooked	½ cup	10	tr	tr	0	1	2	—	79	29	315	22	—	2183
chinese pe-tsai raw shredded	1 cup	12	tr	tr	0	1	2	—	58	7	181	21	60	912
chinese pe-tsai shredded cooked	1 cup	16	tr	tr	0	2	3	—	38	11	268	19	64	1151
danish raw	1 head (2 lbs)	228	2	tr	0	13	49	18	431	164	2231	292	392	1210
danish raw shredded	½ cup (1.2 oz)	9	tr	tr	0	1	2	tr	17	6	86	11	15	47
danish shredded cooked	½ cup (2.6 oz)	17	tr	tr	0	1	3	1	23	6	73	15	15	99
green raw	1 head (2 lbs)	228	2	tr	0	2	49	18	431	164	2231	292	392	1210

FOOD	PORTION	CALORIES	FAT	SAT FAT	CHOL	PROTEIN	CARBO	FIBER	CALCIUM	SOD	POTAS	VIT C	FOLIC	VIT A
green raw shredded	½ cup (1.2 oz)	9	tr	tr	0	1	2	tr	17	6	86	11	15	47
green shredded cooked	½ cup (2.6 oz)	17	tr	tr	0	1	3	1	23	6	73	15	15	99
napa cooked	1 cup (3.8 oz)	13	tr	0	0	1	2	0	32	12	95	0	47	96
red shredded cooked	½ cup	16	tr	tr	0	1	3	—	28	6	105	26	9	20
savoy raw shredded	½ cup	10	tr	tr	0	1	2	—	12	10	81	11	—	350
savoy shredded cooked	½ cup	18	tr	tr	0	1	4	—	22	17	134	12		649
DOLE														
Cabbage	1/12 med head	18	0	—	0	1	3	2	—	30	187	41	—	69
Napa shredded	½ cup	6	tr	—	0	1	1	tr	—	3	90	10	—	456
FRESH EXPRESS														
Cole Slaw	1½ cups (3 oz)	25	0	0	0	1	6	2	40	25	—	36	—	300
TAKE-OUT														
kimchee	½ cup (1.6 oz)	39	2	tr	0	1	5	1	19	177	101	19	18	168

CAKE

(*see also* BROWNIE, CAKE MIX, COOKIE, DANISH PASTRY, DOUGHNUT, PIE)

FOOD	PORTION	CALORIES	FAT	SAT FAT	CHOL	PROTEIN	CARBO	FIBER	CALCIUM	SOD	POTAS	VIT C	FOLIC	VIT A
angelfood	1 cake (11.9 oz)	876	3	tr	0	20	197	5	477	2548	318	0	—	0
angelfood home recipe	1/12 cake (1.9 oz)	142	tr	tr	0	4	32	1	3	96	116	0	2	0
apple crisp home recipe	1 recipe 6 serv (29.6 oz)	1377	31	6	1	15	273	—	239	1537	821	19	42	1154
boston cream pie frzn	1/6 cake (3.2 oz)	232	8	2	34	2	40	1	21	132	36	—	7	74
carrot w/ cream cheese icing home recipe	1 cake 10 in diam	6175	328	66	1183	63	775	—	707	4470	1720	23	—	2240
cheesecake	1/6 cake (2.8 oz)	256	18	9	44	4	20	2	50	165	72	—	12	—
cheesecake	1 cake 9 in diam	3350	213	120	2053	60	317	—	622	2464	1088	56	—	2820
cheesecake home recipe	1/12 cake (4.5 oz)	456	9	18	155	9	32	—	74	362	131	1	16	1354
cherry fudge w/ chocolate frosting	1/8 cake (2.5 oz)	187	9	3	—	2	27	—	34	160	118	10	—	158
chocolate cupcake creme filled w/ frosting home recipe	1 (1.8 oz)	188	7	2	9	2	30	—	37	213	61	—	—	8
chocolate w/o frosting home recipe	2 layers (39.9 oz)	4067	172	62	661	60	608	—	679	3581	1596	2	111	1596
chocolate w/o frosting home recipe	1/12 cake (3.3 oz)	340	14	5	55	5	51	—	57	299	133	tr	9	133

FOOD	PORTION	CALORIES	FAT	SAT FAT	CHOL	PROTEIN	CARBO	FIBER	CALCIUM	SOD	POTAS	VIT C	FOLIC	VIT A
coffeecake creme-filled chocolate frosting home recipe	⅙ cake (3.2 oz)	298	10	3	—	5	49	2	35	290	—	—	—	—
coffeecake crumb topped cinnamon home recipe	1/12 cake (2.1 oz)	240	12	2	36	4	30	2	67	233	144	tr	9	383
coffeecake fruit	⅛ cake (1.8 oz)	156	5	1	—	3	26	—	23	192	45	tr	9	70
cream puff shell home recipe	1 (2.3 oz)	239	17	4	129	6	15	—	24	368	64	0	14	763
devil's food cupcake w/ chocolate frosting	1	120	4	4	19	2	20	—	21	92	46	tr	—	50
devil's food w/ creme filling	1 (1 oz)	105	4	2	15	1	17	—	21	105	34	0	—	20
eclair home recipe	1 (3 oz)	262	16	4	127	6	24	—	63	337	117	tr	14	718
fruitcake	1 piece (1.5 oz)	139	4	tr	2	1	27	—	14	116	66	—	—	—
fruitcake dark home recipe	1 cake 7½ in x 2¼ in	5185	228	48	640	74	738	—	1293	2123	6138	504	—	1720
pound	1 cake (8½ x 3½ x 3 in	1935	94	52	1100	26	257	—	146	1857	443	0	—	2820
pound	1/10 cake (1 oz)	117	6	3	66	2	15	—	11	119	36	—	—	182
pound fat free	1 cake (12 oz)	961	4	1	0	18	208	—	146	1158	373	1	14	327
pound cake home recipe	1 loaf 8½ in x 3½ in	1935	94	21	1100	33	265	—	146	1645	483	1	—	3470
sheet cake w/ white frosting home recipe	1 cake 9 in sq	4020	129	42	636	37	694	—	548	2488	669	2	—	2190
sheet cake w/o frosting home recipe	⅑ cake	315	12	3	61	4	48	—	55	258	68	tr	—	150
sheet cake w/o frosting home recipe	1 cake 9 in sq	2830	108	30	552	35	434	—	497	2331	614	2	—	1320
shortcake home recipe	1 (2.3 oz)	225	9	2	2	4	32	—	133	329	69	tr	7	47
sour cream pound	1/10 cake (1 oz)	117	5	1	17	1	16	tr	19	120	32	—	—	—
sponge	1/12 cake (1.3 oz)	110	1	tr	39	2	23	—	26	93	38	0	5	59
sponge home recipe	1/12 cake (2.2 oz)	140	2	1	80	3	27	—	20	107	66	0	9	121
sponge w/ creme filling	1 (1.5 oz)	155	5	1	7	1	27	—	19	155	—	—	—	—
tiramisu	1 cake (4.4 lbs)	5732	421	217	2395	101	439	3	1602	1107	2953	8.3	221	22095
toaster pastry apple	1 (1¾ oz)	204	5	1	—	2	37	—	14	218	58	—	42	502

FOOD	PORTION	CALORIES	FAT	SAT FAT	CHOL	PROTEIN	CARBO	FIBER	CALCIUM	SOD	POTAS	VIT C	FOLIC	VIT A
toaster pastry blueberry	1 (1¾ oz)	204	5	1	—	2	37	—	14	218	58	—	42	502
toaster pastry brown sugar cinnamon	1 (1¾ oz)	206	7	2	—	3	34	—	17	212	57	—	40	493
toaster pastry cherry	1 (1¾ oz)	204	5	1	—	2	37	—	14	218	58	—	42	502
toaster pastry strawberry	1 (1¾ oz)	204	5	1	—	2	37	—	14	218	58	—	42	502
white w/ coconut frosting home recipe	1/12 cake (3.9 oz)	399	12	4	2	5	71	—	101	318	111	tr	6	43
white w/o frosting home recipe	1/12 cake (2.6 oz)	264	9	2	2	4	42	—	96	242	70	tr	5	42
white w/ white frosting	1 cake 9 in diam	4170	148	33	46	43	670	—	536	2827	832	0	—	640
white w/ white frosting	1/16 cake	260	9	2	3	3	42	—	33	176	52	0	—	40
yellow w/ chocolate frosting	1/8 cake (2.2 oz)	242	11	3	35	2	36	1	24	216	114	—	—	—
yellow w/ chocolate frosting	1 cake 9 diam	3895	175	92	609	40	620	—	366	3080	1972	0	—	1850
yellow w/o frosting home recipe	1/12 cake (2.4 oz)	245	10	3	37	4	36	—	99	233	62	tr	7	94
yellow w/o frosting home recipe	2 layers (28.7 oz)	2947	119	32	443	43	433	—	1192	2803	740	2	85	1135
BABY WATSON														
Cheesecake	1 slice (3.8 oz)	390	30	18	142	6	23	2	92	330	—	1	—	890
Cheesecake Light	1/16 cake (3.9 oz)	280	16	9	33	8	24	3	98	270	—	0	—	390
BAKER MAID														
Creole Royal Pineapple Apricot	3 slices (5 oz)	270	3	1	20	5	61	4	100	230	—	6	—	100
Creole Royal Pineapple Apricot	1 slice (1.7 oz)	90	1	0	5	2	20	1	40	75	—	2	—	0
CAROUSEL														
New York Cheese Cake	1 cake (3 oz)	250	19	11	95	4	16	1	80	180	—	0	—	500
DRAKE'S														
Light & Fruity Apple	1 (1.2 oz)	90	1	—	0	2	20	—	—	110	40	—	—	—
Light & Fruity Blueberry	1 (1.2 oz)	90	1	—	0	1	20	—	—	95	30	—	—	—
Light & Fruity Cinnamon Raisin	1 (1.2 oz)	90	1	—	0	1	19	—	—	105	45	—	—	—
Mini Coffee Cakes	4 (1.83 oz)	220	9	2	18	3	33	1	20	140	—	0	—	0
DUTCH MILL														
Dessert Shells Chocolate Covered	1 (0.5 oz)	80	5	2	0	1	8	0	0	—	—	0	—	0

FOOD	PORTION	CALORIES	FAT	SAT FAT	CHOL	PROTEIN	CARBO	FIBER	CALCIUM	SOD	POTAS	VIT C	FOLIC	VIT A
ENTENMANN'S														
Apple Puffs	1 (3 oz)	280	13	—	—	4	39	—	—	320	—	—	—	—
Apple Strudel Old Fashioned	1 serv (1.5 oz)	120	5	—	—	1	17	—	—	110	—	—	—	—
Cheese Topped Buns	1 (2.3 oz)	240	12	—	—	5	29	—	—	240	—	—	—	—
Cinnamon Buns	1 (2.1 oz)	230	10	—	—	4	31	—	—	200	—	—	—	—
Cinnamon Filbert Ring	1 serv (1.5 oz)	190	12	—	—	3	19	—	—	160	—	—	—	—
Coffee Cake Cheese	1 serv (1.6 oz)	150	7	—	—	3	20	—	—	140	—	—	—	—
Coffee Cake Cheese Filled Crumb	1 serv (1.4 oz)	130	6	—	—	3	18	—	—	140	—	—	—	—
Coffee Cake Crumb	1 serv (1.3 oz)	160	7	—	—	3	21	—	—	160	—	—	—	—
Danish Ring	1 serv (1.5 oz)	180	10	—	—	3	18	—	—	160	—	—	—	—
Danish Ring Pecan	1 serv (1.5 oz)	190	12	—	—	3	19	—	—	130	—	—	—	—
Danish Ring Walnut	1 serv (1.5 oz)	190	12	—	—	3	19	—	—	130	—	—	—	—
Danish Twist Lemon	1 serv (1.2 oz)	140	7	—	—	2	17	—	—	140	—	—	—	—
Danish Twist Raspberry	1 serv (1.2 oz)	140	7	—	—	2	18	—	—	120	—	—	—	—
Devil's Food Cake Fudge Iced	1 serv (1.2 oz)	130	5	—	—	2	19	—	—	120	—	—	—	—
French Crumb Cake All Butter	1 serv (1.6 oz)	180	8	—	—	2	26	—	—	220	—	—	—	—
Louisiana Crunch Cake	1 serv (1.7 oz)	180	8	—	—	2	27	—	—	180	—	—	—	—
Pound Loaf All Butter	1 serv (1 oz)	110	5	—	—	2	15	—	—	150	—	—	—	—
Pound Loaf Sour Cream	1 serv (1 oz)	120	7	—	—	1	14	—	—	90	—	—	—	—
Thick Fudge Golden Cake	1 serv (1.2 oz)	130	6	—	—	2	20	—	—	120	—	—	—	—
FREIHOFER'S														
Angel Food	⅕ cake (2 oz)	150	0	0	0	3	35	0	60	410	—	0	—	0
Cinnamon Swirl Buns	1 (2.8 oz)	290	9	2	30	5	47	1	20	250	—	0	—	0
Coffee Cake Cinnamon Pecan	⅛ cake (2 oz)	220	9	2	25	3	33	1	20	160	—	0	—	0
Crumb	⅛ cake (2 oz)	240	11	2	15	4	33	1	0	260	—	0	—	200
Homestyle Golden Loaf	⅛ cake (1.8 oz)	200	9	2	50	3	28	0	0	190	—	0	—	0
Pound	⅕ cake (2.8 oz)	330	17	4	65	4	41	0	20	330	—	0	—	0

FOOD	PORTION	CALORIES	FAT	SAT FAT	CHOL	PROTEIN	CARBO	FIBER	CALCIUM	SOD	POTAS	VIT C	FOLIC	VIT A
GREENFIELD														
Blondie Apple Spice	1 (1.4 oz)	120	0	0	0	2	28	0	20	65	—	0	—	0
Blondie Chocolate Chip	1 (1.4 oz)	120	0	0	0	2	29	0	20	65	—	0	—	0
HOSTESS														
Angel Food Ring	⅙ cake (1.6 oz)	150	3	2	<5	2	29	0	—	220	50	—	—	—
Apple Twist	1 (2.5 oz)	220	4	2	15	4	42	tr	—	270	70	—	—	—
Baseball Yellow Cakes	1 (1.6 oz)	160	3	1	<5	1	32	0	—	160	80	—	—	—
Choco Licious	1 (1.5 oz)	170	6	3	10	2	28	1	—	190	120	—	—	—
Choco-Diles	1 (1.8 oz)	210	10	7	20	2	31	1	—	160	140	—	—	—
Cinnaminis Original	5 (2.4 oz)	300	17	4	20	3	37	2	—	230	45	—	—	—
Cinnamon Roll	1 (2.3 oz)	220	6	3	25	4	39	1	150	260	75	—	—	—
Crumb Cake	1 (1.9 oz)	210	8	3	15	2	33	1	20	135	40	—	—	—
Cup Cakes Chocolate	1 (1.6 oz)	170	5	3	<5	2	28	tr	100	160	70	—	—	—
Cup Cakes Chocolate Light	1 (1.4 oz)	120	2	0	0	2	26	tr	—	170	110	—	—	—
Cup Cakes Orange	1 (1.5 oz)	160	5	2	10	1	28	0	80	160	35	—	—	—
Dessert Cups	1 (1 oz)	90	2	0	10	2	18	0	—	170	30	—	—	—
Ding Dongs	1 (1.3 oz)	160	9	6	5	1	21	tr	—	110	140	—	—	—
Fruit Cake Holiday	⅙ cake (5.3 oz)	490	14	2	10	4	93	3	40	410	230	—	—	—
Fruit Loaf	1 (3.8 oz)	350	10	1	5	3	67	2	40	290	170	—	—	—
Ho Ho's	1 (1 oz)	130	6	4	10	1	17	tr	—	75	90	—	—	—
Holiday Cakes	1 (1.6 oz)	160	3	1	<5	1	32	0	—	160	80	—	—	—
Honey Bun Glazed	1 (2.7 oz)	320	19	9	15	5	35	2	100	90	35	—	—	—
Honey Bun Iced	1 (3.4 oz)	390	20	9	15	5	49	2	80	220	85	—	—	—
Hopper Cakes	1 (1.6 oz)	160	3	1	<5	1	32	0	—	160	80	—	—	—
Lights Low Fat Cinnamon Crumb Cake	1 (1 oz)	90	1	0	0	1	19	0	0	100	—	0	—	0
Lil Angels	1 (1 oz)	90	2	1	<5	1	17	0	—	130	30	—	—	—
Pecan Spinners	1 (1 oz)	110	5	1	0	2	15	tr	20	65	35	—	—	—
Pound Cake	⅕ cake (3.2 oz)	350	16	4	55	5	48	1	60	360	95	—	—	—
Sno Balls	1 (1.6 oz)	160	5	3	0	2	29	1	—	180	60	—	—	—
Suzy Q's	1 (2 oz)	220	9	4	10	2	35	2	20	270	85	—	—	—
Suzy Q's Banana	1 (2 oz)	220	10	1	25	3	32	tr	60	280	60	—	—	—
Swirls Caramel Pecan	1 (2 oz)	140	15	6	15	3	25	1	—	55	130	—	—	—
Tiger Tails	1 (1.5 oz)	160	6	3	15	2	26	tr	—	150	50	—	—	—
Twinkies	1 (1.4 oz)	140	4	2	15	1	25	0	—	180	30	—	—	—
Twinkies Banana	2 (2.7 oz)	300	13	2	35	4	42	tr	60	370	—	—	—	—

FOOD	PORTION	CALORIES	FAT	SAT FAT	CHOL	PROTEIN	CARBO	FIBER	CALCIUM	SOD	POTAS	VIT C	FOLIC	VIT A
HOSTESS (CONT.)														
Twinkies Devil Food	2 (2.7 oz)	300	12	5	15	3	47	2	20	360	110	—	—	—
Twinkies Lights	1 (1.4 oz)	120	2	0	0	2	24	0	—	200	50	—	—	—
Twinkies Strawberry Fruit 'n Creme	1 (1.6 oz)	150	3	1	20	2	30	tr	—	200	40	—	—	—
JELL-O														
Cheesecake Snack Original	1 (3.3 oz)	160	6	3	10	3	23	0	80	130	110	0	—	200
Cheesecake Snack Strawberry	1 (3.3 oz)	150	5	3	10	2	26	0	60	125	90	0	—	100
KELLOGG'S														
Pop-Tarts Apple Cinnamon	1 (1.8 oz)	210	5	1	0	2	38	1	0	170	—	0	40	500
Pop-Tarts Blueberry	1 (1.8 oz)	210	7	1	0	2	36	1	0	210	—	0	40	500
Pop-Tarts Brown Sugar Cinnamon	1 (1.8 oz)	220	9	1	0	3	32	1	0	210	—	0	40	500
Pop-Tarts Cherry	1 (1.8 oz)	200	5	1	0	2	37	1	0	220	—	0	40	500
Pop-Tarts Chocolate Graham	1 (1.8 oz)	210	6	1	0	3	36	1	0	220	—	0	40	500
Pop-Tarts Frosted Blueberry	1 (1.8 oz)	200	5	1	0	2	37	1	0	210	—	0	40	500
Pop-Tarts Frosted Brown Sugar Cinnamon	1 (1.8 oz)	210	7	1	0	3	34	1	0	180	—	0	40	500
Pop-Tarts Frosted Cherry	1 (1.8 oz)	200	5	1	0	2	37	1	0	220	—	0	40	500
Pop-Tarts Frosted Chocolate Vanilla Creme	1 (1.8 oz)	200	5	1	0	3	37	1	0	230	—	0	40	500
Pop-Tarts Frosted Chocolate Fudge	1 (1.8 oz)	200	5	1	0	3	37	1	0	220	—	0	40	500
Pop-Tarts Frosted Grape	1 (1.8 oz)	200	5	1	0	2	38	1	0	200	—	0	40	500
Pop-Tarts Frosted Raspberry	1 (1.8 oz)	210	6	1	0	2	37	1	0	210	—	0	40	500
Pop-Tarts Frosted S'mores	1 (1.8 oz)	200	5	1	0	3	37	1	0	200	—	0	40	500
Pop-Tarts Frosted Strawberry	1 (1.8 oz)	200	5	2	0	2	38	1	0	170	—	0	40	500
Pop-Tarts Strawberry	1 (1.8 oz)	200	5	2	0	2	37	1	0	180	—	0	40	500
Pop-Tarts Minis Frosted Chocolate	1 pkg (1.5 oz)	170	4	1	0	2	30	1	0	200	—	0	40	500
Pop-Tarts Minis Frosted Grape	1 pkg (1.5 oz)	170	4	1	0	2	32	0	0	180	—	0	40	500

FOOD	PORTION	CALORIES	FAT	SAT FAT	CHOL	PROTEIN	CARBO	FIBER	CALCIUM	SOD	POTAS	VIT C	FOLIC	VIT A
KELLOGG'S (CONT.)														
Pop-Tarts Minis Frosted Strawberry	1 pkg (1.5 oz)	170	4	1	0	2	32	0	0	180	—	0	40	500
Rice Krispies Treats	1 (0.8 oz)	90	2	0	0	1	18	0	0	75	—	0	40	200
LANCE														
Apple Oatmeal	1 pkg (51 g)	200	9	3	10	3	35	—	—	210	70	—	—	—
Dunking Sticks	1 (39 g)	190	10	3	5	2	22	—	—	130	—	—	—	—
Fig Cake	1 pkg (60 g)	210	3	1	0	2	43	—	—	90	50	—	—	—
Honey Buns	1 (85 g)	330	14	4	0	4	48	—	40	210	70	—	—	0.1
Oatmeal Cake	1 (57 g)	240	11	3	0	4	35	—	—	250	5	—	—	300
Pecan Twirls	1 pkg (57 g)	220	8	—	0	2	34	—	—	190	30	—	—	—
Raisin Cake	1 (57 g)	230	10	3	0	3	35	—	—	200	20	—	—	—
LITTLE DEBBIE														
Apple Delights	1 pkg (1.2 oz)	140	5	2	5	1	24	1	0	115	—	0	—	0
Apple-Roos	1 pkg (1.5 oz)	150	3	0	0	0	32	1	0	80	—	0	—	0
Banana Nut Muffin Loaves	1 pkg (1.9 oz)	210	9	2	10	2	30	1	20	210	—	1	—	0
Banana Twins	1 pkg (2.2 oz)	250	10	2	10	15	40	0	60	180	—	0	—	0
Be My Valentine	1 pkg (2.2 oz)	280	14	3	0	1	39	1	0	150	—	0	—	0
Cherry Cordials	1 pkg (1.3 oz)	160	8	2	0	0	23	1	0	100	—	0	—	0
Choc-o-Jel	1 pkg (1.2 oz)	150	7	2	0	0	21	1	0	95	—	0	—	0
Choco-Cakes	1 pkg (2.1 oz)	250	13	3	0	2	35	1	0	170	—	0	—	0
Choco-Cakes	1 pkg (2.2 oz)	240	12	3	0	2	35	1	0	180	—	0	—	0
Chocolate	1 pkg (3 oz)	360	17	4	0	2	52	1	20	220	—	0	—	0
Chocolate Chip	1 pkg (2.4 oz)	290	15	3	0	2	42	1	0	190	—	0	—	0
Chocolate Twins	1 pkg (2.4 oz)	240	9	2	20	2	42	1	20	280	—	0	—	0
Christmas Tree Cakes	1 pkg (1.5 oz)	190	9	2	0	0	27	0	0	90	—	0	—	0
Coconut	1 pkg (2.1 oz)	270	13	3	5	2	38	1	0	180	—	0	—	0
Coconut	1 pkg (2.4 oz)	300	14	4	5	2	42	0	0	200	—	0	—	0
Coconut Rounds	1 pkg (1.2 oz)	140	7	3	0	0	22	1	0	85	—	0	—	0
Coffee Cake Apple	1 pkg (1.9 oz)	220	7	1	10	2	36	1	20	190	—	0	—	0
Coffee Cake Apple Streusel	1 pkg (2 oz)	220	7	1	10	3	37	1	20	200	—	0	—	0
Devil Cremes	1 pkg (1.6 oz)	190	8	2	0	1	28	0	0	160	—	0	—	0
Devil Cremes	1 pkg (3.2 oz)	380	17	3	5	2	57	1	20	310	—	0	—	0
Devil Squares	1 pkg (2.2 oz)	260	13	3	0	2	39	1	20	180	—	0	—	0
Easter Basket Cakes	1 pkg (2.5 oz)	310	15	3	0	2	44	1	0	180	—	0	—	0
Fancy Cakes	1 pkg (2.4 oz)	300	15	3	0	1	42	0	0	160	—	0	—	0
Fudge Crispy	1 pkg (1.1 oz)	170	10	3	0	1	20	1	0	50	—	0	—	0
Fudge Round	1 pkg (2.5 oz)	290	12	3	5	2	49	2	20	170	—	0	—	0
Fudge Round	1 pkg (3 oz)	350	14	4	5	3	59	2	20	210	—	0	—	0
Fudge Rounds	1 pkg (1.2 oz)	140	5	1	5	1	23	1	0	80	—	0	—	0
Golden Cremes	1 pkg (1.5 oz)	170	7	2	0	2	25	0	20	180	—	0	—	0
Golden Cremes	1 pkg (3 oz)	330	15	3	10	3	50	0	40	350	—	2	—	750

FOOD	PORTION	CALORIES	FAT	SAT FAT	CHOL	PROTEIN	CARBO	FIBER	CALCIUM	SOD	POTAS	VIT C	FOLIC	VIT A
LITTLE DEBBIE (CONT.)														
Holiday Cake Chocolate	1 pkg (2.4 oz)	290	14	3	0	2	43	1	0	180	—	0	—	0
Holiday Cake Vanilla	1 pkg (2.5 oz)	310	15	3	0	2	44	1	0	180	—	0	—	0
Honey Bun	1 pkg (4 oz)	510	31	8	0	6	53	5	150	250	—	0	—	0
Honey Bun	1 pkg (3 oz)	380	23	6	0	4	39	4	100	190	—	0	—	0
Jelly Rolls	1 pkg (2.1 oz)	230	7	2	15	1	41	0	0	160	—	0	—	0
Lemon Stix	1 pkg (1.5 oz)	210	10	3	0	2	30	1	20	45	—	1	—	0
Marshmallow Supremes	1 pkg (1.1 oz)	130	5	1	0	0	22	1	0	70	—	0	—	0
Mint Sprints	1 pkg (1.5 oz)	230	13	3	0	1	28	1	0	70	—	0	—	0
Nutty Bar	1 pkg (2 oz)	290	17	3	0	4	34	1	0	115	—	0	—	0
Pecan Twins	1 pkg (2 oz)	220	9	1	0	3	32	1	20	200	—	0	—	0
Pumpkin Delights	1 pkg (1.1 oz)	130	5	1	5	1	21	1	0	115	—	0	—	500
Smiley Faces Cherry	1 pkg (1.2 oz)	140	5	1	5	1	23	1	0	115	—	0	—	0
Smiley Faces Pumpkin	1 pkg (1 oz)	130	5	1	0	2	20	1	20	215	—	0	—	0
Snack Cake Chocolate	1 pkg (2.5 oz)	300	15	3	0	2	43	1	0	180	—	0	—	0
Snack Cake Vanilla	1 pkg (2.6 oz)	320	16	3	0	2	45	1	0	180	—	0	—	0
Spice	1 pkg (2.5 oz)	300	15	3	10	2	43	1	0	230	—	0	—	0
Star Crunch	1 pkg (1.1 oz)	140	6	1	0	0	21	1	20	85	—	0	—	0
Star Crunch	1 pkg (2.6 oz)	330	14	3	0	3	51	1	20	240	—	0	—	0
Swiss Rolls	1 pkg (2.1 oz)	250	12	3	15	1	38	1	20	160	—	0	—	0
Swiss Rolls	1 pkg (2.7 oz)	320	15	4	15	2	47	1	20	210	—	0	—	0
Swiss Rolls	1 pkg (3.2 oz)	380	18	4	20	2	57	1	20	250	—	0	—	0
Teddy Berries	1 pkg (1.2 oz)	130	4	1	5	1	23	1	0	105	—	0	—	0
Vanilla	1 pkg (3 oz)	370	18	4	0	2	53	0	0	210	—	0	—	0
Vanilla Cremes	1 pkg (1.4 oz)	170	7	2	0	1	25	0	0	125	—	0	—	0
Zebra Cakes	1 pkg (2.6 oz)	150	16	3	0	2	45	1	0	180	—	0	—	0
NABISCO														
Frosted Strawberry	1 (1.7 oz)	190	5	2	0	2	35	1	—	190	45	2	—	500
NATURE'S CHOICE														
Toaster Pastries Fat Free Apple Cinnamon	1 (1.9 oz)	180	0	0	0	3	41	4	—	180	—	—	—	—
Toaster Pastries Fat Free Blueberry	1 (1.9 oz)	180	0	0	0	3	41	4	—	180	—	—	—	—
Toaster Pastries Fat Free Raspberry	1 (1.9 oz)	180	0	0	0	3	41	3	—	190	—	—	—	—
Toaster Pastries Fat Free Strawberry	1 (1.9 oz)	180	0	0	0	3	41	3	—	190	—	—	—	—
Toaster Pastries Low Fat Cherry	1 (1.9 oz)	180	3	0	0	3	36	3	—	30	—	—	—	—

FOOD	PORTION	CALORIES	FAT	SAT FAT	CHOL	PROTEIN	CARBO	FIBER	CALCIUM	SOD	POTAS	VIT C	FOLIC	VIT A
NATURE'S CHOICE (CONT.)														
Toaster Pastries Low Fat Frosted Blueberry	1 (1.9 oz)	190	2	0	0	3	42	3	—	40	—	—	—	—
Toaster Pastries Low Fat Frosted Chocolate	1 (1.9 oz)	200	3	0	0	3	42	3	—	45	—	—	—	—
Toaster Pastries Low Fat Frosted Cinnamon	1 (1.9 oz)	190	2	0	0	3	42	3	—	40	—	—	—	—
Toaster Pastries Low Fat Frosted Strawberry	1 (1.9 oz)	190	2	0	0	3	42	3	—	40	—	—	—	—
Toaster Pastries Low Fat Peach Apricot	1 (1.9 oz)	180	3	0	0	3	36	3	—	30	—	—	—	—
PEPPERIDGE FARM														
Amhurst Apple Crumb Coffee Cake	1	220	11	7	20	2	30	—	40	150	—	—	—	—
Apple 'N Spice Bake Dessert Lights	1 piece (4¼ oz)	170	2	0	10	2	37	—	60	105	—	—	—	—
Apple Turnover	1	300	17	—	—	2	34	—	—	210	—	2	—	—
Berkshire Apple Crisp	1	250	8	4	40	2	43	1	40	130	—	—	—	—
Blueberry Turnovers	1	310	19	—	—	3	32	—	—	230	—	6	—	—
Boston Cream Supreme	1 piece (2⅞ oz)	290	14	6	50	3	39	—	40	190	—	—	—	—
Butter Pound	1 slice (1 oz)	130	7	3	60	1	16	—	—	150	—	—	—	—
Carrot Classic	1 cake	260	16	6	50	2	32	—	—	280	—	1	—	1000
Carrot w/ Cream Cheese Icing	1 slice (1½ oz)	150	9	3	15	1	19	—	—	160	—	—	—	750
Charleston Peach Melba Shortcake	1	220	5	3	135	2	41	—	20	170	—	—	—	—
Cherries Supreme Dessert Lights	1 piece (3¼ oz)	170	11	0	80	0	38	—	40	35	—	1	—	400
Cherry Turnover	1	310	19	—	—	3	32	—	—	280	—	5	—	—
Chocolate Supreme	1 piece (2⅞ oz)	300	16	7	25	3	37	—	40	140	—	—	—	—
Chocolate Fudge Large Layer	1 slice (1⅝ oz)	180	10	3	20	1	23	—	—	140	—	—	—	—
Chocolate Fudge Strip Large Layer	1 piece (1⅝ oz)	170	9	3	20	2	20	—	—	140	—	—	—	—
Chocolate Mousse Cake Dessert Lights	1 piece (2½ oz)	190	9	3	5	3	25	—	20	260	—	9	—	—

FOOD	PORTION	CALORIES	FAT	SAT FAT	CHOL	PROTEIN	CARBO	FIBER	CALCIUM	SOD	POTAS	VIT C	FOLIC	VIT A
PEPPERIDGE FARM (CONT.)														
Cholesterol Free Pound	1 slice (1 oz)	110	6	—	0	1	13	—	—	85	—	—	—	—
Coconut Classic	1 cake	230	11	4	20	2	31	—	—	160	—	—	—	—
Coconut Large Layer	1 slice (1⅝ oz)	180	8	3	20	1	24	—	20	120	—	—	—	—
Devil's Food Large Layer	1 slice (1⅝ oz)	180	9	3	20	1	24	—	—	135	—	—	—	—
Double Chocolate Classic	1 cake	250	13	4	35	2	31	—	—	180	—	—	—	—
Fruit Squares Apple	1	220	12	—	—	2	27	—	—	170	—	1	—	—
Fruit Squares Cherry	1	230	12	—	—	2	28	—	—	180	—	5	—	—
Fudge Golden Classic	1 cake	260	14	4	40	2	34	—	20	160	—	—	—	—
German Chocolate Classic	1 cake	250	13	4	45	2	29	—	—	230	—	—	—	—
German Chocolate Large Layer	1 slice (1⅝ oz)	180	10	4	20	1	22	—	20	170	—	—	—	—
Golden Large Layer	1 slice (1⅝ oz)	180	9	3	20	1	24	—	20	110	—	—	—	—
Lemon Cake Supreme Dessert Lights	1 piece (2¾ oz)	170	5	1	50	4	26	—	40	100	—	9	—	100
Lemon Coconut Supreme	1 piece (3 oz)	280	13	6	30	3	38	—	20	220	—	2	—	—
Lemon Cream Supreme	1 piece (1⅝ oz)	170	9	3	20	2	21	—	—	120	—	—	—	—
Manhattan Strawberry Cheesecake	1	300	9	5	150	6	49	—	60	250	—	1	—	—
Peach Melba Supreme	1 (3⅛ oz)	270	7	3	35	2	50	—	20	135	—	—	—	—
Peach Parfait Dessert Lights	1 piece (4¼ oz)	150	5	1	10	3	24	—	20	70	—	24	—	300
Peach Turnover	1	310	18	—	—	3	34	—	—	260	—	36	—	300
Pineapple Cream Supreme	1 piece (2 oz)	190	7	2	20	2	28	—	20	130	—	—	—	—
Raspberry Turnovers	1	310	17	—	—	4	36	—	—	260	—	2	—	—
Raspberry Vanilla Swirl Dessert Lights	1 piece (3¼ oz)	160	5	1	15	4	25	—	40	140	—	9	—	—
Strawberry Shortcake Dessert Lights	1 piece (3 oz)	170	5	1	70	2	30	1	40	50	—	12	—	200
Strawberry Cream Supreme	1 piece (2 oz)	190	7	3	20	1	30	—	20	120	—	—	—	—
Strawberry Strip Large Layer	1 piece (1½ oz)	160	8	3	20	1	21	—	—	120	—	—	—	—

FOOD	PORTION	CALORIES	FAT	SAT FAT	CHOL	PROTEIN	CARBO	FIBER	CALCIUM	SOD	POTAS	VIT C	FOLIC	VIT A
PEPPERIDGE FARM (CONT.)														
Toaster Tart Apple Cinnamon	1	170	7	2	0	3	25	—	20	120	—	—	—	—
Toaster Tart Cheese	1	190	10	3	14	5	22	—	60	180	—	—	—	—
Toaster Tart Strawberry	1	190	7	2	0	3	28	—	40	120	—	—	—	—
Vanilla Fudge Swirl Classic	1 cake	250	11	4	35	2	33	—	—	160	—	—	—	—
Vanilla Large Layer	1 slice (1⅝ oz)	190	8	3	20	1	25	—	—	120	—	—	—	—
PERUGINA														
Pannettone Au Beurre	⅙ cake (2.9 oz)	310	12	5	110	5	47	2	20	140	—	0	—	100
PET-RITZ														
Cobbler Apple	⅙ cake (4.33 oz)	290	9	—	—	1	50	—	—	—	—	1	—	—
Cobbler Blackberry	⅙ cake (4.33 oz)	250	10	—	—	2	39	—	—	—	—	2	—	—
Cobbler Blueberry	⅙ cake (4.33 oz)	270	12	—	—	3	50	—	20	—	—	3	—	—
Cobbler Cherry	⅙ cake (4.33 oz)	280	10	—	—	2	46	—	—	—	—	2	—	450
Cobbler Peach	⅙ cake (4.33 oz)	260	10	—	—	2	46	—	—	—	—	7	—	300
Cobbler Strawberry	⅙ cake (4.33 oz)	290	9	—	—	1	50	—	—	—	—	7	—	—
SARA LEE														
Banana	⅙ cake (2.3 oz)	230	8	3	20	2	37	0	—	210	—	—	—	—
Banana Sundae	1/10 cake (2.8 oz)	270	14	10	20	3	32	tr	—	140	—	—	—	—
Carrot	⅙ cake (3.2 oz)	320	17	4	30	4	39	2	—	340	—	—	—	—
Cheesecake Cherry	¼ cake (4.7 oz)	350	12	5	35	6	55	2	—	310	—	—	—	—
Cheesecake Chocolate Chip	¼ cake (4.2 oz)	410	21	14	65	8	47	2	—	300	—	—	—	—
Cheesecake Chocolate Mousse	⅕ cake	400	25	20	30	5	37	2	—	190	—	—	—	—
Cheesecake French	⅙ cake	350	21	13	20	5	34	1	—	280	—	—	—	—
Cheesecake Singles Fudge Brownie Crumble	1 slice (4 oz)	400	22	15	90	6	43	2	—	250	—	—	—	—
Cheesecake Singles Strawberry Drizzle	1 slice (4 oz)	380	20	13	85	5	46	2	—	240	—	—	—	—
Cheesecake Strawberry	¼ pie (4.7 oz)	330	12	5	40	6	49	2	—	310	—	—	—	—
Cheesecake Strawberry French	⅙ cake	320	14	9	20	4	43	1	—	230	—	—	—	—

FOOD	PORTION	CALORIES	FAT	SAT FAT	CHOL	PROTEIN	CARBO	FIBER	CALCIUM	SOD	POTAS	VIT C	FOLIC	VIT A
SARA LEE (CONT.)														
Cheesecake Bars Chocolate Dipped Original	1 bar (2.7 oz)	190	14	11	20	2	14	0	—	50	—	—	—	—
Cheesecake Bites Chocolate Praline Pecan	5 pieces (4 oz)	480	31	21	80	6	44	3	—	290	—	—	—	—
Cheesecake Bites Chocolate Praline Pecan	1 piece (0.8 oz)	100	6	4	15	1	9	tr	—	60	—	—	—	—
Cheesecake Bites Chocolate Dipped Original	5 pieces (4 oz)	500	34	25	75	6	41	2	—	290	—	—	—	—
Cheesecake Bites Chocolate Dipped Original	1 piece (0.8 oz)	100	7	5	15	1	8	0	—	60	—	—	—	—
Cheesecake Bites Toasted Almond Crunch	5 pieces (4 oz)	470	30	22	80	6	43	2	—	310	—	—	—	—
Cheesecake Bits Toasted Almond Crunch	1 (0.8 oz)	90	6	5	15	1	9	0	—	65	—	—	—	—
Coffee Cake Butter Streusel	1/6 cake (1.9 oz)	220	12	6	35	4	25	tr	—	240	—	—	—	—
Coffee Cake Cheese	1/6 cake (1.9 oz)	180	6	2	20	3	28	0	40	230	—	0	—	0
Coffee Cake Crumb	1/8 cake (2 oz)	220	9	2	15	3	32	tr	—	210	—	—	—	—
Coffee Cake Pecan	1/6 cake (1.9 oz)	230	12	5	25	4	24	tr	—	170	—	—	—	—
Coffee Cake Raspberry	1/6 cake (1.9 oz)	200	8	3	15	3	27	tr	—	220	—	0	—	—
Harvest Pumpkin Spice	1/8 cake (2.9 oz)	270	14	9	25	3	33	1	—	200	—	—	—	—
Layer Cake Coconut	1/8 cake (2.8 oz)	280	14	12	30	3	34	2	—	170	—	—	—	—
Layer Cake Double Chocolate	1/8 cake (2.8 oz)	260	13	11	25	3	33	2	—	180	—	—	—	—
Layer Cake Fudge Golden	1/8 cake (2.8 oz)	270	13	10	15	3	36	1	—	160	—	—	—	—
Layer Cake German Chocolate	1/8 cake (2.9 oz)	280	15	11	30	4	34	2	—	160	—	—	—	—
Layer Cake Vanilla	1/8 cake (2.8 oz)	250	13	10	35	2	31	0	—	140	—	—	—	—
Pound Cake	1/4 cake (2.7 oz)	320	16	9	85	4	38	1	—	280	—	—	—	—
Pound Cake Chocolate Swirl	1 slice (1 oz)	110	5	3	25	2	14	0	20	115	—	0	—	0
Pound Cake Family Size	1/6 cake (2.7 oz)	310	177	9	75	4	36	1	—	360	—	—	—	—

FOOD	PORTION	CALORIES	FAT	SAT FAT	CHOL	PROTEIN	CARBO	FIBER	CALCIUM	SOD	POTAS	VIT C	FOLIC	VIT A
SARA LEE (CONT.)														
Pound Cake Free & Light	¼ cake (2.5 oz)	200	4	1	0	3	39	1	—	290	—	—	—	—
Pound Cake Golden	1 slice (1 oz)	120	5	1	41	tr	15	0	—	90	—	—	—	—
Pound Cake Reduced Fat	1 slice (1 oz)	100	4	1	25	2	15	0	0	125	—	0	—	100
Pound Cake Strawberry	¼ cake (2.9 oz)	290	11	3	60	4	44	1	—	140	—	—	—	—
Red White & Blueberry	¹/₁₀ cake (3 oz)	210	8	6	15	2	31	1	—	135	—	—	—	—
Slice Chocolate	1 (3 oz)	320	16	4	40	3	42	tr	—	115	—	—	—	—
Strawberry Shortcake	⅛ cake (2.5 oz)	180	7	5	15	2	27	1	—	140	—	—	—	—
SINBAD														
Baklava	1 piece (2 oz)	337	20	4	10	5	44	2	0	153	—	0	—	0
TASTYKAKE														
Butter Cream Cream Filled Cupcake	1 (32 g)	120	4	1	5	1	20	1	—	120	—	—	—	—
Chocolate Cream Filled Cupcake	1 (34 g)	130	5	1	5	2	21	1	—	130	—	—	—	—
Chocolate Cupcake	1 (30 g)	100	3	1	5	2	19	1	—	120	—	—	—	—
Honeybun Glazed	1 pkg (92 g)	360	20	4	0	6	42	4	—	220	—	—	—	—
Honeybun Iced	1 pkg (92 g)	350	15	3	50	5	50	1	80	250	—	—	—	—
Junior Chocolate	1 pkg (94 g)	340	12	3	60	4	57	4	100	220	—	—	—	—
Junior Coconut	1 pkg (94 g)	300	6	3	50	4	60	3	80	300	—	—	—	—
Junior Lemon	1 pkg (94 g)	310	7	3	75	3	75	1	40	330	—	—	—	—
Junior Orange	1 pkg (94 g)	340	9	3	50	3	61	1	40	240	—	—	—	—
Kandy Kake Chocolate	1 (19 g)	80	3	2	0	1	13	1	—	35	—	—	—	—
Kandy Kake Coconut	1 (19 g)	80	4	3	0	1	11	1	—	40	—	—	—	—
Kandy Kake Peanut Butter	1 (19 g)	90	4	2	5	2	11	1	—	40	—	—	—	—
Koffee Kake Cream Filled	1 (29 g)	110	4	1	15	1	18	0	—	80	—	—	—	—
Koffee Kake Junior	1 pkg (71 g)	260	8	2	40	3	44	1	40	210	—	—	—	—
Kreme Kup	1 (25 g)	90	3	1	5	1	15	1	—	115	—	—	—	—
Krimpet Butterscotch	1 (28 g)	100	1	3	19	1	19	0	—	85	—	—	—	—
Krimpet Jelly	1 (28 g)	90	1	1	20	1	19	1	40	80	—	—	—	—
Krimpet Strawberry	1 (28 g)	100	2	1	20	1	20	0	—	85	—	—	—	—
Pastry Pocket Apple	1 (85 g)	320	18	4	10	4	38	—	—	220	—	—	—	—
Pastry Pocket Cheese	1 (85 g)	330	19	5	10	4	38	1	—	230	—	—	—	300
Pastry Pocket Cherry	1 (85 g)	330	17	4	10	4	41	1	—	230	—	—	—	—

FOOD	PORTION	CALORIES	FAT	SAT FAT	CHOL	PROTEIN	CARBO	FIBER	CALCIUM	SOD	POTAS	VIT C	FOLIC	VIT A
TASTYKAKE (CONT.)														
Pecan Twirls	1 (28 g)	110	1	—	—	1	17	—	80	75	—	—	—	—
Royale Chocolate Cupcake	1 (46 g)	170	7	2	5	2	28	2	—	130	—	—	—	—
Tasty Too Chocolate Cream Filled Cupcake	1 (32 g)	100	1	1	0	1	21	1	—	115	—	—	—	—
Tasty Too Vanilla Cream Filled Cupcake	1 (32 g)	100	1	1	0	1	21	1	—	120	—	—	—	—
Tasty Twists	1 (4 g)	18	1	—	—	0	3	—	—	—	—	—	—	—
THOMAS'														
Date Nut Loaf	1 oz	90	2	—	<5	1	18	1	—	170	—	—	—	—
TOAST-R-CAKES														
Blueberry	1	110	3	—	—	2	18	—	4	158	18	tr	—	105
Bran	1	103	3	—	—	2	18	—	12	163	55	tr	—	59
Corn	1	120	4	—	—	2	19	—	6	142	17	tr	—	32
TOASTETTES														
Frosted Blueberry	1 (1.7 oz)	190	5	2	0	2	45	1	—	190	45	—	—	500
Frosted Brown Sugar Cinnamon	1 (1.7 oz)	190	5	2	0	2	35	1	—	180	60	—	—	500
Frosted Cherry	1 (1.7 oz)	190	5	2	0	2	35	1	—	190	45	—	—	500
Frosted Fudge	1 (1.7 oz)	190	5	2	0	2	34	3	20	280	75	—	—	500
Strawberry	1 (1.7 oz)	190	5	2	0	2	35	1	—	200	45	2	—	500
WEIGHT WATCHERS														
Chocolate Raspberry Royale	1 (3.5 oz)	190	3	1	15	5	39	2	100	190	—	0	—	0
Chocolate Chip Cookie Dough Sundae	1 (2.64 oz)	180	4	2	5	3	33	2	80	115	—	0	—	200
Chocolate Eclair	1 (2.1 oz)	150	5	1	30	2	25	2	40	160	—	0	—	0
Coffee Cake Apple Cinnamon Danish	1 piece (1.9 oz)	160	3	1	0	3	30	1	0	170	—	0	—	0
Coffee Cake Cheese Danish	1 piece (1.9 oz)	160	3	1	5	4	29	1	20	200	—	0	—	0
Coffee Cake Raspberry Danish	1 piece (1.9 oz)	160	3	1	0	4	30	1	0	170	—	0	—	0
Double Fudge	1 piece (2.75 oz)	190	5	1	0	4	36	2	80	200	—	0	—	0
French Style Cheesecake	1 piece (3.9 oz)	180	5	2	15	7	28	2	80	230	—	2	—	200
New York Style Cheesecake	1 piece (2.5 oz)	150	5	2	10	6	21	0	80	140	—	0	—	300
Strawberry Parfait Royale	1 (5.24 oz)	180	2	1	10	5	35	0	250	100	—	0	—	0
Triple Chocolate Eclair	1 (2.14 oz)	160	5	1	30	3	25	1	40	190	—	0	—	0

FOOD	PORTION	CALORIES	FAT	SAT FAT	CHOL	PROTEIN	CARBO	FIBER	CALCIUM	SOD	POTAS	VIT C	FOLIC	VIT A
WELL-BRED LOAF														
Banana Bread	1 slice (3.5 oz)	330	11	5	60	4	52	tr	40	380	—	0	—	750
Banana Nut	1 slice (4.3 oz)	440	19	8	85	6	59	2	40	350	—	0	—	400
Blueberry	1 slice (4.3 oz)	440	16	10	110	6	69	1	40	330	—	0	—	500
Carrot	1 slice (4.3 oz)	480	24	11	125	6	64	2	40	125	—	0	—	8000
Carrot Traditional	1 slice (4.3 oz)	440	16	6	40	4	71	2	20	280	—	0	—	8500
Chocolate Chip	1 slice (4.3 oz)	490	19	11	105	6	74	2	40	320	—	0	—	500
Cinnamon Walnut	1 slice (4.3 oz)	480	18	10	110	7	72	1	40	340	—	0	—	500
Coconut Rum	1 slice (4.3 oz)	490	23	13	95	6	64	tr	40	330	—	0	—	400
Cranberry	1 slice (4.3 oz)	460	15	9	100	6	77	1	40	320	—	0	—	500
Marble	1 slice (4.3 oz)	530	18	11	115	7	83	1	60	390	—	0	—	500
Pound All Butter	1 slice (4.3 oz)	470	17	10	115	7	73	tr	40	360	—	0	—	500
Pound Mandarin Orange	1 slice (4 oz)	460	18	5	70	6	68	tr	40	310	—	0	—	0
Raisin	1 slice (4.3 oz)	460	15	9	105	6	76	2	40	310	—	0	—	500
TAKE-OUT														
angelfood	1/12 cake (1 oz)	73	tr	tr	0	2	16	1	40	212	26	0	—	0
apple crisp	1/2 cup (5 oz)	230	5	1	0	37	46	—	40	257	137	3	7	193
boston cream pie	1/6 cake (3.3 oz)	293	12	4	43	4	43	1	93	309	95	tr	8	180
carrot w/ cream cheese icing	1/12 cake (3.9 oz)	484	29	5	60	5	52	—	27	273	124	1	14	3827
cheesecake w/ cherry topping	1/12 cake (5 oz)	359	23	13	106	6	33	—	54	254	116	1	12	1122
chocolate w/ chocolate frosting	1/8 cake (2.2 oz)	235	11	3	—	3	35	2	28	213	128	—	—	—
coffeecake cheese	1/6 cake (2.7 oz)	258	12	4	—	5	38	1	45	257	—	—	—	—
coffeecake crumb topped cheese	1/6 cake (2.7 oz)	258	12	4	—	5	38	1	45	257	—	—	—	—
coffeecake crumb topped cinnamon	1/9 cake (2.2 oz)	263	15	4	20	4	29	2	34	221	77	—	20	—
cream puff w/ custard filling	1 (4.6 oz)	336	20	5	174	9	30	—	86	444	149	tr	20	968
eclair w/ chocolate icing & custard filling	1	205	10	—	35	—	—	—	10	—	—	—	—	—
fruitcake	1/36 cake (2.9 oz)	302	10	1	24	3	54	3	55	121	259	4	8	60
gingerbread	1/9 cake (2.6 oz)	264	12	3	24	3	36	2	52	242	325	tr	6	36
panettone dal forno	1/9 cake (1.9 oz)	212	8	4	25	4	31	0	15	120	—	0	—	25
pineapple upside down	1/9 cake (4 oz)	367	14	3	25	4	58	—	137	367	129	1	8	291
pound fat free	1 oz	80	tr	tr	0	2	17	—	12	96	31	0	1	27
pound cake	1 slice (1 oz)	120	5	1	32	2	15	—	20	96	28	tr	—	200

FOOD	PORTION	CALORIES	FAT	SAT FAT	CHOL	PROTEIN	CARBO	FIBER	CALCIUM	SOD	POTAS	VIT C	FOLIC	VIT A
sheet cake w/ white frosting	⅑ cake	445	14	5	70	4	77	—	61	275	74	tr	—	240
strudel apple	1 piece (2½ oz)	195	8	2	—	2	29	2	11	191	—	1	—	21
tiramisu	1 piece (5.1 oz)	409	30	15	171	7	31	tr	114	79	211	1	16	1580
yellow w/ vanilla frosting	⅛ cake (2.2 oz)	239	9	2	—	2	38	—	39	220	34	—	—	12

CAKE ICING

FOOD	PORTION	CALORIES	FAT	SAT FAT	CHOL	PROTEIN	CARBO	FIBER	CALCIUM	SOD	POTAS	VIT C	FOLIC	VIT A
chocolate as prep w/ butter	1/12 box (1.5 oz)	161	6	—	10	1	30	—	—	63	60	—	—	143
chocolate as prep w/ butter	1 box (13.7 oz)	1908	65	—	121	6	357	—	—	754	713	—	—	1695
chocolate as prep w/ butter home recipe	1/12 recipe (1.8 oz)	200	6	4	15	1	39	—	9	95	45	0	1	203
chocolate as prep w/ butter home recipe	1 recipe (21.1 oz)	2409	69	43	176	8	467	—	104	1144	544	tr	14	2445
chocolate as prep w/ margarine	1 box (13.7 oz)	1909	65	—	0	6	357	—	—	819	722	—	—	1834
chocolate as prep w/ margarine	1/12 box (1.5 oz)	161	6	—	0	1	30	—	—	69	61	—	—	154
chocolate as prep w/ margarine home recipe	1/12 recipe (1.8 oz)	200	6	1	0	1	39	—	9	103	46	0	1	219
chocolate as prep w/ margarine home recipe	1 recipe (21.1 oz)	2411	69	16	5	8	468	—	106	1235	557	1	12	2640
chocolate ready-to-use	1/12 pkg (1.3 oz)	151	7	2	0	tr	24	—	3	70	74	—	0	249
chocolate ready-to-use	1 pkg (16 oz)	1834	81	26	0	5	292	—	37	845	905	—	0	3026
coconut ready-to-use	1 pkg (16 oz)	1903	111	32	0	7	244	—	62	899	858	—	—	0
coconut ready-to-use	1/12 pkg (1.3 oz)	157	9	3	0	1	20	—	5	74	71	—	—	0
cream cheese ready-to-use	1 pkg (16 oz)	1906	80	23	0	tr	308	—	15	1094	163	—	0	1769
cream cheese ready-to-use	1/12 pkg (1.3 oz)	157	7	2	0	0	25	—	1	90	13	—	0	146
glaze home recipe	1 recipe (11.5 oz)	1173	26	6	7	2	240	—	73	307	97	1	3	1039
glaze home recipe	1/12 recipe (1 oz)	97	2	tr	1	tr	20	—	6	25	8	0	0	86
seven minute home recipe	1 recipe (13.6 oz)	1231	0	0	0	6	312	—	9	859	246	0	2	3
seven minute home recipe	1/12 recipe (1.1 oz)	102	0	0	0	1	26	—	1	55	20	0	0	0

FOOD	PORTION	CALORIES	FAT	SAT FAT	CHOL	PROTEIN	CARBO	FIBER	CALCIUM	SOD	POTAS	VIT C	FOLIC	VIT A
sour cream ready-to-use	¹/₁₂ pkg (1.3 oz)	157	7	2	—	0	26	—	1	78	74	—	—	152
sour cream ready-to-use	1 pkg (16 oz)	1904	80	23	—	1	312	—	11	943	896	—	—	1853
vanilla as prep w/ butter	¹/₁₂ pkg (1.5 oz)	182	7	—	10	tr	30	—	4	90	9	—	—	199
vanilla as prep w/ butter	1 pkg (14.5 oz)	2188	86	—	126	1	366	—	45	1082	102	—	—	2396
vanilla as prep w/ butter home recipe	¹/₁₂ recipe (1.7 oz)	165	2	1	6	tr	38	—	11	31	14	tr	0	73
vanilla as prep w/ butter home recipe	1 recipe (20.1 oz)	1972	24	14	67	4	448	—	128	366	168	1	6	872
vanilla as prep w/ margarine	1 pkg (14.5 oz)	2190	86	—	0	1	366	—	48	1149	112	—	—	2539
vanilla as prep w/ margarine	¹/₁₂ pkg (1.5 oz)	182	7	—	0	tr	30	—	4	96	9	—	—	211
vanilla as prep w/ margarine home recipe	¹/₁₂ recipe (1.7 oz)	195	5	1	0	tr	38	—	6	98	9	0	0	211
vanilla as prep w/ margarine home recipe	1 recipe (20.1 oz)	2326	62	13	5	2	454	—	75	1175	103	1	3	2518
vanilla ready-to-use	¹/₁₂ pkg (1.3 oz)	159	6	2	0	tr	26	—	1	34	14	0	0	284
vanilla ready-to-use	1 pkg (16 oz)	1936	78	23	0	1	321	—	14	418	169	0	0	3448
white as prep w/ water	¹/₁₂ pkg (0.9 oz)	64	0	—	—	tr	16	—	1	40	20	0	—	—
white as prep w/ water	1 pkg (11.1 oz)	770	0	—	—	5	197	—	11	490	243	0	—	—
BETTY CROCKER														
Butter Pecan Ready-to-Spread	¹/₁₂ tub	170	7	2	0	0	26	—	—	50	20	—	—	200
Cherry Ready-to-Spread	¹/₁₂ tub	160	6	2	0	0	27	—	—	50	15	—	—	200
Chocolate Ready-to-Spread	¹/₁₂ tub	160	7	2	0	tr	24	—	—	60	85	—	—	200
Chocolate Chip Ready-to-Spread	¹/₁₂ tub	170	7	3	0	tr	27	—	—	30	30	—	—	200
Chocolate Fudge as prep	¹/₁₂ mix	180	6	2	0	tr	30	—	—	70	60	—	—	100
Chocolate Light Ready-to-Spread	¹/₁₂ tub	130	2	1	0	tr	28	—	—	60	95	—	—	—
Chocolate With Candy Coated Chocolate Chips Ready-to-Spread	¹/₁₂ tub	160	7	2	0	tr	24	—	—	60	90	—	—	200

FOOD	PORTION	CALORIES	FAT	SAT FAT	CHOL	PROTEIN	CARBO	FIBER	CALCIUM	SOD	POTAS	VIT C	FOLIC	VIT A
BETTY CROCKER (CONT.)														
Chocolate With Dinosaurs Ready-to-Spread	1/12 tub	160	7	2	0	tr	24	—	—	60	90	—	—	200
Chocolate With Turbo Racers Ready-to-Spread	1/12 tub	160	7	2	0	tr	24	—	—	60	90	—	—	200
Coconut Pecan Ready-to-Spread	1/12 tub	160	9	3	0	tr	20	—	—	80	80	—	—	—
Coconut Pecan as prep	1/12 mix	180	8	2	0	tr	19	—	—	50	35	—	—	100
Cream Cheese Ready-to-Spread	1/12 tub	170	7	2	0	tr	26	—	—	70	15	—	—	200
Creamy Milk Chocolate as prep	1/12 mix	170	5	1	0	1	29	—	—	40	90	—	—	100
Creamy Vanilla as prep	1/12 mix	170	5	1	0	0	32	—	—	50	5	—	—	100
Dark Dutch Fudge Ready-to-Spread	1/12 tub	160	7	2	0	1	22	—	—	70	150	—	—	200
Lemon Ready-to-Spread	1/12 tub	170	6	2	0	0	28	—	—	70	15	—	—	200
Milk Chocolate Light Ready-to-Spread	1/12 tub	140	2	1	0	tr	29	—	—	50	65	—	—	—
Milk Chocolate Ready-to-Spread	1/12 tub	160	6	2	0	tr	25	—	—	55	85	—	—	200
Rainbow Chip Ready-to-Spread	1/12 tub	170	7	3	0	tr	27	—	—	30	20	—	—	200
Sour Cream Chocolate Ready-to-Spread	1/12 tub	160	7	2	0	tr	23	—	—	100	115	—	—	200
Sour Cream White Ready-to-Spread	1/12 tub	160	6	2	0	0	27	—	—	50	15	—	—	200
Vanilla Ready-to-Spread	1/12 tub	160	6	2	0	0	27	—	—	30	15	—	—	200
Vanilla Light Ready-to-Spread	1/12 tub	140	2	1	0	0	30	—	—	30	15	—	—	—
Vanilla With Teddy Bears Ready-to-Spread	1/12 tub	160	6	2	0	0	27	—	—	25	15	—	—	200
White Fluffy as prep	1/12 mix	70	0	0	0	tr	16	—	—	40	20	—	—	—
DUNCAN HINES														
Chocolate Creamy Homestyle	2 tbsp	130	5	2	0	0	20	2	—	95	—	—	—	—
Milk Chocolate Creamy Homestyle	2 tbsp	130	5	2	0	0	20	1	—	95	—	—	—	—
Vanilla Creamy Homestyle	2 tbsp	140	5	2	0	0	22	1	—	60	—	—	—	—

FOOD	PORTION	CALORIES	FAT	SAT FAT	CHOL	PROTEIN	CARBO	FIBER	CALCIUM	SOD	POTAS	VIT C	FOLIC	VIT A
ESTEE														
Lite Frosting as prep	3 tbsp (0.7 oz)	100	3	0	0	0	20	0	20	0	0	0	—	0
JIFFY														
Fudge	¼ cup (1.2 oz)	150	4	2	0	1	28	tr	0	150	—	0	—	0
White	¼ cup (1.2 oz)	150	5	1	0	0	27	0	0	150	—	0	—	0

CAKE MIX

(see also CAKE*)*

FOOD	PORTION	CALORIES	FAT	SAT FAT	CHOL	PROTEIN	CARBO	FIBER	CALCIUM	SOD	POTAS	VIT C	FOLIC	VIT A
angelfood	10 in cake (20.9 oz)	1535	2	tr	0	36	350	9	503	3036	808	0	—	0
angelfood	¹⁄₁₂ cake (1.8 oz)	129	tr	tr	0	3	29	1	42	255	68	0	—	0
carrot w/o frosting	2 layers (29.6 oz)	2886	133	22	—	43	395	—	927	3001	1011	—	—	9521
carrot w/o frosting	¹⁄₁₂ cake (2.5 oz)	239	11	2	—	4	33	—	77	249	64	—	—	790
cheesecake no-bake	⅛ cake (3.5 oz)	271	13	7	—	6	35	2	170	377	209	1	17	363
chocolate pudding type w/o frosting	2 layers (32.4 oz)	3234	172	35	—	43	409	—	765	4815	1926	—	—	—
chocolate pudding type w/o frosting	¹⁄₁₂ cake (2.7 oz)	270	14	3	—	4	34	—	64	402	161	—	—	—
chocolate w/o frosting	2 layers (26.8 oz)	2393	92	21	425	44	384	—	843	4464	1851	0	—	—
chocolate w/o frosting	¹⁄₁₂ cake (2.3 oz)	198	8	2	35	4	32	—	70	370	153	0	—	—
chocolate w/o frosting low sodium	¹⁄₁₀ cake (1.3 oz)	116	3	1	0	1	23	—	11	130	82	0	2	0
coffeecake crumb topped cinnamon	⅛ cake (2 oz)	178	5	1	28	3	30	2	76	236	63	—	—	78
devil's food w/o frosting	¹⁄₁₂ cake (2.3 oz)	198	8	2	35	4	32	—	70	370	153	0	—	—
devil's food w/ chocolate frosting	¹⁄₁₆ cake	235	8	4	37	3	40	—	41	181	90	tr	—	100
devil's food w/ chocolate frosting	1 cake 9 in diam	3755	136	56	598	49	645	—	653	2900	1439	1	—	1660
fudge w/o frosting	¹⁄₁₂ cake (2.3 oz)	198	8	2	35	4	32	—	70	370	153	0	—	—
german chocolate pudding type w/ coconut nut frosting	¹⁄₁₂ cake (3.9 oz)	404	21	5	53	4	55	—	54	369	151	0	—	—
gingerbread	1 cake 8 in sq	1575	39	10	6	18	291	—	513	1733	1562	1	—	0
gingerbread	¹⁄₉ cake (2.4 oz)	207	7	2	24	3	34	2	46	307	162	—	—	—

FOOD	PORTION	CALORIES	FAT	SAT FAT	CHOL	PROTEIN	CARBO	FIBER	CALCIUM	SOD	POTAS	VIT C	FOLIC	VIT A
lemon w/o frosting no sugar low sodium	1/10 cake (1.3 oz)	118	3	tr	0	1	23	—	8	83	50	0	2	0
marble pudding type w/o frosting	1/12 cake (2.6 oz)	253	12	2	53	3	35	—	40	242	68	0	—	—
marble pudding type w/o frosting	2 layers (30.6 oz)	3021	148	27	638	36	412	—	475	2884	816	0	—	—
white pudding type w/o frosting	1/12 cake (2.4 oz)	244	10	2	—	3	36	—	35	305	42	—	—	—
white pudding type w/o frosting	2 layers (29 oz)	2915	123	23	—	30	427	—	417	3654	508	—	—	—
white w/o frosting	1/12 cake (2.2 oz)	190	5	1	—	3	34	—	85	301	59	—	—	—
white w/o frosting	2 layer cake (26 oz)	2265	57	9	—	30	410	—	1016	3593	700	—	—	—
white w/o frosting no sugar low sodium	1/10 cake (1.3 oz)	118	3	tr	0	1	23	—	8	83	50	0	2	0
yellow pudding-type w/o frosting	1/12 cake (2.6 oz)	257	12	2	—	3	35	—	57	317	42	—	—	—
yellow pudding-type w/o frosting	2 layers (31 oz)	3084	139	28	—	40	421	—	681	3800	509	—	—	—
yellow w/ chocolate frosting	1/16 cake	235	8	3	36	3	40	—	63	157	75	tr	—	100
yellow w/o frosting	1/12 cake (2.2 oz)	202	6	1	37	3	34	—	64	299	46	—	—	—
yellow w/o frosting	2 layers (26.5 oz)	2415	71	12	437	35	411	—	761	3580	552	—	—	—
yellow w/ chocolate frosting	1 cake 9 in diam	3895	175	92	609	40	620	—	366	3080	1972	0	—	1850
AUNT JEMIMA														
Coffee Cake Easy Mix	1/3 cup (1.4 oz)	170	5	1	0	2	30	1	40	240	25	—	0	—
BETTY CROCKER														
Angel Food Confetti	1/12 cake	150	0	0	0	3	34	—	60	300	50	—	—	—
Angel Food Traditional	1/12 cake	130	0	0	0	3	30	—	40	170	80	—	—	—
Angel Food White	1/12 cake	150	0	0	0	3	34	—	60	300	50	—	—	—
Angel Food Lemon Custard	1/12 cake	150	0	0	0	3	34	—	60	300	50	—	—	—
Apple Streusel MicroRave	1/6 cake	240	11	3	45	2	33	—	40	190	50	—	—	—
Apple Streusel MicroRave No Cholesterol Recipe	1/6 cake	210	8	2	0	2	33	—	40	200	50	—	—	—
Butter Chocolate	1/12 cake	280	14	7	75	4	35	—	40	400	170	—	—	300

BETTY CROCKER (CONT.)

FOOD	PORTION	CALORIES	FAT	SAT FAT	CHOL	PROTEIN	CARBO	FIBER	CALCIUM	SOD	POTAS	VIT C	FOLIC	VIT A
Butter Pecan No Cholesterol Recipe	1/12 cake	220	7	2	0	3	35	—	80	320	45	—	—	—
Butter Pecan SuperMoist	1/12 cake	250	11	1	55	1	35	—	80	320	40	—	—	—
Butter Yellow	1/12 cake	260	11	6	75	3	37	—	60	340	35	—	—	300
Carrot	1/12 cake	250	10	2	55	3	36	—	40	300	70	—	—	—
Carrot No Cholesterol Recipe	1/12 cake	210	6	2	0	3	36	—	40	300	75	—	—	—
Cherry Chip	1/12 cake	190	3	1	0	3	37	—	—	270	35	—	—	—
Chocolate Chocolate Chip	1/12 cake	260	12	3	55	3	34	—	60	400	115	—	—	—
Chocolate Pudding Classic Dessert	1/6 cake	230	5	—	—	3	44	—	40	250	170	—	—	—
Chocolate Chip	1/12 cake	290	15	3	55	3	35	—	80	300	60	—	—	—
Chocolate Chip No Cholesterol Recipe	1/12 cake	220	8	2	0	3	35	—	80	300	65	—	—	—
Chocolate Fudge	1/12 cake	260	12	3	55	3	35	—	60	450	120	—	—	—
Cinnamon Pecan Streusel Microwave	1/6 cake	280	12	3	35	2	40	—	60	220	40	—	—	—
Cinnamon Pecan Streusel Microwave No Cholesterol	1/6 cake	230	7	2	0	2	40	—	60	220	45	—	—	—
Devil's Food	1/12 cake	260	12	3	55	4	35	—	20	430	145	—	—	—
Devil's Food Chocolate Frosting MicroRave	1/6 cake	310	17	5	35	2	37	—	40	250	180	—	—	100
Devil's Food No Cholesterol Recipe	1/12 cake	220	7	2	0	3	35	—	20	430	150	—	—	—
Devil's Food SuperMoist Light	1/12 cake	200	4	2	55	4	36	—	60	340	190	—	—	—
Devil's Food SuperMoist Light No Cholesterol Recipe	1/12 cake	180	3	1	0	3	36	—	60	370	200	—	—	—
Devil's Food With Chocolate Frosting MicroRave Single	1	440	18	6	50	5	64	—	100	480	480	—	—	300
German Chocolate	1/12 cake	260	12	3	55	3	35	—	20	420	80	—	—	—
German Chocolate Chocolate Frosting MicroRave	1/6 cake	320	18	5	35	3	37	—	40	250	70	—	—	—

FOOD	PORTION	CALORIES	FAT	SAT FAT	CHOL	PROTEIN	CARBO	FIBER	CALCIUM	SOD	POTAS	VIT C	FOLIC	VIT A
BETTY CROCKER (CONT.)														
German Chocolate No Cholesterol Recipe	1/12 cake	220	8	2	0	3	35	—	20	420	85	—	—	—
Gingerbread Classic Dessert	1/9 cake	22	7	2	30	3	35	—	20	330	150	—	—	—
Gingerbread Classic Dessert No Cholesterol Recipe	1/9 cake	210	6	2	0	3	35	—	20	330	150	—	—	—
Golden Pound Classic Dessert	1/12 cake	200	9	3	35	2	28	—	20	170	25	—	—	—
Golden Vanilla	1/12 cake	280	14	3	55	3	36	—	60	270	35	—	—	—
Golden Vanilla No Cholesterol Recipe	1/12 cake	220	7	2	0	3	36	—	60	270	40	—	—	—
Golden Vanilla Rainbow Chip Frosting MicroRave	1/6 cake	320	18	5	35	2	40	—	60	230	40	—	—	—
Lemon	1/12 cake	260	11	3	55	3	37	—	80	280	35	—	—	—
Lemon Chiffon Classic Dessert	1/12 cake	200	5	—	—	4	36	—	20	200	60	—	—	—
Lemon No Cholesterol Recipe	1/12 cake	220	7	2	0	3	37	—	80	280	40	—	—	—
Lemon Pudding Classic Dessert	1/6 cake	230	5	—	—	2	45	—	40	270	35	—	—	—
Marble	1/12 cake	260	11	3	55	3	36	—	80	290	60	—	—	—
Marble No Cholesterol Recipe	1/12 cake	220	7	2	0	3	36	—	80	290	65	—	—	—
Milk Chocolate	1/12 cake	260	12	3	55	4	34	—	60	340	130	—	—	—
Milk Chocolate No Cholesterol Recipe	1/12 cake	210	7	2	0	3	34	—	60	340	135	—	—	—
Pineapple Upsidedown Classic Dessert	1/9 cake	250	10	4	40	2	39	—	40	210	70	—	—	100
Rainbow Chip	1/12 cake	250	11	3	55	3	35	—	100	320	45	—	—	—
Sour Cream Chocolate	1/12 cake	260	12	3	55	3	35	—	20	430	115	—	—	—
Sour Cream Chocolate No Cholesterol Recipe	1/12 cake	220	8	2	0	3	35	—	20	430	120	—	—	—
Sour Cream White	1/12 cake	180	3	1	0	3	36	—	20	290	35	—	—	—
Spice	1/12 cake	260	11	2	55	3	36	—	100	320	45	—	—	—

FOOD	PORTION	CALORIES	FAT	SAT FAT	CHOL	PROTEIN	CARBO	FIBER	CALCIUM	SOD	POTAS	VIT C	FOLIC	VIT A
BETTY CROCKER (CONT.)														
Spice No Cholesterol Recipe	1/12 cake	220	7	2	0	3	36	—	100	320	50	—	—	—
White	1/12 cake	240	9	2	0	3	36	—	60	270	40	—	—	—
White No Cholesterol Recipe	1/12 cake	220	7	2	0	3	36	—	60	270	40	—	—	—
White SuperMoist Light	1/12 cake	180	3	1	0	2	37	—	80	330	350	—	—	—
Yellow	1/12 cake	260	11	3	55	3	36	—	80	300	35	—	—	—
Yellow Chocolate Frosting MicroRave	1/6 cake	300	17	4	35	2	36	—	60	220	60	—	—	—
Yellow No Cholesterol Recipe	1/12 cake	220	7	3	0	3	36	—	80	300	40	—	—	—
Yellow SuperMoist Light	1/12 cake	200	4	2	55	3	37	—	60	310	40	—	—	—
Yellow SuperMoist Light No Cholesterol Recipe	1/12 cake	190	3	1	0	3	37	—	60	330	45	—	—	—
Yellow With Chocolate Frosting MicroRave Single	1	440	19	6	50	4	64	—	150	500	140	—	—	300
BISQUICK														
Mix	1/2 cup (2 oz)	240	8	2	0	4	37	—	80	700	80	—	—	—
Reduced Fat	1/2 cup (2 oz)	210	4	1	0	5	39	—	60	660	80	—	—	—
DROMEDARY														
Carrot	1/12 cake	232	15	—	—	3	23	—	40	292	—	—	—	350
Cobbler Apple Crumb	1/8 cake	237	6	—	—	3	41	—	20	490	—	—	—	100
Cobbler Cherry Crumb	1/8 cake	231	6	—	—	3	42	—	20	160	—	—	—	100
Date Nut	1/12 cake	183	8	—	—	2	26	—	40	248	—	—	—	—
Date Nut Roll	1/2 in slice	80	2	—	—	1	13	—	20	160	60	—	—	—
Gingerbread	1 piece (2 in x 2 in)	100	2	—	—	1	19	—	20	190	90	—	—	—
Pound	1/2 in slice	150	6	—	—	2	21	—	20	160	65	—	—	—
DUNCAN HINES														
Angel Food as prep	1/12 pkg (1.3 oz)	140	0	0	0	4	31	1	15	310	—	0	—	0
Butter Recipe Golden as prep	1/12 cake	320	16	7	80	3	42	—	60	190	—	—	—	—
Cupcake Yellow as prep	1	180	0	2	6	1	29	—	20	140	—	—	—	—

FOOD	PORTION	CALORIES	FAT	SAT FAT	CHOL	PROTEIN	CARBO	FIBER	CALCIUM	SOD	POTAS	VIT C	FOLIC	VIT A
DUNCAN HINES (CONT.)														
Dark Chocolate Fudge as prep	1/12 cake	290	15	3	55	4	34	—	60	360	—	—	—	—
Devil's Food Moist Deluxe as prep	1/12 cake (1.5 oz)	290	15	3	55	4	34	1	60	360	—	0	—	0
French Vanilla	1/12 cake (1.5 oz)	250	11	2	55	3	—	—	80	290	—	—	—	—
Fudge Marble Moist Deluxe as prep	1/12 cake (1.5 oz)	250	17	2	45	3	36	0	80	290	—	0	—	0
Lemon Supreme Moist Deluxe	1/12 cake (1.5 oz)	250	17	2	55	3	36	0	80	290	—	0	—	0
White Moist Deluxe as prep	1/12 cake	190	6	1	0	3	34	—	60	300	—	—	—	—
Yellow Moist Deluxe as prep	1/12 cake (1.5 oz)	250	17	11	55	3	36	—	—	270	—	—	—	—
Yellow Moist Deluxe as prep	1/12 cake	250	11	2	55	3	36	—	80	290	—	—	—	—
ESTEE														
Lite White as prep	1/5 cake (1.7 oz)	200	4	2	0	2	38	tr	0	170	70	0	—	0
Lite Chocolate	1/5 cake (1.7 oz)	190	4	2	0	2	36	1	0	264	240	0	—	0
Lite Pound as prep	1/5 cake (1.7 oz)	200	4	2	0	2	38	tr	0	170	70	0	—	0
HAIN														
Whole Wheat Baking Mix	1 1/2 oz	150	1	—	—	6	30	5	40	680	170	—	—	—
JELL-O														
No Bake Cherry Cheesecake as prep	1/8 cake (4.8 oz)	340	12	5	5	5	52	tr	150	400	280	0	—	400
No Bake Double Layer Chocolate as prep	1/8 cake (4.4 oz)	260	12	5	<5	4	34	1	100	410	220	0	—	400
No Bake Double Layer Cookies And Creme as prep	1/8 cake (4.5 oz)	390	19	7	<5	5	51	1	80	480	150	0	—	500
No Bake Double Layer Lemon as prep	1/8 cake (4.4 oz)	260	12	4	<5	4	36	tr	80	370	125	0	—	400
No Bake Homestyle Cheesecake as prep	1/6 cake (4.6 oz)	360	15	4	10	7	50	tr	200	550	280	0	—	500
No Bake Peanut Butter Cup as prep	1/8 cake (3.8 oz)	380	23	10	<5	5	41	1	100	380	180	0	—	400

FOOD	PORTION	CALORIES	FAT	SAT FAT	CHOL	PROTEIN	CARBO	FIBER	CALCIUM	SOD	POTAS	VIT C	FOLIC	VIT A
JELL-O (CONT.)														
No Bake Reduced Fat Strawberry Swirl Cheesecake as prep	⅛ cake (4 oz)	250	6	2	5	7	44	0	200	430	310	1	—	200
No Bake Strawberry Cheesecake as prep	⅛ cake (4.8 oz)	340	12	5	5	5	52	tr	150	400	270	2	—	400
Real Cheesecake as prep	⅛ cake (4.6 oz)	360	16	6	5	7	47	1	200	510	320	0	—	500
JIFFY														
Devil's Food as prep	⅕ cake	220	6	2	42	3	40	1	20	528	—	0	—	0
Golden Yellow as prep	⅕ cake	220	5	1	36	2	41	1	20	340	—	0	—	0
White as prep	⅕ cake	210	5	1	0	2	41	tr	0	320	—	0	—	0
PILLSBURY														
Strawberry	1/12 cake	260	11	—	—	3	37	—	40	300	85	0	—	100
ROYAL														
Cheese Cake Lite No-Bake	⅛ pie	130	3	0	5	4	22	—	150	230	190	—	—	—
Cheese Cake Real No-Bake	⅛ pie	160	3	—	—	4	29	—	80	250	115	—	—	—
WANDA'S														
Double Chocolate	¼ cup mix per serv (1.4 oz)	170	2	1	0	4	35	2	40	460	—	4	—	0
CALABAZA														
fresh	½ cup	32	tr	—	—	1	8	—	—	3	246	18	—	5460
CALZONE														
TAKE-OUT														
cheese	1 (12 oz)	1020	54	24	100	48	86	8	700	1760	—	1	—	500
CANADIAN BACON														
grilled	1 pkg (6 oz)	257	12	4	81	34	2	0	14	2149	—	0	6	0
HORMEL														
Canadian Bacon	2 oz	70	3	2	30	10	0	0	0	640	—	0	—	0
JONES														
Slices	1	30	1	—	7	3	tr	—	—	160	—	—	—	—
OSCAR MAYER														
Canandian Bacon	2 slices (1.6 oz)	50	2	1	25	8	0	0	0	620	—	0	—	0
CANDY														
(*see also* CHEWING GUM and MARSHMALLOW)														
butterscotch	1 piece (6 g)	24	tr	tr	1	0	6	—	0	3	0	0	0	8
butterscotch	1 oz	112	1	tr	3	0	27	—	1	12	1	0	0	39
candy corn	1 oz	105	0	0	0	tr	27	—	2	57	1	0	—	0
caramels	1 pkg (2.5 oz)	271	6	5	5	3	55	—	98	174	152	—	4	23

FOOD	PORTION	CALORIES	FAT	SAT FAT	CHOL	PROTEIN	CARBO	FIBER	CALCIUM	SOD	POTAS	VIT C	FOLIC	VIT A
caramels	1 piece (8 g)	31	1	1	1	tr	6	—	11	20	17	—	0	3
caramels chocolate	1 piece (6 g)	22	tr	tr	0	tr	6	—	—	—	—	—	—	—
caramels chocolate	1 bar (2.3 oz)	231	2	tr	0	1	56	—	—	—	—	—	—	—
carob bar	1 (3.1 oz)	453	28	7	—	11	42	—	391	—	785	—	27	39
crisped rice bar almond	1 bar (1 oz)	130	6	1	0	2	18	1	21	66	65	—	0	750
crisped rice bar chocolate chip	1 bar (1 oz)	115	4	1	0	4	21	1	6	79	48	—	40	500
dark chocolate	1 oz	150	10	6	0	1	16	—	7	5	86	tr	—	10
fondant chocolate coated	1 sm (0.4 oz)	40	1	1	0	tr	9	—	2	3	18	—	—	2
fondant chocolate coated	1 lg (1.2 oz)	128	3	2	0	1	28	—	6	9	59	—	—	7
fondant mint	1 oz	105	0	0	0	tr	27	—	2	57	1	0	—	0
gumdrops	10 sm (0.4 oz)	135	0	0	0	0	35	—	1	15	2	—	—	—
gumdrops	10 lg (3.8 oz)	420	0	0	0	0	108	—	3	48	5	—	—	—
hard candy	1 oz	106	0	0	0	0	28	—	1	11	1	—	—	0
jelly beans	10 sm (0.4 oz)	40	tr	—	0	0	10	—	0	3	4	0	—	0
jelly beans	10 lg (1 oz)	104	tr	—	0	0	26	—	1	7	11	0	—	0
lollipop	1 (6 g)	22	0	0	0	0	6	—	0	2	0	—	—	0
milk chocolate	1 bar (1.55 oz)	226	14	8	10	3	26	—	84	36	169	tr	4	82
milk chocolate crisp	1 bar (1.45 oz)	203	11	7	8	3	28	—	70	59	141	tr	3	23
milk chocolate w/ almonds	1 bar (1.45 oz)	215	14	7	8	4	22	—	92	30	182	tr	—	30
peanut bar	1 (1.4 oz)	209	14	2	—	6	19	—	31	91	163	—	—	—
peanuts chocolate covered	10 (1.4 oz)	208	13	6	4	5	20	—	42	16	201	0	3	0
peanuts chocolate covered	1 cup (5.2 oz)	773	50	22	13	19	74	—	155	61	748	0	12	0
pretzels chocolate covered	1 oz	130	5	2	—	2	20	—	21	—	—	tr	—	—
pretzels chocolate covered	1 (0.4 oz)	50	2	1	—	1	8	—	8	10	—	tr	—	—
sesame crunch	1 oz	146	9	1	0	3	14	—	—	—	—	—	—	—
sesame crunch	20 pieces (1.2 oz)	181	12	2	0	4	18	—	—	—	—	—	—	—
sweet chocolate	1 bar (1.45 oz)	201	14	8	0	2	25	—	10	7	119	—	—	8
sweet chocolate	1 oz	143	10	6	0	1	17	—	7	5	82	—	—	6
100 GRAND														
Bar	1 bar (1.5 oz)	200	8	5	10	2	30	tr	40	75	—	—	—	—
3 MUSKETEERS														
Bar	2 fun size (1.2 oz)	140	4	3	5	1	25	0	—	60	—	—	—	—
Bar	1 (2.1 oz)	260	8	4	5	2	46	1	20	110	—	—	—	—
BABY RUTH														
Bar	1 (2.1 oz)	270	13	7	0	4	36	2	20	130	—	0	—	0
Fun Size	2 pieces	200	9	5	—	3	27	1	—	95	—	—	—	—

FOOD	PORTION	CALORIES	FAT	SAT FAT	CHOL	PROTEIN	CARBO	FIBER	CALCIUM	SOD	POTAS	VIT C	FOLIC	VIT A
BARRICINI														
Dark Chocolate Raspberry Creme Shells	1 piece (0.3 oz)	47	3	1	0	0	5	0	0	4	—	0	—	0
BITS O BRICKLE														
Candy	1 tbsp (0.5 oz)	80	5	2	5	0	9	0	0	85	—	0	—	100
BONUS														
Bar	1 bar (2.1 oz)	290	16	7	0	6	34	2	60	140	—	0	—	0
BREATH SAVERS														
Sugar Free Mint Cinnamon	1 piece (2 g)	10	0	0	0	0	2	—	—	0	0	—	—	—
Sugar Free Peppermint	1 piece (2 g)	10	0	0	0	0	2	—	—	0	0	—	—	—
Sugar Free Spearmint	1 piece (2 g)	10	0	—	—	0	2	—	—	0	0	—	—	—
Sugar Free Wintergreen	1 piece (2 g)	10	0	—	—	0	2	—	—	0	0	—	—	—
BROCK														
Butterscotch Discs	3 pieces (0.6 oz)	70	0	0	0	0	17	—	—	80	—	—	—	—
Candy Corn	21 pieces (1.4 oz)	150	0	0	0	0	37	—	—	85	—	—	—	—
Candy Rolls	2 rolls (0.5 oz)	50	0	0	0	0	12	—	—	0	—	—	—	—
Caramel Dots	3 pieces (1.3 oz)	140	3	1	—	2	25	tr	20	50	—	0	—	100
Cinnamon Discs	3 pieces (0.6 oz)	70	0	0	0	0	17	—	—	5	—	—	—	—
Circus Peanuts	11 pieces (2.5 oz)	260	0	0	0	1	65	—	—	25	—	—	—	—
Coconut Mountains	4 pieces (1.4 oz)	170	6	1	—	1	29	—	—	80	—	—	—	—
Fruit Basket	3 pieces (0.6 oz)	60	0	0	0	0	15	—	—	0	—	—	—	—
Fruit Kisses	3 pieces (0.6 oz)	70	0	0	0	0	17	—	—	5	—	—	—	—
Glitters	2 pieces (0.5 oz)	50	0	0	0	0	13	—	—	15	—	—	—	—
Gummy Bears	5 pieces (1.4 oz)	130	0	0	0	0	30	—	—	15	—	—	—	—
Gummy Squirms	5 pieces (1.3 oz)	120	0	0	0	0	28	—	—	15	—	—	—	—
Jelly Beans	12 pieces (1.4 oz)	140	0	0	0	0	36	—	—	15	—	—	—	—
Lemon Drops	3 pieces (0.5 oz)	60	0	0	0	0	14	—	—	5	—	—	—	—
Orange Slices	4 pieces (1.5 oz)	140	0	0	0	0	36	—	—	20	—	—	—	—
Party Mints	9 pieces (0.5 oz)	60	0	0	0	0	15	—	—	0	—	—	—	—

FOOD	PORTION	CALORIES	FAT	SAT FAT	CHOL	PROTEIN	CARBO	FIBER	CALCIUM	SOD	POTAS	VIT C	FOLIC	VIT A
BROCK (CONT.)														
Peanut Butter Crunch	3 pieces (0.6 oz)	80	2	—	—	tr	15	—	—	45	—	—	—	—
Pops Assorted	2 (0.5 oz)	60	0	0	0	0	15	—	—	5	—	—	—	—
Sour Balls	3 pieces (0.6 oz)	70	0	0	0	0	17	—	—	5	—	—	—	—
Sour Sharks	23 pieces (2.5 oz)	30	3	2	—	0	60	—	—	45	—	—	—	—
Spearmint Starlights	3 pieces (0.6 oz)	60	0	0	0	0	16	—	—	5	—	—	—	—
Spice Drops	12 pieces (1.4 oz)	130	0	0	0	0	33	—	—	20	—	—	—	—
Starlight Mints	3 pieces (0.6 oz)	60	0	0	0	0	16	—	—	5	—	—	—	—
Toffee	6 pieces (1.5 oz)	170	5	2	—	1	31	—	—	45	—	—	—	—
BUTTERFINGER														
BB's	1 pkg (1.7 oz)	230	10	7	0	2	34	1	—	90	—	—	—	—
Bar	1 (2.1 oz)	280	11	6	0	4	41	1	—	120	—	—	—	—
Fun Size	2 bars (1.6 oz)	200	8	4	—	3	30	1	—	85	—	—	—	—
CELLAS														
Chocolate Covered Cherries Dark Chocolate	2 pieces (1 oz)	100	4	3	—	—	—	—	—	—	—	—	—	—
Chocolate Covered Cherries Milk Chocolate	2 pieces (1 oz)	110	4	3	0	tr	18	2	20	15	—	0	—	0
CERTS														
Breath Mints	1 piece (1.67 g)	6	0	0	0	0	2	—	—	—	—	—	—	—
Mini Sugar Free	1 piece (0.365 g)	1	0	0	0	0	tr	—	—	—	—	—	—	—
Sugar Free	1 piece (1.67 g)	7	0	0	0	0	2	—	—	—	—	—	—	—
CHARLESTON CHEW														
Candy	1 pkg (1.9 oz)	230	7	6	—	—	—	—	—	—	—	—	—	—
CHARMS														
Blow Pop	1 (0.6 oz)	70	0	0	0	0	17	—	100	0	—	—	—	—
Lollipop Sour	1 (0.6 oz)	70	0	0	0	0	18	—	—	0	—	—	—	—
Lollipop Sweet	1 (0.6 oz)	70	0	0	0	0	18	—	—	0	—	—	—	—
CHUCKLES														
Candy	4 pieces (1.4 oz)	140	0	0	0	0	34	—	—	15	—	—	—	—
CHUNKY														
Bar	1 (1.4 oz)	200	11	6	<5	3	22	2	60	20	—	—	—	—
CLORETS														
Mints	1 piece (1.67 g)	6	0	0	0	0	2	—	—	—	—	—	—	—

FOOD	PORTION	CALORIES	FAT	SAT FAT	CHOL	PROTEIN	CARBO	FIBER	CALCIUM	SOD	POTAS	VIT C	FOLIC	VIT A
CRUNCH														
Fun Size	4 bars (1.5 oz)	200	10	6	5	2	25	1	60	55	—	—	—	—
DOVE														
Dark Chocolate	¼ bar (1.5 oz)	230	14	8	5	2	26	3	—	0	—	—	—	—
Dark Chocolate	1 bar (1.3 oz)	200	12	7	5	2	22	2	—	0	—	—	—	—
Dark Chocolate Minatures	7 (1.5 oz)	220	14	8	5	2	26	2	—	0	—	—	—	—
Milk Chocolate	1 bar (1.3 oz)	200	12	7	5	2	22	1	60	25	—	—	—	100
Milk Chocolate	¼ bar (1.5 oz)	230	13	8	10	3	25	1	60	30	—	—	—	100
Milk Chocolate Miniatures	7 (1.5 oz)	230	13	8	10	3	25	1	60	30	—	—	—	100
Truffles	3 (1.2 oz)	200	13	9	5	2	19	1	40	15	—	—	—	—
DREAM														
Caramel & Nougat In Milk Chocolate	1 bar (1 oz)	90	3	2	<5	1	21	1	0	70	—	0	—	0
ESTEE														
Caramels Chocolate & Vanilla No Sugar Added	5 (1.3 oz)	150	5	1	0	1	26	0	40	65	155	0	—	0
Dark Chocolate	½ bar (1.4 oz)	200	14	8	10	2	23	0	0	10	140	0	—	0
Gum Drops Assorted Fruit Sugar Free	23 (1.4 oz)	140	0	0	0	0	36	0	—	0	0	—	—	—
Gum Drops Licorice	23 (1.4 oz)	140	0	0	0	0	36	—	—	0	0	—	—	—
Gummy Bears Sugar Free	16 (1.4 oz)	140	0	0	0	4	31	—	—	0	0	—	—	—
Hard Candies Assorted Fruit Sugar Free	5 (0.5 oz)	60	0	0	0	0	16	0	—	0	0	—	—	—
Hard Candies Assorted Mint Sugar Free	5 (0.5 oz)	60	0	0	0	0	16	0	—	0	0	—	—	—
Hard Candies Butterscotch Sugar Free	2 (0.4 oz)	50	0	0	0	0	12	—	—	50	0	—	—	—
Hard Candies Peppermint Swirls Sugar Free	3 (0.5 oz)	60	0	0	0	0	14	—	—	0	0	—	—	—
Hard Candies Tropical Fruit Sugar Free	5 (0.5 oz)	60	0	0	0	0	16	0	—	0	0	—	—	—
Lollipops Assorted Fruit Sugar Free	2 (0.5 oz)	60	0	0	0	0	16	—	—	0	0	—	—	—
Milk Chocolate	½ bar (1.4 oz)	230	17	10	20	4	17	0	80	65	210	0	—	0
Milk Chocolate With Almonds	½ bar (1.4 oz)	230	17	9	20	4	16	0	80	65	220	0	—	0

FOOD	PORTION	CALORIES	FAT	SAT FAT	CHOL	PROTEIN	CARBO	FIBER	CALCIUM	SOD	POTAS	VIT C	FOLIC	VIT A
ESTEE (CONT.)														
Milk Chocolate With Crisp Rice	1 bar (2.3 oz)	370	26	15	30	7	29	0	150	110	340	0	—	0
Milk Chocolate With Fruit & Nuts	½ bar (1.4 oz)	220	16	9	20	4	18	0	80	65	220	0	—	0
Mint Chocolate	½ bar (1.4 oz)	200	14	8	10	2	23	0	0	10	140	0	—	0
Peanut Brittle No Sugar Added	⅓ box (1.5 oz)	210	9	2	10	4r	28	1	0	115	90	0	—	0
Peanut Butter Cups	1 (0.3 oz)	40	3	4	0	1	3	0	20	0	35	0	—	0
Peanut Butter Cups	5 (1.3 oz)	200	12	7	5	5	19	1	100	70	240	0	—	0
Toffee Sugar Free	5 (0.5 oz)	60	0	0	0	0	16	—	—	0	0	—	—	—
FAVORITE BRANDS														
Candy Corn	24 pieces (1.4 oz)	150	0	0	—	0	37	—	—	110	—	—	—	—
Cinnamon Imperials	52 (0.5 oz)	80	0	0	—	0	14	—	—	5	—	—	—	—
Circus Peanuts	5 pieces (1.6 oz)	160	0	0	—	1	39	—	—	10	—	—	—	—
Gummallo Apple Ring	5 pieces (1.4 oz)	120	0	0	—	2r	27	—	—	0	—	—	—	—
Gummallo Peach Ring	5 pieces (1.4 oz)	120	0	0	—	2	27	—	—	5	—	—	—	—
Gummi Bears	18 pieces (1.4 oz)	130	0	0	—	2	30	—	—	15	—	—	—	—
Gummi Dinos	7 pieces (1.3 oz)	120	0	0	—	2	28	—	—	15	—	—	—	—
Gummi Worms	4 pieces (1.4 oz)	130	0	0	—	2	29	—	—	15	—	—	—	—
Jelly Beans	13 (1.4 oz)	150	0	0	—	0	37	—	—	20	—	—	—	—
Marshmallow Eggs	3 (1.3 oz)	140	0	0	—	0r	34	—	—	10	—	—	—	—
Neon Worms	4 pieces (1.4 oz)	120	0	0	—	2	28	—	—	0	—	—	—	—
Sour Gummi Bears	16 pieces (1.4 oz)	110	0	0	—	2	26	—	—	0	—	—	—	—
Sour Gummi Worms	4 pieces (1.6 oz)	130	0	0	—	2	29	—	—	0	—	—	—	—
FERRERO ROCHER														
Candy	2 pieces (0.9 oz)	150	10	3	0	2	11	0	40	24	—	0	—	0
FRANKLIN														
Crunch 'N Munch Candied	1.25 oz	170	7	—	0	2	28	1	—	200	—	—	—	—
Crunch 'N Munch Caramel	1.25 oz	160	5	—	13	2	28	1	—	130	—	—	—	400
Crunch 'N Munch Maple Walnut	1.25 oz	160	6	—	6	1	28	1	—	180	—	—	—	400

FOOD	PORTION	CALORIES	FAT	SAT FAT	CHOL	PROTEIN	CARBO	FIBER	CALCIUM	SOD	POTAS	VIT C	FOLIC	VIT A
FRANKLIN (CONT.)														
Crunch 'N Munch Toffee	1.25 oz	160	5	—	6	2	28	1	—	210	—	—	—	400
GLENNY'S														
Brown Rice Treats Carob & Mint With Oat Bran	1 bar (1.75 oz)	180	2	—	—	3	37	2	—	20	—	—	—	—
Brown Rice Treats Cinnamon & Raisin	1 bar (1.75 oz)	170	1	—	—	2	38	—	—	30	—	—	—	—
Brown Rice Treats Peanut & Raisin	1 bar (2 oz)	210	5	—	—	4	39	—	—	29	—	—	—	—
Brown Rice Treats Plain & Fancy	1 bar (1.25 oz)	120	1	—	—	1	28	—	—	29	—	—	—	—
Brown Rice Treats Raisin Bran	1 bar (1.75 oz)	170	1	—	—	2	38	—	—	17	—	—	—	—
Brown Rice Treats Toasted Almond With Oat Bran	1 bar (1.75 oz)	200	5	—	34	4	34	2	—	20	—	—	—	—
Fruit Drops Black Cherry	1	6	tr	—	—	tr	1	—	—	tr	—	—	—	—
Fruit Drops Gentle Mint	1	6	tr	—	—	tr	1	—	—	tr	—	—	—	—
Fruit Drops Mandarin Orange	1	6	tr	—	—	tr	1	—	—	tr	—	—	—	—
Fruit Drops Mixed Fruit	1	6	tr	—	—	tr	1	—	—	tr	—	—	—	—
Fruit Drops Twist Of Lemon	1	6	tr	—	—	tr	1	—	—	tr	—	—	—	—
Hard Candies Fruit	1	19	tr	—	—	tr	4	—	—	tr	—	—	—	—
Hard Candies Peppermint	1	19	tr	—	—	tr	4	—	—	tr	—	—	—	—
Lollipops C Pops	1	35	tr	—	—	tr	8	—	—	tr	—	—	—	—
Lollipops Fruit	1	21	tr	—	—	tr	5	—	—	tr	—	—	—	—
Moist & Chewy Coconut Almondine Bar	1 bar (1.5 oz)	190	10	—	—	3	22	—	—	20	—	—	—	—
Moist & Chewy Oatmeal Raisin Bar	1 bar (1.5 oz)	160	3	—	—	3	30	—	—	25	—	—	—	—
Moist & Chewy Peanut Bar	1 bar (1.5 oz)	180	7	—	—	5	24	—	—	20	—	—	—	—
Moist & Chewy Sunflower Bar	1 bar (1.5 oz)	180	7	—	—	5	24	—	—	15	—	—	—	—
Snack Bar Fat-Free Apple-Cinnamon	1 (1.25 oz)	120	1	—	—	1	28	—	—	15	—	—	—	—
Snack Bar Fat-Free Caramel	1 (1.25 oz)	120	tr	—	—	1	29	—	—	70	—	—	—	—

FOOD	PORTION	CALORIES	FAT	SAT FAT	CHOL	PROTEIN	CARBO	FIBER	CALCIUM	SOD	POTAS	VIT C	FOLIC	VIT A
GLENNY'S (CONT.)														
Snack Bar Fat-Free Chocolate	1 (1.25 oz)	120	tr	—	—	1	28	—	—	10	—	—	—	—
Snack Bar Fat-Free Raspberry	1 (1.25 oz)	120	tr	—	—	1	29	—	—	15	—	—	—	—
GODIVA														
Almond Butter Dome	3 pieces (1.5 oz)	240	17	6	5	4	19	0	80	20	—	0	—	0
Bouchee Au Chocolat	1 piece (1.5 oz)	210	11	6	5	3	25	0	20	40	—	0	—	0
Bouchee Ivory Raspberry	1 pieces (1 oz)	160	9	3	5	2	17	0	20	25	—	0	—	0
Gold Ballotin	3 pieces (1.5 oz)	210	10	4	5	2	27	0	40	15	—	0	—	0
Truffle Amaretto Di Saronno	2 pieces (1.5 oz)	210	12	6	5	2	24	0	40	25	—	0	—	0
Truffle Deluxe Liqueur	2 pieces (1.5 oz)	210	13	6	5	2	23	0	20	25	—	0	—	0
GOLDENBERG'S														
Peanut Chews	3 pieces (1.3 oz)	180	9	2	0	4	22	1	0	40	—	0	—	0
GOO GOO SUPREME														
With Pecans	1 pkg (1.5 oz)	188	5	2	0	2	34	4	20	51	—	0	—	0
GOOBERS														
Peanuts	1 pkg (1.38 oz)	210	13	5	<5	5	19	3	40	20	—	—	—	—
GOOD & FRUITY														
Candy	1 box (1.8 oz)	140	1	—	—	0	35	2	—	75	—	—	—	—
GOOD & PLENTY														
Snacksize	3 boxes (1.5 oz)	140	0	0	0	1	34	—	20	80	—	—	—	—
HAVILAND														
Chocolate Covered Thin Mints	6 (1.5 oz)	170	5	3	0	1	33	1	0	5	—	0	—	0
HEATH														
Bar	1 (1.4 oz)	210	13	7	20	2	25	0	40	180	—	0	—	300
HERSHEY														
Amazin' Fruit Gummy Candy	2 snack pkg (1.4 oz)	130	0	0	0	2	30	—	—	45	—	—	—	—
JOLLY RANCHER														
Candies	3 pieces (0.6 oz)	60	0	0	0	0	14	—	—	5	—	—	—	—
JOYVA														
Halvah	1.5 oz	240	16	3	0	4	16	2	0	80	—	0	—	0
Halvah Chocolate Covered	1 bar (2 oz)	380	23	5	0	5	20	3	0	95	—	0	—	0
Jells Raspberry	3 pieces (1.6 oz)	200	3	2	0	0	25	tr	0	15	—	0	—	0

FOOD	PORTION	CALORIES	FAT	SAT FAT	CHOL	PROTEIN	CARBO	FIBER	CALCIUM	SOD	POTAS	VIT C	FOLIC	VIT A
JOYVA (CONT.)														
Joys Raspberry	1 (1.6 oz)	200	3	2	0	0	25	1	0	15	—	0	—	0
Marshmallow Twists Chocolate Covered	2 (1.5 oz)	190	4	2	0	1	21	0	0	20	—	0	—	0
Rings Orange & Raspberry	3 pieces (1.5 oz)	190	3	2	0	0	23	tr	0	15	—	0	—	0
Sesame Crunch	3 pieces (0.5)	80	4	1	0	1	7	0	0	25	—	0	—	0
Sticks Orange	3 pieces (1.6 oz)	200	3	2	0	0	25	tr	0	15	—	0	—	0
Twists Vanilla & Cherry	2 pieces (1.5 oz)	190	4	2	0	1	21	0	0	20	—	0	—	0
JUICEFULS														
Candy	3 pieces (0.5 oz)	60	0	0	0	0	15	—	—	0	—	—	—	—
JUNIOR MINTS														
Candies	1 pkg (1.6 oz)	190	4	3	—	—	—	—	—	—	—	—	—	—
JUST BORN														
Hot Tamales	1 pkg (2.1 oz)	220	0	0	0	0	55	—	—	25	—	—	—	—
Mike and Ike Berry Fruits	1 pkg (2.1 oz)	220	0	0	0	0	55	—	—	85	—	—	—	—
Mike and Ike Cherry & Bubble Gum	1 pkg (2.1 oz)	220	0	0	0	0	55	—	—	25	—	—	—	—
Mike and Ike Chewy Grape	1 pkg (2.1 oz)	220	0	0	0	0	55	—	—	25	—	—	—	—
Mike and Ike Lemon Watermelon	1 pkg (2.1 oz)	220	0	0	0	0	55	—	—	25	—	—	—	—
Mike and Ike Original	1 pkg (1.2 oz)	220	0	0	0	0	55	—	—	25	—	—	—	—
Mike and Ike Strawberry & Banana	1 pkg (2.1 oz)	220	0	0	0	0	55	—	—	25	—	—	—	—
Mike and Ike Tropical Fruits	1 pkg (2.1 oz)	220	0	0	0	0	55	—	—	25	—	—	—	—
Super Hot Tamales	1 pkg (2.1 oz)	220	0	0	0	0	55	—	—	25	—	—	—	—
Teenee Beanee Assorted Fruits	36 pieces (1.4 oz)	150	0	0	0	0	36	—	—	15	—	—	—	—
Teenee Beanee Berry Berry	36 pieces (1.4 oz)	150	0	0	0	0	36	—	—	15	—	—	—	—
Teenee Beanee Tropical Mix	36 pieces (1.4 oz)	150	0	0	0	0	36	—	—	15	—	—	—	—
LANCE														
Chocolaty Peanut Bar	1 (57 g)	320	18	6	0	9	29	—	40	40	50	—	—	—
Peanut Bar	1 pkg (50 g)	260	14	3	0	9	24	—	—	80	35	—	—	—
Popscotch	1 pkg (35 g)	160	6	1	0	3	24	—	—	120	85	—	—	—

FOOD	PORTION	CALORIES	FAT	SAT FAT	CHOL	PROTEIN	CARBO	FIBER	CALCIUM	SOD	POTAS	VIT C	FOLIC	VIT A
LIFESAVERS														
Big Tablet Candy Cane	4 pieces (0.5 oz)	60	0	0	0	0	16	—	—	0	0	—	—	—
Cards 'N Candy	4 pieces (0.4 oz)	40	0	0	0	0	10	—	—	0	0	—	—	—
Christmas Tin	4 pieces (0.5 oz)	60	0	0	0	0	16	—	—	20	0	—	—	—
Egg-Sortment	1 roll (0.4 oz)	40	0	0	0	0	10	—	—	0	0	—	—	—
Fruit Juicers Lollipops	1	40	0	0	0	0	10	0	—	0	10	—	—	—
Gummi Bunnies	3 pkg (1.6 oz)	140	0	0	0	3	34	—	—	0	5	—	—	—
Gummi Savers Five Flavor	1 roll (1.5 oz)	130	0	0	0	2	32	—	—	0	5	—	—	—
Gummi Savers Five Flavor	1 pkg (1.8 oz)	160	0	0	0	3	38	—	—	0	5	—	—	—
Gummi Savers Mixed Berry	1 roll (1.5 oz)	130	0	0	0	2	32	—	—	0	5	—	—	—
Gummi Savers Mixed Berry	1 pkg (1.8 oz)	160	0	0	0	3	38	—	—	0	5	—	—	—
Gummi Savers Tangy Fruits	1 pkg (1.8 oz)	160	0	0	0	3	38	—	—	0	5	—	—	—
Gummi Savers Tangy Fruits	1 roll (1.5 oz)	130	0	0	0	2	32	—	—	0	5	—	—	—
Gummi Savers Variety	2 pkg (1.3 oz)	120	0	0	0	2	27	—	—	0	5	—	—	—
Gummi Savers Wacky Frootz	1 roll (1.5 oz)	130	0	0	0	2	32	—	—	0	5	—	—	—
Gummi Savers Wacky Frootz	1 pkg (1.8 oz)	160	0	0	0	3	38	—	—	0	5	—	—	—
Holes Five Flavor	20 pieces (5 g)	20	0	0	0	0	5	—	—	0	0	—	—	—
Holes Island Fruit	20 pieces (5 g)	20	0	0	0	0	5	—	—	0	0	—	—	—
Holes Sour 'N Sweet	16 pieces (5 g)	20	0	0	0	0	5	—	—	0	0	—	—	—
Holes Sunshine Fruits	20 pieces (0.2 oz)	20	0	0	0	0	5	—	—	0	0	—	—	—
Holes Super Tart	20 pieces (5 g)	20	0	0	0	0	5	—	—	0	0	—	—	—
Holes Tangerine	1 candy	2	0	0	0	0	1	0	—	0	0	—	—	—
Holes Wild Fruits	20 pieces (5 g)	20	0	—	<5	0	5	—	—	0	0	—	—	—
Lollipops Candy Cane	1 (0.4 oz)	40	0	0	0	0	10	—	—	0	0	—	—	—
Lollipops Christmas	1 (0.4 oz)	40	0	0	0	0	10	—	—	0	0	—	—	—
Lollipops Easter	1 (0.4 oz)	40	0	0	0	0	10	—	—	0	0	—	—	—
Lollipops Fruit Flavors	1 (0.4 oz)	45	0	0	0	0	11	0	—	0	0	—	—	—
Lollipops Swirled Flavors	1 (0.4 oz)	40	0	0	0	0	10	—	—	0	0	—	—	—
Lollipops Valentine	1 (0.4 oz)	40	0	0	0	0	10	—	—	0	0	—	—	—

FOOD	PORTION	CALORIES	FAT	SAT FAT	CHOL	PROTEIN	CARBO	FIBER	CALCIUM	SOD	POTAS	VIT C	FOLIC	VIT A
LIFESAVERS (CONT.)														
Roll Butter Rum	2 pieces (5 g)	20	0	0	0	0	5	—	—	20	0	—	—	—
Roll Candy Cane	4 pieces (0.4 oz)	40	0	0	0	0	10	—	—	0	0	—	—	—
Roll Cryst-O-Mint	2 pieces (5 g)	20	0	0	0	0	5	—	—	0	0	—	—	—
Roll Five Flavor	2 pieces (5 g)	20	0	0	0	0	5	—	—	0	0	—	—	—
Roll Fruits On Fire	2 pieces (5 g)	20	0	0	0	0	5	—	—	0	0	—	—	—
Roll Pep-O-Mint	3 pieces (5 g)	20	0	0	0	0	5	—	—	0	0	—	—	—
Roll Spear-O-Mint	3 pieces (5 g)	20	0	0	0	0	5	—	—	0	0	—	—	—
Roll Sunshine Fruits	2 pieces (5 g)	20	0	0	0	0	5	—	—	0	0	—	—	—
Roll Tangy Fruit Swirl	2 pieces (5 g)	20	0	0	0	0	5	—	—	0	0	—	—	—
Roll Tangy Fruit Watermelon	1 pieces (5 g)	20	0	0	0	0	5	—	—	0	0	—	—	—
Roll Tangy Fruits	2 pieces (5 g)	20	0	0	0	0	5	—	—	0	0	—	—	—
Roll Tropical Fruits	2 pieces (5 g)	20	0	0	0	0	5	—	—	0	0	—	—	—
Roll Wild Cherry	1 pieces (5 g)	20	0	0	0	0	5	—	—	0	0	—	—	—
Roll Wild Flavors	2 pieces (5 g)	20	0	0	0	0	5	—	—	0	0	—	—	—
Roll Wild Sour Berries	2 pieces (5 g)	20	0	0	0	0	5	—	—	0	0	—	—	—
Roll Wint-O-Green	3 pieces (5 g)	20	0	0	0	0	5	—	—	0	0	—	—	—
Sack'it Butter Rum	4 pieces (0.5 oz)	60	0	0	0	0	15	—	—	65	0	—	—	—
Sack'it Five Flavor	4 pieces (0.5 oz)	60	0	0	0	0	16	—	—	0	0	—	—	—
Sack'it Holiday Tin	4 pieces (0.5 oz)	60	0	0	0	0	16	—	—	65	0	—	—	—
Sack'it Pep-O-Mint	4 pieces (0.5 oz)	60	0	0	0	0	16	—	—	0	0	—	—	—
Sack'it Tangy Fruits	4 pieces (0.5 oz)	60	0	0	0	0	16	—	—	0	0	—	—	—
Sack'it Wild Cherry	4 pieces (0.5 oz)	60	0	0	0	0	16	—	—	0	0	—	—	—
Sack'it Wint-O-Green	4 pieces (0.5 oz)	60	0	0	0	0	16	—	—	0	0	—	—	—
Sugar Free Iced Mint	1 pieces (2 g)	10	0	0	0	0	2	—	—	0	0	—	—	—
Sugar Free Vanilla Mint	1 pieces (2 g)	10	0	0	0	0	2	—	—	0	0	—	—	—
Valentine Book	2 pieces (5 g)	20	0	0	0	0	5	—	—	20	0	—	—	—
LINDT														
Truffles	3 pieces (1.3 oz)	220	18	14	5	1	14	0	20	10	—	0	—	0
M&M'S														
Almond	1.5 oz	220	12	4	5	4	24	2	60	20	—	—	—	—
Almond	1 pkg (1.3 oz)	200	11	4	5	3	21	2	40	20	—	—	—	—
Mint	1 pkg (1.7 oz)	230	10	6	10	2	34	1	40	35	—	—	—	—

FOOD	PORTION	CALORIES	FAT	SAT FAT	CHOL	PROTEIN	CARBO	FIBER	CALCIUM	SOD	POTAS	VIT C	FOLIC	VIT A
M&M'S (CONT.)														
Mint	1.5 oz	200	9	5	5	2	30	1	40	30	—	—	—	—
Peanut	½ bag king size (1.6 oz)	240	12	5	5	4	28	2	40	25	—	—	—	—
Peanut	1 fun size (0.7 oz)	110	5	2	5	2	13	1	20	10	—	—	—	—
Peanut	1 pkg (1.7 oz)	250	13	5	5	5	30	2	40	25	—	—	—	—
Peanut	1.5 oz	220	11	5	5	4	25	2	40	20	—	—	—	—
Peanut Butter	1 fun size (0.7 oz)	110	6	4	0	2	12	1	—	45	—	—	—	—
Peanut Butter	1.5 oz	220	12	8	5	4	25	2	20	90	—	—	—	—
Peanut Butter	1 pkg (1.6 oz)	240	13	8	5	5	27	2	40	100	—	—	—	—
Plain	1 pkg fun size (0.7 oz)	100	4	3	5	1	15	0	20	15	—	—	—	—
Plain	½ pkg king size (1.6 oz)	220	9	6	5	2	32	1	40	30	—	—	—	—
Plain	1 pkg (1.7 oz)	230	10	10	6	2	34	1	40	35	—	—	—	—
Plain	1.5 oz	200	9	5	5	2	30	1	40	30	—	—	—	—
MARS														
Almond Bar	2 fun size (1.3 oz)	190	10	3	5	3	23	1	40	55	—	—	—	—
Almond Bar	1 bar (1.8 oz)	240	13	4	5	3	31	1	60	70	—	—	—	—
MAYFAIR														
Mints	5 pieces (1.3 oz)	180	9	5	0	1	26	tr	0	5	—	0	—	0
MILK DUDS														
Pieces	1 box (1.8 oz)	230	8	6	0	1	38	0	20	120	—	0	—	0
Snack Size	4 boxes (1.3 oz)	160	5	4	0	1	26	0	20	85	—	0	—	0
MILKSHAKE														
Bar	1 bar (1.8 oz)	220	7	4	0	2	38	0	60	120	—	0	—	0
MILKY WAY														
Bar	2 fun size (1.4 oz)	180	7	4	5	2	28	0	40	60	—	—	—	—
Bar	⅓ king size (1.2 oz)	160	6	3	5	1	24	0	20	50	—	—	—	—
Bar	1 (2.1 oz)	280	11	5	5	2	43	1	60	90	—	—	—	—
Dark	1 fun size (0.7 oz)	90	3	2	0	1	14	0	—	35	—	—	—	—
Dark	1 bar (1.8 oz)	220	8	5	5	1	36	1	20	85	—	—	—	—
Miniature	5 (1.5 oz)	190	7	4	5	2	30	0	40	65	—	—	—	—
NECCO														
Mint	1 piece	12	tr	—	0	—	—	—	—	—	—	—	—	—
NESTLE														
Areo Bar	1 bar (1.45 oz)	210	13	7	10	<1	26	2	60	20	—	—	—	—
Buncha Crunch	1 pkg (1.4 oz)	90	10	5	5	2	26	tr	40	95	—	—	—	—
Crunch	1 bar (1.55 oz)	230	12	7	5	3	28	1	80	60	—	—	—	—

FOOD	PORTION	CALORIES	FAT	SAT FAT	CHOL	PROTEIN	CARBO	FIBER	CALCIUM	SOD	POTAS	VIT C	FOLIC	VIT A
NESTLE (CONT.)														
Milk Chocolate	1 bar (1.45 oz)	220	13	7	10	4	23	2	—	30	—	—	—	—
Turtles Pecan Caramel Candy	2 pieces (1.2 oz)	160	9	3	<5	2	20	1	40	30	—	—	—	—
NEWMAN'S OWN														
Organics Espresso Sweet Dark Chocolate	1 bar (1.2 oz)	190	12	7	0	2	19	0	0	10	—	0	—	0
NIPS														
Butter Rum	2 pieces (0.5 oz)	60	2	2	—	0	12	—	—	35	—	—	—	—
Caramel	2 pieces (0.5 oz)	60	2	2	—	0	12	—	—	40	—	—	—	—
Chocolate Mint	2 pieces (0.5 oz)	60	2	2	—	tr	11	—	—	40	—	—	—	—
Chocolate Parfait	2 pieces (0.5 oz)	60	2	2	—	tr	11	—	—	35	—	—	—	—
Peanut Butter Parfait	2 pieces (0.5 oz)	60	2	2	—	tr	11	—	—	40	—	—	—	—
OCEAN SPRAY														
Fruit Waves Assorted	3 pieces (0.3 oz)	35	0	0	0	0	9	—	—	0	—	—	—	—
OH HENRY!														
Bar	1 (1.8 oz)	230	9	4	<5	6	32	2	40	125	—	—	—	—
PALMER														
Milk Chocolate Lollipop	1 (0.9 oz)	130	7	4	4	1	16	2	100	35	—	0	—	0
PAYDAY														
Bar	1 (1.85 oz)	240	12	2	0	7	28	2	40	170	—	0	—	0
PEARSON														
Licorice	2 pieces (0.5 oz)	60	2	2	—	0	12	—	—	40	—	—	—	—
PEZ														
Candy	1 roll (0.3 oz)	30	0	0	0	0	8	—	—	0	—	—	—	—
Sugar Free	1 roll (0.3 oz)	30	0	0	0	0	8	0	—	0	—	21	—	—
PLANTERS														
Original Peanut Bar	1 pkg (1.6 oz)	230	14	2	0	6	22	2	20	70	210	—	—	—
POM POM														
Candies	1 pkg (1.6 oz)	200	6	5	—	—	—	—	—	—	—	—	—	—
RAISINETS														
Candy	1 pkg (1.58 oz)	200	8	4	<5	2	31	2	40	15	—	—	—	—
Fun Size	3 pkg (1.7 oz)	210	8	5	<5	2	33	1	40	15	—	0	—	0
REESE'S														
Sticks	1 (0.7 oz)	120	7	3	—	2	11	—	—	55	—	—	—	—

FOOD	PORTION	CALORIES	FAT	SAT FAT	CHOL	PROTEIN	CARBO	FIBER	CALCIUM	SOD	POTAS	VIT C	FOLIC	VIT A
RIESEN														
Candy	5 pieces (1.4 oz)	180	7	3	<5	3	29	3	40	30	—	0	—	0
RUSSELL STOVER														
Assorted Creams	3 pieces (1.4 oz)	180	7	4	<5	1	29	0	20	50	—	0	—	0
Pecan Roll	1 (2 oz)	300	20	3	5	3	26	3	40	95	—	2	—	100
SIMPLY LITE														
Sugar Free Lil'l Bits Chocolately	36 pieces (1.4 oz)	130	5	5	0	3	28	1	0	55	—	0	—	0
Sugar Free Lil'l Bits Peanut Buttery	36 pieces (1.4 oz)	140	5	5	0	4	26	1	0	50	—	0	—	0
Sugar Free Patteez	5 pieces (1.3 oz)	110	3	2	0	1	29	1	0	10	—	0	—	0
SKITTLES														
Original	2 pkg fun size (1.6 oz)	180	2	0	0	0	41	0	—	5	—	21	—	—
Original	1 pkg (2.8 oz)	250	3	1	0	0	55	0	—	10	—	30	—	—
Original	½ king size (1.3 oz)	150	2	0	0	0	34	0	—	5	—	18	—	—
Original	1.5 oz	170	2	0	0	0	38	0	—	5	—	21	—	—
Tropical	1 bag (2.2 oz)	250	3	1	0	0	56	0	—	10	—	30	—	—
Tropical	1.5 oz	170	2	0	0	0	38	0	—	5	—	21	—	—
Tropical	2 bags fun size (1.4 oz)	160	2	0	0	0	36	0	—	5	—	18	—	—
Wild Berry	2 bags fun size (1.4 oz)	160	2	0	0	0	36	0	—	5	—	18	—	—
Wild Berry	1 bag (2.2 oz)	250	3	1	0	0	56	0	—	10	—	30	—	—
Wild Berry	1.5 oz	170	2	0	0	0	38	0	—	5	—	21	—	—
SMUCKER'S														
Jelly Beans	1 pkg (0.7 oz)	70	0	0	0	0	18	0	0	10	—	0	—	0
SNICKERS														
Bar	1 bar (2.1 oz)	280	14	5	10	4	36	1	40	150	—	—	—	—
Bar	2 bars fun size (1.4 oz)	190	9	4	5	3	24	1	20	100	—	—	—	—
Bar	⅓ king size (1.2 oz)	170	8	3	5	3	21	1	20	85	—	—	—	—
Miniatures	4 (1.3 oz)	170	8	3	5	3	22	1	20	90	—	—	—	—
Munch Bar	1 (1.4 oz)	230	15	4	10	6	17	2	20	150	—	—	—	100
Peanut Butter	1 bar (2 oz)	310	20	7	5	6	28	1	60	150	—	—	—	—
SNO-CAPS														
Candies	1 pkg (2.3 oz)	300	13	8	—	2	48	3	—	0	—	—	—	—
SOUR PUNCH														
Candy Straws Sour Apple	6 pieces (1.4 oz)	130	1	—	0	1	31	—	—	10	—	—	—	—

FOOD	PORTION	CALORIES	FAT	SAT FAT	CHOL	PROTEIN	CARBO	FIBER	CALCIUM	SOD	POTAS	VIT C	FOLIC	VIT A
SPICE STIX														
And Drops	14 pieces (1.6 oz)	140	0	0	0	0	35	—	—	15	—	—	—	—
STARBURST														
California Fruits	8 pieces (1.4 oz)	160	3	1	0	0	33	0	—	20	—	21	—	—
California Fruits	1 stick (2.1 oz)	240	5	1	2	0	48	0	—	35	—	30	—	—
Original Fruits	⅓ king size (1.2 oz)	140	3	1	0	0	28	0	—	20	—	18	—	—
Original Fruits	8 pieces (1.4 oz)	160	3	1	0	0	33	0	—	20	—	21	—	—
Original Fruits	1 stick (2.1 oz)	240	5	1	0	0	48	0	—	35	—	30	—	—
Strawberry Fruits	8 pieces (1.4 oz)	160	3	1	0	0	33	0	—	20	—	21	—	—
Strawberry Fruits	1 stick (2.1 oz)	240	5	1	0	0	48	0	—	35	—	30	—	—
Tropical Fruits	1 stick (2.1 oz)	240	5	1	0	0	48	0	—	35	—	30	—	—
Tropical Fruits	8 pieces (1.4 oz)	160	3	1	0	0	33	0	—	20	—	21	—	—
SUGAR BABIES														
Candies	1 pkg (1.7 oz)	190	2	2	—	—	—	—	—	—	—	—	—	—
SWEDISH FISH														
Original	19 pieces (1.4 oz)	160	0	0	0	0	39	0	0	25	—	0	—	0
SWEET ESCAPES														
Triple Chocolate Wafer Bars	1 (0.7 oz)	80	3	2	0	tr	14	—	—	30	—	—	—	—
SWEET'N LOW														
Sugar Free Butter Toffee	4 pieces (0.5 oz)	30	1	1	<5	0	15	—	—	80	—	—	—	—
Sugar Free Butterscotch	1 piece	7	0	0	0	0	4	—	—	0	—	—	—	—
Sugar Free Cinnamon	1 piece	7	0	0	0	0	4	—	—	0	—	—	—	—
Sugar Free Fancy Fruit	1 piece	7	0	0	0	0	4	—	—	0	—	—	—	—
Sugar Free Fruit Flavors	1 piece	7	0	0	0	0	4	—	—	0	—	—	—	—
Sugar Free Hard Candy Coffee	4 pieces (0.5 oz)	30	0	0	0	0	14	—	—	20	—	—	—	—
Sugar Free Peppermint	1 piece	7	0	0	0	0	4	—	—	0	—	—	—	—
Sugar Free Soft Candy Fruitie Flavors	1 piece	11	tr	—	—	tr	4	—	—	0	—	—	—	—

FOOD	PORTION	CALORIES	FAT	SAT FAT	CHOL	PROTEIN	CARBO	FIBER	CALCIUM	SOD	POTAS	VIT C	FOLIC	VIT A
SWEET'N LOW (CONT.)														
Sugar Free Soft Candy Tropical Flavors	1 piece	11	tr	—	—	tr	4	—		0	—	—	—	—
Sugar Free Watermelon	1 piece	7	0	0	0	0	4	—	—	0	—	—	—	—
Sugar Free Wild Cherry	1 piece	7	0	0	0	0	4	—	—	0	—	—	—	—
SWITZER														
Cherry Bites	12 pieces (1.6 oz)	50	0	0	0	1	11	—	—	25	—	—	—	—
Licorice Bites	12 pieces (1.6 oz)	46	0	0	0	0	11	—	20	56	—	—	—	—
TERRY'S														
Orange Milk Chocolate	5 pieces (1.5 oz)	240	14	9	10	3	26	1	80	40	—	0	—	100
TOOTSIE ROLL														
Candy	1 (1 oz)	110	2	0	—	—	—	—	—	—	—	—	—	—
Dots	12 (1.5 oz)	160	0	0	0	—	—	—	—	—	—	—	—	—
Midgees	6 (1.4 oz)	160	3	1	—	—	—	—	—	—	—	—	—	—
Pop	1 (0.6 oz)	60	0	0	0	—	—	—	—	—	—	—	—	—
TWIX														
Caramel	1 pkg (2 oz)	280	14	5	5	3	37	0	40	115	—	—	—	—
Caramel	1 (1 oz)	140	7	3	0 ·	1	19	0	20	60	—	—	—	—
Caramel	1 fun size (0.5 oz)	80	4	2	0	1	10	0	—	30	—	—	—	—
Caramel	1 king size (0.8 oz)	120	6	2	0	1	15	1	20	45	—	—	—	—
Peanut Butter	1 (0.9 oz)	130	8	3	0	3	13	1	—	70	—	—	—	—
TWIZZLERS														
Candy	4 pieces (1.4 oz)	130	1	—	—	1	30	—	—	95	—	—	—	—
Pull-N-Peel Cherry	1 piece (1.1 oz)	110	0	0	0	1	23	—	0	80	—	0	—	0
VELAMINTS														
Cocoamint	1 piece (1.7 g)	5	0	0	0	0	2	—	—	0	—	—	—	—
Peppermint	1 piece (1.7 g)	5	0	0	0	0	2	—	—	0	—	—	—	—
Spearmint	1 piece (1.7 g)	5	0	0	0	0	2	—	—	0	—	—	—	—
Wintergreen	1 piece (1.7 g)	5	0	0	0	0	2	—	—	0	—	—	—	—
VERY SPECIAL														
Chocolate Bottles Liquor Filled	3 pieces (1 oz)	150	6	4	0	1	24	2	0	10	—	0	—	0
WHITMAN'S														
Assorted	3 pieces (1.4 oz)	190	8	5	5	2	27	0	20	50	—	0	—	0
Dark Chocolate	3 pieces (1.4 oz)	200	10	6	<5	2	25	1	20	55	—	0	—	0

FOOD	PORTION	CALORIES	FAT	SAT FAT	CHOL	PROTEIN	CARBO	FIBER	CALCIUM	SOD	POTAS	VIT C	FOLIC	VIT A
WHITMAN'S (CONT.)														
Little Ambassadors	7 pieces (1.4 oz)	190	9	5	5	2	26	1	20	50	—	0	—	0
Pecan Delight	1 bar (2 oz)	310	20	7	10	3	27	2	60	75	—	0	—	100
Pecan Roll	1 bar (2 oz)	300	20	3	5	3	26	1	40	95	—	2	—	100
Sampler	3 pieces (1.4 oz)	200	11	6	5	2	25	1	40	60	—	0	—	0
WHOPPERS														
Candy	1 pkg (1.8 oz)	230	10	8	0	2	36	1	20	130	—	0	—	0
YORK														
Peppermint Patty	1 snack size (0.5 oz)	57	1	1	0	tr	11	—	—	3	—	—	—	—
ZERO														
Bar	2 pieces (1.4 oz)	170	6	3	0	2	28	0	40	85	—	0	—	0
HOME RECIPE														
divinity	1 recipe 48 pieces (19 oz)	1891	tr	—	0	7	486	—	13	247	103	0	1	24
divinity	1 (11 g)	38	0	0	0	tr	10	—	0	5	2	0	0	0
fondant	1 recipe 60 pieces (32.6 oz)	3327	tr	—	0	tr	863	—	14	374	148	0	0	18
fondant	1 piece (0.6 oz)	57	0	—	0	0	15	—	0	6	3	0	0	0
fudge brown sugar w/ nuts	1 piece (0.5 oz)	56	1	tr	1	tr	11	—	16	14	52	tr	1	11
fudge brown sugar w/ nuts	1 recipe 60 pieces (30.7 oz)	3453	88	15	49	25	676	—	967	852	3256	5	92	677
fudge chocolate	1 piece (0.6 oz)	65	1	1	2	tr	14	—	7	10	17	0	0	32
fudge chocolate	1 recipe 48 pieces (29 oz)	3161	70	43	120	14	660	—	351	511	852	2	15	1581
fudge chocolate marshmallow	1 recipe (43.1 oz)	5182	207	125	304	29	880	—	554	1273	1750	3	27	4052
fudge chocolate marshmallow	1 piece (0.7 oz)	84	3	2	5	1	14	—	9	21	28	0	0	66
fudge chocolate marshmallow w/ nuts	1 piece (0.8 oz)	96	4	2	5	1	15	—	11	21	37	tr	1	67
fudge chocolate marshmallow w/ nuts	1 recipe 60 pieces (43.1 oz)	5182	207	125	304	29	880	—	554	1273	1750	3	27	4052
fudge chocolate marshmallow w/ nuts	1 recipe 60 pieces (46.1 oz)	5742	258	127	291	42	903	—	636	1234	2199	5	86	3983

FOOD	PORTION	CALORIES	FAT	SAT FAT	CHOL	PROTEIN	CARBO	FIBER	CALCIUM	SOD	POTAS	VIT C	FOLIC	VIT A
fudge chocolate w/ nuts	1 recipe 48 pieces (32.7 oz)	3967	150	52	130	32	678	—	464	562	1470	5	95	1877
fudge chocolate w/ nuts	1 piece (0.7 oz)	81	3	1	3	1	14	—	9	11	30	tr	2	38
fudge peanut butter	1 piece (0.6 oz)	59	1	tr	1	1	13	—	7	12	21	0	2	6
fudge peanut butter	1 recipe 36 pieces (20.4 oz)	2161	38	9	25	21	456	—	247	424	761	1	66	247
fudge vanilla	1 piece (0.6 oz)	59	1	1	3	tr	13	—	6	11	8	0	0	33
fudge vanilla	1 recipe 48 pieces (27.5 oz)	2893	42	26	125	8	644	—	305	525	393	2	11	1567
fudge vanilla w/ nuts	1 recipe 60 pieces (31 oz)	3666	117	33	125	26	665	—	419	538	1000	5	91	1751
fudge vanilla w/ nuts	1 piece (0.5 oz)	62	2	1	2	tr	11	—	7	9	17	tr	2	30
peanut brittle	1 recipe (17.6 oz)	2288	95	25	66	38	347	—	149	2269	1040	0	348	958
peanut brittle	1 oz	128	5	1	4	2	20	—	8	128	59	0	20	54
praline	1 recipe 23 pieces (31.8 oz)	4116	220	17	0	26	562	—	282	559	1910	7	128	416
praline	1 piece (1.4 oz)	177	10	1	0	1	24	—	12	24	82	tr	6	18
taffy	1 piece (0.5 oz)	56	1	tr	1	0	14	—	0	13	1	0	0	20
taffy	1 recipe 48 pieces (25 oz)	2677	24	15	63	1	651	—	20	636	29	0	1	950
toffee	1 piece (0.4 oz)	65	4	2	13	tr	8	—	4	22	6	0	0	152
toffee	1 recipe 48 pieces (19.4 oz)	2997	182	113	580	6	356	—	185	1036	277	1	10	7023
truffles	1 piece (0.4 oz)	59	4	3	6	1	5	—	19	8	37	tr	0	62
truffles	1 recipe 49 pieces (21.5 oz)	2985	210	132	318	35	275	—	950	433	1867	3	5	3161

CANTALOUPE

BIG VALLEY

Balls frzn	¾ cup (4.9 oz)	40	0	0	0	1	10	0	0	16	—	33	—	3000

DOLE

Fresh	¼	50	0	—	0	1	11	0	—	35	120	63	—	6382

FOOD	PORTION	CALORIES	FAT	SAT FAT	CHOL	PROTEIN	CARBO	FIBER	CALCIUM	SOD	POTAS	VIT C	FOLIC	VIT A
CAPERS														
PROGRESSO														
Capers	1 tsp (5 g)	0	0	0	0	0	0	0	0	105	—	0	—	0
REESE														
Capers	1 tsp (5 g)	0	0	0	0	0	0	—	—	105	—	—	—	—
CARAWAY														
seed	1 tsp	7	tr	tr	0	tr	1	—	14	tr	28	—	—	8
CARDAMON														
ground	1 tsp	6	tr	tr	0	tr	1	—	8	tr	22	—	—	—
CARDOON														
fresh cooked	3½ oz	22	tr	tr	0	1	5	—	72	176	392	2	—	118
raw shredded	½ cup	36	tr	tr	0	1	4	—	62	151	356	2	—	107
CARIBOU														
roasted	3 oz	142	4	1	93	25	0	—	19	51	264	3	4	—
CARISSA														
fresh	1	12	tr	—	0	tr	3	—	2	1	52	8	—	8
CAROB														
carob mix	3 tsp	45	0	0	0	tr	11	—	—	12	—	0	—	—
carob mix as prep w/ whole milk	9 oz	195	8	5	33	8	23	—	291	132	370	2	12	307
flour	1 cup	185	1	tr	0	5	92	—	359	36	852	tr	30	15
flour	1 tbsp	14	tr	tr	0	tr	7	—	28	3	66	0	2	1
CARP														
fresh cooked	3 oz	138	6	1	72	19	0	—	44	54	363	1	—	27
fresh cooked	1 fillet (6 oz)	276	12	2	143	39	0	—	89	107	726	3	—	54
raw	3 oz	108	5	1	56	15	0	—	15	42	283	1	—	25
roe raw	3½ oz	130	2	—	360	24	2	—	—	—	—	14	—	—
CARROT JUICE														
canned	6 oz	73	tr	tr	0	2	17	—	44	54	538	16	7	47381
HAIN														
Juice	6 fl oz	80	0	0	0	1	17	—	60	170	490	—	—	25000
HOLLYWOOD														
Juice	6 fl oz	80	0	0	0	1	17	2	60	170	490	4	—	25000
ODWALLA														
Juice	8 fl oz	70	0	0	0	2	18	2	40	200	—	4	—	10500
CARROTS														
CANNED														
ALLEN														
Sliced	½ cup (4.5 oz)	35	1	0	0	0	8	3	60	230	—	1	—	15500
CREST TOP														
Sliced	½ cup (4.5 oz)	35	1	0	0	0	8	3	60	230	—	1	—	15500
DEL MONTE														
Cut	½ cup (4.3 oz)	35	0	0	0	0	8	3	20	300	—	4	—	15000

FOOD	PORTION	CALORIES	FAT	SAT FAT	CHOL	PROTEIN	CARBO	FIBER	CALCIUM	SOD	POTAS	VIT C	FOLIC	VIT A
DEL MONTE (CONT.)														
Sliced	½ cup (4.3 oz)	35	0	0	0	0	8	3	20	300	—	4	—	15000
GREEN GIANT														
Sliced	½ cup (4.2 oz)	25	0	0	0	tr	6	2	40	380	—	12	—	5000
LESUEUR														
Baby Whole	½ cup (4.2 oz)	35	0	0	0	tr	8	3	40	410	—	0	—	4000
SENECA														
Diced	½ cup	30	0	0	0	1	6	2	20	264	210	2	—	11500
Sliced	½ cup	30	0	0	0	1	6	2	20	264	210	2	—	11500
FRESH														
slices cooked	½ cup	35	tr	tr	0	1	8	—	24	52	177	2	11	19152
DOLE														
Medium	1	40	1	—	0	1	8	1	—	40	311	6	—	16065
FROZEN														
slices cooked	½ cup	26	tr	tr	0	1	6	—	21	43	115	2	8	12922
BIG VALLEY														
Carrots	½ cup (3 oz)	35	0	0	0	tr	8	2	20	40	—	5	—	10000
BIRDS EYE														
Baby Whole	⅔ cup (3 oz)	35	0	0	0	tr	6	2	20	45	—	1	—	5000
FRESH LIKE														
Carrots	3.5 oz	42	tr	—	—	1	10	—	33	42	194	5	—	19856
GREEN GIANT														
Harvest Fresh Baby	⅔ cup (3 oz)	20	0	0	0	0	5	2	20	70	—	0	—	4000
Select Baby Cut	¾ cup (2.8 oz)	30	0	0	0	tr	7	3	20	40	—	0	—	7000
CASABA														
cubed	1 cup	45	tr	—	0	2	11	—	9	20	357	27	—	51
fresh	1/10	43	tr	—	0	1	10	—	8	20	344	26	—	49
CASHEWS														
cashew butter w/o salt	1 tbsp	94	8	2	0	3	4	—	7	2	87	0	11	0
dry roasted	1 oz	163	13	3	0	4	9	—	13	4	160	0	20	0
dry roasted salted	1 oz	163	13	3	0	4	9	—	13	213	160	0	20	0
oil roasted	1 oz	163	14	3	0	5	8	—	12	5	151	0	19	0
oil roasted salted	1 oz	163	14	3	0	5	8	—	12	209	151	0	19	0
BEER NUTS														
Cashews	1 pkg (1 oz)	170	13	—	0	5	8	—	—	65	—	—	—	—
FISHER														
Honey Roasted Halves	1 oz	150	13	3	0	4	7	—	—	—	—	—	—	—
Honey Roasted Whole	1 oz	150	13	3	0	4	7	—	—	90	—	—	—	—
Oil Roasted Halves	1 oz	170	15	3	0	5	8	—	—	160	—	—	—	—
Oil Roasted Whole	1 oz	170	15	3	0	5	8	—	—	140	—	—	—	—
FRITO LAY														
Cashews	1 oz	170	14	—	0	4	9	—	—	115	—	—	—	—

FOOD	PORTION	CALORIES	FAT	SAT FAT	CHOL	PROTEIN	CARBO	FIBER	CALCIUM	SOD	POTAS	VIT C	FOLIC	VIT A
GUY'S														
Whole Salted	1 oz	170	14	—	0	5	5	—	—	140	170	—	—	—
HAIN														
Cashew Butter Raw	2 tbsp	190	15	3	0	6	8	—	0	125	—	0	—	400
Cashew Butter Raw Unsalted	2 tbsp	210	19	3	—	5	8	—	—	170	—	—	—	—
Cashew Butter Toasted	2 tbsp	210	17	3	0	7	7	—	—	190	—	—	—	—
LANCE														
Cashews	1 pkg (32 g)	190	15	3	0	6	8	—	—	95	100	—	—	—
PLANTERS														
Fancy Oil Roasted	1 oz	170	14	3	0	5	8	1	—	120	150	—	—	—
Fancy Oil Roasted	1 pkg (2 oz)	340	29	6	0	9	16	3	20	240	310	—	—	—
Halves Lightly Salted Oil Roasted	1 oz	160	13	3	0	4	9	2	—	55	150	—	—	—
Halves Oil Roasted	1 oz	170	14	3	0	5	8	2	—	120	150	—	—	—
Honey Roasted	1 oz	150	12	2	0	4	11	1	—	120	130	—	—	—
Honey Roasted	1 pkg (2 oz)	310	24	4	0	9	23	3	20	240	270	—	—	—
Munch'N Go Honey Roasted	1 pkg (2 oz)	310	24	4	0	9	23	3	20	240	270	—	—	—
Munch'N Go Singles Oil Roasted	1 pkg (2 oz)	330	28	6	0	10	16	3	60	240	310	—	—	—
Oil Roasted	1 pkg (1 oz)	160	14	3	0	5	8	1	20	120	150	—	—	—
Oil Roasted	1 pkg (1.5 oz)	250	21	4	0	7	12	2	20	240	250	—	—	—
CASSAVA														
raw	3½ oz	120	tr	tr	0	3	27	—	91	8	764	48	—	10
CATFISH														
channel breaded & fried	3 oz	194	11	3	69	15	7	—	37	238	289	0	—	—
channel raw	3 oz	99	4	1	49	15	0	—	34	54	296	—	—	—
CATSUP														
(*see* KETCHUP)														
CAULIFLOWER														
FRESH														
cooked	½ cup (2.2 oz)	14	tr	tr	0	1	3	1	10	9	88	28	27	19
flowerets cooked	3 (2 oz)	12	tr	tr	0	1	2	1	9	8	76	24	24	9
flowerets raw	3 (2 oz)	14	tr	tr	0	1	3	1	12	17	170	26	32	11
green cooked	1½ cup (3.2 oz)	29	tr	tr	0	3	6	3	29	21	250	0	40	127
green raw	1 cup (2.2 oz)	20	tr	tr	0	2	4	2	21	15	192	22	36	97
green raw	1 head 7 in diam (18 oz)	158	2	tr	0	15	31	16	169	118	1533	450	291	777
green raw floweret	1 (0.9 oz)	8	tr	tr	0	1	2	1	8	6	75	22	14	38
raw	½ cup (1.8 oz)	13	tr	tr	0	1	3	1	11	15	151	23	28	10

FOOD	PORTION	CALORIES	FAT	SAT FAT	CHOL	PROTEIN	CARBO	FIBER	CALCIUM	SOD	POTAS	VIT C	FOLIC	VIT A
DOLE														
Cauliflower	⅙ med head	18	0	—	0	2	3	2	—	45	250	53	—	17
FROZEN														
cooked	½ cup	17	tr	tr	0	1	3	—	15	16	125	28	37	20
BIG VALLEY														
Florets	¾ cup (3 oz)	25	0	0	0	2	4	1	20	15	—	42	—	0
BIRDS EYE														
Frzn	⅔ cup	25	0	0	0	2	5	2	20	20	190	48	—	—
In Cheese Sauce	½ cup (4.1 oz)	80	5	2	5	3	7	1	60	630	—	18	—	0
FRESH LIKE														
Cauliflower	3.5 oz	26	tr	—	—	2	5	1	21	48	195	52	—	23
GREEN GIANT														
Cheese Sauce	½ cup (3.5 oz)	60	3	1	<5	2	8	2	60	510	—	18	—	1000
Florets	1 cup (2.8 oz)	25	0	0	0	2	4	2	0	25	—	24	—	0
JARRED														
VLASIC														
Hot & Spicy	1 oz	4	0	0	0	0	1	—	—	435	—	—	—	—
Sweet	1 oz	35	0	0	0	0	9	—	tr	225	—	—	—	—
CAVIAR														
black	1 oz	71	5	—	165	7	1	—	—	420	—	—	—	—
black	1 tbsp	40	3	—	94	4	1	—	—	240	—	—	—	—
red	1 tbsp	40	3	—	94	4	1	—	—	240	—	—	—	—
red	1 oz	71	5	—	165	7	1	—	—	420	—	—	—	—
CELERIAC														
fresh cooked	3½ oz	25	tr	—	0	1	6	—	26	61	173	4	—	0
raw	½ cup	31	tr	—	0	1	7	—	34	78	234	6	—	0
CELERY														
DRIED														
seed	1 tsp	8	tr	tr	0	tr	1	—	35	3	28	—	—	1
FRESH														
DOLE														
Stalks	2 med	20	0	—	0	1	2	4	—	140	355	9	—	156
FROZEN														
FRESH LIKE														
Celery	3.5 oz	14	tr	—	—	1	3	1	31	88	239	6	—	230
CELTUCE														
raw	3½ oz	22	tr	—	0	1	4	—	39	11	330	20	—	3500
CEREAL														
bran flakes	¾ cup (1 oz)	90	1	tr	0	4	22	—	14	264	180	0	—	1250
corn flakes	1¼ cup (1 oz)	110	tr	tr	0	2	24	—	1	351	26	15	—	1250
farina	¾ cup	87	tr	tr	0	3	19	3	3	1	22	—	4	—
farina not prep	1 tbsp	40	0	0	0	1	9	tr	2	0	10	—	3	—
oatmeal	1 cup	145	2	tr	0	6	25	—	20	1	132	—	9	38
oatmeal instant cooked w/o salt	1 cup	145	2	tr	0	6	25	—	19	2	131	0	—	40

FOOD	PORTION	CALORIES	FAT	SAT FAT	CHOL	PROTEIN	CARBO	FIBER	CALCIUM	SOD	POTAS	VIT C	FOLIC	VIT A
oatmeal not prep	1 cup	311	5	tr	0	13	54	9	42	3	284	—	26	82
oatmeal quick cooked w/o salt	1 cup	145	2	tr	0	6	25	—	19	2	131	0	—	40
oatmeal regular cooked w/o salt	1 cup	145	2	tr	0	6	25	—	19	2	131	0	—	40
sugar-coated corn flakes	¾ cup (1 oz)	110	1	tr	0	1	26	—	1	230	18	15	—	1250
ALBERS														
Hominy Quick Grits uncooked	¼ cup	140	1	—	0	3	31	1	—	0	—	—	—	—
ARROWHEAD														
4 Grain + Flax	¼ cup (1.6 oz)	150	2	0	0	6	28	6	20	0	190	0	—	0
7 Grain	⅓ cup (1.4 oz)	140	2	0	0	6	25	5	40	0	140	0	—	0
Amaranth Flakes	1 cup (1.2 oz)	130	2	0	0	4	25	3	0	0	210	0	—	0
Apple Corns	1 cup (1.5 oz)	150	2	0	0	3	35	4	0	110	75	0	—	0
Bear Mush	¼ cup (1.6 oz)	160	1	0	0	5	33	2	150	0	40	0	—	0
Bran Flakes	1 cup (1 oz)	100	1	0	0	5	22	4	0	80	105	0	—	0
Kamut Flakes	1 cup (1.1 oz)	120	1	0	0	4	25	3	0	65	190	0	—	0
Maple Corns	1 cup (1.9 oz)	190	3	1	0	5	43	6	20	140	105	0	—	0
Multi Grain Flakes	1 cup (1.2 oz)	140	2	0	0	33	29	3	20	130	110	0	—	0
Nature O's	1 cup (1.1 oz)	130	2	1	0	4	24	3	0	5	120	0	—	0
Oat Bran Flakes	1 cup (1.2 oz)	110	2	1	0	6	22	4	0	60	120	0	—	0
Oat Flakes Rolled	⅓ cup (1.2 oz)	130	3	1	0	5	23	4	20	0	120	0	—	0
Oat Groats	¼ cup (1.5 oz)	160	3	1	0	6	29	4	20	0	150	0	—	0
Oatmeal Instant Original	1 oz	100	0	—	—	3	22	—	—	15	70	—	—	—
Puffed Corn	1 cup (0.8 oz)	80	0	0	0	3	16	1	0	0	70	0	—	0
Puffed Kamut	1 cup (0.6 oz)	50	0	0	0	2	11	2	0	0	70	0	—	0
Puffed Millet	1 cup (0.9 oz)	90	1	0	0	3	19	1	0	0	70	0	—	0
Puffed Rice	1 cup (0.8 oz)	90	0	0	0	2	19	1	0	0	70	0	—	0
Puffed Wheat	1 cup (0.9)	90	1	0	0	3	20	2	0	0	105	0	—	0
Rice & Shine	¼ cup (1.5 oz)	150	1	0	0	3	32	2	0	0	90	0	—	0
Spelt Flakes	1 cup (1.1 oz)	100	1	0	0	5	22	3	0	60	140	0	—	0
Wheat Flakes Rolled	⅓ cup (1.2 oz)	110	1	0	0	4	24	5	20	0	125	0	—	0
BARBARA'S														
Apple Cinnamon Toasted O's	¾ cup	110	1	0	0	3	24	2	—	90	—	—	—	—
Bite Size Shredded Oats	1¼ cups (2 oz)	220	3	1	0	6	46	6	—	260	—	—	—	—
Breakfast O's	1 cup (1 oz)	120	2	0	0	5	22	3	—	115	—	—	—	—
Brown Rice Crisps	1 cup (1 oz)	120	1	0	0	2	25	1	—	125	—	—	—	—
Cocoa Crunch Stars	1 cup (1 oz)	110	1	0	0	2	26	1	—	140	—	—	—	—
Corn Flakes	1 cup (1 oz)	110	0	0	0	2	26	2	—	130	—	—	—	—
Frosted Corn Flakes	1 cup (1 oz)	110	0	0	0	2	27	4	—	100	—	—	—	—

FOOD	PORTION	CALORIES	FAT	SAT FAT	CHOL	PROTEIN	CARBO	FIBER	CALCIUM	SOD	POTAS	VIT C	FOLIC	VIT A
BARBARA'S (CONT.)														
Honey Crunch Stars	1 cup (1 oz)	110	0	0	0	2	26	2	—	50	—	—	—	—
Honey Nut Toasted O's	¾ cup	120	2	1	0	2	23	2	—	90	—	—	—	—
Organic Ultra Minis Frosted	¾ cup (1.9 oz)	190	1	0	0	4	46	7	—	200	—	—	—	—
Organic Ultra Minis Original	¾ cup (1.9 oz)	190	1	0	0	5	45	8	—	240	—	—	—	—
Organic Fruity Punch	1 cup (1 oz)	110	1	0	0	2	26	0	—	120	—	—	—	—
Puffins	¾ cup (0.9 oz)	90	1	0	0	2	23	5	—	150	—	—	—	—
Shredded Spoonfuls	¾ cup (1.1 oz)	120	2	0	0	5	23	4	—	200	—	—	—	—
Shredded Wheat	2 biscuits (1.4 oz)	140	1	0	0	4	31	5	—	0	—	—	—	—
BETTY CROCKER														
Dutch Apple	1 cup (1.9 oz)	220	2	0	0	4	47	1	40	330	90	15	100	750
Streusel	¾ cup (1 oz)	120	2	0	0	2	25	1	20	170	60	15	100	750
ESTEE														
Corn Flakes	1 pkg (1 oz)	90	0	0	0	2	24	4	0	310	50	15	100	1250
Raisin Bran	1 pkg (1 oz)	90	1	0	0	4	21	3	0	100	210	0	60	750
GENERAL MILLS														
Apple Cinnamon Cheerios	¾ cup (1 oz)	120	2	0	0	2	25	1	20	160	65	6	100	500
Basic 4	1 cup (1.9 oz)	200	2	0	0	4	43	3	250	320	160	0	100	1250
Berry Berry Kix	¾ cup (1 oz)	120	2	0	0	1	26	0	40	180	25	15	100	750
Body Buddies Natural Fruit	1 cup (1 oz)	120	2	0	0	2	26	0	40	290	30	15	100	750
Booberry	1 cup (1 oz)	120	1	0	0	1	27	0	20	220	15	15	100	0
Cheerios	1 cup (1 oz)	110	2	0	0	3	22	3	40	280	95	15	100	1250
Cinnamon Grahams	¾ cup (1 oz)	120	1	0	0	1	26	1	0	240	45	15	100	750
Cinnamon Toast Crunch	¾ cup (1 oz)	130	4	1	0	1	24	1	40	210	45	15	100	750
Cocoa Puffs	1 cup (1 oz)	120	1	0	0	1	27	0	20	190	55	15	100	0
Cookie Crisp	1 cup (1 oz)	120	2	0	0	1	25	0	0	115	40	0	100	0
Corn Chex	1 cup (1 oz)	110	0	0	0	2	26	0	0	300	30	6	100	0
Count Chocula	1 cup (1 oz)	120	1	0	0	1	26	0	20	180	50	15	100	0
Country Corn Flakes	1 cup (1 oz)	120	1	0	0	2	26	0	40	290	35	15	100	750
Crispy Wheaties 'n Raisins	1 cup (1.9 oz)	190	1	0	0	4	44	4	40	270	220	0	100	1250
Fiber One	½ cup (1 oz)	60	1	0	0	2	24	13	40	135	250	0	100	1250
Frankenberry	1 cup (1 oz)	120	1	0	0	1	27	0	20	210	15	15	100	0
French Toast Crunch	¾ cup (1 oz)	120	2	0	0	1	26	0	60	170	20	15	100	750

GENERAL MILLS (CONT.)

FOOD	PORTION	CALORIES	FAT	SAT FAT	CHOL	PROTEIN	CARBO	FIBER	CALCIUM	SOD	POTAS	VIT C	FOLIC	VIT A
Frosted Cheerios	1 cup (1 oz)	120	1	0	0	2	25	1	20	210	60	15	100	750
Golden Grahams	¾ cup (1 oz)	120	1	0	0	1	25	1	0	280	55	15	100	750
Honey Frosted Wheaties	¾ cup (1 oz)	110	1	0	0	1	27	0	20	200	35	15	100	750
Honey Nut Cheerios	1 cup (1 oz)	120	2	0	0	3	24	2	40	270	95	9	100	0
Honey Nut Clusters	1 cup (1.9 oz)	210	3	0	0	4	46	3	40	270	130	9	100	0
Jurassic Park Crunch	1 cup (1 oz)	120	1	0	0	2	26	1	20	200	50	15	100	750
Kaboom	1¼ cup (1 oz)	120	2	0	0	3	24	1	40	280	65	15	100	750
Kix	1⅓ cup (1 oz)	120	1	0	0	2	26	1	40	270	45	15	100	1250
Lucky Charms	1 cup (1 oz)	120	1	0	0	2	25	1	20	210	60	15	100	750
Multi-Bran Chex	1 cup (2 oz)	200	2	0	0	4	49	7	0	360	230	6	100	0
Multi-Grain Cheerios	1 cup (1 oz)	110	1	0	0	3	24	3	100	210	85	60	400	1250
Oatmeal Crisp Almond	1 cup (1.9 oz)	220	5	1	0	6	42	4	20	250	190	9	100	0
Oatmeal Crisp Apple Cinnamon	1 cup (1.9 oz)	210	2	0	0	4	46	4	20	280	160	9	100	0
Oatmeal Crisp Raisin	1 cup (1.9 oz)	210	3	0	0	4	44	3	20	210	220	0	100	750
Raisin Nut Bran	¾ cup (1.9 oz)	200	4	1	0	4	41	5	60	250	220	0	100	0
Reese's Peanut Butter Puffs	¾ cup (1 oz)	130	3	1	0	2	24	0	20	210	45	15	100	750
Rice Chex	1¼ cup (1.1 oz)	120	0	0	0	2	27	0	0	280	35	6	100	0
S'Mores Grahams	¾ cup (1 oz)	120	1	0	0	1	26	0	0	370	130	15	100	750
Sun Crunchers	1 cup (1.9 oz)	220	3	0	0	5	45	2	80	370	130	15	100	750
Team Cheerios	1 cup (1 oz)	120	1	0	0	2	25	1	20	220	65	15	100	750
Total Corn Flakes	1⅓ cup (1 oz)	110	1	0	0	2	25	0	200	210	30	60	400	1250
Total Raisin Bran	1 cup (1.9 oz)	180	1	0	0	4	43	5	200	240	280	0	400	1250
Total Whole Grain	¾ cup (1 oz)	110	1	0	0	3	24	3	250	200	100	60	400	1250
Trix	1 cup (1 oz)	120	2	0	0	1	26	1	20	200	20	15	100	750
Wheat Chex	1 cup (1.9 oz)	180	1	0	0	5	41	5	0	420	200	6	100	0
Wheat Hearts not prep	¼ cup (1.3 oz)	130	1	0	0	5	26	2	0	0	130	0	—	0
Wheaties	1 cup (1 oz)	110	1	0	0	3	24	3	0	220	110	15	100	1250

GLENNY'S

FOOD	PORTION	CALORIES	FAT	SAT FAT	CHOL	PROTEIN	CARBO	FIBER	CALCIUM	SOD	POTAS	VIT C	FOLIC	VIT A
Maple Frosted Corn	1 oz	109	tr	—	—	4	20	—	—	50	—	—	—	—
Oat Mini Puffs	1 oz	108	tr	—	—	5	22	—	—	30	—	—	—	—
Oat Mini Puffs No Salt No Sugar	1 oz	108	tr	—	—	5	22	—	—	7	—	—	—	—
Rice Mini Puffs	1 oz	109	tr	—	—	4	20	—	—	30	—	—	—	—

FOOD	PORTION	CALORIES	FAT	SAT FAT	CHOL	PROTEIN	CARBO	FIBER	CALCIUM	SOD	POTAS	VIT C	FOLIC	VIT A
GOOD SHEPHERD														
Millet Rice Flakes Wheat Free	1 oz	95	1	—	0	3	19	1	—	30	160	—	—	—
Spelt	1 oz	90	tr	—	0	4	20	3	—	0	110	—	—	—
Spelt Flakes	1 oz	100	6	—	0	3	21	2	—	80	106	—	—	—
GRIST MILL														
Apple Cinnamon Natural	½ cup (1.9 oz)	260	10	2	0	6	36	3	60	20	—	0	—	0
Bran	½ cup (1.9 oz)	250	8	6	0	7	37	11	60	40	380	9	—	2000
Oat & Honey Natural	½ cup (1.9 oz)	270	12	3	0	7	34	4	60	10	—	0	—	0
Oat Honey & Raisin Natural	½ cup (1.9 oz)	260	10	2	0	6	35	4	40	10	—	0	—	0
H-O														
Farina Instant	1 pkg	110	0	0	0	3	22	3	—	235	100	—	—	—
Farina not prep	3 tbsp	120	0	0	0	3	26	3	—	0	100	—	—	—
Oatmeal Instant	½ cup	130	2	0	0	5	22	3	—	<5	100	—	—	—
Oatmeal Instant	1 pkg	110	2	0	0	4	18	3	20	230	100	—	—	—
Oatmeal Instant Apple Cinnamon	1 pkg	130	2	0	0	4	26	3	20	220	95	—	—	—
Oatmeal Instant Maple Brown Sugar	1 pkg	160	2	0	0	4	32	3	20	285	110	—	—	—
Oatmeal Instant Raisin & Spice	1 pkg	150	2	0	0	4	32	3	20	140	140	—	—	—
Oatmeal Instant Sweet 'n Mellow	1 pkg	150	2	0	0	4	30	3	20	270	110	—	—	—
Oats 'n Fiber	⅓ cup	100	2	0	0	5	15	3	—	5	100	—	—	—
Oats 'n Fiber	1 pkg	110	2	0	0	5	18	3	20	140	100	—	—	—
Oats 'n Fiber Apple & Bran	1 pkg	130	2	0	0	4	26	3	20	140	100	—	—	—
Oats 'n Fiber Raisin & Bran	1 pkg	150	2	0	0	4	32	3	20	140	100	—	—	—
Oats Gourmet	⅓ cup	100	2	0	0	3	18	3	—	0	110	—	—	—
Oats Quick	½ cup	130	2	0	0	5	22	3	—	<5	100	—	—	—
HEALTH VALLEY														
100% Natural Bran With Apples & Cinnamon	¼ cup (1 oz)	100	1	—	0	3	22	5	13	10	80	1	11	tr
Amaranth Cereal With Bananas	½ cup (1 oz)	110	2	—	0	4	20	4	29	5	110	1	4	160
Amaranth Crunch With Raisins	¼ cup (1 oz)	110	3	—	0	3	20	3	20	10	100	tr	13	7
Amaranth Flakes 100% Organic	½ cup (1 oz)	90	tr	—	0	3	21	3	50	5	65	1	3	26
Blue Corn Flakes 100% Organic	½ cup (1 oz)	90	tr	—	0	3	19	3	2	10	80	0	tr	203

FOOD	PORTION	CALORIES	FAT	SAT FAT	CHOL	PROTEIN	CARBO	FIBER	CALCIUM	SOD	POTAS	VIT C	FOLIC	VIT A
HEALTH VALLEY (CONT.)														
Bran Cereal With Dates 100% Organic	¼ cup (1 oz)	100	1	—	0	4	20	5	13	5	100	1	18	0
Bran Cereal With Raisins 100% Organic	¼ cup (1 oz)	100	1	—	0	4	20	5	13	5	100	1	18	0
Fiber 7 Flakes 100% Organic	½ cup (1 oz)	90	tr	—	0	3	20	5	2	0	95	1	17	73
Fiber 7 Flakes With Raisins 100% Organic	½ cup (1 oz)	90	tr	—	0	3	20	5	2	0	95	1	17	73
Fruit & Fitness	1 cup (2 oz)	220	4	—	0	9	37	11	56	5	460	—	—	333
Fruit Lites Corn	½ cup (0.5 oz)	45	0	0	0	2	10	tr	21	2	50	tr	2	40
Fruit Lites Rice	½ cup (0.5 oz)	45	1	—	0	1	11	tr	22	2	65	1	tr	1
Fruit Lites Wheat	½ cup (0.5 oz)	45	1	—	0	1	11	2	6	2	90	tr	5	1
Healthy Crunch Almond Date	¼ cup (1 oz)	110	3	—	0	4	18	4	13	5	70	3	18	1
Healthy Crunch Apple Cinnamon	¼ cup (1 oz)	110	3	—	0	4	18	4	14	10	70	3	17	tr
Healthy O's 100% Organic	¾ cup (1 oz)	90	1	—	0	3	18	3	15	1	90	1	11	1
Lites Puffed Corn	½ cup (1 oz)	50	0	0	0	3	11	tr	2	0	35	tr	3	72
Lites Puffed Rice	½ cup (1 oz)	50	0	0	0	1	12	tr	5	0	45	1	0	0
Lites Puffed Wheat	½ cup (1 oz)	50	0	0	0	2	11	1	7	0	75	1	8	0
Oat Bran Flakes 100% Organic	½ cup (1 oz)	100	tr	—	0	3	20	4	11	0	105	tr	13	5
Oat Bran Flakes Almonds/Dates 100% Organic	½ cup (1 oz)	100	tr	—	0	3	20	4	20	0	105	tr	—	8
Oat Bran Flakes With Raisins 100% Organic	½ cup (1 oz)	100	tr	—	0	3	20	4	17	0	105	tr	12	8
Oat Bran Natural Apples & Cinnamon	¼ cup (1 oz)	100	tr	—	0	3	19	4	16	10	100	tr	24	tr
Oat Bran Natural Raisins & Spice	¼ cup	100	tr	—	0	3	19	4	16	10	100	1	24	tr
Oat Bran O's 100% Organic	½ cup (1 oz)	110	tr	—	0	3	20	3	12	0	115	1	23	10
Oat Bran O's Fruit & Nuts	½ cup (1 oz)	110	3	—	0	3	19	3	21	0	130	1	21	40
Orangeola Almonds & Dates	¼ cup	110	3	—	0	3	18	4	25	5	60	2	21	3
Orangeola Bananas & Hawaiian Fruit	¼ cup (1 oz)	120	4	—	0	3	20	4	32	10	80	2	20	200
Raisin Bran Flakes 100% Organic	½ cup (1 oz)	100	tr	—	0	3	21	6	19	5	110	1	32	tr

FOOD	PORTION	CALORIES	FAT	SAT FAT	CHOL	PROTEIN	CARBO	FIBER	CALCIUM	SOD	POTAS	VIT C	FOLIC	VIT A
HEALTH VALLEY (CONT.)														
Real Oat Bran Almond Crunch	¼ cup (1 oz)	110	3	—	0	5	17	4	14	2	150	2	20	277
Real Oat Bran Hawaiian Fruit	¼ cup (1 oz)	130	3	—	0	5	22	5	26	2	240	2	22	494
Real Oat Bran Raisin Nut	¼ cup (1 oz)	130	3	—	0	5	21	5	14	2	190	2	20	144
Rice Bran O's	½ cup	110	1	—	0	2	22	2	11	5	180	1	tr	8
Rice Bran With Almonds & Dates	½ cup (1 oz)	110	3	—	0	2	19	2	17	2	130	2	1	4
Sprouts 7 Bananas & Hawaiian Fruit	¼ cup (1 oz)	90	1	—	0	3	16	4	15	5	170	1	4	65
Sprouts 7 Raisin	¼ cup	90	1	—	0	4	16	5	1	5	170	1	4	97
Swiss Breakfast Raisin Nut	¼ cup (1 oz)	100	3	—	0	4	19	3	1	10	60	1	15	1
Swiss Breakfast Tropical Fruit	¼ cup (1 oz)	100	3	—	0	3	19	3	1	10	60	1	17	2
HEALTHY CHOICE														
Multi-Grain Flakes	1 cup (1.1 oz)	100	0	0	0	3	26	3	0	210	—	0	—	500
Multi-Grain Raisins & Almonds	1¼ cup (2 oz)	200	2	0	0	4	44	4	20	240	—	0	—	500
Multi-Grain Squares	1¼ cup (2 oz)	190	1	0	0	5	45	6	0	0	—	0	—	500
HEARTLAND														
Coconut	1 oz	130	5	—	0	3	18	2	—	80	103	—	—	—
Plain	1 oz	130	4	—	0	3	18	2	—	80	101	—	—	—
Raisin	1 oz	130	4	—	0	3	18	2	—	80	113	—	—	—
KELLOGG'S														
All-Bran	½ cup (1 oz)	80	1	0	0	4	22	10	100	280	340	15	100	750
All-Bran With Extra Fiber	½ cup (1 oz)	50	1	0	0	4	22	15	100	150	350	15	100	750
Apple Cinnamon Rice Krispies	¾ cup (1 oz)	110	0	0	0	2	27	1	0	220	25	15	100	750
Apple Cinnamon Squares	¾ cup (1.9 oz)	180	1	0	0	4	44	0	20	15	170	0	100	0
Apple Jacks	1 cup (1 oz)	110	0	0	0	2	26	1	0	135	30	15	100	750
Apple Raisin Crisp	1 cup (1.9 oz)	180	0	0	0	3	46	4	0	340	160	0	100	750
Blueberry Squares	¾ cup (1.9 oz)	180	1	0	0	4	44	5	0	15	160	0	100	0
Bran Buds	⅓ cup (1 oz)	70	1	0	0	3	24	11	20	210	320	15	100	750
Cinnamon Mini Buns	¾ cup (1 oz)	120	1	0	0	1	27	1	0	210	35	15	100	750
Cocoa Krispies	¾ cup (1 oz)	120	1	0	0	2	27	0	0	190	25	15	100	750
Common Sense Oat Bran	¾ cup (1 oz)	110	1	0	0	4	23	4	0	270	135	0	100	750
Complete Bran Flakes	¾ cup (1 oz)	100	1	0	0	3	25	5	0	230	180	15	100	750

FOOD	PORTION	CALORIES	FAT	SAT FAT	CHOL	PROTEIN	CARBO	FIBER	CALCIUM	SOD	POTAS	VIT C	FOLIC	VIT A
KELLOGG'S (CONT.)														
Corn Flakes	1 cup (1 oz)	110	0	0	0	2	26	1	0	330	35	15	100	750
Corn Pops	1 cup (1 oz)	110	0	0	0	1	27	1	0	95	20	15	100	750
Cracklin' Oat Bran	¾ cup (1.9 oz)	230	8	3	0	4	40	6	20	180	240	15	100	750
Crispix	1 cup (1 oz)	110	0	0	0	2	26	1	0	230	35	15	100	750
Double Dip Crunch	¾ cup (1 oz)	110	0	0	0	2	27	0	0	160	20	15	100	750
Froot Loops	1 cup (1 oz)	120	1	1	0	1	26	1	0	150	30	15	100	750
Frosted Bran	¾ cup (1 oz)	100	0	0	0	2	26	3	0	200	120	15	100	750
Frosted Flakes	¾ cup (1 oz)	120	0	0	0	1	28	0	0	200	20	15	100	750
Frosted Krispies	¾ cup (1 oz)	110	0	0	0	1	27	0	0	230	30	15	100	750
Frosted Mini-Wheats	1 cup (1.9 oz)	190	1	0	0	5	45	6	0	0	160	0	100	0
Frosted Mini-Wheats Bite Size	1 cup (1.9 oz)	190	1	0	0	5	45	6	0	0	160	0	100	0
Fruitful Bran	1¼ cup (1.9 oz)	170	1	0	0	4	44	6	20	330	260	0	100	750
Fruity Marshmallow Krispies	¾ cups (1 oz)	110	0	0	0	1	27	0	0	180	20	15	100	750
Just Right Crunchy Nuggets	1 cup (1.9 oz)	200	2	0	0	4	46	3	0	340	120	0	100	1250
Just Right Fruit & Nut	1 cup (1.9 oz)	210	2	0	0	4	46	3	0	260	140	0	100	1250
Mueslix Golden Crunch	¾ cup (1.9 oz)	210	5	1	0	6	40	6	40	280	190	0	100	750
Nut & Honey Crunch	1¼ cup (1.9 oz)	220	4	1	0	4	45	1	0	370	75	15	100	750
Oatbake Raisin Nut	⅓ cup (1 oz)	110	3	1	0	2	21	3	—	190	110	15	100	750
Pop-Tart Crunch Frosted Brown Sugar Cinnamon	¾ cup (1 oz)	120	1	0	0	1	26	0	0	160	40	15	100	750
Pop-Tart Crunch Frosted Strawberry	¾ cup (1 oz)	120	1	0	0	1	27	0	0	125	35	0	100	750
Product 19	1 cup (1 oz)	110	0	0	0	3	25	1	0	280	40	60	400	750
Raisin Bran	1 cup (1.9 oz)	170	1	0	0	5	43	7	40	310	400	0	100	750
Raisin Squares	¾ cup (1.9 oz)	180	1	0	0	4	44	5	0	0	210	0	100	0
Rice Krispies	1¼ cup (1 oz)	110	0	0	0	2	26	1	0	320	35	15	100	750
Smart Start	1 cup (1.8 oz)	180	1	0	0	3	43	2	0	310	100	15	400	750
Special K	1 cup (1 oz)	110	0	0	0	6	21	1	0	250	55	15	100	750
Strawberry Squares	¾ cup (1.9 oz)	180	1	0	0	4	44	5	20	10	170	0	100	0
Temptations French Vanilla Almond	¾ cup (1 oz)	120	2	1	0	2	24	1	0	210	45	15	100	750
Temptations Honey Roasted Pecan	1 cup (1 oz)	120	3	0	0	2	24	0	0	240	30	15	100	750

FOOD	PORTION	CALORIES	FAT	SAT FAT	CHOL	PROTEIN	CARBO	FIBER	CALCIUM	SOD	POTAS	VIT C	FOLIC	VIT A
KOLLN														
Crispy Oats	1 cup (1.8 oz)	190	3	1	0	5	40	2	20	210	—	0	—	0
Oat Bran Crunch	⅔ cup (2.1 oz)	220	5	1	0	10	41	9	60	0	—	0	—	500
Oat Muesli Fruit	¾ cup (2 oz)	200	5	1	0	6	39	4	20	15	—	0	—	0
LITTLE CROW														
Coco Wheat	3 tbsp (36 g)	130	1	—	0	4	28	4	—	12	42	6	—	—
MALTEX														
Cereal	1 oz	105	1	tr	0	3	21	3	—	0	105	—	—	—
MAYPO														
30 Second	1 oz	100	1	tr	0	4	19	2	80	0	95	18	—	1500
Vermont Style	1 oz	105	1	tr	0	4	20	2	80	0	95	18	—	1500
With Oat Bran	1 oz	130	2	tr	0	5	26	4	100	1	130	24	—	2000
MCCANN'S														
Irish Oatmeal	1 oz	110	2	—	0	5	20	3	20	0	105	—	—	—
MORNING TRADITIONS														
Banana Nut Crunch	1 cup (2 oz)	250	6	1	0	5	43	4	0	240	170	0	100	750
Blueberry Morning	1¼ cup (1.9 oz)	220	3	1	0	4	43	2	20	250	95	0	100	750
Cranberry Almond Crunch	1 cup (1.9 oz)	220	3	0	0	4	44	3	0	200	100	0	100	750
Great Grains Crunchy Pecan	⅔ cup (1.9 oz)	220	6	1	0	5	38	4	0	190	150	0	100	750
Great Grains Raisins Dates & Pecans	⅔ cup (1.9 oz)	210	5	1	0	4	39	4	0	160	120	0	120	750
MOTHER'S														
Oatmeal Instant	½ cup (1.4 oz)	150	3	1	0	5	27	4	0	0	150	—	8	0
Whole Wheat Natural	½ cup (1.4 oz)	130	1	0	0	5	30	4	0	0	170	—	16	0
MUESLIX														
Crispy Blend	⅔ cup (1.9 oz)	200	2	0	0	4	42	4	20	190	200	0	100	200
NABISCO														
100% Bran	⅓ cup (1 oz)	80	1	0	0	4	23	8	20	120	270	0	100	750
Cream Of Rice	1 oz	100	0	0	0	2	23	—	—	0	—	—	—	—
Cream Of Wheat Instant as prep	1 cup	120	0	—	—	3	25	1	100	0	—	0	—	0
Cream Of Wheat Quick as prep	1 cup	120	0	—	—	3	25	1	100	—	—	0	—	0
Cream Of Wheat Regular as prep	1 cup	120	0	—	—	3	25	1	100	0	—	0	—	0
Frosted Shredded Wheat Bite Size	1 cup (1.8 oz)	190	1	0	0	4	44	5	0	10	170	0	100	0
Honey Nut Shredded Wheat Bite Size	1 cup (1.8 oz)	200	2	0	0	5	43	4	0	40	200	0	100	0

FOOD	PORTION	CALORIES	FAT	SAT FAT	CHOL	PROTEIN	CARBO	FIBER	CALCIUM	SOD	POTAS	VIT C	FOLIC	VIT A
NABISCO (CONT.)														
Mix'n Eat Cream Of Wheat Apple & Cinnamon	1 pkg (1¼ oz)	130	0	0	0	2	29	1	40	250	45	—	—	1250
Mix'n Eat Cream Of Wheat Brown Sugar Cinnamon	1 pkg (1¼ oz)	130	0	0	0	2	29	1	40	230	65	—	—	1250
Mix'n Eat Cream Of Wheat Maple Brown Sugar	1 pkg (1¼ oz)	130	0	0	0	2	29	1	40	180	40	—	—	1250
Mix'n Eat Cream Of Wheat Our Original	1 pkg (1¼ oz)	100	0	0	0	3	21	1	40	170	30	—	—	1250
Original Shredded Wheat	2 biscuits (1.6 oz)	160	1	0	0	5	38	5	20	0	200	0	16	0
Original Shredded Wheat 'N Bran	1¼ cup (2.1 oz)	200	1	0	0	7	47	8	20	0	250	0	24	0
Original Shredded Wheat Spoon Size	1 cup (1.7 oz)	170	1	0	0	5	41	5	20	0	200	0	16	0
NUT & HONEY														
Crunch O's	¾ cup (1 oz)	120	3	0	0	3	23	2	0	200	70	15	100	750
NUTRI-GRAIN														
Almond Raisin	1¼ cup (2 oz)	200	3	0	0	4	43	4	150	200	200	0	100	0
Golden Wheat	¾ cup (1.1 oz)	100	1	0	0	3	24	4	0	220	110	0	100	0
Golden Wheat & Raisin	1¼ cup (2 oz)	180	1	0	0	4	45	6	20	280	240	0	100	0
POST														
Alpha-Bits	1 cup (1 oz)	130	2	0	0	3	27	1	0	210	60	0	100	750
Bran Flakes	¾ cup (1 oz)	100	1	0	0	3	24	5	0	220	190	0	100	750
Cocoa Pebbles	¾ cup (1 oz)	120	1	1	0	1	26	0	0	160	40	0	100	750
Fruit & Fibre Dates Raisins & Walnuts	1 cup (1.9 oz)	210	3	1	0	4	42	5	20	250	250	0	120	750
Fruit & Fibre Peaches Raisins & Almonds	1 cup (1.9 oz)	210	3	1	0	4	42	5	20	260	260	0	120	750
Fruity Pebbles	¾ cup (1 oz)	110	1	0	0	tr	24	0	0	160	30	0	100	750
Golden Crisp	¾ cup (1 oz)	110	0	0	0	1	25	0	0	40	35	0	100	750
Grape-Nuts	½ cup (2 oz)	200	1	0	0	6	47	5	20	350	160	0	100	750
Grape-Nuts	¾ cup (1 oz)	100	1	0	0	3	24	3	0	140	80	0	100	750
Honey Bunches Of Oats	¾ cup (1 oz)	120	2	1	0	2	25	1	0	190	50	0	100	750
Honey Bunches Of Oats With Almonds	¾ cup (1.1 oz)	130	3	1	0	3	24	1	0	180	65	0	100	750
Honeycomb	1⅓ cups (1 oz)	110	1	0	0	2	26	tr	0	220	35	0	100	750
Marshmallow Alpha-Bits	1 cup (1 oz)	120	1	0	0	2	25	0	0	160	30	0	100	750

FOOD	PORTION	CALORIES	FAT	SAT FAT	CHOL	PROTEIN	CARBO	FIBER	CALCIUM	SOD	POTAS	VIT C	FOLIC	VIT A
POST (CONT.)														
Post Toasties	1 cup (1 oz)	100	0	0	0	2	24	1	0	270	30	0	100	750
Raisin Bran	1 cup (2 oz)	190	1	0	0	4	47	8	20	300	340	0	140	750
Waffle Crisp	1 cup (1 oz)	130	3	0	0	2	24	0	0	120	35	0	100	750
Waffle Crisp	1 cup (1 oz)	130	3	0	0	2	24	0	0	120	35	0	100	750
PRITIKIN														
Apple Raisin Spice	1 pkg (1.6 oz)	170	3	1	0	—	34	—	—	5	200	—	—	—
Multigrain	1 pkg	160	2	0	0	—	33	—	—	0	180	—	—	—
QUAKER														
Instant Grits Original	1 pkg (1 oz)	100	0	0	0	2	22	1		300	—	—	40	—
Multigrain	½ cup	130	2	0	0	5	29	5	0	10	160	—	8	0
Oatmeal Instant	1 pkg (1.2 oz)	130	3	1	0	5	22	3	250	95	125	—	140	1500
Oatmeal Instant Apples & Cinnamon	1 pkg (1.2 oz)	130	2	1	0	4	26	3	150	105	110	—	80	750
Oatmeal Instant Cinnamon Graham Cookie	1 pkg (1.4 oz)	150	3	1	0	4	30	3	150	170	105	—	100	1250
Oatmeal Instant Cinnamon Spice	1 pkg (1.6 oz)	170	2	0	0	4	36	3	150	290	115	—	120	1000
Oatmeal Instant Cinnamon Toast	1 pkg (1.2 oz)	130	2	0	0	3	27	2	150	160	90	—	100	1000
Oatmeal Instant Fruit & Cream Blueberry	1 pkg (1.2 oz)	130	3	1	0	3	27	2	100	140	110	—	100	1000
Oatmeal Instant Honey Nut	1 pkg (1.2 oz)	130	3	1	0	3	25	2	100	210	100	—	80	1000
Oatmeal Instant Kids Choice Radical Raspberry	1 pkg (1.4 oz)	150	3	1	0	4	29	3	150	170	115	—	100	1250
Oatmeal Instant Maple Brown Sugar	1 pkg (1.5 oz)	160	2	1	0	4	33	3	190	240	115	—	100	1000
Oatmeal Instant Peaches & Cream	1 pkg (1.2 oz)	130	2	1	0	3	27	2	100	150	125	—	100	1000
Oatmeal Instant Raisin & Walnut	1 pkg (1.3 oz)	140	3	1	0	3	27	3	150	160	130	—	80	1000
Oatmeal Instant Raisin Date Walnut	1 pkg (1.3 oz)	130	3	1	0	3	27	3	150	240	130	—	80	1000
Oatmeal Instant Raisin Spice	1 pkg (1.5 oz)	160	2	1	0	5	32	3	150	250	160	—	100	1000
Oatmeal Instant Strawberries & Cream	1 pkg (1.2 oz)	130	2	1	0	3	27	2	150	160	135	—	80	750
Oatmeal Instant Strawberries 'N Stuff	1 pkg (1.4 oz)	150	2	1	0	3	30	3	150	170	115	—	100	1250

FOOD	PORTION	CALORIES	FAT	SAT FAT	CHOL	PROTEIN	CARBO	FIBER	CALCIUM	SOD	POTAS	VIT C	FOLIC	VIT A
QUAKER (CONT.)														
Oats Old Fashion	½ cup	150	3	1	0	5	27	4	—	0	140	—	16	0
Oats Quick	½ cup	150	3	1	0	5	27	4	0	0	140	—	16	0
RALSTON														
Almond Delight	1 cup (1.8 oz)	210	3	0	0	5	41	4	20	410	—	6	100	0
Bran Flakes	¾ cup (1.1 oz)	110	1	0	0	3	24	5	0	220	—	0	100	1250
Chex Multi-Bran	1¼ cup (2 oz)	220	2	0	0	5	46	7	0	320	—	6	100	0
Cocoa Crispy Rice	1 cup (1.8 oz)	200	1	0	0	3	45	tr	0	340	—	27	180	1250
Cocoa Crunchies	¾ cup (1.1 oz)	120	1	0	0	1	26	0	0	170	—	15	100	0
Cookie Crisp	1 cup (1 oz)	120	2	0	0	1	25	0	0	110	—	0	100	0
Corn Flakes	1¼ cup (1.1 oz)	120	0	0	0	2	27	1	0	280	—	15	—	1250
Crisp Crunch	¾ cup (1.1 oz)	120	1	0	0	1	26	tr	0	240	—	0	100	0
Crisp Rice	1¼ cup (1.2 oz)	130	0	0	0	2	28	0	0	330	—	15	160	1250
Frosted Flakes	¾ cup (1.1 oz)	120	0	0	0	1	28	1	0	180	—	15	100	1250
Fruit Rings	¾ cup (0.9 oz)	100	1	0	0	1	23	0	0	115	—	60	80	1000
Magic Stair	¾ cup (1.1 oz)	120	1	0	0	2	26	tr	20	160	—	15	100	1250
Muesli Blueberry	1 cup (1.9 oz)	200	3	2	0	5	41	4	0	170	—	0	120	1500
Muesli Cranberry	¾ cup (1.9 oz)	200	3	0	0	5	40	4	0	180	—	0	120	1500
Muesli Peach	¾ cup (1.9 oz)	200	3	0	0	5	39	4	0	170	—	0	120	1500
Muesli Raspberry	¾ cup (2 oz)	220	3	0	0	5	44	4	0	170	—	0	140	1750
Muesli Strawberry	1 cup (1.9 oz)	210	3	2	0	5	41	4	0	170	—	0	120	1500
Multi Vitamin Whole Grain Flakes	1 cup (1.1 oz)	120	1	0	0	3	25	3	200	300	—	60	400	5000
Nutty Nuggets	½ cup (1.7 oz)	180	2	0	0	6	38	5	0	220	—	0	160	2000
Raisin Bran	¾ cup (1.9 oz)	190	1	0	0	5	41	6	20	290	—	0	120	1500
Tasteeos	1¼ cup (1.1 oz)	130	3	0	0	5	22	3	60	260	—	15	100	1250
Tasteeos Apple Cinnamon	1 cup (1.2 oz)	130	2	0	0	2	27	1	20	150	—	15	100	1250
Tasteeos Honey Nut	1 cup (1.2 oz)	130	2	0	0	3	28	1	40	250	—	15	100	1250
RICE KRISPIES														
Treats	¾ cup (1 oz)	120	1	0	0	1	25	0	0	170	20	15	100	750
ROMAN MEAL														
Apple Cinnamon	1.2 oz	105	2	tr	0	3	18	6	16	6	179	tr	—	1
Cream Of Rye	1.3 oz	111	1	tr	0	5	20	5	12	2	97	0	—	0
Oats Wheat Dates Raisins Almonds	1.3 oz	129	2	tr	0	5	24	3	19	3	151	tr	—	1
Oats Wheat Honey Coconuts Almonds	1.3 oz	155	5	3	0	4	22	3	31	8	143	tr	—	tr
Original	1 oz	83	1	tr	0	4	15	5	10	tr	138	0	—	0
Original With Oats	1.2 oz	108	1	tr	0	5	19	5	15	1	148	0	—	0

FOOD	PORTION	CALORIES	FAT	SAT FAT	CHOL	PROTEIN	CARBO	FIBER	CALCIUM	SOD	POTAS	VIT C	FOLIC	VIT A
SMACKS														
Cereal	¾ cup (1 oz)	110	1	0	0	2	26	1	0	75	40	15	100	750
STONE-BUHR														
4 Grain	⅓ cup (1.6 oz)	140	2	0	0	6	31	5	20	0	—	0	—	0
7 Grain	⅓ cup (1.6 oz)	140	2	0	0	6	31	7	20	0	—	0	—	0
Bran Flakes	¼ cup (0.6 oz)	64	0	0	0	2	14	2	0	160	—	0	—	0
Cracked Wheat	¼ cup (2.4 oz)	210	1	0	0	8	48	6	40	0	—	0	—	0
Manna Golden	6 tsp (1.6 oz)	160	0	0	0	5	35	1	0	0	—	0	—	0
Rolled Oats Old Fashion	6 tsp (1.6 oz)	150	3	1	0	8	28	5	20	0	—	0	—	0
Scotch Oats	¼ cup (1.6 oz)	150	4	1	0	7	28	4	20	0	—	0	—	0
SUNBELT														
Muesli	1.9 oz	210	2	1	1	4	44	3	20	70	—	4	—	300
UNCLE ROY'S														
Muesli Swiss Style	½ cup (1.6 oz)	170	5	1	0	5	32	3	—	20	—	—	—	—
WHEATENA														
Cereal	⅓ cup (1.4 oz)	150	1	0	0	5	32	5	0	0	200	0	—	0

CEREAL BARS

(*see also* GRANOLA BARS, NUTRITIONAL SUPPLEMENTS)

FOOD	PORTION	CALORIES	FAT	SAT FAT	CHOL	PROTEIN	CARBO	FIBER	CALCIUM	SOD	POTAS	VIT C	FOLIC	VIT A
CAP'N CRUNCH														
Bar	1 (0.8 oz)	90	2	1	0	1	17	—	—	105	—	—	40	—
Berries Bar	1 (0.8 oz)	90	2	—	0	—	17	—	—	110	—	—	—	—
GOLDEN GRAHAMS TREATS														
Chocolate Chunk	1 bar (0.8 oz)	90	3	1	0	1	17	tr	—	110	—	6	40	300
Honey Graham	1 bar (0.8 oz)	90	2	0	0	1	17	tr	—	120	—	6	40	300
NATURE'S CHOICE														
Fat Free Apple	1 bar (1.3 oz)	110	0	0	0	2	27	2	—	90	—	—	—	—
Fat Free Blueberry	1 bar (1.3 oz)	110	0	0	0	2	27	2	—	90	—	—	—	—
Fat Free Cranberry	1 bar (1.3 oz)	110	0	0	0	2	27	2	—	110	—	—	—	—
Fat Free Peach	1 bar (1.3 oz)	110	0	0	0	2	27	2	—	90	—	—	—	—
Fat Free Raspberry	1 bar (1.3 oz)	110	0	0	0	2	27	2	—	110	—	—	—	—
Fat Free Strawberry	1 bar (1.3 oz)	110	0	0	0	2	27	2	—	110	—	—	—	—
Low Fat Triple Berry	1 bar (1.3 oz)	130	2	0	0	2	28	2	—	190	—	—	—	—
Low Fat Very Cherry	1 bar (1.3 oz)	130	2	0	0	2	28	2	—	190	—	—	—	—
RICE KRISPIES														
Treats	1 bar (0.8 oz)	90	2	1	0	1	17	0	0	105	—	0	24	200
Treats Chocolate Chip	1 (1 oz)	120	4	2	0	1	20	1	0	60	—	0	40	500

CHAMPAGNE

FOOD	PORTION	CALORIES	FAT	SAT FAT	CHOL	PROTEIN	CARBO	FIBER	CALCIUM	SOD	POTAS	VIT C	FOLIC	VIT A
sekt german champagne	3.5 fl oz	84	0	—	0	tr	5	—	—	—	—	—	—	—
ANDRE														
Blush	1 fl oz	22	0	0	0	0	1	—	—	1	—	—	—	—
Brut	1 fl oz	21	0	0	0	0	1	—	—	1	—	—	—	—

FOOD	PORTION	CALORIES	FAT	SAT FAT	CHOL	PROTEIN	CARBO	FIBER	CALCIUM	SOD	POTAS	VIT C	FOLIC	VIT A
ANDRE (CONT.)														
Cold Duck	1 fl oz	25	0	0	0	0	2	—	—	1	—	—	—	—
Extra Dry	1 fl oz	23	0	0	0	0	1	—	—	1	—	—	—	—
BALLATORE														
Spumante	1 fl oz	23	0	0	0	0	2	—	—	2	—	—	—	—
EDEN ROC														
Brut	1 fl oz	21	0	0	0	0	1	—	—	1	—	—	—	—
Brut Rosé	1 fl oz	22	0	0	0	0	2	—	—	1	—	—	—	—
Extra Dry	1 fl oz	21	0	0	0	0	1	—	—	1	—	—	—	—
TOTT'S														
Blanc de Noir	1 fl oz	22	0	0	0	0	2	—	—	1	—	—	—	—
Brut	1 fl oz	20	0	0	0	0	tr	—	—	1	—	—	—	—
Extra Dry	1 fl oz	21	0	0	0	0	1	—	—	1	—	—	—	—

CHAYOTE

FOOD	PORTION	CALORIES	FAT	SAT FAT	CHOL	PROTEIN	CARBO	FIBER	CALCIUM	SOD	POTAS	VIT C	FOLIC	VIT A
fresh cooked	1 cup	38	1	—	0	1	8	—	21	1	276	13	—	75
raw	1 (7 oz)	49	1	—	0	2	11	—	39	8	305	22	—	114
raw cut up	1 cup	32	tr	—	0	1	7	—	25	198	34	15	—	74

CHEESE

(*see also* CHEESE DISHES, CHEESE SUBSTITUTES, COTTAGE CHEESE, CREAM CHEESE)

FOOD	PORTION	CALORIES	FAT	SAT FAT	CHOL	PROTEIN	CARBO	FIBER	CALCIUM	SOD	POTAS	VIT C	FOLIC	VIT A
american	1 oz	93	7	4	18	6	2	—	163	337	79	0	—	259
american cheese food	1 pkg (8 oz)	745	56	35	145	45	17	—	1303	2700	633	0	—	2073
american cheese spread	1 jar (5 oz)	412	30	19	78	23	12	—	798	1910	343	0	10	1119
american cold pack	1 pkg (8 oz)	752	56	35	144	45	19	—	1129	2193	824	0	12	1600
american cheese spread	1 oz	82	6	4	16	5	2	—	159	381	69	0	2	223
blue	1 oz	100	8	6	21	6	1	—	150	396	73	0	10	204
blue crumbled	1 cup (4.7 oz)	477	39	25	102	29	3	—	712	1884	346	0	49	973
brick	1 oz	105	8	5	27	7	1	—	191	159	38	0	6	307
brie	1 oz	95	8	—	28	8	tr	—	52	178	43	0	18	189
cacio di roma sheep's milk cheese	1 oz	130	10	6	30	8	0	—	300	170	—	—	—	—
camembert	1 oz	85	7	4	20	6	tr	—	110	239	53	0	18	262
camembert	1 wedge (1⅓ oz)	114	9	6	27	8	tr	—	147	320	71	0	24	351
caraway	1 oz	107	8	—	—	7	1	—	191	196	—	0	—	299
cheddar	1 oz	114	9	6	30	7	tr	—	204	176	28	0	5	300
cheddar low fat	1 oz	49	2	1	6	9	1	—	118	174	19	0	3	68
cheddar low sodium	1 oz	113	9	6	28	7	1	—	200	6	32	0	5	297
cheddar shredded	1 cup	455	37	24	119	28	1	—	815	701	111	0	21	1197
cheshire	1 oz	110	9	—	29	7	1	—	182	198	27	0	—	279
colby	1 oz	112	9	6	27	7	1	—	194	171	36	0	—	293
colby low fat	1 oz	49	2	1	6	9	1	—	118	174	19	0	3	68

FOOD	PORTION	CALORIES	FAT	SAT FAT	CHOL	PROTEIN	CARBO	FIBER	CALCIUM	SOD	POTAS	VIT C	FOLIC	VIT A
colby low sodium	1 oz	113	9	6	28	7	1	—	200	6	32	0	5	297
edam	1 oz	101	8	5	25	7	tr	—	207	274	53	0	5	260
feta	1 oz	75	6	4	25	4	1	—	140	316	18	0	—	—
fontina	1 oz	110	9	5	33	7	tr	—	156	—	—	0	—	333
gjetost	1 oz	132	8	5	—	3	12	—	113	170	—	0	1	—
gouda	1 oz	101	8	5	32	7	1	—	198	232	34	0	6	183
gruyere	1 oz	117	9	5	31	8	tr	—	287	95	23	0	3	346
limburger	1 oz	93	8	5	26	8	tr	—	141	227	36	0	16	363
monterey	1 oz	106	9	—	—	7	tr	—	212	152	23	0	—	269
mozzarella	1 oz	80	6	4	22	6	1	—	147	106	19	0	1	225
mozzarella	1 lb	1276	98	60	356	88	10	—	2345	1692	304	0	32	3593
mozzarella low moisture	1 oz	90	7	4	25	6	1	—	163	118	21	0	2	256
mozzarella low moisture part skim	1 oz	79	5	3	15	8	1	—	207	150	27	0	3	178
mozzarella part skim	1 oz	72	5	3	16	7	1	—	183	132	24	0	2	166
muenster	1 oz	104	9	5	27	7	tr	—	203	178	38	0	3	318
parmesan grated	1 tbsp (5 g)	23	2	1	4	2	tr	—	69	93	5	0	tr	35
parmesan grated	1 oz	129	9	5	22	12	1	—	390	528	30	0	2	199
parmesan hard	1 oz	111	7	5	19	10	1	—	336	454	26	0	2	171
pimento	1 oz	106	9	6	27	6	tr	—	174	405	46	—	2	358
port du salut	1 oz	100	8	5	35	7	tr	—	184	151	—	0	5	378
provolone	1 oz	100	8	5	20	7	1	—	214	248	39	0	3	231
queso anego	1 oz	106	9	5	30	6	1	—	193	321	25	0	0	63
queso asadero	1 oz	101	8	5	30	6	1	—	188	186	25	0	2	63
queso chichuahua	1 oz	106	8	5	30	6	2	—	185	175	15	0	1	64
ricotta part skim	½ cup (4.4 oz)	171	10	6	38	14	6	—	337	155	155	0	—	536
ricotta part skim	1 cup (8.6 oz)	340	19	12	76	28	13	—	669	307	308	0	—	1063
ricotta whole milk	1 cup (8.6 oz)	428	32	20	124	28	7	—	509	207	257	0	—	1205
ricotta whole milk	½ cup (4.4 oz)	216	16	10	63	14	4	—	257	104	130	0	—	608
romano	1 oz	110	8	—	29	9	1	—	302	340	—	0	2	162
roquefort	1 oz	105	9	5	26	6	1	—	188	513	26	0	14	297
swiss	1 oz	107	8	5	26	8	1	—	272	74	31	0	2	240
swiss cheese food	1 pkg (8 oz)	734	55	—	186	50	10	—	1642	3523	645	0	—	1943
swiss processed	1 oz	95	7	5	24	7	1	—	219	388	61	0	—	229
tilsit	1 oz	96	7	5	29	7	1	—	198	213	18	0	—	296
whey cheese	3.5 oz	440	27	18	—	15	33	0	340	511	—	1	—	1245
yogurt cheese	1 oz	20	0	—	7	—	—	—	70	—	—	—	—	—
ALOUETTE														
Brie Baby	1 oz	110	9	5	30	5	2	0	150	180	—	0	—	300
Brie Baby With Herbs	1 oz	110	9	5	30	5	2	0	150	180	—	0	—	300
French Onion	2 tbsp (0.8 oz)	70	7	5	30	2	1	0	20	160	—	0	—	100
Garlic	2 tbsp (0.8 oz)	70	7	5	30	1	1	0	20	135	—	0	—	200
Light Dill	2 tbsp (0.8 oz)	50	4	3	20	2	2	0	20	120	—	0	—	100

FOOD	PORTION	CALORIES	FAT	SAT FAT	CHOL	PROTEIN	CARBO	FIBER	CALCIUM	SOD	POTAS	VIT C	FOLIC	VIT A
ALOUETTE (CONT.)														
Light Garlic	2 tbsp (0.8 oz)	50	4	3	20	2	1	1	20	120	—	0	—	100
Light Herb	2 tbsp (0.8 oz)	50	4	3	20	2	2	0	20	125	—	0	—	100
Light Herbs & Garlic	2 tbsp (0.8 oz)	50	4	3	20	2	1	0	20	120	—	0	—	100
Light Spring Vegetable	2 tbsp (0.8 oz)	50	4	3	20	2	1	0	20	110	—	0	—	400
Salmon	2 tbsp (0.8 oz)	60	5	3	15	3	1	0	20	95	—	0	—	100
Scallions	2 tbsp (0.8 oz)	70	7	5	30	1	1	0	20	120	—	0	—	200
Spinach	2 tbsp (0.8 oz)	60	6	4	25	1	1	0	20	85	—	0	—	400
ALPINE LACE														
American	1 slice (0.66 oz)	50	3	2	10	4	1	0	80	260	—		0	—	100
American Fat Free	1 piece (1 oz)	45	tr	tr	<5	8	2	0	200	280	—	—	—	300
American Hot Pepper Less Fat Less Sodium	1 piece (1 oz)	80	20	4	6	6	2	0	250	260	—	—	—	300
American Less Fat Less Sodium	1 piece (1 oz)	80	6	4	20	6	2	0	250	200	—	—	—	300
Cheddar Fat Free	1 piece (1 oz)	45	tr	tr	<5	8	2	0	200	280	—	—	—	300
Cheddar Reduced Fat	1 piece (1 oz)	80	5	3	15	9	1	0	250	135	—	—	—	300
Colby Reduced Fat	1 piece (1 oz)	80	5	3	15	9	1	0	350	115	—	—	—	300
Fat Free For Parmesan Lovers	2 tsp (5 g)	10	0	0	0	1	0	0	40	65	—	—	—	—
Fat Free Mexican Macho	2 tbsp (1 oz)	30	tr	tr	3	5	1	0	100	165	—	—	—	200
Fat Free Singles	1 slice (0.66 oz)	25	0	0	<5	5	tr	0	150	280	—	—	—	200
Feta Reduced Fat	1 piece (1 oz)	60	4	3	10	5	1	0	50	370	—	—	—	250
Goat	1 oz	40	3	2	5	2	tr	—	—	130	—	—	—	—
Mozzarella Fat Free	1 piece (1 oz)	45	tr	tr	<5	8	2	0	200	280	—	—	—	300
Mozzarella Reduced Sodium Part Skim	1 piece (1 oz)	70	5	3	15	7	1	0	300	75	—	—	—	200
Muenster Reduced Sodium	1 piece (1 oz)	100	9	5	25	7	1	0	300	85	—	—	—	300
Provolone Smoked Reduced Fat	1 piece (1 oz)	70	5	3	15	9	1	0	350	120	—	—	—	300
Swiss Reduced Fat	1 piece (1 oz)	90	6	4	20	8	1	0	250	35	—	—	—	300
BABYBEL														
Mini Light	1 (0.7 oz)	45	3	2	5	6	0	0	190	180	—	0	—	250
BONGRAIN														
Chavrie	2 tbsp (0.8 oz)	40	3	2	15	2	1	0	0	110	—	0	—	0
Montrachet	1 oz	70	6	4	30	4	tr	0	20	135	—	0	—	100
Montrachet Chive	1 oz	70	6	4	30	4	tr	0	20	135	—	0	—	100
Montrachet Classic	1 oz	70	6	4	30	4	tr	0	20	130	—	0	—	200

FOOD	PORTION	CALORIES	FAT	SAT FAT	CHOL	PROTEIN	CARBO	FIBER	CALCIUM	SOD	POTAS	VIT C	FOLIC	VIT A
BONGRAIN (CONT.)														
Montrachet Classic Herb	1 oz	70	6	4	30	4	tr	0	20	150	—	0	—	100
Montrachet Herbs & Garlic	1 oz	70	6	4	30	4	tr	0	20	150	—	0	—	100
Montrachet In Oil drained	1 oz	70	6	4	30	4	tr	0	20	130	—	0	—	200
Montrachet With Ash	1 oz	70	6	4	30	4	tr	0	20	125	—	0	—	200
BORDEN														
American Slices	1 oz	110	9	5	25	6	1	—	150	490	20	—	—	200
American Very Sharp	1 oz	110	9	—	25	6	1	—	150	490	20	—	—	200
Swiss Slices	1 oz	100	8	4	20	7	1	—	200	380	25	—	—	100
BREAKSTONE'S														
Ricotta	¼ cup (2.2 oz)	110	8	5	25	7	3	0	250	90	105	0	—	200
BRESSE														
Brie	1 oz	110	9	5	30	5	2	0	150	180	—	0	—	300
Brie Light	1 oz	70	4	3	20	8	1	tr	150	160	—	0	—	200
Brie With Herbs	1 oz	110	9	5	30	5	2	0	150	180	—	0	—	300
Creme De Brie	2 tbsp (1 oz)	90	8	5	25	4	tr	0	80	220	—	0	—	200
Creme De Brie Herb	2 tbsp (1 oz)	90	8	5	25	4	tr	0	80	220	—	0	—	200
BRIER RUN														
Cherve	1 oz	61	5	—	18	3	—	—	—	70	—	—	—	—
Quark	1 oz	34	3	—	10	2	—	—	—	15	—	—	—	—
BRISTOL GOLD														
Cheddar Light	1 oz	70	4	—	15	5	3	—	150	150	—	—	—	—
French Onion Light	1 oz	70	4	—	15	5	3	—	150	150	—	—	—	—
Garlic & Herb Light	1 oz	70	4	—	15	5	3	—	150	150	—	—	—	—
Horseradish Light	1 oz	70	4	—	15	5	3	—	150	150	—	—	—	—
Smoke Light	1 oz	70	4	—	15	5	3	—	150	150	—	—	—	—
Wine Light	1 oz	70	4	—	15	5	3	—	150	150	—	—	—	—
CABOT														
Cheddar	1 oz	110	9	6	30	7	0	—	204	175	—	—	—	300
Mediterranean Cheddar		110	9	5	30	7	1	0	200	180	—	0	—	300
Monterey Jack	1 oz	80	5	5	15	8	1	—	150	200	—	—	—	200
Vermont Cheddar 50% Light	1 oz	70	5	3	15	6	1	0	200	170	—	0	—	300
Vitalait	1 oz	70	4	2	15	8	1	—	254	170	—	—	—	200
Vitalait Jalapeno	1 oz	70	4	2	15	8	1	—	254	170	—	—	—	200
CHEEZ WHIZ														
Light	2 tbsp (1.2 oz)	80	3	2	15	6	6	0	150	540	110	0	—	750
CHURNEY														
Feta	1 oz	80	6	4	20	5	tr	0	60	320	—	0	—	200

FOOD	PORTION	CALORIES	FAT	SAT FAT	CHOL	PROTEIN	CARBO	FIBER	CALCIUM	SOD	POTAS	VIT C	FOLIC	VIT A
CRACKER BARREL														
Baby Swiss	1 oz	110	9	6	25	7	0	0	200	110	15	0	—	300
Cheddar Extra Sharp	1 oz	120	10	7	30	6	0	0	200	180	30	0	—	300
Cheddar Marbled Sharp	1 oz	110	9	6	30	7	tr	0	200	180	30	0	—	300
Cheddar New York Aged	1 oz	120	10	7	30	6	0	0	200	180	30	0	—	300
Cheddar Sharp	1 oz	120	10	7	30	6	0	0	200	180	30	0	—	300
Cheddar Vermont Sharp	1 oz	110	9	6	30	7	tr	0	200	180	30	0	—	300
Reduced Fat Cheddar Extra Sharp	1 oz	90	6	4	20	7	tr	0	200	240	45	0	—	300
Reduced Fat Cheddar Sharp	1 oz	90	6	4	20	7	tr	0	200	240	45	0	—	300
Reduced Fat Cheddar Vermont Sharp	1 oz	90	6	4	20	7	tr	0	200	240	45	0	—	300
Whipped Spreadable Cream Cheese & Extra Sharp Cheddar	2 tbsp (0.9 oz)	80	8	5	20	3	tr	0	80	180	25	0	—	300
Whipped Spreadable Cream Cheese & Sharp Cheddar	2 tbsp (0.9 oz)	80	8	5	20	3	tr	0	80	180	20	0	—	300
Whipped Spreadable Cream Cheese & Sharp Cheddar w/ Herbs	2 tbsp (0.9 oz)	80	8	5	20	3	tr	0	80	180	25	0	—	300
DELICE DE FRANCE														
Cheese	1 oz	110	9	5	30	5	2	0	150	180	—	0	—	300
With Herbs	1 oz	110	9	5	30	5	2	0	150	180	—	0	—	300
DELICO														
Alouette Cajun	2 tbsp (0.8 oz)	70	7	5	30	1	1	0	20	120	—	0	—	200
Alouette French Onion	2 tbsp (0.8 oz)	70	7	5	30	2	1	0	20	160	—	0	—	100
Alouette Garden Vegetable	2 tbsp (0.8 oz)	60	6	4	30	1	1	0	20	130	—	0	—	400
Alouette Garlic	2 tbsp (0.8 oz)	70	7	5	30	1	1	0	20	135	—	0	—	200
Alouette Horseradish & Chive	2 tbsp (0.8 oz)	60	7	4	30	1	1	0	20	100	—	0	—	200
Alouette Spinach	2 tbsp (0.8 oz)	60	6	4	25	1	1	0	20	85	—	1	—	300
DI GIORNO														
Parmesan Grated	2 tsp (5 g)	25	2	1	5	2	0	0	60	85	10	0	0	0
Parmesan Shredded	2 tsp (5 g)	20	2	1	<5	2	0	0	40	75	0	0	—	0
Parmesan Shredded	2 tsp (5 g)	20	2	1	5	2	0	0	40	75	0	0	0	0

FOOD	PORTION	CALORIES	FAT	SAT FAT	CHOL	PROTEIN	CARBO	FIBER	CALCIUM	SOD	POTAS	VIT C	FOLIC	VIT A
DI GIORNO (CONT.)														
Romano Grated	2 tsp (5 g)	25	2	1	5	2	0	0	60	90	0	0	0	0
Romano Shredded	2 tsp (5 g)	20	2	1	5	2	0	0	40	70	0	0	0	0
EASY CHEESE														
Spread American	2 tbsp (1.2 oz)	100	7	4	25	6	2	0	150	400	65	—	—	200
Spread Cheddar	2 tbsp (1.2 oz)	100	7	4	25	5	3	0	150	410	85	—	—	200
Spread Cheddar'n Bacon	2 tbsp (1.2 oz)	100	7	4	25	5	3	0	150	410	75	—	—	200
Spread Nacho	2 tbsp (1.2 oz)	100	7	4	25	5	3	0	150	390	75	2	—	300
Spread Sharp Cheddar	2 tbsp (1.2 oz)	100	7	4	25	5	3	0	150	440	70	—	—	200
FATHER TIME														
Cheddar Extra-Sharp Premium	1 oz	110	9	5	30	7	1	0	200	180	—	0	—	300
FORMAGG														
Formaggio D'Oro	1 oz	70	5	3	15	6	1	0	350	450	—	0	—	200
FRIENDSHIP														
Farmer	2 tbsp (1 oz)	50	3	2	10	5	0	0	0	120	—	0	—	0
Farmer No Salt Added	2 tbsp (1 oz)	50	3	2	10	5	0	0	0	10	—	0	—	0
Hoop	2 tbsp (1 oz)	20	0	0	0	5	0	0	0	10	—	0	—	0
FRIGO														
Asiago	1 oz	110	9	—	—	7	1	—	150	400	—	—	—	300
Blue	1 oz	100	8	—	—	6	1	—	150	400	—	—	—	200
Cheddar	1 oz	110	9	6	30	7	1	—	200	200	—	—	—	200
Cheddar Lite	1 oz	80	5	3	17	8	1	—	250	190	—	—	—	500
Feta	1 oz	100	8	—	—	6	1	—	150	400	—	—	—	200
Impastata	1 oz	60	5	—	15	4	1	—	100	50	—	—	—	—
Mozzarella Part Skim Low Moisture	1 oz	80	5	3	10	7	1	—	200	190	—	—	—	100
Mozzarella Whole Milk Low Moisture	1 oz	90	7	4	15	6	1	—	150	190	—	—	—	200
Mozzarella Lite Whole Milk Low Moisture	1 oz	60	2	2	8	9	1	—	250	140	—	—	—	200
Parmazest	1 oz	120	7	—	—	10	5	—	400	410	—	—	—	200
Parmesan & Romano Dry Grated	1 oz	130	9	—	—	12	1	—	400	510	—	—	—	200
Parmesan & Romano Grated	1 oz	110	7	—	—	10	1	—	350	350	—	—	—	200
Parmesan Dry Grated	1 oz	130	9	—	—	12	1	—	400	510	—	—	—	200
Parmesan Grated	1 oz	110	7	—	—	10	1	—	350	350	—	—	—	200
Parmesan Whole	1 oz	110	7	—	—	10	1	—	350	350	—	—	—	200

FOOD	PORTION	CALORIES	FAT	SAT FAT	CHOL	PROTEIN	CARBO	FIBER	CALCIUM	SOD	POTAS	VIT C	FOLIC	VIT A
FRIGO (CONT.)														
Pizza Shredded	1 oz	65	3	—	10	9	1	—	200	150	—	—	—	100
Provolone	1 oz	100	7	5	20	7	1	—	200	230	—	—	—	200
Provolone Lite	1 oz	70	4	2	10	8	1	—	250	205	—	—	—	200
Ricotta Low Fat Low Salt	1 oz	30	1	—	5	3	1	—	60	10	—	—	—	100
Ricotta Part Skim	1 oz	40	3	—	10	3	1	—	60	30	—	—	—	100
Ricotta Whole Milk	1 oz	60	5	—	15	3	1	—	60	40	—	—	—	100
Romano Dry Grated	1 oz	130	9	—	35	12	1	—	400	510	—	—	—	200
Romano Grated	1 oz	110	8	—	30	9	1	—	300	350	—	—	—	200
Romano Whole	1 oz	110	8	—	30	9	1	—	300	350	—	—	—	200
String	1 oz	80	5	—	10	7	1	—	200	190	—	—	—	100
String Lite	1 oz	60	2	—	8	9	1	—	250	140	—	—	—	200
Swiss	1 oz	110	8	—	—	8	1	—	250	80	—	—	—	200
Taco Shredded	1 oz	110	9	—	—	7	1	—	200	200	—	—	—	200
GERARD														
Brie	1 oz	90	7	5	25	5	2	0	100	180	—	0	—	200
HANDI-SNACKS														
Cheez'n Breadsticks	1 pkg (1.1 oz)	120	6	3	15	4	12	0	60	320	55	0	—	200
Cheez'n Crackers	1 pkg (1.1 oz)	110	7	3	15	3	9	0	60	300	45	0	—	200
Cheez'n Pretzels	1 pkg (1 oz)	100	5	3	15	4	11	tr	60	410	50	0	—	200
Mozzarella String Cheese	1 piece (1 oz)	80	6	4	20	7	0	0	150	240	35	0	—	200
Nacho Stix'n Cheez	1 pkg (1.1 oz)	110	6	3	15	4	11	0	60	320	55	0	—	200
HEALTHY CHOICE														
American Singles White	1 slice (0.7 oz)	30	0	0	<5	5	2	—	150	290	—	0	—	400
American Singles Yellow	1 slice (0.7 oz)	30	0	0	<5	5	2	—	150	290	—	0	—	500
Cheddar Fancy Shreds	¼ cup (1 oz)	45	0	0	<5	9	2	—	250	200	—	0	—	750
Cheddar Shreds	¼ cup (1 oz)	45	0	0	<5	9	2	—	250	200	—	0	—	750
Loaf	1 in cube (1 oz)	35	0	0	<5	8	3	—	200	390	—	0	—	750
Mexican Shreds	¼ cup (1 oz)	45	0	0	<5	9	2	—	250	200	—	0	—	750
Mozzarella	1 oz	45	0	0	<5	10	1	—	250	200	—	0	—	300
Mozzarella Fancy Shreds	¼ cup (1 oz)	45	0	0	<5	9	2	—	250	200	—	0	—	750
Mozzarella Shreds	¼ cup (1 oz)	45	0	0	<5	9	2	—	250	200	—	0	—	750
Mozzarella String Cheese	1 stick (1 oz)	45	0	0	<5	9	1	—	250	200	—	0	—	300
Pizza Fancy Shreds	¼ cup (1 oz)	45	0	0	<5	9	2	—	250	200	—	0	—	750
Pizza String	1 stick (1 oz)	45	0	0	<5	10	1	—	200	200	—	0	—	100
HELUVA GOOD CHEESE														
American	1 slice (0.7)	45	5	3	15	4	2	0	150	390	—	0	—	300

FOOD	PORTION	CALORIES	FAT	SAT FAT	CHOL	PROTEIN	CARBO	FIBER	CALCIUM	SOD	POTAS	VIT C	FOLIC	VIT A
HELUVA GOOD CHEESE (CONT.)														
Cheddar Curds Snack	1 oz	113	9	5	28	7	1	0	250	179	—	0	—	400
Cheddar Extra-Sharp	1 oz	110	9	5	30	7	1	0	200	180	—	0	—	300
Cheddar Mild	1 oz	110	9	5	30	7	1	0	200	180	—	0	—	300
Cheddar Mild Reduced Fat	1 oz	80	6	4	15	7	1	0	300	200	—	0	—	300
Cheddar Mild White	1 oz	110	9	5	30	7	1	0	200	180	—	0	—	300
Cheddar Sharp	1 oz	110	9	5	30	7	1	0	200	180	—	0	—	300
Cheddar Sharp White	1 oz	110	9	5	30	7	1	0	200	180	—	0	—	300
Cheddar Shredded	¼ cup (1 oz)	110	9	5	30	7	1	0	200	180	—	0	—	300
Cheddar Very Low Sodium	1 oz	110	9	6	25	7	0	0	200	140	—	0	—	300
Cheddar White Extra-Sharp	1 oz	110	9	5	30	7	1	0	200	180	—	0	—	300
Cheddar White Very Low Sodium	1 oz	110	9	6	25	7	0	0	200	140	—	0	—	300
Cheddar White Shredded	¼ cup (1 oz)	110	9	5	30	7	1	0	200	180	—	0	—	300
Colby	1 oz	117	9	6	30	7	0	0	200	186	—	0	—	350
Colby-Jack	1 oz	110	9	6	30	6	0	0	200	200	—	0	—	200
Cold Pack Cheddar Sharp	2 tbsp (1 oz)	90	7	3	20	5	3	0	150	210	—	0	—	300
Cold Pack Cheddar Sharp With Bacon	2 tbsp (1 oz)	90	7	3	20	5	3	0	150	210	—	0	—	300
Cold Pack Cheddar Sharp With Horseradish	2 tbsp (1 oz)	90	7	3	20	5	3	0	150	210	—	0	—	300
Cold Pack Cheddar Sharp With Jalapenos	2 tbsp (1 oz)	90	7	3	20	5	3	0	150	210	—	0	—	300
Cold Pack Cheddar Sharp With Port Wine	2 tbsp (1 oz)	90	7	3	20	5	3	0	150	210	—	0	—	300
Monterey Jack	1 oz	100	8	6	25	6	0	0	200	180	—	0	—	300
Monterey Jack Shredded	¼ cup (1 oz)	100	8	5	30	8	1	0	200	170	—	0	—	300
Monterey Jack With Jalapenos	1 oz	100	8	6	25	7	0	0	200	180	—	2	—	300
Mozzarella Part Skim Low Moisture Shredded	¼ cup (1 oz)	80	5	3	15	8	1	0	200	170	—	0	—	200
Mozzarella Whole Milk	1 oz	80	6	4	20	6	tr	0	100	220	—	0	—	200
Muenster	1 oz	100	8	6	25	6	0	0	200	180	—	0	—	300

FOOD	PORTION	CALORIES	FAT	SAT FAT	CHOL	PROTEIN	CARBO	FIBER	CALCIUM	SOD	POTAS	VIT C	FOLIC	VIT A
HELUVA GOOD CHEESE (CONT.)														
Swiss	1 oz	112	8	5	28	9	0	0	200	62	—	0	—	300
Washed Curd Cheese	1 oz	110	9	5	30	7	1	0	200	170	—	0	—	300
HOFFMAN														
American Yellow	1 oz	110	9	6	25	6	1	0	150	400	—	0	—	750
Hot Pepper	1 oz	90	7	5	20	5	2	0	150	460	—	0	—	300
Super Sharp	1 oz	110	9	6	25	6	1	0	150	380	—	0	—	750
KELLER'S														
Chub	2 tbsp (1 oz)	100	10	6	35	2	1	0	20	120	—	0	—	300
KRAFT														
Cheddar Extra Sharp	1 oz	120	10	7	30	6	0	0	200	180	30	0	—	300
Cheddar Medium	1 oz	110	9	6	30	7	tr	0	200	180	30	0	—	300
Cheddar Mild	1 oz	110	9	6	30	7	tr	0	200	180	30	0	—	300
Cheddar Sharp	1 oz	120	10	7	30	6	0	0	200	180	30	0	—	300
Cheddary Melts Medium Cheddar	1 oz	110	9	6	30	5	2	0	150	390	50	0	—	300
Cheddary Melts Mild Cheddar	1 oz	110	9	6	30	5	2	0	150	390	50	0	—	300
Cheddary Melts Shreds Medium Cheddar	1/4 cup (1.1 oz)	120	9	6	30	6	2	0	150	420	55	0	—	300
Cheddary Melts Shreds Mild Cheddar	1/4 cup (1.1 oz)	120	9	6	30	6	2	0	150	420	55	0	—	300
Cheese Food w/ Garlic	1 oz	90	7	5	20	5	2	0	150	370	75	0	—	300
Cheese Food w/ Jalapeno Peppers	1 oz	90	7	5	20	5	2	0	150	370	80	0	—	300
Colby	1 oz	110	9	6	30	7	tr	0	200	180	15	0	—	300
Colby Monterey Jack	1 oz	110	9	6	30	7	0	0	200	180	15	0	—	300
Deluxe American	1 oz	100	9	6	25	6	tr	0	150	430	25	0	—	400
Deluxe American White	1 oz	100	9	6	25	6	tr	0	150	430	25	0	—	300
Deluxe Singles American	1 (0.7 oz)	70	6	4	15	4	tr	0	100	310	15	0	—	200
Deluxe Singles American	1 (1 oz)	110	9	6	30	6	tr	0	150	460	25	0	—	300
Deluxe Singles Pimento	1 (1 oz)	100	8	6	25	6	tr	0	150	430	25	0	—	300
Deluxe Singles Swiss	1 slice (0.7 oz)	70	5	4	20	5	0	0	150	310	15	0	—	200
Deluxe Singles Swiss	1 (1 oz)	90	7	5	25	6	0	0	200	410	20	0	—	300
Free Grated	2 tsp (5 g)	15	0	0	0	tr	3	0	0	75	10	0	—	0

FOOD	PORTION	CALORIES	FAT	SAT FAT	CHOL	PROTEIN	CARBO	FIBER	CALCIUM	SOD	POTAS	VIT C	FOLIC	VIT A
Free Shredded Cheddar	¼ cup (0.9 oz)	40	0	0	<5	9	1	0	250	270	35	0	—	500
Free Shredded Mozzarella	¼ cup (1 oz)	45	0	0	<5	9	2	tr	250	340	30	0	—	400
Grated Parm Plus! Garlic Herb	2 tsp (5 g)	15	0	0	0	tr	2	0	0	110	20	0	—	0
Grated Parm Plus! Zesty Red Pepper	2 tsp (5 g)	15	0	0	0	tr	2	0	20	110	15	0	—	0
Grated Parmesan	2 tsp (5 g)	20	2	1	5	2	0	0	60	85	10	0	—	0
Grated Romano	2 tsp (5 g)	20	2	1	<5	2	0	0	60	70	10	0	—	0
Marbled Cheddar Mild	1 oz	110	9	6	30	7	tr	0	200	180	30	0	—	300
Marbled Cheddar & Monterey Jack	1 oz	110	9	6	30	7	tr	0	200	190	20	0	—	300
Marbled Cheddar & Whole Milk Mozzarella	1 oz	100	8	5	25	6	tr	0	200	190	25	0	—	300
Marbled Colby Monterey Jack	1 oz	110	9	6	30	7	0	0	200	180	15	0	—	300
Monterey Jack	1 oz	110	9	6	30	6	0	0	200	190	15	0	—	300
Monterey Jack w/ Jalapeno Peppers	1 oz	110	9	6	30	7	tr	0	200	190	15	0	—	400
Mozzarella Part Skim Low Moisture	1 oz	80	5	4	15	8	tr	0	200	200	20	0	—	200
Mozzarella String Cheese Low Moisture Part Skim	1 piece (1 oz)	80	6	4	20	7	0	0	150	240	35	0	—	200
Pizza Shredded Four Cheese	¼ cup (0.9 oz)	90	7	5	20	6	tr	0	200	220	20	0	—	200
Pizza Shredded Mozzarella & Cheddar	⅓ cup (1.1 oz)	120	9	6	30	7	1	0	200	220	30	0	—	300
Pizza Shredded Mozzarella & Provolone w/ Smoke Flavor	¼ cup (0.9 oz)	90	7	5	20	6	tr	0	150	200	20	0	—	200
Reduced Fat Cheddar Mild	1 oz	90	6	4	20	7	tr	0	200	240	45	0	—	300
Reduced Fat Cheddar Sharp	1 oz	90	6	4	20	7	tr	0	200	240	45	0	—	300
Reduced Fat Colby	1 oz	80	6	4	20	7	0	0	200	220	50	0	—	400
Reduced Fat Monterey Jack	1 oz	80	6	4	20	7	tr	0	200	240	45	0	—	400
Shredded Cheddar Medium	¼ cup (0.9 oz)	100	8	6	30	6	tr	0	200	170	25	0	—	300

FOOD	PORTION	CALORIES	FAT	SAT FAT	CHOL	PROTEIN	CARBO	FIBER	CALCIUM	SOD	POTAS	VIT C	FOLIC	VIT A
KRAFT (CONT.)														
Shredded Cheddar Mild	¼ cup (0.9 oz)	100	8	6	30	6	tr	0	200	170	25	0	—	300
Shredded Cheddar Sharp	1 oz (0.9 oz)	110	9	6	25	6	tr	0	150	170	25	0	—	300
Shredded Cheddar & Monterey Jack	¼ cup (0.9 oz)	100	8	6	25	6	tr	0	200	170	20	0	—	300
Shredded Colby & Monterey Jack	¼ cup (0.9 oz)	100	8	6	25	6	tr	0	150	170	15	0	—	300
Shredded Hearty Italian	⅓ cup (1.1 oz)	100	8	5	25	7	2	0	200	230	35	0	—	200
Shredded Italian Style Classic Garlic	⅓ cup (1.1 oz)	100	8	5	25	7	2	tr	200	240	45	0	—	300
Shredded Italian Style Mozzarelle & Parmesan	⅓ cup (1.1 oz)	100	8	5	25	7	1	0	200	240	25	0	—	300
Shredded Lower Fat Cheddar Mild	¼ cup (0.9 oz)	80	6	4	20	7	tr	0	200	220	40	0	—	300
Shredded Lower Fat Cheddar Sharp	¼ cup (0.9 oz)	80	6	4	20	7	tr	0	200	220	40	0	—	300
Shredded Lower Fat Colby & Monterey Jack	¼ cup (0.9 oz)	80	5	4	15	7	tr	0	200	210	40	0	—	400
Shredded Lower Fat Mozzarella	⅓ cup (1.1 oz)	80	5	3	15	9	tr	0	250	210	25	0	—	400
Shredded Lower Fat Pizza Cheese	⅓ cup (1.1 oz)	90	6	4	20	9	1	0	250	240	40	0	—	400
Shredded Mexican Style Cheddar & Monterey Jack	⅓ cup (1.1 oz)	120	10	7	30	7	tr	0	200	200	25	0	—	400
Shredded Mexican Style Cheddar & Monterey Jack w/ Jalapeno Peppers	⅓ cup (1.1 oz)	120	10	6	30	7	tr	0	200	200	25	0	—	400
Shredded Mexican Style Four Cheese	⅓ cup (1.1 oz)	120	10	7	30	7	tr	0	200	210	25	0	—	400
Shredded Mexican Style Taco Cheese	⅓ cup (1.1 oz)	120	10	7	30	7	1	0	200	240	25	0	—	400
Shredded Monterey Jack	¼ cup (0.9 oz)	100	8	6	25	6	tr	0	150	170	15	0	—	300
Shredded Parmesan	2 tsp (5 g)	20	2	1	2	2	0	0	40	75	0	0	—	0
Shredded Part Skim Mozzarella	¼ cup (1.1 oz)	90	6	4	20	8	tr	0	250	220	20	0	—	200
Shredded Swiss	¼ cup (0.9 oz)	100	8	5	25	7	tr	0	250	25	45	0	—	300

FOOD	PORTION	CALORIES	FAT	SAT FAT	CHOL	PROTEIN	CARBO	FIBER	CALCIUM	SOD	POTAS	VIT C	FOLIC	VIT A
KRAFT (CONT.)														
Shredded Whole Milk Mozzarella	¼ cup (1.1 oz)	100	8	5	25	7	1	0	200	220	25	0	—	300
Shredded Finely Cheddar Mild	¼ cup (1.1 oz)	120	10	6	30	7	tr	0	200	190	30	0	—	400
Shredded Finely Cheddar Sharp	¼ cup (1.1 oz)	120	10	7	30	7	tr	0	200	190	30	0	—	400
Shredded Finely Colby & Monterey Jack	¼ cup (1 oz)	110	9	6	30	7	tr	0	200	190	15	0	—	300
Shredded Finely Lower Fat Cheddar Milk	⅓ cup (1.1 oz)	100	7	5	20	8	1	0	200	260	50	0	—	400
Shredded Finely Lower Fat Cheddar Sharp	⅓ cup (1.1 oz)	100	7	5	20	8	1	0	200	260	50	0	—	400
Shredded Finely Part Skim Mozzarella	¼ cup (1.1 oz)	90	6	4	20	8	tr	0	250	220	20	0	—	200
Shredded Finely Swiss	¼ cup (0.9 oz)	110	8	6	25	7	tr	0	250	45	20	0	—	300
Singles American	1 (0.6 oz)	60	5	3	15	3	2	0	150	260	45	0	—	200
Singles American	1 (0.7 oz)	60	5	3	15	3	2	0	100	260	45	0	—	100
Singles American	1 (1.2 oz)	110	8	6	25	6	3	0	200	460	80	0	—	400
Singles Mild Mexican	1 (0.7 oz)	70	5	4	15	4	2	0	100	280	50	0	—	300
Singles Monterey	1 slice (0.7 oz)	70	5	4	15	4	2	0	100	290	55	0	—	100
Singles Pimento	1 (0.7 oz)	60	5	3	15	4	1	0	100	260	50	0	—	300
Singles Reduced Fat American	1 (0.7 oz)	50	3	2	10	5	2	0	150	320	60	0	—	300
Singles Reduced Fat American White	1 (0.7 oz)	50	3	2	10	4	2	0	150	320	60	0	—	200
Singles Sharp	1 slice (0.7 oz)	70	6	4	20	4	tr	0	100	300	25	0	—	300
Singles Swiss	1 slice (0.7 oz)	70	5	4	15	4	1	0	150	320	55	0	—	200
Singles Nonfat American	1 (0.7 oz)	30	0	0	<5	4	3	0	150	270	60	0	—	300
Singles Nonfat Sharp Cheddar	1 (0.7 oz)	35	0	0	<5	5	3	0	150	300	65	0	—	300
Singles Nonfat Swiss	1 slice (0.7 oz)	30	0	0	<5	5	3	0	150	270	55	0	—	200
Slices Cheddar Mild	1 (1 oz)	110	9	6	30	7	tr	0	200	180	30	0	—	300
Slices Colby	1 (1.6 oz)	180	14	10	45	11	tr	0	300	290	25	0	—	500
Slices Part Skim Mozzarella	1 (1.5 oz)	120	8	5	25	12	tr	0	350	310	30	0	—	300
Slices Part Skim Mozzarella	1 (1.6 oz)	130	8	6	25	12	tr	0	350	320	30	0	—	300

FOOD	PORTION	CALORIES	FAT	SAT FAT	CHOL	PROTEIN	CARBO	FIBER	CALCIUM	SOD	POTAS	VIT C	FOLIC	VIT A
KRAFT (CONT.)														
Slices Provolone Smoke Flavor	1 (1.5 oz)	150	11	8	35	11	tr	0	300	370	35	0	—	400
Slices Swiss	1 (0.8 oz)	90	7	5	25	6	0	0	200	40	15	0	—	200
Slices Swiss	1 (1.3 oz)	150	12	8	40	10	tr	0	350	65	25	0	—	400
Slices Swiss	1 (1.5 oz)	170	13	9	45	12	tr	0	400	45	75	0	—	500
Slices Swiss	1 (1.6 oz)	180	14	9	45	12	tr	0	400	45	75	0	—	500
Slices Swiss Aged	1 (1.5 oz)	170	13	9	45	12	tr	0	400	75	30	0	—	500
Slices Deli-Thin Part Skim Mozzarella	1 (1 oz)	80	5	4	15	8	tr	0	200	200	20	0	—	200
Slices Deli-Thin Swiss	1 (0.8 oz)	90	7	5	25	6	0	0	200	40	15	0	—	200
Slices Deli-Thin Swiss Aged	1 (0.8 oz)	90	7	5	25	6	0	0	200	40	15	0	—	200
Slices Reduced Fat Swiss	1 (1.3 oz)	130	9	6	25	11	tr	0	400	90	55	0	—	400
Spread Bacon	2 tbsp (1.1 oz)	90	8	5	25	5	tr	0	150	570	20	0	—	500
Spread Olive & Pimento	2 tbsp (1.1 oz)	70	6	4	20	2	3	0	20	220	50	0	—	300
Spread Pimento	2 tbsp (1.1 oz)	80	6	4	20	2	3	0	20	170	60	0	—	300
Spread Pineapple	2 tbsp (1.1 oz)	70	5	4	15	2	4	0	20	120	55	0	—	200
Spread Pineapple	2 tbsp (1.1 oz)	70	5	4	15	2	4	0	20	115	55	0	—	300
Spread Roka Brand Blue	2 tbsp (1.1 oz)	90	8	5	25	5	tr	0	150	520	15	0	—	500
Swiss	1 oz	110	9	6	30	8	0	0	250	50	20	0	—	300
LACTAID														
American	3.5 oz	328	25	15	64	20	7	0	574	1189	279	0	0	913
LAND O'LAKES														
American	1 slice (0.75 oz)	80	6	5	20	4	tr	0	100	340	—	0	—	300
American	2 slices (1 oz)	100	9	6	25	5	1	0	150	460	—	0	—	400
American	1 oz	110	9	6	30	5	tr	0	200	430	—	0	—	300
American Less Salt	1 oz	110	9	6	30	6	tr	0	150	270	—	0	—	400
American Light	1 oz	70	5	3	20	7	2	0	200	400	—	0	—	500
American Sharp	1 oz	110	9	6	30	6	tr	0	200	360	—	0	—	400
American & Swiss	1 oz	100	8	6	35	6	0	0	200	380	—	0	—	300
Baby Swiss	1 oz	110	8	5	25	7	0	0	250	125	—	0	—	400
Brick	1 oz	100	8	5	30	7	tr	0	200	160	—	0	—	300
Chedarella	1 oz	100	8	5	25	7	0	0	200	200	—	0	—	300
Cheddar Light	1 oz	70	4	3	10	8	tr	0	250	230	—	0	—	300
Gouda	1 oz	110	8	5	30	7	1	—	200	230	35	—	—	200
Jalapeno Light	1 oz	70	4	3	15	7	1	0	200	400	—	0	—	400
Monterey Jack	1 oz	110	9	5	30	6	tr	0	200	160	—	0	—	300
Mozzarella	1 oz	80	6	4	15	7	tr	0	200	190	—	0	—	200
Muenster	1 oz	100	8	5	25	6	0	0	200	220	—	0	—	300
Provolone	1 oz	100	8	5	20	7	tr	0	200	240	—	0	—	200

FOOD	PORTION	CALORIES	FAT	SAT FAT	CHOL	PROTEIN	CARBO	FIBER	CALCIUM	SOD	POTAS	VIT C	FOLIC	VIT A
LAND O'LAKES (CONT.)														
Swiss	1 oz	110	8	6	25	8	tr	0	250	75	—	0	—	400
Swiss Light	1 oz	80	4	3	15	9	tr	0	250	60	—	0	—	200
LAUGHING COW														
Assorted Wedge	1 (1 oz)	70	6	4	20	4	1	0	120	370	—	0	—	100
Babybel	1 oz	90	7	5	10	7	0	0	240	230	—	0	—	100
Babybel Mini	1 (0.7 oz)	70	6	4	15	5	0	0	150	170	—	0	—	200
Bonbel	1 oz	100	8	5	25	6	0	0	200	230	—	0	—	400
Bonbel Mini	1 (0.7 oz)	70	6	4	15	5	0	0	150	170	—	0	—	200
Cheesebits	6 pieces (1 oz)	70	6	4	20	4	1	0	120	370	—	0	—	100
Gouda Mini	1 (0.7 oz)	80	6	4	20	5	0	0	150	170	—	0	—	200
Original Wedge	1 (1 oz)	70	6	4	20	4	1	0	120	370	—	0	—	100
Wedge Light	1 (1 oz)	50	3	2	10	5	1	0	150	370	—	0	—	100
LIFETIME														
Cheddar Fat Free	1 oz	40	0	0	<5	8	1	0	400	220	—	—	—	300
Cheddar Fat Free Lactose Free	1 oz	40	0	0	<5	8	1	0	400	220	—	—	—	300
Garden Vegetable Fat Free	1 oz	40	0	0	<5	8	1	0	400	220	—	—	—	300
Jalapeno Jack Fat Free	1 oz	40	0	0	<5	8	1	0	400	220	—	—	—	300
Jalapeno Jack Fat Free Lactose Free	1 oz	40	0	0	<5	8	1	0	400	220	—	—	—	300
Mild Mexican Fat Free	1 oz	40	0	0	<5	8	1	0	400	220	—	—	—	300
Monterey Jack Fat Free	1 oz	40	0	0	<5	8	1	0	400	220	—	—	—	300
Mozzarella Fat Free	1 oz	40	0	0	<5	8	1	0	400	220	—	—	—	300
Mozzarella Fat Free Lactose Free	1 oz	40	0	0	<5	8	1	0	400	220	—	—	—	300
Onions & Chives Fat Free	1 oz	40	0	0	<5	8	1	0	400	220	—	—	—	300
Sharp Cheddar Fat Free	1 oz	40	0	0	<5	8	1	0	400	220	—	—	—	300
Smoked Cheddar Fat Free	1 oz	40	0	0	<5	8	1	0	400	220	—	—	—	300
Swiss Fat Free	1 oz	40	0	0	<5	8	1	0	400	220	—	—	—	300
LIGHT N'LIVELY														
Singles American	1 (0.7 oz)	45	3	2	10	5	2	0	150	280	50	0	—	300
MAYBUD														
Edam	1 oz	100	8	6	25	7	1	0	200	210	—	0	—	300
Gouda	1 oz	100	8	6	25	7	1	0	200	210	—	0	—	200
Gouda Round	1 oz	100	8	6	25	7	1	0	200	210	—	0	—	300
NEW HOLLAND														
Cheese	1 oz	90	7	5	30	7	0	0	150	105	—	0	—	100
Garlic	1 oz	90	7	5	30	7	tr	0	150	105	—	0	—	100

FOOD	PORTION	CALORIES	FAT	SAT FAT	CHOL	PROTEIN	CARBO	FIBER	CALCIUM	SOD	POTAS	VIT C	FOLIC	VIT A
NEW HOLLAND (CONT.)														
Havarti Lower Fat Garden Vegetable	1 oz	80	6	4	25	6	0	0	150	145	—	0	—	400
Jalapeno	1 oz	80	6	4	25	6	tr	0	100	140	—	1	—	100
Natural Vegetable	1 oz	80	6	4	25	6	0	0	150	110	—	0	—	400
OLD ENGLISH														
American Sharp	1 slice (1 oz)	100	9	6	30	6	tr	0	150	460	20	0	—	300
POLLY-O														
Mozzarella Free	1 oz	35	0	0	<5	7	tr	—	—	220	—	—	—	—
Mozzarella Lite	1 oz	60	3	2	10	7	tr	—	—	230	—	—	—	—
Mozzarella Part Skim	1 oz	70	5	3	15	6	tr	—	—	220	—	—	—	—
Mozzarella Part Skim Shredded	¼ cup	80	5	4	15	8	tr	—	—	200	—	—	—	—
Mozzarella Shredded Free	¼ cup	45	0	0	<5	10	1	—	—	270	—	—	—	—
Mozzarella Shredded Lite	¼ cup	60	3	2	15	8	1	—	—	220	—	—	—	—
Mozzarella Whole Milk	1 oz	80	6	4	20	6	tr	—	—	220	—	—	—	—
Mozzarella Whole Milk Shredded	¼ cup	90	7	5	20	6	tr	—	—	200	—	—	—	—
Ricotta Free	¼ cup	50	0	0	<5	10	2	—	—	80	—	—	—	—
Ricotta Lite	¼ cup	70	3	2	10	8	3	—	—	80	—	—	—	—
Ricotta Part Skim	¼ cup	90	6	4	20	8	2	—	—	65	—	—	—	—
Ricotta Whole Milk	¼ cup	110	8	5	25	7	2	—	—	60	—	—	—	—
String	1 oz	80	6	—	15	7	1	—	—	200	—	—	—	—
String Lite	1 piece (1 oz)	60	3	2	10	7	tr	0	150	230	—	0	—	300
PRESIDENT														
Feta Fat Free	1 oz	30	0	0	0	6	2	0	100	450	—	0	—	1000
PRICE'S														
Cheese & Bacon Spread	2 tbsp (1.1 oz)	90	7	3	15	3	2	0	80	340	—	0	—	200
Jalapeno Nacho Dip Hot	2 tbsp (1.1 oz)	80	7	3	15	3	2	0	80	370	—	0	—	100
Jalapeno Nacho Dip Mild	2 tbsp (1.1 oz)	80	7	3	15	3	2	0	80	370	—	0	—	100
Pimento Cheese Spread	2 tbsp (1.1 oz)	80	7	3	15	3	2	0	80	320	—	0	—	100
Pimento Cheese Spread Light	2 tbsp (1.1 oz)	60	4	1	10	4	3	0	100	260	—	0	—	300
Vegetable Garden	2 tbsp (1.1 oz)	70	5	2	15	3	3	0	100	290	—	0	—	300
QUAKER														
Chub	2 tbsp (1 oz)	100	10	6	35	2	1	0	20	120	—	0	—	300
RONDELE														
Light Soft Spreadable Garlic & Herb	2 tbsp (0.9 oz)	60	4	3	10	4	2	0	40	190	—	0	—	400

FOOD	PORTION	CALORIES	FAT	SAT FAT	CHOL	PROTEIN	CARBO	FIBER	CALCIUM	SOD	POTAS	VIT C	FOLIC	VIT A
RONDELE (CONT.)														
Soft Spreadable Garlic & Herbs	2 tbsp (1 oz)	100	9	6	25	2	1	0	20	180	—	0	—	300
SARGENTO														
4 Cheese Mexican Recipe Blend Shredded	¼ cup (1 oz)	110	9	6	25	6	tr	0	200	200	—	0	—	300
6 Cheese Italian Recipe Blend Shredded	¼ cup (1 oz)	90	7	4	20	7	0	0	200	180	—	0	—	200
Blue Crumbled	¼ cup (1 oz)	100	8	5	20	6	1	0	150	350	—	0	—	200
Cheddar	1 slice (1 oz)	110	9	6	30	6	1	0	200	160	—	0	—	400
Cheddar Mild Shredded Classic Supreme	¼ cup (1 oz)	110	9	6	30	6	1	0	200	160	—	0	—	400
Cheddar Mild Shredded Fancy Supreme	¼ cup (1 oz)	110	9	6	30	6	1	0	200	160	—	0	—	400
Cheddar Mild Shredded Preferred Light	¼ cup (1 oz)	70	5	3	10	8	tr	0	250	200	—	0	—	400
Cheddar Mild White Shredded Classic Supreme	¼ cup (1 oz)	110	9	6	30	6	1	0	200	160	—	0	—	400
Cheddar New York Sharp Shredded Classic Supreme	¼ cup (1 oz)	110	9	6	30	6	1	0	200	160	—	0	—	400
Cheddar Sharp Shredded Classic Supreme	¼ cup (1 oz)	110	9	6	30	6	1	0	200	160	—	0	—	400
Cheddar Sharp Shredded Fancy Supreme	¼ cup (1 oz)	110	9	6	30	6	1	0	200	160	—	0	—	400
Cheese For Nachos & Tacos Shredded	¼ cup (1 oz)	110	9	5	25	6	1	0	200	240	—	0	—	300
Cheese For Pizza Shredded	¼ cup (1 oz)	90	6	4	20	7	0	0	200	210	—	0	—	300
Cheese For Tacos Shredded	¼ cup (1 oz)	110	9	6	25	6	1	0	200	220	—	0	—	500
Cheese For Tacos Shredded Preferred Light	¼ cup (1 oz)	70	5	3	15	8	tr	0	250	240	—	0	—	500
Colby	1 slice (1 oz)	110	9	6	30	6	0	0	200	190	—	0	—	400
Colby-Jack Shredded Fancy Supreme	¼ cup (1 oz)	110	9	6	25	6	tr	0	200	190	—	0	—	300
Gourmet Parm	1 tbsp	20	1	—	5	3	tr	—	—	95	—	—	—	—
Jarlsberg	1 slice (1.2 oz)	120	9	5	20	9	1	0	300	50	—	0	—	400
Monterey Jack	1 slice (1 oz)	100	9	5	30	6	0	0	200	190	—	0	—	300

FOOD	PORTION	CALORIES	FAT	SAT FAT	CHOL	PROTEIN	CARBO	FIBER	CALCIUM	SOD	POTAS	VIT C	FOLIC	VIT A
SARGENTO (CONT.)														
MooTown Snackers Cheddar	1 piece (0.8 oz)	100	8	5	25	5	1	0	150	130	—	0	—	400
MooTown Snackers Cheddar Mild Light	1 piece (0.8 oz)	60	4	3	10	7	tr	0	200	170	—	0	—	400
MooTown Snackers Cheese & Pretzels	1 pkg (1 oz)	90	3	2	10	3	12	0	60	320	—	0	—	200
MooTown Snackers Cheese & Sticks	1 pkg (1 oz)	100	4	3	10	3	13	0	60	260	—	0	—	200
MooTown Snackers Colby-Jack	1 piece (0.8 oz)	90	8	5	20	5	tr	0	150	160	—	0	—	200
MooTown Snackers Pizza Cheese & Sticks	1 pkg (1 oz)	100	4	3	10	3	13	0	60	260	—	0	—	200
MooTown Snackers String	1 piece (0.8 oz)	70	5	3	15	6	tr	0	150	170	—	0	—	200
MooTown Snackers String Light	1 piece (0.8 oz)	60	3	2	10	7	tr	0	200	200	—	0	—	200
Mozzarella	1 slice (1.5 oz)	130	9	6	25	11	2	0	300	230	—	0	—	400
Mozzarella Preferred Light	1 slice (1.5 oz)	100	5	3	15	13	0	0	350	210	—	0	—	500
Mozzarella Shredded Classic Supreme	1/4 cup (1 oz)	80	6	4	15	7	1	0	200	150	—	0	—	300
Mozzarella Shredded Fancy Supreme	1/4 cup (1 oz)	80	6	4	15	7	1	0	200	150	—	0	—	300
Mozzarella Shredded Preferred Light	1/4 cup (1 oz)	70	3	2	10	8	tr	0	200	140	—	0	—	400
Muenster	1 slice (1 oz)	100	9	6	25	6	tr	0	200	200	—	0	—	300
Parmesan Fresh	1 oz	111	7	—	19	10	1	—	336	454	—	0	—	171
Parmesan Shredded	1/4 cup (1 oz)	110	7	5	25	9	1	0	250	300	—	0	—	300
Parmesan & Romano Shredded	1/4 cup (1 oz)	110	7	5	25	9	1	0	250	340	—	0	—	200
Pizza Double Cheese Shredded	1/4 cup (1 oz)	90	6	5	20	7	1	0	200	150	—	0	—	300
Provolone	1 slice (1 oz)	100	8	6	25	7	0	0	200	190	—	0	—	200
Ricotta Light	1/4 cup (2.2 oz)	60	3	2	15	5	3	0	100	55	—	0	—	100
Ricotta Old Fashioned	1/4 cup (2.2 oz)	90	6	4	25	7	3	0	150	75	—	0	—	400
Ricotta Part Skim	1/4 cup (2.2 oz)	80	5	3	20	7	2	0	150	75	—	0	—	300
Swiss	1 slice (0.7 oz)	80	6	4	20	6	0	0	200	30	—	0	—	200
Swiss Preferred Light	1 slice (1 oz)	80	4	3	15	9	tr	0	300	50	—	0	—	500
Swiss Shredded Fancy Supreme	1/4 cup (1 oz)	110	8	5	30	8	0	0	250	40	—	0	—	300
Swiss Wafer Thin	2 slices (1 oz)	110	9	5	25	5	0	0	250	40	—	0	—	300

FOOD	PORTION	CALORIES	FAT	SAT FAT	CHOL	PROTEIN	CARBO	FIBER	CALCIUM	SOD	POTAS	VIT C	FOLIC	VIT A
SMART BEAT														
American Fat Free	1 slice (0.6 oz)	25	0	0	0	4	3	—	—	180	95	—	—	200
Lactose Free Fat Free	1 slice (0.6 oz)	25	0	0	0	4	3	—	—	180	95	—	—	200
Mellow Cheddar Fat Free	1 slice (0.6 oz)	25	0	0	0	4	3	—	—	180	110	—	—	200
Sharp Cheddar Fat Free	1 slice (0.6 oz)	25	0	0	0	4	3	—	—	220	81	—	—	200
TREASURE CAVE														
Blue Crumbled	1 oz	110	9	6	25	6	tr	0	150	400	—	0	—	300
Feta Crumbled	1 oz	80	6	4	20	5	tr	0	100	370	—	0	—	400
TREE OF LIFE														
Cheddar 33% Reduced Fat Organic Milk	1 oz	90	6	4	15	8	1	—	250	135	—	1	—	300
Cheddar Low Sodium Raw Milk	1 oz	110	9	6	24	7	0	—	200	110	—	—	—	300
Cheddar Mild Organic Milk	1 oz	110	9	6	25	7	1	—	200	190	—	1	—	750
Cheddar Mild Raw Milk	1 oz	110	9	6	25	7	0	—	200	180	—	—	—	300
Cheddar Razor Sharp Raw Milk	1 oz	110	9	6	25	7	0	—	200	180	—	—	—	300
Cheddar Sharp Organic Milk	1 oz	110	9	6	25	7	0	—	200	190	—	1	—	750
Cheddar Sharp Raw Milk	1 oz	110	9	6	25	7	0	—	200	180	—	—	—	300
Colby Organic Milk	1 oz	120	10	6	30	7	1	—	200	190	—	—	—	300
Colby Raw Milk	1 oz	110	9	6	30	7	1	—	200	170	—	—	—	300
Farmer Part-Skim Organic Milk	1 oz	90	6	4	15	7	1	—	200	110	—	1	—	300
Jalapeno Jack Organic Milk	1 oz	110	9	6	20	6	1	—	200	190	—	—	—	400
Jalapeno Jack Semi-Soft Organic Milk	1 oz	110	9	6	25	7	0	—	200	150	—	—	—	300
Monterey Jack 35% Reduced Fat Organic Milk	1 oz	80	5	3	15	8	1	—	250	190	—	1	—	300
Monterey Jack Organic Milk	1 oz	100	8	6	20	6	1	—	200	185	—	—	—	300
Monterey Jack Semi-Soft Raw Milk	1 oz	110	9	6	25	7	0	—	200	150	—	—	—	300
Mozzarella Low Moisture Part Skim	1 oz	80	5	3	15	8	1	—	200	150	—	—	—	200
Mozzarella Low Moisture Part Skim Organic Milk	1 oz	80	5	3	16	8	1	—	200	170	—	—	—	200

FOOD	PORTION	CALORIES	FAT	SAT FAT	CHOL	PROTEIN	CARBO	FIBER	CALCIUM	SOD	POTAS	VIT C	FOLIC	VIT A
TREE OF LIFE (CONT.)														
Muenster Organic Milk	1 oz	100	8	5	25	6	1	—	200	185	—	—	—	200
Muenster Semi-Soft Raw Milk	1 oz	100	9	5	30	7	0	—	200	180	—	—	—	300
Provolone	1 oz	100	8	5	20	7	1	—	200	250	—	—	—	300
Swiss Raw Milk	1 oz	110	8	5	25	8	1	—	200	75	—	—	—	300
VELVEETA														
Light	1 oz	60	3	2	10	5	3	0	150	440	90	0	—	300
Shredded	¼ cup (1.3 oz)	130	9	6	30	8	3	0	200	500	100	0	—	750
Shredded Mild Mexican w/ Jalapeno Pepper	¼ cup (1.3 oz)	120	9	6	30	8	3	0	200	520	95	0	—	1000
Spread	1 oz	90	6	4	25	5	3	0	150	420	95	0	—	300
Spread Hot Mexican	1 oz	90	6	4	20	5	3	0	150	420	90	0	—	300
Spread Mild Mexican	1 oz	90	6	4	25	5	3	0	150	420	90	0	—	300
WEIGHT WATCHERS														
Cheddar Mild Yellow	1 oz	80	5	3	15	8	1	0	200	180	—	0	—	300
Cheddar Sharp Yellow	1 oz	80	5	3	15	8	1	0	200	180	—	0	—	300
Fat Free Grated Italian Topping	1 tbsp	20	0	0	0	2	2	0	20	60	—	0	—	0
Fat Free Reduced Sodium American Yellow	2 slices (0.75 oz)	30	0	0	0	5	3	0	150	160	—	0	—	300
Fat Free Sharp Cheddar	2 slices (0.75 oz)	30	0	0	0	5	3	0	150	320	—	0	—	300
Fat Free Swiss	2 slices (0.75 oz)	30	0	0	0	5	2	0	150	320	—	0	—	300
Fat Free White	2 slices (0.75 oz)	30	0	0	0	5	3	0	150	320	—	0	—	300
Fat Free Yellow	2 slices (0.75 oz)	30	0	0	0	5	3	0	150	320	—	0	—	300
WISPRIDE														
Chunk	1 oz	110	8	3	20	5	4	0	100	180	—	0	—	200
Garlic & Herb Cup	2 tbsp (1.1 oz)	100	7	4	20	4	4	0	150	270	—	0	—	300
Hickory Smoked Cup	2 tbsp (1.1 oz)	100	7	4	20	4	4	0	150	230	—	0	—	300
Port Wine Ball	2 tbsp (1.1 oz)	100	8	4	20	4	4	0	150	190	—	0	—	300
Port Wine Cup	2 tbsp (1.1 oz)	100	7	4	20	4	4	0	150	230	—	0	—	300
Port Wine Light Cup	2 tbsp (1.1 oz)	80	3	2	10	5	5	0	150	200	—	0	—	200
Sharp Ball	2 tbsp (1.1 oz)	100	8	4	20	4	4	0	150	190	—	0	—	300
Sharp Cheddar Ball	2 tbsp (1.1 oz)	100	8	4	20	4	4	0	150	190	—	0	—	300

FOOD	PORTION	CALORIES	FAT	SAT FAT	CHOL	PROTEIN	CARBO	FIBER	CALCIUM	SOD	POTAS	VIT C	FOLIC	VIT A
WISPRIDE (CONT.)														
Sharp Cup	2 tbsp (1.1 oz)	100	7	4	20	4	4	0	150	230	—	0	—	300
Sharp Light Cup	2 tbsp (1.1 oz)	80	3	2	10	5	5	0	150	200	—	0	—	200
Swiss Ball	2 tbsp (1.1 oz)	110	8	3	20	5	5	0	150	125	—	0	—	200

CHEESE DISHES

FROZEN

STOUFFER'S

FOOD	PORTION	CALORIES	FAT	SAT FAT	CHOL	PROTEIN	CARBO	FIBER	CALCIUM	SOD	POTAS	VIT C	FOLIC	VIT A
Welsh Rarebit	½ cup (2.5 oz)	120	9	4	20	5	5	0	150	280	90	0	—	0
TAKE-OUT														
fondue	1 cup (7.5 oz)	492	29	19	97	31	8	—	1023	283	225	0	9	891
fondue	½ cup (3.8 oz)	247	15	9	49	15	4	—	514	142	113	0	5	447

CHEESE SUBSTITUTES

BORDEN

FOOD	PORTION	CALORIES	FAT	SAT FAT	CHOL	PROTEIN	CARBO	FIBER	CALCIUM	SOD	POTAS	VIT C	FOLIC	VIT A
Cheese Two	1 oz	90	7	1	<5	5	2	—	150	360	25	—	—	200
Taco-Mate	1 oz	100	7	2	10	6	2	—	200	360	25	—	—	500
FORMAGG														
American White	1 slice (0.66 oz)	60	4	1	0	4	tr	0	200	260	—	0	16	400
American Yellow	1 slice (0.66 oz)	60	4	1	0	4	tr	0	200	260	—	0	16	400
Caesar's Italian Garden American	1 oz	60	3	0	0	7	1	0	300	240	—	0	—	500
Cheddar	1 slice (0.66 oz)	60	4	tr	0	4	tr	0	200	260	—	0	16	400
Cheddar Shredded	1 oz	60	3	0	0	7	1	0	300	190	—	0	—	500
Classic American	1 oz	60	3	0	0	7	1	0	200	290	—	0	—	500
Macaroni And Cheese Sauce	⅔ cup (5 oz)	190	2	0	0	7	35	0	200	470	—	0	—	500
Mozzarella Shredded	1 oz	60	3	0	0	7	1	0	300	140	—	0	—	500
Old World Mozzarella	1 oz	60	3	0	0	7	1	0	300	140	—	0	—	500
Parmesan Grated	2 tsp (5 g)	15	1	0	0	2	tr	tr	60	80	—	0	—	100
Swiss	1 oz	60	3	0	0	7	1	0	300	240	—	0	—	500
Swiss White	1 slice (0.66 oz)	60	4	1	0	4	tr	0	200	260	—	0	16	400
Vintage Provolone	1 oz	60	3	0	0	7	1	0	300	190	—	0	—	500
Zesty Jalapeno American	1 oz	60	3	0	0	7	1	0	300	290	—	0	—	500
FRIGO														
Imitation Cheddar	1 oz	90	7	1	—	5	1	—	300	280	—	—	—	—
Imitation Mozzeralla	1 oz	90	7	1	—	6	1	—	200	240	—	—	—	400
GEORGIO'S														
Imitation Cheddar Shredded	¼ cup (1 oz)	90	7	1	0	6	1	0	150	450	—	0	—	100

FOOD	PORTION	CALORIES	FAT	SAT FAT	CHOL	PROTEIN	CARBO	FIBER	CALCIUM	SOD	POTAS	VIT C	FOLIC	VIT A
GEORGIO'S (CONT.)														
Imitation Mozzarella Shredded	¼ cup (1 oz)	90	7	1	0	6	1	0	150	350	—	0	—	100
SARGENTO														
Classic Supreme Cheddar Shredded	¼ cup (1 oz)	90	6	1	0	5	2	0	150	470	—	0	—	1000
Classic Supreme Mozzarella Shredded	¼ cup (1 oz)	80	6	1	0	6	tr	0	150	320	—	0	40	400
Fancy Supreme Cheddar Shredded	¼ cup (1 oz)	90	6	1	0	5	2	0	150	470	—	0	—	1000
WHITE WAVE														
Soy A Melt Cheddar	1 oz	80	5	1	0	8	1	—	140	170	—	—	—	—
Soy A Melt Fat Free Cheddar	1 oz	40	tr	—	0	7	3	—	250	370	—	—	—	—
Soy A Melt Fat Free Mozzarella	1 oz	40	tr	—	0	7	3	—	250	370	—	—	—	—
Soy A Melt Garlic Herb	1 oz	80	5	1	0	8	1	—	140	170	—	—	—	—
Soy A Melt Jalapeno Jack	1 oz	80	5	1	0	8	1	—	140	170	—	—	—	—
Soy A Melt Monterey Jack	1 oz	80	5	1	0	8	1	—	140	170	—	—	—	—
Soy A Melt Mozzarella	1 oz	80	5	1	0	8	1	—	140	170	—	—	—	—
Soy A Melt Singles American	1 slice (¾ oz)	60	4	1	0	5	1	—	150	280	—	—	—	—
Soy A Melt Singles Mozzarella	1 slice (¾ oz)	60	4	1	0	5	1	—	150	280	—	—	—	—
CHERIMOYA														
fresh	1	515	2	—	0	7	131	—	126	—	—	49	—	55
CHERRIES														
CANNED														
sour in heavy syrup	½ cup	232	tr	tr	0	2	60	—	26	18	238	5	19	1827
sour in light syrup	½ cup	189	tr	tr	0	2	49	—	26	18	238	5	19	—
sour water packed	1 cup	87	tr	tr	0	2	22	—	26	17	240	5	20	1840
sweet in heavy syrup	½ cup	107	tr	tr	0	1	27	—	12	3	187	5	—	199
sweet in light syrup	½ cup	85	tr	tr	0	1	22	—	12	3	186	5	—	197
sweet juice pack	½ cup	68	tr	tr	0	1	17	—	17	3	163	3	—	156
sweet water pack	½ cup	57	tr	tr	0	1	15	—	13	2	162	3	—	198
DEL MONTE														
Dark Pitted In Heavy Syrup	½ cup (4.2 oz)	120	0	0	0	tr	24	tr	0	10	—	12	—	0

FOOD	PORTION	CALORIES	FAT	SAT FAT	CHOL	PROTEIN	CARBO	FIBER	CALCIUM	SOD	POTAS	VIT C	FOLIC	VIT A
DEL MONTE (CONT.)														
Sweet Dark Whole Unpitted In Heavy Syrup	½ cup (4.2 oz)	120	0	0	0	tr	24	tr	0	10	—	12	—	0
DRIED														
SONOMA														
Pitted	¼ cup (1.4 oz)	140	0	0	0	1	34	2	0	0	—	9	—	0
FRESH														
sour	1 cup	51	tr	tr	0	1	13	—	16	3	178	10	8	1321
sweet	10	49	1	tr	0	1	11	—	10	0	152	5	3	146
DOLE														
Cherries	1 cup	90	1	—	0	1	19	3	—	0	270	11	—	64
FROZEN														
sour unsweetened	1 cup	72	1	tr	0	1	17	—	20	1	192	3	7	1349
sweet sweetened	1 cup	232	tr	tr	0	3	58	—	31	3	514	3	—	489
BIG VALLEY														
Dark Sweet	¾ cup (4.9 oz)	90	0	0	0	1	20	3	20	0	—	6	—	0

CHERRY JUICE

FOOD	PORTION	CALORIES	FAT	SAT FAT	CHOL	PROTEIN	CARBO	FIBER	CALCIUM	SOD	POTAS	VIT C	FOLIC	VIT A
AFTER THE FALL														
Black Cherry	1 can (12 oz)	170	0	0	0	0	42	0	20	20	340	1	—	0
CAPRI SUN														
Wild Cherry Drink	1 pkg (7 oz)	100	0	0	0	0	30	0	0	20	25	0	—	0
HI-C														
Box	8.45 fl oz	140	0	0	0	0	35	—	—	30	—	60	—	—
Drink	8 fl oz	130	0	0	0	0	33	—	—	30	—	60	—	—
JUICY JUICE														
Drink	1 bottle (6 fl oz)	90	0	0	0	1	23	—	20	10	140	60	—	—
Drink	1 box (8.45 fl oz)	130	0	0	0	1	30	—	20	10	200	60	—	—
KOOL-AID														
Black Cherry Drink as prep w/ sugar	1 serv (8 oz)	100	0	0	0	0	25	0	0	15	0	6	—	—
Bursts Cherry Drink	1 (7 oz)	100	0	0	0	0	25	0	0	30	15	0	—	0
Drink as prep w/ sugar	1 serv (8 oz)	100	0	0	0	0	25	0	0	5	0	6	—	0
Splash Drink	1 serv (8 oz)	110	0	0	0	0	29	0	0	35	15	0	—	0
Sugar Free Drink Mix as prep	1 serv (8 oz)	5	0	0	0	0	0	0	0	5	0	6	—	0
TREE OF LIFE														
Concentrate	8 tsp (1.4 oz)	110	0	0	0	0	28	—	20	0	—	14	—	—
VERYFINE														
Juice-Ups	8 fl oz	130	0	0	0	0	33	0	0	15	—	60	—	0

CHERVIL

FOOD	PORTION	CALORIES	FAT	SAT FAT	CHOL	PROTEIN	CARBO	FIBER	CALCIUM	SOD	POTAS	VIT C	FOLIC	VIT A
seed	1 tsp	1	tr	—	0	tr	tr	—	8	tr	28	—	—	—

FOOD	PORTION	CALORIES	FAT	SAT FAT	CHOL	PROTEIN	CARBO	FIBER	CALCIUM	SOD	POTAS	VIT C	FOLIC	VIT A
CHESTNUTS														
chinese cooked	1 oz	44	tr	tr	0	1	10	—	3	1	87	—	—	—
chinese dried	1 oz	103	tr	tr	0	2	23	—	8	2	206	—	—	—
chinese raw	1 oz	64	tr	tr	0	1	14	—	5	1	127	10	—	57
chinese roasted	1 oz	68	tr	tr	0	1	15	—	5	1	135	—	—	1
cooked	1 oz	37	tr	tr	0	1	8	—	13	8	203	—	—	—
dried peeled	1 oz	105	1	tr	0	1	22	—	18	11	281	—	—	—
japanese cooked	1 oz	16	tr	tr	0	tr	4	—	3	1	34	—	—	4
japanese dried	1 oz	102	tr	tr	0	1	23	—	20	10	218	17	—	24
japanese raw	1 oz	44	tr	tr	0	1	10	—	9	4	94	8	—	10
japanese roasted	1 oz	57	tr	tr	0	1	13	—	10	—	—	8	—	21
raw peeled	1 oz	56	tr	tr	0	tr	13	—	5	1	137	—	—	—
roasted	2 to 3 (1 oz)	70	1	tr	0	1	15	—	8	1	168	7	10	7
roasted	1 cup	350	3	1	0	5	76	—	42	3	846	37	100	35
CHEWING GUM														
bubble gum	1 block (8 g)	27	0	0	0	0	8	—	—	0	0	0	—	0
stick	1 (3 g)	10	0	0	0	0	3	—	—	0	0	0	—	0
BAZOOKA														
Fruit Chunk	1 piece (6 g)	25	0	0	0	0	5	—		0	—	—	—	—
Fruit Soft	1 piece (6 g)	25	0	0	0	0	5	—		0	—	—	—	—
Gum	1 piece (4 g)	15	0	0	0	0	4	—		0	—	—	—	—
Gum	1 piece (6 g)	25	0	0	0	0	5	—		0	—	—	—	—
BEECH-NUT														
Peppermint	1 stick (3 g)	10	0	0	0	0	2	0	—	0	0	—	—	—
Spearmint	1 stick (3 g)	10	0	0	0	0	2	0	—	0	0	—	—	—
BROCK														
Bubble Gum	1 piece (0.2 oz)	20	0	0	0	0	4	—	—	0	—	—	—	—
BUBBLE YUM														
Bananaberry Split	1 piece (0.3 oz)	25	0	0	0	0	6	—	—	0	0	—	—	—
Cotton Candy	1 piece (0.3 oz)	25	0	0	0	0	6	—	—	0	0	—	—	—
Grape	1 piece (0.3 oz)	25	0	0	0	0	6	—	—	0	0	—	—	—
Luscious Lime	1 piece (0.3 oz)	25	0	0	0	0	6	—	—	0	0	—	—	—
Regular	1 piece (0.3 oz)	25	0	0	0	0	6	0	—	0	0	—	—	—
Sour Apple	1 piece (0.3 oz)	25	0	0	0	0	6	1	—	0	0	—	—	—
Sour Cherry	1 piece (0.3 oz)	25	0	0	0	0	6	0	—	0	0	—	—	—
Sugarless	1 piece (0.2 oz)	15	0	—	—	0	3	—	—	0	0	—	—	—
Sugarless Grape	1 piece (0.2 oz)	15	0	—	—	0	3	—	—	0	0	—	—	—

FOOD	PORTION	CALORIES	FAT	SAT FAT	CHOL	PROTEIN	CARBO	FIBER	CALCIUM	SOD	POTAS	VIT C	FOLIC	VIT A
BUBBLE YUM (CONT.)														
Sugarless Peppermint	1 piece (0.2 oz)	15	0	—	—	0	3	—	—	0	0	—	—	—
Sugarless Strawberry	1 piece (0.2 oz)	15	0	—	—	0	3	—	—	0	0	—	—	—
Sugarless Variety	1 piece (0.2 oz)	15	0	—	—	0	3	—	—	0	0	—	—	—
Variety Pack	1 piece (0.3 oz)	25	0	0	0	0	6	0	—	0	0	—	—	—
Watermelon	1 piece (0.3 oz)	25	0	0	0	0	6	0	—	0	0	—	—	—
Wild Strawberry	1 piece (0.3 oz)	25	0	0	0	0	6	0	—	0	0	—	—	—
BUBBLICIOUS														
Gum	1 piece (7.9 g)	25	0	0	0	0	6	—	—	—	—	—	—	—
CARE*FREE														
Sugarless Bubble Gum	1 stick (3 g)	10	0	—	—	0	2	—	—	0	0	—	—	—
Sugarless Cinnamon	1 piece (3 g)	5	0	—	—	0	2	—	—	0	0	—	—	—
Sugarless Peppermint	1 piece (3 g)	5	0	—	—	0	2	—	—	0	0	—	—	—
Sugarless Spearmint	1 piece (3 g)	5	0	—	—	0	2	—	—	0	0	—	—	—
Sugarless Wild Cherry	1 stick (3 g)	10	0	0	0	0	2	—	—	0	0	—	—	—
CHICLETS														
Original	1 piece (1.59 g)	6	0	0	0	0	2	—	—	—	—	—	—	—
Tiny Size	8 pieces (0.13 g)	tr	0	0	0	0	tr	—	—	—	—	—	—	—
CLORETS														
Clorets	1 piece (1.59 g)	6	0	0	0	0	2	—	—	—	—	—	—	—
DENTYNE														
Cinn-A-Burst	1 piece (3.2 g)	9	0	0	0	0	2	—	—	—	—	—	—	—
Gum	1 piece (1.88 g)	6	0	0	0	0	1	—	—	—	—	—	—	—
Sugar Free	1 piece (1.88 g)	5	0	0	0	0	1	—	—	—	—	—	—	—
FRESHEN-UP														
Gum	1 piece (4.2 g)	13	0	0	0	0	3	—	—	—	—	—	—	—
FRUIT STRIPE														
Bubble Gum Jumbo Pack	1 stick (3 g)	10	0	0	0	0	2	0	—	0	0	—	—	—
Variety Pack Chewing & Bubble Gum	1 stick (3 g)	10	0	0	0	0	2	0	—	0	0	—	—	—

FOOD	PORTION	CALORIES	FAT	SAT FAT	CHOL	PROTEIN	CARBO	FIBER	CALCIUM	SOD	POTAS	VIT C	FOLIC	VIT A
RAIN-BLO														
Bubble Gum Balls	1 piece (2 g)	5	0	0	0	0	2	—	—	0	—	—	—	—
*STICK*FREE*														
Sugarless Peppermint	1 stick (3 g)	10	0	—	—	0	2	—	—	0	0	—	—	—
Sugarless Spearmint	1 stick (3 g)	10	0	—	—	0	2	—	—	0	0	—	—	—
SWELL														
Bubble Gum	1 piece (3 g)	10	0	0	0	0	2	—	—	0	—	—	—	—
TRIDENT														
Gum	1 piece (1.88 g)	5	0	0	0	0	1	—	—	—	—	—	—	—
Soft Bubble Gum	1 piece (3.3 g)	9	0	0	0	0	2	—	—	—	—	—	—	—
WINTERFRESH														
Stick	1 stick (3 g)	10	0	0	0	0	2	—	—	0	—	—	—	—
CHIA SEEDS														
dried	1 oz	134	7	3	0	5	14	—	150	—	—	—	—	10
CHICKEN														
(*see also* CHICKEN DISHES, CHICKEN SUBSTITUTES, DINNER, HOT DOGS)														
CANNED														
chicken spread	1 tbsp	25	2	—	—	2	1	—	16	—	—	—	—	—
chicken spread	1 oz	55	3	—	—	4	2	—	35	—	—	—	—	—
chicken spread barbeque flavored	1 oz	55	3	—	—	4	2	—	35	—	—	1	—	373
w/ broth	½ can (2.5 oz)	117	6	2	—	15	0	—	10	357	98	1	—	—
w/ broth	1 can (5 oz)	234	11	3	—	31	0	—	20	714	196	3	—	—
SWANSON														
Chunk Style Mixin' Chicken	2½ oz	130	8	—	—	13	1	—	20	230	—	—	—	—
White	2½ oz	100	4	—	—	15	0	—	—	235	—	—	—	—
White & Dark	2½ oz	100	4	—	—	16	0	—	—	240	—	—	—	—
UNDERWOOD														
Chunky	2.08 oz	150	9	3	40	10	2	—	—	440	95	—	—	—
Chunky Light	2.08 oz	80	3	1	30	11	2	—	100	330	100	—	—	—
Smoky	2.08 oz	150	8	2	40	10	10	—	—	290	115	—	—	—
FRESH														
broiler/fryer back w/ skin batter dipped & fried	½ back (2.5 oz)	238	16	4	63	16	7	—	17	228	130	0	6	85
broiler/fryer back w/ skin floured & fried	1.5 oz	146	9	2	39	12	3	—	10	40	100	0	3	54
broiler/fryer back w/ skin roasted	1 oz	96	7	2	28	8	0	—	7	28	67	0	2	111
broiler/fryer back w/ skin stewed	½ back (2.1 oz)	158	11	3	48	14	0	—	11	39	89	0	3	188

FOOD	PORTION	CALORIES	FAT	SAT FAT	CHOL	PROTEIN	CARBO	FIBER	CALCIUM	SOD	POTAS	VIT C	FOLIC	VIT A
broiler/fryer back w/o skin fried	½ back (2 oz)	167	9	2	54	17	3	—	15	58	146	0	5	57
broiler/fryer breast w/ skin batter dipped & fried	½ breast (4.9 oz)	364	18	5	119	35	13	—	28	385	282	0	8	94
broiler/fryer breast w/ skin batter dipped & fried	2.9 oz	218	11	3	72	21	8	—	17	231	169	0	5	56
broiler/fryer breast w/ skin roasted	½ breast (3.4 oz)	193	8	2	83	29	0	—	14	69	240	0	3	91
broiler/fryer breast w/ skin roasted	2 oz	115	5	1	49	17	0	—	8	41	142	0	2	54
broiler/fryer breast w/ skin stewed	½ breast (3.9 oz)	202	8	2	83	30	0	—	14	68	195	0	3	90
broiler/fryer breast w/o skin fried	½ breast (3 oz)	161	4	1	78	29	tr	—	14	68	237	0	4	20
broiler/fryer breast w/o skin roasted	½ breast (3 oz)	142	3	1	73	27	0	—	13	63	220	0	3	18
broiler/fryer breast w/o skin stewed	2 oz	86	2	tr	44	17	0	—	7	36	107	0	2	11
broiler/fryer dark meat w/ skin batter dipped & fried	5.9 oz	497	31	8	149	36	16	—	36	493	309	0	15	172
broiler/fryer dark meat w/ skin floured & fried	3.9 oz	313	19	5	101	30	4	—	19	98	254	0	9	114
broiler/fryer dark meat w/ skin roasted	3.5 oz	256	16	4	92	26	0	—	15	88	222	0	7	203
broiler/fryer dark meat w/ skin stewed	3.9 oz	256	16	4	90	26	0	—	15	77	182	0	7	205
broiler/fryer dark meat w/o skin fried	1 cup (5 oz)	334	16	4	135	41	4	—	25	136	354	0	12	110
broiler/fryer dark meat w/o skin roasted	1 cup (5 oz)	286	14	4	130	38	0	—	21	130	336	0	11	101
broiler/fryer dark meat w/o skin stewed	1 cup (5 oz)	269	13	3	123	36	0	—	20	104	253	0	10	97
broiler/fryer dark meat w/o skin stewed	3 oz	165	8	2	76	22	0	—	12	64	155	0	6	59
broiler/fryer drumstick w/ skin batter dipped & fried	1 (2.6 oz)	193	11	3	62	16	6	—	12	194	134	0	6	62

FOOD	PORTION	CALORIES	FAT	SAT FAT	CHOL	PROTEIN	CARBO	FIBER	CALCIUM	SOD	POTAS	VIT C	FOLIC	VIT A
broiler/fryer drumstick w/ skin floured & fried	1 (1.7 oz)	120	7	2	44	13	1	—	6	44	112	0	4	41
broiler/fryer drumstick w/ skin roasted	1 (1.8 oz)	112	6	2	48	14	0	—	6	47	119	0	4	52
broiler/fryer drumstick w/ skin stewed	1 (2 oz)	116	6	2	48	14	0	—	7	43	105	0	4	52
broiler/fryer drumstick w/o skin fried	1 (1.5 oz)	82	3	1	40	12	0	—	5	40	105	0	4	26
broiler/fryer drumstick w/o skin roasted	1 (1.5 oz)	76	2	1	41	12	0	—	5	42	108	0	4	26
broiler/fryer drumstick w/o skin stewed	1 (1.6 oz)	78	3	1	40	13	0	—	5	37	92	0	4	26
broiler/fryer leg w/ skin batter dipped & fried	1 (5.5 oz)	431	26	7	142	34	14	—	28	442	299	0	14	144
broiler/fryer leg w/ skin floured & fried	1 (3.9 oz)	285	16	4	105	30	3	—	15	99	261	0	9	103
broiler/fryer leg w/ skin roasted	1 (4 oz)	265	15	4	105	30	0	—	14	99	256	0	8	154
broiler/fryer leg w/ skin stewed	1 (4.4 oz)	275	16	4	105	30	0	—	14	92	220	0	8	156
broiler/fryer leg w/o skin fried	1 (3.3 oz)	195	9	2	93	27	1	—	12	90	239	0	8	62
broiler/fryer leg w/o skin roasted	1 (3.3 oz)	182	8	2	89	26	0	—	12	87	230	0	8	60
broiler/fryer leg w/o skin stewed	1 (3.5 oz)	187	8	2	90	26	0	—	11	78	192	0	8	60
broiler/fryer light meat w/ skin batter dipped & fried	4 oz	312	17	5	94	27	11	—	22	324	209	0	7	89
broiler/fryer light meat w/ skin floured & fried	2.7 oz	192	9	3	68	24	1	—	12	60	186	0	3	53
broiler/fryer light meat w/ skin roasted	2.8 oz	175	9	2	67	23	0	—	12	59	179	0	3	87
broiler/fryer light meat w/ skin stewed	3.2 oz	181	9	3	66	9	0	—	11	57	150	0	3	86
broiler/fryer light meat w/o skin fried	1 cup (5 oz)	268	8	2	125	46	1	—	22	114	368	0	6	42

FOOD	PORTION	CALORIES	FAT	SAT FAT	CHOL	PROTEIN	CARBO	FIBER	CALCIUM	SOD	POTAS	VIT C	FOLIC	VIT A
broiler/fryer light meat w/o skin roasted	1 cup (5 oz)	242	6	2	118	43	0	—	21	108	345	0	5	41
broiler/fryer light meat w/o skin stewed	1 cup (5 oz)	223	6	2	107	40	0	—	18	91	252	0	5	37
broiler/fryer neck w/ skin stewed	1 (1.3 oz)	94	7	2	27	7	0	—	10	20	41	0	1	61
broiler/fryer neck w/o skin stewed	1 (.6 oz)	32	1	tr	14	4	0	—	8	12	25	0	tr	22
broiler/fryer skin batter dipped & fried	from ½ chicken (6.7 oz)	748	55	14	140	20	44	—	49	1105	143	0	17	263
broiler/fryer skin batter dipped & fried	4 oz	449	33	9	84	12	26	—	29	663	86	0	10	158
broiler/fryer skin floured & fried	1 oz	166	14	4	24	6	3	—	5	18	41	0	1	77
broiler/fryer skin floured & fried	from ½ chicken (2 oz)	281	24	7	41	24	5	—	8	30	70	0	2	130
broiler/fryer skin roasted	from ½ chicken (2 oz)	254	23	6	46	11	0	—	8	36	76	0	1	146
broiler/fryer skin stewed	from ½ chicken (2.5 oz)	261	24	7	45	11	0	—	9	40	84	0	1	143
broiler/fryer thigh w/ skin batter dipped & fried	1 (3 oz)	238	14	4	80	19	8	—	16	248	165	0	8	82
broiler/fryer thigh w/ skin floured & fried	1 (2.2 oz)	162	9	3	60	17	2	—	8	55	147	0	5	61
broiler/fryer thigh w/ skin roasted	1 (2.2 oz)	153	10	3	58	16	0	—	8	52	137	0	4	102
broiler/fryer thigh w/ skin stewed	1 (2.4 oz)	158	10	3	57	16	0	—	8	49	115	0	4	103
broiler/fryer thigh w/o skin fried	1 (1.8 oz)	113	5	1	53	15	1	—	7	49	134	0	4	37
broiler/fryer thigh w/o skin roasted	1 (1.8 oz)	109	6	2	49	13	0	—	6	46	124	0	4	34
broiler/fryer thigh w/o skin stewed	1 (1.9 oz)	107	5	1	49	14	0	—	6	41	101	0	4	34
broiler/fryer w/ skin floured & fried	½ chicken (11 oz)	844	47	13	283	90	10	—	52	264	735	0	20	280
broiler/fryer w/ skin floured & fried	½ breast (3.4 oz)	218	9	2	88	31	2	—	16	75	253	0	4	49
broiler/fryer w/ skin fried	½ chicken (16.4 oz)	1347	81	22	404	81	44	—	97	1360	863	0	35	434

FOOD	PORTION	CALORIES	FAT	SAT FAT	CHOL	PROTEIN	CARBO	FIBER	CALCIUM	SOD	POTAS	VIT C	FOLIC	VIT A
broiler/fryer w/ skin roasted	½ chicken (10.5 oz)	715	41	11	263	82	0	—	45	244	667	0	16	482
broiler/fryer w/ skin stewed	½ chicken (11.7 oz)	730	42	12	262	82	0	—	44	224	556	0	16	488
broiler/fryer w/ skin neck & giblets batter dipped & fried	1 chicken (2.3 lbs)	2987	180	48	1054	235	93	—	218	2921	1951	4	241	6202
broiler/fryer w/ skin neck & giblets roasted	1 chicken (1.5 lbs)	1598	90	25	730	183	tr	—	105	536	1447	4	201	4340
broiler/fryer w/ skin neck & giblets stewed	1 chicken (1.6 lbs)	1625	93	26	726	184	tr	—	104	494	1224	4	200	4350
broiler/fryer w/o skin fried	1 cup	307	13	3	131	43	2	—	24	127	360	0	10	82
broiler/fryer w/o skin roasted	1 cup (5 oz)	266	10	3	125	41	0	—	21	120	340	0	8	74
broiler/fryer w/o skin stewed	1 cup (5 oz)	248	9	3	116	38	0	—	19	98	252	0	8	70
broiler/fryer w/o skin stewed	1 oz	54	3	1	22	7	0	—	6	18	41	0	2	23
broiler/fryer wing w/ skin batter dipped & fried	1 (1.7 oz)	159	11	3	39	10	5	—	10	157	68	0	3	55
broiler/fryer wing w/ skin floured & fried	1 (1.1 oz)	103	7	2	26	8	1	—	5	25	57	0	1	40
broiler/fryer wing w/ skin roasted	1 (1.2 oz)	99	7	2	29	9	0	—	5	28	62	0	1	54
broiler/fryer wing w/ skin stewed	1 (1.4 oz)	100	7	2	28	9	0	—	5	27	56	0	1	53
capon w/ skin neck & giblets roasted	1 chicken (3.1 lbs)	3211	165	46	1458	402	1	—	211	704	3439	6	367	10408
cornish hen w/ skin roasted	1 hen (8 oz)	595	42	12	299	51	0	—	31	146	562	1	5	241
cornish hen w/o skin & bone roasted	1 hen (3.8 oz)	144	4	1	113	25	0	—	14	67	268	1	2	70
cornish hen w/o skin & bone roasted	½ hen (2 oz)	72	2	1	57	13	0	—	7	34	134	tr	1	35
cornish hen w/skin roasted	½ hen (4 oz)	296	21	6	149	25	0	—	15	73	280	1	3	120
roaster dark meat w/o skin roasted	1 cup (5 oz)	250	12	3	104	33	0	—	15	133	313	0	9	76
roaster light meat w/o skin roasted	1 cup (5 oz)	214	6	2	105	38	0	—	18	71	330	0	5	35

FOOD	PORTION	CALORIES	FAT	SAT FAT	CHOL	PROTEIN	CARBO	FIBER	CALCIUM	SOD	POTAS	VIT C	FOLIC	VIT A
roaster w/ skin neck & giblets roasted	1 chicken (2.4 lbs)	2363	140	39	1003	257	1	—	136	760	2183	4	251	6400
roaster w/ skin roasted	½ chicken (1.1 lbs)	1071	64	18	365	115	0	—	58	349	1014	0	22	399
roaster w/o skin roasted	1 cup (5 oz)	469	28	3	160	9	0	—	25	105	321	0	7	57
stewing dark meat w/o skin stewed	1 cup (5 oz)	361	21	6	132	39	0	—	17	133	285	0	12	203
stewing w/ skin neck & giblets stewed	1 chicken (1.3 lbs)	1636	107	29	603	157	tr	—	78	419	1052	3	211	5487
stewing w/ skin stewed	½ chicken (9.2 oz)	744	49	13	205	70	0	—	33	190	476	0	13	343
stewing w/ skin stewed	6.2 oz	507	34	9	140	34	0	—	22	130	325	0	9	234
PERDUE														
Boneless Breasts Cooked	3 oz	120	2	1	70	25	0	—	—	10	—	—	—	—
Boneless Breast Tenderloins Cooked	3 oz	100	1	1	55	23	0	—	—	25	—	—	—	—
Boneless Thighs Roasted	2 (3.5 oz)	200	11	3	130	25	0	—	—	60	—	—	—	—
Breast Quarters Cooked	3 oz	180	10	3	90	21	0	—	—	35	—	—	—	—
Burger Cooked	1 (3 oz)	170	11	3	120	17	0	—	20	35	—	—	—	—
Chicken Breast Seasoned Barbecue Cooked	3 oz	110	1	1	60	22	5	—	—	420	—	—	—	—
Chicken Breast Seasoned Italian Cooked	3 oz	100	1	1	55	20	2	—	—	520	—	—	—	—
Chicken Breast Seasoned Lemon Pepper Cooked	3 oz	90	1	1	55	19	2	—	—	520	—	—	—	—
Chicken Breast Seasoned Oriental Cooked	3 oz	100	1	1	55	20	3	—	—	550	—	—	—	—
Cornish Hen Split Dark Meat Roasted	1 half (6.5 oz)	210	15	5	130	18	0	0	—	45	—	—	—	200
Cornish Hen White Meat Cooked	3 oz	170	9	3	100	21	0	—	—	40	—	—	—	100
Drumsticks Roasted	1 (2 oz)	110	6	2	85	14	0	—	—	50	—	—	—	—
Drumsticks Skinless Roasted	2 (3.5 oz)	150	6	2	135	25	0	—	—	85	—	—	—	—
Ground Cooked	3 oz	180	12	4	145	17	0	—	40	55	—	—	—	—

FOOD	PORTION	CALORIES	FAT	SAT FAT	CHOL	PROTEIN	CARBO	FIBER	CALCIUM	SOD	POTAS	VIT C	FOLIC	VIT A
PERDUE (CONT.)														
Jumbo Drumsticks Roasted	1 (2 oz)	110	6	2	85	14	0	—	—	50	—	—	—	—
Jumbo Split Breast Roasted	1 (7 oz)	370	20	6	175	48	0	—	—	80	—	—	—	200
Jumbo Thighs Roasted	1 (3 oz)	240	18	5	125	19	0	—	—	60	—	—	—	100
Jumbo Whole Leg Roasted	2 (5.5 oz)	360	25	7	205	33	0	—	—	110	—	—	—	200
Jumbo Wings Roasted	2 (3 oz)	210	15	5	125	20	0	—	—	75	—	—	—	100
Leg Quarters Cooked	3 oz	210	16	5	115	18	0	—	—	55	—	—	—	—
Oven Stuffer Boneless Breast Cooked	3 oz	120	2	1	70	24	0	—	—	25	—	—	—	—
Oven Stuffer Boneless Breast Thin Sliced Cooked	1 slice (2 oz)	80	1	1	50	17	0	—	—	10	—	—	—	—
Oven Stuffer Boneless Thighs Roasted	1 (3.5 oz)	170	8	3	125	25	0	—	—	40	—	—	—	—
Oven Stuffer Dark Meat Roasted	3 oz	200	14	4	105	19	0	—	—	50	—	—	—	100
Oven Stuffer Drumstick Roasted	1 (3.5 oz)	190	11	3	135	25	0	—	—	80	—	—	—	100
Oven Stuffer White Meat Roasted	3 oz	160	8	3	80	22	0	—	—	45	—	—	—	0
Oven Stuffer Whole Breast Cooked	3 oz	150	7	2	75	22	0	—	—	35	—	—	—	—
Oven Stuffer Wing Drummettes Roasted	2 (2.5 oz)	170	11	4	90	17	0	—	—	45	—	—	—	100
Split Breast Skinless Roasted	1 (6 oz)	250	8	3	140	46	0	—	—	55	—	—	—	—
Split Breasts Roasted	1 (7 oz)	370	20	6	175	48	0	—	—	80	—	—	—	200
Thighs Roasted	1 (3 oz)	240	18	5	125	19	0	—	—	60	—	—	—	100
Thighs Skinless Roasted	1 (2.5 oz)	160	9	3	100	18	0	—	—	55	—	—	—	—
Whole White Meat Cooked	3 oz	160	9	3	85	20	0	0	—	40	—	—	—	100
Whole Leg Roasted	1 (5.5 oz)	360	25	7	200	33	0	—	—	110	—	—	—	200
Wingettes Roasted	3 (3 oz)	200	14	4	120	19	0	0	—	65	—	—	—	100
Wings Roasted	2 (3 oz)	210	15	5	125	20	0	—	—	75	—	—	—	100

FOOD	PORTION	CALORIES	FAT	SAT FAT	CHOL	PROTEIN	CARBO	FIBER	CALCIUM	SOD	POTAS	VIT C	FOLIC	VIT A
TYSON														
Breast	3 oz	116	2	—	72	24	0	—	—	63	—	—	—	—
Cornish Hen	3.5 oz	250	15	—	155	27	1	—	—	80	—	—	—	—
Drumstick	3 oz	131	4	—	79	23	0	—	—	81	—	—	—	—
Thigh	3 oz	152	7	—	81	21	0	—	—	75	—	—	—	—
Whole	3 oz	134	4	—	76	23	0	—	—	73	—	—	—	—
Wing	3 oz	147	6	—	72	23	0	—	—	78	—	—	—	—
WAMPLER LONGACRE														
Ground raw	1 oz	50	4	—	30	4	0	—	—	20	—	—	—	—
FROZEN														
BANQUET														
Country Fried	1 serv (3 oz)	270	18	5	65	14	13	1	80	620	—	4	—	0
Drum Snackers	2.25 oz	190	13	3	25	9	12	1	0	460	—	0	—	0
Fried Breast	1 piece (4.45 oz)	240	26	13	85	23	18	4	60	600	—	5	—	—
Fried Hot & Spicy	1 serv (3 oz)	260	18	5	65	14	13	1	80	590	—	4	—	0
Fried Original	1 serv (3 oz)	270	18	5	65	14	13	1	80	620	—	4	—	0
Fried Thigh & Drumsticks	1 serv (3 oz)	260	18	5	65	15	10	2	20	540	—	5	—	0
Hot & Spicy Nuggets	2.5 oz	230	17	4	25	9	11	1	0	320	—	0	—	0
Hot Popcorn Chicken	1 pkg (3 oz)	290	19	4	35	11	18	2	60	790	—	0	—	0
Nuggets	3 oz	240	15	3	35	14	12	1	0	540	—	0	—	0
Nuggets Chicken & Cheddar	2.7 oz	280	19	6	25	12	13	1	0	560	—	0	—	0
Nuggets Chicken & Mozzarella	6 (2.8 oz)	210	11	4	10	9	20	2	150	1060	—	0	—	0
Nuggets Southern Fried	6 (4.5 oz)	340	20	4	45	16	22	2	20	840	—	2	—	0
Nuggets Sweet & Sour	6 (4.5 oz)	320	18	4	45	16	25	2	20	670	—	1	—	0
Patties	1 (2.5 oz)	180	11	3	25	10	10	tr	0	360	—	0	—	0
Patties Southern Fried	1 (2.5 oz)	190	12	3	25	11	12	tr	0	480	—	1	—	0
Skinless Fried	1 serv (3 oz)	210	13	3	55	18	7	2	20	480	—	6	—	0
Skinless Fried Honey BBQ	1 serv (3 oz)	210	13	3	55	18	7	2	20	480	—	6	—	0
Southern Fried	1 serv (3 oz)	270	18	5	65	14	13	1	80	590	—	4	—	0
Tenders	3 pieces (3 oz)	260	16	4	25	12	16	2	0	490	—	1	—	0
Tenders Southern Fried	3 pieces (3 oz)	260	16	4	15	12	16	1	0	480	—	1	—	0
Wings Hot & Spicy	4 pieces (5 oz)	230	16	5	85	15	5	1	20	280	—	4	—	0
COUNTRY SKILLET														
Chicken Chunks	5 (3.1 oz)	270	17	3	20	12	18	1	20	720	—	0	—	0
Chicken Nuggets	10 (3.3 oz)	280	18	4	24	14	16	1	20	620	—	0	—	0
Chicken Patties	2.5 oz	190	12	3	20	9	12	1	0	500	—	0	—	0

FOOD	PORTION	CALORIES	FAT	SAT FAT	CHOL	PROTEIN	CARBO	FIBER	CALCIUM	SOD	POTAS	VIT C	FOLIC	VIT A
COUNTRY SKILLET (CONT.)														
Southern Fried Chicken Chunks	5 (3.1 oz)	250	15	3	20	12	16	1	20	550	—	0	—	0
Southern Fried Chicken Patties	1 (2.5 oz)	190	12	3	20	9	12	1	0	450	—	1	—	0
EMPIRE														
Nuggets	5 (3 oz)	180	9	2	15	13	12	1	0	370	—	0	—	0
Stix	4 (3.1 oz)	180	9	2	25	18	6	2	0	420	—	0	—	0
OZARK VALLEY														
Nuggets	4 (2.9 oz)	210	10	2	25	13	16	2	0	590	—	0	—	0
Patties	1 (3 oz)	210	11	3	30	14	14	1	0	550	—	1	—	0
SENSIBLE CHEF														
Fried Breast	1 (3 oz)	200	10	3	55	21	8	2	0	310	—	2	—	0
SWANSON														
Chicken Nibbles	3¼ oz	300	19	—	—	12	19	—	20	690	—	—	—	—
Chicken Nuggets	3 oz	230	14	—	—	13	14	—	—	360	—	—	—	—
Fried Chicken Breast Portion	4½ oz	360	20	—	—	23	21	—	40	800	—	—	—	—
Pre-Fried Chicken Parts	3¼ oz	270	16	—	—	15	16	—	—	650	—	—	—	—
Thighs & Drumsticks	3¼ oz	290	18	—	—	15	17	—	—	610	—	—	—	—
TYSON														
BBQ Breast Fillets	3 oz	110	2	—	50	14	13	—	—	200	—	—	—	—
Boneless Breasts	3.5 oz	210	12	—	80	26	0	—	—	50	—	—	—	—
Boneless Skinless Breast	3.5 oz	130	2	—	55	27	0	—	—	50	—	—	—	—
Boneless Skinless Thighs	3.5 oz	200	10	—	105	26	0	—	—	70	—	—	—	—
Breaded Patties	3 oz	300	20	—	—	14	15	—	—	—	—	—	—	—
Breast Chunks	3 oz	240	17	—	30	13	10	—	—	430	—	—	—	—
Breast Fillets	3 oz	190	9	—	25	13	15	—	—	400	—	—	—	—
Breast Patties	2.6 oz	220	15	—	35	10	11	—	—	640	—	—	—	—
Breast Tenders	3 oz	220	12	—	—	14	13	—	—	500	—	—	—	—
Chick'n Cheddar	2.6 oz	220	15	—	40	11	11	—	—	310	—	—	—	—
Chick'n Chunks	2.6 oz	220	15	—	35	10	11	—	—	500	—	—	—	—
Cordon Blue Mini	1	90	4	—	17	8	5	—	—	210	—	—	—	—
Diced	3 oz	130	3	—	70	24	1	—	—	40	—	—	—	—
Drums & Thighs	3.5 oz	270	17	—	130	28	0	—	—	110	—	—	—	—
Grilled Sandwich	3.5 oz	200	5	—	32	15	25	—	—	470	—	—	—	—
Hors D'Oeuvres Mesquite Chunks	3.5 oz	100	1	—	45	22	1	—	—	600	—	—	—	—
Hot BBQ Breast Tenders	2.75 oz	110	3	—	45	16	4	—	—	580	—	—	—	—
Mesquite Breast Fillets	2.75 oz	100	2	—	50	16	3	—	—	250	—	—	—	—

FOOD	PORTION	CALORIES	FAT	SAT FAT	CHOL	PROTEIN	CARBO	FIBER	CALCIUM	SOD	POTAS	VIT C	FOLIC	VIT A
TYSON (CONT.)														
Mesquite Breast Strips	2.75 oz	100	2	—	50	17	2	—	—	240	—	—	—	—
Mesquite Breast Tenders	2.75 oz	110	2	—	55	18	2	—	—	290	—	—	—	—
Microwave Chunks	3.5 oz	220	15	—	—	10	11	—	—	—	—	—	—	—
Microwave Chunks BBQ Sandwich	4 oz	230	6	—	30	16	27	—	—	600	—	—	—	—
Microwave Tenders	3.5 oz	230	11	—	—	16	19	—	—	600	—	—	—	—
Roasted Breast Fillets	1 oz	50	2	—	15	6	—	—	—	160	—	—	—	—
Roasted Breasts	1 oz	50	3	—	15	6	—	—	—	160	—	—	—	—
Roasted Drumsticks	1 oz	50	3	—	40	7	—	—	—	190	—	—	—	—
Roasted Half Chicken	1 oz	60	4	—	30	7	—	—	—	150	—	—	—	—
Roasted Thighs	1 oz	70	5	—	40	5	—	—	—	180	—	—	—	—
Roasted Whole Chicken	1 oz	60	4	—	30	7	—	—	—	150	—	—	—	—
Skinless Breast Tenders	3.5 oz	120	1	—	50	28	0	—	—	55	—	—	—	—
Southern Fried Breast Fillets	3 oz	220	11	—	25	14	15	—	—	630	—	—	—	—
Southern Fried Breast Patties	2.6 oz	220	15	—	35	11	9	—	—	460	—	—	—	—
Southern Fried Chick'n Chunks	2.6 oz	220	15	—	35	10	11	—	—	540	—	—	—	—
Thick & Crispy Patties	2.6 oz	220	14	—	40	11	13	—	—	490	—	—	—	—
WEAVER														
Batter Dipped Breast	4.4 oz	310	20	—	—	20	13	—	—	220	—	—	—	—
Batter Dipped Drums & Thighs	3 oz	210	14	—	—	11	11	—	—	220	—	—	—	—
Batter Dipped Wings	4 oz	400	28	—	—	16	20	—	—	520	—	—	—	—
Breast Fillets	4.5 oz	270	13	—	—	20	18	—	—	520	—	—	—	—
Breast Fillets Strips	3.3 oz	200	10	—	—	13	14	—	—	500	—	—	—	—
Breast Patties	3 oz	205	11	—	—	12	14	—	—	640	—	—	—	—
Chicken Nuggets	2.6 oz	190	12	—	—	10	10	—	—	450	—	—	—	—
Crispy Dutch Frye Assorted	3.6 oz	290	18	—	—	16	16	—	—	550	—	—	—	—
Crispy Dutch Frye Breasts	4.5 oz	350	22	—	—	22	17	—	—	520	—	—	—	—
Crispy Dutch Frye Drums & Thighs	3.5 oz	290	19	—	—	16	14	—	—	640	—	—	—	—
Crispy Dutch Frye Wings	4 oz	400	28	—	—	16	20	—	—	520	—	—	—	—

FOOD	PORTION	CALORIES	FAT	SAT FAT	CHOL	PROTEIN	CARBO	FIBER	CALCIUM	SOD	POTAS	VIT C	FOLIC	VIT A
WEAVER (CONT.)														
Crispy Light Skinless	2.9 oz	170	9	—	—	14	9	—	—	320	—	—	—	—
Croquettes	2 pieces	280	16	—	—	14	22	—	—	780	—	—	—	—
Croquettes With Gravy	2 pieces + ½ cup gravy	282	18	—	—	15	26	—	—	1040	—	—	—	—
Honey Batter Tenders	3 oz	220	12	—	—	13	14	—	—	500	—	—	—	—
Hot Wings	2.7 oz	170	11	—	—	17	1	—	—	670	—	—	—	—
Mini Drums Crispy	3 oz	210	12	—	—	13	13	—	—	480	—	—	—	—
Mini Drums Herbs & Spice	3 oz	200	11	—	—	13	13	—	—	320	—	—	—	—
Premium Tenders	3 oz	170	9	—	—	12	11	—	—	500	—	—	—	—
Rondelets Cheese	1 (2.6 oz)	190	11	—	—	11	12	—	—	520	—	—	—	—
Rondelets Italian	1 (2.6 oz)	190	11	—	—	11	11	—	—	560	—	—	—	—
Rondelets Original	1 (3 oz)	190	10	—	—	13	13	—	—	610	—	—	—	—
READY-TO-EAT														
chicken roll light meat	1 pkg (6 oz)	271	13	3	85	33	4	—	73	992	388	—	—	—
chicken roll light meat	2 oz	90	4	1	28	11	1	—	24	331	129	—	—	—
poultry salad sandwich spread	1 tbsp (13 g)	109	2	tr	4	2	1	—	1	49	24	0	1	18
poultry salad sandwich spread	1 oz	238	4	1	9	3	2	—	3	107	52	0	1	39
BANQUET														
Breast Tenders Fat Free	3 (3.2 oz)	130	0	0	30	13	20	2	0	480	—	0	—	0
CARL BUDDIG														
Chicken	1 oz	50	3	2	20	5	1	0	20	320	55	0	—	0
CHICKEN BY GEORGE														
Cajun	1 breast (4 oz)	130	4	1	60	21	3	0	0	700	—	1	—	100
Caribbean Grill	1 breast (4 oz)	150	4	1	60	22	8	0	0	550	—	2	—	0
Garlic & Herb	1 breast (4 oz)	120	3	1	60	21	3	0	0	600	—	0	—	0
Italian Bleu Cheese	1 breast (4 oz)	130	5	1	60	20	2	0	20	790	—	1	—	0
Lemon Herb	1 breast (4 oz)	120	3	1	60	20	3	0	0	800	—	1	—	0
Lemon Oregano	1 breast (4 oz)	130	4	1	50	20	3	0	0	600	—	2	—	0
Mesquite Barbecue	1 breast (4 oz)	130	3	1	60	21	5	0	0	700	—	1	—	100
Mustard Dill	1 breast (4 oz)	140	5	1	60	20	2	0	20	650	—	1	—	0
Roasted	1 breast (4 oz)	110	3	1	55	20	1	0	0	500	—	1	—	0
Teriyaki	1 breast (4 oz)	130	3	1	55	21	6	0	0	530	—	1	—	0
Tomato Herb With Basil	1 breast (4 oz)	140	5	1	60	20	5	0	0	630	—	1	—	100
EMPIRE														
Barbarcue Whole	5 oz	280	17	5	110	31	1	0	0	460	—	0	—	500
Battered & Breaded Cutlets	1 (3.3 oz)	200	9	2	25	18	11	2	—	320	—	—	—	—

FOOD	PORTION	CALORIES	FAT	SAT FAT	CHOL	PROTEIN	CARBO	FIBER	CALCIUM	SOD	POTAS	VIT C	FOLIC	VIT A
EMPIRE (CONT.)														
Battered & Breaded Fried Breasts	3 oz	170	8	2	45	21	3	tr	20	440	—	0	—	0
Battered & Breaded Nuggets	5 (3 oz)	200	13	3	30	13	9	1	0	650	—	0	—	0
Bologna	3 slices (1.8 oz)	200	7	2	40	7	2	0	20	360	—	0	—	0
Fried Drum & Thigh	3 oz	240	16	4	80	16	7	2	0	260	—	0	—	0
FALLS														
BBQ	3 oz	150	8	—	75	18	—	—	—	310	—	—	—	—
HEALTHY CHOICE														
Deli-Thin Oven Roasted Breast	6 slices (2 oz)	45	0	0	25	11	0	0	0	410	—	0	—	0
Deli-Thin Smoked Breast	6 slices (2 oz)	60	2	1	30	11	1	0	0	420	—	0	—	0
Fresh-Trak Oven Roasted Breast	1 slice (1 oz)	30	1	0	15	6	0	0	0	290	—	0	—	0
Oven Roasted Breast	1 slice (1 oz)	25	0	0	15	6	0	0	0	220	—	0	—	0
Smoked Breast	1 slice (1 oz)	35	1	0	15	6	0	0	0	220	—	0	—	0
HEBREW NATIONAL														
Deli Thin Oven Roasted	1.8 oz	45	1	—	20	10	—	—	—	460	—	—	—	—
HILLSHIRE														
Deli Select Oven Roasted Breast	1 slice	10	tr	—	—	2	tr	—	—	115	—	—	—	—
Deli Select Smoked Breast	1 slice	10	tr	—	—	2	tr	—	—	95	—	—	—	—
Flavor Pack 90-99% Fat Free Smoked Breast	1 slice (0.75 oz)	20	tr	—	—	4	tr	—	—	220	—	—	—	—
Lunch 'N Munch Smoked Chicken/ Monterey Jack	1 pkg (4.5 oz)	350	20	—	—	22	19	—	—	1260	—	—	—	—
Lunch 'N Munch Smoked Chicken/ Monterey/ Snickers	1 pkg (4.25 oz)	400	23	—	—	19	31	—	—	1080	—	—	—	—
LOUIS RICH														
Carving Board Classic Baked	2 slices (1.6 oz)	45	1	0	25	9	2	0	0	510	—	0	—	0
Carving Board Grilled	2 slices (1.6 oz)	45	1	0	25	9	2	0	0	510	—	0	—	0
Deli-Thin Oven Roasted Breast	4 slices (1.8 oz)	50	1	1	25	10	1	0	0	620	—	0	—	0
Oven Roasted Deluxe Breast	1 slice (1 oz)	30	1	0	15	5	1	0	0	330	—	0	—	0

FOOD	PORTION	CALORIES	FAT	SAT FAT	CHOL	PROTEIN	CARBO	FIBER	CALCIUM	SOD	POTAS	VIT C	FOLIC	VIT A
MR. TURKEY														
Deli Cuts Hardwood Smoked	3 slices	30	tr	—	13	5	2	—	—	305	—	—	—	—
Deli Cuts Oven Roasted	3 slices	25	0	—	15	5	2	—	—	220	—	—	—	—
OSCAR MAYER														
Free Oven Roasted Breast	4 slices (1.8 oz)	45	0	0	25	10	1	0	0	650	—	0	—	0
Lunchables Chicken/ Monterey Jack	1 pkg (4.5 oz)	350	21	10	75	20	20	1	250	1690	—	0	—	200
Lunchables Deluxe Chicken/Turkey	1 pkg (5.1 oz)	380	22	11	70	22	24	1	200	1840	—	0	—	300
Lunchables Dessert Chocolate Pudding/ Chicken/ Jack	1 pkg (6.2 oz)	370	18	9	55	19	33	0	200	1490	—	0	—	200
PERDUE														
Cafe Meal Kit Stir Fry	1 serv (8.2 oz)	360	2	—	25	19	65	3	—	1180	—	—	—	—
Cornish Hen Dark Meat Cooked	3 oz	200	15	5	130	17	0	—	—	45	—	—	—	200
Cornish Hen Split White Meat Roasted	½ hen (6.5 oz)	200	11	4	115	24	0	0	—	45	—	—	—	100
Nuggets Chicken & Cheese	5 (3 oz)	220	15	4	95	11	11	2	—	550	—	—	—	200
Nuggets Chik-Tac-Toe Cooked	5 (3 oz)	200	12	3	35	9	15	2	—	390	—	—	—	—
Nuggets Football Basketball Baseball	4 (3 oz)	230	15	4	35	11	14	—	80	500	—	—	—	—
Nuggets Original	5 (3 oz)	200	12	3	35	9	15	2	—	390	—	—	—	—
Nuggets Star & Drumstick	4 (3 oz)	200	12	3	35	9	15	2	—	390	—	—	—	—
Original Tenderloins Cooked	3 oz	160	7	3	65	18	7	2	—	320	—	—	—	—
Original Cutlets Cooked	1 (3.5 oz)	230	13	4	40	10	18	2	—	450	—	—	—	100
Oven Roasted Breast	1 (5 oz)	190	6	2	115	34	0	0	20	540	—	—	—	100
Oven Roasted Drumsticks	2 (2.5 oz)	100	4	1	95	17	0	0	—	350	—	—	—	—
Oven Roasted Half Dark Meat	3 oz	170	11	3	110	17	0	0	—	320	—	—	—	100
Oven Roasted Half White Meat	3 oz	140	7	2	80	19	0	0	—	320	—	—	—	—

FOOD	PORTION	CALORIES	FAT	SAT FAT	CHOL	PROTEIN	CARBO	FIBER	CALCIUM	SOD	POTAS	VIT C	FOLIC	VIT A
PERDUE (CONT.)														
Oven Roasted Thighs	1 (3 oz)	170	12	4	105	16	0	0	—	360	—	—	—	100
Oven Roasted Whole Chicken Dark Meat	3 oz	170	11	3	110	17	0	0	—	320	—	—	—	100
Oven Roasted Whole Chicken White Meat	3 oz	140	7	2	60	19	0	0	—	320	—	—	—	—
Seasoned Whole Chicken White Meat	3 oz	160	9	3	75	19	1	—	—	320	—	—	—	—
Short Cuts Italian	3 oz	110	2	1	55	22	1	0	—	540	—	—	—	—
Short Cuts Lemon Pepper	½ cup (2.5 oz)	90	2	1	50	19	2	—	—	530	—	—	—	—
Short Cuts Mesquite	3 oz	110	2	1	50	21	2	0	—	510	—	—	—	—
Short Cuts Oven Roasted	3 oz	110	2	1	55	22	2	0	—	765	—	—	—	—
Wings Barbecued	3 oz	200	13	4	105	16	3	1	40	600	—	—	—	100
Wings Hot & Spicy	3 oz	190	13	4	110	16	2	1	20	610	—	—	—	100
SHADY BROOK														
Slow Roasted Breast	2 oz	60	1	0	30	12	—	—	—	400	—	—	—	—
TYSON														
Bologna	1 slice	44	1	—	—	2	4	—	—	185	—	—	—	—
Hickory Smoked Breast	1 slice	25	1	—	—	4	1	—	—	195	—	—	—	—
Honey Flavored Breast	1 slice	25	1	—	—	4	1	—	—	—	—	—	—	—
Oven Roasted Breast	1 slice	25	1	—	—	4	1	—	—	185	—	—	—	—
Oven Roasted Mesquite Breast	1 slice	25	1	—	—	4	1	—	—	—	—	—	—	—
Roasted Drumsticks w/ Skin	2 (3.8 oz)	220	12	4	150	27	1	—	—	580	—	—	—	—
Roll	1 slice	26	1	—	—	3	1	—	—	153	—	—	—	—
Wings Barbecue	6-7 (3.5 oz)	218	14	—	—	23	0	—	—	400	—	—	—	—
Wings Hot & Spicy	6-7 (3.5 oz)	218	14	—	—	23	0	—	—	400	—	—	—	—
Wings Roasted	6-7 (3.5 oz)	218	14	—	—	23	0	—	—	400	—	—	—	—
Wings Teriyaki	6-7 (3.5 oz)	218	14	—	—	23	0	—	—	400	—	—	—	—
WAMPLER LONGACRE														
Breast	1 oz	35	1	—	15	5	1	—	—	200	—	—	—	—
Chef's Select Breast	1 oz	35	1	—	15	6	tr	—	—	320	—	—	—	—
Premium Oven Roasted Breast	1 oz	50	3	—	20	4	2	—	—	350	—	—	—	—
Roll	1 oz	65	5	—	25	5	tr	—	—	240	—	—	—	—

FOOD	PORTION	CALORIES	FAT	SAT FAT	CHOL	PROTEIN	CARBO	FIBER	CALCIUM	SOD	POTAS	VIT C	FOLIC	VIT A
WAMPLER LONGACRE (CONT.)														
Roll Sliced	1 slice (0.8 oz)	50	4	—	20	4	1	—	—	170	—	—	—	—
WEAVER														
Roasted Wings	1 oz	70	5	—	45	6	—	—	—	180	—	—	—	—
WEIGHT WATCHERS														
Roasted & Smoked Breast	2 slices (¾ oz)	25	1	—	15	4	tr	—	—	220	—	—	—	—
Roasted Ham	2 slices (¾ oz)	25	1	—	10	4	tr	—	—	210	—	—	—	—
TAKE-OUT														
boneless breaded & fried w/ barbecue sauce	6 pieces (4.6 oz)	330	18	6	61	17	25	—	21	830	319	tr	28	342
boneless breaded & fried w/ honey	6 pieces (4 oz)	339	18	5	61	17	27	—	17	537	255	tr	11	101
boneless breaded & fried w/ mustard sauce	6 pieces (4.6 oz)	323	17	6	62	17	21	—	25	791	280	tr	12	110
boneless breaded & fried w/ sweet & sour sauce	6 pieces (4.6 oz)	346	18	6	61	17	29	—	20	791	280	tr	12	242
breast & wing breaded & fried	2 pieces (5.7 oz)	494	30	8	149	36	20	—	60	975	566	0	9	192
drumstick breaded & fried	2 pieces (5.2 oz)	430	27	7	165	30	16	—	36	756	446	0	10	222
oven roasted breast of chicken	2 oz	60	1	0	25	11	0	—	—	470	—	—	—	—
thigh breaded & fried	2 pieces (5.2 oz)	430	27	7	165	30	16	—	36	756	446	0	10	222

CHICKEN DISHES

(*see also* CHICKEN SUBSTITUTES, DINNER)

FOOD	PORTION	CALORIES	FAT	SAT FAT	CHOL	PROTEIN	CARBO	FIBER	CALCIUM	SOD	POTAS	VIT C	FOLIC	VIT A
CANNED														
DINTY MOORE														
Noodles & Chicken	1 can (7.5 oz)	180	8	2	30	7	19	1	20	1010	—	0	—	500
Stew	1 cup (8.5 oz)	220	11	3	40	12	16	2	20	980	—	1	—	2000
SWANSON														
Chicken & Dumplings	7½ oz	220	11	—	—	11	19	—	20	980	—	—	—	400
Chicken Ala King	5¼ oz	190	12	—	—	10	9	—	40	690	—	—	—	—
Chicken Stew	7⅝ oz	160	7	—	—	9	15	—	20	990	—	6	—	5500
FROZEN														
CROISSANT POCKET														
Stuffed Sandwich Chicken Broccoli & Cheddar	1 piece (4.5 oz)	300	11	4	35	14	37	5	80	640	—	9	—	500
HOT POCKET														
Stuffed Sandwich Chicken & Cheddar With Broccoli	1 (4.5 oz)	300	12	5	30	12	37	tr	250	620	—	0	—	300

FOOD	PORTION	CALORIES	FAT	SAT FAT	CHOL	PROTEIN	CARBO	FIBER	CALCIUM	SOD	POTAS	VIT C	FOLIC	VIT A
JIMMY DEAN														
Grilled Breast Sandwich	1 (5.5 oz)	330	11	4	70	28	27	1	—	730	—	—	—	—
LEAN POCKETS														
Stuffed Sandwich Chicken Fajita	1 (4.5 oz)	260	8	3	40	12	36	3	200	770	—	2	—	400
Stuffed Sandwich Chicken Parmesan	1 (4.5 oz)	260	8	3	25	12	34	1	200	630	—	0	—	300
Stuffed Sandwich Glazed Chicken Supreme	1 (4.5 oz)	240	7	3	30	10	34	1	150	600	—	1	—	1000
LUIGINO'S														
Chicken A La King With Noodles	1 pkg (8 oz)	240	7	3	60	18	28	2	100	660	—	0	—	200
Noodles With Chicken Peas & Carrots	1 cup (6.3 oz)	260	10	3	40	11	33	2	60	560	—	0	—	200
Noodles With Chicken Peas & Carrots	1 pkg (8 oz)	300	11	3	50	13	38	2	60	640	—	0	—	200
Sweet & Sour Chicken With Rice	1 pkg (8 oz)	300	6	3	20	12	50	2	40	480	—	0	—	400
MRS. PATERSON'S														
Aussie Pie Chicken	1 (5.5 oz)	460	25	8	90	12	45	2	20	770	—	0	—	1000
Aussie Pie Chicken Low Fat	1 (5.5 oz)	380	17	6	35	13	44	1	20	930	—	0	—	500
TYSON														
Microwave Breast Sandwich	4.25 oz	328	14	—	—	16	33	—	—	520	—	—	—	—
WHITE CASTLE														
Grilled Chicken Sandwich	2 (4 oz)	250	9	3	20	17	24	5	40	490	—	0	—	0
Grilled Chicken Sandwich w/ Sauce	2 (4.8 oz)	290	9	3	20	17	33	5	40	600	—	0	—	0
MIX														
CHICKEN SKILLET HELPER														
Stir-Fried Chicken as prep	1 cup	270	9	2	110	18	30	1	60	810	210	0	60	300
HAMBURGER HELPER														
Cheddar Spirals Reduced Sodium Chicken Recipe as prep	1 cup	240	6	2	40	21	27	1	100	630	720	0	60	500
Italian Herb Reduced Sodium Chicken Recipe as prep	1 cup	200	2	1	35	19	29	2	20	630	570	0	60	500

FOOD	PORTION	CALORIES	FAT	SAT FAT	CHOL	PROTEIN	CARBO	FIBER	CALCIUM	SOD	POTAS	VIT C	FOLIC	VIT A
HAMBURGER HELPER (CONT.)														
Southwestern Beef Reduced Sodium Chicken Recipe as prep	1 cup	220	3	1	35	20	32	2	20	630	610	0	60	500
READY-TO-EAT														
SHADY BROOK														
Chicken Breast w/ Rice Pilaf	1 serv (12 oz)	350	13	4	120	46	—	—	—	270	—	—	—	—
Teriyaki Breast	1 serv (12 oz)	490	3	1	15	34	—	—	—	1600	—	—	—	—
WAMPLER LONGACRE														
Cacciatore	1 serv (4 oz)	118	3	—	40	14	5	—	—	267	—	—	—	—
Salad	1 oz	70	3	—	15	3	3	—	—	125	—	—	—	—
Salad Lite	1 oz	45	2	—	10	3	3	—	—	95	—	—	—	—
Smokey Barbecue	1 serv (4 oz)	175	7	—	65	17	11	—	—	460	—	—	—	—
Sweet N Sour	1 serv (4 oz)	106	tr	—	25	9	16	—	—	231	—	—	—	—
Szechwan With Peanuts	1 serv (4 oz)	112	4	—	22	13	6	—	—	560	—	—	—	—
SHELF-STABLE														
DINTY MOORE														
Microwave Cup Chicken & Dumpling	1 pkg (7.5 oz)	200	6	2	35	15	21	1	20	890	—	0	—	0
Microwave Cup Stew	1 pkg (7.5 oz)	180	8	2	30	10	18	2	20	920	—	5	—	2000
LUNCH BUCKET														
Dumplings'n Chicken	1 pkg (7.5 oz)	140	2	—	—	4	25	—	—	880	—	—	—	—
Light'n Healthy Chicken Fiesta	1 pkg (7.5 oz)	170	3	—	10	7	28	—	—	600	—	—	—	—
TAKE-OUT														
chicken & noodles	1 cup	365	18	5	103	22	26	—	26	600	149	tr	—	430
chicken a la king	1 cup	470	34	13	221	27	12	—	127	760	404	12	—	1130
chicken paprikash	1½ cups	296	10	—	90	—	—	—	99	—	—	—	—	—
fillet sandwich plain	1	515	29	9	60	24	39	—	60	957	358	9	28	100
fillet sandwich w/ cheese lettuce mayonnaise & tomato	1	632	39	12	76	29	42	—	258	1238	334	3	46	620

CHICKEN SUBSTITUTES

FOOD	PORTION	CALORIES	FAT	SAT FAT	CHOL	PROTEIN	CARBO	FIBER	CALCIUM	SOD	POTAS	VIT C	FOLIC	VIT A
HARVEST DIRECT														
TVP Poultry Chunks	3.5 oz	280	1	tr	0	52	32	18	—	15	2200	—	—	—
TVP Poultry Ground	3.5 oz	280	1	tr	0	52	32	18	—	15	2200	—	—	—
KNOX MOUNTAIN FARM														
Chick'N Wheat Mix	1 serv (⅑ pkg)	110	1	—	—	13	3	2	40	220	—	—	—	—

FOOD	PORTION	CALORIES	FAT	SAT FAT	CHOL	PROTEIN	CARBO	FIBER	CALCIUM	SOD	POTAS	VIT C	FOLIC	VIT A
LOMA LINDA														
Chicken Supreme Mix not prep	⅓ cup (0.9 oz)	90	1	0	0	15	6	4	20	720	450	0	—	0
Chik Nuggets	5 pieces (3 oz)	240	16	3	0	12	13	5	40	710	150	0	—	0
Fried Chik'n w/ Gravy	2 pieces (2.8 oz)	210	17	3	5	12	3	2	0	440	35	0	—	0
MORNINGSTAR FARMS														
Chik Nuggets	4 pieces (3 oz)	160	4	1	0	13	17	5	40	670	330	0	—	0
Chik Patties	1 (2.5 oz)	150	6	1	0	9	15	2	0	570	150	0	—	0
SOY IS US														
Chicken Not!	½ cup (1.75 oz)	140	2	1	0	24	15	9	160	5	—	0	—	0
WHITE WAVE														
Meatless Sandwich Slices	2 slices (1.6 oz)	80	0	0	0	12	8	0	0	260	—	0	—	0
WORTHINGTON														
Chic-Ketts	2 slices (1.9 oz)	120	7	1	0	13	2	2	0	390	30	0	—	0
Chicken Sliced	2 slices (2 oz)	80	5	1	0	9	1	tr	0	270	280	0	—	0
ChikStiks	1 (1.6 oz)	110	7	1	0	9	3	2	0	360	60	0	—	0
CrispyChik Patties	1 (2.5 oz)	170	9	2	0	8	15	4	0	600	200	0	—	0
Cutlets	1 slice (2.1 oz)	70	1	0	0	11	3	2	0	340	30	0	—	0
Diced Chik	¼ cup (1.9 oz)	40	0	0	0	7	1	1	0	270	100	0	—	0
FriChik	2 pieces (3.2 oz)	120	8	1	0	10	1	1	0	430	150	0	—	0
FriChik Low Fat	2 pieces (3 oz)	80	3	0	0	10	2	1	0	430	150	0	—	0
Golden Croquettes	4 pieces (3 oz)	210	10	2	0	14	14	6	40	600	190	0	—	0
Sliced Chik	3 slices (3.2 oz)	70	1	0	0	14	2	2	20	430	170	0	—	0

CHICKPEAS

FOOD	PORTION	CALORIES	FAT	SAT FAT	CHOL	PROTEIN	CARBO	FIBER	CALCIUM	SOD	POTAS	VIT C	FOLIC	VIT A
CANNED														
chickpeas	1 cup	285	3	tr	0	12	54	—	78	718	413	9	160	58
ALLEN														
Garbanzo	½ cup (4.4 oz)	120	3	1	0	5	19	8	20	330	—	0	—	0
EAST TEXAS FAIR														
Garbanzo	½ cup (4.4 oz)	120	3	1	0	5	19	8	20	330	—	0	—	0
EDEN														
Organic	½ cup (4.6 oz)	120	2	—	—	7	19	5	60	10	250	—	—	—
GOYA														
Spanish Style	7.5 oz	150	2	—	0	9	32	9	90	890	480	2	—	460
GREEN GIANT														
Garbanzo	½ cup (4.4 oz)	110	2	0	0	6	18	5	40	380	—	0	—	0
OLD EL PASO														
Garbanzo	½ cup (4.6 oz)	120	3	0	0	5	20	7	40	280	—	0	—	0
PROGRESSO														
Chick Peas	½ cup (4.6 oz)	120	3	0	0	5	20	7	40	280	—	0	—	0

FOOD	PORTION	CALORIES	FAT	SAT FAT	CHOL	PROTEIN	CARBO	FIBER	CALCIUM	SOD	POTAS	VIT C	FOLIC	VIT A
DRIED														
cooked	1 cup	269	4	tr	0	15	45	—	80	11	477	2	282	44
BEAN CUISINE														
Garbanzo	½ cup	115	1	—	0	8	—	5	—	5	310	—	62	—
CHICORY														
greens raw chopped	½ cup	21	tr	tr	0	2	4	—	90	41	378	22	—	3600
root raw	1 (2.1 oz)	44	tr	tr	0	1	11	—	25	30	174	3	—	4
roots raw cut up	½ cup (1.6 oz)	33	tr	tr	0	1	8	—	18	23	131	2	—	3
witloof head raw	1 (1.9 oz)	9	tr	tr	0	tr	2	—	10	1	112	2	20	15
witloof raw	½ cup (1.6 oz)	8	tr	tr	0	tr	2	—	9	1	95	1	17	13
CHILI														
CANNED														
chili w/ beans	1 cup	286	14	6	43	15	30	—	119	1330	932	4	—	860
ALLEN														
Mexican Chili Beans	½ cup (4.5 oz)	120	1	0	0	6	22	8	60	300	—	0	—	200
ARMOUR														
Chili No Beans	1 cup (8.7 oz)	470	38	—	85	14	18	—	—	1200	—	—	—	—
Chili With Beans	1 cup (8.9 oz)	440	28	—	50	14	34	—	—	1270	—	—	—	—
Chili With Beans Hot	1 cup (8.9 oz)	440	28	—	50	14	34	—	—	1270	—	—	—	—
Chili With Beans Western Style	1 cup (8.8 oz)	460	32	—	60	14	29	—	—	1130	—	—	—	—
BROWN BEAUTY														
Mexican Chili Beans	½ cup (4.5 oz)	120	1	0	0	6	22	8	60	300	—	0	—	200
DEL MONTE														
Sauce	1 tbsp (0.6 oz)	20	0	0	0	1	0	0	0	480	—	1	—	500
EDEN														
Organic Chili Beans w/ Jalapeno & Red Peppers	½ cup (4.6 oz)	130	0	0	0	9	21	7	60	250	400	—	—	—
GEBHARDT														
Hot With Beans	1 cup	470	27	10	65	16	47	6	95	1000	1450	40	—	293
Plain	1 cup	530	43	16	70	21	20	1	59	990	680	11	—	39
With Beans	1 cup	495	28	10	92	20	47	6	96	1010	1470	40	—	86
HAIN														
Spicy Tempeh	7½ oz	160	4	—	0	7	24	—	80	1350	410	15	—	1500
Spicy Vegetarian	7½ oz	160	1	—	0	7	29	—	80	1060	440	15	—	1250
Spicy Vegetarian Reduced Sodium	7½ oz	170	1	—	0	7	31	—	80	200	440	18	—	1500
Spicy With Chicken	7½ oz	130	2	—	40	11	19	—	60	1030	460	1	—	500
HEALTH VALLEY														
Mild Vegetarian With Beans	5 oz	160	3	—	0	10	21	12	3	290	580	2	3	750

FOOD	PORTION	CALORIES	FAT	SAT FAT	CHOL	PROTEIN	CARBO	FIBER	CALCIUM	SOD	POTAS	VIT C	FOLIC	VIT A
HEALTH VALLEY (CONT.)														
Mild Vegetarian With Beans No Salt Added	5 oz	160	3	—	0	10	21	12	59	30	580	2	3	750
Mild Vegetarian With Lentils	5 oz	140	4	—	0	8	15	7	60	290	490	12	7	1050
Mild Vegetarian With Lentils No Salt Added	5 oz	140	4	—	0	8	15	7	60	50	490	12	7	1050
Spicy Vegetarian With Beans	5 oz	160	4	—	0	10	21	12	52	280	580	2	3	950
HORMEL														
Chunky With Beans	1 cup (8.7 oz)	270	7	3	35	18	34	7	60	1240	—	0	—	500
Hot No Beans	1 cup (8.3 oz)	210	9	3	35	16	17	3	40	910	—	0	—	1000
Hot With Beans	1 cup (8.7 oz)	270	7	3	35	18	33	7	60	1240	—	0	—	500
No Beans	1 cup (8.3 oz)	210	9	3	35	16	17	3	40	910	—	0	—	1000
Turkey No Beans	1 cup (8.3 oz)	190	3	1	75	24	17	3	100	1250	—	0	—	1250
Turkey With Beans	1 cup (8.7 oz)	210	3	1	35	17	30	5	80	1180	—	1	—	1250
Vegetarian	1 cup (8.7 oz)	200	1	0	0	12	38	7	60	780	—	0	—	1250
With Beans	1 cup (8.7 oz)	270	7	3	35	18	33	7	60	1240	—	0	—	500
With Beans	1 cup (8.7 oz)	270	7	3	35	18	33	7	60	1240	—	0	—	500
HUNT'S														
Chili Beans	½ cup (4.5 oz)	87	1	0	0	6	17	6	4	597	—	2	—	21
JUST RITE														
Hot With Beans	4 oz	195	10	4	33	11	16	1	39	495	450	4	—	13
With Beans	4 oz	200	11	4	33	10	16	1	38	500	435	4	—	7
Without Beans	4 oz	180	11	4	41	13	9	tr	31	515	375	5	—	8
NATURAL TOUCH														
Vegetarian	1 cup (8.1 oz)	170	1	0	0	18	21	11	40	870	480	0	—	500
OLD EL PASO														
Chili With Beans	1 cup (8 oz)	200	7	2	30	19	15	6	60	420	—	0	—	0
VAN CAMP'S														
Chilee Beanee Weenee	1 can (8 oz)	240	12	3	35	14	27	9	40	1090	510	—	140	1250
Chili With Beans	1 cup (8.9 oz)	350	21	8	45	19	28	7	40	1020	620	—	100	1750
WORTHINGTON														
Chili	1 cup (8.1 oz)	290	15	3	0	19	21	9	40	1130	420	0	—	0
Low Fat	1 cup (8.1 oz)	170	1	0	0	18	21	11	40	870	480	0	—	500
DRIED														
powder	1 tsp	8	tr	—	0	tr	1	—	7	26	50	2	—	908
GEBHARDT														
Chili Powder	1 tsp	15	tr	—	0	tr	3	tr	—	0	90	—	—	—
Chili Quik Seasoning	1 tsp	10	tr	—	0	tr	2	tr	5	165	40	—	—	—
HAIN														
Hot Chili	¼ pkg	30	1	—	0	1	5	—	20	370	125	1	—	400

FOOD	PORTION	CALORIES	FAT	SAT FAT	CHOL	PROTEIN	CARBO	FIBER	CALCIUM	SOD	POTAS	VIT C	FOLIC	VIT A
HAIN (CONT.)														
Medium Chili	¼ pkg	30	1	—	0	1	5	—	40	300	120	6	—	—
Mild Chili	¼ pkg	30	1	—	0	1	5	—	20	330	105	1	—	500
HURST														
HamBeens Chili Beans	1 serv	130	1	0	0	8	22	10	40	170	—	0	—	0
NILE SPICE														
Chili'n Beans Original	1 pkg	150	2	0	0	8	25	6	80	670	—	6	—	300
Chili'n Beans Spicy	1 pkg	150	2	0	0	8	25	6	80	720	—	9	—	300
OLD EL PASO														
Chili Seasoning Mix	1 tbsp (0.3 oz)	25	1	—	0	tr	4	1	0	770	—	0	—	300
WATKINS														
Chili Seasoning	1¼ tsp (4 g)	15	0	0	0	0	2	0	0	110	—	0	—	200
Powder	¼ tsp (0.5 g)	0	0	0	0	0	0	0	0	10	—	0	—	0
FROZEN														
AMY'S ORGANIC														
Whole Meals Chili & Cornbread	1 pkg (10.5 oz)	320	6	2	10	11	59	8	—	780	—	—	—	—
LEAN CUISINE														
Three Bean w/ Rice	1 pkg (10 oz)	250	6	2	5	10	38	9	150	590	700	6	—	2000
LIGHTLIFE														
Chili	4.3 oz	110	3	tr	0	7	14	—	—	360	—	—	—	—
LUIGINO'S														
Chili-Mac	1 pkg (8 oz)	230	7	3	25	14	29	3	60	770	—	0	—	200
STOUFFER'S														
With Beans	1 pkg (8.75 oz)	270	10	4	35	15	29	8	100	1130	610	4	—	750
SWANSON														
Homestyle Chili Con Carne	8¼ oz	270	10	—	—	20	26	—	60	740	—	4	—	1250
TABATCHNICK														
Vegetarian	7.5 oz	210	6	1	0	12	28	10	150	530	—	5	—	0
TYSON														
Chicken Chili	3.5 oz	105	3	—	—	8	11	—	—	420	—	—	—	—
SHELF-STABLE														
HORMEL														
Microcup Meals Chili Mac	1 cup (7.5 oz)	200	9	4	25	11	17	2	0	980	—	0	—	750
Microcup Meals Hot With Beans	1 cup (7.3 oz)	220	6	3	30	15	27	6	40	1050	—	0	—	400
Microcup Meals No Beans	1 cup (7.3 oz)	190	8	3	30	14	15	2	20	800	—	0	—	750
Microcup Meals With Beans	1 cup (7.3 oz)	220	6	3	30	15	27	6	40	1050	—	0	—	400

FOOD	PORTION	CALORIES	FAT	SAT FAT	CHOL	PROTEIN	CARBO	FIBER	CALCIUM	SOD	POTAS	VIT C	FOLIC	VIT A
LUNCH BUCKET														
Chili With Beans	1 pkg (7.5 oz)	300	14	—	45	16	26	—	—	1120	—	—	—	—
WAMPLER LONGACRE														
Turkey	1 serv (4 oz)	118	3	—	32	10	10	—	—	850	—	—	—	—
TAKE-OUT														
con carne w/ beans	8.9 oz	254	8	3	133	25	22	—	67	1008	691	2	30	1663

CHINESE CABBAGE

(_see_ CABBAGE)

CHINESE FOOD

(_see_ ASIAN FOOD)

CHINESE PRESERVING MELON

FOOD	PORTION	CALORIES	FAT	SAT FAT	CHOL	PROTEIN	CARBO	FIBER	CALCIUM	SOD	POTAS	VIT C	FOLIC	VIT A
cooked	½ cup	11	tr	tr	0	tr	3	—	16	93	5	9	—	0

CHIPS

(_see also_ POPCORN, PRETZELS, SNACKS)

FOOD	PORTION	CALORIES	FAT	SAT FAT	CHOL	PROTEIN	CARBO	FIBER	CALCIUM	SOD	POTAS	VIT C	FOLIC	VIT A
CORN														
barbecue	1 oz	148	9	1	0	2	16	1	37	216	67	1	—	173
barbecue	1 bag (7 oz)	1036	65	9	0	14	111	10	259	1511	468	3	—	1210
cones nacho	1 oz	152	9	8	—	2	17	—	10	270	35	—	—	—
cones plain	1 oz	145	8	6	0	2	18	—	1	290	23	—	—	—
onion	1 oz	142	6	1	0	2	19	—	8	278	40	—	—	34
plain	1 bag (7 oz)	1067	66	9	0	13	113	9	251	1248	281	0	40	186
plain	1 oz	153	10	1	0	2	16	1	36	179	40	0	6	27
puffs cheese	1 bag (8 oz)	1256	78	15	9	17	122	2	131	2383	376	tr	272	601
puffs cheese	1 oz	157	10	2	1	2	15	tr	16	298	47	0	34	75
twists cheese	1 bag (8 oz)	1256	78	15	9	17	122	2	131	2383	376	tr	272	601
twists cheese	1 oz	157	10	2	1	2	15	tr	16	298	47	0	34	75
ENERGY FOOD FACTORY														
Corn Pops Fat Free	½ oz	50	0	0	0	1	11	1	0	110	—	0	—	0
Corn Pops Nacho	½ oz	50	1	0	0	1	12	1	0	150	—	0	—	0
Corn Pops Original	½ oz	50	1	0	0	1	11	1	0	110	—	0	—	0
FRITOS														
Chili Cheese	34 pieces (1 oz)	160	10	—	0	2	15	1	40	300	55	—	—	—
Crisp 'N Thin	18 pieces (1 oz)	160	10	—	0	2	16	1	40	240	55	—	—	—
Dip Size	13 pieces (1 oz)	150	10	—	0	1	16	1	40	240	55	—	—	—
Non-Stop Nacho Cheese	34 pieces (1 oz)	150	9	—	tr	2	16	1	40	220	55	—	—	—
Rowdy Rustlers Bar-B-Q	34 pieces (1 oz)	150	9	—	0	2	17	1	40	300	45	—	—	—
Wild 'N Mild	32 pieces (1 oz)	160	9	—	0	2	16	1	40	240	55	—	—	—
HEALTH VALLEY														
Chips	1 oz	160	11	—	0	1	13	1	6	90	30	2	5	97

FOOD	PORTION	CALORIES	FAT	SAT FAT	CHOL	PROTEIN	CARBO	FIBER	CALCIUM	SOD	POTAS	VIT C	FOLIC	VIT A
HEALTH VALLEY (CONT.)														
No Salt Added	1 oz	160	11	—	0	1	13	1	4	1	30	2	5	97
With Cheddar Cheese	1 oz	160	10	—	2	3	15	1	18	120	60	2	5	114
LANCE														
BBQ	1 pkg (50 g)	260	16	3	0	3	25	—	40	360	30	—	—	—
Chips	1 pkg (50 g)	270	17	4	0	3	26	—	40	350	50	—	—	—
PLANTERS														
Corn Chips	34 chips (1 oz)	170	10	2	0	2	17	2	40	180	45	—	—	200
King Size	17 chips (1 oz)	160	10	2	0	2	16	2	40	180	45	—	—	200
Snacks To Go	1 pkg (1.5 oz)	240	15	2	0	3	23	3	60	260	65	—	—	100
SNYDER'S														
BBQ	1 oz	160	11	—	0	2	14	2	20	200	—	—	—	—
Chips	1 oz	160	11	—	0	2	14	2	20	150	—	—	—	—
WISE														
Corn Crunchies	1 oz	160	10	—	0	2	15	—	20	180	40	—	—	—
Crispy Corn	1 oz	160	10	—	0	2	15	—	20	125	35	—	—	—
Crispy Corn Nacho Cheese	1 oz	160	10	—	0	2	16	—	20	190	45	—	—	—
Dipsy Doodles	1 pkg (1.5 oz)	240	15	3	0	2	24	1	40	270	—	0	—	0
MULTIGRAIN														
BARBARA'S														
Pinta Chips	13 (1 oz)	130	6	2	0	2	19	2	—	70	—	—	—	—
Pinta Chips Salsa	12 (1 oz)	130	6	1	0	2	19	2	—	210	—	—	—	—
SUNCHIPS														
Chips	12 pieces (1 oz)	150	8	—	0	2	18	—	—	100	45	—	—	—
French Onion	12 pieces (1 oz)	140	7	—	tr	3	18	—	—	120	60	—	—	—
POTATO														
barbecue	1 oz	139	9	2	0	2	15	—	14	213	358	10	24	62
barbecue	1 bag (7 oz)	971	64	16	0	15	105	—	96	1486	2498	67	164	430
cheese	1 oz	140	8	2	—	2	16	—	20	225	433	15	—	—
cheese	1 bag (6 oz)	842	46	15	—	14	98	—	122	1348	2597	92	—	—
light	1 oz	134	6	1	0	2	19	—	6	139	495	7	—	—
light	1 bag (6 oz)	801	35	7	0	12	114	—	35	836	2955	44	—	—
potato	1 oz	152	10	3	0	2	15	—	7	168	361	9	13	0
potato	1 bag (8 oz)	1217	79	25	0	16	120	—	54	1347	2894	71	103	0
sour cream & onion	1 bag (7 oz)	1051	67	18	14	16	102	—	143	1237	2634	74	122	336
sour cream & onion	1 oz	150	10	3	2	2	15	—	20	177	377	11	18	48
sticks	1 oz	148	10	3	0	2	15	1	5	71	351	13	11	0
sticks	½ cup (0.6 oz)	94	6	2	0	1	10	1	3	45	223	9	7	0
sticks	1 pkg (1 oz)	148	10	3	0	2	15	—	5	71	351	13	11	0

FOOD	PORTION	CALORIES	FAT	SAT FAT	CHOL	PROTEIN	CARBO	FIBER	CALCIUM	SOD	POTAS	VIT C	FOLIC	VIT A
BARBARA'S														
No Salt Added	1¼ cups (1 oz)	150	10	1	0	2	15	0	—	20	—	—	—	—
Regular	1¼ cups (1 oz)	150	10	1	0	2	15	0	—	180	—	—	—	—
Ripple	1¼ cups (1 oz)	150	10	1	0	2	15	1	—	180	—	—	—	—
Yogurt & Green Onion	1¼ cups (1 oz)	150	9	1	0	2	15	1	—	240	—	—	—	—
BARREL O' FUN														
Barbeque	1 oz	145	9	2	0	2	16	0	20	250	—	6	—	0
Chips	1 oz	150	9	2	0	2	15	0	60	160	—	6	—	0
Sour Cream & Onion	1 oz	150	9	2	0	2	15	0	—	230	—	—	—	—
BUTTERFIELD														
Sticks	1 pkg (1.7 oz)	250	15	5	1	3	26	3	0	150	—	15	—	0
Sticks	⅔ cup (1 oz)	150	9	3	0	2	16	2	0	90	—	9	—	0
CAPE COD														
Chips	19 chips (1 oz)	150	8	2	0	2	17	1	0	110	—	6	—	0
COTTAGE FRIES														
No Salt Added	1 oz	160	11	—	0	2	14	—	—	5	340	6	—	—
ENERGY FOOD FACTORY														
Potato Pops Au Gratin	½ oz	60	2	1	<5	1	12	1	0	110	—	5	—	0
Potato Pops Fat Free	½ oz	50	0	0	0	1	13	1	0	110	—	5	—	0
Potato Pops Herb & Garlic	½ oz	50	1	0	0	1	11	1	0	110	—	5	—	0
Potato Pops Mesquite	½ oz	50	1	0	0	1	12	1	0	110	—	5	—	0
Potato Pops Original	½ oz	50	1	0	0	1	11	1	0	110	—	5	—	0
Potato Pops Salt N' Vinegar	½ oz	50	1	0	0	1	11	1	0	110	—	5	—	0
HEALTH VALLEY														
Country Ripple	1 oz	160	10	—	0	2	15	1	7	60	320	2	13	—
Country Ripple No Salt Added	1 oz	160	10	—	0	2	15	1	7	1	320	2	13	—
Dip Chips	1 oz	160	10	—	0	2	15	1	7	60	320	2	13	—
Dip Chips No Salt Added	1 oz	160	10	—	0	2	15	1	7	1	320	2	13	—
Natural	1 oz	160	10	—	0	2	15	1	7	60	320	2	13	—
Natural No Salt Added	1 oz	160	10	—	0	2	15	1	7	1	320	2	13	—
HERR'S														
Potato	1 oz	140	8	2	0	2	16	1	7	180	361	10	—	—

FOOD	PORTION	CALORIES	FAT	SAT FAT	CHOL	PROTEIN	CARBO	FIBER	CALCIUM	SOD	POTAS	VIT C	FOLIC	VIT A
LANCE														
BBQ	1 pkg (32 g)	190	12	3	0	3	18	—	—	270	420	6	—	—
Cajun Style	1 pkg (32 g)	160	11	2	0	2	16	—	—	250	—	7	—	400
Chips	1 pkg (32 g)	190	15	4	0	2	12	—	—	220	260	8	—	—
Hot Fries	1 pkg (28 g)	160	10	2	0	2	14	—	—	220	160	1	—	600
Ripple	1 pkg (32 g)	190	15	4	0	2	12	—	—	220	260	8	—	—
Sour Cream & Onion	1 pkg (32 g)	190	12	3	0	3	18	—	20	390	370	6	—	0.1
LAY'S														
Baked KC Masterpiece	11 pieces (1 oz)	110	2	tr	0	2	23	2	40	200	160	4	—	0
Baked Original	12 chips (1 oz)	110	2	tr	0	2	23	2	40	150	160	2	—	0
Baked Sour Cream & Onion	12 chips (1 oz)	110	2	tr	0	2	23	2	40	170	160	4	—	0
Bar-B-Q	17 pieces (1 oz)	150	9	—	0	1	15	1	—	270	350	6	—	—
Cheddar Cheese	17 pieces (1 oz)	150	10	—	tr	2	14	1	—	300	410	6	—	—
Crunch Tators	16 pieces (1 oz)	150	8	—	0	2	17	1	—	120	400	6	—	—
Crunch Tators Amazin' Cajun	16 pieces (1 oz)	150	8	—	0	2	17	—	—	150	370	6	—	—
Crunch Tators Hoppin' Jalapeno	16 pieces (1 oz)	140	7	—	0	1	18	1	—	200	400	6	—	—
Crunch Tators Mighty Mesquite	16 pieces (1 oz)	150	8	—	0	2	17	—	—	135	390	6	—	—
Crunch Tators Supreme Sour Cream	16 pieces (1 oz)	150	8	—	0	2	16	—	20	180	430	6	—	—
Flamin' Hot	17 pieces (1 oz)	150	9	—	0	2	15	1	—	190	380	6	—	—
Reduced Fat Original	21 chips (1 oz)	150	8	1	0	2	18	1	0	160	430	6	—	0
Salt & Vinegar	17 pieces (1 oz)	150	10	—	0	1	14	1	—	390	360	3	—	—
Tangy Ranch	17 pieces (1 oz)	160	10	—	0	2	15	1	—	210	340	6	—	—
Unsalted	17 pieces (1 oz)	150	10	—	0	2	15	1	—	10	410	6	—	—
Wow Original	25 chips (1 oz)	80	0	0	0	2	19	1	—	180	380	8	—	—
Wow Original	1 pkg (0.75 oz)	55	0	0	0	1	13	1	0	130	—	5	—	0
LOUISE'S														
"1g" Mesquite BBQ	1 oz	110	1	—	0	2	24	2	—	180	—	—	—	—
"1g" Original	1 oz	110	1	—	0	2	24	2	—	180	—	—	—	—

FOOD	PORTION	CALORIES	FAT	SAT FAT	CHOL	PROTEIN	CARBO	FIBER	CALCIUM	SOD	POTAS	VIT C	FOLIC	VIT A
LOUISE'S (CONT.)														
70% Less Fat Mesquite BBQ	1 oz	110	3	—	0	2	21	2	—	180	—	—	—	—
70% Less Fat Original	1 oz	110	3	—	0	2	21	2	—	200	—	—	—	—
Fat-Free Maui Onion	1 oz	110	0	0	0	3	23	2	—	180	—	—	—	—
Fat-Free Mesquite BBQ	1 oz	110	0	0	0	3	23	2	—	180	—	—	—	—
Fat-Free No Salt	1 oz	110	0	0	0	3	24	2	—	10	—	—	—	—
Fat-Free Original	1 oz	110	0	0	0	3	23	2	—	180	—	—	—	—
Fat-Free Vinegar & Salt	1 oz	110	0	0	0	3	23	2	—	300	—	—	—	—
MR. PHIPPS														
Tater Crisps Bar-B-Que	21 (1 oz)	130	4	1	0	2	21	1	20	270	200	1	—	200
Tater Crisps Original	23 (1 oz)	120	7	1	0	2	20	1	40	220	200	1		
Tater Crisps Sour Cream 'n Onion	22 (1 oz)	130	4	1	0	1	21	1	40	210	210	1		
NEW YORK DELI														
Chips	1 oz	160	11	—	0	2	14	—	—	120	340	6	—	—
PRINGLES														
BBQ	14 chips (1 oz)	150	6	3	0	2	15	—	—	200	—	4	—	—
Cheez-ums	14 chips (1 oz)	150	10	3	1	2	—	—	—	190	—	4	—	—
Fat Free	15 chips (1 oz)	75	0	0	0	2	17	2	—	170	—	1	—	—
Original	14 chips (1 oz)	160	11	3	0	2	—	—	—	170	—	4	—	—
Ranch	14 chips (1 oz)	150	10	3	0	2	—	—	—	130	—	4	—	—
Ridges Cheddar & Sour Cream	12 chips (1 oz)	150	10	3	0	1	—	—	—	200	—	4	—	—
Ridges Mesquite BBQ	12 chips (1 oz)	150	10	3	0	1	—	—	—	220	—	4	—	—
Ridges Original	12 chips (1 oz)	150	10	3	0	1	—	—	—	150	—	4	—	—
Right BBQ	16 chips (1 oz)	140	7	2	0	2	18	—	—	160	—	4	—	—
Right Original	16 chips (1 oz)	140	7	2	0	1	—	—	—	135	—	4	—	—
Right Ranch	16 chips (1 oz)	140	7	2	0	2	18	—	—	120	—	4	—	—
Right Sour Cream 'N Onion	16 chips (1 oz)	140	7	2	0	2	18	—	—	120	—	4	—	—
Rippled Original	10 chips (1 oz)	160	11	3	0	2	15	—	—	150	—	4	—	—

FOOD	PORTION	CALORIES	FAT	SAT FAT	CHOL	PROTEIN	CARBO	FIBER	CALCIUM	SOD	POTAS	VIT C	FOLIC	VIT A
PRINGLES (CONT.)														
Sour Cream N'Onion	14 chips (1 oz)	160	10	3	1	2	15	—	—	135	—	4	—	—
RUFFLES														
Cheddar Cheese & Sour Cream	18 chips (1 oz)	160	10	—	tr	2	15	1	—	250	360	3	—	—
Chips	18 chips (1 oz)	150	10	—	0	2	15	1	—	135	400	6	—	—
Mesquite Grille B-B-Q	18 chips (1 oz)	160	10	—	0	2	15	1	—	270	370	6	—	—
Monterey Jack Cheese Attack	18 chips (1 oz)	160	10	—	tr	2	15	1	—	200	390	3	—	—
Ranch	18 chips (1 oz)	160	10	—	0	2	15	1	—	220	360	3	—	—
Reduced Fat	16 chips (1 oz)	140	7	1	0	2	18	1	0	130	450	6	—	0
Sour Cream & Onion	18 chips (1 oz)	160	10	—	tr	2	15	1	—	220	370	3	—	—
SNYDER'S														
BBQ	1 oz	150	10	—	0	2	13	1	—	370	16	6	16	—
Cheddar Bacon	1 oz	150	10	—	0	2	13	1	—	260	16	6	16	—
Chips	1 oz	150	10	—	0	2	13	1	—	130	16	6	16	—
Coney Island	1 oz	150	10	—	0	2	13	1	—	280	16	6	16	—
Grilled Steak & Onion	1 oz	150	10	—	0	2	13	1	—	260	16	6	16	—
Hot Buffalo Wings	1 oz	150	10	—	0	2	13	1	—	200	16	6	16	—
Kosher Dill	1 oz	150	10	—	0	2	13	1	—	400	16	6	16	—
No Salt	1 oz	150	10	—	0	2	13	1	—	0	16	6	16	—
Salt & Vinegar	1 oz	150	10	—	0	2	13	1	—	200	16	6	16	—
Sausage Pizza	1 oz	150	10	—	0	2	13	1	—	230	16	6	16	—
Sour Cream & Onion	1 oz	150	10	—	0	2	13	1	—	190	16	6	16	—
Sour Cream & Onion Unsalted	1 oz	150	10	—	0	2	13	1	—	10	16	6	16	—
STATE LINE														
Chips	1 pkg (0.5 oz)	80	5	1	0	1	7	tr	0	70	—	4	—	0
SUPRIMOS														
Cheddar & Jack	1 oz	140	6	—	tr	4	17	—	—	180	55	—	—	—
Cool Onion	1 oz	140	6	—	tr	4	17	—	—	170	60	—	—	—
UTZ														
Wavy	20 chips (1 oz)	150	9	2	0	2	14	1	0	95	370	9	—	0
WISE														
Natural	1 oz	160	11	—	0	2	14	—	—	190	340	6	—	—
Ridgies Barbecue	1 oz	150	10	—	0	2	14	—	—	240	370	—	—	—
TORTILLA														
nacho	1 oz	141	7	1	0	2	18	2	42	201	61	1	4	105

FOOD	PORTION	CALORIES	FAT	SAT FAT	CHOL	PROTEIN	CARBO	FIBER	CALCIUM	SOD	POTAS	VIT C	FOLIC	VIT A
nacho	1 bag (8 oz)	1131	58	11	0	18	142	12	354	1606	491	4	32	841
nacho light	1 oz	126	4	1	0	3	20	—	45	284	77	tr	—	108
nacho light	1 bag (6 oz)	757	26	5	0	15	122	—	270	1705	462	tr	—	646
plain	1 bag (7.5 oz)	1067	56	11	0	15	134	14	327	1124	419	0	—	418
plain	1 oz	142	7	1	0	2	18	2	44	150	56	0	—	56
ranch	1 oz	139	7	1	0	2	18	—	40	174	69	tr	—	73
ranch	1 bag (7 oz)	969	47	9	1	15	128	—	280	1212	483	2	—	507
taco	1 bag (8 oz)	1089	55	11	—	18	143	—	352	1788	492	—	—	2055
taco	1 oz	136	7	1	—	2	18	—	44	223	61	—	—	257
BARBARA'S														
Blue Corn	15 (1 oz)	140	7	tr	0	3	16	1	—	40	—	—	—	—
Blue Corn No Salt Added	15 (1 oz)	140	7	tr	0	3	16	1	—	0	—	—	—	—
BARREL O' FUN														
Nacho	1 oz	140	6	2	0	2	19	1	80	160	—	—	—	—
Tostada Yellow	1 oz	140	6	2	0	2	19	0	20	40	—	—	—	—
White	1 oz	140	6	2	0	2	20	0	—	50	—	—	—	—
DORITOS														
Reduced Fat Cooler Ranch	13 chips (1 oz)	130	5	1	0	2	20	1	40	200	55	0	—	0
Reduced Fat Nacho Cheesier	13 chips (1 oz)	130	5	1	0	3	19	1	40	210	50	0	—	0
Wow Nacho Cheese	11 chips (1 oz)	97	1	—	—	3	21	1	—	260	60	tr	—	—
Wow Nacho Cheesier	1 pkg (0.75 oz)	70	1	0	0	2	13	1	40	180	—	0	—	0
FRITO LAY														
Salsa 'N Cheese	16 (1 oz)	150	8	—	0	2	17	2	40	180	75	—	—	—
GUILTLESS GOURMET														
Baked	22-26 chips (1 oz)	110	1	—	0	3	21	1	—	119	55	—	—	—
HAIN														
Sesame	1 oz	140	7	—	0	2	19	—	—	190	—	—	—	—
Sesame Cheese	1 oz	160	8	—	<5	2	20	—	—	270	—	—	—	—
Sesame No Salt Added	1 oz	140	7	—	0	2	19	—	—	<5	—	—	—	—
Taco Style	1 oz	160	11	—	<5	2	15	—	—	320	—	—	—	—
LA FAMOUS														
No Salt Added	1 oz	140	7	—	0	2	18	—	20	5	50	—	—	—
Tortilla	1 oz	140	7	—	0	2	18	—	20	180	50	—	—	—
LANCE														
Nacho	1 pkg (32 g)	160	8	2	0	3	19	—	20	240	35	—	—	—
LOUISE'S														
95% Fat-Free	1 oz	120	2	—	0	2	23	1	—	170	—	—	—	—
MR. PHIPPS														
Nacho	28 (1 oz)	130	4	1	0	2	20	3	40	150	100	1	—	400

FOOD	PORTION	CALORIES	FAT	SAT FAT	CHOL	PROTEIN	CARBO	FIBER	CALCIUM	SOD	POTAS	VIT C	FOLIC	VIT A
MR. PHIPPS (CONT.)														
Original	28 (1 oz)	130	4	1	0	2	21	3	20	130	85	—	—	100
OLD EL PASO														
NACHIPS	9 chips (1 oz)	150	8	2	0	3	17	2	40	85	—	0	—	0
White Corn	11 chips (1 oz)	140	8	1	0	2	18	1	40	60	—	0	—	0
SANTITAS														
Cantina Style	1 oz	140	6	—	0	2	19	2	20	75	50	—	—	—
Cantina Style Fajita	1 oz	140	7	—	0	2	19	2	20	95	60	—	—	—
Chips	1 oz	140	7	—	0	2	19	2	40	50	60	—	—	—
Strips	1 oz	140	7	—	0	2	19	2	40	65	50	—	—	—
SNYDER'S														
Chips	1 oz	140	7	—	0	2	18	2	30	130	—	—	—	—
Enchilada	1 oz	140	7	—	0	2	18	2	30	220	—	—	—	—
Nacho Cheese	1 oz	140	7	—	0	2	18	2	30	130	—	—	—	—
No Salt	1 oz	140	7	—	0	2	18	2	30	0	—	—	—	—
Ranch	1 oz	140	7	—	0	2	18	2	30	150	—	—	—	—
TOSTITOS														
Baked Cool Ranch	11 chips (1 oz)	120	3	0	0	2	21	1	40	170	60	0	—	0
Baked Original	9 chips (1 oz)	110	tr	0	0	2	24	2	40	200	60	0	—	0
Baked Unsalted	13 chips (1 oz)	110	1	0	0	3	24	2	40	10	60	0	—	0
Bite Size	16 pieces (1 oz)	150	8	—	0	2	18	2	40	110	45	—	—	—
Chips	11 pieces (1 oz)	140	8	—	0	2	18	2	40	160	50	—	—	—
Restaurant Style Lime 'N Chili	7 pieces (1 oz)	150	7	—	0	2	18	2	40	190	50	—	—	—
Restaurant Style White Corn	7 pieces (1 oz)	150	6	—	0	2	20	2	40	75	60	—	—	—
TYSON														
Nacho Cheese	1 oz	140	7	—	0	2	17	—	—	145	—	—	—	—
Ranch Flavor	1 oz	140	2	—	0	2	17	—	—	—	—	—	—	—
Traditional	1 oz	140	7	—	0	2	17	—	—	95	—	—	—	—
Unsalted	1 oz	140	7	—	0	2	17	—	—	7	—	—	—	—
WISE														
Bravos	1 oz	150	8	—	0	2	18	—	40	180	55	—	—	—
VEGETABLE														
taro	10 (0.8 oz)	115	6	1	0	1	16	—	14	79	174	1	—	0
taro	1 oz	141	7	2	0	1	19	—	17	97	214	1	—	0
EDEN														
Vegetable Chips	50 (1 oz)	130	4	2	0	tr	24	0	0	260	35	0	—	0
Wasabi Chip Hot & Spicy	50 (1 oz)	130	4	2	0	tr	24	0	0	260	35	0	—	0
HAIN														
Carrot Chips	1 oz	150	9	—	—	2	16	0	20	160	150	—	—	750

FOOD	PORTION	CALORIES	FAT	SAT FAT	CHOL	PROTEIN	CARBO	FIBER	CALCIUM	SOD	POTAS	VIT C	FOLIC	VIT A
HAIN (CONT.)														
Carrot Chips Barbecue	1 oz	140	8	—	—	2	16	0	20	160	150	—	—	750
Carrot Chips No Salt Added	1 oz	150	7	—	0	2	16	0	20	30	140	—	—	750
HEALTH VALLEY														
Carrot Lites	0.5 oz	75	4	—	0	1	9	tr	—	5	25	—	—	500
TERRA CHIPS														
Sweet Potato	1 oz	140	7	1	0	1	18	1	20	10	—	0	—	1000
Sweet Potato Spiced	1 oz	140	7	1	0	1	16	3	60	105	—	5	—	4000
Taro Spiced	1 oz	130	5	1	0	1	20	2	20	170	—	0	—	0
Vegetable	1 oz	140	7	1	0	1	18	3	20	70	—	2	—	0
TOP BANANA														
Plantain Chips	1 oz	150	8	—	0	1	17	—	—	85	200	4	—	—

CHITTERLINGS

FOOD	PORTION	CALORIES	FAT	SAT FAT	CHOL	PROTEIN	CARBO	FIBER	CALCIUM	SOD	POTAS	VIT C	FOLIC	VIT A
pork cooked	3 oz	258	24	9	122	9	0	0	23	33	—	0	3	0

CHIVES

FOOD	PORTION	CALORIES	FAT	SAT FAT	CHOL	PROTEIN	CARBO	FIBER	CALCIUM	SOD	POTAS	VIT C	FOLIC	VIT A
freeze-dried	1 tbsp	1	tr	tr	0	tr	tr	—	2	—	6	1	—	137

CHOCOLATE

(*see also* CANDY, CAROB, COCOA, ICE CREAM TOPPINGS, MILK DRINKS)

FOOD	PORTION	CALORIES	FAT	SAT FAT	CHOL	PROTEIN	CARBO	FIBER	CALCIUM	SOD	POTAS	VIT C	FOLIC	VIT A
BAKING														
baking	1 oz	145	15	9	0	3	8	—	22	1	235	0	—	10
grated unsweetened	1 cup (4.6 oz)	690	73	43	0	14	37	18	98	18	1100	0	9	129
liquid unsweetened	1 oz	134	14	7	0	3	10	—	15	3	331	—	—	—
squares unsweetened	1 square (1 oz)	148	16	9	0	3	8	4	21	4	236	0	2	28
BAKER'S														
Bittersweet	½ square (0.5 oz)	70	6	3	0	1	7	1	0	0	75	0	—	0
German's Sweet	2 squares (0.5 oz)	60	4	2	0	1	8	tr	0	0	50	0	—	0
Semi-Sweet	½ square (0.5 oz)	70	5	3	0	1	8	1	0	0	70	0	—	0
Unsweetened	½ square (0.5 oz)	70	7	5	0	2	4	2	0	0	140	0	—	0
White	½ square (0.5 oz)	80	5	3	<5	1	8	0	20	15	45	0	—	0
NESTLE														
Choco Bake	½ oz	80	8	5	—	1	5	3	—	0	—	—	—	—
Premier White	½ oz	80	5	3	<5	1	8	—	40	15	—	—	—	—
Semi-Sweet	½ oz	70	4	3	—	<1	9	2	—	0	—	—	—	—
Unsweetened	½ oz	80	7	2	—	2	5	3	—	0	—	—	—	—
CHIPS														
milk chocolate	1 cup (6 oz)	862	52	31	38	12	100	—	321	138	646	1	14	312
semisweet	1 cup (6 oz)	804	50	30	0	7	106	—	54	19	614	0	4	35

FOOD	PORTION	CALORIES	FAT	SAT FAT	CHOL	PROTEIN	CARBO	FIBER	CALCIUM	SOD	POTAS	VIT C	FOLIC	VIT A
semisweet	60 pieces (1 oz)	136	9	5	0	1	18	—	9	3	104	0	1	6
BAKER'S														
Chips	1 oz	143	8	—	5	2	18	—	47	25	93	—	2	46
Real Milk Chocolate	½ oz	70	4	2	0	1	9	0	20	10	50	0	—	0
Real Semi-Sweet	½ oz	60	4	2	0	1	9	1	0	0	60	0	—	0
Semi-Sweet	½ oz	70	4	3	0	0	10	0	0	15	55	0	—	0
M&M'S														
Baking Bits Milk Chocolate	0.5 oz	70	3	2	5	7	10	0	—	0	—	—	—	—
Baking Bits Semi-Sweet	0.5 oz	70	4	2	0	1	9	1	—	0	—	—	—	—
NESTLE														
Morsels Milk Chocolate	1 tbsp	70	4	—	—	0	10	—	—	0	—	—	—	—
Morsels Mint Chocolate	1 tbsp	70	4	2	—	0	9	2	—	0	—	—	—	—
Morsels Rainbow	1 tbsp	70	3	2	—	0	10	1	—	0	—	—	—	—
Morsels Mini Semi-Sweet	1 tbsp	70	4	—	—	0	9	2	—	0	—	—	—	—
Semi-Sweet Morsels	1 tbsp	40	4	—	—	0	9	2	—	0	—	—	—	—
MIX														
powder	2-3 heaping tsp	75	1	tr	0	1	20	—	8	45	128	tr	—	4
powder as prep w/ whole milk	9 oz	226	9	5	33	9	31	—	300	165	498	3	12	312
QUIK														
Chocolate Powder	2 tbsp (0.8 oz)	90	1	1	0	1	19	1	0	30	150	0	—	0
Chocolate Powder No Sugar Added	2 tbsp (0.4 oz)	40	1	1	0	1	7	2	0	45	170	0	—	0

CHOCOLATE MILK

(*see* CHOCOLATE, COCOA, MILK DRINKS, MILKSHAKE)

CHOCOLATE SYRUP

FOOD	PORTION	CALORIES	FAT	SAT FAT	CHOL	PROTEIN	CARBO	FIBER	CALCIUM	SOD	POTAS	VIT C	FOLIC	VIT A
chocolate fudge	1 cup (11.9 oz)	1176	46	19	—	15	200	—	340	442	731	—	—	306
chocolate fudge	1 tbsp (0.7 oz)	73	3	1	—	1	12	—	21	27	45	—	—	19
syrup	1 cup	653	3	2	0	6	177	—	42	287	672	1	12	89
syrup	2 tbsp	82	tr	tr	0	1	22	—	5	36	84	tr	2	11
syrup as prep w/ whole milk	9 oz	232	9	5	33	9	34	—	297	156	455	2	14	319
ESTEE														
Choco-Syp	2 tbsp (1.2 oz)	50	0	0	0	tr	11	—	—	15	50	—	—	—
MARZETTI														
Syrup	2 tbsp	40	4	1	0	1	21	0	20	50	—	0	—	0

FOOD	PORTION	CALORIES	FAT	SAT FAT	CHOL	PROTEIN	CARBO	FIBER	CALCIUM	SOD	POTAS	VIT C	FOLIC	VIT A
QUIK														
Chocolate	2 tbsp (1.3 oz)	100	1	0	0	1	23	tr	0	30	75	0	—	0
RED WING														
Syrup	2 tbsp (1.4 oz)	110	1	1	0	1	25	0	0	10	—	0	—	0
TOLLHOUSE														
Mint-Chocolate	2 tbsp (1.5 oz)	130	3	2	0	1	25	1	0	30	0	0	—	0
Semi-Sweet	2 tbsp (1.5 oz)	130	4	2	0	1	24	1	0	30	0	0	—	0
CHUTNEY														
coconut	¼ cup	74	7	6	0	1	4	2	—	5	—	—	—	—
SONOMA														
Dried Tomato	1 tbsp (0.7 g)	35	0	0	0	0	9	0	0	0	—	0	—	0
CILANTRO														
fresh	1 tsp (2 g)	tr	tr	0	0	tr	tr	tr	1	1	8	1	1	98
fresh	1 cup (1.6 oz)	11	tr	tr	0	1	2	1	31	25	235	1	29	2820
WATKINS														
Dried	¼ tsp (0.5 oz)	0	0	0	0	0	0	0	0	0	—	0	—	200
CINNAMON														
ground	1 tsp	6	tr	tr	0	tr	2	—	28	1	11	1	—	6
sticks	0.5 oz	39	tr	tr	—	1	8	3	175	4	—	4	—	20
WATKINS														
Ground	¼ tsp (0.5 g)	0	0	0	0	0	0	0	0	0	—	0	—	0
CISCO														
raw	3 oz	84	2	tr	—	16	0	—	—	47	301	—	—	—
smoked	3 oz	151	10	1	27	14	0	—	22	409	249	—	2	802
smoked	1 oz	50	3	tr	9	5	0	—	7	135	82	—	1	264
CLAM JUICE														
DOXSEE														
Canned	3 fl oz	4	0	0	—	tr	0	—	—	110	15	—	—	—
CLAMS														
CANNED														
liquid only	1 cup	6	tr	—	—	1	tr	—	31	516	—	—	—	—
liquid only	3 oz	2	tr	—	—	tr	tr	—	11	183	—	—	—	—
meat only	1 cup	236	3	tr	107	41	8	—	148	179	1005	—	158	912
meat only	3 oz	126	2	tr	57	22	4	—	78	95	534	—	—	484
DOXSEE														
Chopped	6.5 oz	90	tr	—	—	16	6	—	40	1020	120	—	—	—
GORTON'S														
Minced & Chopped	½ can	70	1	—	—	12	4	—	—	640	—	—	—	—
PROGRESSO														
Creamy Clam	½ cup (4.2 oz)	100	6	2	10	5	8	0	0	560	—	0	—	0
Minced	¼ cup (2 oz)	25	0	0	10	4	2	0	0	250	—	0	—	0
Red Clam	½ cup (4.4 oz)	80	3	1	5	6	8	1	20	620	—	0	—	200
White Clam Sauce	½ cup (4.4 oz)	120	9	2	15	10	1	0	20	310	—	2	—	0

FOOD	PORTION	CALORIES	FAT	SAT FAT	CHOL	PROTEIN	CARBO	FIBER	CALCIUM	SOD	POTAS	VIT C	FOLIC	VIT A
SNOW'S														
Minced	6.5 oz	90	tr	—	—	16	6	—	40	1020	120	—	—	—
FRESH														
cooked	3 oz	126	2	tr	57	22	4	—	78	95	534	—	—	—
cooked	20 sm	133	2	tr	60	23	5	—	83	100	565	—	—	513
raw	20 sm (180 g)	133	2	tr	60	23	5	—	83	100	565	—	—	540
raw	3 oz	63	1	tr	29	11	2	—	39	47	267	—	—	255
raw	9 lg (180 g)	133	2	tr	60	23	5	—	83	100	565	—	—	540
FROZEN														
GORTON'S														
Microwave Crunchy Clam Strips	3.5 oz	330	22	6	30	10	24	—	20	430	—	—	—	—
MRS. PAUL'S														
Fried	2½ oz	200	9	—	15	10	21	—	—	450	—	—	—	—
TAKE-OUT														
breaded & fried	20 sm	379	21	5	115	27	19	—	119	684	612	—	—	568
CLOVES														
ground	1 tsp	7	tr	tr	0	tr	1	—	14	5	23	2	—	11
COCOA														
(see also CHOCOLATE*)*														
hot cocoa	1 cup	218	9	6	33	9	26	—	298	123	480	2	12	318
mix as prep w/ water	7 oz	103	1	1	—	3	23	—	96	149	203	1	tr	4
mix w/ equal as prep w/ water	7 oz	48	tr	tr	—	4	9	—	90	173	405	0	2	—
powder unsweetened	1 tbsp (5 g)	11	1	tr	0	1	3	2	6	1	76	0	2	1
powder unsweetened	1 cup (3 oz)	197	12	7	0	17	47	29	110	18	1310	0	27	17
NESTLE														
Cocoa	1 tbsp	15	1	0	0	1	3	2	—	0	—	—	—	—
SWISS MISS														
Cocoa Diet	6 oz	20	tr	—	1	2	3	0	80	180	170	—	—	—
Hot Cocoa Bavarian Chocolate	6 oz	110	3	1	2	1	20	0	40	170	150	—	—	—
Hot Cocoa Double Rich	6 oz	110	1	1	0	2	22	0	60	150	125	—	—	—
Hot Cocoa Milk Chocolate	6 oz	110	1	tr	5	2	24	0	40	125	150	—	—	—
Hot Cocoa Milk Chocolate	1 serv	110	1	tr	1	1	24	1	33	139	—	0	—	0
Hot Cocoa Mini-Marshmallow	1 serv	109	1	tr	1	1	24	1	36	149	—	0	—	0
Hot Cocoa Rich Chocolate	1 serv	110	1	tr	1	2	24	1	2	166	—	0	—	0

FOOD	PORTION	CALORIES	FAT	SAT FAT	CHOL	PROTEIN	CARBO	FIBER	CALCIUM	SOD	POTAS	VIT C	FOLIC	VIT A
SWISS MISS (CONT.)														
Hot Cocoa Sugar Free	1 serv	67	tr	tr	1	3	13	1	107	242	—	0	—	0
Hot Cocoa Sugar Free Milk Chocolate	1 serv	49	tr	tr	tr	2	10	1	79	179	—	0	—	0
Hot Cocoa Sugar Free Mini-Marshmallow	1 serv	51	1	tr	1	1	11	1	28	159	—	0	—	0
Hot Cocoa White Chocolate	1 serv	109	1	tr	1	3	21	tr	33	128	—	0	—	0
Hot Cocoa With Mini Marshmallows	6 oz	110	1	tr	5	1	23	0	20	170	200	—	—	—
Hot Cocoa Lite	1 serv	74	tr	tr	tr	1	17	2	5	197	—	0	—	0
Lite as prep	6 oz	70	tr	—	1	1	17	0	40	160	200	—	—	—
Sugar Free With Sugar Free Marshmallows as prep	6 oz	50	tr	—	2	3	9	0	80	120	200	—	—	—
Sugar Free as prep	6 oz	60	tr	—	2	3	10	0	80	125	170	—	—	—
ULTRA SLIM-FAST														
Hot Cocoa as prep w/ water	8 oz	190	tr	—	8	14	35	5	500	140	750	21	120	1750
WEIGHT WATCHERS														
Hot Cocoa Mix as prep	1 pkg	70	0	0	0	6	7	1	250	160	—	0	—	300
COCONUT														
coconut water	1 tbsp	3	tr	tr	0	tr	1	—	4	16	38	tr	—	0
coconut water	1 cup	46	tr	tr	0	2	9	—	58	252	600	6	—	0
cream canned	1 cup	568	52	47	0	8	25	—	4	149	299	—	—	—
cream canned	1 tbsp	36	3	3	0	1	2	—	0	10	19	—	—	—
dried sweetened flaked	1 cup	351	24	21	0	2	35	—	10	189	234	0	—	0
dried sweetened flaked	7 oz pkg	944	64	57	0	7	95	—	28	509	629	0	—	0
dried sweetened flaked canned	1 cup	341	24	22	0	3	32	—	11	15	249	—	—	0
dried sweetened shredded	7 oz pkg	997	71	63	0	6	95	—	30	522	670	1	—	0
dried sweetened shredded	1 cup	466	33	29	0	2	44	—	14	244	313	1	—	0
dried toasted	1 oz	168	13	12	0	2	13	—	8	11	157	—	—	—
dried unsweetened	1 oz	187	18	16	0	2	7	—	7	11	154	tr	3	0
milk canned	1 cup	445	48	43	0	5	6	—	40	29	497	2	—	—
milk canned	1 tbsp	30	3	3	0	tr	tr	—	3	2	33	tr	—	—
milk frozen	1 cup	486	50	44	0	4	13	—	11	29	556	—	—	—
milk frozen	1 tbsp	30	3	3	0	tr	1	—	1	2	35	—	—	—

FOOD	PORTION	CALORIES	FAT	SAT FAT	CHOL	PROTEIN	CARBO	FIBER	CALCIUM	SOD	POTAS	VIT C	FOLIC	VIT A
BAKER'S														
Angel Flake	1 tbsp (0.5 oz)	70	5	5	0	1	6	1	0	45	55	0	—	0
Angel Flake (canned)	2 tbsp (0.5 oz)	70	6	5	0	1	6	1	0	0	65	0	—	0
Premium Shred	2 tbsp (0.5 oz)	70	5	5	0	1	6	1	0	45	60	0	—	0
COCO LOPEZ														
Cream Of Coconut	2 tbsp	120	5	—	—	0	20	—	—	10	15	—	—	—
COD														
CANNED														
atlantic	3 oz	89	1	tr	47	19	0	—	18	185	449	1	—	39
atlantic	1 can (11 oz)	327	3	1	171	71	0	—	66	680	1647	1	—	144
roe	3.5 oz	118	3	—	—	22	tr	—	15	—	—	—	—	—
DRIED														
atlantic	3 oz	246	2	tr	129	53	0	—	136	5973	1239	3	—	120
FRESH														
atlantic cooked	1 fillet (6.3 oz)	189	2	tr	99	41	0	—	25	141	440	2	—	83
atlantic cooked	3 oz	89	1	tr	47	19	0	—	12	66	208	1	—	39
atlantic raw	3 oz	70	1	tr	37	15	0	—	13	46	351	1	—	34
roe baked w/ butter & lemon juice	3.5 oz	126	3	—	—	22	2	—	13	73	132	—	—	—
roe raw	3½ oz	130	2	—	360	24	2	—	—	—	—	14	—	—
FROZEN														
GORTON'S														
Fishmarket Fresh	5 oz	110	1	—	—	26	0	—	—	90	—	—	—	—
MRS. PAUL'S														
Light Fillets	1 fillet	240	11	—	50	15	22	—	20	430	—	—	—	—
VAN DE KAMP'S														
Lightly Breaded Fillets	1 (4 oz)	220	10	2	35	14	19	0	20	410	—	0	—	0
COFFEE														
(see also COFFEE BEVERAGES, COFFEE SUBSTITUTES*)*														
INSTANT														
cappuccino mix as prep	7 oz	62	2	2	—	tr	11	—	7	104	119	0	0	0
decaffeinated	1 rounded tsp (1.8 g)	4	0	0	0	tr	1	—	3	0	63	0	0	0
decaffeinated as prep	6 oz	4	0	0	0	tr	1	—	6	6	63	0	0	0
french mix as prep	7 oz	57	3	3	—	1	7	—	8	—	137	—	—	—
mocha mix as prep	7 oz	51	2	2	—	1	8	—	7	36	119	0	0	0
regular	1 rounded tsp	4	0	0	0	tr	1	—	3	1	64	0	0	0
regular as prep	6 oz	4	0	0	0	tr	1	—	6	6	64	0	0	0
regular w/ chicory	1 rounded tsp	6	0	0	0	tr	1	—	2	5	61	—	—	—

FOOD	PORTION	CALORIES	FAT	SAT FAT	CHOL	PROTEIN	CARBO	FIBER	CALCIUM	SOD	POTAS	VIT C	FOLIC	VIT A
regular w/ chicory as prep	6 oz	6	0	0	0	tr	1	—	6	10	61	—	—	—
REGULAR														
FOLGERS														
Colombian Supreme	1 tbsp	16	tr	—	0	tr	3	—	5	tr	71	0	—	2
Custom Roast	1 tbsp	16	tr	—	0	tr	3	—	5	tr	71	0	—	2
Decaffeinated	1 tbsp	17	tr	—	0	1	3	—	5	tr	73	0	—	2
French Roast	1 tbsp	16	tr	—	0	tr	3	—	5	tr	71	0	—	2
Gourmet Supreme	1 tbsp	16	tr	—	0	tr	3	—	5	tr	71	0	—	2
Instant	1 tsp	8	tr	—	0	tr	1	—	37	1	86	0	—	0
Instant Decaffeinated	1 tsp	8	tr	—	0	tr	2	—	12	2	113	0	—	0
Singles	1 bag	21	tr	—	0	1	4	—	37	1	137	0	—	2
Singles Decaffeinated	1 bag	21	tr	—	0	1	4	—	15	2	164	0	—	2
Special Roast	1 tbsp	16	tr	—	0	tr	3	—	5	tr	71	0	—	2
Vacuum Pack	1 tbsp	16	tr	—	0	tr	3	—	5	tr	71	0	—	2
MARYLAND CLUB														
Ground	1 tbsp	16	tr	—	0	tr	3	—	5	tr	71	0	—	2
TAKE-OUT														
cafe au lait	1 cup (8 fl oz)	77	4	3	17	4	6	—	148	62	249	1	6	230
cafe brulot	1 cup (4.8 fl oz)	48	0	0	0	tr	3	—	2	2	64	0	tr	0
cappuccino	1 cup (8 fl oz)	77	4	3	17	4	6	—	148	62	249	1	6	230
coffee con leche	1 cup (8 fl oz)	77	4	3	17	4	6	—	148	62	249	1	6	230
espresso	1 cup (3 fl oz)	2	0	0	0	tr	tr	—	2	2	48	0	tr	0
irish coffee	1 serv (9 fl oz)	107	3	2	12	1	3	—	20	25	151	0	1	206
latte w/ skim milk	13 oz	88	tr	tr	4	8	12	0	304	128	470	2	13	750
latte w/ whole milk	13 oz	152	8	5	33	8	12	0	293	122	434	2	12	460
mocha	1 mug (9.6 fl oz)	202	15	9	40	3	17	—	67	28	228	tr	2	655

COFFEE BEVERAGES

(*see also* COFFEE SUBSTITUTES)

GENERAL FOODS

FOOD	PORTION	CALORIES	FAT	SAT FAT	CHOL	PROTEIN	CARBO	FIBER	CALCIUM	SOD	POTAS	VIT C	FOLIC	VIT A
Cappuccino Coolers French Vanilla as prep w/ 2% milk	1 serv	180	5	3	21	—	27	0	300	120	—	1	—	500
International Coffee Sugar Free Cafe Vienna as prep	1 serv (8 oz)	30	2	1	0	tr	3	0	0	75	110	0	—	0
International Coffee Sugar Free Fat Free Suisse Mocha as prep	1 serv (8 oz)	25	0	0	0	0	5	tr	0	35	110	0	—	0

FOOD	PORTION	CALORIES	FAT	SAT FAT	CHOL	PROTEIN	CARBO	FIBER	CALCIUM	SOD	POTAS	VIT C	FOLIC	VIT A
GENERAL FOODS (CONT.)														
International Coffees Cafe Francais as prep	1 serv (8 oz)	60	4	1	0	tr	7	0	0	95	130	0	—	0
International Coffees Cafe Vienna as prep	1 serv (8 oz)	70	3	1	0	tr	11	tr	0	110	130	0	—	0
International Coffees Decaffeinated French Vanilla Cafe as prep	1 serv (8 oz)	60	3	1	0	tr	10	0	0	55	75	0	—	0
International Coffees Decaffeinated Suisse Mocha as prep	1 serv (8 oz)	60	2	1	0	tr	9	0	0	35	110	0	—	0
International Coffees French Vanilla Cafe as prep	1 serv (8 oz)	60	3	1	0	tr	10	0	0	55	80	0	—	0
International Coffees Hazelnut Belgain Cafe as prep	1 serv (8 oz)	70	2	1	0	tr	12	0	0	60	115	0	—	0
International Coffees Irish Creme Cafe as prep	1 serv (8 oz)	60	2	1	0	tr	10	0	0	45	70	0	—	0
International Coffees Italian Cappuccino as prep	1 serv (8 oz)	60	2	1	0	tr	10	0	0	50	85	0	—	0
International Coffees Kahlua Cafe as prep	1 serv (8 oz)	60	2	1	0	tr	10	0	0	55	80	0	—	0
International Coffees Orange Cappuccino as prep	1 serv (8 oz)	70	2	1	0	tr	11	tr	0	100	140	0	—	0
International Coffees Suisse Mocha as prep	1 serv (8 oz)	60	2	1	0	tr	8	0	0	35	115	0	—	0
International Coffees Viennese Chocolate Cafe as prep	1 serv (8 oz)	50	2	1	0	tr	10	0	0	30	70	0	—	0
International Coffees Sugar Free Fat Free Decaffeinated French Vanilla	1 serv (8 oz)	25	0	0	0	0	5	0	0	65	65	0	—	0

FOOD	PORTION	CALORIES	FAT	SAT FAT	CHOL	PROTEIN	CARBO	FIBER	CALCIUM	SOD	POTAS	VIT C	FOLIC	VIT A
GENERAL FOODS (CONT.)														
International Coffees Sugar Free Fat Free Decaffeinated Suisse Mocha	1 serv (8 oz)	25	0	0	0	0	5	tr	0	35	105	0	—	0
International Coffees Sugar Free Fat Free French Vanilla Cafe as prep	1 serv (8 oz)	25	0	0	0	0	5	0	0	65	70	0	—	0
MAXWELL HOUSE														
Cafe Cappuccino Amaretto as prep	1 serv (8 oz)	90	1	0	0	1	19	0	60	65	95	0	—	0
Cafe Cappuccino Decaffeinated Mocha as prep	1 serv (8 oz)	100	3	1	0	2	17	0	80	70	160	0	—	0
Cafe Cappuccino Decaffeinated Vanilla as prep	1 serv (8 oz)	90	1	0	0	1	19	0	60	65	90	0	—	0
Cafe Cappuccino Irish Cream as prep	1 serv (8 oz)	90	1	0	0	1	19	0	60	65	105	0	—	0
Cafe Cappuccino Mocha as prep	1 serv (8 oz)	100	3	1	0	2	17	0	80	65	170	0	—	0
Cafe Cappuccino Sugar Free Mocha as prep	1 serv (8 oz)	60	3	1	0	1	7	tr	0	80	90	0	—	0
Cafe Cappuccino Sugar Free Vanilla as prep	1 serv (8 oz)	60	3	1	0	tr	7	0	0	85	65	0	—	0
Cafe Cappuccino Vanilla as prep	1 serv (8 oz)	90	1	0	0	1	19	0	60	65	105	0	—	0
Iced Cappuccino as prep w/ 2% milk	1 serv (8 oz)	180	5	3	20	8	27	tr	300	125	460	1	—	500
STARBUCKS														
Frappuccino	1 bottle (9.5 fl oz)	190	3	2	12	6	39	0	220	110	—	0	—	100

COFFEE SUBSTITUTES

FOOD	PORTION	CALORIES	FAT	SAT FAT	CHOL	PROTEIN	CARBO	FIBER	CALCIUM	SOD	POTAS	VIT C	FOLIC	VIT A
powder	1 tsp	9	tr	tr	0	tr	2	—	1	2	42	—	—	—
powder as prep	6 oz	9	tr	tr	0	tr	2	—	5	7	43	—	—	—
powder as prep w/ milk	6 oz	121	6	4	25	6	10	—	219	91	319	2	9	230
KAVA														
Instant	1 tsp	2	0	0	0	0	1	—	—	<5	115	—	—	—
NATURAL TOUCH														
Kaffree Roma	1 tsp (2 g)	10	0	0	0	0	2	0	0	0	20	0	—	0
Roma Cappuccino	3 tbsp (0.4 oz)	50	3	3	0	1	5	0	0	15	70	0	—	0

FOOD	PORTION	CALORIES	FAT	SAT FAT	CHOL	PROTEIN	CARBO	FIBER	CALCIUM	SOD	POTAS	VIT C	FOLIC	VIT A
PERO														
Instant Grain Beverage	1 tsp (1.5 g)	5	0	0	0	0	1	—	—	0	—	—	—	—
POSTUM														
Instant Coffee Flavor as prep	1 serv (8 oz)	10	0	0	0	0	3	0	0	0	110	0	—	0
Instant as prep	1 serv (8 oz)	10	0	0	0	0	3	0	0	0	110	0	—	0

COFFEE WHITENERS

(*see also* MILK SUBSTITUTES)

FOOD	PORTION	CALORIES	FAT	SAT FAT	CHOL	PROTEIN	CARBO	FIBER	CALCIUM	SOD	POTAS	VIT C	FOLIC	VIT A
liquid nondairy frzn	1 tbsp (0.5 oz)	20	2	tr	0	tr	2	—	1	12	29	0	0	13
powder nondairy	1 tsp	11	tr	1	0	tr	1	—	tr	4	16	0	0	4
COFFEE-MATE														
Liquid	1 tbsp (0.5 fl oz)	16	1	tr	0	0	2	—	—	5	20	—	—	—
Powder	1 tsp (2 g)	10	1	1	0	tr	1	—	—	5	15	—	—	—
CREMORA														
Whitener	1 tsp	12	1	—	—	0	1	—	—	5	15	—	—	—
HOOD														
Non Dairy	1 tbsp (0.5 oz)	20	2	0	0	0	2	0	0	0	—	0	—	0
INTERNATIONAL DELIGHT														
Amaretto	1 tbsp (0.6 fl oz)	45	2	0	0	0	7	0	0	5	—	0	—	0
Cinnamon Hazelnut	1 tbsp (0.6 fl oz)	45	2	0	0	0	7	0	0	5	—	0	—	0
Irish Creme	1 tbsp (0.6 fl oz)	45	2	0	0	0	7	0	0	5	—	0	—	0
No Fat Amaretto	1 tbsp (0.5 fl oz)	30	0	0	0	0	7	0	0	5	—	0	—	0
No Fat French Vanilla Royale	1 tbsp (0.5 fl oz)	30	0	0	0	0	7	0	0	5	—	0	—	0
No Fat Hawaiian Macadamia	1 tbsp (0.5 fl oz)	30	0	0	0	0	7	0	0	5	—	0	—	0
No Fat Irish Creme	1 tbsp (0.5 fl oz)	30	0	0	0	0	7	0	0	5	—	0	—	0
Suisse Chocolate Mocha	1 tbsp (0.6 fl oz)	45	2	0	0	0	7	0	0	10	—	0	—	0
MOCHA MIX														
Fat-Free	1 tbsp (0.5 fl oz)	10	0	0	0	0	1	0	0	0	—	0	—	0
Lite	1 tbsp (0.5 fl oz)	10	tr	0	0	0	tr	0	0	0	—	0	—	0
Lite	4 fl oz	80	7	2	0	1	3	0	0	24	—	0	—	0
Original	1 tbsp (0.5 fl oz)	20	2	0	0	0	1	0	0	5	—	0	—	0
Signature Flavors French Vanilla	1 tbsp (0.5 fl oz)	35	0	0	0	0	8	—	—	5	—	—	—	—
Signature Flavors Irish Creme	1 tbsp (0.5 fl oz)	35	0	0	0	0	8	—	—	5	—	—	—	—

FOOD	PORTION	CALORIES	FAT	SAT FAT	CHOL	PROTEIN	CARBO	FIBER	CALCIUM	SOD	POTAS	VIT C	FOLIC	VIT A
MOCHA MIX (CONT.)														
Signature Flavors Kahlua	1 tbsp (0.5 fl oz)	35	0	0	0	0	8	—	—	5	—	—	—	—
Signature Flavors Mauna Loa Macadamia Nut	1 tbsp (0.5 fl oz)	35	0	0	0	0	8	—	—	5	—	—	—	—
N-RICH CREAMER														
Whitener	1 tsp	10	tr	—	0	tr	1	0	—	0	21	—	—	—
COLESLAW														
HOME RECIPE														
coleslaw w/ dressing	¾ cup	147	11	2	5	1	13	—	34	267	177	8	39	337
TAKE-OUT														
vinegar & oil coleslaw	3.5 oz	150	9	1	0	1	16	—	20	480	—	30	—	500
COLLARDS														
CANNED														
ALLEN														
Collards	½ cup (4.1 oz)	30	1	0	0	1	5	3	150	20	—	12	—	5500
SUNSHINE														
Collards	½ cup (4.1 oz)	30	1	0	0	1	5	3	150	20	—	12	—	5500
FROZEN														
chopped cooked	½ cup	31	tr	—	0	3	6	—	179	42	214	23	65	5084
COOKIES														
(*see also* BROWNIE, CAKE, DOUGHNUT, PIE)														
HOME RECIPE														
chocolate chip as prep w/ butter	1 (0.42 oz)	78	5	2	11	1	9	—	6	55	35	0	2	95
chocolate chip as prep w/ margarine	1 (0.56 oz)	78	5	1	5	1	9	—	6	58	36	0	2	102
macaroons	1 (0.8 oz)	97	3	3	0	1	17	—	12	59	38	0	1	0
oatmeal	1 (0.5 oz)	67	3	1	5	1	10	—	18	90	27	0	2	107
oatmeal w/ raisins	1 (0.52 oz)	65	2	tr	5	1	10	—	15	81	36	tr	2	96
peanut butter	1 (0.7 oz)	95	5	1	6	2	12	—	8	104	460	0	4	120
shortbread as prep w/ butter	1 (0.38 oz)	60	4	2	10	1	6	—	2	51	8	0	1	136
shortbread as prep w/ margarine	1 (0.38 oz)	60	4	1	0	1	6	—	2	56	8	0	1	—
sugar as prep w/ butter	1 (0.49 oz)	66	3	2	12	1	8	—	10	64	10	0	2	125
sugar as prep w/ margarine	1 (0.49 oz)	66	3	1	4	1	8	—	10	69	11	0	2	135
MIX														
chocolate chip	1 (0.56 oz)	79	4	1	7	1	10	—	7	47	34	0	—	—
oatmeal	1 (0.6 oz)	74	3	1	7	1	10	tr	5	75	30	—	—	—
oatmeal raisin	1 (0.6 oz)	74	3	1	7	1	10	tr	5	75	30	—	—	—

FOOD	PORTION	CALORIES	FAT	SAT FAT	CHOL	PROTEIN	CARBO	FIBER	CALCIUM	SOD	POTAS	VIT C	FOLIC	VIT A
BETTY CROCKER														
Chocolate Chip Big Batch	2	120	6	—	—	1	16	—	—	100	75	—	—	100
Date Bar Classic Dessert	1	60	2	1	0	1	9	—	—	35	35	—	—	—
ESTEE														
Chocolate Chip	3	130	7	2	0	1	17	0	0	120	70	0	—	0
READY-TO-EAT														
animal	11 crackers (1 oz)	126	4	1	—	2	21	—	12	112	28	0	4	—
animal crackers	1 box (2.4 oz)	299	9	4	11	4	51	—	11	274	57	tr	22	27
animal crackers	1 (2.5 g)	11	tr	tr	—	tr	2	—	1	10	2	0	0	—
butter	1 (5 g)	23	1	1	—	tr	3	tr	1	18	6	0	0	0
chocolate chip	1 (0.4 oz)	48	2	1	—	1	7	tr	2	32	14	0	1	—
chocolate chip	1 box (1.9 oz)	233	12	5	12	3	36	—	20	188	82	tr	16	52
chocolate chip low fat	1 (0.25 oz)	45	2	tr	0	1	7	—	2	38	12	—	—	0
chocolate chip low sugar low sodium	1 (0.24 oz)	31	1	1	0	tr	5	—	—	1	14	0	—	—
chocolate chip soft-type	1 (0.5 oz)	69	4	1	0	1	9	tr	2	49	14	0	1	—
chocolate w/ creme filling	1 (0.35 oz)	47	2	tr	—	1	7	tr	3	36	18	0	0	0
chocolate w/ creme filling chocolate coated	1 (0.60 oz)	82	5	1	—	1	11	—	6	55	41	—	—	—
chocolate w/ creme filling sugar free low sodium	1 (0.35 oz)	46	2	1	—	1	7	—	—	24	29	—	—	—
chocolate w/ extra creme filling	1 (0.46 oz)	65	3	1	—	1	9	—	3	64	16	0	—	—
chocolate wafer	1 (0.2 oz)	26	1	tr	0	tr	4	—	2	35	13	—	—	—
chocolate wafer cookie crumbs	½ cup (5.9 oz)	728	25	6	0	11	120	—	56	980	364	—	—	—
fig bars	1 (0.56 oz)	56	1	tr	—	1	11	1	10	56	33	—	2	—
fortune	1 (0.28 oz)	30	tr	tr	—	tr	7	tr	1	22	3	0	1	—
fudge	1 (0.73 oz)	73	1	tr	—	1	17	tr	7	40	29	—	—	—
gingersnaps	1 (0.24 oz)	29	1	tr	0	tr	5	—	5	48	24	0	—	—
graham	1 squares (0.24 oz)	30	1	tr	0	1	5	—	2	42	9	0	1	0
graham chocolate covered	1 (0.49 oz)	68	3	2	0	1	9	—	8	41	29	0	—	—
graham honey	1 (0.24 oz)	30	1	tr	0	1	5	tr	2	42	9	0	1	0
ladyfingers	1 (0.38 oz)	40	1	tr	40	1	7	—	5	16	12	tr	4	61
marshmallow chocolate coated	1 (0.46 oz)	55	2	1	—	1	9	—	6	22	24	—	—	—
marshmallow pie chocolate coated	1 (1.4 oz)	165	7	2	—	2	26	—	18	66	72	—	—	—

FOOD	PORTION	CALORIES	FAT	SAT FAT	CHOL	PROTEIN	CARBO	FIBER	CALCIUM	SOD	POTAS	VIT C	FOLIC	VIT A
molasses	1 (0.5 oz)	65	2	tr	0	1	11	—	11	69	52	0	—	—
oatmeal	1 (0.6 oz)	81	3	1	0	1	12	1	7	69	26	—	—	—
oatmeal	1 (0.52 oz)	71	4	1	0	1	9	tr	5	62	25	0	—	—
oatmeal soft-type	1 (0.5 oz)	61	2	tr	—	1	10	tr	13	52	20	—	—	—
oatmeal raisin	1 (0.6 oz)	81	3	1	0	1	12	1	7	69	26	—	—	—
oatmeal raisin low sugar no sodium	1 (0.24 oz)	31	1	1	0	tr	5	—	—	1	12	—	—	—
oatmeal raisin soft-type	1 (0.5 oz)	61	2	tr	—	1	10	tr	13	52	20	—	—	—
peanut butter sandwich	1 (0.5 oz)	67	3	1	0	1	9	—	7	52	27	0	—	—
peanut butter sandwich sugar free low sodium	1 (0.35 oz)	54	3	1	—	1	5	—	—	41	29	0	—	—
peanut butter soft-type	1 (0.5 oz)	69	4	1	0	1	9	tr	2	50	16	0	1	0
raisin soft-type	1 (0.5 oz)	60	2	1	0	1	10	—	7	51	21	—	—	—
shortbread	1 (0.28 oz)	40	2	tr	2	1	5	—	3	36	8	0	—	—
shortbread pecan	1 (0.49 oz)	79	5	1	5	1	8	tr	4	39	10	—	—	—
sugar	1 (0.52 oz)	72	3	1	8	1	10	—	3	53	9	—	—*	13
sugar low sugar sodium free	1 (0.24 oz)	30	1	tr	0	1	5	—	—	0	7	0	—	0
sugar wafers w/ creme filling	1 (0.12 oz)	18	1	tr	0	tr	3	—	1	5	2	0	—	—
sugar wafers w/ creme filling sugar free sodium free	1 (0.14 oz)	20	1	tr	0	tr	3	—	2	0	2	0	0	0
vanilla sandwich	1 (0.35 oz)	48	2	tr	0	tr	7	tr	3	35	9	0	0	0
vanilla wafers	1 (0.21 oz)	28	1	tr	—	tr	4	—	2	18	6	—	—	—
ARCHWAY														
Almond Crescents	2 (0.8 oz)	100	4	1	<5	1	17	tr	0	75	—	0	—	0
Apple N' Raisin	1 (1.1 oz)	130	52	1	<5	2	20	1	0	105	—	0	—	0
Apricot Filled	1 (1 oz)	110	4	1	5	1	18	tr	0	90	—	0	—	0
Bells And Stars	3 (1 oz)	150	7	2	5	1	19	tr	0	100	—	0	—	0
Blueberry Filled	1 (1 oz)	110	4	2	5	1	19	tr	0	115	—	0	—	0
Carrot Cake	1 (1 oz)	120	5	1	<5	1	18	0	0	180	—	0	—	0
Cherry Filled	1 (1 oz)	110	4	2	10	1	19	tr	0	100	—	0	—	0
Cherry Nougat	3 (1 oz)	150	9	2	0	1	18	0	0	40	—	0	—	0
Chocolate Chip	1 (1 oz)	130	6	2	tr	1	19	0	0	150	—	0	—	0
Chocolate Chip & Toffee	1 (1 oz)	140	7	2	<5	1	19	tr	0	120	—	0	—	0
Chocolate Chip Bag	3 (0.9 oz)	130	7	2	10	1	17	0	0	70	—	0	—	0
Chocolate Chip Drop	1 (1 oz)	140	10	3	10	2	11	tr	0	105	—	0	—	0
Chocolate Chip Ice Box	1 (1 oz)	140	7	3	5	1	19	0	0	80	—	0	—	0

FOOD	PORTION	CALORIES	FAT	SAT FAT	CHOL	PROTEIN	CARBO	FIBER	CALCIUM	SOD	POTAS	VIT C	FOLIC	VIT A
ARCHWAY (CONT.)														
Chocolate Chip Mini	12 (1.1 oz)	150	7	2	5	1	20	0	0	95	—	0	—	0
Cinnamon Snaps	12 (1.1 oz)	150	7	1	5	1	19	0	0	115	—	0	—	0
Coconut Macaroon	1 (0.8 oz)	90	5	4	0	1	14	2	0	55	—	0	—	0
Cookie Jar Hermits	1 (1 oz)	110	3	1	<5	1	19	tr	0	160	—	0	—	0
Dark Chocolate	1 (1 oz)	110	4	1	<5	1	20	tr	40	150	—	0	—	0
Dutch Chocolate	1 (1 oz)	120	4	1	<5	1	19	0	0	110	—	0	—	0
Fig Bars Low Fat	2 (1.1 oz)	100	1	0	0	2	23	1	36	105	—	1	—	0
Frosty Lemon	1 (1 oz)	120	5	1	0	1	19	0	0	110	—	0	—	0
Frosty Orange	1 (1 oz)	120	4	1	0	1	19	1	0	140	—	0	—	0
Fruit And Honey Bar	1 (1 oz)	110	4	1	5	1	18	tr	0	120	—	0	—	0
Fruit Bar No Fat	1 (1 oz)	90	0	0	0	tr	21	0	0	95	—	0	—	0
Fruit Cake	1 (1.1 oz)	140	7	2	0	2	20	2	20	100	—	0	—	0
Fudge Nut Bar	1 (1 oz)	110	5	1	<5	2	17	tr	0	120	—	0	—	0
Fun Chip Mini	12 (1.1 oz)	140	6	1	5	1	21	0	0	100	—	0	—	0
Gingersnaps	5 (1.1 oz)	130	5	1	0	1	22	0	0	110	—	0	—	0
Granola No Fat	1 (0.5 oz)	50	0	0	0	1	11	tr	0	60	—	0	—	0
Holiday Pak	3 (1.1 oz)	150	8	2	<5	1	19	tr	0	95	—	0	—	0
Iced Gingerbread	3 (1.1 oz)	140	5	1	5	1	23	0	20	130	—	0	—	0
Iced Molasses	1 (1 oz)	110	5	1	0	1	19	tr	20	170	—	0	—	0
Iced Oatmeal	1 (1 oz)	120	5	1	<5	2	19	1	0	85	—	0	—	0
Lemon Snaps	12 (1.1 oz)	150	7	1	5	1	19	0	0	120	—	0	—	0
New Orleans Cake	1 (1 oz)	110	4	1	<5	1	18	tr	0	105	—	0	—	0
Nutty Nougat	3 (1.1 oz)	160	10	2	0	1	18	0	0	60	—	0	—	0
Oatmeal	1 (0.9 oz)	110	3	1	<5	2	19	tr	0	95	—	0	—	0
Oatmeal Apple Filled	1 (1 oz)	110	3	1	<5	1	18	0	0	105	—	0	—	0
Oatmeal Date Filled	1 (1 oz)	110	4	1	<5	2	18	tr	0	120	—	0	—	0
Oatmeal Mini	12 (1.1 oz)	150	8	2	5	2	19	1	0	130	—	0	—	0
Oatmeal Pecan	1 (1 oz)	120	5	2	<5	2	18	1	0	100	—	0	—	0
Oatmeal Raisin	1 (1 oz)	110	4	1	<5	2	19	tr	0	115	—	0	—	0
Oatmeal Raisin Bran	1 (1 oz)	110	4	1	<5	2	19	tr	0	100	—	0	—	0
Old Fashioned Molasses	1 (1 oz)	120	3	1	5	1	20	0	0	150	—	0	—	0
Old Fashioned Windmill	1 (0.7 oz)	100	4	1	0	1	15	0	0	95	—	0	—	0
Party Treats	3 (1.1 oz)	140	7	2	15	2	20	0	0	105	—	0	—	0
Peanut Butter	1 (1 oz)	140	7	—	10	3	16	tr	0	125	—	0	—	0
Peanut Butter & Chip	3 (0.9 oz)	130	7	2	10	2	16	0	0	125	—	0	—	0
Peanut Butter N' Chips	1 (1 oz)	140	7	2	10	3	16	tr	0	115	—	0	—	0

FOOD	PORTION	CALORIES	FAT	SAT FAT	CHOL	PROTEIN	CARBO	FIBER	CALCIUM	SOD	POTAS	VIT C	FOLIC	VIT A
ARCHWAY (CONT.)														
Peanut Butter Nougat	3 (1.1 oz)	160	9	2	0	2	18	1	0	140	—	0	—	0
Pecan Crunch	6 (1.1 oz)	150	8	2	10	2	18	0	0	120	—	0	—	0
Pecan Ice Box	1 (1 oz)	140	7	2	10	1	18	0	0	100	—	0	—	0
Pecan Malted Nougat	3 (1.1 oz)	160	10	2	0	2	17	2	0	60	—	0	—	0
Pfeffernusse	2 (1.3 oz)	140	1	0	0	1	32	tr	0	100	—	0	—	0
Pineapple Filled	1 (0.9 oz)	100	4	1	5	1	16	1	0	75	—	0	—	0
Raisin Oatmeal	1 (1 oz)	130	5	1	5	2	19	1	0	40	—	0	—	0
Raisin Oatmeal Bag	3 (1 oz)	130	6	2	10	1	19	1	0	55	—	0	—	0
Raspberry Filled	1 (1 oz)	110	4	1	5	1	18	tr	0	90	—	0	—	0
Rocky Road	1 (1 oz)	130	6	2	10	1	18	tr	0	85	—	0	—	0
Ruth's Golden Oatmeal	1 (1 oz)	120	5	1	<5	2	19	tr	0	135	—	0	—	0
Select Assortment	3 (0.9 oz)	130	6	2	10	1	18	0	0	80	—	0	—	0
Soft Molasses Drop	1 (1 oz)	110	4	1	<5	1	18	1	0	160	—	0	—	0
Soft Sugar	1 (1 oz)	110	4	1	5	1	18	0	0	110	—	0	—	0
Strawberry Filled	1 (1 oz)	110	4	1	<5	1	18	tr	0	90	—	0	—	0
Sugar	1 (1 oz)	120	4	1	<5	2	20	0	0	190	—	0	—	0
Vanilla Wafer	5 (1.1 oz)	130	4	1	5	2	22	0	0	130	—	0	—	0
Wedding Cakes	3 (1.1 oz)	160	8	2	0	1	20	0	0	45	—	0	—	0
BAKERY WAGON														
Apple Walnut Raisin	1	100	4	1	0	2	16	1	—	130	—	—	—	—
Cobbler Apple Cranberry Fat Free	1	70	0	0	0	1	16	1	—	60	—	—	—	—
Cobbler Apple Fat Free	1	70	0	0	0	1	17	1	—	55	—	—	—	—
Cobbler Mixed Fruit Fat Free	1	70	0	0	0	1	16	1	—	65	—	—	—	—
Cobbler Raspberry Fat Free	1	70	0	0	0	1	17	1	—	60	—	—	—	—
Ginger Snaps	5	160	7	2	0	1	22	1	—	140	—	—	—	—
Honey Fruit Bars	1	100	3	1	5	1	17	1	—	80	—	—	—	—
Iced Molasses	1	100	3	1	2	1	18	1	—	120	—	—	—	—
Iced Molasses Mini	3	130	3	1	0	1	18	1	—	170	—	—	—	—
Oatmeal Apple Filled	1	90	3	1	0	1	14	1	—	65	—	—	—	—
Oatmeal Chocolate Chunk	1	100	3	1	0	1	16	1	—	75	—	—	—	—
Oatmeal Date Filled	1	90	3	1	0	1	17	1	—	90	—	—	—	—
Oatmeal Raspberry Filled	1	100	3	1	0	1	16	1	—	105	—	—	—	—
Oatmeal Soft	1	100	4	1	0	2	16	1	—	90	—	—	—	—

FOOD	PORTION	CALORIES	FAT	SAT FAT	CHOL	PROTEIN	CARBO	FIBER	CALCIUM	SOD	POTAS	VIT C	FOLIC	VIT A
BAKERY WAGON (CONT.)														
Oatmeal Walnut Raisin	1	100	4	1	0	2	17	1	—	125	—	—	—	—
Vanilla Wafers Cholesterol Free	6	130	6	2	0	2	22	1	—	140	—	—	—	—
BAKING ON THE LITE SIDE														
Oatmeal Crunchy	2 (0.6 oz)	60	0	0	0	1	13	0	0	20	—	0	—	0
Raspberry Linzer	1 (0.6 oz)	55	0	0	0	1	12	0	0	20	—	0	—	0
BARNUM'S														
Animal Crackers	12 (1.1 oz)	140	4	1	0	2	23	1	—	160	30	—	—	—
BISCOS														
Sugar Wafers	8 (1 oz)	140	6	2	0	tr	21	tr	—	40	10	—	—	—
Waffle Cremes	4 (1.2 oz)	180	9	2	0	tr	24	tr	—	35	10	—	—	—
CADBURY														
Fingers	3	85	4	3	2	1	11	tr	25	30	—	tr	—	0
CHIP-A-ROOS														
Cookies	3 (1.3 oz)	190	10	4	0	2	23	1	—	150	—	—	—	—
CHIPS AHOY!														
Bit Size Chocolate Chip	14 (1.1 oz)	170	7	3	0	2	21	tr	—	105	45	—	—	—
Chewy Chocolate Chip	3 (1.3 oz)	170	8	3	<5	1	23	tr	—	125	40	—	—	—
Chunky Chocolate Chip	1 (0.5 oz)	80	4	3	10	1	11	tr	—	60	40	—	—	—
Real Chocolate Chip	3 (1.1 oz)	160	8	3	0	2	21	1	—	105	45	—	—	—
Reduced Fat	3 (1.1 oz)	150	6	2	0	2	23	1	—	150	40	—	—	—
Sprinkled Real Chocolate Chip	3 (1.3 oz)	170	8	3	0	2	24	tr	—	120	55	—	—	—
Striped Chocolate Chip	1 (0.5 oz)	80	4	2	0	1	10	tr	—	45	25	—	—	—
CHORTLES														
Cookies	½ pkg. (1 oz)	125	3	1	0	2	23	1	<10	109	—	tr	—	<100
COOKIE LOVER'S														
Blue Ribbon Brownies	1 (0.8 oz)	90	3	1	11	2	14	0	—	75	—	—	—	—
Classic Shortbread	1 (0.8 oz)	110	7	2	15	1	12	0	—	75	—	—	—	—
Dutch Chocolate Chip	1 (0.8 oz)	90	4	1	14	1	12	0	—	65	—	—	—	—
Fancy Peanut Butter	1 (0.8 oz)	100	6	1	7	2	10	0	—	90	—	—	—	—
Grahams Cinnamon Honey	2 (1 oz)	110	1	0	0	2	24	1	0	130	—	0	—	0
Grahams Honey	2 (1 oz)	100	2	0	0	2	22	1	0	130	—	0	—	0
Old-Time Raisin	1 (0.8 oz)	90	3	1	15	1	14	0	—	60	—	—	—	—
DELACRE														
Cookie Assortment	4 (1.1 oz)	130	<5	6	8	3	18	1	20	35	—	0	—	0

FOOD	PORTION	CALORIES	FAT	SAT FAT	CHOL	PROTEIN	CARBO	FIBER	CALCIUM	SOD	POTAS	VIT C	FOLIC	VIT A
DUTCH MILL														
Chocolate Chip	3 (1.1 oz)	160	10	3	0	1	18	1	0	85	—	0	—	0
Coconut Macaroons	3 (1 oz)	120	7	6	0	1	14	0	20	115	—	0	—	0
Oatmeal Raisin	3 (1 oz)	130	6	2	0	2	18	1	0	75	—	0	—	0
ENTENMANN'S														
Chocolate Chip	3 (0.9 oz)	140	7	—	—	1	19	—	—	85	—	—	—	—
ESTEE														
Chocolate Chip	4 (1.1 oz)	150	7	2	0	2	21	tr	0	30	55	0	—	0
Coconut	4 (1 oz)	140	6	2	0	2	19	tr	0	25	25	0	—	0
Creme Wafers Chocolate	7 (1.1 oz)	160	8	2	0	tr	21	tr	0	0	100	0	—	0
Creme Wafers Lemon	5 (1.2 oz)	170	8	2	0	1	23	0	0	10	20	0	—	0
Creme Wafers Peanut Butter	5 (1.2 oz)	170	9	2	0	3	21	0	0	85	20	0	—	0
Creme Wafers Triple Decker Banana Split	3 (0.9 oz)	140	7	2	0	1	18	0	0	0	35	0	—	0
Creme Wafers Triple Decker Chocolate Caramel & Peanut Butter	3 (0.9 oz)	140	7	1	0	2	17	0	0	45	35	0	—	0
Creme Wafers Vanilla	7 (1.1 oz)	160	7	1	0	tr	22	0	0	0	20	0	—	0
Creme Wafers Vanilla & Strawberry	5 (1.2 oz)	170	8	1	0	1	23	0	0	0	25	0	—	0
Fig Bars Apple Low Fat	2 (1 oz)	100	1	0	0	1	22	3	0	25	45	0	—	0
Fig Bars Cranberry Low Fat	2 (1 oz)	100	1	0	0	1	22	3	0	20	40	0	—	0
Fig Bars Low Fat	2 (1 oz)	100	0	0	0	1	23	3	0	20	80	0	—	0
Fudge	4 (1 oz)	150	7	2	0	2	19	1	0	45	55	0	—	0
Lemon	4 (1 oz)	140	6	1	0	2	19	tr	0	25	15	0	—	0
Oatmeal Raisin	4 (1 oz)	130	5	1	0	2	19	1	40	25	45	0	—	0
Sandwich Chocolate	3 (1.2 oz)	160	6	2	0	2	24	1	0	60	45	0	—	0
Sandwich Original	3 (1.2 oz)	160	6	2	0	2r	24	1	0	45	25	0	—	0
Sandwich Peanut Butter	3 (1.2 oz)	160	7	1	0	4	22	1	0	55	85	0	—	0
Sandwich Vanilla	3 (1.2 oz)	160	5	1	0	2	25	tr	0	35	20	0	—	0
Shortbread Reduced Fat	4 (1 oz)	130	4	1	0	2	22	tr	0	150	30	0	—	0
Vanilla	4 (1 oz)	140	6	1	0	2	19	tr	0	25	15	0	—	0
FAMOUS AMOS														
Chocolate Chip	3 (1 oz)	140	6	—	—	2	20	—	—	100	—	—	—	—

FOOD	PORTION	CALORIES	FAT	SAT FAT	CHOL	PROTEIN	CARBO	FIBER	CALCIUM	SOD	POTAS	VIT C	FOLIC	VIT A
FAMOUS AMOS (CONT.)														
Chocolate Chip Pecan	3 (1 oz)	150	8	—	—	2	18	—	60	98	—	1	—	300
Oatmeal Raisin	3 (1 oz)	134	6	—	—	2	19	—	60	137	—	6	—	300
FREIHOFER'S														
Chocolate Chip	2 (0.9 oz)	120	6	3	10	1	16	1	0	75	—	0	—	0
FRITO LAY														
Peanut Butter Bar	1.75 oz	270	16	—	0	2	30	—	—	65	100	—	—	—
GENERAL MILLS														
Dunkaroos	1 pkg (1 oz)	130	5	1	0	1	19	—	—	70	—	—	—	—
FundaMiddles Vanilla Creme In Chocolate Graham Shells	1 pkg (0.8 oz)	110	4	1	—	1	18	—	—	120	—	—	—	—
GIRL SCOUT														
Chalet Cremes Sugar Free	4 (1 oz)	150	6	1	0	2	22	1	0	55	—	0	—	0
Do-si-dos	3 (1.2 oz)	170	8	1	0	3	22	1	0	105	—	0	—	0
Samoas	2 (1 oz)	160	9	6	0	2	17	2	0	45	—	2	—	0
Snaps	7 (1.1 oz)	130	2	0	0	2	26	1	0	210	—	0	—	0
Striped Chocolate Chip	3 (1.2 oz)	180	10	4	0	2	20	1	0	100	—	0	—	0
Tagalongs	2 (0.9 oz)	150	10	4	0	3	13	2	0	85	—	0	—	0
Thin Mints	4 (1 oz)	140	8	2	0	1	18	1	20	80	—	0	—	0
Trefoils	5 (1.1 oz)	160	8	1	0	2	20	1	0	90	—	0	—	0
GLENNY'S														
Noah'N Friends Animal Peanut Butter	0.5 oz	65	3	—	—	1	9	—	—	35	—	—	—	—
Noah'N Friends Animal Vanilla	0.5 oz	65	2	—	—	1	10	—	—	35	—	—	—	—
Noah'N Friends Animal Wheat-Free Oatmeal	0.5 oz	65	2	—	—	1	10	—	—	20	—	—	—	—
Nookie Bar	1 (1.15 oz)	138	3	—	—	2	18	—	—	—	—	—	—	—
Sesame Nookie	1 pkg (1.5 oz)	180	12	—	—	3	18	—	—	24	—	—	—	—
Sesame Nookie	1 (0.5 oz)	60	4	—	—	1	6	—	—	8	—	—	—	—
GOLDEN FRUIT														
Apple	1 (0.7 oz)	80	2	0	0	1	15	tr	—	55	—	—	—	—
Cranberry	1 (0.7 oz)	70	1	0	0	1	15	tr	—	55	—	—	—	—
Cranberry Low Fat	1 (0.7 oz)	70	1	0	0	1	15	tr	—	55	—	—	—	—
Raisin	1 (0.7 oz)	80	2	0	0	1	15	tr	—	40	—	—	—	—
GRANDMA'S														
Animal Cookies Candied	5 (1 oz)	140	6	—	0	1	20	—	—	80	25	—	—	—
Chocolate Chip	2 (2.75 oz)	370	17	—	5	4	50	—	20	270	160	—	—	—

FOOD	PORTION	CALORIES	FAT	SAT FAT	CHOL	PROTEIN	CARBO	FIBER	CALCIUM	SOD	POTAS	VIT C	FOLIC	VIT A
GRANDMA'S (CONT.)														
Chocolate Chip Rich'N Chewy	3 (1 oz)	140	6	—	5	1	20	—	—	80	40	—	—	—
Fudge Chocolate Chip	2 (2.75 oz)	350	13	—	5	4	54	—	—	380	160	—	—	—
Grab Cookie Bits Chocolate	8 (1 oz)	140	6	—	0	2	19	—	—	180	65	—	—	—
Grab Cookie Bits Peanut Butter	8 (1 oz)	140	6	—	0	3	19	—	—	125	55	—	—	—
Grab Cookie Bits Vanilla	8 (1 oz)	140	6	—	5	2	20	—	—	75	40	—	—	—
Oatmeal Apple Spice	2 (2.75 oz)	330	12	—	10	5	51	—	60	570	180	—	—	—
Old Time Molasses	2 (2.75 oz)	320	9	—	5	4	58	—	—	520	190	—	—	—
Peanut Butter	2 (2.75 oz)	410	30	—	10	7	43	—	—	410	160	—	—	—
Raisin Soft	2 (2.75 oz)	320	10	—	10	3	54	—	40	280	135	—	—	—
HANDI-SNACK														
Cookie Jammers Cookies & Fruit Spread	1 pkg (1.3 oz)	130	3	0	0	1	26	tr	0	125	15	0	—	0
HEALTH VALLEY														
Amaranth Cookies	1	70	3	—	0	2	12	2	20	30	40	3	4	88
Fancy Fruit Chunks Apricot Almond	2	90	4	—	0	2	12	2	17	45	135	3	6	217
Fancy Fruit Chunks Date Pecan	2	90	4	—	0	2	13	2	21	45	135	3	6	6
Fancy Fruit Chunks Raisin Oat Bran	2	70	2	—	0	2	13	2	16	95	120	2	5	4
Fancy Fruit Chunks Tropical Fruit	2	90	3	—	0	2	15	2	16	45	140	3	8	216
Fancy Peanut Chunks	2	90	3	—	0	2	12	2	12	55	90	3	8	4
Fat Free Apple Spice	3	75	tr	—	0	2	17	3	20	40	190	2	—	—
Fat Free Apricot Delight	3	75	tr	—	0	2	16	3	20	40	190	4	—	300
Fat Free Date Delight	3	75	tr	—	0	2	17	3	20	40	190	4	—	—
Fat Free Hawaiian Fruit	3	75	tr	—	0	2	16	3	20	40	190	4	—	200
Fat Free Jumbos Apple Raisin	1	70	tr	—	0	2	16	3	20	35	160	2	—	—
Fat Free Jumbos Raisin	1	70	tr	—	0	2	16	3	20	35	160	2	—	—
Fat Free Jumbos Raspberry	1	70	tr	—	0	2	16	3	20	35	160	2	—	—
Fat Free Raisin Oatmeal	3	75	tr	—	0	2	17	3	20	40	190	2	—	—

FOOD	PORTION	CALORIES	FAT	SAT FAT	CHOL	PROTEIN	CARBO	FIBER	CALCIUM	SOD	POTAS	VIT C	FOLIC	VIT A
HEALTH VALLEY (CONT.)														
Fiber Jumbos Blueberry Nut	1	100	3	—	0	2	14	3	20	45	110	2	—	—
Fiber Jumbos Chunky Pecan	1	100	3	—	0	2	14	3	20	45	110	2	—	—
Fiber Jumbos Raisin Nut	1	100	3	—	0	2	14	3	20	45	110	2	—	—
Fruit & Fitness	5	200	6	—	0	4	34	6	39	115	520	3	tr	1257
Fruit Jumbos Almond Date	1	70	3	—	0	2	10	1	8	30	40	3	4	1
Fruit Jumbos Oat Bran	1	70	2	—	0	2	12	2	6	35	45	tr	5	8
Fruit Jumbos Raisin Nut	1	70	3	—	0	2	10	1	8	35	45	3	4	1
Fruit Jumbos Tropical Fruit	1	70	3	—	0	1	10	2	10	35	25	3	4	513
Graham Amaranth	7	110	3	—	0	3	25	3	31	110	850	5	11	0
Graham Honey	7	100	4	—	0	3	18	2	20	125	115	4	9	1
Graham Oat Bran	7	120	3	—	0	3	20	5	15	45	85	4	12	1
Honey Jumbos Crisp Cinnamon	1	70	4	—	0	2	9	1	20	35	55	3	4	3
Honey Jumbos Crisp Peanut Butter	1	70	2	—	0	2	11	1	20	35	55	2	5	tr
Honey Jumbos Fancy Oat Bran	2	130	4	—	0	4	20	4	20	50	110	tr	13	1
Oat Bran Animal Cookies	7	110	4	—	0	2	17	3	13	50	80	3	1	2
Oat Bran Fruit & Nut	2	110	4	—	0	3	17	3	23	70	150	3	10	3
The Great Tofu	2	90	3	—	0	2	14	4	9	30	25	3	1	99
The Great Wheat Free	2	80	3	—	0	2	14	3	36	35	95	4	1	3
HEYDAY														
Caramel & Peanut	1 (0.8 oz)	110	5	1	0	2	13	tr	—	40	70	—	—	—
Fudge	1 (0.8 oz)	110	5	1	0	2	13	tr	—	40	70	—	—	—
HONEY MAID														
Cinnamon Grahams	10 (1.1 oz)	140	3	1	0	2	26	1	20	210	40	—	—	—
Honey Grahams	8 (1 oz)	120	3	1	0	2	22	1	—	180	30	—	—	—
HYDROX														
Original	3	150	7	2	0	2	21	1	—	125	—	—	—	—
Reduced Fat	3 (1.1 oz)	130	4	1	0	1	24	1	—	140	—	—	—	—
KEEBLER														
Buttercup	3	70	3	tr	0	1	11	—	—	110	20	—	—	—
Chocolate Fudge Sandwich	1	80	4	1	0	tr	12	—	—	70	25	—	—	—
Commodore	1	60	2	tr	0	1	10	—	—	65	20	—	—	—

FOOD	PORTION	CALORIES	FAT	SAT FAT	CHOL	PROTEIN	CARBO	FIBER	CALCIUM	SOD	POTAS	VIT C	FOLIC	VIT A
KEEBLER (CONT.)														
Cookies Mates	2	50	2	1	0	tr	8	—	—	55	20	—	—	—
French Vanilla Creme	1	80	4	tr	0	tr	12	—	—	80	15	—	—	—
Graham Honey Fiber Enriched	2	90	2	1	0	2	16	—	2	110	30	—	—	—
Graham Kitchen Rich	2	60	2	1	0	1	9	—	—	55	30	—	—	—
Homeplate	1	60	2	—	1	1	10	—	—	130	20	—	—	—
Keebies	1	80	3	tr	0	1	12	—	—	80	25	—	—	—
Krisp Kreem Wafers	2	50	3	1	0	tr	7	—	—	20	10	—	—	—
Old Fashion Chocolate Chip	1	80	4	1	0	tr	11	—	—	75	25	—	—	—
Old Fashion Double Fudge	1	80	4	1	0	tr	11	—	—	65	22	—	—	—
Old Fashion Oatmeal	1	80	4	1	0	1	13	—	—	110	30	—	—	—
Old Fashion Peanut Butter	1	80	4	1	0	1	10	—	—	100	35	—	—	—
Old Fashion Sugar	1	80	3	1	0	1	13	—	—	70	10	—	—	—
Pitter Patter	1	90	4	tr	0	2	12	—	—	115	40	—	—	—
Vanilla Wafers	4	80	4	—	1	tr	10	—	—	60	15	—	—	—
LU														
Chocolatiers	4 (1.1 oz)	170	8	4	0	2	20	2	0	35	—	0	—	0
Chocolatiers Dipped	3 (1 oz)	170	11	9	0	2	17	1	20	15	—	0	—	0
Le Petit Ecolier Dark Chocolate	2 (0.9 oz)	130	6	4	5	2	17	1	0	55	—	0	—	0
Little Schoolboy Milk Chocolate	2 (0.9 oz)	130	7	3	5	2	15	0	0	85	—	0	—	0
Marie Lu	3 (1.2 oz)	170	6	2	5	2	25	1	0	170	—	0	—	0
Truffle Lu	4 (1.2 oz)	180	11	7	0	2	18	1	20	410	—	0	—	0
LA CHOY														
Fortune	1	15	tr	—	0	tr	4	tr	tr	1	2	0	—	tr
LANCE														
Choc-O-Lunch	1 pkg (37 g)	180	7	2	0	3	26	—	—	150	60	—	—	—
Choc-O-Mint	1 pkg (35 g)	180	10	3	0	2	22	—	—	90	35	—	—	—
Chocolate Chip Fudge	1 (28 g)	130	5	2	5	2	20	—	—	130	35	—	—	—
Chocolate Chip Soft	1 (28 g)	130	5	2	5	2	19	—	—	100	40	1	—	200
Coated Graham	1 pkg (50 g)	200	10	4	0	3	24	—	80	60	40	—	—	—
Fig Bar	1 pkg (42 g)	150	2	1	0	2	30	—	60	85	60	—	—	—
Lem-O-Lunch	1 pkg (48 g)	240	11	2	0	3	32	—	—	190	60	1	—	—
Lemon Nekot	1 pkg (42 g)	220	11	4	5	2	28	—	—	100	45	2	—	—
Malt	1 pkg (35 g)	190	11	2	0	5	16	—	60	125	45	—	—	—

FOOD	PORTION	CALORIES	FAT	SAT FAT	CHOL	PROTEIN	CARBO	FIBER	CALCIUM	SOD	POTAS	VIT C	FOLIC	VIT A
LANCE (CONT.)														
Oatmeal	1 (57 g)	130	5	1	0	2	20	—	—	70	65	—	—	—
Peanut Butter Creme Filled Wafer	1 pkg (50 g)	240	10	3	0	4	34	—	40	80	40	—	—	—
Van-O-Lunch	1 pkg (37 g)	180	7	2	0	2	26	—	—	150	20	—	—	—
LITTLE DEBBIE														
Animal	1 pkg (1.5 oz)	190	5	2	0	3	33	0	0	110	—	0	—	0
Apple Flips	1 (1.2 oz)	150	5	2	5	1	24	tr	0	115	—	0	—	0
Caramel Cookie Bars	1 pkg (1.2 oz)	160	8	2	0	0	23	1	20	90	—	0	—	0
Chocolate Chip Chewy	1 pkg (2 oz)	370	19	6	10	3	47	1	20	280	—	0	—	0
Chocolate Chip Crisp	1 pkg (1.5 oz)	210	12	4	5	2	26	1	20	150	—	0	—	0
Cookie Wreaths	1 pkg (0.6 oz)	90	5	1	0	1	11	0	0	45	—	0	—	0
Creme Filled Chocolate	1 pkg (1.2 oz)	180	8	2	0	2	24	1	0	115	—	0	—	0
Creme Filled Chocolate	1 pkg (1.8 oz)	260	11	3	0	3	36	1	0	230	—	0	—	0
Easter Puffs	1 pkg (1.2 oz)	140	5	1	0	0	25	0	0	65	—	0	—	0
Figaroos	1 pkg (1.5 oz)	160	4	1	0	1	31	3	0	115	—	0	—	0
Figaroos	1 pkg (2 oz)	200	5	1	0	2	40	2	20	160	—	0	—	0
Fudge Macaroons	1 pkg (1 oz)	140	8	4	0	1	18	1	0	65	—	0	—	0
Ginger	1 pkg (0.7 oz)	90	3	1	5	0	14	1	20	55	—	0	—	0
Oatmeal Crisp	1 pkg (1.5 oz)	210	11	3	5	2	27	1	20	230	—	0	—	0
Oatmeal Lights	1 pkg (1.3 oz)	140	4	1	0	2	28	1	0	190	—	0	—	0
Oatmeal Raisin	1 pkg (2.7 oz)	320	13	3	0	4	50	2	20	330	—	0	—	0
Peanut Butter	1 pkg (1.5 oz)	210	10	3	5	2	27	1	0	230	—	0	—	0
Peanut Butter & Jelly Sandwich	1 pkg (1.1 oz)	130	5	1	0	2	22	1	0	100	—	0	—	0
Peanut Butter Bars	1 pkg (1.9 oz)	270	15	3	0	4	33	1	20	190	—	0	—	0
Peanut Clusters	1 pkg (1.4 oz)	190	11	2	0	3	23	1	20	125	—	0	—	0
Pecan Spinwheels	1 pkg (1 oz)	110	4	1	0	1	16	1	0	100	—	0	—	0
Pecan Shortbread	1 pkg (1.5 oz)	220	13	3	5	2	26	0	0	170	—	0	—	0
LORNA DOONE														
Cookies	4 (1 oz)	140	7	1	5	2	19	tr	—	130	25	—	—	—
MALLOMARS														
Cookies	2 (0.9 oz)	120	5	3	0	1	17	1	—	35	40	—	—	—
MALLOPUFFS														
Cookies	1 (0.6 oz)	70	2	2	0	1	12	tr	—	35		—	—	—
MANISCHEWITZ														
Macaroons Chocolate	2 (0.9 oz)	90	4	4	0	2	15	4	0	80	—	0	—	0
MOTHER'S														
Almond Shortbread	3	180	11	4	0	2	19	1	—	115	—	—	—	—
Butter	5	140	6	3	10	2	21	—	—	95	—	—	—	—

FOOD	PORTION	CALORIES	FAT	SAT FAT	CHOL	PROTEIN	CARBO	FIBER	CALCIUM	SOD	POTAS	VIT C	FOLIC	VIT A
MOTHER'S (CONT.)														
Checkerboard Wafers	8	150	8	5	0	1	20	1	—	40	—	—	—	—
Chocolate Chip	2	160	8	3	10	2	20	0	—	105	—	—	—	—
Chocolate Chip Angel	3	180	9	4	0	2	21	1	—	70	—	—	—	—
Chocolate Chip Bag	4	140	5	—	2	1	23	1	—	85	—	—	—	—
Chocolate Chip Parade	4	130	5	2	0	1	19	1	—	100	—	—	—	—
Circus Animals	6	140	6	5	0	1	20	0	—	55	—	—	—	—
Cocadas	5	150	7	3	5	2	20	2	—	140	—	—	—	—
Cookie Parade	4	140	7	3	0	1	18	2	—	95	—	—	—	—
Dinosaur Grrrahams	2	130	3	1	0	2	24	—	—	130	—	—	—	—
Double Fudge	3	170	8	4	0	2	22	2	—	100	—	—	—	—
Duplex Creme	3	170	8	4	0	2	23	1	—	130	—	—	—	—
English Tea	2	180	7	4	0	2	26	1	—	100	—	—	—	—
Fig Bar	2	130	4	1	0	1	24	0	—	105	—	—	—	—
Fig Bar Fat Free	1	70	0	0	0	1	16	1	—	65	—	—	—	—
Fig Bar Whole Wheat	2	130	5	2	0	1	20	3	—	140	—	—	—	—
Fig Bar Whole Wheat Fat Free	1	70	0	0	0	1	17	1	—	60	—	—	—	—
Flaky Flix Fudge	2	140	7	5	0	1	17	2	—	50	—	—	—	—
Flaky Flix Vanilla	2	140	8	5	0	1	17	1	—	40	—	—	—	—
Frosted Holiday	4	130	6	5	0	1	19	0	—	50	—	—	—	—
Fudge Bowl Crowns	2	140	6	4	0	1	21	1	—	55	—	—	—	—
Fudge Bowl Nuggets	2	140	6	4	0	1	21	1	—	70	—	—	—	—
Gaucho Peanut Butter	2	190	10	3	0	3	22	2	—	200	—	—	—	—
Gingerbread Man	6	140	6	2	5	2	21	1	—	160	—	—	—	—
Iced Oatmeal	2	120	4	2	0	1	20	1	—	150	—	—	—	—
Iced Oatmeal Bag	4	120	4	2	0	1	20	1	—	150	—	—	—	—
Iced Raisin	2	180	8	7	0	1	24	1	—	110	—	—	—	—
MLB Double Header Duplex	3	170	8	4	5	2	23	1	—	130	—	—	—	—
Macaroon	2	150	8	4	0	1	18	2	—	80	—	—	—	—
Marias	3	170	6	2	5	2	28	1	—	150	—	—	—	—
North Poles	2	140	7	6	0	1	17	0	—	30	—	—	—	—
Oatmeal	2	110	5	2	0	1	17	1	—	150	—	—	—	—
Oatmeal Chocolate Chip	2	120	5	2	0	2	19	1	—	140	—	—	—	—
Oatmeal Raisin	5	150	7	2	5	2	20	2	—	125	—	—	—	—
Oatmeal Walnut Chocolate Chip	2	130	6	2	0	2	17	1	—	135	—	—	—	—

FOOD	PORTION	CALORIES	FAT	SAT FAT	CHOL	PROTEIN	CARBO	FIBER	CALCIUM	SOD	POTAS	VIT C	FOLIC	VIT A
MOTHER'S (CONT.)														
Pecan Goldens	2	170	11	2	0	2	17	5	—	110	—	—	—	—
Rainbow Wafers	8	150	8	5	0	1	20	1	—	40	—	—	—	—
Striped Shortbread	3	170	8	5	0	2	22	1	—	75	—	—	—	—
Sugar	2	140	6	2	0	1	19	1	—	75	—	—	—	—
Taffy	2	180	8	2	0	2	25	2	—	160	—	—	—	—
Triplet Assortment	2	140	7	3	0	1	18	1	—	112	—	—	—	—
Vanilla Wafers	6	150	6	2	4	2	24	1	—	85	—	—	—	—
Walnut Fudge	2	130	7	3	0	1	16	1	—	90	—	—	—	—
Zoo Pals	14	140	5	2	0	2	23	1	—	120	—	—	—	—
MYSTIC MINT														
Cookies	1 (0.5 oz)	90	4	1	0	1	11	0	—	65	30	—	—	—
NABISCO														
Brown Edge Wafers	5 (1 oz)	140	6	2	<5	1	21	tr	—	80	30	—	—	—
Bugs Bunny Chocolate Graham	13 (1.1 oz)	140	5	1	0	2	22	1	—	180	45	—	—	—
Bugs Bunny Cinnamon Graham	13 (1.1 oz)	140	5	1	0	2	23	tr	—	160	30	—	—	—
Bugs Bunny Graham	13 (1.1 oz)	140	7	1	0	2	23	1	20	160	30	—	—	—
Cameo	2 (1 oz)	130	5	1	0	1	21	tr	—	105	30	—	—	—
Chocolate Grahams	3 (1.1 oz)	160	8	5	0	2	21	1	—	90	85	—	—	—
Chocolate Chip Snaps	7 (1.1 oz)	150	5	2	0	2	24	tr	—	115	30	—	—	—
Chocolate Snaps	7 (1.1 oz)	140	5	2	0	2	23	1	—	180	60	—	—	—
Cookie Break	3 (1.1 oz)	160	6	2	0	1	23	tr	—	115	20	—	—	—
Danish Imported	5 (1.1 oz)	170	8	2	0	2	22	1	40	80	25	—	—	—
Family Favorites Fudge Covered Grahams	3 (1 oz)	140	7	2	0	2	19	1	—	125	50	—	—	—
Family Favorites Fudge Striped Shortbread	3 (1.1 oz)	160	8	2	0	2	22	1	—	140	45	—	—	—
Family Favorites Oatmeal	1 (0.5 oz)	80	3	1	0	1	12	tr	—	65	20	—	—	—
Family Favorites Vanilla Sandwich	3 (1.2 oz)	170	8	2	0	2	25	0	—	120	35	—	—	—
Famous Chocolate Wafers	5 (1.1 oz)	140	4	2	<5	2	24	1	—	230	80	—	—	—
Ginger Snaps Old Fashioned	4 (1 oz)	120	3	1	0	tr	22	tr	20	170	130	—	—	—
Grahams	8 (1 oz)	120	3	1	0	2	22	1	20	180	50	—	—	—
Marshmallow Puffs	1 (0.75 oz)	90	4	1	0	1	14	0	—	45	25	—	—	—
Marshmallow Twirls	1 (1 oz)	130	6	2	0	1	20	tr	—	75	50	—	—	—
Nilla Wafers	8 (1.1 oz)	140	5	1	5	2	24	0	20	105	30	—	—	—

FOOD	PORTION	CALORIES	FAT	SAT FAT	CHOL	PROTEIN	CARBO	FIBER	CALCIUM	SOD	POTAS	VIT C	FOLIC	VIT A
NABISCO (CONT.)														
Pecan Passion	1 (0.5 oz)	90	5	1	<5	tr	9	0	—	35	15	—	—	—
Pinwheels	1 (1 oz)	130	5	3	0	1	21	tr	—	35	25	—	—	—
NATIONAL														
Arrowroot	1 (5 g)	20	1	0	0	0	3	tr	—	15	5	—	—	—
NEWTONS														
Apple Fat Free	2 (1 oz)	100	0	0	0	1	24	1	—	60	35	—	—	—
Cranberry Fat Free	2 (1 oz)	100	0	0	0	1	23	1	—	95	20	—	—	—
Fig	2 (1.1 oz)	110	3	1	0	1	20	1	—	120	80	—	—	—
Fig Fat Free	1 (1 oz)	100	0	0	0	1	22	2	20	115	80	—	—	—
Raspberry Fat Free	2 (1 oz)	100	0	0	0	1	23	tr	—	115	25	1	—	—
Strawberry Fat Free	2 (1 oz)	100	0	0	0	1	23	tr	—	115	30	5	—	—
NUTRA/BALANCE														
Chocolate Chip	1 (2 oz)	260	14	—	—	3	34	8	—	81	114	—	—	—
Oatmeal Raisin	1 (2 oz)	240	9	—	—	4	36	8	—	50	150	—	—	—
NUTTER BUTTER														
Bites Peanut Butter Sandwich	10 (1.1 oz)	150	7	2	<5	3	20	1	—	125	55	—	—	—
Peanut Butter Sandwich	2 (1 oz)	130	6	1	<5	3	19	1	—	110	55	—	—	—
Peanut Creme Patties	5 (1.1 oz)	160	9	2	0	4	17	1	—	80	90	—	—	—
OREO														
Cookies	3 (1.2 oz)	160	7	2	0	2	23	1	—	220	60	—	—	—
Double Stuf	2 (1 oz)	140	7	1	0	1	19	tr	—	150	40	—	—	—
Fudge Covered	1 (0.75 oz)	110	6	2	0	1	14	tr	—	85	80	—	—	—
Halloween Treats	2 (1 oz)	140	7	2	0	1	19	1	—	125	40	—	—	—
Reduced Fat	3 (1.2 oz)	140	5	1	0	2	24	1	—	190	60	—	—	—
White Fudge Covered	1 (0.75 oz)	110	6	2	0	1	14	tr	20	70	55	—	—	—
PALLY														
Butter	4 (0.88 oz)	100	3	2	7	2	17	—	—	95	—	—	—	34
PEPPERIDGE FARM														
Beacon Hill Chocolate Chocolate Walnut	1	120	7	2	5	2	14	1	—	65	—	—	—	—
Blondie Chocolate Chip Fat Free	1 (1.4 oz)	120	0	0	0	2	29	tr	20	65	—	0	—	0
Bordeaux	2	70	3	1	0	1	11	0	—	40	—	—	—	—
Brownie Chocolate Nut	2	110	7	2	<5	1	11	—	—	45	—	—	—	—
Brownie Nut Large	1	140	8	3	5	1	15	—	—	65	—	—	—	—
Brussels	2	110	5	2	0	1	13	0	—	65	—	—	—	—
Brussels Mint	2	130	7	2	0	1	17	—	—	40	—	—	—	—
Butter Chessman	2	90	4	2	10	1	12	—	—	60	—	—	—	—
Cappucino	1	50	3	1	<5	0	6	—	—	20	—	—	—	—

FOOD	PORTION	CALORIES	FAT	SAT FAT	CHOL	PROTEIN	CARBO	FIBER	CALCIUM	SOD	POTAS	VIT C	FOLIC	VIT A
PEPPERIDGE FARM (CONT.)														
Capri	1	80	5	1	0	0	10	—	—	45	—	—	—	—
Chantilly	1	80	2	1	<5	1	14	—	—	35	—	—	—	—
Cheasapeake Chocolate Chunk Pecan	1	120	7	2	5	1	14	1	—	60	—	—	—	—
Cheyenne Peanut Butter Milk Chocolate Chunk	1	110	6	2	5	2	13	1	—	80	—	—	—	—
Chocolate Chip	2	100	5	2	5	1	12	0	—	45	—	—	—	—
Chocolate Chip Large	1	130	6	2	5	2	16	—	—	60	—	—	—	—
Chocolate Chunk Pecan	1	70	4	1	12	0	8	—	—	25	—	—	—	—
Dakota Milk Chocolate Oatmeal	1	110	6	2	5	1	15	1	—	70	—	—	—	—
Date Pecan	2	110	5	2	10	1	15	—	—	40	—	—	—	—
Fruit Filled Apricot- Raspberry	2	100	4	2	10	1	15	—	—	50	—	—	—	—
Fruit Filled Strawberry	2	100	5	2	10	1	15	—	—	50	—	—	—	—
Geneva	2	130	6	2	0	1	14	—	—	50	—	—	—	—
Gingerman	2	70	3	0	5	1	10	—	—	50	—	—	—	—
Hazelnut	2	110	6	2	0	1	15	—	—	75	—	—	—	—
Irish Oatmeal	2	90	5	1	5	1	13	—	—	80	—	—	—	—
Lemon Nut Crunch	2	110	7	2	<5	1	13	—	—	50	—	—	—	—
Lido	1	90	5	1	<5	1	10	—	—	30	—	—	—	—
Linzer	1	120	4	1	<5	2	20	—	—	55	—	—	—	—
Milano	2	120	6	2	15	1	15	—	—	45	—	—	—	—
Mint Milano	2	150	7	2	5	1	17	—	—	60	—	—	—	—
Molasses Crisps	2	70	3	0	0	1	8	—	—	50	—	—	—	—
Nantucket Chocolate Chunk	1	120	6	2	5	1	15	1	20	60	—	—	—	—
Nassau	1	80	5	1	<5	1	9	—	—	45	—	—	—	—
Oatmeal Large	1	120	6	1	5	1	18	—	—	105	—	—	—	—
Oatmeal Raisin	2	110	5	2	10	1	15	—	—	115	—	—	—	—
Old Fashioned Chocolate Chip	2	100	5	2	5	1	12	0	—	45	—	—	—	—
Orange Milano	2	150	7	2	5	1	17	—	—	60	—	—	—	—
Orleans	3	90	6	2	0	0	11	—	—	30	—	—	—	—
Orleans Sandwich	2	120	8	2	0	1	14	—	—	40	—	—	—	—
Pecan Shortbread	1	70	5	2	0	1	7	—	—	15	—	—	—	—
Pirouettes Chocolate Laced	2	70	4	1	<5	1	8	—	—	20	—	—	—	—
Pirouettes Original	2	70	4	1	<5	0	9	—	—	35	—	—	—	—
Raisin Bran	2	110	5	2	<5	1	13	—	—	55	—	—	—	—

FOOD	PORTION	CALORIES	FAT	SAT FAT	CHOL	PROTEIN	CARBO	FIBER	CALCIUM	SOD	POTAS	VIT C	FOLIC	VIT A
PEPPERIDGE FARM (CONT.)														
Ripple Milk Chocolate Fat Free	1 (0.6 oz)	60	0	0	0	1	13	tr	0	60	—	0	—	0
Sante Fe Oatmeal Raisin	1	100	4	1	<5	1	16	1	—	70	—	—	—	—
Sausalito Milk Chocolate Macadamia	1	120	7	2	5	1	14	0	—	65	—	—	—	—
Shortbread	2	150	8	2	<5	1	17	—	—	85	—	—	—	—
Sugar	2	100	5	2	10	1	13	—	—	55	—	—	—	—
Tahiti	1	90	6	2	5	0	9	—	—	25	—	—	—	—
Zurich	1	60	2	1	0	1	10	—	—	30	—	—	—	—
RITZ														
Chocolate Covered	3 (1 oz)	150	9	5	0	2	17	1	20	95	60	—	—	—
SARGENTO														
MooTown Snackers Cookies & Creme Honey Graham Sticks & Vanilla Creme w/Sprinkle	1 pkg (1.1 oz)	140	7	1	0	2	19	0	40	60	—	0	—	0
MooTown Snackers Cookies & Creme Vanilla Sticks & Chocolate Fudge Creme	1 pkg (1.1 oz)	140	7	2	0	1	20	0	0	65	—	0	—	0
SNACKWELL'S														
Fat Free Double Fudge	1 (0.5 oz)	50	0	0	0	1	12	tr	—	70	25	—	—	—
Golden Devil's Food	1 (0.5 oz)	50	1	0	0	1	12	0	0	30	—	0	—	0
Reduced Fat Chocolate Chip	13 (1 oz)	130	4	2	0	2	22	1	—	170	40	—	—	—
Reduced Fat Chocolate Sandwich With Chocolate Creme	2 (0.9 oz)	100	3	1	0	1	20	1	—	190	40	—	—	—
Reduced Fat Oatmeal Raisin	2 (1 oz)	110	3	0	0	2	20	1	20	135	75	—	—	—
Reduced Fat Vanilla Sandwich	2 (0.9 oz)	110	3	1	0	1	21	1	20	95	—	0	—	0
SOCIAL TEA														
Cookies	6 (1 oz)	120	4	1	5	2	20	tr	—	105	35	—	—	—
STELLA D'ORO														
Almond Toast Mandel	1	60	1	—	tr	1	10	—	—	43	—	—	—	—
Angel Bars	1	80	5	—	tr	1	7	—	—	15	—	—	—	—
Angel Wings	1	70	5	—	1	1	7	—	—	40	—	—	—	—
Angelica Goodies	1	110	4	—	tr	2	16	—	—	45	—	—	—	—

FOOD	PORTION	CALORIES	FAT	SAT FAT	CHOL	PROTEIN	CARBO	FIBER	CALCIUM	SOD	POTAS	VIT C	FOLIC	VIT A
STELLA D'ORO (CONT.)														
Anginetti	1	30	1	—	tr	1	5	—		3	—	—	—	—
Anisette Sponge	1	50	1	—	tr	1	10	—		40	—	—	—	—
Anisette Toast	1	50	1	—	tr	1	9	—		50	—	—	—	—
Anisette Toast Jumbo	1	110	1	—	tr	2	23	—		65	—	—	—	—
Apple Pastry Low Sodium	1	80	3	—	>5	1	14	—		5	—	—	—	—
Biscottini Cashews	1	110	6	—	—	2	14	—		50	—	—	—	—
Breakfast Treats	1	100	4	—	tr	2	15	—		80	—	—	—	—
Castelets Chocolate	1	60	3	—	tr	1	9	—		33	—	—	—	—
Chinese Dessert Cookies	1	170	9	—	tr	2	19	—		90	—	—	—	—
Como Delight	1	150	7	—	1	2	18	—		60	—	—	—	—
Deep Night Fudge	1	65	4	—	2	1	8	—		33	—	—	—	—
Dutch Apple Bars	1	110	3	—	1	1	19	—		35	—	—	—	—
Egg Biscuits Low Sodium	3	120	3	—	40	4	20	—		15	—	—	—	—
Egg Biscuits Sugared	1	80	1	—	1	2	14	—		45	—	—	—	—
Egg Jumbo	1	50	1	—	tr	1	9	—		30	—	—	—	—
Fruit Delight Apple Cinnamon Fat Free	1	70	0	0	0	tr	17	—		50	—	—	—	—
Fruit Delight Peach Apricot Fat Free	1	70	0	0	0	tr	17	—		35	—	—	—	—
Fruit Delight Raspberry Fat Free	1	70	0	0	0	tr	17	—		40	—	—	—	—
Fruit Slices	1	60	2	—	tr	2	9	—		45	—	—	—	—
Fruit Slices Fat Free	1	50	0	0	0	1	12	—		60	—	—	—	—
Golden Bars	1	110	4	—	tr	2	16	—		65	—	—	—	—
Holiday Rings & Stars	1	47	1	—	0	tr	7	—		12	—	—	—	—
Holiday Trinkets	1	40	2	—	tr	1	5	—		31	—	—	—	—
Hostess Assortment	1	40	2	—	tr	1	6	—		20	—	—	—	—
Indulgente Cashew Biscottini	1 (1.1 oz)	150	8	2	10	2	19	tr	0	70	—	0	—	0
Kichel Low Sodium	21	150	9	—	80	4	13	—		25	—	—	—	—
Lady Stella Assortment	1	40	2	—	tr	1	6	—		22	—	—	—	—
Margherite Chocolate	1	70	3	—	tr	1	10	—		40	—	—	—	—
Margherite Vanilla	1	70	3	—	tr	1	11	—		45	—	—	—	—
Peach Apricot Pastry Sodium Free	1	80	3	—	>5	1	13	—		0	—	—	—	—

FOOD	PORTION	CALORIES	FAT	SAT FAT	CHOL	PROTEIN	CARBO	FIBER	CALCIUM	SOD	POTAS	VIT C	FOLIC	VIT A
STELLA D'ORO (CONT.)														
Pfeffernusse Spice Drops	1	40	1	—	tr	1	7	—	—	18	—	—	—	—
Prune Pastry Dietetic	1	90	3	—	>5	1	14	—	—	0	—	—	—	—
Roman Egg Biscuits	1	140	5	—	tr	3	20	—	—	125	—	—	—	—
Royal Nuggets	1	2	tr	—	tr	tr	tr	—	—	—	—	—	—	—
Sesame Regina	1	50	2	—	tr	1	6	—	—	28	—	—	—	—
Swiss Fudge	1	70	3	—	tr	1	9	—	—	33	—	—	—	—
SUNSHINE														
Almond Crescents	4 (1.1 oz)	150	6	2	0	2	22	tr	—	105	—	—	—	—
Animal Crackers	1 box (2 oz)	260	7	2	0	4	43	1	—	230	—	—	—	—
Animal Crackers	14 (1.1 oz)	140	4	1	0	2	24	tr	—	125	—	—	—	—
Classics Chocolate Chip With Pecans	1 (0.7 oz)	110	7	2	3	1	11	tr	—	45	—	—	—	—
Classics Chocolate Chip With Walnuts	1 (0.7 oz)	100	6	3	5	2	11	1	—	70	—	—	—	—
Classics Premier Chocolate Chip	1 (0.7 oz)	100	5	3	5	1	13	tr	—	75	—	—	—	—
Dixie Vanilla	2 (0.9 oz)	120	5	1	0	2	19	tr	—	105	—	—	—	—
Fig Bars	2 (1 oz)	110	3	1	0	1	20	1	tr	60	—	—	—	—
Fudge Family Bears Vanilla	2 (1 oz)	140	6	2	0	1	20	tr	—	115	—	—	—	—
Fudge Mint Patties	2 (0.8 oz)	130	7	4	0	1	16	tr	—	60	—	—	—	—
Fudge Striped Shortbread	3 (1.1 oz)	160	8	5	0	2	20	1	—	85	—	—	—	—
Ginger Snaps	7 (1 oz)	130	5	1	0	2	22	tr	—	150	—	—	—	—
Grahams Cinnamon	2 (1.1 oz)	140	6	2	0	2	22	tr	20	150	—	0	—	—
Grahams Fudge Dipped	4 (1.2 oz)	170	9	6	0	2	21	1	—	75	—	—	—	—
Grahams Honey	2 (1 oz)	120	4	1	0	2	20	1	20	130	—	—	—	—
Grahamy Bears	1 pkg (2 oz)	260	10	2	0	4	41	2	—	230	—	—	—	—
Grahamy Bears	10 (1.1 oz)	140	5	1	0	2	22	1	—	125	—	—	—	—
Iced Gingerbread	5 (1 oz)	130	6	2	5	2	19	tr	—	135	—	—	—	—
Iced Oatmeal	2 (0.9 oz)	120	5	1	0	2r	18	tr	—	90	—	—	—	—
Jingles	6 (1.1 oz)	150	5	1	0	2	22	tr	—	115	—	—	—	—
Lemon Coolers	5 (1 oz)	140	6	2	0	1	21	tr	—	100	—	—	—	—
Mini Chocolate Chip Cookies	5 (1.1 oz)	160	8	3	0	2	20	tr	—	120	—	—	—	—
Mini Fudge Royals	15 (1.1 oz)	160	8	5	0	2	20	1	—	90	—	—	—	—
Oatmeal Chocolate Chip	3 (1.3 oz)	170	8	3	0	3	23	2	—	130	—	—	—	—
Oatmeal Country Style	3 (1.2 oz)	170	7	2	0	2	24	1	—	160	—	—	—	0.1
School House Cookies	20 (1.1 oz)	140	5	1	0	2	23	tr	—	115	—	—	—	—

FOOD	PORTION	CALORIES	FAT	SAT FAT	CHOL	PROTEIN	CARBO	FIBER	CALCIUM	SOD	POTAS	VIT C	FOLIC	VIT A
SUNSHINE (CONT.)														
Sugar Wafers Chocolate	3 (0.9 oz)	130	7	2	0	2	17	tr	20	30	—	—	—	—
Sugar Wafers Peanut Butter	4 (1.1 oz)	170	9	2	0	3	19	1	—	75	—	—	—	—
Sugar Wafers Vanilla	3 (0.9 oz)	130	6	2	0	1	18	tr	—	20	—	—	—	—
Tru Blu Chocolate	1 (0.6 oz)	80	3	1	0	1	11	tr	—	64	—	—	—	—
Tru Blu Lemon	1 (0.6 oz)	80	3	1	0	1	11	tr	—	65	—	—	—	—
Tru Blu Vanilla	1 (0.5 oz)	80	3	1	0	1	11	tr	—	65	—	—	—	—
Vanilla Wafers	7 (1.1 oz)	150	7	2	3	2	20	tr	—	110	—	—	—	—
Vienna Fingers	2 (1 oz)	140	6	2	0	2	21	tr	—	105	—	—	—	—
TASTYKAKE														
Chocolate Chip Bar	1 (43 g)	190	8	2	5	3	28	1	—	95	—	—	—	0.1
Chocolate Chunk Macadamia Nut	1 pkg (56 g)	310	14	5	40	2	42	2	—	180	—	—	—	—
Fudge Bar	1 (50 g)	200	7	2	5	2	35	1	20	160	—	—	—	—
Oatmeal Raisin Bar	1 (50 g)	210	8	2	15	3	32	1	20	250	—	—	—	—
Soft'n Chewy Chocolate Chip	1 (39 g)	170	7	2	10	2	25	1	—	170	—	—	—	—
Soft'n Chewy Chocolate Chocolate Chip	1 (32 g)	170	7	2	5	2	26	1	—	110	—	—	—	—
Soft'n Chewy Oatmeal Raisin	1 (39 g)	160	5	1	5	3	27	1	—	160	—	—	—	—
Vanilla Sugar Wafer	1 (6 g)	36	2	0	0	0	4	0	—	10	—	—	—	—
TEDDY GRAHAMS														
Chocolate	24 (1 oz)	140	5	1	0	2	22	1	—	150	95	—	—	—
Cinnamon	24 (1 oz)	140	4	1	0	2	23	1	—	150	30	—	—	—
Honey	24 (1 oz)	140	4	1	0	2	22	1	—	150	30	—	—	—
TREE OF LIFE														
Creme Supremes	2 (0.9 oz)	120	5	0	0	1	18	1	20	90	—	0	—	0
Creme Supremes Mint	2 (0.9 oz)	120	5	0	0	1	18	1	20	90	—	0	—	0
Fat Free Classic Carrot Cake	1 (0.8 oz)	60	0	0	0	1	14	1	0	50	—	0	—	0
Fat Free Devil's Food Chocolate	1 (0.8 oz)	70	0	0	0	2	15	1	20	80	—	0	—	0
Fat Free Golden Oatmeal Raisin	1 (0.8 oz)	70	0	0	0	2	16	1	—	40	—	—	—	—
Fat Free Harvest Fruit & Nut	1 (0.8 oz)	70	0	0	0	1	16	1	—	45	—	—	—	—
Fat Free Toasted Almond Butter	1 (0.8 oz)	70	0	0	0	2	16	1	—	35	—	—	—	—
Fruit Bars Apple Spice	2 (1.3 oz)	120	3	1	0	1	22	2	20	120	—	—	—	—
Fruit Bars Fat Free Fig	1 (0.8 oz)	70	0	0	0	1	16	2	20	100	—	—	—	—

FOOD	PORTION	CALORIES	FAT	SAT FAT	CHOL	PROTEIN	CARBO	FIBER	CALCIUM	SOD	POTAS	VIT C	FOLIC	VIT A
TREE OF LIFE (CONT.)														
Fruit Bars Fat Free Peach Apricot	1 (0.8 oz)	70	0	0	0	1	17	1	20	110	—	—	—	—
Fruit Bars Fat Free Wildberry	1 (0.8 oz)	70	0	0	0	1	16	2	20	170	—	—	—	—
Fruit Bars Fig	2 (1.3 oz)	120	3	1	0	2	21	3	20	100	—	—	—	—
Fruit Bars Peach Apricot	2 (1.3 oz)	120	3	1	0	2	22	2	20	105	—	—	—	—
Honey-Sweet Colossal Carrot Cake	1 (0.8 oz)	110	5	0	0	1	16	1	0	105	—	0	—	200
Honey-Sweet Lemon Burst	1 (0.8 oz)	110	5	0	0	1	15	1	0	25	—	0	—	0
Honey-Sweet Oh-So-Oatmeal	1 (0.8 oz)	110	5	0	0	2	14	1	0	140	—	2	—	0
Honey-Sweet Pecans-A-Plenty	1 (0.8 oz)	125	7	1	0	1	14	1	0	30	—	0	—	0
Monster Fat Free Carrot Cake	¼ cookie (0.9 oz)	60	0	0	0	1	15	1	20	30	—	1	—	1000
Monster Fat Free Devil's Food Chocolate	¼ cookie (0.9 oz)	80	0	0	0	2	20	2	0	45	—	1	—	0
Monster Fat Free Gingerbread	¼ cookie (0.9 oz)	80	0	0	0	2	19	2	0	50	—	1	—	0
Monster Fat Free Maple Pecan	¼ cookie (0.9 oz)	90	0	0	0	2	20	2	0	50	—	1	—	0
Royal Vanilla	2 (0.9 oz)	120	5	0	0	1	17	0	20	115	—	0	—	0
Small World Animal Grahams	7 (1 oz)	120	3	0	0	2	21	3	0	60	—	1	—	0
Small World Chocolate Chip	7 (1 oz)	120	4	1	0	2	20	3	0	60	—	1	—	0
Soft-Bake Chocolate Chip	1 (0.8 oz)	125	7	2	0	1	15	1	0	15	—	2	—	0
Soft-Bake Double Fudge	1 (0.8 oz)	110	5	0	0	1	16	2	0	20	—	2	—	0
Soft-Bake Maui Macaroon	1 (0.8 oz)	135	10	6	0	2	12	2	0	0	—	2	—	0
Soft-Bake Oatmeal	1 (0.8 oz)	115	5	0	0	2	16	2	0	20	—	1	—	0
Soft-Bake Peanut Butter	1 (0.8 oz)	125	7	1	0	3	13	1	0	60	—	2	—	0
Wheat-Free American Oatmeal	1 (0.8 oz)	90	5	0	0	1	11	1	60	25	—	0	—	0
Wheat-Free California Carob	1 (0.8 oz)	105	5	0	0	1	14	6	0	75	—	0	—	0
Wheat-Free Georgia Peanut Butter	1 (0.8 oz)	95	6	1	0	2	8	1	20	110	—	0	—	0

FOOD	PORTION	CALORIES	FAT	SAT FAT	CHOL	PROTEIN	CARBO	FIBER	CALCIUM	SOD	POTAS	VIT C	FOLIC	VIT A
TREE OF LIFE (CONT.)														
Wheat-Free Mountain Maple Walnut	1 (0.8 oz)	100	6	0	0	2	9	6	60	50	—	0	—	0
VIENNA FINGERS														
Low Fat	2 (1 oz)	130	4	1	0	1	23	tr	—	95	—	—	—	—
WEIGHT WATCHERS														
Apple Raisin Bar	1 (0.75 oz)	70	2	1	0	1	14	2	0	60	—	0	—	0
Chocolate Chip	2 (1.06 oz)	140	5	2	0	2	22	1	20	90	—	0	—	0
Chocolate Sandwich	2 (1.06)	140	4	1	0	2	23	1	0	160	—	0	—	0
Fruit Filled Fig	1 (0.7 oz)	70	0	0	0	1	16	0	20	50	—	0	—	0
Fruit Filled Raspberry	1 (0.7 oz)	70	0	0	0	1	16	0	0	45	—	0	—	0
Oatmeal Raisin	2 (1.06 oz)	120	2	0	0	2	22	1	0	90	—	0	—	0
Vanilla Sandwich	2 (1.06 oz)	140	3	1	0	1	25	1	0	80	—	0	—	0
REFRIGERATED														
chocolate chip	1 (0.42 oz)	59	3	1	3	1	8	—	3	28	24	0	—	7
chocolate chip unbaked	1 oz	126	6	2	7	1	17	—	7	59	51	0	—	17
oatmeal	1 (0.4 oz)	56	3	1	3	1	8	—	4	39	20	—	—	8
oatmeal raisin	1 (0.4 oz)	56	3	1	3	1	8	—	4	39	20	—	—	8
peanut butter	1 (0.4 oz)	60	3	1	4	1	7	—	13	52	41	0	—	6
peanut butter dough	1 oz	130	7	2	8	2	15	—	29	112	87	0	—	13
sugar	1 (0.42 oz)	58	3	1	4	1	8	—	11	56	20	0	—	4
sugar dough	1 oz	124	6	2	8	1	17	—	23	120	42	0	—	10
TAKE-OUT														
biscotti with nuts chocolate dipped	1 (1.3 oz)	117	6	3	18	2	16	1	10	33	—	1	—	100
black & white	1 lg (3 oz)	302	9	5	58	4	52	1	32	72	68	tr	11	465

CORIANDER

leaf dried	1 tsp	2	tr	—	0	tr	tr	—	7	1	27	3	—	—
seed	1 tsp	5	tr	tr	0	tr	1	—	13	1	23	—	—	—

CORN

(*see also* BRAN, CEREAL, CORNMEAL)

CANNED														
cream style	½ cup	93	1	tr	0	2	23	—	4	365	172	6	57	124
w/ red & green peppers	½ cup	86	1	tr	0	3	21	—	5	396	174	10	—	265
white	½ cup	66	1	tr	0	2	15	—	—	—	—	—	—	tr
DEL MONTE														
Cream Style Golden	½ cup (4.4 oz)	90	1	0	0	2	20	2	0	360	—	6	—	0

FOOD	PORTION	CALORIES	FAT	SAT FAT	CHOL	PROTEIN	CARBO	FIBER	CALCIUM	SOD	POTAS	VIT C	FOLIC	VIT A
DEL MONTE (CONT.)														
Cream Style Golden 50% Less Salt	½ cup (4.4 oz)	90	1	0	0	2	20	2	0	180	—	6	—	0
Cream Style Golden No Salt Added	½ cup (4.4 oz)	90	1	0	0	2	20	2	0	10	—	6	—	0
Cream Style Supersweet Golden	½ cup (4.4 oz)	60	1	0	0	1	14	2	0	360	—	6	—	0
Cream Style White	½ cup (4.4 oz)	100	0	0	0	2	21	2	0	360	—	4	—	0
Whole Kernel Golden	½ cup (4.4 oz)	90	0	0	0	2	18	3	0	360	—	6	—	0
Whole Kernel Golden Supersweet 50% Less Salt	½ cup (4.4 oz)	60	1	0	0	2	11	3	0	130	—	6	—	0
Whole Kernel Golden Supersweet No Salt Added	½ cup (4.4 oz)	60	1	0	0	2	11	3	0	10	—	6	—	0
Whole Kernel Golden Supersweet No Sugar	½ cup (4.4 oz)	60	0	0	0	2	11	3	0	360	—	6	—	0
Whole Kernel Golden Supersweet Vacuum Packed	½ cup (3.7 oz)	70	1	0	0	2	13	3	0	270	—	6	—	0
Whole Kernel Golden Supersweet Vacuum Packed No Salt Added	½ cup (3.7 oz)	70	1	0	0	2	13	3	0	10	—	6	—	0
Whole Kernel White Sweet	½ cup (4.4 oz)	80	0	0	0	2	17	2	0	360	—	9	—	0
GREEN GIANT														
Cream Style	½ cup (4.5 oz)	100	1	0	0	2	22	1	0	430	—	2	—	200
Mexicorn	⅓ cup (2.7 oz)	60	0	0	0	2	14	2	0	430	—	1	—	0
Niblets	⅓ cup (2.7 oz)	70	0	0	0	2	15	2	0	230	—	0	—	100
Niblets 50% Less Sodium	⅓ cup (2.7 oz)	60	0	0	0	2	14	1	0	115	—	2	—	0
Niblets Extra Sweet	⅓ cup (2.6 oz)	50	1	0	0	2	10	2	0	200	—	0	—	0
Niblets No Added Sugar or Salt	⅓ cup (2.7 oz)	60	0	0	0	2	13	2	0	0	—	2	—	0
White Shoepeg	⅓ cup	80	1	0	0	2	16	1	0	220	—	4	—	0
Whole Sweet	½ cup (4.3 oz)	80	1	0	0	2	18	2	0	360	—	2	—	0
Whole Sweet 50% Less Sodium	½ cup (4.2 oz)	80	1	0	0	2	17	2	0	180	—	2	—	0

FOOD	PORTION	CALORIES	FAT	SAT FAT	CHOL	PROTEIN	CARBO	FIBER	CALCIUM	SOD	POTAS	VIT C	FOLIC	VIT A
KA-ME														
Baby	½ cup (4.5 oz)	20	0	0	0	1	3	2	—	10	—	—	—	—
Stir Fry	½ cup (4.5 oz)	20	0	0	0	1	3	2	—	10	—	—	—	—
SENECA														
Cream Style	½ cup	80	0	0	0	2	18	1	0	288	140	6	—	0
Whole Kernel	½ cup	90	0	0	0	2	21	2	0	288	175	6	—	0
Whole Kernel Natural Pack	½ cup	80	1	0	0	3	18	2	0	0	175	6	—	0
DRIED														
GOYA														
Giant White	⅓ cup (1.6 oz)	160	2	1	0	2	35	4	0	10	—	0	—	0
FRESH														
on-the-cob w/ butter cooked	1 ear	155	3	2	6	4	32	—	5	30	360	7	44	391
white cooked	½ cup	89	1	tr	0	3	21	—	2	14	204	5	38	tr
white raw	½ cup	66	1	tr	0	2	15	—	2	12	208	5	35	tr
yellow cooked	1 ear (2.7 oz)	83	1	tr	0	3	19	—	2	13	192	5	36	167
yellow cooked	½ cup	89	1	tr	0	3	21	—	2	14	204	5	38	178
yellow raw	1 ear (3 oz)	77	1	tr	0	3	17	—	2	14	243	6	41	253
yellow raw	½ cup	66	1	tr	0	2	15	—	2	12	208	5	35	216
FROZEN														
cooked	½ cup	67	tr	tr	0	2	17	—	2	4	114	2	19	204
on-the-cob cooked	1 ear (2.2 oz)	59	tr	tr	0	2	14	—	2	3	158	3	19	133
BIRDS EYE														
Baby Corn Blend	⅔ cup (2.9 oz)	60	1	0	0	2	11	2	0	15	—	12	—	500
Baby Gold & White	⅔ cup (3.3 oz)	80	1	tr	0	3	15	2	0	10	—	2	—	0
In Butter Sauce	½ cup (4.6 oz)	110	3	2	5	3	23	2	0	230	—	5	—	300
FRESH LIKE														
Cob Corn	1 ear (3 in)	96	1	—	—	3	24	1	4	4	304	6	—	208
Cob Corn	1 ear (5 in)	96	1	—	—	3	23	1	4	4	303	6	—	208
Cut	3.5 oz	85	1	—	—	3	21	1	5	5	196	5	—	242
GREEN GIANT														
Butter Sauce Niblets	⅔ cup (4.3 oz)	130	3	2	<5	3	23	3	0	350	—	4	—	100
Butter Sauce Shoepeg White	¾ cup (4 oz)	120	3	2	<5	3	21	3	0	320	—	1	—	200
Cream Corn	½ cup (4.1 oz)	110	1	0	0	2	23	2	0	330	—	2	—	0
Extra Sweet Niblets	⅔ cup (3.1 oz)	70	1	0	0	2	13	2	0	0	—	0	—	0
Harvest Fresh Niblets	⅔ cup (3.4 oz)	80	1	0	0	3	17	3	0	60	—	1	—	0
Harvest Fresh Shoepeg White	½ cup (2.6 oz)	70	1	0	0	2	14	2	0	45	—	2	—	0
Niblets	⅔ cup (2.9 oz)	80	1	0	0	2	17	2	0	5	—	2	—	0
On The Cob Extra Sweet	1 ear (4.4 oz)	120	2	0	0	4	22	3	0	0	—	4	—	200
On The Cob Nibblers	1 ear (2.1 oz)	70	1	0	0	2	14	1	0	0	—	2	—	0

FOOD	PORTION	CALORIES	FAT	SAT FAT	CHOL	PROTEIN	CARBO	FIBER	CALCIUM	SOD	POTAS	VIT C	FOLIC	VIT A
GREEN GIANT (CONT.)														
On The Cob Niblets	1 ear (5 oz)	160	2	0	0	4	32	3	0	10	—	6	—	200
Select Extra Sweet White	⅔ cup (2.9 oz)	50	1	0	0	2	10	3	0	0	—	5	—	0
Select Shoepeg White	¾ cup (3.2 oz)	100	1	0	0	3	20	3	0	0	—	6	—	0
MRS. PAUL'S														
Fritters	2	240	9	—	10	5	35	—	20	560	—	—	—	200
ORE IDA														
Cob Corn	1 ear (6.1 oz)	180	3	0	0	6	33	4	0	5	460	2	—	200
Cob Corn Mini-Gold	1 ear (3.1 oz)	90	1	0	0	3	16	2	0	0	230	1	—	100
STOUFFER'S														
Souffle	½ cup (6 oz)	170	7	2	65	5	21	1	40	490	230	2	—	100
TREE OF LIFE														
Corn	⅔ cup (3.2 oz)	80	1	0	0	3	19	1	0	10	—	2	—	0

CORN CHIPS

(*see* CHIPS)

CORNISH HENS

(*see* CHICKEN)

CORNMEAL

FOOD	PORTION	CALORIES	FAT	SAT FAT	CHOL	PROTEIN	CARBO	FIBER	CALCIUM	SOD	POTAS	VIT C	FOLIC	VIT A
corn grits cooked	1 cup	146	tr	tr	0	4	31	—	1	0	54	—	1	—
corn grits uncooked	1 cup	579	2	tr	0	14	124	—	3	1	213	—	7	—
degermed	1 cup	506	2	tr	0	12	107	7	7	5	224	0	66	570
self-rising degermed	1 cup	489	2	tr	0	12	103	—	482	1860	235	0	43	—
white	1 cup (4.8 oz)	505	2	tr	0	12	107	10	7	4	224	0	258	0
whole grain	1 cup	442	4	tr	0	10	94	13	7	43	350	0	—	573
ALBERS														
White	3 tbsp	110	0	0	0	2	34	tr	—	0	—	—	—	—
Yellow	3 tbsp	110	0	0	0	2	34	tr	—	0	—	—	—	—
ARROWHEAD														
Yellow	¼ cup (1.2 oz)	120	1	0	0	3	27	3	0	0	100	0	—	200
MIX														
ARROWHEAD														
Corn Bread	¼ cup (1.2 oz)	120	1	0	0	5	24	4	100	270	90	0	—	0
GOLDEN DIPT														
Corny Dog Batter Mix	1 oz	100	0	0	0	3	22	—	40	490	—	—	—	—
Hush Puppy Deluxe Mix	1¼ oz	120	0	0	0	3	26	—	20	520	—	—	—	—
Hush Puppy Jalapeno Mix	1¼ oz	120	0	0	0	3	27	—	80	570	—	—	—	200
Hush Puppy With Onion	1¼ oz	120	0	0	0	3	27	—	20	520	—	—	—	—

FOOD	PORTION	CALORIES	FAT	SAT FAT	CHOL	PROTEIN	CARBO	FIBER	CALCIUM	SOD	POTAS	VIT C	FOLIC	VIT A
HODGSON MILL														
Yellow	¼ cup (1 oz)	100	1	0	0	3	22	3	0	0	—	0	—	100
Yellow Self Rising	¼ cup (1 oz)	90	1	0	0	3	21	3	100	260	—	0	—	100
KENTUCKY KERNAL														
White Corn Meal Mix	¼ cup (1 oz)	100	1	0	0	3	22	2	60	210	—	0	—	0
MIRACLE MAIZE														
Complete as prep	1 piece (1.5 oz)	193	3	—	0	4	34	2	—	193	—	—	—	—
Country Style as prep	1 piece 2 in x 2 in (1.8 oz)	230	5	—	0	5	38	2	—	406	—	—	—	—
Sweet as prep	1 piece 2 in x 2 in (1.8 oz)	236	5	—	0	5	41	1	—	260	—	—	—	—
STONE-BUHR														
Yellow Corn Meal	¼ cup (1 oz)	100	0	0	0	2	23	1	—	0	—	—	—	—
READY-TO-EAT														
AURORA														
Polenta	½ cup (5 oz)	110	0	0	0	2	24	1	10	470	—	5	—	200
TAKE-OUT														
hush puppies	5 (2.7 oz)	256	12	3	135	5	35	4	69	965	188	0	21	94
hush puppies	1 (0.75 oz)	74	3	tr	10	3	10	1	61	147	32	0	4	31
CORNSALAD														
raw	1 cup	12	tr	—	0	1	2	—	—	—	—	—	—	—
CORNSTARCH														
cornstarch	⅓ cup	164	tr	tr	0	tr	39	tr	1	4	1	0	—	—
HODGSON MILL														
Cornstarch	2 tsp (0.4 oz)	35	0	0	0	0	9	—	—	0	—	—	—	—
COTTAGE CHEESE														
creamed	1 cup (7.4 oz)	217	9	6	31	26	6	—	126	850	177	tr	26	342
creamed	4 oz	117	5	3	17	14	3	—	68	457	95	tr	14	184
creamed w/ fruit	4 oz	140	4	2	13	11	15	—	54	457	76	tr	11	139
dry curd	1 cup (5.1 oz)	123	1	tr	10	25	3	—	46	19	47	0	21	44
dry curd	4 oz	96	tr	tr	8	20	2	—	36	14	37	0	17	34
lowfat 1%	1 cup (7.9 oz)	164	2	1	10	28	6	—	138	918	193	tr	28	84
lowfat 1%	4 oz	82	1	1	5	14	3	—	69	459	97	tr	14	42
lowfat 2%	4 oz	101	2	1	9	16	4	—	77	459	109	tr	15	79
lowfat 2%	1 cup (7.9 oz)	203	4	3	19	31	8	—	155	918	217	tr	30	158
AXELROD														
Nonfat	½ cup (4.4 oz)	90	0	0	10	15	7	0	100	500	—	0	—	0
BORDEN														
4%	½ cup	120	5	—	—	14	4	—	60	400	90	—	—	—
Dry Curd 0.5%	½ cup	80	1	—	—	18	3	—	20	20	25	—	—	—
Unsalted 4%	½ cup	120	5	—	—	14	4	—	60	40	75	—	—	—
BREAKSTONE'S														
2% Fat Large Curd	½ cup (4.2 oz)	90	3	2	15	13	4	0	80	390	110	0	—	0

FOOD	PORTION	CALORIES	FAT	SAT FAT	CHOL	PROTEIN	CARBO	FIBER	CALCIUM	SOD	POTAS	VIT C	FOLIC	VIT A
BREAKSTONE'S (CONT.)														
2% Fat Small Curd	½ cup (4.2 oz)	90	3	2	15	13	4	0	80	390	110	0	—	0
4% Fat Large Curd	½ cup (4.2 oz)	120	5	3	25	13	5	0	80	400	120	0	—	200
4% Fat Small Curd	½ cup (4.2 oz)	120	5	3	25	13	5	0	80	400	125	0	—	200
Dry Curd	¼ cup (1.9 oz)	45	0	0	<5	8	3	0	80	30	95	0	—	0
Free	½ cup (4.4 oz)	80	0	0	5	13	6	0	80	440	150	0	—	200
Snack 2% Fat Small Curd	1 pkg (4 oz)	90	2	2	15	12	4	0	80	370	105	0	—	0
Snack 4% Fat Small Curd	1 pkg (4 oz)	110	5	3	25	12	4	0	80	380	115	0	—	200
Snack Free	1 pkg (4 oz)	70	0	0	5	12	6	0	80	400	135	0	—	200
CABOT														
Cottage Cheese	4 oz	120	5	3	17	14	3	—	68	455	—	—	—	200
Light	4 oz	90	1	1	5	14	3	—	69	360	—	—	—	—
FRIENDSHIP														
California Style	½ cup (4 oz)	115	5	3	25	15	4	0	100	380	—	0	—	200
Lowfat No Salt Added	½ cup (4 oz)	90	1	1	10	16	4	0	100	40	—	0	—	100
Lowfat Pineapple	½ cup (4 oz)	120	1	1	10	12	17	0	80	300	—	0	—	100
Lowfat 1%	½ cup (4 oz)	90	1	1	10	16	4	0	100	360	—	0	—	100
Nonfat	½ cup (4 oz)	80	0	0	0	15	5	0	100	380	—	0	—	0
Nonfat Plus Peach	½ cup (4 oz)	110	0	0	0	12	15	0	100	300	—	0	—	0
Pot Style	½ cup (4 oz)	90	3	2	15	15	3	0	80	430	—	0	—	100
With Pineapple	½ cup (4 oz)	140	4	3	15	16	15	0	80	310	—	0	—	100
HOOD														
1% Fat	½ cup (4 oz)	90	2	1	10	13	6	0	100	390	—	0	—	0
1% Fat Chive & Onion	½ cup (4 oz)	90	2	1	10	13	6	0	100	390	—	1	—	100
1% Fat No Salt Added	½ cup (4 oz)	90	2	1	10	13	6	0	100	65	—	0	—	0
1% Fat Pepper & Herb	½ cup (4 oz)	90	2	1	10	13	6	0	100	450	—	0	—	0
1% Fat Pineapple Cherry	½ cup (4 oz)	110	1	1	10	10	15	0	80	290	—	1	—	0
4% Fat	½ cup (4 oz)	120	4	3	25	13	5	0	100	390	—	0	—	200
4% Fat Chive	½ cup (4 oz)	130	4	3	25	13	5	0	100	380	—	1	—	200
4% Fat Pineapple	½ cup (4 oz)	130	4	3	20	10	15	0	80	290	—	1	—	100
Nonfat	½ cup (4 oz)	80	0	0	5	13	6	0	100	330	—	0	—	0
Nonfat Pineapple	½ cup (4 oz)	110	0	0	<5	10	16	0	80	250	—	1	—	0
KNUDSEN														
1.5% Fat Small Curd Pineapple	½ cup (4.6 oz)	120	2	1	10	11	14	0	80	330	110	0	—	0
2% Fat Small Curd	½ cup (4.2 oz)	100	3	2	15	14	5	0	100	400	115	0	—	0
4% Fat Large Curd	½ cup (4.5 oz)	130	5	4	30	16	4	0	80	330	90	0	—	200
4% Fat Small Curd	½ cup (4.3 oz)	120	5	4	25	14	4	0	80	400	95	0	—	200
Free	½ cup (4.2 oz)	80	0	0	5	14	4	0	80	380	90	0	—	200

FOOD	PORTION	CALORIES	FAT	SAT FAT	CHOL	PROTEIN	CARBO	FIBER	CALCIUM	SOD	POTAS	VIT C	FOLIC	VIT A
KNUDSEN (CONT.)														
On The Go! 1.5% Fat Peach	1 pkg (4 oz)	110	2	1	10	10	13	0	60	300	105	0	—	0
On The Go! 1.5% Fat Pineapple	1 pkg (4 oz)	110	2	1	10	10	13	0	60	300	100	0	—	0
On The Go! 1.5% Fat Strawberry	1 pkg (4 oz)	110	2	1	10	10	13	0	60	290	105	0	—	0
On The Go! 1.5% Fat Tropical Fruit	1 pkg (4 oz)	110	2	2	10	10	13	0	60	300	110	0	—	0
On The Go! 2% Fat	1 pkg (4 oz)	90	2	2	15	13	5	0	100	370	110	0	—	0
On The Go! Free	1 pkg (4 oz)	70	0	0	5	13	4	0	80	350	85	0	—	200
LACTAID														
1%	4 oz	72	1	1	4	12	3	—	61	406	866	—	12	37
LIGHT N'LIVELY														
1% Fat	½ cup (4 oz)	80	1	1	10	12	5	0	200	370	140	0	—	0
1% Fat Garden Salad	½ cup (4.2 oz)	80	2	1	10	12	5	0	200	390	150	0	—	100
1% Fat Peach & Pineapple	½ cup (4.3 oz)	110	1	1	10	11	15	0	200	340	140	0	—	0
Fat Free	½ cup (4.4 oz)	80	0	0	5	13	6	0	200	440	140	0	—	200
LITE LINE														
Lowfat 1½%	½ cup	90	2	—	—	14	4	0	60	400	90	—	—	—
VIVA														
Nonfat	½ cup	70	0	0	5	13	5	—	80	430	—	—	—	—
WEIGHT WATCHERS														
1%	½ cup	90	1	1	5	14	4	0	60	460	80	0	—	0
2%	½ cup	90	2	2	15	12	4	0	80	460	12	0	—	100
COTTONSEED														
kernels roasted	1 tbsp	51	4	1	0	3	2	—	10	3	135	1	—	—
COUGH DROPS														
HALLS														
Cough Drops	1 (3.8 g)	15	0	0	0	0	4	—	—	—	—	—	—	—
Plus	1 (4.7 g)	18	0	0	0	0	5	—	—	—	—	—	—	—
With Vitamin C	1 (3.8 g)	14	0	0	0	0	4	—	—	—	—	—	—	—
LIFESAVERS														
Menthol	2 (0.5 oz)	60	0	0	0	0	14	—	—	0	0	—	—	—
COUSCOUS														
cooked	½ cup	101	tr	tr	0	3	21	—	8	4	52	—	13	—
dry	½ cup	346	tr	tr	0	12	71	—	22	9	152	0	16	—
CASBAH														
Almond Chicken Vegetarian	1 pkg (1.5 oz)	160	2	0	0	5	29	tr	550	470	—	1	—	1300
Asparagus Au Gratin Organic	1 pkg (1.5 oz)	150	2	0	<5	14	28	1	50	400	—	17	—	2150
Cheddar Broccoli	1 pkg (1.3 oz)	130	2	1	<5	11	23	tr	50	470	—	20	—	2150

FOOD	PORTION	CALORIES	FAT	SAT FAT	CHOL	PROTEIN	CARBO	FIBER	CALCIUM	SOD	POTAS	VIT C	FOLIC	VIT A
CASBAH (CONT.)														
Hearty Harvest Zestful Organic as prep	1 pkg (10 fl oz)	180	1	—	0	6	36	2	100	460	400	8	—	50
Moroccan Stew	1 pkg (2 oz)	180	1	0	0	5	36	1	50	430	—	8	—	1900
Pilaf as prep	1 cup	200	tr	0	0	8	40	tr	20	480	—	1	—	2600
Tomato Parmesan	1 pkg (1.8 oz)	170	2	0	<5	7	34	2	90	460	—	36	—	2450
KITCHEN DEL SOL														
Aegean Citrus as prep	½ cup (1.1 oz)	110	3	tr	0	3	20	1	0	290	—	18	—	750
Moroccan Ginger as prep	½ cup (1.1 oz)	120	3	tr	0	3	21	1	0	290	—	4	—	300
Spicy Vegetable as prep	½ cup (1.1 oz)	120	3	tr	0	3	20	1	0	290	—	2	—	100
Tomato & Olive	½ cup (1 oz)	120	4	1	0	3	19	1	0	290	—	2	—	0
Tomato & Olive	½ cup (1.1 oz)	120	4	1	0	3	19	1	0	290	—	2	—	0
MELTING POT														
Calypso Cranberry	1 cup	200	0	0	0	7	42	1	20	220	—	0	—	0
Lentil Curry	1 cup	170	0	0	0	7	35	1	0	290	—	0	—	100
Lucky Seven	1 cup	190	1	0	0	7	38	1	0	300	—	1	—	200
Mango Salsa	1 cup	190	0	0	0	6	40	1	20	270	—	0	—	0
Roasted Garlic	1 cup	170	0	0	0	7	34	1	0	370	—	0	—	0
Sesame Ginger	1 cup	180	1	0	0	7	36	0	20	350	—	0	—	100
Sun-Dried Tomatoes	1 cup	190	1	0	0	8	36	1	20	230	—	0	—	0
Wild Mushroom	1 cup	190	0	0	0	8	38	1	0	370	—	0	—	100
NEAR EAST														
As Prep	1¼ cup	260	6	2	0	8	46	2	—	65	150	—	8	300
COWPEAS														
catjang dried cooked	1 cup	200	1	tr	0	14	35	—	44	32	641	1	242	17
common canned	1 cup	184	1	tr	0	11	33	—	48	718	413	7	123	32
frozen cooked	½ cup	112	tr	tr	0	7	20	—	20	5	319	2	120	64
leafy tips chopped cooked	1 cup	12	tr	tr	0	2	1	—	36	3	186	10	—	305
leafy tips raw chopped	1 cup	10	tr	tr	0	1	2	—	23	2	164	13	—	256
CRAB														
CANNED														
blue	1 cup	133	2	tr	120	28	0	—	137	5	450	—	—	—
blue	3 oz	84	1	tr	76	17	0	—	86	283	318	—	—	—
FRESH														
alaska king cooked	1 leg (4.7 oz)	129	2	tr	72	26	0	—	80	1436	350	—	—	39
alaska king cooked	3 oz	82	1	tr	45	16	0	—	50	911	222	—	—	25
alaska king raw	3 oz	71	1	—	35	16	0	—	39	711	173	—	—	20
alaska king raw	1 leg (6 oz)	144	1	—	72	32	0	—	80	1438	351	—	—	41

FOOD	PORTION	CALORIES	FAT	SAT FAT	CHOL	PROTEIN	CARBO	FIBER	CALCIUM	SOD	POTAS	VIT C	FOLIC	VIT A
blue cooked	3 oz	87	2	tr	85	17	0	—	88	237	275	—	—	—
blue cooked	1 cup	138	2	tr	135	27	0	—	140	376	437	—	—	—
blue raw	1 crab (7 oz)	18	tr	tr	16	4	tr	—	19	62	69	—	—	—
blue raw	3 oz	74	1	tr	66	15	tr	—	76	249	280	—	—	—
dungeness raw	3 oz	73	1	tr	50	15	1	—	39	251	301	—	—	—
dungeness raw	1 crab (5.7 oz)	140	2	tr	97	28	1	—	75	481	577	—	—	—
FROZEN														
MRS. PAUL'S														
Deviled Crab	1 cake	180	9	—	20	8	18	—	60	480		—	—	—
Deviled Crab Miniatures	3½ oz	240	12	—	20	9	25	—	60	540		—	—	—
TAKE-OUT														
crab cakes	1 (2.1 oz)	93	5	1	90	12	tr	—	63	198	195	—	—	—
soft-shell fried	1 (4.4 oz)	334	18	4	45	11	31	—	55	1118	163	tr	20	15

CRACKER CRUMBS

FOOD	PORTION	CALORIES	FAT	SAT FAT	CHOL	PROTEIN	CARBO	FIBER	CALCIUM	SOD	POTAS	VIT C	FOLIC	VIT A
cracker meal	1 cup (4 oz)	440	2	tr	0	11	93	—	27	32	132	0	—	0
graham cracker crumbs	½ cup (4.4 oz)	540	13	3	0	9	97	3	36	756	162	0	18	0
GOLDEN DIPT														
Cracker Meal	1 oz	100	0	0	0	3	22	—	—	0		—	—	—
HONEY MAID														
Graham Cracker	0.5 oz	70	2	0	0	1	13	tr	—	90	15	—	—	—
KEEBLER														
Cracker Meal	1 cup	100	3	tr	0	3	23	—	—	5	40	—	—	—
Graham Crumbs	1 cup	520	14	tr	0	8	90	—	—	630	170	—	—	—
Zesty Meal	1 cup	85	10	2	0	8	61	—	—	100	110	—	—	—
KELLOGG'S														
Corn Flake Crumbs	2 tbsp (0.4 oz)	40	0	0	0	1	9	0	0	120	—	5	32	0
LANCE														
Cracker Meal	1 oz	100	1	—	0	3	21	—	—	1	25	—	—	—
NABISCO														
Nilla Cookie Crumbs	2 tbsp (0.5 oz)	70	3	1	<5	1	13	tr	—	55	15	—	—	—
OREO														
Cookie Crumbs	2 tbsp (0.5 oz)	80	3	1	0	1	13	1	—	140	45	—	—	—
PREMIUM														
Fat Free Cracker Crumbs	¼ cup (1 oz)	100	0	0	0	3	23	1	—	0	30	—	—	—
RITZ														
Cracker Crumbs	⅓ cup (1 oz)	140	7	1	0	2	17	1	40	270	20	—	—	—
SUNSHINE														
Graham	3 tbsp (0.6 oz)	80	2	1	0	2	13	tr	—	150		—	—	—

CRACKERS

(*see also* CRACKER CRUMBS)

FOOD	PORTION	CALORIES	FAT	SAT FAT	CHOL	PROTEIN	CARBO	FIBER	CALCIUM	SOD	POTAS	VIT C	FOLIC	VIT A
cheese	1 (1 in sq) (1 g)	5	tr	tr	0	tr	1	—	2	10	1	0	0	2

FOOD	PORTION	CALORIES	FAT	SAT FAT	CHOL	PROTEIN	CARBO	FIBER	CALCIUM	SOD	POTAS	VIT C	FOLIC	VIT A
cheese	14 (½ oz)	71	4	1	2	1	8	—	21	141	21	0	4	23
cheese low sodium	1 (1 in sq) (1 g)	5	tr	tr	0	tr	1	—	2	5	1	0	0	2
cheese low sodium	14 (½ oz)	71	4	1	2	1	8	—	21	68	15	0	4	23
cheese w/ peanut butter filling	1 (0.24 oz)	34	2	tr	0	1	4	tr	6	69	17	0	2	—
crispbread rye	1 (0.35 oz)	37	tr	tr	0	1	8	2	3	26	32	0	2	0
melba toast plain	1 (5 g)	19	tr	tr	0	1	4	tr	5	41	10	0	1	0
melba toast pumpernickel	1 (5 g)	19	tr	tr	0	1	4	tr	4	45	10	—	1	—
melba toast rye	1 (5 g)	19	tr	tr	0	1	4	tr	4	45	10	—	1	—
melba toast wheat	1 (5 g)	19	tr	tr	0	1	4	tr	2	42	7	0	1	0
milk	1 (0.42 oz)	55	2	tr	—	1	8	—	21	71	14	—	—	—
oyster cracker	1 (1 g)	4	tr	tr	0	tr	1	tr	1	13	1	0	tr	0
peanut butter sandwich	1 (7 g)	34	2	tr	—	1	4	—	7	66	16	—	—	—
rusk toast	1 (0.35 oz)	41	1	tr	—	1	7	—	3	25	25	0	—	—
rye w/ cheese filling	1 (0.24 oz)	34	2	tr	1	1	4	—	16	73	24	—	—	—
rye wafers plain	1 (0.9 oz)	84	tr	tr	0	2	20	—	10	199	124	—	11	—
rye wafers seasoned	1 (0.8 oz)	84	2	tr	0	2	16	—	10	195	100	—	12	—
saltines	1 (3 g)	13	tr	tr	0	tr	2	tr	4	38	4	0	1	0
saltines fat free low sodium	3 (0.5 oz)	59	tr	tr	0	2	12	—	3	95	17	0	2	0
saltines fat free low sodium	6 (1 oz)	118	tr	tr	0	3	25	—	7	191	34	0	4	0
saltines low salt	1 (3 g)	13	tr	tr	0	tr	2	tr	4	19	22	0	1	0
snack cracker	1 (3 g)	15	1	tr	0	tr	2	tr	4	25	4	0	0	0
snack cracker low salt	1 (3 g)	15	1	tr	0	tr	2	tr	4	11	11	0	0	0
snack cracker w/ cheese filling	1 (7 g)	33	2	tr	0	1	4	—	18	98	30	—	—	—
soup cracker	1 (1 g)	4	tr	tr	0	tr	1	tr	1	13	1	0	tr	0
wheat w/ cheese filling	1 (0.24 oz)	35	2	tr	1	1	4	—	14	64	21	tr	—	5
wheat w/ peanut butter filling	1 (0.24 oz)	35	2	tr	0	1	4	—	12	57	21	0	—	—
wheat thins	1 (2 g)	9	tr	tr	0	tr	1	—	1	16	4	0	0	0
wheat thins	7 (0.5 oz)	67	3	1	0	1	9	1	7	113	26	0	3	0
wheat thins low salt	7 (0.5 oz)	67	3	1	0	1	9	1	7	40	28	0	3	0
whole wheat	1 (4 g)	18	1	tr	0	tr	3	—	2	26	12	0	1	tr
whole wheat low salt	1 (4 g)	18	1	tr	0	tr	3	—	2	10	12	0	1	tr
ADRIENNE'S														
Gourmet Flatbread Caraway & Rye	2	20	tr	—	<5	1	4	—	—	45	15	—	—	—
Gourmet Flatbread Classic Island	2	20	tr	—	<5	1	3	—	—	45	10	—	—	—

FOOD	PORTION	CALORIES	FAT	SAT FAT	CHOL	PROTEIN	CARBO	FIBER	CALCIUM	SOD	POTAS	VIT C	FOLIC	VIT A
ADRIENNE'S (CONT.)														
Gourmet Flatbread Slightly Onion	2	20	tr	—	<5	tr	3	—	—	45	10	—	—	—
Gourmet Flatbread Ten Grain	2	20	tr	0	0	1	3	1	—	45	20	—	—	—
AK-MAK														
100% Whole Wheat	5 (1 oz)	116	2	tr	0	5	19	4	0	214	—	0	—	0
Armenian Cracker Bread	1 sheet (1 oz)	100	2	1	0	4	19	2	0	200	—	0	—	0
Armenian Cracker Bread Whole Wheat	1 sheet (1 oz)	116	2	tr	0	5	19	4	0	214	—	0	—	0
Round Cracker Bread No Seeds	1 (1 oz)	100	1	1	0	4	20	1	0	170	—	0	—	0
Round Cracker Bread Seeded	1 (1 oz)	100	2	1	0	4	19	2	0	200	—	0	—	0
Round Cracker Bread Whole Wheat	1 (1 oz)	116	2	tr	0	5	19	4	0	214	—	0	—	0
AMERICAN HERITAGE														
Sesame	9 (1.1 oz)	160	9	2	0	4	17	1	40	300	—	—	—	—
Wheat & Bran	9 (1 oz)	140	7	2	0	3	17	2	20	280	—	—	—	—
BARBARA'S														
Cheese Bites	26 (1 oz)	120	2	0	0	3	24	1	—	290	—	—	—	—
French Onion	3	60	1	0	0	1	12	tr	—	140	—	—	—	—
Rite Lite Rounds	5 (0.5 oz)	55	tr	0	0	1	12	0	—	150	—	—	—	—
Roasted Garlic & Herb	3	60	1	0	0	1	12	tr	—	140	—	—	—	—
Sundried Tomato & Basil	3	60	1	0	0	1	12	tr	—	140	—	—	—	—
Toasted Sesame	3	60	2	0	0	1	11	tr	—	135	—	—	—	—
Wheatines All Flavors	1 lg sq (0.5 oz)	50	2	0	0	1	10	1	—	110	—	—	—	—
BETTER CHEDDARS														
Crackers	22 (1 oz)	70	8	2	<5	4	17	tr	40	290	45	—	—	200
Low Sodium	22 (1 oz)	150	7	2	<5	3	18	tr	20	75	135	—	—	—
Reduced Fat	24 (1 oz)	140	6	2	<5	3	19	tr	40	350	40	—	—	100
BURNS & RICKER														
Bagel Crisps Garlic	5 (1 oz)	100	0	0	0	5	22	1	10	280	—	0	—	0
CHEEZ-IT														
Crackers	27 (1 oz)	160	8	2	0	4	16	tr	40	240	—	—	—	—
Crackers	1 pkg (1.5 oz)	220	12	3	3	6	23	1	60	340	—	—	—	—
Crackers	1 pkg (2 oz)	290	16	4	3	7	31	2	80	450	—	—	—	—
Hot & Spicy	26 (1 oz)	160	8	2	0	3	17	1	—	220	—	—	—	—
Hot & Spicy	1 pkg (1.5 oz)	220	12	2	0	4	25	1	20	310	—	—	—	—
Low Sodium	27 (1 oz)	160	8	2	0	4	16	tr	40	70	—	—	—	—

FOOD	PORTION	CALORIES	FAT	SAT FAT	CHOL	PROTEIN	CARBO	FIBER	CALCIUM	SOD	POTAS	VIT C	FOLIC	VIT A
CHEEZ-IT (CONT.)														
Party Mix	½ cup (1 oz)	140	5	1	0	4	19	1	20	270	—	—	—	—
Reduced Fat	30 (1 oz)	130	5	1	0	4	19	tr	40	280	—	—	—	—
White Cheddar	1 pkg (1.5 oz)	220	12	3	3	4	24	tr	20	400	—	—	—	—
White Cheddar	26 (1 oz)	160	9	2	3	3	17	tr	—	280	—	—	—	—
CROWN PILOT														
Crackers	1 (0.5 oz)	70	2	0	0	1	13	tr	—	85	20	—	—	—
DEVONSHEER														
Melba Rounds Garlic	½ oz	56	1	—	0	2	9	1	6	132	—	—	—	—
Melba Rounds Honey Bran	½ oz	52	1	—	0	2	9	1	4	98	—	—	—	—
Melba Rounds Onion	½ oz	51	1	—	0	2	10	1	7	120	—	—	—	—
Melba Rounds Plain	½ oz	53	1	—	0	2	10	1	4	111	—	—	—	—
Melba Rounds Plain Unsalted	½ oz	52	1	—	0	2	10	1	10	<5	—	—	—	—
Melba Rounds Rye	½ oz	53	1	—	0	2	10	1	9	130	—	—	—	—
Melba Rounds Sesame	½ oz	57	2	—	0	2	8	1	14	131	—	—	—	—
EDEN														
Brown Rice	5 (1 oz)	120	2	0	0	3	22	2	27	230	110	0	—	0
ESCORT														
Crackers	3 (0.5 oz)	70	4	tr	0	1	9	—	—	115	15	—	—	—
ESTEE														
Unsalted	1 (0.5 oz)	70	2	1	0	1	10	0	0	0	15	0	—	0
FRITO LAY														
Cheese Filled	6 (1.5 oz)	210	10	—	5	4	24	—	60	470	170	—	—	—
Cracker Snacks Cheddar	13-16 (1 oz)	70	4	—	0	1	8	—	20	150	20	—	—	—
Cracker Snacks Zesty Italian	13-16 (1 oz)	70	3	—	0	1	9	—	20	115	20	—	—	—
Peanut Butter Filled	6 (1.5 oz)	210	10	—	0	6	24	—	60	450	120	—	—	—
GOYA														
Butter Crackers	1	40	1	—	—	0	6	—	2	60	15	0	—	<100
Crackers	1	30	0	—	—	1	5	—	1	45	10	0	—	<100
HAIN														
Cheese	1 oz	130	6	—	—	3	17	—	20	180	80	1	—	200
Onion	1 oz	130	6	—	—	3	17	—	20	160	75	2	—	—
Onion No Salt Added	1 oz	130	6	—	—	3	17	—	20	5	75	2	—	—
Rich	1 oz	130	5	—	—	3	18	—	—	160	200	1	—	—
Rich No Salt Added	1 oz	130	5	—	—	3	18	—	—	15	200	1	—	—
Rye	1 oz	120	4	—	—	3	19	—	20	200	80	2	—	—
Rye No Salt Added	1 oz	120	4	—	—	3	19	—	20	10	80	2	—	—

FOOD	PORTION	CALORIES	FAT	SAT FAT	CHOL	PROTEIN	CARBO	FIBER	CALCIUM	SOD	POTAS	VIT C	FOLIC	VIT A
HAIN (CONT.)														
Sesame	1 oz	140	7	—	—	3	16	—	—	210	85	1	—	—
Sesame No Salt Added	1 oz	140	7	—	—	3	16	—	—	5	85	1	—	—
Sour Cream & Chive	1 oz	130	6	—	—	3	15	—	20	150	85	—	—	100
Sour Cream & Chive No Salt Added	1 oz	130	6	—	—	3	15	—	20	25	85	—	—	100
Sourdough	½ oz	65	3	—	—	2	9	—	—	100	30	—	—	100
Sourdough Low Salt	1 oz	130	5	—	—	3	18	—	20	10	60	1	—	200
Vegetable	1 oz	130	5	—	—	3	10	—	20	180	60	2	—	200
Vegetable No Salt Added	1 oz	130	5	—	—	3	10	—	20	50	60	2	—	200
HARVEST CRISPS														
5 Grain	13 (1.1 oz)	130	4	1	0	3	23	1	20	300	60	4	—	400
Oat	13 (1.1 oz)	140	5	1	0	3	22	1	20	300	65	—	—	—
HEALTH VALLEY														
Herb Stoned Wheat	13	55	2	—	0	1	9	2	10	80	75	1	—	—
Herb Stoned Wheat No Salt	13	55	2	—	0	1	9	2	10	30	75	1	—	50
Rice Bran	7	130	4	—	0	4	19	2	22	65	75	2	tr	15
Sesame Stoned Wheat	13	55	2	—	0	1	9	2	10	80	75	1	—	50
Sesame Stoned Wheat No Salt Added	13	55	2	—	0	1	9	2	10	30	75	1	—	—
Seven Grain Vegetable Stoned Wheat	13	55	2	—	0	1	9	2	10	80	75	1	—	—
Seven Grain Vegetable Stoned Wheat No Salt Added	13	55	2	—	0	1	9	2	10	30	75	1	—	—
Stoned Wheat	13	55	2	—	0	1	9	2	10	80	75	1	—	50
Stoned Wheat No Salt Added	13	55	2	—	0	1	9	2	10	30	75	1	—	—
HEALTHY CHOICE														
Bread Crisps Garlic Herb	11 (1 oz)	110	2	0	0	3	22	2	100	115	—	0	—	0
HI HO														
Butter Flavored	9 (1.1 oz)	160	9	2	3	2	19	tr	—	280	—	—	—	—
Cracked Pepper	9 (1.1 oz)	160	9	2	3	2	18	tr	20	280	—	—	—	—
Crackers	9	160	9	2	0	2	18	tr	20	280	—	—	—	—
Low Salt	9 (1.1 oz)	160	9	2	0	2	18	tr	20	135	—	—	—	—
Multi Grain	9 (1.1 oz)	160	9	2	0	2	18	1	20	370	—	—	—	—

FOOD	PORTION	CALORIES	FAT	SAT FAT	CHOL	PROTEIN	CARBO	FIBER	CALCIUM	SOD	POTAS	VIT C	FOLIC	VIT A
HI HO (CONT.)														
Reduced Fat	10 (1.1 oz)	140	5	1	0	2	21	tr	20	280	—	—	—	—
Whole Wheat	9 (1.1 oz)	150	8	2	0	3	18	2	—	280	—	—	—	—
J.J. FLATS														
Breadflats Caraway	1	52	1	—	tr	2	10	1	6	126	—	—	—	—
Breadflats Caraway And Salt	1	51	1	—	tr	2	9	1	6	213	—	—	—	—
Breadflats Cinnamon	1	53	1	—	tr	2	10	1	4	126	—	—	—	—
Breadflats Flavorall	1	52	1	—	tr	2	10	1	11	139	—	—	—	—
Breadflats Garlic	1	52	1	—	tr	2	10	1	3	127	—	—	—	—
Breadflats Oat Bran	1	49	1	—	0	2	8	2	5	141	—	—	—	—
Breadflats Onion	1	53	1	—	tr	2	10	1	4	140	—	—	—	—
Breadflats Plain	1	53	1	—	tr	1	10	1	3	143	—	—	—	—
Breadflats Poppy	1	53	1	—	tr	2	9	1	13	126	—	—	—	—
Breadflats Sesame	1	55	2	—	tr	2	9	1	20	124	—	—	—	—
KAVLI														
Crackers	1 piece	40	tr	—	0	1	10	2	—	40	—	—	—	—
KEEBLER														
Club	2	30	2	tr	0	tr	4	—	—	75	10	—	—	—
Melba Toast Garlic	2	25	tr	tr	0	1	4	—	—	35	9	—	—	—
Melba Toast Long	2	30	tr	tr	0	1	7	—	—	10	12	—	—	—
Melba Toast Onion	2	25	tr	tr	0	1	4	—	—	35	9	—	—	—
Melba Toast Plain	2	25	tr	tr	0	1	4	—	—	35	9	—	—	—
Melba Toast Sesame	2	25	tr	tr	0	1	4	—	—	35	9	—	—	—
Oyster Crackers Large	26	80	2	tr	0	2	13	—	—	175	25	—	—	—
Oyster Crackers Small	50	80	2	tr	0	2	13	—	—	175	25	—	—	—
Snack Crackers Toasted Rye	2	30	2	tr	0	tr	4	—	—	70	10	—	—	—
Snack Crackers Toasted Sesame	2	30	2	tr	0	tr	4	—	—	65	10	—	—	—
Snack Crackers Toasted Wheat	2	30	2	tr	0	tr	4	—	—	60	10	—	—	—
Toasted Snack Bacon	2	30	2	tr	0	tr	4	—	—	65	10	—	—	—
Toasted Snack Onion	2	30	2	tr	0	tr	4	—	—	70	10	—	—	—
Toasted Snack Pumpernickel	2	30	2	tr	0	tr	4	—	—	55	10	—	—	—
Wholegrain Wheat	2	30	1	tr	0	1	5	—	—	70	10	—	—	—
KRISPY														
Cracked Pepper	5 (0.5 oz)	60	2	0	0	2	10	tr	—	180	—	—	—	—
Fat Free	5 (0.5 oz)	60	0	0	0	2	12	tr	—	135	—	—	—	—
Mild Cheddar	5 (0.5 oz)	60	2	1	0	2	10	tr	—	180	—	—	—	—

FOOD	PORTION	CALORIES	FAT	SAT FAT	CHOL	PROTEIN	CARBO	FIBER	CALCIUM	SOD	POTAS	VIT C	FOLIC	VIT A
KRISPY (CONT.)														
Original	5 (0.5 oz)	60	2	0	0	2	10	tr	—	180	—	—	—	—
Soup & Oyster Crackers	17 (0.5 oz)	60	2	0	0	2	11	tr	—	200	—	—	—	—
Unsalted Tops	5 (0.5 oz)	60	2	0	0	2	10	tr	—	120	—	—	—	—
Whole Wheat	5 (0.5 oz)	60	2	0	0	2	10	tr	—	130	—	—	—	—
LANCE														
Bonnie	1 pkg (34 g)	160	7	2	5	2	24	—	—	170	40	1	—	—
Captain Wafers	2	30	1	0	0	1	5	—	—	60	5	—	—	—
Captain Wafers Very Low Sodium	2	30	1	0	0	1	5	—	—	25	10	—	—	—
Captain Wafers w/ Cream Cheese & Chives	1 pkg (37 g)	170	9	2	0	4	23	—	60	260	60	—	—	—
Cheese-On-Wheat	1 pkg (37 g)	180	9	2	5	4	22	—	60	260	65	—	—	—
Lanchee	1 pkg (35 g)	180	11	2	5	5	19	—	20	110	—	—	—	—
Melba Toast Oblong	2	30	0	0	0	1	7	—	20	50	15	—	—	—
Melba Toast Plain	2	20	0	0	0	1	4	—	—	30	10	—	—	—
Melba Toast Round Garlic	2	20	0	0	0	1	4	—	—	35	10	—	—	—
Melba Toast Round Onion	2	20	0	0	0	1	4	—	—	30	10	—	—	—
Melba Toast Sesame	2	25	0	0	0	1	4	—	—	35	10	—	—	—
Nekot	1 pkg (42 g)	210	10	2	5	6	24	—	—	95	80	—	—	—
Nip-Chee	1 pkg (37 g)	180	8	2	5	4	21	—	60	320	40	—	—	—
Oyster Crackers	1 pkg (14 g)	70	2	1	0	2	10	—	—	170	10	—	—	—
Peanut Butter Wheat	1 pkg (37 g)	190	11	2	0	6	18	—	—	210	120	—	—	—
Rye Twins	2	30	1	0	0	1	5	—	—	65	10	—	—	—
Rye-Chee	1 pkg (41 g)	190	9	2	5	4	22	—	60	320	40	—	—	—
Saltines	2	25	1	0	0	1	4	—	—	65	—	—	—	—
Saltines Slug Pack	4 crackers	50	1	0	0	1	8	—	—	130	—	—	—	—
Sesame Twins	2	40	1	0	0	1	6	—	20	65	5	—	—	—
Toastchee	1 pkg (39 g)	190	11	2	5	6	19	—	—	310	60	—	—	—
Toasty	1 pkg (35 g)	180	10	2	0	5	17	—	60	160	65	—	—	—
Wheat Twins	2	30	1	0	0	1	5	—	—	70	10	—	—	—
Wheatswafer	2	30	1	0	0	1	4	—	—	50	20	—	—	—
LAVASH														
Bread Crisp Original	2 (0.5 oz)	60	1	tr	0	2	11	—	—	90	25	—	—	—
Bread Crisp Sesame	2 (0.5 oz)	60	1	tr	0	2	10	—	—	70	40	—	—	—
LITTLE DEBBIE														
Cheese Crackers With Peanut Butter	1 pkg (0.9 oz)	140	7	2	0	3	16	1	0	290	—	0	—	0

FOOD	PORTION	CALORIES	FAT	SAT FAT	CHOL	PROTEIN	CARBO	FIBER	CALCIUM	SOD	POTAS	VIT C	FOLIC	VIT A
LITTLE DEBBIE (CONT.)														
Cheese Crackers With Peanut Butter	1 pkg (1.4 oz)	210	10	3	0	5	23	1	0	430	—	0	—	0
Toasty Crackers With Peanut Butter	1 pkg (0.9 oz)	140	7	2	0	3	16	1	0	290	—	0	—	0
Toasty Crackers With Peanut Butter	1 pkg (1.4 oz)	200	10	2	0	5	20	1	40	350	—	0	—	0
Wheat Crackers With Cheddar Cheese	1 pkg (0.9 oz)	140	7	2	5	3	16	0	40	270	—	0	—	0
MCCRACKENS														
Cracker Crisp Country Butter	1 oz	140	8	—	tr	2	18	—	40	170	65	—	—	—
Cracker Crisp Sour Cream & Chives	1 oz	140	8	—	tr	2	18	—	40	170	65	—	—	—
Cracker Crisp Tangy Cheddar	1 oz	140	8	—	tr	2	18	—	40	170	65	—	—	—
Cracker Crisp Toasted Wheat	1 oz	140	8	—	0	2	18	—	40	170	65	—	—	—
NABS														
Cheese Peanut Butter Sandwich	6 (1.4 oz)	190	10	2	0	4	24	1	20	390	90	—	—	—
Peanut Butter Toast Sandwich	6 (1.4 oz)	190	10	2	0	4	24	1	—	380	90	—	—	—
NABISCO														
Bacon Flavored	15 (1.1 oz)	160	8	2	0	3	19	tr	—	460	55	—	—	—
Chicken In A Biskit	14 (1 oz)	160	9	2	0	2	17	tr	—	270	30	—	—	—
Garden Crisps	15 (1 oz)	130	4	1	0	2	22	1	40	290	85	—	—	500
Oat Thins	18 (1 oz)	140	1	1	0	3	20	2	—	190	65	—	—	—
Royal Lunch	1 (0.4 oz)	50	2	0	0	tr	8	0	20	65	10	—	—	—
Swiss	15 (1 oz)	140	7	2	0	2	18	tr	60	350	80	—	—	—
Tid-Bit Cheese	32 (1 oz)	150	8	2	0	2	17	tr	40	420	40	—	—	—
Vegetable Thins	14 (1.1 oz)	160	9	2	0	2	19	1	40	310	70	—	—	750
Wheat Thins Original	16 (1 oz)	140	6	1	0	2	19	2	20	170	60	—	—	—
Wheat Thins Reduced Fat	18 (1 oz)	120	4	1	0	2	21	2	20	220	65	—	—	—
Zings!	1 pkg (1.8 oz)	240	11	2	0	3	34	2	—	420	160	1	—	—
NIPS														
Cheese	29 (1 oz)	150	6	2	0	3	18	tr	20	310	55	—	—	—
OLD LONDON														
Melba Toast Pumpernickel	½ oz	54	1	—	0	2	10	1	5	156	—	—	—	—
Melba Toast Rye	½ oz	52	1	—	0	2	10	—	4	132	—	—	—	—

FOOD	PORTION	CALORIES	FAT	SAT FAT	CHOL	PROTEIN	CARBO	FIBER	CALCIUM	SOD	POTAS	VIT C	FOLIC	VIT A
OLD LONDON (CONT.)														
Melba Toast Sesame	½ oz	55	2	—	0	2	8	1	16	148	—	—	—	—
Melba Toast Sesame Unsalted	½ oz	55	2	—	0	2	8	1	14	5	—	—	—	—
Melba Toast Wheat	½ oz	51	1	—	0	2	10	1	60	121	—	—	—	—
Melba Toast White	½ oz	51	1	—	0	2	10	1	4	111	—	—	—	—
Melba Toast White Unsalted	½ oz	51	1	—	0	2	10	1	20	4	—	—	—	—
Melba Toast Whole Grain	½ oz	52	1	—	0	2	9	1	5	116	—	—	—	—
Melba Toast Whole Grain Unsalted	½ oz	53	1	—	0	2	10	1	4	4	—	—	—	—
Rounds Bacon	½ oz	53	1	—	0	2	9	1	7	126	—	—	—	—
Rounds Garlic	½ oz	56	1	—	0	2	9	1	30	132	—	—	—	—
Rounds Onion	½ oz	52	1	—	0	2	10	1	4	121	—	—	—	—
Rounds Rye	½ oz	52	1	—	0	2	10	—	4	132	—	—	—	—
Rounds Sesame	½ oz	56	2	—	0	2	8	1	16	149	—	—	—	—
Rounds White	½ oz	48	1	—	0	2	9	1	40	111	—	—	—	—
Rounds Whole Grain	½ oz	54	1	—	0	2	9	1	4	102	—	—	—	—
OYSTERETTES														
Crackers	19 (0.5 oz)	60	3	1	0	1	10	tr	—	150	20	—	—	—
PARTNERS														
Walla Walla Sweet Onion Perservative Free	0.5 oz	65	3	2	3	2	8	tr	—	60	—	—	—	100
PEPPERIDGE FARM														
Butter Thins	4	70	3	1	<5	1	10	0	—	115	—	—	—	—
Cracked Wheat	3	100	4	1	0	2	14	1	—	180	—	—	—	—
Crispy Graham	4	70	2	0	0	1	13	—	—	115	—	—	—	—
English Water Biscuits	4	70	1	0	0	2	13	0	—	100	—	—	—	—
Flutters Garden Herb	¾ oz	100	4	1	0	2	14	—	—	190	—	—	—	—
Flutters Golden Sesame	¾ oz	110	5	1	0	2	13	—	—	150	—	—	—	—
Flutters Original Butter	¾ oz	100	4	1	5	2	15	—	—	150	—	—	—	—
Flutters Toasted Wheat	¾ oz	110	5	1	0	2	13	—	—	170	—	—	—	—
Garden Vegetable	5	60	2	0	0	1	10	—	—	125	—	—	—	—
Goldfish Cheddar Cheese	1 pkg (1½ oz)	190	6	2	5	6	28	1	80	340	—	—	—	100
Goldfish Cheddar Cheese	1 oz	120	4	1	5	4	19	1	40	230	—	—	—	—
Goldfish Cheese Thins	4	50	2	0	0	18	—	0	—	160	—	—	—	—

FOOD	PORTION	CALORIES	FAT	SAT FAT	CHOL	PROTEIN	CARBO	FIBER	CALCIUM	SOD	POTAS	VIT C	FOLIC	VIT A
PEPPERIDGE FARM (CONT.)														
Goldfish Original	1 oz	130	5	1	0	3	18	1	—	190	—	—	—	—
Goldfish Parmesan Cheese	1 oz	120	4	1	<5	4	19	1	60	330	—	—	—	—
Goldfish Pizza Flavored	1 oz	130	5	1	<5	4	19	1	—	220	—	1	—	—
Goldfish Pretzel	1 oz	110	3	—	0	3	20	1	—	160	—	1	—	—
Hearty Wheat	4	100	5	1	0	2	13	1	—	140	—	—	—	—
Multi Grain	4	70	2	0	0	1	12	—	—	115	—	—	—	—
Sesame	4	80	4	1	0	2	12	2	—	140	—	—	—	—
Snack Mix Classic	1 oz	140	8	1	0	4	14	1	40	360	—	—	—	—
Snack Mix Lightly Smoked	1 oz	150	9	1	0	4	13	1	40	350	—	—	—	—
Snack Sticks Cheese	8	130	5	2	0	4	19	1	40	400	—	—	—	—
Snack Sticks Pretzel	8	120	3	0	0	3	23	1	—	430	—	—	—	—
Snack Sticks Pumpernickel	8	140	6	1	0	3	20	1	—	330	—	—	—	—
Snack Sticks Sesame	8	140	5	1	0	4	19	1	60	280	—	—	—	—
Spicy Lightly Smoked	1 oz	140	8	2	<5	4	14	1	20	340	—	—	—	—
Toasted Rice	4	60	2	0	0	2	10	—	—	140	—	—	—	—
Toasted Wheat With Onion	4	80	3	1	0	2	12	0	—	140	—	—	—	—
PLANTERS														
Cheese Peanut Butter Sandwiches	1 pkg (1.4 oz)	190	10	2	0	4	24	1	20	390	80	—	—	—
Toast Peanut Butter Sandwiches	1 pkg (1.4 oz)	190	10	2	0	4	24	1	—	380	80	—	—	—
PREMIUM														
Saltine Bits	34 (1 oz)	150	7	1	0	2	19	tr	40	340	30	—	—	—
Saltine Fat Free	5 (0.5 oz)	50	0	0	0	1	11	0	—	130	15	—	—	—
Saltine Low Sodium	5 (0.5 oz)	60	1	0	0	1	10	tr	20	35	100	—	—	—
Saltine Original	5 (0.5 oz)	60	2	0	0	1	10	tr	20	180	15	—	—	—
Saltine Unsalted Tops	5 (0.5 oz)	60	2	0	0	1	10	tr	20	135	15	—	—	—
Soup & Oyster	23 (0.5 oz)	60	2	0	0	1	11	tr	—	230	15	—	—	—
RITZ														
Bits	48 (1 oz)	160	9	2	0	2	18	1	40	250	25	—	—	—
Bits Sandwiches With Peanut Butter	13 (1 oz)	150	8	2	0	4	17	1	40	130	60	—	—	—
Bits Sanwiches With Real Cheese	14 (1.1 oz)	160	10	3	5	3	17	1	80	300	50	—	—	—
Crackers	5 (0.5 oz)	80	4	1	0	1	10	tr	20	135	10	—	—	—
Low Sodium	5 (0.5 oz)	80	4	1	0	1	10	tr	—	35	35	—	—	—

FOOD	PORTION	CALORIES	FAT	SAT FAT	CHOL	PROTEIN	CARBO	FIBER	CALCIUM	SOD	POTAS	VIT C	FOLIC	VIT A
RITZ (CONT.)														
Sandwiches With Real Cheese	1 pkg (1.4 oz)	210	12	3	5	4	21	1	100	450	70	—	—	—
SAVORY THINS														
Toasted Onion & Garlic	15 (1 oz)	110	1	0	0	3	23	2	0	90	—	0	—	0
SESMARK														
Brown Rice	15 (1 oz)	120	2	0	0	2	25	tr	0	85	—	0	—	0
Cheese Thins	15 (1 oz)	130	3	0	0	2	26	tr	0	110	—	0	—	0
Rice Thins Original	15 (1 oz)	130	3	0	0	2	24	tr	40	150	—	0	—	0
Rice Thins Teriyaki Flavored	13 (1 oz)	130	3	0	0	2	24	tr	20	170	—	0	—	0
Savory Thins Original	15 (1 oz)	125	2	0	0	3	25	1	40	125	—	0	—	0
Sesame Thins Cheddar	9 (1 oz)	150	8	1	0	5	15	3	80	400	—	0	—	50
Sesame Thins Garlic	9 (1 oz)	150	8	1	0	4	16	3	60	340	—	0	—	0
Sesame Thins Original	9 (1 oz)	150	8	1	0	5	16	2	70	380	—	0	—	0
Sesame Thins Unsalted	11 (1 oz)	150	8	1	0	5	17	3	60	1	—	0	—	0
SNACKWELL'S														
Cracked Pepper	7 (0.5 oz)	60	0	0	0	2	13	tr	20	150	20	—	—	—
Fat Free Wheat	5 (0.5 oz)	60	0	0	0	2	12	1	20	170	45	—	—	—
Reduced Fat Cheese	38 (1 oz)	130	2	1	0	4	23	1	20	340	45	—	—	—
Reduced Fat Classic Golden	6 (0.5 oz)	60	1	0	0	1	11	0	20	140	15	—	—	—
Salsa Cheddar	32 (1 oz)	120	2	0	0	2	23	1	40	340	—	0	—	0
SNORKLES														
Cheddar	56 (1 oz)	140	5	2	5	4	19	1	20	200	50	—	—	100
SOCIABLES														
Crackers	7 (0.5 oz)	80	4	1	0	1	9	tr	20	150	20	—	—	—
SUNSHINE														
Saltines Cracked Pepper	5 (0.5 oz)	60	2	0	0	2	10	tr	—	180	—	—	—	—
TOWN HOUSE														
Crackers	2	35	2	tr	0	tr	4	—	—	60	5	—	—	—
TREE OF LIFE														
Bite Size Fat Free Corn & Salsa	12	60	0	0	0	1	12	0	0	90	—	0	—	100
Bite Size Fat Free Cracked Pepper	12	55	0	0	0	1	12	0	0	80	—	0	—	0
Bite Size Fat Free Garden Vegetable	12	55	0	0	0	2	12	0	0	80	—	1	—	100
Bite Size Fat Free Garlic & Herb	12	55	0	0	0	2	12	0	0	80	—	0	—	0

FOOD	PORTION	CALORIES	FAT	SAT FAT	CHOL	PROTEIN	CARBO	FIBER	CALCIUM	SOD	POTAS	VIT C	FOLIC	VIT A
TREE OF LIFE (CONT.)														
Bite Size Fat Free Soya Nut	12	60	0	0	0	2	12	0	0	80	—	0	—	0
Bite Size Fat Free Toasted Onion	12	60	0	0	0	2	12	0	0	80	—	0	—	0
Bite Size Fat Free Whole Wheat	12	60	0	0	0	2	12	2	0	85	—	0	—	0
Fat Free Oyster	40 (0.5 oz)	60	0	0	0	2	13	0	0	130	—	0	—	0
Saltine Cracked Pepper Fat Free	4 (0.5 oz)	60	0	0	0	2	13	1	0	130	—	0	—	0
Saltine Fat Free	4 (0.5 oz)	50	0	0	0	2	11	0	—	140	—	—	—	—
TRISCUIT														
Crackers	7 (1.1 oz)	140	5	1	0	3	21	4	—	170	95	—	—	—
Deli-Style Rye	7 (1.1 oz)	140	5	1	0	3	22	4	—	180	125	—	—	—
Garden Herb	6 (1 oz)	130	5	1	0	3	20	3	—	120	20	—	—	200
Low Sodium	7 (1.1 oz)	150	6	1	0	3	21	3	—	50	95	—	—	—
Reduced Fat	8 (1.1 oz)	130	3	1	0	3	24	4	—	180	140	—	—	—
Wheat 'n Bran	7 (1.1 oz)	140	5	1	0	3	22	4	—	170	115	—	—	—
TWIGS														
Sesame & Cheese Sticks	15 (1 oz)	150	7	2	0	4	17	tr	80	300	60	—	—	100
UNEEDA BISCUIT														
Unsalted Tops	2 (0.5 oz)	60	2	0	0	1	11	tr	—	110	20	—	—	—
VENUS														
Armenian Thin Bread	2 (0.9 oz)	100	1	tr	0	3	19	—	—	165	—	—	—	—
Bran Wafers Salt Free	5 (0.5 oz)	60	1	—	0	1	11	2	—	0	60	—	—	—
Corn Crackers Salt Free	5 (0.5 oz)	60	1	tr	0	2	10	2	—	0	50	—	—	—
Cracked Wheat Wafers Salt Free	5 (0.5 oz)	60	1	tr	0	1	11	—	—	0	30	—	—	—
Cracker Bread	5 (0.5 oz)	60	1	tr	0	2	11	—	—	90	25	—	—	—
Hors D'oeuvre	3 (0.5 oz)	60	2	tr	0	1	11	—	—	20	—	—	—	—
Oat Bran Wafers	5 (0.5 oz)	60	1	—	0	2	11	2	—	105	40	—	—	—
Oat Bran Wafers Salt Free	5 (0.5 oz)	60	1	tr	0	2	11	1	—	0	40	—	—	—
Old Brussels Cheddar Waferettes	5 (0.5 oz)	80	5	1	1	1	7	—	20	160	80	—	—	—
Old Brussels Jalapeno Waferettes	5 (0.5 oz)	80	5	1	1	1	7	1	20	160	80	—	—	—
Rye Wafers Low Salt	5 (0.5 oz)	60	1	tr	0	2	11	—	—	110	25	—	—	—
Stoned Wheat Wafers Bite Size	7 (0.5 oz)	60	1	tr	0	1	11	—	—	180	25	—	—	—

FOOD	PORTION	CALORIES	FAT	SAT FAT	CHOL	PROTEIN	CARBO	FIBER	CALCIUM	SOD	POTAS	VIT C	FOLIC	VIT A
VENUS (CONT.)														
Water Crackers Fat Free	5 (0.5 oz)	55	0	0	0	2	11	—	—	70	25	—	—	—
Wheat Wafers Low Salt	5 (0.5 oz)	60	2	tr	0	2	10	1	—	110	50	—	—	—
WALDORF														
Sodium Free	2	30	1	tr	0	tr	5	—	—	0	10	—	—	—
WASA														
Crisp	3 (0.5 oz)	50	0	—	0	2	11	2	—	100	—	—	—	—
Crisp'N Light Sourdough Rye	3 (0.6 oz)	60	0	0	0	2	12	1	20	120	—	0	—	0
Crisp'N Light Wheat	2 (0.5 oz)	50	0	0	0	2	10	1	20	100	—	0	—	0
Crispbread Cinnamon Toast	1 (0.6 oz)	60	1	0	0	2	11	1	0	65	—	0	—	0
Crispbread Fiber Rye	1 (0.4 oz)	30	1	0	0	1	4	2	20	60	—	0	—	0
Crispbread Gluten & Wheat Free Corn	1 (0.4 oz)	40	1	0	0	tr	7	0	20	90	—	0	—	0
Crispbread Hearty Rye	1 (0.5 oz)	45	0	0	0	1	9	2	0	40	—	0	—	0
Crispbread Light Rye	1 (0.3 oz)	25	0	0	0	tr	5	1	0	40	—	0	—	0
Crispbread Multi Grain	1 (0.5 oz)	45	0	0	0	2	8	2	0	85	—	0	—	0
Crispbread Organic Rye	1 (0.3 oz)	25	0	0	0	tr	7	1	0	50	—	0	—	0
Crispbread Sodium Free Rye	1 (0.3 oz)	30	0	0	0	tr	7	2	0	0	—	0	—	0
Crispbread Sourdough Rye	1 (0.4 oz)	35	0	0	0	1	7	1	0	55	—	0	—	0
Crispbread Toasted Wheat	1 (0.5 oz)	50	2	0	0	2	8	1	20	85	—	0	—	0
Crispbread Whole Wheat	1 (0.5 oz)	50	1	0	0	2	11	1	0	55	—	0	—	0
WAVERLY														
Crackers	5 (0.5 oz)	70	4	1	0	1	10	0	—	135	20	—	—	—
WHEAT THINS														
Low Salt	16 (1 oz)	140	6	1	0	2	20	2	—	75	60	—	—	—
Multi-Grain	17 (1 oz)	130	4	1	0	2	21	2	40	290	70	—	—	—
WHEATWORTH														
Stone Ground	5 (0.5 oz)	80	4	1	0	2	10	1	—	170	35	—	—	—
ZESTA														
Saltine	2	25	1	tr	0	tr	4	—	—	75	10	—	—	—
Saltine Unsalted Top	2	25	1	tr	0	tr	4	—	—	35	10	—	—	—

FOOD	PORTION	CALORIES	FAT	SAT FAT	CHOL	PROTEIN	CARBO	FIBER	CALCIUM	SOD	POTAS	VIT C	FOLIC	VIT A
ZWIEBACK														
Crackers	1 (8 g)	35	1	1	0	1	5	tr	—	10	10	—	—	—
CRANBERRIES														
CANNED														
cranberry sauce sweetened	½ cup	209	tr	—	0	tr	54	—	5	40	35	3	—	28
OCEAN SPRAY														
CranOrange	¼ cup	120	0	0	0	0	30	1	—	35	0	0	—	0
Cranberry Sauce Jellied	¼ cup	110	0	0	0	0	27	tr	—	35	0	0	—	0
Whole Berry Sauce	¼ cup	110	0	0	0	0	28	1	—	35	0	0	—	0
DRIED														
OCEAN SPRAY														
Craisins	⅓ cup (1.4 oz)	130	0	0	0	0	33	2	—	2	16	0	—	0
FRESH														
chopped	1 cup	54	tr	—	0	tr	14	—	8	1	78	15	2	50
CRANBERRY BEANS														
canned	1 cup	216	1	tr	0	14	39	—	67	863	675	2	201	0
dried cooked	1 cup	240	1	tr	0	17	43	—	44	1	685	0	366	0
BEAN CUISINE														
Dried	½ cup	115	1	—	0	8	—	5	—	5	310	—	62	—
CRANBERRY JUICE														
cocktail	1 cup	147	tr	—	0	tr	38	—	8	10	61	108	1	—
cranberry juice cocktail	6 oz	108	tr	—	0	0	27	—	7	4	34	67	1	7
cranberry juice cocktail low calorie	6 oz	33	0	0	0	0	9	—	16	6	39	57	—	—
cranberry juice cocktail frzn	12 oz can	821	0	0	0	tr	210	—	48	13	213	148	0	148
cranberry juice cocktail frzn as prep	6 oz	102	0	0	0	0	26	—	9	6	27	18	0	18
AFTER THE FALL														
Cape Cod Cranberry	1 bottle (10 oz)	130	0	0	0	0	30	—	20	25	310	2	—	0
Cranberry Ginger Ale	1 can (12 oz)	140	0	0	0	1	35	0	20	65	90	1	—	0
APPLE & EVE														
Juice	6 fl oz	100	0	0	0	0	25	—	13	10	80	1	—	90
CRYSTAL LIGHT														
Cranberry Breeze Drink	1 serv (8 oz)	5	0	0	0	0	0	0	0	20	150	0	—	0
Cranberry Breeze Drink Mix as prep	1 serv (8 oz)	5	0	0	0	0	0	0	0	0	10	6	—	0
EVERFRESH														
Cranberry Cocktail	1 can (8 oz)	140	0	0	0	0	36	0	—	0	—	—	—	—

FOOD	PORTION	CALORIES	FAT	SAT FAT	CHOL	PROTEIN	CARBO	FIBER	CALCIUM	SOD	POTAS	VIT C	FOLIC	VIT A
OCEAN SPRAY														
Cocktail	8 fl oz	140	0	0	0	0	34	0	—	35	—	60	—	0
Lightstyle Low Calorie Cranberry Juice Cocktail	8 fl oz	40	0	0	0	0	10	0	—	35	45	60	—	0
Reduced Calorie Cocktail	8 fl oz	50	0	0	0	0	13	0	—	35	45	60	—	0
SENECA														
Cocktail frzn as prep	8 fl oz	140	0	0	0	0	36	0	0	0	35	60	—	0
SNAPPLE														
Cranberry Royal	10 fl oz	150	0	0	0	0	37	—	20	25	140	0	—	0
TREE OF LIFE														
Concentrate	8 tsp (1.4 oz)	110	0	0	0	0	28	—	0	0	—	6	—	—
TROPICANA														
Twister Ruby Red	8 fl oz	120	0	0	0	0	30	—	—	25	—	—	—	—
Twister Ruby Red	1 bottle (10 fl oz)	150	0	0	0	0	37	—	—	30	—	—	—	—
VERYFINE														
Cocktail	1 bottle (10 oz)	180	0	0	0	0	45	0	0	30	—	36	—	0

CRAYFISH

(*see also* LOBSTER)

FOOD	PORTION	CALORIES	FAT	SAT FAT	CHOL	PROTEIN	CARBO	FIBER	CALCIUM	SOD	POTAS	VIT C	FOLIC	VIT A
cooked	3 oz	97	1	tr	151	20	0	—	26	58	298	3	—	—
raw	8	24	tr	tr	37	5	0	—	6	14	74	1	—	—
raw	3 oz	76	1	tr	118	16	0	—	20	45	233	3	—	—

CREAM

(*see also* SOUR CREAM, SOUR CREAM SUBSTITUTES, WHIPPED TOPPINGS)

FOOD	PORTION	CALORIES	FAT	SAT FAT	CHOL	PROTEIN	CARBO	FIBER	CALCIUM	SOD	POTAS	VIT C	FOLIC	VIT A
LIQUID														
half & half	1 tbsp (0.5 oz)	20	2	1	6	tr	1	—	16	6	19	tr	tr	65
half & half	1 cup (8.5 oz)	315	28	17	89	7	10	—	254	98	314	2	6	1050
heavy whipping	1 tbsp (0.5 oz)	52	6	3	21	tr	tr	—	10	6	11	tr	1	220
light coffee	1 tbsp (0.5 oz)	29	3	2	10	tr	1	—	14	6	18	tr	tr	108
light coffee	1 cup (8.4 oz)	496	46	29	159	6	9	—	14	95	292	2	6	1728
light whipping	1 tbsp (0.5 oz)	44	5	3	17	tr	tr	—	10	5	15	tr	1	169
FARMLAND														
Half & Half	2 tbsp	40	3	2	0	1	2	0	40	15	—	0	—	100
Light Cream	2 tbsp	30	3	2	0	1	1	0	0	10	—	0	—	100
HOOD														
Half & Half	2 tbsp (1 oz)	40	4	2	15	1	1	0	40	15	—	0	—	100
Heavy	1 tbsp (0.5 oz)	50	5	4	20	0	0	0	0	0	—	0	—	200
Light	1 tbsp (0.5 oz)	30	3	2	10	1	tr	0	0	10	—	0	—	100
Whipping Cream	1 tbsp (0.5 oz)	45	5	3	20	0	tr	0	0	5	—	0	—	200
PARMALAT														
Half & Half	2 tbsp (1 oz)	40	3	2	15	1	2	0	40	20	—	0	—	100

FOOD	PORTION	CALORIES	FAT	SAT FAT	CHOL	PROTEIN	CARBO	FIBER	CALCIUM	SOD	POTAS	VIT C	FOLIC	VIT A
WHIPPED														
heavy whipping	1 cup (4.1 oz)	411	44	27	163	5	7	—	77	89	179	1	9	3499
light whipping	1 cup (4.2 oz)	345	37	23	132	5	7	—	83	82	231	1	9	2694
CREAM CHEESE														
cream cheese	1 oz	99	10	6	31	2	1	—	23	84	34	0	4	405
cream cheese	1 pkg (3 oz)	297	30	19	93	6	2	—	68	251	101	0	11	1213
ALPINE LACE														
Fat Free Garden Vegetable	2 tbsp (1 oz)	30	tr	tr	3	5	1	0	100	165	—	—	—	300
Fat Free Garlic & Herbs	2 tbsp (1 oz)	30	tr	tr	3	5	1	0	100	165	—	—	—	300
BREAKSTONE'S														
Temp-Tee Whipped	2 tbsp (0.8 oz)	80	8	5	25	2	tr	0	0	70	25	0	—	300
FLEUR DE LAIT														
Bermuda Onion & Chives	2 tbsp (0.9 oz)	90	8	5	30	1	2	0	20	130	—	0	—	200
Cinnamon Raisin	2 tbsp (0.9 oz)	90	8	5	25	1	6	0	20	90	—	0	—	200
Date Nut Rum	2 tbsp (0.9 oz)	90	8	5	30	2	4	0	20	90	—	0	—	200
Fresh Cut Garden Vegetable	2 tbsp (0.9 oz)	80	8	5	30	2	1	0	20	200	—	0	—	400
Garden Vegetable	2 tbsp (0.9 oz)	80	8	5	30	2	1	0	20	200	—	0	—	400
Garlic & Spice	2 tbsp (0.9 oz)	90	9	6	30	2	1	0	20	160	—	0	—	200
Herb & Spice	2 tbsp (0.9 oz)	90	9	6	30	2	2	0	20	190	—	0	—	200
Irish Creme	2 tbsp (0.9 oz)	100	9	5	30	2	2	0	20	95	—	0	—	200
Lemon	2 tbsp (0.9 oz)	90	7	4	25	1	5	0	0	90	—	0	—	200
Lox	2 tbsp (0.9 oz)	90	8	5	30	2	1	0	20	125	—	0	—	200
Mandarin Orange	2 tbsp (0.9 oz)	90	7	5	30	1	3	0	20	90	—	0	—	200
Peach	2 tbsp (0.9 oz)	90	7	5	25	1	3	0	20	90	—	2	—	200
Pineapple	2 tbsp (0.9 oz)	90	8	5	30	1	3	0	20	95	—	2	—	200
Plain	2 tbsp (1 oz)	100	10	6	35	2	1	0	20	60	—	0	—	300
Strawberry	2 tbsp (0.9 oz)	90	8	5	30	1	3	0	20	90	—	1	—	200
Toasted Onion	2 tbsp (0.9 oz)	90	9	6	30	2	2	0	20	190	—	0	—	200
Wildberry	2 tbsp (0.9 oz)	90	7	5	25	1	4	0	0	90	—	0	—	200
FRESH CUT														
Bac'n & Horseradish	2 tbsp (0.9 oz)	90	9	5	30	2	1	0	20	135	—	0	—	200
Bermuda Onion & Chives	2 tbsp (0.9 oz)	90	8	5	30	1	2	0	20	130	—	0	—	200
Date Nut & Rum	2 tbsp (0.9 oz)	90	8	5	30	2	4	0	20	90	—	0	—	200
Garlic & Spice	2 tbsp (0.9 oz)	90	9	6	35	2	1	0	20	160	—	0	—	200
Herb & Spice	2 tbsp (0.9 oz)	90	9	6	30	2	2	0	20	190	—	0	—	200
Lox	2 tbsp (0.9 oz)	90	8	5	30	2	1	0	20	125	—	0	—	200
Peaches & Cream	2 tbsp (0.9 oz)	90	7	5	25	1	3	0	20	90	—	2	—	200
Strawberry	2 tbsp (0.9 oz)	90	8	5	30	1	3	0	20	90	—	1	—	200

FOOD	PORTION	CALORIES	FAT	SAT FAT	CHOL	PROTEIN	CARBO	FIBER	CALCIUM	SOD	POTAS	VIT C	FOLIC	VIT A
FRIENDSHIP														
NY Style Reduced Fat	2 tbsp (1 oz)	50	3	2	10	5	0	0	0	120	—	0	—	0
HEALTHY CHOICE														
Herbs & Garlic	2 tbsp (1 oz)	25	0	0	<5	4	2	—	20	200	—	0	—	100
Plain	2 tbsp (1 oz)	25	0	0	<5	4	2	—	20	200	—	0	—	100
Strawberry	2 tbsp (1 oz)	30	0	0	<5	4	5	—	20	200	—	0	—	50
HELUVA GOOD CHEESE														
Cream Cheese	1 tbsp (1 oz)	100	10	6	30	2	1	0	200	85	—	0	—	500
PHILADELPHIA														
Free	1 oz	30	0	0	<5	4	2	0	80	140	60	0	—	400
Regular	1 oz	100	10	6	30	2	tr	0	0	90	25	0	—	300
Soft	2 tbsp (1 oz)	100	10	7	30	2	1	0	20	100	40	0	—	300
Soft Apple Cinnamon	2 tbsp (1.1 oz)	100	8	5	25	1	5	0	20	100	40	0	—	300
Soft Cheesecake	2 tbsp (1 oz)	110	9	6	25	2	4	0	20	95	35	0	—	300
Soft Chives & Onions	2 tbsp (1.1 oz)	110	10	7	30	1	2	0	40	135	60	0	—	400
Soft Garden Vegetable	2 tbsp (1.1 oz)	110	11	7	30	1	1	0	20	170	35	0	—	400
Soft Honey Nut	2 tbsp (1.1 oz)	110	10	6	30	2	4	0	20	150	35	0	—	300
Soft Pineapple	2 tbsp (1.1 oz)	100	9	6	25	1	4	0	40	100	60	0	—	300
Soft Salmon	3 tbsp (1.1 oz)	100	9	6	30	2	2	0	20	200	45	0	—	200
Soft Strawberry	2 tbsp (1.1 oz)	100	9	6	25	1	5	0	40	100	55	0	—	300
Soft Free	2 tbsp (1.2 oz)	30	0	0	<5	5	2	0	150	200	75	0	—	500
Soft Free Garden Vegetable	2 tbsp (1.2 oz)	30	0	0	<5	5	2	0	150	220	80	0	—	500
Soft Free Strawberries	2 tbsp (1.2 oz)	45	0	0	<5	4	6	0	100	180	70	0	—	400
Soft Light	2 tbsp (1.1 oz)	70	5	4	15	3	2	0	40	150	55	0	—	400
Soft Light Jalapeno	2 tbsp (1.1 oz)	60	5	3	15	3	2	0	40	210	55	0	—	400
Soft Light Raspberry	2 tbsp (1.1 oz)	70	5	3	15	3	6	0	40	125	50	0	—	300
Soft Light Roasted Garlic	2 tbsp (1.1 oz)	70	5	3	15	3	2	0	40	180	550	0	—	400
Whipped	2 tbsp (0.7 oz)	70	7	5	25	1	tr	0	0	85	25	0	—	200
Whipped Chives	2 tbsp (0.7 oz)	70	6	4	20	1	tr	0	20	130	30	0	—	200
Whipped Smoked Salmon	2 tbsp (0.7 oz)	70	6	4	20	2	1	0	20	140	35	0	—	200
With Chives	1 oz	90	9	6	30	2	tr	0	0	135	25	0	—	300
ULTRA DELIGHT														
Cheddar Cream Cheese	2 tbsp (0.9 oz)	60	4	3	20	3	2	1	60	150	—	0	—	100
Chive	2 tbsp (0.9 oz)	60	4	3	20	3	2	1	40	130	—	0	—	100
Garlic	2 tbsp (0.9 oz)	60	4	3	20	3	2	1	40	130	—	0	—	100
Mixed Berry	2 tbsp (0.9 oz)	70	4	3	20	2	5	1	20	70	—	2	—	100
Nacho	2 tbsp (0.9 oz)	60	4	3	20	3	2	1	40	190	—	0	—	200

FOOD	PORTION	CALORIES	FAT	SAT FAT	CHOL	PROTEIN	CARBO	FIBER	CALCIUM	SOD	POTAS	VIT C	FOLIC	VIT A
ULTRA DELIGHT (CONT.)														
Salsa	2 tbsp (0.9 oz)	60	4	3	20	2	2	1	20	140	—	1	—	300
Shrimp	2 tbsp (0.9 oz)	60	4	3	30	3	2	1	40	130	—	4	—	100
Strawberry	2 tbsp (0.9 oz)	60	4	3	20	2	4	1	20	80	—	1	—	100
Vegetable	2 tbsp (0.9 oz)	50	4	3	20	2	2	1	40	150	—	0	—	400
WEIGHT WATCHERS														
Light	2 tbsp	40	3	2	10	3	1	0	20	105	44	0	—	400

CREAM CHEESE SUBSTITUTES

FOOD	PORTION	CALORIES	FAT	SAT FAT	CHOL	PROTEIN	CARBO	FIBER	CALCIUM	SOD	POTAS	VIT C	FOLIC	VIT A
TOFUTTI														
Better Than Cream Cheese French Onion	1 oz	80	8	2	0	1	1	—	—	135	—	—	—	—
Better Than Cream Cheese Herb & Chive	1 oz	80	8	2	0	1	1	—	—	135	—	—	—	—
Better Than Cream Cheese Plain	1 oz	80	8	2	0	1	1	—	—	135	—	—	—	—

CREAM OF TARTAR

FOOD	PORTION	CALORIES	FAT	SAT FAT	CHOL	PROTEIN	CARBO	FIBER	CALCIUM	SOD	POTAS	VIT C	FOLIC	VIT A
cream of tartar	1 tsp	8	0	0	0	0	2	—	0	2	495	0	0	0

CREPES

FOOD	PORTION	CALORIES	FAT	SAT FAT	CHOL	PROTEIN	CARBO	FIBER	CALCIUM	SOD	POTAS	VIT C	FOLIC	VIT A
basic crepe unfilled	1	75	2	—	55	—	—	—	38	—	—	—	—	—

CRESS

(see also WATERCRESS)

FOOD	PORTION	CALORIES	FAT	SAT FAT	CHOL	PROTEIN	CARBO	FIBER	CALCIUM	SOD	POTAS	VIT C	FOLIC	VIT A
garden cooked	½ cup	16	tr	tr	0	1	3	—	41	5	240	16	—	5236
garden raw	½ cup	8	tr	tr	0	tr	1	—	20	4	152	17	—	2325

CROAKER

FOOD	PORTION	CALORIES	FAT	SAT FAT	CHOL	PROTEIN	CARBO	FIBER	CALCIUM	SOD	POTAS	VIT C	FOLIC	VIT A
atlantic breaded & fried	3 oz	188	11	3	71	15	6	—	27	296	289	—	—	—
atlantic raw	3 oz	89	3	1	52	15	0	—	13	47	293	—	—	—

CROISSANT

FOOD	PORTION	CALORIES	FAT	SAT FAT	CHOL	PROTEIN	CARBO	FIBER	CALCIUM	SOD	POTAS	VIT C	FOLIC	VIT A
apple	1 (2 oz)	145	5	3	—	4	21	1	17	156	51	—	7	—
cheese	1 (2 oz)	236	12	5	—	5	27	2	30	316	76	—	19	—
plain	1 (2 oz)	232	12	7	—	5	26	2	21	424	67	—	16	—
plain	1 mini (1 oz)	115	6	3	—	2	13	1	10	211	34	—	8	—
PEPPERIDGE FARM														
Croissant Sandwich Quartet	1	170	7	—	—	4	22	tr	40	250	—	—	—	300
Petite All Butter	1	120	6	—	—	3	13	—	20	170	—	—	—	—
RUDY'S FARM														
Ham & Swiss Sandwich	1 (3.4 oz)	310	18	5	25	12	27	1	—	830	—	—	—	—
TAKE-OUT														
w/ egg & cheese	1	369	25	14	216	13	24	—	244	551	174	tr	36	1000
w/ egg cheese & bacon	1	413	28	15	215	16	24	—	151	889	210	2	35	472

FOOD	PORTION	CALORIES	FAT	SAT FAT	CHOL	PROTEIN	CARBO	FIBER	CALCIUM	SOD	POTAS	VIT C	FOLIC	VIT A
w/ egg cheese & ham	1	475	34	17	213	19	24	—	144	1080	272	11	36	451
w/ egg cheese & sausage	1	524	38	18	216	20	25	—	144	1115	283	tr	38	422

CROUTONS

FOOD	PORTION	CALORIES	FAT	SAT FAT	CHOL	PROTEIN	CARBO	FIBER	CALCIUM	SOD	POTAS	VIT C	FOLIC	VIT A
plain	1 cup (1 oz)	122	2	tr	0	4	22	2	23	209	37	0	7	0
seasoned	1 cup (1.4 oz)	186	7	2	—	4	25	2	38	495	72	—	16	—
ARNOLD														
Crispy Cheddar Romano	½ oz	64	3	—	3	2	8	tr	16	154	—	—	—	—
Crispy Cheese Garlic	½ oz	60	2	tr	0	2	9	tr	—	130	—	—	—	—
Crispy Fine Herbs	½ oz	50	1	0	0	2	10	1	—	150	—	—	—	—
Crispy Italian	½ oz	60	3	tr	0	2	8	tr	—	150	—	—	—	—
Crispy Onion & Garlic	½	60	2	tr	0	2	9	—	—	190	—	—	—	—
Crispy Seasoned	½ oz	60	3	tr	0	2	8	—	—	160	—	—	—	—
BROWNBERRY														
Ceasar Salad	½ oz	62	3	—	tr	2	8	1	20	165	—	—	—	—
Cheddar Cheese	½ oz	63	3	—	3	2	8	tr	14	155	—	—	—	—
Onion & Garlic	½ oz	60	2	—	1	2	9	tr	6	190	—	—	—	—
Seasoned	½ oz	59	2	—	1	2	8	1	8	155	—	—	—	—
Toasted	½ oz	56	1	—	0	2	10	tr	7	145	—	—	—	—
PEPPERIDGE FARM														
Cheddar & Romano Cheese	½ oz	60	2	0	0	2	10	—	20	200	—	—	—	—
Cheese & Garlic	½ oz	70	3	1	0	2	9	—	20	180	—	—	—	—
Onion & Garlic	½ oz	70	3	0	0	2	9	—	—	160	—	—	—	—
Seasoned	½ oz	70	3	1	0	2	9	—	20	180	—	—	—	—
Sour Cream & Chive	½ oz	70	3	1	0	2	9	—	20	170	—	—	—	—

CUCUMBER

FOOD	PORTION	CALORIES	FAT	SAT FAT	CHOL	PROTEIN	CARBO	FIBER	CALCIUM	SOD	POTAS	VIT C	FOLIC	VIT A
FRESH														
raw	1 (11 oz)	38	tr	tr	0	2	8	3	43	6	434	16	38	647
raw sliced	½ cup (1.8 oz)	7	tr	tr	0	tr	1	1	7	1	76	3	7	112
JARRED														
ROSOFF'S														
Salad	3 slices (1 oz)	12	0	0	0	0	3	—	—	220	—	—	—	—
SCHORR'S														
Cucumber Garden Salad	3 slices (1 oz)	12	0	0	0	0	3	—	—	220	—	—	—	—
TAKE-OUT														
cucumber salad	3.5 oz	50	tr	tr	0	1	11	—	—	480	—	9	—	750
kimchee	½ cup (1.8 oz)	36	2	tr	0	tr	4	tr	10	173	79	6	6	158
tzatziki	½ cup (3.4 oz)	72	6	1	5	2	4	1	59	197	146	3	10	83

FOOD	PORTION	CALORIES	FAT	SAT FAT	CHOL	PROTEIN	CARBO	FIBER	CALCIUM	SOD	POTAS	VIT C	FOLIC	VIT A
CUMIN														
seed	1 tsp	8	tr	—	0	tr	1	—	20	4	38	tr	—	27
CURRANTS														
black fresh	½ cup	36	tr	tr	0	1	9	—	31	1	180	101	—	129
zante dried	½ cup	204	tr	tr	0	3	53	—	62	6	642	3	7	52
CUSTARD														
HOME RECIPE														
baked	1 recipe 4 serv (19.8 oz)	549	26	13	491	29	60	—	632	436	880	3	55	1249
flan	1 recipe 10 serv (53.7 oz)	2206	63	30	1408	70	349	—	1321	864	1850	8	—	3138
MIX														
as prep w/ 2% milk	½ cup (4.7 oz)	148	4	2	74	7	24	—	197	200	287	1	10	296
as prep w/ 2% milk	1 recipe 4 serv (18.7 oz)	595	15	8	297	22	95	—	788	801	1152	4	42	1185
as prep w/ whole milk	½ cup (4.7 oz)	163	5	3	—	6	23	—	194	—	—	1	—	200
as prep w/ whole milk	1 recipe 4 serv (18.7 oz)	652	22	12	—	22	94	—	777	—	—	4	—	801
flan as prep w/ 2% milk	½ cup (4.7 oz)	135	2	1	9	4	26	—	153	68	194	1	3	249
flan as prep w/ 2% milk	1 recipe 4 serv (18.7 oz)	542	9	6	57	16	102	—	613	265	779	4	21	999
flan as prep w/ whole milk	½ cup (4.7 oz)	150	4	3	17	4	25	—	150	65	191	1	5	183
flan as prep w/ whole milk	1 recipe 4 serv (18.7 oz)	600	16	10	66	16	102	—	602	291	765	4	21	614
JELL-O														
Americana Custard Dessert as prep w/ 2% milk	½ cup (5 oz)	140	3	2	10	5	25	0	200	190	300	0	—	200
Flan as prep w/ 2% milk	½ cup (5.1 oz)	140	3	2	10	4	26	0	150	65	200	0	—	200
ROYAL														
Custard	mix for 1 serv	60	0	—	—	0	16	—	—	75	—	—	—	—
Flan Caramel Custard	mix for 1 serv	60	0	—	—	0	15	—	—	55	25	—	—	—
READY-TO-EAT														
KOZY SHACK														
Flan	1 pkg (4 oz)	150	4	2	40	4	25	0	100	90	—	0	—	200
TAKE-OUT														
baked	½ cup (5 oz)	148	7	3	123	7	15	—	158	109	216	1	44	313
flan	½ cup (5.4 oz)	220	6	3	140	7	35	—	132	86	185	1	—	314
zabaione	½ cup (57.2 g)	135	5	2	213	3	13	0	23	9	16	0	24	485

FOOD	PORTION	CALORIES	FAT	SAT FAT	CHOL	PROTEIN	CARBO	FIBER	CALCIUM	SOD	POTAS	VIT C	FOLIC	VIT A
DANDELION GREENS														
fresh cooked	½ cup	17	tr	—	0	1	3	—	73	23	121	9	—	6084
raw chopped	½ cup	13	tr	—	0	1	3	—	52	21	111	10	—	3920
DANISH PASTRY														
FROZEN														
MORTON														
Honey Buns	1 (2.28 oz)	250	10	3	0	3	35	2	0	160	—	0	—	0
Honey Buns Mini	1 (1.23 oz)	160	8	2	0	2	19	tr	0	100	—	0	—	0
PEPPERIDGE FARM														
Apple	1	220	8	—	—	2	35	—	40	130	—	—	—	—
Cheese	1	240	14	—	—	3	25	—	40	230	—	—	—	—
Cinnamon Raisin	1	250	11	—	—	3	35	—	40	170	—	—	—	—
Raspberry	1	220	9	—	—	3	31	—	40	140	—	—	—	—
READY-TO-EAT														
plain ring	1 (12 oz)	1305	71	22	292	21	152	—	360	1302	316	tr	—	360
HOSTESS														
Apple	1 (3.8 oz)	400	22	10	20	4	47	2	40	340	115	—	—	—
Apple Fruit Roll	1 (2 oz)	180	4	2	<5	4	33	1	—	170	80	—	—	—
Coffee Cake Raspberry	1 (1.2 oz)	110	3	1	<5	2	21	tr	—	110	35	—	—	—
TAKE-OUT														
almond	1 (4¼ in) (2.3 oz)	280	16	4	30	5	30	2	61	236	62	1	—	34
apple	1 (4¼ in) (2.5 oz)	264	13	3	—	4	34	1	33	251	59	3	12	27
cheese	1 (3 oz)	353	25	5	20	6	29	—	70	320	116	3	15	155
cheese	1 (4¼ in) (2.5 oz)	266	16	5	—	6	26	—	25	319	70	—	—	—
cinnamon	1 (3 oz)	349	17	3	28	5	47	—	37	326	96	3	14	18
cinnamon	1 (4¼ in) (2.3 oz)	262	15	4	—	5	29	1	46	241	81	—	—	—
cinnimon nut	1 (4¼ in) (2.3 oz)	280	16	4	30	5	30	2	61	236	62	1	—	34
fruit	1 (3.3 oz)	335	16	3	19	5	45	—	22	333	110	2	15	86
lemon	1 (4¼ in) (2.5 oz)	264	13	3	—	4	34	1	33	251	59	3	12	124
raisin	1 (4¼ in) (2.5 oz)	264	13	3	—	4	34	1	33	251	59	3	12	27
raisin nut	1 (4¼ in) (2.3 oz)	280	16	4	30	5	30	2	61	236	62	1	—	34
raspberry	1 (4¼ in) (2.5 oz)	264	13	3	—	4	34	1	33	251	59	3	12	142
strawberry	1 (4¼ in) (2.5 oz)	264	13	3	—	4	34	1	33	251	59	3	12	37
DATES														
DRIED														
chopped	1 cup	489	1	—	0	4	131	—	58	5	1161	0	22	89

FOOD	PORTION	CALORIES	FAT	SAT FAT	CHOL	PROTEIN	CARBO	FIBER	CALCIUM	SOD	POTAS	VIT C	FOLIC	VIT A
deglet noor	10	240	0	—	0	—	—	—	40	—	—	—	—	—
whole	10	228	tr	—	0	2	61	—	27	2	541	0	10	42
BORDO														
Diced	2 oz	203	1	—	0	1	48	—	40	5	396	12	—	tr
DOLE														
Chopped	½ cup	230	0	0	0	0	56	—	—	5	390	—	—	—
Pitted	½ cup	280	0	0	0	8	62	—	—	0	560	—	—	—
DROMEDARY														
Chopped	¼ cup	130	0	0	0	1	31	—	20	0	190	—	—	—
Pitted	5	100	0	0	0	1	23	—	20	0	190	—	—	—
SONOMA														
Dried	5-6 (1.4 oz)	110	0	0	0	1	30	5	0	15	—	0	—	0

DEER

(*see* VENISON)

DELI MEATS/COLD CUTS

(*see also* CHICKEN, HAM, MEAT SUBSTITUTES, TURKEY)

FOOD	PORTION	CALORIES	FAT	SAT FAT	CHOL	PROTEIN	CARBO	FIBER	CALCIUM	SOD	POTAS	VIT C	FOLIC	VIT A
barbecue loaf pork & beef	1 oz	49	3	1	11	4	2	—	13	378	93	5	—	—
beerwurst beef	1 slice (4 in x ⅛ in)	75	7	3	13	3	tr	—	2	214	42	3	1	—
beerwurst pork	1 slice (2¾ in x 1/16 in)	14	1	tr	4	1	tr	—	0	74	15	2	0	—
beerwurst pork	1 slice (4 in x ⅛ in)	55	4	1	13	4	tr	—	2	285	58	7	1	—
berliner pork & beef	1 oz	65	4	2	13	4	1	—	3	368	80	2	—	—
blood sausage	1 oz	95	9	3	30	4	tr	—	—	—	—	—	—	—
bologna beef & pork	1 oz	89	8	3	16	3	1	—	3	289	51	6	1	—
bologna pork	1 oz	70	6	2	17	4	tr	—	3	336	80	10	1	—
braunschweiger pork	1 slice (2½ in x ¼ in)	65	6	2	28	2	1	—	2	206	36	2	—	2529
braunschweiger pork	1 oz	102	9	3	44	4	1	—	2	324	57	3	—	3984
dried beef	1 oz	47	1	—	—	—	tr	—	2	—	—	—	—	—
dried beef	5 slices (21 g)	35	tr	—	—	—	tr	—	1	—	—	—	—	—
dutch brand loaf pork & beef	1 oz	68	5	2	13	4	2	—	24	354	107	5	—	—
honey loaf pork & beef	1 oz	36	1	tr	10	4	2	—	5	374	97	6	—	—
honey roll sausage beef	1 oz	42	2	1	12	4	1	—	2	304	67	4	—	—
luncheon meat pork & beef	1 oz	100	9	3	15	4	1	—	5	367	57	4	2	—
luncheon sausage pork & beef	1 oz	74	6	2	18	4	tr	—	3	335	70	5	—	—

FOOD	PORTION	CALORIES	FAT	SAT FAT	CHOL	PROTEIN	CARBO	FIBER	CALCIUM	SOD	POTAS	VIT C	FOLIC	VIT A
mortadella beef & pork	1 oz	88	7	3	16	5	1	—	5	353	46	7	—	—
mother's loaf pork	1 oz	80	6	2	13	3	2	—	12	320	64	0	—	—
new england sausage pork & beef	1 oz	46	2	1	14	5	1	—	2	346	91	6	2	—
peppered loaf pork & beef	1 oz	42	2	1	13	5	1	—	15	432	112	7	—	—
pepperoni pork & beef	1 slice (0.2 oz)	27	2	1	—	1	tr	—	1	112	19	—	—	—
pepperoni pork & beef	1 (9 oz)	1248	110	40	—	53	7	—	25	5120	871	—	—	—
picnic loaf pork & beef	1 oz	66	5	2	11	4	1	—	13	330	76	5	—	—
salami cooked beef & pork	1 oz	71	6	2	18	4	1	—	4	302	56	3	1	—
salami hard pork	1 slice (⅓ oz)	41	4	1	—	2	3	—	1	226	—	—	—	—
salami hard pork	1 pkg (4 oz)	460	38	13	—	26	2	—	15	2554	—	—	—	—
salami hard pork & beef	1 pkg (4 oz)	472	39	14	89	26	3	—	8	2101	427	29	—	—
salami hard pork & beef	1 slice (⅓ oz)	42	3	1	8	2	tr	—	1	186	38	3	—	—
sandwich spread pork & beef	1 tbsp	35	3	1	6	1	2	—	2	152	16	0	—	—
sandwich spread pork & beef	1 oz	67	5	2	11	2	3	—	3	287	31	0	—	—
summer sausage thuringer cervelat	1 oz	98	8	3	19	5	1	—	2	412	65	7	—	—
CARL BUDDIG														
Beef	1 oz	40	2	1	20	5	1	0	0	430	75	0	—	0
Corned Beef	1 oz	40	2	1	20	5	1	0	0	380	75	0	—	0
Pastrami	1 oz	40	2	0	20	5	1	0	0	320	75	0	—	0
HEALTHY CHOICE														
Bologna	1 slice (1 oz)	30	1	0	15	4	1	0	0	290	—	5	—	0
Bologna Beef	1 slice (1 oz)	35	1	0	10	4	3	0	0	280	—	4	—	0
Deli-Thin Bologna	4 slices (1.8 oz)	60	2	1	25	8	3	0	20	560	—	6	—	0
Well-Pack Bologna	1 slice (1 oz)	30	1	0	15	4	1	0	0	290	—	5	—	0
HEBREW NATIONAL														
Bologna Beef	2 oz	180	16	—	40	7	—	—	—	440	—	—	—	—
Bologna Beef Reduced Fat	2 oz	130	12	—	35	6	—	—	—	320	—	—	—	—
Bologna Lean Chub	2 oz	90	6	—	25	8	—	—	—	430	—	—	—	—
Bologna Midget	2 oz	180	16	—	40	7	—	—	—	440	—	—	—	—
Deli Pastrami	2 oz	80	3	—	30	12	—	—	—	510	—	—	—	—
Deli Express Corned Beef	2 oz	80	3	—	35	15	—	—	—	450	—	—	—	—

FOOD	PORTION	CALORIES	FAT	SAT FAT	CHOL	PROTEIN	CARBO	FIBER	CALCIUM	SOD	POTAS	VIT C	FOLIC	VIT A
HEBREW NATIONAL (CONT.)														
Deli Express Tongue Sliced	2 oz	120	9	—	50	10	—	—	—	330	—	—	—	—
Salami Beef	2 oz	170	14	—	40	8	—	—	—	420	—	—	—	—
Salami Beef Reduced Fat	2 oz	110	8	—	30	8	—	—	—	380	—	—	—	—
Salami Sean Chub	2 oz	90	6	—	30	9	—	—	—	340	—	—	—	—
Salami Midget	2 oz	170	14	—	40	8	—	—	—	420	—	—	—	—
HILLSHIRE														
Bologna Large	1 oz	90	8	—	—	3	tr	—	—	260	—	—	—	—
Bologna Ring	1 oz	90	8	—	—	3	tr	—	—	230	—	—	—	—
Brunschweiger	1 oz	95	8	—	—	4	2	—	—	270	—	—	—	—
Deli Select Corned Beef	1 slice	10	tr	—	—	2	tr	—	—	100	—	—	—	—
Deli Select Light Bologna	1 slice	12	1	—	—	1	tr	—	—	85	—	—	—	—
Deli Select Oven Roasted Cured Beef	1 slice	10	tr	—	—	2	tr	—	—	95	—	—	—	—
Deli Select Pastrami	1 slice	10	tr	—	—	2	tr	—	—	100	—	—	—	—
Deli Select Roast Beef	1 slice	10	tr	—	—	2	tr	—	—	135	—	—	—	—
Deli Select Smoked Beef	1 slice	10	tr	—	—	2	tr	—	—	100	—	—	—	—
Flavor Pack 90-99% Fat Free Light Bologna	1 slice (0.73 oz)	30	2	—	—	3	1	—	—	190	—	—	—	—
Flavor Pack 90-99% Fat Free Pastrami	1 slice (0.6 oz)	18	tr	—	—	4	tr	—	—	180	—	—	—	—
Lunch 'N Munch Bologna/ American/ Snickers	1 pkg (4.25 oz)	490	34	—	—	15	31	—	—	1110	—	—	—	—
Lunch 'N Munch Bologna/ American/ Snickers/Hi-C	1 pkg (4.25 oz + 6 fl oz)	590	34	—	—	15	55	—	—	1130	—	—	—	—
Lunch 'N Munch Bologna/American	1 pkg (4.5 oz)	480	37	—	—	17	20	—	—	1390	—	—	—	—
Lunch 'N Munch Cotto Salami/ Monterey Jack	1 pkg (4.5 oz)	440	32	—	—	18	21	—	—	1270	—	—	—	—
Lunch 'N Munch Pepperoni/ American	1 pkg (4.5 oz)	570	46	—	—	22	20	—	—	1670	—	—	—	—
Pepperoni	1 oz	110	10	—	—	5	0	—	—	450	—	—	—	—
Salami Hard	1 oz	100	9	—	—	5	0	—	—	450	—	—	—	—
Salami Hard	1 oz	90	7	—	—	5	1	—	—	470	—	—	—	—

FOOD	PORTION	CALORIES	FAT	SAT FAT	CHOL	PROTEIN	CARBO	FIBER	CALCIUM	SOD	POTAS	VIT C	FOLIC	VIT A
HILLSHIRE (CONT.)														
Summer Sausage	2 oz	180	16	—	—	9	1	—	—	670	—	—	—	—
Summer Sausage Beef	2 oz	190	17	—	—	9	1	—	—	612	—	—	—	—
Summer Sausage Light	2 oz	150	12	—	—	10	1	—	—	630	—	—	—	—
Summer Sausage w/ Cheddar Cheese	2 oz	200	18	—	—	9	1	—	—	605	—	—	—	—
HORMEL														
Liverwurst Spread	4 tbsp (2 oz)	130	10	4	70	8	2	0	0	650	—	1	—	5000
Pepperoni Chunk	1 oz	140	13	6	35	5	0	0	0	470	—	0	—	0
Pepperoni Sliced	15 slices (1 oz)	140	13	6	35	5	0	0	0	470	—	0	—	0
Pepperoni Twin	1 oz	140	13	5	35	5	0	0	0	500	—	6	—	0
Pillow Pack Genoa Salami	2 oz	160	18	7	50	12	0	0	0	940	—	0	—	0
Pillow Pack Pepperoni	16 slices (1 oz)	140	13	6	35	5	0	0	0	470	—	0	—	0
JONES														
Liver Sausage	1 slice	80	7	—	43	3	tr	—	—	180	—	—	—	—
Liver Sausage Chub	1 slice	80	7	—	43	5	tr	—	—	230	—	—	—	—
JORDAN'S														
Healthy Trim 95% Fat Free Macaroni & Cheese Loaf	2 slices (1.6 oz)	50	2	1	15	6	3	0	0	290	—	1	—	0
Healthy Trim 95% Fat Free Olive Loaf	2 slices (1.6 oz)	50	2	1	15	6	2	0	0	290	—	4	—	0
Healthy Trim 95% Fat Free Pickle & Pepper Loaf	2 slices (1.6 oz)	50	2	1	15	6	2	0	0	290	—	1	—	0
Healthy Trim 97% Fat Free Corned Beef	2 slices (1.6 oz)	45	2	1	30	9	0	0	0	290	—	0	—	0
Healthy Trim Low Fat Cooked Salami	3 slices (2 oz)	70	3	1	25	8	2	0	0	360	—	0	—	0
Healthy Trim Low Fat German Brand Bologna	3 slices (2 oz)	70	3	1	25	6	3	0	0	360	—	0	—	0
OSCAR MAYER														
Bologna	1 slice (1 oz)	90	8	3	30	3	1	0	0	290	—	0	—	0
Bologna Beef	1 slice (1 oz)	90	8	4	20	3	1	0	0	310	—	0	—	0
Bologna Garlic	1 slice (1.4 oz)	110	12	5	40	4	1	0	20	420	—	0	—	0
Bologna Wisconsin Made Ring	2 oz	180	16	6	35	6	2	0	0	460	—	0	—	0
Braunschweiger Spread	2 oz	190	17	6	90	8	2	0	0	630	—	5	—	9500

FOOD	PORTION	CALORIES	FAT	SAT FAT	CHOL	PROTEIN	CARBO	FIBER	CALCIUM	SOD	POTAS	VIT C	FOLIC	VIT A
OSCAR MAYER (CONT.)														
Brunschweiger	1 slice (1 oz)	100	9	3	40	4	1	0	0	320	—	2	—	4500
Free Bologna	1 slice (1 oz)	20	0	0	5	4	2	0	0	280	—	0	—	0
Head Cheese	1 slice (1 oz)	50	4	2	25	5	0	0	0	360	—	0	—	0
Light Bologna	1 slice (1 oz)	60	4	2	15	3	2	0	0	310	—	0	—	0
Light Bologna Beef	1 slice (1 oz)	60	4	2	15	3	2	0	0	310	—	0	—	0
Liver Cheese	1 slice (1.3 oz)	120	10	4	80	6	1	0	0	420	—	0	—	8500
Lunchables Bologna/American	1 pkg (4.5 oz)	450	34	15	85	18	19	0	300	1620	—	0	—	300
Lunchables Deluxe Turkey/Ham	1 pkg (5.1 oz)	360	19	10	60	23	23	1	300	1930	—	0	—	300
Lunchables Dessert Jello/Honey Turkey/Cheddar	1 pkg (5.7 oz)	320	16	9	50	17	27	tr	200	1360	—	0	—	400
Lunchables Fun Pack Bologna/ Wild Cherry	1 pkg (11.2 oz)	530	29	14	60	13	58	tr	200	1120	—	0	—	400
Lunchables Fun Pack Ham/Fruit Punch	1 pkg (11.2 oz)	450	20	10	50	15	53	tr	200	1260	—	0	—	400
Lunchables Ham/ Swiss	1 pkg (4.5 oz)	320	17	8	60	22	19	0	300	1770	—	0	—	400
Lunchables Pepperoni/ American	1 pkg (4.5 oz)	480	36	17	95	20	19	0	250	1840	—	0	—	300
Lunchables Salami/ American	1 pkg (4.5 oz)	430	32	15	80	18	18	0	250	1740	—	0	—	300
Luncheon Loaf Spiced	1 slice (1 oz)	70	5	2	20	4	2	0	40	340	—	0	—	0
New England Brand Sausage	2 slices (1.6 oz)	60	3	1	25	8	1	0	0	570	—	0	—	0
Old Fashioned Loaf	1 slice (1 oz)	70	5	2	15	4	2	0	40	330	—	0	—	0
Olive Loaf	1 slice (1 oz)	70	6	2	20	3	2	0	40	370	—	0	—	0
Pepperoni	15 slices (1 oz)	140	13	5	25	6	0	0	0	550	—	0	—	0
Pickle And Pimiento Loaf	1 slice (1 oz)	80	6	2	20	3	3	0	40	360	—	0	—	0
Salami Cotto	1 slice (1 oz)	70	5	2	25	3	1	0	0	280	—	0	—	0
Salami Cotto Beef	1 slice (1 oz)	60	5	2	25	4	1	0	0	370	—	0	—	0
Salami For Beer	1 slices (1.6 oz)	110	9	3	30	6	1	0	0	580	—	0	—	0
Salami Genoa	3 slices (1 oz)	100	9	3	25	5	0	0	0	490	—	0	—	0
Salami Hard	3 slices (1 oz)	100	9	3	25	6	0	0	0	510	—	0	—	0
Salami Machaich Brand Beef	2 slices (1.6 oz)	120	10	5	30	6	1	0	0	510	—	0	—	0
Sandwich Spread	2 oz	130	10	4	25	4	8	0	0	460	—	0	—	0
Summer Sausage	2 slices (1.6 oz)	140	13	5	40	7	0	0	0	650	—	0	—	0

FOOD	PORTION	CALORIES	FAT	SAT FAT	CHOL	PROTEIN	CARBO	FIBER	CALCIUM	SOD	POTAS	VIT C	FOLIC	VIT A
OSCAR MAYER (CONT.)														
Summer Sausage Beef	2 slices (1.6 oz)	140	12	5	35	7	1	0	0	640	—	0	—	0
RUSSER														
Bologna	2 oz	180	15	7	30	6	3	—	—	540	—	—	—	—
Bologna Jalapeno Pepper	2 oz	170	14	6	25	6	3	—	—	600	—	—	—	—
Bologna Wunderbar German Brand	2 oz	190	16	6	20	6	5	—	40	600	—	—	—	—
Bologna Beef	2 oz	180	15	7	30	6	3	—	—	600	—	—	—	—
Bologna Garlic	2 oz	180	16	6	30	6	3	—	—	520	—	—	—	—
Bologna Italian Brand Sweet Red Pepper	2 oz	180	15	6	30	6	3	—	—	540	—	—	—	—
Braunschweiger	2 oz	170	14	6	90	8	3	—	—	600	—	—	—	—
Cooked Salami	2 oz	120	8	3	50	8	3	—	—	600	—	—	—	—
Dutch Brand	2 oz	130	8	3	25	7	6	—	—	600	—	—	—	—
Hot Cooked Salami	2 oz	110	7	3	45	8	3	—	—	600	—	—	—	—
Italian Brand Loaf	2 oz	130	8	3	25	7	5	—	—	600	—	—	—	—
Jalapeno Loaf With Monterey Jack Cheese	2 oz	160	13	5	25	6	4	—	—	650	—	—	—	—
Kielbasa Loaf	2 oz	120	8	3	35	7	5	—	—	600	—	—	—	—
Light Bologna	2 oz	120	8	4	30	8	3	—	—	400	—	—	—	—
Light Bologna Beef	2 oz	120	8	4	30	8	3	—	—	400	—	—	—	—
Light Braunschweiger	2 oz	120	8	3	60	8	3	—	—	400	—	—	—	—
Light Old Fashioned Loaf	2 oz	90	4	3	30	8	4	—	—	430	—	—	—	—
Light P&P Loaf	2 oz	100	6	3	30	8	4	—	—	430	—	—	—	—
Light Salami Cooked	2 oz	90	5	3	40	8	4	—	—	400	—	—	—	—
Olive Loaf	2 oz	160	13	5	20	6	4	—	—	600	—	—	—	—
P&P Loaf	2 oz	160	13	5	25	6	4	—	—	600	—	—	—	—
Pepper Loaf	2 oz	90	3	2	30	8	6	—	—	600	—	—	—	—
Polish Loaf	2 oz	140	10	4	25	7	7	—	—	600	—	—	—	—
SARA LEE														
Pastrami Beef	2 oz	100	6	3	25	10	1	1	—	540	—	6	—	—
Peppered Beef	2 oz	70	2	1	25	12	1	—	—	200	—	—	—	—
SHOFAR														
Salami Beef	2 oz	160	15	6	40	7	0	0	0	410	—	0	—	0
SPAM														
Less Salt	2 oz	170	16	6	40	7	0	0	0	560	—	18	—	0
Lite	2 oz	110	8	3	45	9	0	0	0	560	—	18	—	0
Original	2 oz	170	16	6	40	7	0	0	0	750	—	0	—	0
Smoked	2 oz	170	16	6	40	7	0	0	0	750	—	0	—	0

FOOD	PORTION	CALORIES	FAT	SAT FAT	CHOL	PROTEIN	CARBO	FIBER	CALCIUM	SOD	POTAS	VIT C	FOLIC	VIT A
UNDERWOOD														
Liverwurst	2.08 oz	180	15	—	90	8	4	—	—	470	—	—	—	650
WEIGHT WATCHERS														
Bologna	2 slices (¾ oz)	35	2	—	15	3	1	—	—	220	—	—	—	—
TAKE-OUT														
corned beef	2 oz	70	2	1	40	12	0	—	—	390	—	12	—	—
corned beef brisket	2 oz	90	5	2	35	11	0	—	—	370	—	12	—	—

DIETING AIDS

(*see* NUTRITIONAL SUPPLEMENTS)

DILL

seed	1 tsp	6	tr	tr	0	tr	1	—	32	tr	25	—	—	1
weed dry	1 tsp	3	tr	—	0	tr	1	—	18	2	33	—	—	—
WATKINS														
Liquid Spice	1 tbsp (0.5 oz)	120	14	2	0	0	0	0	0	0	—	0	—	0

DINNER

(*see also* ASIAN FOOD, PASTA DISHES, POT PIES, SPANISH FOOD)

FROZEN

AMY'S ORGANIC														
Whole Meals Country Dinner	1 pkg (11 oz)	380	12	4	15	11	60	9	—	570	—	—	—	—
ARMOUR														
Classics Chicken Parmigiana	1 meal (10.75 oz)	360	18	6	45	24	25	7	100	1020	—	9	—	500
Classics Chicken & Noodles	1 meal (11 oz)	280	9	5	60	19	30	6	80	550	—	36	—	3000
Classics Chicken Mesquite	1 meal (9.5 oz)	280	13	4	65	21	39	5	20	630	—	18	—	200
Classics Chicken w/ Wine & Mushroom	1 meal (10 oz)	260	11	5	50	20	20	4	60	540	—	12	—	3000
Classics Glazed Chicken	1 meal (10.75 oz)	280	14	4	55	19	20	4	20	740	—	9	—	300
Classics Meatloaf	1 meal (11.25 oz)	300	10	5	65	19	33	7	40	600	—	12	—	200
Classics Salisbury Steak	1 meal (11.25 oz)	330	18	8	50	23	20	4	100	1310	—	24	—	300
Classics Swedish Meatballs	1 meal (10 oz)	300	17	7	40	18	20	4	80	940	—	0	—	2500
Classics Turkey and Dressing	1 meal (11.25 oz)	270	7	4	60	17	34	5	60	1020	—	6	—	2250
Classics Veal Parmigiana	1 meal (11.25 oz)	400	22	11	65	16	35	5	150	1050	—	30	—	750
Classics Lite Beef Pepper	1 meal (11 oz)	210	4	2	60	16	29	5	40	870	—	12	—	750
Classics Lite Chicken Burgundy	1 meal (10 oz)	210	5	2	45	20	20	4	40	760	—	9	—	2500

FOOD	PORTION	CALORIES	FAT	SAT FAT	CHOL	PROTEIN	CARBO	FIBER	CALCIUM	SOD	POTAS	VIT C	FOLIC	VIT A
ARMOUR (CONT.)														
Classics Lite Salisbury Steak	1 meal (11.5 oz)	260	7	4	55	22	26	6	60	860	—	18	—	300
Classics Lite Shrimp Creole	1 meal (10 oz)	220	1	0	20	6	49	16	40	720	—	120	—	400
Classics Lite Sweet & Sour Chicken	1 meal (11 oz)	220	1	0	30	16	38	4	40	520	—	27	—	750
BANQUET														
BBQ Style Chicken	1 meal (9 oz)	320	12	2	60	18	36	3	60	800	—	6	—	300
Beef	1 meal (9 oz)	240	7	3	70	26	19	12	40	660	—	6	—	200
Chicken Parmigiana	1 pkg (9.5 oz)	290	15	4	50	14	27	3	60	900	—	60	—	300
Chicken & Dumplings	1 meal (10 oz)	260	8	3	35	13	35	16	40	780	—	0	—	2000
Chicken Fried Steak	1 pkg (10 oz)	400	20	6	30	15	39	4	100	1180	—	0	—	100
Chicken Nuggets	1 pkg (6.75 oz)	410	21	5	45	18	38	11	20	650	—	6	—	0
Extra Helping All White Chicken	1 meal (18 oz)	820	41	9	95	40	72	8	150	1890	—	0	—	0
Extra Helping Chicken Parmigiana	1 meal (19 oz)	650	33	8	65	24	64	9	150	1770	—	108	—	2250
Extra Helping Chicken Fried Steak	1 meal (18.5 oz)	800	44	14	55	29	73	6	250	2050	—	0	—	0
Extra Helping Fried Chicken	1 meal (18 oz)	790	39	9	110	37	72	8	150	1820	—	0	—	0
Extra Helping Meatloaf	1 meal (19 oz)	650	38	16	85	29	49	10	100	2140	—	102	—	4500
Extra Helping Mexican Style	1 meal (22 oz)	820	34	14	50	28	100	20	300	2060	—	6	—	1500
Extra Helping Salisbury Steak	1 meal (19 oz)	740	46	19	75	31	52	11	100	1860	—	6	—	100
Extra Helping Southern Fried Chicken	1 meal (17.5 oz)	750	37	9	120	38	67	9	150	2140	—	0	—	0
Extra Helping Turkey Dinner	1 meal (18.8 oz)	560	20	5	75	32	63	7	100	1910	—	0	—	0
Family Entree Beef Stew	1 serv (8.13 oz)	160	4	2	25	14	17	4	20	1120	—	9	—	500
Family Entree Chicken Parmigiana	1 serv (4.67 oz)	240	13	5	20	11	18	2	100	690	—	36	—	200
Family Entree Chicken & Dumplings	1 serv (7.47 oz)	290	14	5	2	12	30	2	40	1270	—	0	—	0

FOOD	PORTION	CALORIES	FAT	SAT FAT	CHOL	PROTEIN	CARBO	FIBER	CALCIUM	SOD	POTAS	VIT C	FOLIC	VIT A
BANQUET (CONT.)														
Family Entree Gravy & Sliced Turkey	1 serv (4.8 oz)	100	5	2	25	8	5	tr	0	590	—	0	—	0
Family Entree Gravy w/ Charbroiled Beef	1 serv (4.67 oz)	180	13	6	25	8	7	2	20	640	—	0	—	0
Family Entree Onion Gravy w/ Beef	1 serv (4.67 oz)	180	14	6	20	8	7	2	20	630	—	0	—	0
Family Entree Salisbury Steak	1 serv (4.67 oz)	200	14	6	25	12	7	2	20	610	—	0	—	0
Family Entree Veal Parmigiana	1 serv (4.67 oz)	230	14	4	20	9	19	2	40	740	—	54	—	200
Family Entrees Dumplings & Chicken	7 oz	280	14	—	—	12	28	—	—	—	—	—	—	—
Family Entrees Gravy & Sliced Beef	1 serv (5.6 oz)	100	3	2	40	13	7	tr	0	850	—	0	—	0
Family Entrees Gravy & Sliced Turkey	6 oz	120	6	—	—	9	6	—	—	—	—	—	—	—
Fried Chicken	1 meal (9 oz)	470	27	9	105	21	35	6	80	980	—	5	—	0
Gravy w/ Beef Patty	1 pkg (9.5 oz)	300	20	8	35	11	21	2	40	1060	—	4	—	3000
Hot Sandwich Toppers Chicken Ala King	1 pkg (4.5 oz)	100	4	2	40	9	7	1	60	480	—	1	—	500
Hot Sandwich Toppers Creamed Chipped Beef	1 pkg (4 oz)	100	3	2	25	9	8	0	80	700	—	0	—	0
Hot Sandwich Toppers Gravy & Sliced Beef	1 pkg (4 oz)	70	2	1	25	8	5	tr	0	440	—	0	—	0
Hot Sandwich Toppers Gravy & Sliced Turkey	1 pkg (5 oz)	90	4	2	30	8	7	tr	20	670	—	0	—	0
Hot Sandwich Toppers Salisbury Steak	1 pkg (5 oz)	220	16	7	25	9	8	2	20	790	—	1	—	0
Hot Sandwich Toppers Sloppy Joe	1 meal (4 oz)	140	7	3	25	7	12	1	20	530	—	0	—	300
Meatloaf	1 meal (9.5 oz)	280	17	7	40	12	23	2	40	1100	—	42	—	3000
Mexican Style Combo Meal	1 pkg (11 oz)	380	11	5	15	15	55	9	150	1370	—	4	—	750
Mexican Style Meal	1 pkg (11 oz)	340	13	5	15	14	56	10	150	1520	—	0	—	750
Oriental Style Chicken	1 pkg (9 oz)	260	9	3	40	12	34	4	40	610	—	18	—	1250

FOOD	PORTION	CALORIES	FAT	SAT FAT	CHOL	PROTEIN	CARBO	FIBER	CALCIUM	SOD	POTAS	VIT C	FOLIC	VIT A
BANQUET (CONT.)														
Salisbury Steak	1 meal (9.5 oz)	310	16	7	35	14	28	2	40	910	—	4	—	0
Southern Fried Chicken Meal	1 pkg (8.75 oz)	260	30	8	85	22	44	4	80	1610	—	6	—	0
Turkey	1 meal (9.25 oz)	270	10	3	45	15	31	3	80	1100	—	2	—	0
Veal Parmagiana	1 pkg (9 oz)	530	14	5	25	13	35	7	60	960	—	27	—	300
Western Style Meal	1 meal (9.5 oz)	210	20	9	30	14	28	5	40	1400	—	2	—	0
White Meat Chicken Meal	1 pkg (8.75 oz)	470	28	11	100	22	33	2	40	1100	—	5	—	0
BIRDS EYE														
Easy Recipe Meal Starter Cacciatore as prep	1 serv	280	8	2	69	6	30	2	40	336	—	27	—	1000
Easy Recipe Meal Starter Orange Glaze Chicken as prep	1 serv	280	8	2	69	6	30	2	40	336	—	27	—	1000
Easy Recipe Meal Starter Southwestern	1 serv	280	8	2	69	7	30	2	40	336	—	27	—	1000
Easy Recipe Meal Starter Sweet & Sour as prep	1 serv	280	8	2	69	4	30	2	40	336	—	27	—	1000
BUDGET GOURMET														
Beef Cantonese	1 meal (9.1 oz)	270	9	—	40	15	31	—	20	880	470	30	—	2250
Beef Stroganoff	1 meal (8.75 oz)	260	10	5	50	19	27	—	60	840	260	4	—	500
Chicken And Egg Noodles	1 meal (10 oz)	440	26	—	90	24	28	—	200	880	300	9	—	1000
Chicken Au Gratin	1 meal (9.1 oz)	230	8	5	40	18	23	—	150	820	400	9	—	3500
Chicken Breast Parmigiana	1 pkg (11 oz)	270	9	3	50	22	30	—	100	530	530	5	—	1000
Chicken Marsala	1 meal (9 oz)	260	8	—	90	17	31	—	40	730	210	4	—	1750
Chicken With Fettucini	1 meal (10 oz)	400	21	—	85	24	29	—	200	700	340	4	—	1000
Chinese Style Vegetables & Chicken	1 meal (10 oz)	280	7	1	10	11	47	—	60	590	320	15	—	1250
French Recipe Chicken	1 meal (10 oz)	220	9	4	40	17	21	—	60	870	650	9	—	2500
Glazed Turkey	1 meal (9 oz)	260	5	2	30	16	38	—	20	710	240	1	—	200
Ham & Asparagus Au Gratin	1 meal (8.7 oz)	300	14	7	50	17	26	—	150	860	610	15	—	100

BUDGET GOURMET (CONT.)

FOOD	PORTION	CALORIES	FAT	SAT FAT	CHOL	PROTEIN	CARBO	FIBER	CALCIUM	SOD	POTAS	VIT C	FOLIC	VIT A
Herbed Chicken Breast With Fettucini	1 pkg (11 oz)	240	6	2	45	21	30	—	150	430	380	30	—	4000
Italian Style Vegetables & Chicken	1 meal (10.25 oz)	310	8	2	30	14	50	—	80	690	260	9	—	2000
Mandarin Chicken	1 meal (10 oz)	240	5	1	40	15	38	—	20	710	260	15	—	1250
Mesquite Chicken Breast	1 pkg (11 oz)	250	6	1	40	23	33	—	60	550	710	15	—	4500
Orange Glazed Chicken	1 meal (9 oz)	270	3	1	25	17	46	—	20	870	360	9	—	500
Oriental Beef	1 meal (10 oz)	290	8	3	30	18	36	—	40	840	500	15	—	1250
Oriental Chicken With Vegetables	1 meal (9 oz)	280	6	1	20	19	44	—	40	690	250	4	—	500
Pepper Steak With Rice	1 meal (10 oz)	300	8	—	35	18	40	—	20	720	330	12	—	1250
Pot Roast Beef	1 meal (10.5 oz)	230	7	3	60	25	19	—	20	510	590	12	—	5000
Roast Chicken With Homestyle Gravy	1 meal (11 oz)	280	8	2	35	20	36	—	100	560	620	12	—	3500
Roast Sirloin Supreme	1 meal (9 oz)	320	15	—	85	19	28	—	40	630	250	5	—	200
Sirloin Salisbury Steak	1 meal (11 oz)	280	9	4	40	21	30	—	100	530	630	21	—	3000
Sirloin Salisbury Steak	1 meal (9 oz)	220	8	3	25	16	24	—	60	730	520	9	—	2000
Sirloin Cheddar Melt	1 meal (9.4 oz)	380	21	—	85	18	29	—	150	950	800	12	—	500
Sirloin Of Beef In Herb Sauce	1 meal (9.5 oz)	250	9	3	30	20	21	—	40	860	650	4	—	400
Sirloin Of Beef In Wine Sauce	1 pkg (11 oz)	280	8	2	25	21	36	—	40	560	440	9	—	5000
Sirloin Tips And Country Vegetables	1 meal (10 oz)	290	17	—	40	17	19	—	60	810	430	15	—	1750
Special Recipe Sirloin Of Beef	1 meal (11 oz)	250	9	3	60	18	29	—	60	560	450	6	—	5000
Stuffed Turkey Breast	1 pkg (11 oz)	250	6	2	35	21	31	—	—	570	520	60	—	3000
Swedish Meatballs With Noodles	1 meal (10 oz)	590	38	—	145	24	37	—	100	920	350	4	—	1000
Sweet And Sour Chicken	1 meal (10 oz)	340	5	—	30	17	55	—	60	620	240	12	—	2250
Teriyaki Beef	1 pkg (10.75 oz)	260	7	2	30	19	37	—	40	530	390	21	—	2500
Teriyaki Chicken Breast	1 meal (11 oz)	300	8	1	30	18	41	—	40	480	480	27	—	1250

FOOD	PORTION	CALORIES	FAT	SAT FAT	CHOL	PROTEIN	CARBO	FIBER	CALCIUM	SOD	POTAS	VIT C	FOLIC	VIT A
GREEN GIANT														
Create A Meal Broccoli Stir Fry as prep	1⅓ cups (9.9 oz)	290	13	3	60	27	16	4	60	1160	—	54	—	750
Create A Meal Cheese & Herb Primavera as prep	1¼ cups (10 oz)	330	11	4	65	30	27	4	150	920	—	30	—	750
Create A Meal Garlic Herb as prep	1¼ cups (10 oz)	340	14	6	145	24	30	4	150	670	—	24	—	2500
Create A Meal Hearty Vegetable Stew as prep	1¼ cups (10 oz)	280	9	2	55	23	25	3	40	1000	—	15	—	3000
Create A Meal Lemon Herb as prep	1½ cups (10 oz)	360	11	4	65	28	37	3	100	830	—	24	—	500
Create A Meal Mushroom & Wine as prep	1¼ cups (10 oz)	390	16	6	75	28	31	4	40	910	—	6	—	2000
Create A Meal Vegetable Almond Stir Fry as prep	1⅓ cups (10 oz)	320	11	2	65	32	22	6	80	1190	—	9	—	5500
HEALTHY CHOICE														
Beef & Peppers Cantonese	1 meal (11.5 oz)	270	5	3	35	16	40	5	40	560	—	21	—	500
Beef Pepper Steak Oriental	1 meal (9.5 oz)	250	4	2	35	19	34	3	20	470	—	9	—	200
Beef Tips Francais	1 meal (9.5 oz)	280	5	2	30	20	40	4	20	520	—	0	—	0
Beef Tips With Sauce	1 meal (11 oz)	290	6	3	40	19	40	5	20	270	—	21	—	500
Chicken Cantonese	1 meal (11.25)	210	1	0	30	19	31	5	20	360	—	30	—	500
Chicken Parmigiana	1 meal (11.5 oz)	300	2	1	35	23	47	6	100	490	—	30	—	5000
Chicken & Vegetables Marsala	1 meal (11.5 oz)	220	1	0	30	22	32	3	60	440	—	4	—	500
Chicken Bangkok	1 meal (9.5 oz)	270	4	1	45	25	35	5	20	390	—	0	—	100
Chicken Dijon	1 meal (11 oz)	280	4	2	30	21	41	9	40	410	—	18	—	500
Chicken Imperial	1 meal (9 oz)	230	4	1	40	17	31	3	20	470	—	9	—	750
Chicken Picante	1 meal (11.25 oz)	220	2	2	35	19	30	6	100	330	—	30	—	300
Chicken Teriyaki	1 meal (12.25 oz)	270	2	1	40	21	42	5	20	420	—	27	—	1500
Classics Beef Broccoli Beijing	1 meal (12 oz)	330	3	1	20	20	55	5	40	500	—	18	—	1000
Classics Cacciatore Chicken	1 meal (12.5 oz)	260	3	1	25	22	36	6	40	510	—	4	—	750

FOOD	PORTION	CALORIES	FAT	SAT FAT	CHOL	PROTEIN	CARBO	FIBER	CALCIUM	SOD	POTAS	VIT C	FOLIC	VIT A
HEALTHY CHOICE (CONT.)														
Classics Chicken Fransesca	1 meal (12.5 oz)	360	5	2	30	27	51	5	100	500	—	6	—	400
Classics Country Inn Roast Turkey	1 meal (10 oz)	250	4	1	30	26	29	6	40	530	—	0	—	1500
Classics Ginger Chicken Hunan	1 meal (12.6 oz)	350	3	1	25	24	59	5	60	430	—	0	—	750
Classics Mesquite Beef Barbecue	1 meal (11 oz)	310	4	2	45	23	45	6	40	490	—	0	—	200
Classics Salisbury Steak	1 meal (11 oz)	260	6	3	30	18	32	5	40	500	—	5	—	200
Classics Sesame Chicken Shanghai	1 meal (12 oz)	310	5	1	30	24	42	5	40	460	—	5	—	500
Classics Shrimp & Vegetables Maria	1 meal (12.5 oz)	260	2	1	35	15	46	5	40	540	—	21	—	500
Country Glazed Chicken	1 meal (8.5 oz)	200	2	1	30	17	30	3	20	480	—	0	—	0
Country Herb Chicken	1 meal (11.5 oz)	270	4	2	35	20	40	6	40	340	—	21	—	1500
Country Roast Turkey With Mushroom	1 meal (8.5 oz)	220	4	1	25	19	28	3	20	440	—	0	—	750
Country Turkey & Pasta	1 meal (12.6 oz)	300	4	2	35	22	42	6	80	450	—	114	—	200
Homestyle Turkey With Vegetables	1 meal (9.5 oz)	260	2	1	35	26	34	3	40	490	—	6	—	400
Honey Mustard Chicken	1 meal (9.5 oz)	260	2	0	30	21	40	4	20	550	—	0	—	1500
Lemon Pepper Fish	1 meal (10.7 oz)	290	5	1	25	14	47	7	20	360	—	30	—	500
Mandarin Chicken	1 meal (10 oz)	280	3	0	25	20	44	4	20	520	—	15	—	1500
Mesquite Chicken Barbecue	1 meal (10.5 oz)	320	2	1	35	19	55	6	20	290	—	390	—	500
Shrimp Marinara	1 meal (10.5 oz)	220	1	0	50	10	44	5	60	220	—	27	—	300
Smoky Chicken Barbecue	1 meal (12.75 oz)	380	5	2	50	25	57	7	40	450	—	60	—	750
Southwestern Glazed Chicken	1 meal (12.5 oz)	300	3	1	45	20	48	6	20	430	—	156	—	2500
Sweet & Sour Chicken	1 meal (11.5 oz)	310	5	1	50	23	42	5	40	250	—	84	—	750
Traditional Breast Of Turkey	1 meal (10.5 oz)	280	3	1	45	22	40	7	20	460	—	60	—	400
Traditional Meat Loaf	1 meal (12 oz)	320	8	4	35	16	46	7	40	460	—	54	—	750
Traditional Beef Tips	1 meal (11.25 oz)	260	5	2	40	20	32	6	20	390	—	42	—	3000
Tradtional Salisbury Steak	1 meal (11.5 oz)	320	6	3	45	18	48	7	40	470	—	156	—	1500

FOOD	PORTION	CALORIES	FAT	SAT FAT	CHOL	PROTEIN	CARBO	FIBER	CALCIUM	SOD	POTAS	VIT C	FOLIC	VIT A
HEALTHY CHOICE (CONT.)														
Yankee Pot Roast	1 meal (11 oz)	280	5	2	45	19	38	5	40	460	—	42	—	3000
KID CUISINE														
Chicken Sandwiche	1 pkg (9.43 oz)	480	15	4	20	17	71	4	150	770	—	0	—	0
Chicken Nuggets	1 pkg (9.1 oz)	440	16	5	30	18	54	5	100	1070	—	—	—	—
Fish Sticks	1 pkg (8.25 oz)	370	12	3	15	11	55	4	60	550	—	0	—	0
Fried Chicken	1 pkg (10.1 oz)	440	19	5	40	18	49	5	80	940	—	0	—	0
Hot Dogs w/ Buns	6.7 oz	450	19	—	40	13	57	—	100	880	430	4	—	—
Macaroni & Beef	1 pkg (9.6 oz)	370	9	4	30	12	58	5	—	900	—	0	—	100
LE MENU														
Beef Sirlion Tips	11½ oz	400	18	—	—	30	29	—	60	760	—	15	—	300
Beef Stroganoff	10 oz	430	24	—	—	26	28	—	100	980	—	1	—	500
Chicken Parmigiana	11¾ oz	410	20	—	—	26	31	—	100	1030	—	6	—	400
Chicken A La King	10¼ oz	330	13	—	—	23	29	—	80	830	—	4	—	300
Chicken Cordon Bleu	11 oz	460	20	—	—	23	47	—	100	850	—	4	—	7000
Chicken In Wine Sauce	10 oz	280	7	—	—	26	27	—	60	680	—	4	—	4000
Chopped Sirloin Beef	12¼ oz	430	24	—	—	25	28	—	150	1010	—	5	—	100
Entree LightStyle Chicken A La King	8¼ oz	240	5	—	30	19	29	—	80	670	—	—	—	100
Entree LightStyle Chicken Dijon	8 oz	240	7	—	40	22	21	—	80	500	—	6	—	1250
Entree LightStyle Empress Chicken	8¼ oz	210	5	—	30	16	26	—	20	690	—	9	—	1500
Entree LightStyle Glazed Turkey	8¼ oz	260	6	—	35	18	34	—	20	720	—	4	—	100
Entree LightStyle Herb Roast Chicken	7¾ oz	260	6	—	45	22	29	—	20	500	—	1	—	350
Entree LightStyle Swedish Meatballs	8 oz	260	8	—	40	18	30	—	60	700	—	—	—	1250
Entree LightStyle Traditional Turkey	8 oz	200	5	—	25	19	19	—	40	610	—	12	—	1500
Ham Steak	10 oz	300	11	—	—	19	31	—	60	1500	—	18	—	6000
LightStyle Glazed Chicken Breast	10 oz	230	3	—	55	25	25	—	60	480	—	—	—	3500
LightStyle Herb Roasted Chicken	10 oz	240	7	—	70	27	18	—	60	400	—	18	—	400
LightStyle Salisbury Steak	10 oz	280	9	—	35	18	31	—	100	400	—	—	—	5000

FOOD	PORTION	CALORIES	FAT	SAT FAT	CHOL	PROTEIN	CARBO	FIBER	CALCIUM	SOD	POTAS	VIT C	FOLIC	VIT A
LE MENU (CONT.)														
LightStyle Sliced Turkey	10 oz	210	5	—	30	21	21	—	60	540	—	36	—	3500
LightStyle Sweet & Sour Chicken	10 oz	250	7	—	—	18	29	—	20	530	—	36	—	2000
LightStyle Turkey Divan	10 oz	260	7	—	60	25	23	—	100	420	—	36	—	750
LightStyle Veal Marsala	10 oz	230	3	—	75	22	28	—	40	700	—	—	—	2000
Pepper Steak	11½ oz	370	13	—	—	26	36	—	40	1020	—	6	—	1000
Salisbury Steak	10½ oz	370	20	—	—	20	28	—	100	880	—	—	—	300
Sliced Breast Of Turkey w/ Mushroom Gravy	10½ oz	300	7	—	—	22	38	—	40	1020	—	9	—	2500
Sweet & Sour Chicken	11¼ oz	400	18	—	—	19	41	—	60	1020	—	4	—	1000
Veal Parmigiana	11½ oz	390	17	—	—	24	36	—	200	840	—	6	—	750
Yankee Pot Roast	10 oz	330	13	—	—	26	27	—	40	700	—	6	—	6000
LEAN CUISINE														
American Favorite Baked Chicken	1 pkg (8.6 oz)	230	4	2	35	18	31	5	60	520	500	1	—	300
American Favorite Baked Fish	1 pkg (9 oz)	270	6	2	45	17	36	3	150	540	470	6	—	1500
American Favorite Beef Pot Roast	1 pkg (9 oz)	210	6	2	30	13	25	6	40	570	630	2	—	1000
American Favorite Beef Tips Barbecue	1 pkg (8.75 oz)	290	6	2	30	13	47	7	40	560	1130	2	—	200
American Favorite Chicken Medallions w/ Creamy Cheese	1 pkg (9.37 oz)	260	8	3	50	16	31	4	200	590	610	18	—	1500
American Favorite Country Vegetables & Beef	1 pkg (9 oz)	210	4	1	25	11	33	3	40	590	610	6	—	1000
American Favorite Honey Roasted Chicken	1 pkg (8.5 oz)	290	6	2	25	14	46	5	40	590	750	12	—	300
American Favorite Meatloaf & Whipped Potatoes	1 pkg (9.4 oz)	250	6	3	50	18	30	4	60	590	650	0	—	100
American Favorite Oven Roasted Beef	1 pkg (9.25 oz)	260	8	3	50	18	28	4	150	590	670	15	—	300
American Favorite Roasted Turkey Breast	1 pkg (9.75 oz)	270	3	1	20	13	49	5	40	590	460	48	—	0
American Favorite Salisbury Steak	1 pkg (9.5 oz)	280	8	4	60	24	29	4	150	590	600	0	—	200

FOOD	PORTION	CALORIES	FAT	SAT FAT	CHOL	PROTEIN	CARBO	FIBER	CALCIUM	SOD	POTAS	VIT C	FOLIC	VIT A
LEAN CUISINE (CONT.)														
American Favorite Scalloped Potatoes w/ Turkey Ham	1 pkg (10 oz)	250	6	3	25	10	38	6	150	590	560	6	—	4000
Cafe Classics Chicken Carbonara	1 pkg (9 oz)	280	8	2	30	18	33	2	100	580	370	9	—	200
Cafe Classics Chicken Mediterranean	1 pkg (10.5 oz)	270	4	1	25	18	40	2	60	590	730	4	—	500
Cafe Classics Chicken Breast In Wine Sauce	1 pkg (8.1 oz)	210	6	2	35	7	23	2	100	560	520	0	—	1000
Cafe Classics Chicken Parmesan	1 meal (10.9 oz)	220	5	2	50	18	27	4	150	560	580	5	—	1500
Cafe Classics Chicken Piccata	1 pkg (9 oz)	270	6	2	25	13	41	2	60	530	260	12	—	300
Cafe Classics Chicken w/ Basil Cream Sauce	1 pkg (8.5 oz)	270	7	2	35	16	35	3	100	580	300	21	—	500
Cafe Classics Glazed Turkey	1 pkg (9 oz)	240	5	1	30	19	37	5	100	590	550	0	—	4500
Cafe Classics Grilled Chicken Salsa	1 pkg (8.9 oz)	270	7	3	45	15	36	4	100	570	480	5	—	300
Cafe Classics Herb Roasted Chicken	1 pkg (8 oz)	210	5	1	40	13	27	3	60	540	710	42	—	500
Cafe Classics Honey Mustard Chicken	1 pkg (8 oz)	250	5	2	35	12	39	3	20	520	250	9	—	1000
Cafe Classics Mesquite Beef w/ Rice	1 pkg (9 oz)	290	6	2	25	16	42	5	60	510	640	12	—	400
Cafe Classics Sirlion Beef Peppercorn	1 pkg (8.75 oz)	220	7	2	35	15	23	2	80	580	770	0	—	750
Chicken & Vegetables	1 pkg (10.5 oz)	250	6	1	30	17	31	4	100	590	400	5	—	1250
Chicken A L'Orange	1 pkg (9 oz)	250	2	1	40	19	40	3	20	340	400	18	—	1250
Chicken In Peanut Sauce	1 pkg (9 oz)	290	6	1	30	23	35	4	100	550	490	5	—	750
Fiesta Chicken w/ Rice & Vegetables	1 pkg (8.5 oz)	250	5	1	35	17	34	3	20	540	410	30	—	1000
Glazed Chicken w/ Vegetable Rice	1 pkg (8.5 oz)	240	6	1	55	22	25	0	0	480	340	4	—	100
Homestyle Turkey	1 pkg (9.4 oz)	230	5	1	40	17	30	3	100	590	340	0	—	1500
Mandarin Chicken	1 pkg (9 oz)	250	4	1	25	15	38	3	40	590	380	0	—	2000

FOOD	PORTION	CALORIES	FAT	SAT FAT	CHOL	PROTEIN	CARBO	FIBER	CALCIUM	SOD	POTAS	VIT C	FOLIC	VIT A
LEAN CUISINE (CONT.)														
Oriental Beef	1 pkg (9.25 oz)	220	5	2	30	13	33	2	20	590	350	9	—	1000
Stuffed Cabbage w/ Whipped Potatoes	1 pkg (9.5 oz)	170	5	2	15	8	24	5	60	380	440	2	—	400
Swedish Meatballs w/ Pasta	1 pkg (9.1 oz)	280	7	3	50	20	33	3	60	590	360	0	—	100
LIFE CHOICE														
Garden Potato Casserole	1 meal (13.4 oz)	160	1	0	5	8	37	9	200	590	—	27	—	2000
MORTON														
Breaded Chicken Pattie	1 meal (6.75 oz)	280	15	3	20	11	24	4	40	840	—	0	—	3000
Chicken Nugget	1 meal (7 oz)	320	17	4	30	13	30	3	40	460	—	2	—	2000
Fried Chicken	1 meal (9 oz)	420	25	8	85	20	30	4	60	1000	—	9	—	2250
Meatloaf	1 meal (9 oz)	250	13	4	20	9	24	5	40	1110	—	0	—	500
Mexican	1 meal (10 oz)	260	7	3	5	8	40	8	80	1000	—	6	—	500
Salisbury Steak	1 meal (9 oz)	210	9	4	20	9	23	3	40	950	—	2	—	2000
Turkey	1 meal (9 oz)	230	8	3	35	14	27	5	40	1090	—	0	—	2500
Veal Parmagiana	1 meal (8.75 oz)	280	13	4	20	8	30	4	40	950	—	18	—	2250
Western	1 meal (9 oz)	290	16	7	25	11	26	6	40	1210	—	2	—	0
PATIO														
Chili	1 cup (8 oz)	260	13	1	55	23	13	4	40	1010	—	0	—	500
Ranchera	1 pkg (13 oz)	410	15	6	25	13	14	14	100	2400	—	6	—	500
STOUFFER'S														
Baked Chicken Breast w/ Mashed Potatoes	1 serv (12.2 oz)	330	14	5	60	25	25	3	20	1070	716	2	—	200
Beef Stroganoff	1 pkg (9.75 oz)	390	20	7	85	23	30	2	40	1100	610	0	—	100
Chicken A La King	1 pkg (9.5 oz)	350	13	4	40	17	41	2	100	800	310	6	—	100
Creamed Chicken	1 pkg (6.5 oz)	260	19	10	80	15	8	0	60	680	290	0	—	0
Creamed Chipped Beef	½ cup (5.5 oz)	160	11	3	40	10	6	1	100	690	240	0	—	0
Creamy Chicken & Broccoli	1 pkg (8.9 oz)	320	15	5	60	19	26	2	200	820	400	9	—	0
Escalloped Chicken & Noodles	1 pkg (10 oz)	430	27	5	50	17	30	3	100	1120	330	0	—	0
Fish w/ Macaroni & Cheese	1 serv (9.5 oz)	460	20	6	55	22	47	2	250	970	379	4	—	0
Glazed Chicken w/ Rice	1 serv (11.8 oz)	290	6	1	45	21	39	2	20	810	349	0	—	100
Green Pepper Steak	1 pkg (10.5 oz)	330	9	3	35	17	45	3	20	650	680	12	—	200

FOOD	PORTION	CALORIES	FAT	SAT FAT	CHOL	PROTEIN	CARBO	FIBER	CALCIUM	SOD	POTAS	VIT C	FOLIC	VIT A
STOUFFER'S (CONT.)														
Homestyle Beef Pot Roast & Browned Potatoes	1 pkg (8.9 oz)	250	8	3	35	16	29	4	20	780	730	21	—	1000
Homestyle Fish Filet w/ Macaroni & Cheese	1 pkg (9 oz)	430	21	5	70	24	37	2	150	930	450	0	—	100
Homestyle Fried Chicken & Whipped Potatoes	1 pkg (7.5 oz)	310	12	4	45	17	33	5	20	680	430	1	—	100
Homestyle Meatloaf & Whipped Potatoes	1 pkg (9.9 oz)	330	16	6	70	20	26	3	40	850	510	0	—	200
Homestyle Roast Turkey w/ Gravy Stuffing & Whipped Potatoes	1 pkg (9.6 oz)	320	13	4	50	19	31	3	40	950	410	0	—	100
Homestyle Salisbury Steak & Gravy & Macaroni & Cheese	1 pkg (9.6 oz)	350	16	7	70	24	27	2	150	1290	320	0	—	300
Honestyle Baked Chicken & Gravy & Whipped Potatoes	1 pkg (8.9 oz)	270	12	3	75	22	19	2	20	750	570	1	—	0
Meatloaf	1 serv (5.5 oz)	210	12	4	60	16	9	1	40	520	250	0	—	100
Meatloaf w/ Whipped Potatoes	1 serv (11.5 oz)	380	18	7	70	22	33	4	60	950	551	4	—	200
Stuffed Pepper	1 pkg (10 oz)	200	5	2	20	11	27	3	20	820	470	48	—	400
Swedish Meatballs	1 pkg (10.25 oz)	480	24	9	60	24	43	3	60	960	330	0	—	100
SWANSON														
Beans & Franks	10½ oz	440	19	—	—	14	53	—	150	900	—	9	—	300
Beef	11¼ oz	310	6	—	—	26	38	—	40	770	—	5	—	300
Beef In Barbecue Sauce	11 oz	460	17	—	—	30	51	—	80	860	—	5	—	1250
Chopped Sirloin Beef	10¾ oz	340	16	—	—	20	28	—	60	790	—	4	—	5000
Fish 'n' Chips	10 oz	500	21	—	—	20	60	—	60	960	—	2	—	400
Fried Chicken Dark Meat	9¾ oz	560	28	—	—	22	55	—	60	1130	—	4	—	100
Fried Chicken White Meat	10¼ oz	550	25	—	—	22	60	—	60	1460	—	2	—	100
Homestyle Chicken Cacciatore	10.95 oz	260	8	—	—	15	33	—	80	1030	—	21	—	750
Homestyle Chicken Nibbles	4¼ oz	340	20	—	—	10	29	—	20	730	—	—	—	—

FOOD	PORTION	CALORIES	FAT	SAT FAT	CHOL	PROTEIN	CARBO	FIBER	CALCIUM	SOD	POTAS	VIT C	FOLIC	VIT A
SWANSON (CONT.)														
Homestyle Fish & Fries	6½ oz	340	16	—	—	11	37	—	20	670	—	—	—	—
Homestyle Fried Chicken	7 oz	390	21	—	—	18	33	—	40	1100	—	—	—	—
Homestyle Salisbury Steak	10 oz	320	16	—	—	21	22	—	40	980	—	—	—	—
Homestyle Scalloped Potatoes & Ham	9 oz	300	13	—	—	19	26	—	350	1080	—	9	—	200
Homestyle Seafood Creole With Rice	9 oz	240	6	—	—	7	40	—	100	810	—	30	—	750
Homestyle Sirloin Tips In Burgundy Sauce	7 oz	160	5	—	—	12	16	—	40	550	—	27	—	4000
Homestyle Turkey With Dressing & Potatoes	9 oz	290	11	—	—	18	30	—	40	1010	—	2	—	300
Homestyle Veal Parmigiana	10 oz	330	13	—	—	19	33	—	80	960	—	6	—	300
Hungry-Man Boneless Chicken	17¾ oz	700	28	—	—	48	65	—	80	1530	—	6	—	500
Hungry-Man Chopped Beef Steak	16¾ oz	640	37	—	—	35	41	—	60	1600	—	9	—	400
Hungry-Man Fried Chicken Dark Meat	14¼ oz	860	45	—	—	36	77	—	60	1660	—	5	—	—
Hungry-Man Fried Chicken White Meat	14¼ oz	870	46	—	—	35	80	—	80	2150	—	5	—	—
Hungry-Man Salisbury Steak	16½ oz	680	41	—	—	41	37	—	300	1730	—	6	—	400
Hungry-Man Sliced Beef	15¼ oz	450	12	—	—	37	49	—	40	1060	—	6	—	500
Hungry-Man Turkey	17 oz	550	18	—	—	36	61	—	80	1810	—	9	—	400
Hungry-Man Veal Parmigiana	18¼ oz	590	26	—	—	32	57	—	200	1840	—	15	—	1000
Loin Of Pork	10¾ oz	280	12	—	—	20	27	—	40	790	—	6	—	5000
Macaroni & Beef	12 oz	370	15	—	—	12	48	—	100	930	—	12	—	400
Meatloaf	10¾ oz	360	15	—	—	15	41	—	100	960	—	9	—	750
Noodles & Chicken	10½ oz	280	8	—	—	7	45	—	80	740	—	2	—	4000
Salisbury Steak	10¾ oz	400	17	—	—	18	43	—	60	880	—	4	—	200
Swedish Meatballs	8½ oz	360	20	—	—	19	26	—	80	790	—	—	—	300
Swiss Steak	10 oz	350	11	—	—	26	37	—	40	700	—	9	—	300
Turkey	11½ oz	350	11	—	—	21	42	—	60	1090	—	5	—	300
Veal Parmigiana	12¼ oz	430	20	—	—	20	42	—	150	1010	—	6	—	500
Western Style	11½ oz	430	19	—	—	22	43	—	80	1060	—	12	—	500

FOOD	PORTION	CALORIES	FAT	SAT FAT	CHOL	PROTEIN	CARBO	FIBER	CALCIUM	SOD	POTAS	VIT C	FOLIC	VIT A
TYSON														
Beef Champignon	1 pkg (10.5 oz)	370	15	—	51	27	31	—	—	830	—	—	—	—
Chicken Picante	1 pkg (9 oz)	250	4	—	50	28	26	—	—	390	—	—	—	—
Chicken Supreme	1 pkg (9 oz)	230	6	—	51	21	23	—	—	480	—	—	—	—
Francais	1 pkg (9.5 oz)	280	14	—	54	19	20	—	—	1130	—	—	—	—
Glazed Chicken With Sauce	1 pkg (9.25 oz)	240	4	—	44	22	29	—	—	930	—	—	—	—
Grilled Chicken	1 pkg (7.75 oz)	220	3	—	55	26	22	—	—	520	—	—	—	—
Grilled Italian Chicken	1 pkg (9 oz)	210	3	—	40	28	19	—	—	420	—	—	—	—
Healthy Portions BBQ Chicken	1 pkg (12.5 oz)	400	8	—	50	27	56	—	—	600	—	—	—	—
Healthy Portions Chicken Marinara	1 pkg (13.75 oz)	340	7	—	45	31	37	—	—	590	—	—	—	—
Healthy Portions Herb Chicken	1 pkg (13.75 oz)	340	4	—	50	32	43	—	—	550	—	—	—	—
Healthy Portions Honey Mushtard Chicken	1 pkg (13.75 oz)	390	6	—	—	31	52	—	—	520	—	—	—	—
Healthy Portions Italian Style Chicken	1 pkg (13.75 oz)	310	4	—	50	30	38	—	—	600	—	—	—	—
Healthy Portions Mesquite Chicken	1 pkg (13.25 oz)	330	5	—	45	34	38	—	—	600	—	—	—	—
Healthy Portions Salsa Chicken	1 pkg (13.75 oz)	370	6	—	45	27	52	—	—	470	—	—	—	—
Healthy Portions Sesame Chicken	1 pkg (13.5 oz)	400	6	—	45	27	59	—	—	400	—	—	—	—
Honey Roasted Chicken	1 pkg (9 oz)	220	4	—	48	26	23	—	—	500	—	—	—	—
Kiev	1 pkg (9.25 oz)	450	25	—	78	18	39	—	—	950	—	—	—	—
Marsala	1 pkg (9 oz)	200	4	—	52	22	19	—	—	670	—	—	—	—
Mexquite	1 pkg (9 oz)	320	8	—	55	23	39	—	—	660	—	—	—	—
Picatta	1 pkg (9 oz)	200	4	—	60	24	18	—	—	550	—	—	—	—
Roasted Chicken	1 pkg (9 oz)	200	2	—	42	21	21	—	—	430	—	—	—	—
Sweet & Sour	1 pkg (11 oz)	420	15	—	—	22	50	—	—	850	—	—	—	—
Turkey With Gravy	1 pkg (9.5 oz)	320	12	—	35	19	34	—	—	900	—	—	—	—
ULTRA SLIM-FAST														
Beef Pepper Steak	12 oz	270	4	—	45	22	36	0	20	590	360	30	60	400
Chicken Fettucini	12 oz	380	12	—	65	31	38	1	200	980	280	2	40	—
Chicken & Vegetable	12 oz	290	3	—	30	24	45	4	60	850	350	2	60	2000
Country Style Vegetable & Beef Tips	12 oz	230	5	—	45	21	26	4	60	960	520	5	40	4000

FOOD	PORTION	CALORIES	FAT	SAT FAT	CHOL	PROTEIN	CARBO	FIBER	CALCIUM	SOD	POTAS	VIT C	FOLIC	VIT A
ULTRA SLIM-FAST (CONT.)														
Mesquite Chicken	12 oz	360	1	—	65	29	61	5	60	300	780	15	40	1000
Roasted Chicken In Mushroom Sauce	12 oz	280	6	—	55	25	30	0	20	830	470	1	24	1750
Shrimp Creole	12 oz	240	4	—	80	12	45	5	100	730	470	27	40	750
Shrimp Marinara	12 oz	290	3	—	70	17	53	0	100	880	500	12	100	750
Sweet & Sour Chicken	12 oz	330	2	—	45	20	57	0	40	340	350	24	40	250
Turkey Medallions In Herb Sauce	12 oz	280	6	—	40	23	33	0	40	950	450	—	60	—
WEIGHT WATCHERS														
Smart One Grilled Salisbury Steak	1 pkg (8.5 oz)	260	10	5	40	19	24	3	100	620	—	0	—	200
Smart Ones Fiesta Chicken	1 pkg (8.5 oz)	220	2	1	25	12	38	5	40	540	—	12	—	400
Smart Ones Honey Mustard Chicken	1 pkg (8.5 oz)	200	2	1	30	11	37	3	40	370	—	9	—	500
Smart Ones Lemon Herb Chicken Piccata	1 pkg (8.5 oz)	200	2	1	25	11	34	3	20	460	—	1	—	1000
Smart Ones Pepper Steak	1 pkg (10 oz)	240	5	2	35	18	33	4	40	690	—	12	—	2000
Smart Ones Risotto w/ Cheese & Mushrooms	1 pkg (10 oz)	290	8	4	20	11	44	4	200	540	—	9	—	1250
Smart Ones Roast Turkey Medallions & Mushrooms	1 pkg (8.5 oz)	190	2	1	20	10	32	2	20	530	—	5	—	500
Smart Ones Shrimp Marinara	1 pkg (9 oz)	190	2	1	40	9	35	4	100	470	—	6	—	750
Smart Ones Stuffed Turkey Breast	1 pkg (10 oz)	260	7	2	20	13	37	5	80	680	—	6	—	1000
Smart Ones Swedish Meatballs	1 pkg (9 oz)	300	10	4	50	19	33	2	100	510	—	2	—	300
SHELF-STABLE														
MY OWN MEAL														
Beef Stew	1 pkg (10 oz)	260	11	3	55	19	22	4	60	480	—	24	—	3000
Chicken Mediterranean	1 pkg (10 oz)	270	9	2	45	19	28	4	60	320	—	15	—	500
Chicken Noodles	1 pkg (10 oz)	270	8	2	65	20	29	3	40	900	—	4	—	5000
Chicken & Black Beans	1 pkg (10 oz)	240	5	1	40	20	30	6	40	460	—	18	—	750
Old World Stew	1 pkg (10 oz)	310	12	4	55	20	31	3	40	510	—	9	—	300

DIP

FOOD	PORTION	CALORIES	FAT	SAT FAT	CHOL	PROTEIN	CARBO	FIBER	CALCIUM	SOD	POTAS	VIT C	FOLIC	VIT A
BREAKSTONE'S														
Bacon & Onion	2 tbsp (1.1 oz)	60	5	3	20	2	2	0	20	180	50	0	—	100
Chesapeake Clam	2 tbsp (1.1 oz)	50	4	3	20	1	1	0	20	180	30	0	—	100

FOOD	PORTION	CALORIES	FAT	SAT FAT	CHOL	PROTEIN	CARBO	FIBER	CALCIUM	SOD	POTAS	VIT C	FOLIC	VIT A
BREAKSTONE'S (CONT.)														
Free Creamy Salsa	2 tbsp (1.1 oz)	20	0	0	<5	1	3	0	60	240	85	0	—	0
Free French Onion	2 tbsp (1.1 oz)	25	0	0	<5	2	4	0	40	260	85	0	—	0
Free Ranch	2 tbsp (1.1 oz)	25	0	0	<5	2	4	0	60	330	85	0	—	0
French Onion	2 tbsp (1.1 oz)	50	5	3	20	1	2	0	20	160	45	0	—	200
Toasted Onion	2 tbsp (1.1 oz)	50	5	3	20	1	2	0	20	170	45	0	—	200
CHEEZ WHIZ														
Medium Cheese & Salsa	2 tbsp (1.2 oz)	100	8	5	20	3	3	0	80	490	95	0	—	400
Mild Cheese & Salsa	2 tbsp (1.2 oz)	100	8	5	20	3	3	0	80	490	95	0	—	400
CHI-CHI'S														
Fiesta Bean	2 tbsp (0.9 oz)	35	2	1	0	1	4	1	0	140	—	0	—	0
Fiesta Cheese	2 tbsp (0.9 oz)	40	3	1	10	1	3	0	20	270	—	0	—	0
DURKEE														
Sour Cream as prep	2 tbsp	25	1	0	0	1	4	0	40	200	—	0	—	0
FRITO LAY														
Picante Sauce	1 oz	10	0	—	0	0	3	—	—	160	80	—	—	300
GUILTLESS GOURMET														
Black Bean Mild	1 oz	25	0	0	0	2	5	1	—	80	—	—	—	—
Black Bean Spicy	1 oz	25	0	0	0	2	5	1	—	80	—	—	—	—
Pinto Bean	1 oz	25	0	0	0	2	5	1	—	80	—	—	—	—
HAIN														
Hot Bean	4 tbsp	70	1	—	5	4	10	—	20	250	280	2	—	—
Mexican Bean	4 tbsp	60	1	—	5	4	9	—	20	260	260	1	—	—
Onion Bean	4 tbsp	70	1	—	5	4	10	—	20	270	270	1	—	—
Taco Dip & Sauce	4 tbsp	25	1	—	5	5	1	—	—	350	225	—	—	—
HELUVA GOOD CHEESE														
Bacon Horseradish	2 tbsp (1.1 oz)	60	5	3	20	1	2	0	40	200	—	0	—	200
Clam	2 tbsp (1.1 oz)	50	5	3	20	1	2	0	40	130	—	0	—	200
French Onion	2 tbsp (1.1 oz)	50	5	3	20	1	2	0	40	160	—	0	—	200
Homestyle Onion	2 tbsp (1.1 oz)	60	5	3	20	1	3	0	40	290	—	0	—	200
Light French Onion	2 tbsp (1.1 oz)	35	2	1	10	1	3	0	60	180	—	0	—	100
Light Jalapeno Cheddar	2 tbsp (1.1 oz)	40	2	2	10	2	3	0	40	160	—	0	—	100
Ranch	2 tbsp (1.1 oz)	60	5	3	20	1	2	0	40	180	—	0	—	200
KNUDSEN														
Free Creamy Salsa	2 tbsp (1.1 oz)	20	0	0	<5	1	3	0	60	240	85	0	—	0
Free French Onion	2 tbsp (1.1 oz)	25	0	0	<5	2	4	0	40	260	85	0	—	0
Free Ranch	2 tbsp (1.1 oz)	25	0	0	<5	2	4	0	60	330	85	0	—	0
KRAFT														
Avocado	2 tbsp (1.1 oz)	60	4	3	0	1	4	0	0	240	25	0	—	0
Bacon & Horseradish	2 tbsp (1.1 oz)	60	5	3	0	1	3	0	0	220	25	0	—	0
Clam	2 tbsp (1.1 oz)	60	4	3	0	1	3	0	0	250	20	0	—	0
Free French Onion	2 tbsp (1.1 oz)	25	0	0	<5	2	4	0	40	260	85	0	—	0

FOOD	PORTION	CALORIES	FAT	SAT FAT	CHOL	PROTEIN	CARBO	FIBER	CALCIUM	SOD	POTAS	VIT C	FOLIC	VIT A
KRAFT (CONT.)														
Free Ranch	2 tbsp (1.1 oz)	25	0	0	<5	2	4	0	60	330	85	0	—	0
Free Salsa	2 tbsp (1.1 oz)	20	0	0	<5	1	3	0	60	240	85	0	—	0
French Onion	2 tbsp (1.1 oz)	60	4	3	0	1	4	0	0	230	25	0	—	0
Green Onion	2 tbsp (1.1 oz)	60	4	3	0	1	4	0	0	190	20	0	—	0
Jalapeno Cheese	2 tbsp (1.1 oz)	60	4	3	0	1	3	0	0	260	25	0	—	0
Premium Sour Cream	2 tbsp (1.1 oz)	50	4	3	20	1	1	0	20	180	30	0	—	100
Premium Sour Cream Bacon & Horseradish	2 tbsp (1.1 oz)	60	5	3	15	2	2	0	20	240	45	0	—	100
Premium Sour Cream Bacon & Onion	2 tbsp (1.1 oz)	60	5	3	20	2	2	0	20	180	50	0	—	100
Premium Sour Cream Creamy Onion	2 tbsp (1.1 oz)	45	4	3	15	1	2	0	20	160	40	0	—	100
Premium Sour Cream French Onion	2 tbsp (1.1 oz)	45	4	3	15	tr	2	0	20	160	40	0	—	100
Premium Sour Cream Ranch	2 tbsp (1.1 oz)	50	4	3	15	tr	2	0	20	230	40	0	—	100
Ranch	2 tbsp (1.1 oz)	60	5	3	0	1	3	0	0	210	20	0	—	0
LAY'S														
Low Fat Sour Cream & Onion	2 tbsp (1 oz)	40	1	tr	<5	1	6	tr	0	230	14	0	—	0
LOUISE'S														
Fat Free Honey Mustard	1 oz	40	0	0	0	1	9	0	—	170	—	—	—	—
Fat Free Sour Cream & Onion	1 oz	25	0	0	0	1	4	0	—	195	—	—	—	—
Fat Free White Cheese Peppercorn	1 oz	25	0	0	0	1	4	0	—	195	—	—	—	—
MARZETTI														
Blue Cheese Veggie	2 tbsp	200	21	4	20	1	1	0	20	230	—	0	—	0
Lemon Dill Veggie	2 tbsp	140	14	3	25	1	2	0	0	190	—	1	—	0
Light Ranch Veggie	2 tbsp	60	7	2	10	0	5	1	0	290	—	0	—	100
Ranch Veggie	2 tbsp	140	14	3	25	1	1	0	0	200	—	0	—	100
Sour Cream & Onion	2 tbsp	130	14	3	25	1	2	0	0	200	—	1	—	0
Southwestern Veggie	2 tbsp	130	14	3	25	1	1	0	0	170	—	1	—	0
Spinach Veggie	2 tbsp	130	13	3	20	1	1	0	0	220	—	0	—	300
OLD EL PASO														
Black Bean	2 tbsp (1 oz)	20	0	0	0	1	4	1	0	150	—	0	—	0
Cheese 'n Salsa Medium	2 tbsp (1 oz)	40	3	1	<5	tr	3	0	20	300	—	0	—	0

FOOD	PORTION	CALORIES	FAT	SAT FAT	CHOL	PROTEIN	CARBO	FIBER	CALCIUM	SOD	POTAS	VIT C	FOLIC	VIT A
OLD EL PASO (CONT.)														
Cheese 'n Salsa Mild	2 tbsp (1 oz)	40	3	1	<5	tr	3	0	20	300	—	0	—	0
Chunky Salsa Medium	2 tbsp (1 oz)	15	0	0	0	1	3	1	0	230	—	0	—	100
Chunky Salsa Mild	2 tbsp (1 oz)	15	0	0	0	1	3	1	0	230	—	0	—	100
Jalapeno	2 tbsp (1 oz)	30	1	0	<5	1	4	2	0	125	—	0	—	0
RUFFLES														
Low Fat French Onion	1 tbsp (1 oz)	40	1	tr	0	2	6	tr	0	230	18	0	—	0
SNYDER'S														
Mustard Pretzel	2 tbsp (1.2 oz)	90	4	2	20	1	13	1	10	20	—	1	—	0
TACO BELL														
Fat Free Black Bean	2 tbsp (1.2 oz)	30	0	0	0	2	6	2	0	220	—	0	—	0
Salsa Con Queso Medium	2 tbsp (1.2 oz)	45	3	1	<5	tr	5	tr	20	270	—	0	—	100
Salsa Con Queso Mild	2 tbsp (1.2 oz)	45	3	1	<5	tr	5	tr	20	270	—	0	—	100
TOSTITOS														
Low Fat Con Queso	2 tbsp (1 oz)	40	2	1	<5	1	5	tr	40	180	230	0	—	0
WISE														
Jalapeno Bean	2 tbsp	25	0	0	0	1	5	—	—	100	105	—	—	—
Taco	2 tbsp	12	0	0	0	0	3	—	—	115	85	—	—	750
DOCK														
fresh cooked	3½ oz	20	1	—	0	2	3	—	38	3	321	26	—	3474
raw chopped	½ cup	15	tr	—	0	1	2	—	29	3	261	32	—	2680
DOUGHNUTS														
(see also DUNKIN' DONUTS, WINCHELL'S*)*														
cake type unsugared	1 (1.6 oz)	198	11	2	18	2	23	1	21	257	60	—	4	27
chocolate glazed	1 (1.5 oz)	175	8	3	—	2	24	1	89	143	—	—	—	—
chocolate sugared	1 (1.5 oz)	175	8	3	—	2	24	1	89	143	—	—	—	—
chocolate coated	1 (1.5 oz)	204	13	4	—	2	21	1	15	185	—	—	—	—
creme filled	1 (3 oz)	307	21	6	20	6	26	—	22	262	68	—	—	—
french cruller glazed	1 (1.4 oz)	169	8	2	5	1	24	—	11	142	32	—	—	—
frosted	1 (1.5 oz)	204	13	4	—	2	21	1	15	185	—	—	—	—
honey bun	1 (2.1 oz)	242	14	3	4	4	27	1	26	205	65	—	13	—
jelly	1 (3 oz)	289	16	4	22	5	33	—	21	249	67	—	—	—
old fashioned	1 (1.6 oz)	198	11	2	18	2	23	1	21	257	60	—	4	27
sugared	1 (1.6 oz)	192	10	3	14	2	23	1	27	181	46	—	—	4
wheat glazed	1 (1.6 oz)	162	9	1	9	3	19	—	22	160	66	—	—	—
wheat sugared	1 (1.6 oz)	162	9	1	9	3	19	—	22	160	66	—	—	—
yeast glazed	1 (2.1 oz)	242	14	3	4	4	27	1	26	205	65	—	13	—

FOOD	PORTION	CALORIES	FAT	SAT FAT	CHOL	PROTEIN	CARBO	FIBER	CALCIUM	SOD	POTAS	VIT C	FOLIC	VIT A
DUTCH MILL														
Cider	1 (2.1 oz)	240	10	2	15	3	35	1	20	220	—	0	—	0
Cinnamon	1 (1.8 oz)	210	11	5	15	3	26	1	20	250	—	0	—	0
Donut Holes Double-Dipped Chocolate	3 (1.4 oz)	220	16	6	5	2	19	0	20	140	—	0	—	0
Donut Holes Shootin' Stars	3 (1.4 oz)	190	10	3	5	2	23	0	40	110	—	0	—	0
Double-Dipped Chocolate	1 (2.1 oz)	280	17	7	15	3	31	1	40	360	—	0	—	0
Glazed	1 (2.1 oz)	250	12	3	15	3	34	1	20	220	—	0	—	0
Glazed Chocolate	1 (2.4 oz)	270	11	3	15	3	40	1	20	380	—	0	—	0
Plain	1 (1.8 oz)	210	12	5	15	3	25	1	20	270	—	0	—	0
Sugared	1 (1.8 oz)	220	11	5	15	3	27	1	20	260	—	0	—	0
ENTENMANN'S														
Crumb Topped	1 (2.1 oz)	260	12	—	—	3	34	—	—	220	—	—	—	—
Devil's Food Crumb	1 (2.1 oz)	250	12	—	—	3	34	—	—	200	—	—	—	—
Rich Frosted	1 (2 oz)	280	18	—	—	3	27	—	—	210	—	—	—	—
FREIHOFER'S														
Assorted	1 (2 oz)	270	17	4	10	2	26	0	0	170	—	0	—	0
HOSTESS														
Assorted Regular	1 (1.6 oz)	200	11	6	10	3	23	tr	—	230	85	—	—	—
Cinnamon Family Pack	1 (1 oz)	110	5	2	5	2	15	tr	—	140	40	—	—	—
Cinnamon Swirl	1 (1.6 oz)	180	7	3	<5	3	28	tr	40	220	95	—	—	—
Crumb Regular	1 (1 oz)	130	8	4	5	1	14	tr	40	115	30	—	—	—
Frosted Regular	1 (1.4 oz)	180	11	7	5	2	20	1	—	170	125	—	—	—
Gem Donettes Cinnamon	6 (3 oz)	320	11	4	10	5	53	1	80	390	110	—	—	—
Gem Donettes Frosted	6 (3 oz)	390	23	15	10	5	42	2	20	360	260	—	—	—
Gem Donettes Frosted Strawberry Filled	3 (3 oz)	240	13	9	<5	3	29	1	—	210	160	—	—	—
Gem Donettes Powdered	6 (3 oz)	350	16	6	10	4	47	1	—	380	95	—	—	—
Gem Donettes Powdered Strawberry Filled	3 (3 oz)	210	9	4	<5	3	31	tr	—	210	60	—	—	—
Glazed Party	1 (2.3 oz)	260	10	5	5	4	39	1	60	310	135	—	—	—
Jumbo Frosted	1 (2 oz)	260	16	10	10	3	28	1	—	240	180	—	—	—
Jumbo Plain	1 (1.1 oz)	140	7	4	10	2	16	tr	—	190	50	—	—	—
Jumbo Powdered	1 (1.3 oz)	160	9	5	5	2	19	tr	—	170	85	—	—	—
Mini Chocolate	5 (2 oz)	220	9	0	35	4	33	1	20	220	200	—	—	—
O's Raspberry Filled Powdered	1 (2.2 oz)	230	10	4	5	3	35	tr	—	230	70	—	—	—

FOOD	PORTION	CALORIES	FAT	SAT FAT	CHOL	PROTEIN	CARBO	FIBER	CALCIUM	SOD	POTAS	VIT C	FOLIC	VIT A
HOSTESS (CONT.)														
Old Fashioned Glazed	1 (2.1 oz)	250	12	5	15	3	33	tr	100	230	75	—	—	—
Old Fashioned Glazed Honey Wheat	1 (2.1 oz)	250	12	5	25	3	33	1	150	270	75	—	—	—
Old Fashioned Plain	1 (1.5 oz)	170	9	4	10	3	21	tr	20	230	65	—	—	—
Plain Regular	1 (1 oz)	120	6	3	5	2	13	tr	—	160	45	—	—	—
Powdered Family Pack	1 (1 oz)	110	6	3	5	1	15	1	—	135	35	—	—	—
LITTLE DEBBIE														
Donut Sticks	1 pkg (1.6 oz)	210	13	3	5	2	25	1	40	210	—	0	—	0
Donut Sticks	1 pkg (2.5 oz)	320	19	5	10	3	37	1	60	310	—	0	—	0
Donut Sticks	1 pkg (3 oz)	390	23	6	10	4	45	1	80	370	—	0	—	0
Donut Sticks	1 pkg (2 oz)	250	15	4	5	2	30	1	60	250	—	0	—	0
TASTYKAKE														
Cinnamon	1 (47 g)	180	8	2	10	3	26	1	—	210	—	—	—	—
Frosted Rich	1 (57 g)	260	16	8	10	4	28	3	—	200	—	—	—	—
Frosted Rich Mini	1 (14 g)	44	3	2	5	1	8	1	—	60	—	—	—	—
Honey Wheat	1 (57 g)	210	8	2	10	3	32	1	—	200	—	—	—	—
Honey Wheat Mini	1 (12 g)	40	1	0	5	1	7	0	—	50	—	—	—	—
Orange Glazed	1 (57 g)	210	9	3	10	3	32	1	40	180	—	—	—	—
Plain	1 (47 g)	190	10	3	10	3	22	1	60	170	—	—	—	—
Powdered Sugar	1 (46 g)	180	9	2	24	3	24	1	200	220	—	—	—	—
Powdered Sugar Mini	1 (12 g)	40	1	0	5	1	7	0	—	70	—	—	—	—

DRESSING

(*see* STUFFING/DRESSING)

DRINK MIXERS

(*see also* SODA, MINERAL/BOTTLED WATER)

FOOD	PORTION	CALORIES	FAT	SAT FAT	CHOL	PROTEIN	CARBO	FIBER	CALCIUM	SOD	POTAS	VIT C	FOLIC	VIT A
whiskey sour mix	2 oz	55	0	0	0	0	14	—	1	66	18	2	0	14
whiskey sour mix as prep	3.6 oz	169	0	0	0	tr	16	—	47	48	4	1	0	5
BACARDI														
Margarita Mix w/ rum	8 fl oz	160	0	0	—	0	24	—	—	0	25	8	—	—
Margarita Mix w/o liquor	8 fl oz	100	0	0	0	0	25	—	—	0	—	—	—	—
Pina Colada	8 fl oz	140	0	0	0	0	34	—	—	10	—	—	—	—
Rum Runner	8 fl oz	140	0	0	0	0	35	—	—	10	—	—	—	—
Strawberry Daiquiri w/o liquor	8 fl oz	140	0	0	0	0	35	—	—	0	—	—	—	—
CANADA DRY														
Collins Mixer	8 fl oz	120	0	0	0	0	25	0	—	20	—	—	—	—
Sour Mixer	8 fl oz	90	0	0	0	0	22	0	—	25	—	—	—	—

FOOD	PORTION	CALORIES	FAT	SAT FAT	CHOL	PROTEIN	CARBO	FIBER	CALCIUM	SOD	POTAS	VIT C	FOLIC	VIT A
MCILHENNY														
Tabasco Bloody Mary Mix	8 fl oz	56	tr	tr	0	2	11	1	69	1548	—	0	—	1517
SCHWEPPES														
Collins Mixer	8 fl oz	100	0	0	0	0	24	0	—	55	—	—	—	—
TABASCO														
Bloody Mary Mix Extra Spicy	8 fl oz	58	tr	tr	0	3	11	2	76	1645	—	0	—	1548

DUCK

FOOD	PORTION	CALORIES	FAT	SAT FAT	CHOL	PROTEIN	CARBO	FIBER	CALCIUM	SOD	POTAS	VIT C	FOLIC	VIT A
w/ skin roasted	1 cup (4.9 oz)	472	40	14	118	27	0	0	15	83	286	0	8	294
w/ skin w/ bone leg roasted	3 oz	184	10	3	97	23	0	—	9	94	—	1	—	—
w/ skin w/o bone breast roasted	3 oz	172	9	2	116	21	0	—	7	71	—	2	—	—
w/o skin roasted	1 cup (4.9 oz)	281	16	6	125	33	0	0	17	91	353	0	14	108
w/o skin w/ bone leg braised	1 cup (6.1 oz)	310	10	2	183	51	0	—	17	188	—	4	—	—
w/o skin w/o bone breast broiled	1 cup (6.1 oz)	244	4	1	249	48	0	—	16	183	—	6	—	—
wild w/ skin raw	½ duck (9.5 oz)	571	41	14	216	47	0	—	12	152	672	14	—	—
wild w/o skin breast raw	½ breast (2.9 oz)	102	4	1	—	16	0	—	3	47	222	5	—	44

DUMPLING

FROZEN

PEPPERIDGE FARM

FOOD	PORTION	CALORIES	FAT	SAT FAT	CHOL	PROTEIN	CARBO	FIBER	CALCIUM	SOD	POTAS	VIT C	FOLIC	VIT A
Apple Dumpling	1 (3 oz)	260	13	—	—	2	33	—	—	230	—	1	—	—

EEL

FOOD	PORTION	CALORIES	FAT	SAT FAT	CHOL	PROTEIN	CARBO	FIBER	CALCIUM	SOD	POTAS	VIT C	FOLIC	VIT A
fresh cooked	3 oz	200	13	3	137	20	0	—	22	55	297	—	—	3219
fresh cooked	1 fillet (5.6 oz)	375	24	5	257	38	0	—	41	104	555	—	—	6021
raw	3 oz	156	10	2	107	16	0	—	17	43	232	—	—	2954
smoked	3.5 oz	330	28	7	—	19	0	0	—	—	—	—	—	—

EGG

(*see also* EGG DISHES, EGG SUBSTITUTES)

CHICKEN

FOOD	PORTION	CALORIES	FAT	SAT FAT	CHOL	PROTEIN	CARBO	FIBER	CALCIUM	SOD	POTAS	VIT C	FOLIC	VIT A
frozen	1	75	5	2	213	6	1	—	25	63	60	0	23	317
frozen	1 cup	363	24	8	1033	30	3	—	120	307	293	0	114	1543
hard cooked	1	77	5	2	213	6	1	—	25	62	63	0	22	280
hard cooked chopped	1 cup	210	14	4	578	17	2	—	68	169	172	0	60	762
poached	1	74	5	2	212	6	1	—	25	140	60	0	18	316
raw	1	75	5	2	213	6	1	—	25	63	60	0	23	317
scrambled plain	2	200	15	6	400	13	2	—	54	211	138	3	52	835
scrambled w/ whole milk & margarine	1 cup	365	27	8	774	24	5	—	157	616	304	1	66	1500

FOOD	PORTION	CALORIES	FAT	SAT FAT	CHOL	PROTEIN	CARBO	FIBER	CALCIUM	SOD	POTAS	VIT C	FOLIC	VIT A
white only	1 cup	121	0	0	0	26	2	—	15	399	346	0	7	—
white only	1	17	0	0	0	4	tr	—	2	55	48	0	1	—
EGGSPLUS														
Fresh	1 (1.8 oz)	70	5	2	215	6	0	0	20	65	—	0	—	300
OTHER POULTRY														
duck raw	1 (2.5 oz)	130	10	3	619	9	1	0	45	102	156	0	56	930
goose raw	1 (5 oz)	267	19	5	—	20	2	—	—	—	—	0	—	—
quail raw	1 (9 g)	14	1	tr	76	1	tr	—	6	—	—	0	—	27
turkey raw	1 (2.7 oz)	135	9	3	737	9	1	—	78	—	—	0	—	—

EGG DISHES

FROZEN

FOOD	PORTION	CALORIES	FAT	SAT FAT	CHOL	PROTEIN	CARBO	FIBER	CALCIUM	SOD	POTAS	VIT C	FOLIC	VIT A
CHEFWICH														
Cheese Omelet	5 oz	380	17	—	130	—	—	—	40	—	—	—	—	—
DOWNYFLAKE														
Scrambled Eggs With Ham & Hash Browns	1 pkg (6.25 oz)	360	26	—	—	13	17	—	60	730	380	9	—	200
Scrambled Eggs With Ham & Pecan Twirl	1 pkg (6.25 oz)	470	28	—	—	15	40	—	80	670	230	9	—	300
Scrambled Eggs With Hash Browns & Sausage	1 pkg (6.25 oz)	420	34	—	—	12	17	—	60	790	340	2	—	300
Scrambled Eggs With Sausage & Pecan Twirl	1 pkg (6.25 oz)	510	33	—	—	16	39	—	80	710	210	—	—	100
GREAT STARTS														
Egg Sausage & Cheese	5½ oz	460	28	—	—	18	35	—	200	1310	—	—	—	200
Omelets With Cheese & Ham	7 oz	390	29	—	—	19	15	—	300	1220	—	1	—	750
Reduced Cholesterol Eggs With Mini Oatbran Muffins	4¾ oz	250	12	—	—	10	27	—	60	400	—	—	—	500
Scrambled Eggs & Bacon With Home Fries	5.6 oz	340	26	—	—	11	16	—	60	690	—	—	—	—
Scrambled Eggs & Home Fries	4.6 oz	260	19	—	—	7	14	—	60	380	—	—	—	—
Scrambled Eggs & Sausage With Hash Browns	6½ oz	430	34	—	—	13	19	—	60	760	—	—	—	—
Scrambled Eggs With Cheese & Cinnamon Pancakes	3.4 oz	290	23	—	—	7	14	—	60	380	—	—	—	—

FOOD	PORTION	CALORIES	FAT	SAT FAT	CHOL	PROTEIN	CARBO	FIBER	CALCIUM	SOD	POTAS	VIT C	FOLIC	VIT A
QUAKER														
Scrambled Eggs & Sausage With Hash Browns	1 pkg (5.7 oz)	290	20	—	212	12	14	—	80	810	300	4	—	300
Scrambled Eggs & Sausage With Pancakes	1 pkg (5.2 oz)	270	14	—	180	13	21	—	200	880	180	—	—	200
Scrambled Eggs Cheddar Cheese & Fried Potatoes	1 pkg (5.9 oz)	250	13	—	176	11	22	—	100	910	470	9	—	300
WEIGHT WATCHERS														
Handy Ham & Cheese Omelet	1 (4 oz)	220	5	3	30	13	30	2	100	440	—	2	—	200
TAKE-OUT														
sandwich w/ cheese	1	340	19	7	291	16	26	—	225	804	188	2	36	668
sandwich w/ cheese & ham	1	348	16	7	245	19	31	—	212	1005	209	3	43	561
scrambled	2 eggs	202	14	4	430	17	2	—	88	342	168	0	36	832
sunny side up	1	91	7	2	211	6	1	—	25	162	61	0	18	394
EGG ROLLS														
(see also ASIAN FOODS)														
egg roll wrapper fresh	1	83	tr	tr	3	3	16	—	13	162	23	0	5	4
CHUN KING														
Chicken	8 (4.4 oz)	270	9	2	10	8	40	4	40	350	—	2	—	100
Pork & Shrimp	8 (4.4 oz)	290	11	3	15	11	39	4	20	350	—	5	—	200
Shrimp	8 (4.4 oz)	260	8	2	10	7	39	4	20	480	—	5	—	200
EMPIRE														
Large	1 (3 oz)	190	6	1	2	6	28	2	20	350	—	0	—	200
Miniature	6 (4.8 oz)	280	8	2	0	9	43	4	40	740	—	0	—	750
LA CHOY														
Almond Chicken Restaurant Style	1 (3 oz)	170	6	2	5	6	23	3	20	390	—	0	—	400
Chicken Mini	14 (7.25 oz)	430	11	3	15	15	67	6	60	900	—	—	—	200
Chicken Restaurant Style	1 (3 oz)	170	5	3	10	7	25	4	20	450	—	1	—	1000
Lobster Mini	14 (7.25 oz)	410	11	3	0	13	65	9	40	690	—	4	—	100
Meat & Shrimp Mini	15 (3.75 oz)	240	9	2	10	8	31	3	20	350	—	4	—	100
Mu Sho Pork Restaurant Style	1 (3 oz)	190	7	2	15	6	25	2	20	330	—	0	—	300
Pork Restaurant Style	1 (3 oz)	150	5	—	7	7	20	—	100	480	—	18	—	300
Pork & Shrimp Mini	14 (7.25 oz)	430	12	3	15	15	65	7	40	890	—	—	—	200
Shrimp Mini	14 (7.25 oz)	410	9	2	10	14	68	7	60	990	—	0	—	300

FOOD	PORTION	CALORIES	FAT	SAT FAT	CHOL	PROTEIN	CARBO	FIBER	CALCIUM	SOD	POTAS	VIT C	FOLIC	VIT A
LA CHOY (CONT.)														
Shrimp Restaurant Style	1 (3 oz)	150	4	1	10	6	24	3	40	420	—	0	—	200
Sweet & Sour Restaurant Style	1 (3 oz)	180	4	1	5	6	29	3	20	300	—	2	—	100
LEAN CUISINE														
Vegetable	1 pkg (9 oz)	340	6	2	0	7	64	3	40	590	290	12	—	2500
LO-AN														
White Meat Chicken	1 (2.7 oz)	140	4r	1	10	6	20	1	20	400	—	0	—	200
LUIGINO'S														
Chicken	1 pkg (6 oz)	360	13	7	25	12	48	2	80	590	—	0	—	500
Pork & Shrimp	1 pkg (6 oz)	340	9	3	25	14	51	3	60	760	—	0	—	0
Shrimp	1 pkg (6 oz)	350	11	3	20	24	39	4	60	460	—	0	—	0
Sweet & Sour Chicken	1 pkg (6 oz)	400	12	3	25	13	59	4	60	460	—	0	—	200
Sweet & Sour Pork	1 pkg (6 oz)	360	10	3	15	12	56	4	40	270	—	0	—	400
Szechwan Vegetable	1 pkg (6 oz)	350	12	4	10	23	38	3	80	920	—	0	—	0
WORTHINGTON														
Vegetarian Egg Rolls	1 (3 oz)	180	8	2	0	6	20	2	0	380	100	0	—	0
TAKE-OUT														
lobster	1 (4.8 oz)	270	7	2	0	8	43	6	20	460	—	2	—	0
meat & shrimp	1 (4.8 oz)	320	12	3	10	10	41	4	20	470	—	5	—	100
pork & shrimp	1 (5 oz)	300	10	4	15	13	41	7	40	890	—	0	—	400
shrimp	1 (3 oz)	170	5	1	<5	6	24	5	20	420	—	0	—	100
spicy pork	1 (3 oz)	200	9	2	5	6	23	3	20	410	—	0	—	400
vegetable	1 (3 oz)	170	4	1	0	5	28	4	20	520	—	0	—	750
EGG SUBSTITUTES														
frozen	¼ cup	96	7	1	1	7	2	—	44	120	128	—	—	810
frozen	1 cup	384	27	5	5	27	8	—	175	479	512	—	—	3240
liquid	1 cup (8.8 oz)	211	8	2	3	30	2	—	133	444	828	0	—	5422
liquid	1½ oz	40	2	tr	tr	6	tr	—	25	83	155	0	—	1015
powder	0.7 oz	88	3	1	113	11	4	—	32	158	147	tr	—	243
powder	0.35 oz	44	1	tr	57	5	2	—	32	79	74	tr	—	122
EGG BEATERS														
Eggs Substitute	¼ cup	25	0	0	0	5	1	0	20	80	75	—	—	300
Omelette Cheese	½ cup	110	5	2	5	14	2	—	150	480	135	—	—	750
Omelette Vegetable	½ cup	50	0	0	0	7	5	—	80	170	180	—	—	300
HEALTHY CHOICE														
Cholesterol Free	¼ cup (2 oz)	25	0	0	0	6	tr	0	20	95	—	0	—	500
MORNINGSTAR FARMS														
Better'n Eggs	¼ cup (2 oz)	20	0	0	0	5	0	0	20	90	75	0	—	750
Breakfast Sandwich Bagel Scramblers Pattie Cheese	1 (5.9 oz)	320	5	1	10	28	40	4	250	900	360	0	—	750

FOOD	PORTION	CALORIES	FAT	SAT FAT	CHOL	PROTEIN	CARBO	FIBER	CALCIUM	SOD	POTAS	VIT C	FOLIC	VIT A
MORNINGSTAR FARMS (CONT.)														
Breakfast Sandwich English Muffin Scramblers Pattie	1 (5.1 oz)	240	3	1	5	22	32	5	150	700	350	0	—	500
Breakfast Sandwich English Muffin Scramblers Pattie Cheese	1 (6 oz)	280	3	1	10	28	35	5	300	1000	400	0	—	750
Scramblers	¼ cup (2 oz)	35	0	0	0	6	2	0	20	95	60	0	—	750
SECOND NATURE														
No Cholesterol	2 fl oz	60	2	tr	0	6	3	—	40	90	—	0	32	400
No Fat	2 fl oz	40	0	0	0	6	3	—	40	100	—	0	32	600
No Fat With Garden Vegetables	2.5 fl oz	40	0	0	0	6	4	—	40	100	—	0	32	600
SIMPLY EGGS														
Egg Substitute	1.75 fl oz	35	1	tr	30	5	1	1	20	130	—	—	—	0
EGGNOG														
eggnog	1 cup	342	19	11	149	10	34	—	330	138	420	4	2	894
eggnog	1 qt	1368	76	45	596	39	138	—	1321	553	1678	15	9	3576
eggnog flavor mix as prep w/ milk	9 oz	260	8	5	33	8	39	—	291	163	369	2	12	307
BORDEN														
Eggnog	4 fl oz	160	9	—	—	3	16	—	100	80	85	—	—	300
HOOD														
Fat Free	4 fl oz	100	0	0	<5	4	21	0	150	100	—	0	—	300
Golden	4 fl oz	180	8	5	65	4	22	0	150	100	—	0	—	300
Light	4 fl oz	120	2	1	40	4	23	0	150	105	—	0	—	300
Select	4 fl oz	210	12	8	80	4	22	0	150	100	—	0	—	500
EGGPLANT														
CANNED														
PROGRESSO														
Appetizer	2 tbsp (1 oz)	30	2	0	0	0	2	2	0	130	—	0	—	100
FRESH														
cubed cooked	½ cup	13	tr	tr	0	tr	3	—	3	2	119	1	7	31
raw cut up	½ cup (1.4 oz)	11	tr	tr	0	tr	2	—	3	1	89	1	8	35
slices cooked	4 (7 oz)	38	0	0	0	2	0	—	22	—	—	6	—	20
whole peeled raw	1 (1 lb)	117	1	tr	0	5	28	—	34	14	992	8	67	387
FROZEN														
MRS. PAUL'S														
Parmigiana	5 oz	240	16	—	15	6	18	—	10	600	—	60	—	—
TAKE-OUT														
baba ghannouj	¼ cup	55	4	—	0	2	5	—	—	95	—	—	—	—
caponata	2 tbsp (1 oz)	30	2	—	0	1	3	—	—	115	—	4	—	—
indian eggplant runi	1 serv	180	14	4	0	2	13	1	30	228	527	15	13	378

FOOD	PORTION	CALORIES	FAT	SAT FAT	CHOL	PROTEIN	CARBO	FIBER	CALCIUM	SOD	POTAS	VIT C	FOLIC	VIT A
ELDERBERRIES														
fresh	1 cup	105	1	—	0	1	27	—	55	—	406	52	—	870
ELK														
roasted	3 oz	124	2	1	62	26	0	—	4	52	279	—	—	—
ENDIVE														
raw chopped	½ cup	4	tr	tr	0	tr	1	—	13	6	79	2	36	513
ENERGY BARS														
(*see* BREAKFAST BARS, CEREAL BARS, GRANOLA BARS, NUTRITIONAL SUPPLEMENTS)														
ENGLISH MUFFIN														
FROZEN														
GREAT STARTS														
Egg Beefsteak & Cheese	5.9 oz	360	20	—	—	17	27	—	100	730	—	—	—	200
Egg Canadian Bacon & Cheese	4.1 oz	290	15	—	—	15	25	—	150	770	—	—	—	100
WEIGHT WATCHERS														
Sandwich	1 (4 oz)	210	5	3	20	13	28	2	100	420	—	2	—	200
READY-TO-EAT														
apple cinnamon	1	138	2	tr	0	4	28	—	84	255	119	—	—	—
granola	1	155	1	tr	0	6	31	—	129	275	103	0	—	—
mixed grain	1	155	1	tr	0	6	31	—	129	275	103	0	—	—
plain	1	134	1	tr	0	4	26	—	99	265	75	—	—	—
plain toasted	1	133	1	tr	0	4	26	—	99	262	74	—	—	—
raisin cinnamon	1	138	2	tr	0	4	28	—	84	255	119	—	—	—
sourdough	1	134	1	tr	0	4	26	—	99	265	75	—	—	—
wheat	1	127	1	tr	0	5	26	—	101	218	106	—	—	—
whole wheat	1	134	1	tr	0	6	27	4	175	420	139	0	—	0
ARNOLD														
Extra Crisp	1	130	1	0	0	4	26	1	—	230	—	—	—	—
Sourdough	1	130	1	0	0	4	25	1	—	250	—	—	—	—
MATTHEW'S														
9 Grain & Nut	1	140	4	—	0	10	26	5	100	220	—	—	—	—
Cinnamon Raisin	1	160	2	—	0	6	33	4	20	290	—	—	—	—
Golden White	1	140	4	—	0	5	23	1	100	340	—	—	—	—
Whole Wheat	1	150	2	—	0	7	31	4	20	340	—	—	—	—
PEPPERIDGE FARM														
Cinnamon Apple	1	140	1	—	0	4	27	—	40	210	—	—	—	—
Cinnamon Chip	1	160	3	—	0	4	28	—	20	180	—	—	—	—
Cinnamon Raisin	1	150	2	—	0	4	29	—	20	200	—	—	—	—
Plain	1	140	1	—	0	5	27	—	20	220	—	—	—	—
Sourdough	1	135	1	—	0	4	27	—	20	260	—	—	—	—
ROMAN MEAL														
Engish Muffin	1 (2.2 oz)	135	1	tr	0	6	25	3	89	332	72	0	—	0
TASTYKAKE														
Cinnamon Raisin	1 (64 g)	150	1	—	0	4	31	—	—	150	—	—	—	—

FOOD	PORTION	CALORIES	FAT	SAT FAT	CHOL	PROTEIN	CARBO	FIBER	CALCIUM	SOD	POTAS	VIT C	FOLIC	VIT A
TASTYKAKE (CONT.)														
English Muffin	1 (57 g)	130	1	—	0	5	26	—	—	240	—	—	—	—
Sourdough	1 (57 g)	130	1	—	0	5	25	—	—	210	—	—	—	—
THOMAS'														
Honey Wheat	1	128	1	—	—	5	24	—	67	199	71	tr	—	37
Oat Bran	1	116	1	—	0	4	26	3	66	192	—	—	—	—
Raisin Cinnamon	1	151	1	—	—	4	31	—	34	183	95	tr	—	52
Regular	1	130	1	—	—	4	25	—	71	206	48	tr	—	26
Sandwich Size	1 (92 g)	210	2	1	0	7	42	2	150	330	—	—	—	—
Sour Dough	1	131	1	—	—	4	25	—	74	210	63	tr	—	40
WONDER														
English Muffin	1 (2 oz)	120	1	0	0	5	25	1	200	290	55	—	—	—
Raisin Rounds	1 (2.1 oz)	150	2	0	0	5	30	2	150	240	105	—	—	—
Sourdough	1 (2 oz)	120	1	0	0	5	25	1	200	290	60	—	—	—
REFRIGERATED														
ROMAN MEAL														
English Muffin	½ muffin (1.1 oz)	66	tr	tr	0	2	14	1	43	95	37	0	—	0
Honey Nut Oat Bran	½ muffin (1.1 oz)	81	1	tr	0	2	16	1	55	114	56	0	—	0
TAKE-OUT														
w/ butter	1	189	6	2	13	5	30	—	103	386	69	tr	17	136
w/ cheese & sausage	1	394	24	10	58	15	29	—	168	1036	215	1	18	379
w/ egg cheese & bacon	1	487	31	12	274	22	31	—	196	1135	294	1	54	660
w/ egg cheese & canadian bacon	1	383	20	9	234	20	31	—	207	785	213	1	44	594
EPAZOTE														
fresh	1 tbsp (1 g)	tr	0	—	0	0	tr	tr	2	tr	5	0	2	tr
fresh sprig	1 (2 g)	1	tr	—	0	tr	tr	tr	6	1	13	tr	4	1
EPPAW														
raw	½ cup	75	1	—	0	2	16	—	55	6	170	7	—	0
FALAFEL														
CASBAH														
as prep	5	130	3	0	0	6	20	2	70	530	—	2	—	200
NEAR EAST														
as prep	2½ patties	230	15	2	0	10	18	5	—	560	370	—	—	0
TAKE-OUT														
falafel	1 (1.2 oz)	57	3	tr	0	2	5	—	9	50	99	tr	13	2
falafel	3 (1.8 oz)	170	9	1	0	7	16	—	27	150	298	1	40	7

FAST FOODS

(see individual names in Part Two)

FAT

(see also BUTTER, BUTTER BLENDS, BUTTER SUBSTITUTES, MARGARINE, OIL)

FOOD	PORTION	CALORIES	FAT	SAT FAT	CHOL	PROTEIN	CARBO	FIBER	CALCIUM	SOD	POTAS	VIT C	FOLIC	VIT A
beef cooked	1 oz	193	20	8	27	3	0	—	4	12	34	0	1	0

FOOD	PORTION	CALORIES	FAT	SAT FAT	CHOL	PROTEIN	CARBO	FIBER	CALCIUM	SOD	POTAS	VIT C	FOLIC	VIT A
beef suet	1 oz	242	27	15	19	tr	0	—	—	—	5	—	—	—
beef tallow	1 tbsp (13 g)	115	13	6	14	0	0	—	—	0	0	—	—	—
chicken	1 cup	1846	205	61	174	0	0	—	—	—	—	—	—	—
chicken	1 tbsp	115	13	4	11	0	0	—	—	—	—	—	—	—
cocoa butter	1 tbsp	120	14	8	0	0	0	—	—	—	—	—	—	—
duck	1 tbsp (13 g)	115	13	4	13	0	0	0	0	0	0	0	0	0
goose	1 tbsp	115	13	4	13	0	0	—	—	—	—	—	—	—
goose	3.5 oz	900	100	6	—	0	0	—	—	—	—	—	—	—
lamb new zealand raw	1 oz	182	19	10	25	2	0	—	6	6	15	—	—	—
lard	1 tbsp (13 g)	115	13	5	12	0	0	—	tr	0	0	—	—	—
lard	1 cup (205 g)	1849	205	80	195	0	0	—	tr	tr	tr	—	—	—
nutmeg butter	1 tbsp	120	14	12	—	0	0	—	—	—	—	—	—	—
pork backfat	1 oz	230	25	9	16	1	0	0	1	3	—	tr	tr	4
pork cooked	1 oz	178	18	7	26	3	0	0	15	10	—	0	1	4
salt pork	1 oz	212	23	8	25	23	0	—	2	404	19	—	0	0
turkey	1 tbsp	115	13	4	13	0	0	—	—	—	—	—	—	—
ucuhuba butter	1 tbsp	120	14	12	—	0	0	—	—	—	—	—	—	—
CRISCO														
Butter Flavor	1 tbsp	110	12	3	0	0	0	—	—	0	—	—	—	200
Shortening	1 tbsp	110	12	3	0	0	0	—	—	0	—	—	—	—
Shortening	1 tbsp (0.4 oz)	110	12	3	0	0	0	—	—	0	—	—	—	—
Sticks	1 tbsp (0.4 oz)	110	12	3	0	0	0	0	—	0	—	—	—	—
Sticks Butter Flavor	1 tbsp (0.4 oz)	110	12	3	0	0	0	0	—	0	—	—	—	—
EMPIRE														
Chicken Fat Rendered	1 tbsp (0.5 oz)	120	13	4	10	0	tr	0	0	0	—	0	—	0
WESSON														
Shortening	1 tbsp	100	12	3	0	0	0	0	0	0	—	0	—	0

FAT SUBSTITUTES
SOY IS US

FOOD	PORTION	CALORIES	FAT	SAT FAT	CHOL	PROTEIN	CARBO	FIBER	CALCIUM	SOD	POTAS	VIT C	FOLIC	VIT A
Fat Not! Organic	3 tbsp	66	1	tr	0	11	7	4	55	3	—	0	—	3

FAVA BEANS
PROGRESSO

| Fava Beans | ½ cup (4.6 oz) | 110 | 1 | 0 | 0 | 6 | 20 | 5 | 20 | 250 | — | 0 | — | 0 |

FENNEL

| leaves | 3.5 oz | 24 | tr | — | — | 2 | 3 | 4 | 109 | 86 | — | 93 | 100 | 3917 |
| seed | 1 tsp | 7 | tr | tr | 0 | tr | 1 | — | 24 | 2 | 34 | — | — | 3 |

FENUGREEK

| seed | 1 tsp | 12 | tr | — | 0 | 1 | 2 | — | 6 | 2 | 28 | tr | 2 | — |

FIBER
DELTA

| Natural Fiber | ½ cup (1 oz) | 20 | tr | — | 0 | 3 | 2 | 20 | 250 | 20 | — | — | — | — |

FIDDLEHEAD FERNS

| fresh | 3.5 oz | 34 | tr | — | 0 | 5 | 6 | — | 32 | 1 | 370 | 27 | — | 3676 |

FOOD	PORTION	CALORIES	FAT	SAT FAT	CHOL	PROTEIN	CARBO	FIBER	CALCIUM	SOD	POTAS	VIT C	FOLIC	VIT A
FIGS														
CANNED														
in heavy syrup	3	75	tr	tr	0	tr	19	—	23	1	85	1	—	31
in light syrup	3	58	tr	tr	0	tr	15	—	23	1	86	1	—	32
water pack	3	42	tr	—	0	tr	11	—	22	1	83	1	—	31
DRIED														
California	½ cup (3.5 oz)	200	1	—	0	4	58	17	150	11	710	2	24	100
cooked	½ cup	140	1	tr	0	2	16	—	79	6	391	6	1	207
SONOMA														
White Misson	3-4 (1.4 oz)	110	0	0	0	1	26	5	60	0	—	2	—	0
FRESH														
fig	1 med	50	tr	tr	0	tr	10	—	18	1	116	1	—	71
FIREWEED														
leaves chopped	1 cup (0.8 oz)	24	1	—	0	1	4	2	99	8	114	tr	26	828
FISH														
(see also individual names, FISH SUBSTITUTES, SUSHI)														
CANNED														
HOLMES														
Finest Kippered Snacks drained	1 can (3.2 oz)	135	8	1	60	17	0	0	60	470	—	0	—	0
PORT CLYDE														
Fish Steaks In Louisiana Hot Sauce	1 can (3.75 oz)	150	9	2	80	17	2	0	300	960	—	0	—	200
Fish Steaks In Mustard Sauce	1 can (3.75 oz)	140	7	1	70	18	1	0	300	540	—	0	—	100
Fish Steaks In Soybean Oil With Hot Chilies drained	1 can (3.3 oz)	155	8	2	80	20	0	0	350	420	—	0	—	0
Fish Steaks In Soybean Oil drained	1 can (3.3 oz)	220	17	4	115	19	0	0	300	360	—	0	—	100
FROZEN														
breaded fillet	1 (2 oz)	155	7	2	64	9	14	—	11	332	149	—	10	60
sticks	1 stick (1 oz)	76	3	1	31	4	7	—	6	163	73	—	5	30
CAJUN COOKIN'														
Seafood Gumbo	17 oz	330	7	—	—	16	51	—	80	1330	190	—	—	—
GORTON'S														
Crispy Batter Dipped Fillets	2	290	19	8	35	11	18	—	—	550	—	—	—	—
Crispy Batter Sticks	4	260	18	6	25	9	16	—	—	480	—	—	—	—
Crunch Fillets	2	230	13	3	40	13	16	—	—	420	—	—	—	—
Crunchy Sticks	4	210	13	4	25	7	15	—	—	240	—	—	—	—
Grilled Fillets Cajun Blackened	1 piece (3.8 oz)	120	6	1	60	16	1	—	—	320	—	—	—	—

FOOD	PORTION	CALORIES	FAT	SAT FAT	CHOL	PROTEIN	CARBO	FIBER	CALCIUM	SOD	POTAS	VIT C	FOLIC	VIT A
GORTON'S (CONT.)														
Light Recipe Lightly Breaded Fish Fillets	1 fillet	180	8	3	30	11	16	—	—	380	—	—	—	—
Light Recipe Tempura Fillets	1 fillet	200	14	4	30	10	8	—	—	400	—	—	—	—
Microwave Crispy Batter Large Cut Fillets	1	320	21	—	—	12	20	—	—	680	—	—	—	—
Microwave Entree Fillets In Herb Butter	1 pkg	190	8	5	90	26	3	—	60	450	—	—	—	—
Microwave Fillets	2	340	26	12	30	10	17	—	20	400	—	—	—	—
Microwave Larger Cut Fillets	1	320	22	10	35	11	20	—	20	500	—	—	—	—
Microwave Larger Cut Ranch Fillet	1	330	21	—	—	12	24	—	20	520	—	—	—	—
Microwave Sticks	6	340	22	7	35	11	24	—	—	420	—	—	—	—
Potato Crisp Fillets	2	300	20	6	30	12	18	—	—	360	—	—	—	—
Potato Crisp Sticks	4	260	16	5	25	8	21	—	—	390	—	—	—	—
Value Pack Portions	1 portion	180	11	—	—	7	13	—	—	490	—	—	—	—
Value Pack Sticks	4	190	9	—	—	9	17	—	—	420	—	—	—	—
KINERET														
Fish Sticks	5 pieces (4 oz)	280	14	3	20	12	27	1	0	430	—	0	—	0
MRS. PAUL'S														
Entree Light Seafood Dijon	8¾ oz	200	5	2	60	21	17	—	200	650	—	4	—	—
Entree Light Seafood Florentine	8 oz	220	8	—	95	25	10	—	400	820	—	5	—	100
Entree Light Seafood Mornay	9 oz	230	10	4	80	24	12	—	300	670	—	21	—	100
Fish Cakes	2	190	7	—	20	9	24	—	20	690	—	—	—	—
Fish Fillets Batter Dipped	2 fillets	330	17	—	60	16	28	—	20	650	—	—	—	—
Fish Fillets Crispy Crunchy	2 fillets	220	9	—	22	13	23	—	40	380	—	—	—	—
Fish Fillets Crunchy Batter	2 fillets	280	14	—	22	12	26	—	20	730	—	—	—	—
Fish Sticks Crispy Crunchy	4 sticks	190	8	—	25	9	18	—	40	560	—	—	—	—
In Butter Sauce Light Fillet	1 fillets	140	6	—	40	20	1	—	—	520	—	—	—	—
Portions Battered Fish	2 portions	300	19	—	33	11	21	—	20	540	—	—	—	—
Portions Crispy Crunchy Breaded Fish	2 portions	230	15	—	25	10	14	—	20	300	—	—	—	—
Sticks Battered Fish	4 sticks	210	12	—	25	7	15	—	—	590	—	—	—	—

FOOD	PORTION	CALORIES	FAT	SAT FAT	CHOL	PROTEIN	CARBO	FIBER	CALCIUM	SOD	POTAS	VIT C	FOLIC	VIT A
MRS. PAUL'S (CONT.)														
Sticks Crispy Crunchy Breaded Fish	4 sticks	140	6	—	20	7	14	—	20	340	—	—	—	—
VAN DE KAMP'S														
Battered Fish Fillets	1 (2.6 oz)	180	11	2	20	8	12	0	0	340	—	0	—	0
Battered Fish Nuggets	8 (4 oz)	280	18	3	25	11	20	0	20	600	—	0	—	0
Battered Fish Portions	2 pieces (5 oz)	350	22	4	35	13	26	0	40	710	—	0	—	0
Battered Fish Sticks	6 (4 oz)	260	16	3	30	11	18	0	20	540	—	0	—	0
Breaded Fillets	2 (3.5 oz)	280	19	3	35	11	17	0	0	270	—	0	—	0
Breaded Fish Portions	3 pieces (4.5 oz)	330	21	3	35	14	23	0	0	410	—	0	—	0
Breaded Fish Sticks	6 (4 oz)	290	17	3	35	13	23	0	0	390	—	0	—	0
Breaded Mini Fish Sticks	13 (3.3 oz)	250	14	2	30	11	19	0	0	330	—	0	—	0
Crisp & Healthy Breaded Fillets	2 (3.5 oz)	150	3	1	30	12	20	0	20	380	—	0	—	0
Crisp & Healthy Fish Sticks	6 (4 oz)	180	3	1	25	13	26	0	20	440	—	0	—	0
Fish 'n Fries	1 pkg (6.6 oz)	380	18	3	25	13	41	2	0	370	—	0	—	0
MIX														
GOLDEN DIPT														
Beer Batter Fry	1 oz	100	0	0	0	2	22	—	60	650	—	—	—	—
Cajun Style Fish Fry	⅔ oz	60	0	0	0	2	14	—	—	470	—	—	—	—
Fish & Chips Batter Mix	1¼ oz	120	0	0	0	2	27	—	—	910	—	—	—	—
Fish Fry	⅔ oz	60	0	0	0	2	14	—	—	430	—	—	—	—
Seafood Frying Mix	⅔ oz	60	0	0	0	1	14	—	—	600	—	—	—	—
Tempura Batter Mix	1 oz	100	0	0	0	3	22	—	40	130	—	—	—	—
TAKE-OUT														
fish cake	1 (4.7 oz)	166	7	2	—	18	6	—	179	—	—	5	—	140
jamaican brown fish stew	1 serv	426	22	5	84	48	9	2	—	419	—	—	—	—
sandwich w/ tartar sauce	1	431	55	5	—	17	41	—	84	615	339	3	44	110
sandwich w/ tartar sauce & cheese	1	524	29	8	68	21	48	—	185	939	353	3	32	432
stew	1 cup (7.9 oz)	157	4	2	—	19	10	—	32	—	—	11	—	160

FISH SUBSTITUTES

FOOD	PORTION	CALORIES	FAT	SAT FAT	CHOL	PROTEIN	CARBO	FIBER	CALCIUM	SOD	POTAS	VIT C	FOLIC	VIT A
LOMA LINDA														
Ocean Platter not prep	⅓ cup (0.9 oz)	90	1	0	0	14	8	4	0	450	450	0	—	0

FOOD	PORTION	CALORIES	FAT	SAT FAT	CHOL	PROTEIN	CARBO	FIBER	CALCIUM	SOD	POTAS	VIT C	FOLIC	VIT A
WORTHINGTON														
Fillets	2 (3 oz)	180	10	2	0	16	8	4	0	750	130	0	—	0
Tuno	½ cup (1.9 oz)	80	6	1	0	6	2	1	20	290	35	0	—	0
FLAXSEED														
ARROWHEAD														
Flaxseed	3 tbsp (1 oz)	140	10	1	0	5	11	6	80	0	160	0	—	0
STONE-BUHR														
Flaxseed	1 tsp (1 oz)	150	10	1	0	5	11	5	80	20	—	0	—	0
FLOUNDER														
FRESH														
cooked	3 oz	99	1	tr	58	21	0	—	16	89	292	—	—	32
cooked	1 fillet (4.5 oz)	148	2	tr	86	31	0	—	23	133	436	—	—	48
FROZEN														
GORTON'S														
Fishmarket Fresh	5 oz	110	1	—	—	23	1	—	—	170	—	—	—	—
Microwave Entree Stuffed	1 pkg	350	18	7	120	25	21	—	80	850	—	—	—	—
MRS. PAUL'S														
Crunchy Batter Fillets	2 fillets	220	9	—	40	12	23	—	20	560	—	—	—	—
Light Fillets	1 fillet	240	10	—	50	16	20	—	40	450	—	—	—	100
VAN DE KAMP'S														
Lightly Breaded Fillets	1 (4 oz)	230	11	2	40	15	19	0	20	400	—	0	—	0
Natural Fillets	1 (4 oz)	110	2	0	45	22	0	0	0	105	—	0	—	0
TAKE-OUT														
battered & fried	3.2 oz	211	11	3	31	13	15	—	17	484	292	0	51	35
breaded & fried	3.2 oz	211	11	3	31	13	15	—	17	484	292	0	51	35
FLOUR														
corn masa	1 cup (4 oz)	416	4	1	0	11	87	—	161	6	340	0	213	535
cottonseed lowfat	1 oz	94	tr	tr	0	14	10	—	135	10	500	1	—	123
potato	1 cup (6.3 oz)	628	1	tr	0	14	143	—	59	61	2843	34	—	0
rice brown	1 cup	574	4	tr	0	11	121	4	18	12	456	0	25	—
rice white	1 cup	578	2	tr	0	9	127	2	16	1	120	0	6	—
rye dark	1 cup	415	3	tr	0	18	88	—	72	2	934	0	77	—
rye light	1 cup	374	1	tr	0	9	82	7	21	2	238	0	23	—
rye medium	1 cup	361	2	tr	0	10	79	7	24	3	347	0	20	—
sesame lowfat	1 oz	95	tr	tr	0	14	10	—	42	11	113	—	8	18
triticale whole grain	1 cup	440	2	tr	0	17	95	9	45	3	605	0	96	—
white all-purpose	1 cup	455	1	tr	0	13	95	2	19	3	134	0	193	—
white bread	1 cup (4.8 oz)	495	2	tr	0	16	99	3	21	3	137	0	211	0
white cake unsifted	1 cup (4.8 oz)	496	1	tr	0	11	107	2	19	3	144	0	211	0
white self-rising	1 cup (4.4 oz)	443	1	tr	0	12	93	3	423	1588	155	0	193	0
white unbleached	1 cup (4.4 oz)	455	1	tr	0	13	95	3	19	3	134	0	193	0
whole wheat	1 cup	407	2	tr	0	16	87	8	40	6	486	0	52	—

FOOD	PORTION	CALORIES	FAT	SAT FAT	CHOL	PROTEIN	CARBO	FIBER	CALCIUM	SOD	POTAS	VIT C	FOLIC	VIT A
ARROWHEAD														
Kamut	¼ cup (1.2 oz)	110	1	0	0	4	25	4	0	0	150	0	—	0
Pastry	⅓ cup (1.1 oz)	100	1	0	0	4	22	3	20	0	115	0	—	0
Rye Whole Grain	¼ cup (1.6 oz)	160	1	0	0	6	34	6	20	0	220	0	—	0
Spelt	¼ cup (1.2 oz)	100	1	0	0	4	24	5	0	0	150	0	—	0
Teff	¼ cup (1.4 oz)	140	1	0	0	5	29	5	80	5	200	0	—	0
Unbleached White	⅓ cup (1.6 oz)	160	1	0	0	5	33	0	0	0	45	0	—	0
Whole Grain Wheat	¼ cup (1.6 oz)	160	1	0	0	6	34	7	20	0	170	0	—	0
Whole Wheat	¼ cup (1.2 oz)	130	1	0	0	5	25	4	20	0	130	0	—	0
AUNT JEMIMA														
Self-Rising	3 tbsp	90	0	0	0	3	20	1	80	310	35	—	8	—
GOLD MEDAL														
All Purpose	1 cup	400	1	—	—	11	87	—	20	0	130	—	—	—
Oat Blend	1 cup	390	3	—	—	14	81	—	20	0	210	—	—	—
Self-Rising	1 cup	380	1	—	—	10	83	—	200	1520	130	—	—	—
Unbleached	1 cup	400	1	—	—	11	87	—	20	0	140	—	—	—
Whole Wheat	1 cup	350	2	—	—	16	78	10	20	0	410	—	—	—
Whole Wheat Blend	1 cup	380	2	—	—	14	84	8	20	0	340	—	—	—
HODGSON MILL														
50/50 Flour	¼ cup (1 oz)	100	1	0	0	4	21	2	0	0	—	0	—	0
Best For Bread	¼ cup (1 oz)	100	0	0	0	4	22	1	0	0	—	0	—	0
Buckwheat	⅓ cup (1.6 oz)	160	1	0	0	7	33	2	20	10	—	0	—	0
Oat Bran Blend	¼ cup (1 oz)	110	1	0	0	3	24	3	0	120	—	0	—	0
Oat Bran Flour	¼ cup (1 oz)	110	2	1	0	3	23	3	0	4	—	0	—	0
Rye	¼ cup (1 oz)	90	1	0	0	3	22	5	0	0	—	0	—	0
Seasoned Flour	¼ cup (1 oz)	90	0	0	0	3	20	0	0	1360	—	0	—	0
White	¼ cup (1 oz)	100	0	0	0	3	23	3	0	0	—	0	—	0
Whole Wheat	¼ cup (1 oz)	100	1	0	0	3	22	3	0	0	—	0	—	0
KING ARTHUR														
All Purpose Unbleached	¼ cup (1 oz)	100	0	0	0	3	22	tr	—	0	40	—	—	—
ROBIN HOOD														
All Purpose	1 cup	400	1	—	—	13	85	—	20	0	120	—	—	—
Rye Stone Ground	1 cup	360	2	—	—	13	86	13	40	10	130	—	—	—
Self-Rising	1 cup	380	1	—	—	10	83	—	200	1520	130	—	—	—
Unbleached	1 cup	400	1	—	—	13	85	—	20	0	140	—	—	—
STONE GROUND MILLS														
White Unbleached Organic	¼ cup (1.4 oz)	130	0	0	0	5	25	1	0	0	—	0	—	0
Whole Wheat 100% Stone Ground	3 tbsp (1 oz)	90	1	0	0	4	20	3	0	0	—	0	—	0

FRANKFURTER

(see HOT DOG)

FRENCH BEANS

FOOD	PORTION	CALORIES	FAT	SAT FAT	CHOL	PROTEIN	CARBO	FIBER	CALCIUM	SOD	POTAS	VIT C	FOLIC	VIT A
dried cooked	1 cup	228	1	tr	0	12	43	—	111	11	655	2	132	5

FRENCH FRIES

(*see* POTATOES)

FRENCH TOAST

FOOD	PORTION	CALORIES	FAT	SAT FAT	CHOL	PROTEIN	CARBO	FIBER	CALCIUM	SOD	POTAS	VIT C	FOLIC	VIT A
FROZEN														
french toast	1 slice (2 oz)	126	4	1	48	4	19	2	63	292	79	—	14	110
AUNT JEMIMA														
Cinnamon Swirl	2 pieces (4.1 oz)	240	6	2	90	9	37	2	100	330	125	0	—	100
Slices	2 pieces (4.1 oz)	240	6	2	80	9	38	1	100	360	150	0	—	100
DOWNYFLAKE														
Extra Thick	1	150	9	—	—	5	11	—	40	340	70	—	—	—
French Toast	2 slices	270	12	—	73	6	34	—	40	380	110	—	—	—
Texas Style & Sausage	1 pkg (4.25 oz)	400	24	—	—	10	37	—	40	550	150	—	—	—
GREAT STARTS														
Cinnamon Swirl With Sausage	5½ oz	390	21	—	—	12	37	—	100	530	—	—	—	—
French Toast With Sausage	5½ oz	380	21	—	—	12	35	—	100	550	—	—	—	—
Mini French Toast With Sausage	2½ oz	190	9	—	—	6	22	—	40	320	—	—	—	100
Oatmeal French Toast With Lite Links	4.65 oz	310	13	—	—	13	35	—	80	500	—	—	—	—
QUAKER														
French Toast Sticks & Syrup	1 pkg (5.2 oz)	400	20	—	64	7	48	—	80	640	115	—	—	100
French Toast Wedges & Sausage	1 pkg (5.3 oz)	360	17	—	96	13	40	—	100	780	210	—	—	200
HOME RECIPE														
as prep w/ 2% milk	1 slice	149	7	2	75	7	16	—	65	311	87	tr	15	315
as prep w/ whole milk	1 slice	151	7	2	75	7	16	—	64	311	86	tr	15	298
TAKE-OUT														
w/ butter	2 slices	356	19	8	117	10	36	—	73	513	177	tr	30	472

FROSTING

(*see* CAKE ICING)

FRUCTOSE

FOOD	PORTION	CALORIES	FAT	SAT FAT	CHOL	PROTEIN	CARBO	FIBER	CALCIUM	SOD	POTAS	VIT C	FOLIC	VIT A
ESTEE														
Fructose	1 tsp (4 g)	15	0	0	0	0	4	—	—	0	0	—	—	—
Packet	1 pkg (3 g)	10	0	0	0	0	3	—	—	0	0	—	—	—

FRUIT DRINKS

(*see also individual names*, LEMONADE)

FOOD	PORTION	CALORIES	FAT	SAT FAT	CHOL	PROTEIN	CARBO	FIBER	CALCIUM	SOD	POTAS	VIT C	FOLIC	VIT A
FROZEN														
citrus juice drink as prep	1 cup	114	0	0	0	1	28	—	21	7	277	67	5	103

FOOD	PORTION	CALORIES	FAT	SAT FAT	CHOL	PROTEIN	CARBO	FIBER	CALCIUM	SOD	POTAS	VIT C	FOLIC	VIT A
citrus juice drink not prep	1 can (12 fl oz)	684	tr	tr	0	5	171	—	106	12	1660	403	30	618
fruit punch as prep w/water	1 cup	113	tr	tr	0	tr	29	—	9	11	31	108	2	27
fruit punch not prep	1 can (12 fl oz)	678	tr	tr	0	1	173	—	33	34	184	650	14	161
limeade	1 can (6 oz)	408	tr	tr	0	tr	108	—	11	—	129	—	—	—
limeade as prep w/ water	1 cup	102	tr	tr	0	tr	27	—	7	6	33	—	—	—
BRIGHT & EARLY														
Fruit Punch	8 fl oz	130	0	0	0	0	31	—	—	5	—	60	—	—
DOLE														
100% Juice Blend Country Raspberry as prep	8 fl oz	140	0	0	0	1	34	0	20	30	370	60	0	0
100% Juice Blend Orchard Peach as prep	8 fl oz	140	0	0	0	1	34	0	20	30	370	60	0	0
Mountain Cherry 100% Juice Blend as prep	8 fl oz	120	0	0	0	0	30	0	0	30	310	60	0	0
Pineapple Grapefruit as prep	8 fl oz	130	0	0	0	1	29	0	20	20	400	60	—	100
Pineapple Orange as prep	8 fl oz	120	0	0	0	1	29	0	20	20	330	60	—	0
Pineapple Orange Banana as prep	8 fl oz	130	0	0	0	1	31	0	20	20	430	60	—	0
Pineapple Orange Guava as prep	8 fl oz	120	0	0	0	1	30	0	20	20	310	60	—	100
Pineapple Passion Banana as prep	8 fl oz	120	0	0	0	1	30	0	20	20	310	60	—	100
Tropical Fruit as prep	8 fl oz	140	0	0	0	1	34	0	40	30	290	60	0	0
FIVE ALIVE														
Berry Citrus	8 fl oz	120	0	0	0	0	30	—	—	0	—	—	—	—
Citrus	8 fl oz	120	0	0	0	0	30	—	—	0	—	36	—	—
Tropical Citrus	8 fl oz	120	0	0	0	0	29	—	—	25	—	—	—	—
MINUTE MAID														
Berry Punch	8 fl oz	130	0	0	0	0	31	—	—	5	—	—	—	—
Citrus Punch	8 fl oz	120	0	0	0	0	31	—	—	5	—	—	—	—
Fruit Punch	8 fl oz	120	0	0	0	0	31	—	—	5	—	—	—	—
Limeade	8 fl oz	100	0	0	0	0	26	—	—	0	—	—	—	—
Pineapple Orange	8 fl oz	120	0	0	0	0	31	—	—	0	—	36	—	—
Tropical Punch	8 fl oz	120	0	0	0	0	31	—	—	5	—	—	—	—
SENECA														
Cranberry-Apple Juice Cocktail frzn as prep	8 fl oz	140	0	0	0	0	33	0	0	0	35	60	—	0

FOOD	PORTION	CALORIES	FAT	SAT FAT	CHOL	PROTEIN	CARBO	FIBER	CALCIUM	SOD	POTAS	VIT C	FOLIC	VIT A
SENECA (CONT.)														
Raspberry-Cranberry Juice Cocktail frzn as prep	8 fl oz	140	0	0	0	0	36	0	0	35	36	60	—	0
MIX														
fruit punch as prep w/water	9 oz	97	0	0	0	tr	25	—	41	38	2	31	tr	1
CRYSTAL LIGHT														
Fruit Punch as prep	1 serv (8 oz)	5	0	0	0	0	0	0	0	0	45	6	—	0
Lemon-Lime Drink as prep	1 serv (8 oz)	5	0	0	0	0	0	0	0	0	5	6	—	0
Passion Fruit Pineapple Drink as prep	1 serv (8 oz)	5	0	0	0	0	tr	0	0	0	10	0	—	0
Pineapple Orange Drink as prep	1 serv (8 oz)	5	0	0	0	0	0	0	0	0	0	0	—	0
Strawberry Orange Banana as prep	1 serv (8 oz)	5	0	0	0	0	0	0	0	0	35	0	—	0
Strawberry Kiwi as prep	1 serv (8 oz)	5	0	0	0	0	0	0	0	0	0	0	—	0
Watermelon Strawberry as prep	1 serv (8 oz)	5	0	0	0	0	0	0	0	0	15	0	—	0
KOOL-AID														
Cherry as prep	1 serv (8 oz)	60	0	0	0	0	16	0	0	0	0	6	—	0
Grape Berry Splash Drink as prep	1 serv (8 oz)	70	0	0	0	0	17	0	0	0	0	6	—	0
Grape Berry Splash Drink as prep w/ sugar	1 serv (8 oz)	100	0	0	0	0	25	0	0	0	0	6	—	0
Kickin' Kiwi Lime Drink as prep	1 serv (8 oz)	60	0	0	0	0	16	0	0	0	0	6	—	0
Kickin' Kiwi Lime Drink as prep w/ sugar	1 serv (8 oz)	100	0	0	0	0	25	0	0	10	0	6	—	0
Lemon-Lime Drink as prep w/ sugar	1 serv (8 oz)	100	0	0	0	0	25	0	0	5	0	6	—	0
Man-O-Mango Berry Drink as prep w/ sugar	1 serv (8 oz)	100	0	0	0	0	25	0	0	0	0	6	—	0
Man-O-Mango Berry Drink as prep	1 serv (8 oz)	60	0	0	0	0	16	0	0	0	0	6	—	0
Oh Yeah Orange Pinapple Drink as prep w/ sugar	1 serv (8 oz)	100	0	0	0	0	25	0	0	0	0	6	—	0
Oh Yeah Orange Pineapple Drink as prep	1 serv (8 oz)	60	0	0	0	0	16	0	0	0	0	6	—	0

FOOD	PORTION	CALORIES	FAT	SAT FAT	CHOL	PROTEIN	CARBO	FIBER	CALCIUM	SOD	POTAS	VIT C	FOLIC	VIT A
KOOL-AID (CONT.)														
Pina-Pineapple Drink as prep	1 serv (8 oz)	60	0	0	0	0	17	0	0	0	0	6	—	0
Pina-Pineapple Drink as prep w/ sugar	1 serv (8 oz)	100	0	0	0	0	25	0	0	0	0	6	—	0
Rainbow Punch	1 serv (8 oz)	98	0	0	0	0	25	—	24	—	1	6	—	—
Roarin' Raspberry Cranberry Drink as prep	1 serv (8 oz)	70	0	0	0	0	17	0	0	20	0	6	—	0
Roarin' Raspberry Cranberry Drink as prep w/ sugar	1 serv (8 oz)	100	0	0	0	0	25	0	0	10	0	6	—	0
Slammin' Strawberry Kiwi Drink as prep	1 serv (8 oz)	70	0	0	0	0	17	0	0	15	0	6	—	0
Slammin' Strawberry Kiwi Drink as prep w/ sugar	1 serv (8 oz)	100	0	0	0	0	25	0	0	15	0	6	—	0
Strawberry Raspberry Drink as prep	1 serv (8 oz)	60	0	0	0	0	16	0	0	0	0	6	—	0
Strawberry Raspberry Drink as prep w/ sugar	1 serv (8 oz)	100	0	0	0	0	25	0	0	0	0	6	—	0
Sugar Free Tropical Punch as prep	1 serv (8 oz)	5	0	0	0	0	0	0	0	10	10	6	—	0
Tropical Punch as prep	1 serv (8 oz)	60	0	0	0	0	16	0	0	0	0	6	—	0
Tropical Punch as prep w/ sugar	1 serv (8 oz)	100	0	0	0	0	25	0	0	15	0	6	—	0
Watermelon Cherry Drink as prep	1 serv (8 oz)	60	0	0	0	0	16	0	0	0	0	6	—	0
Watermelon Cherry Drink as prep w/ sugar	1 serv (8 oz)	100	0	0	0	0	25	0	0	10	0	6	—	0
TANG														
Orange Pineapple as prep	1 serv (8 oz)	100	0	0	0	0	24	0	60	45	0	60	—	500
READY-TO-DRINK														
cranberry apple drink	6 fl oz	123	0	—	0	tr	32	—	13	4	50	—	—	—
cranberry apricot drink	6 fl oz	118	0	0	0	0	30	—	17	4	113	0	—	—
fruit punch	6 fl oz	87	tr	0	0	tr	22	—	14	41	47	55	2	26
orange grapefruit juice	8 fl oz	107	tr	tr	0	1	25	—	21	8	390	72	—	293
orange & apricot	8 fl oz	128	tr	tr	0	1	32	—	13	—	201	50	—	1450

FOOD	PORTION	CALORIES	FAT	SAT FAT	CHOL	PROTEIN	CARBO	FIBER	CALCIUM	SOD	POTAS	VIT C	FOLIC	VIT A
pineapple & grapefruit	8 fl oz	117	tr	tr	0	1	29	—	18	14	154	115	26	88
pineapple & orange drink	8 fl oz	125	0	0	0	3	29	—	13	9	116	56	27	1320
AFTER THE FALL														
Amaretto Almond	1 can (12 oz)	170	0	0	0	tr	42	0	20	25	60	1	—	0
American Pie Cherry	1 can (12 oz)	190	0	0	0	tr	35	0	20	20	250	1	—	0
Apple Apricot	1 cup (8 oz)	100	0	0	0	1	26	0	0	20	—	6	—	0
Apple Raspberry	1 bottle (10 oz)	110	0	0	0	0	29	—	0	25	290	2	—	0
Apple Strawberry	1 bottle (10 oz)	120	0	0	0	1	30	—	0	23	290	9	—	0
Banana Casablanca	1 bottle (10 oz)	120	0	0	0	1	24	—	0	13	220	6	—	0
Berrymeister	1 can (12 oz)	160	0	0	0	1	40	0	40	25	190	1	—	0
Cranberry Meets Raspberry	1 bottle (10 oz)	120	0	0	0	0	29	—	20	25	310	2	—	0
Georgia Peach Blend	1 bottle (10 oz)	130	0	0	0	1	33	—	0	23	210	9	—	0
Mango Montage	1 bottle (10 oz)	140	0	0	0	1	33	—	0	15	140	15	—	0
Maui Grove	1 bottle (10 oz)	120	0	0	0	1	29	—	0	20	150	5	—	0
Nantucket Ginger Ale	1 can (12 oz)	140	0	0	0	1	35	0	20	25	90	1	—	0
Orange Icicle Cream	1 can (12 oz)	170	0	0	0	tr	42	0	20	25	60	1	—	0
Oregon Berry	1 bottle (10 oz)	130	0	0	0	0	31	—	20	30	310	2	—	0
Passion Of The Islands	1 bottle (10 oz)	125	0	0	0	1	32	—	0	15	120	9	—	0
Peach Vanilla	1 can (12 oz)	170	0	0	0	tr	42	0	20	35	60	1	—	0
Strawberry Vanilla	1 can (12 oz)	160	0	0	0	tr	42	0	20	25	60	1	—	0
Twist O' Strawberry	1 can (12 oz)	190	0	0	0	tr	37	0	20	25	190	1	—	0
Vanilla Bean Cream	1 can (12 oz)	170	0	0	0	tr	42	0	20	25	60	1	—	0
APPLE & EVE														
Apple Cranberry	6 fl oz	80	0	0	0	0	19	—	13	5	160	1	—	64
Apple Grape	6 fl oz	120	0	0	0	1	29	—	18	0	179	67	—	87
Cranberry Grape	6 fl oz	100	0	0	0	1	23	—	17	5	140	0	—	105
Fruit Punch	6 fl oz	78	0	0	0	0	18	—	7	0	154	1	—	161
Raspberry Cranberry	6 fl oz	90	0	0	0	0	21	—	22	10	210	1	—	85
BAMA														
Fruit Punch	8.45 fl oz	130	0	0	0	0	32	—	—	15	30	30	—	—
BOKU														
White Grape Raspberry	16 fl oz	120	0	0	0	0	29	—	—	75	—	30	—	—

FOOD	PORTION	CALORIES	FAT	SAT FAT	CHOL	PROTEIN	CARBO	FIBER	CALCIUM	SOD	POTAS	VIT C	FOLIC	VIT A
CAPRI SUN														
Fruit Punch	1 pkg (7 oz)	100	0	0	0	0	26	0	0	20	25	0	—	0
Maui Punch	1 pkg (7 oz)	100	0	0	0	0	27	0	0	20	20	0	—	0
Mountain Cooler	1 pkg (7 oz)	90	0	0	0	0	24	0	0	25	25	0	—	0
Pacific Cooler	1 pkg (7 oz)	100	0	0	0	0	26	0	0	20	25	0	—	0
Red Berry	1 pkg (7 oz)	100	0	0	0	0	26	0	0	20	25	0	—	0
Safari Punch	1 pkg (7 oz)	100	0	0	0	0	25	0	0	20	25	0	—	0
Strawberry Kiwi Drink	1 pkg (7 oz)	100	0	0	0	0	26	0	0	20	25	0	—	0
Surfer Cooler Drink	1 pkg (7 oz)	100	0	0	0	0	27	0	0	20	30	0	—	0
COCO LOPEZ														
Mango Kiwi	8 fl oz	130	0	0	0	0	33	—	—	0	—	—	—	—
CRYSTAL GEYSER														
Juice Squeeze Citrus Grape	1 bottle (12 fl oz)	145	0	0	0	1	35	—	—	20	—	—	—	—
Juice Squeeze Orange & Passion Fruit	1 bottle (12 fl oz)	130	0	0	0	0	31	—	—	20	—	—	—	—
Juice Squeeze Passion Fruit & Mango	1 bottle (12 fl oz)	125	0	0	0	0	31	—	—	20	—	—	—	—
Juice Squeeze Wild Berry	1 bottle (12 fl oz)	130	0	0	0	1	31	—	—	20	—	—	—	—
CRYSTAL LIGHT														
Fruit Punch	1 serv (8 oz)	5	0	0	0	0	0	0	0	20	105	0	—	0
Kiwi Strawberry	1 serv (8 oz)	5	0	0	0	0	0	0	0	20	110	0	—	0
Orange Strawberry Banana Drink	1 serv (8 oz)	5	0	0	0	0	0	0	0	20	95	0	—	0
DOLE														
Pineapple Orange	6 fl oz	90	0	0	0	0	22	—	—	10	260	—	—	—
Pineapple Orange Banana	6 fl oz	100	0	0	0	0	23	—	—	10	270	—	—	—
Pineapple Orange Guava	6 fl oz	100	0	0	0	tr	21	—	—	10	180	—	—	—
Pineapple Passion Banana	6 fl oz	100	0	0	0	tr	21	—	—	10	220	—	—	—
EVERFRESH														
Cranberry-Apple Drink	1 can (8 oz)	120	0	0	0	0	31	0	—	0	—	—	—	—
Grape-Strawberry	1 can (8 oz)	120	0	0	0	0	31	0	—	0	—	—	—	—
Kiwi-Strawberry	1 can (8 oz)	120	0	0	0	0	30	0	—	0	—	—	—	—
Mandarin Orange Mango Drink	1 can (8 oz)	120	0	0	0	0	29	0	—	0	—	—	—	—
Orange Banana Strawberry Drink	1 can (8 oz)	120	0	0	0	0	30	0	—	19	—	—	—	—
Tropical Fruit Punch	1 can (8 oz)	120	0	0	0	0	30	0	—	0	—	—	—	—

FOOD	PORTION	CALORIES	FAT	SAT FAT	CHOL	PROTEIN	CARBO	FIBER	CALCIUM	SOD	POTAS	VIT C	FOLIC	VIT A
EVERFRESH (CONT.)														
Wild Blackberry Lime Drink	1 can (8 oz)	120	0	0	0	0	29	0	—	0	—	—	—	—
FIVE ALIVE														
Citrus	6 fl oz	90	0	0	0	0	22	—	—	20	130	30	—	—
Citrus	1 bottle (16 fl oz)	120	0	0	0	0	31	—	—	25	—	5	—	—
Citrus	1 can (11.5 fl oz)	170	0	0	0	0	43	—	—	35	—	36	—	—
Citrus Chilled	8 fl oz	120	0	0	0	0	30	—	—	25	—	—	—	—
FRESH SAMANTHA														
Banana Strawberry	1 cup (8 oz)	148	1	tr	0	4	36	2	20	—	—	72	24	300
Beta Yet	1 cup (8 oz)	98	1	0	0	2	24	2	10	0	—	34	20	25750
Carrot Orange	1 cup (8 oz)	107	1	0	0	4	24	1	40	—	—	54	40	21500
Colossal C	1 cup (8 oz)	116	0	0	0	2	30	2	20	—	—	210	8	100
Desperately Seeking C	1 cup (8 oz)	129	1	tr	0	4	30	3	20	0	—	600	40	5000
Protein Blast	1 cup (8 oz)	156	1	tr	0	9	30	2	40	—	—	60	32	300
Spirulina Fruit Blend	1 cup (8 oz)	129	1	0	0	2	30	2	20	—	—	24	16	2000
Strawberry Orange	1 cup (8 oz)	120	1	0	0	5	27	1	20	0	—	132	40	400
The Big Bang	1 cup (8 oz)	97	1	0	0	2	24	2	0	0	—	27	24	200
FRUITOPIA														
Fruit Integration	8 fl oz	110	0	0	0	0	29	—	—	80	—	60	—	—
HI-C														
Boppin' Berry Box	8.45 fl oz	140	0	0	0	0	33	—	—	30	—	60	—	—
Boppin' Berry	8 fl oz	130	0	0	0	0	32	—	—	30	—	60	—	—
Double Fruit Box	8.45 fl oz	130	0	0	0	0	32	—	—	35	—	60	—	—
Double Fruit Cooler	8 fl oz	130	0	0	0	0	31	—	—	30	—	60	—	—
Ecto Cooler	8 fl oz	130	0	0	0	0	32	—	—	25	—	60	—	—
Ecto Cooler	1 can (11.5 fl oz)	180	0	0	0	0	45	—	—	40	—	84	—	—
Ecto Cooler Box	8.45 fl oz	130	0	0	0	0	32	—	—	35	—	60	—	—
Fruit Punch	8 fl oz	130	0	0	0	0	32	—	—	30	—	60	—	—
Fruit Punch	1 can (11.5 fl oz)	190	0	0	0	0	46	—	—	40	—	84	—	—
Fruit Punch Box	8.45 fl oz	140	0	0	0	0	32	—	—	30	—	60	—	—
Fruity Bubble Gum	8 fl oz	120	0	0	0	0	30	—	—	25	—	60	—	—
Fruity Bubble Gum Box	8.45 fl oz	130	0	0	0	0	32	—	—	30	—	60	—	—
Hula Punch	8 fl oz	120	0	0	0	0	29	—	—	30	—	60	—	—
Hula Punch	1 can (11.5 fl oz)	170	0	0	0	0	42	—	—	40	—	84	—	—
Hula Punch Box	8.45 fl oz	120	0	0	0	0	30	—	—	30	—	60	—	—
Jammin' Apple Box	8.45 fl oz	130	0	0	0	0	33	—	—	30	—	60	—	—

FOOD	PORTION	CALORIES	FAT	SAT FAT	CHOL	PROTEIN	CARBO	FIBER	CALCIUM	SOD	POTAS	VIT C	FOLIC	VIT A
HI-C (CONT.)														
Stompin' Banana Berry	8 fl oz	130	0	0	0	0	31	—	—	30	—	60	—	—
Stompin' Banana Berry Box	8.45 fl oz	130	0	0	0	0	32	—	—	30	—	60	—	—
Wild Berry	8 fl oz	120	0	0	0	0	30	—	—	30	—	60	—	—
Wild Berry Box	8.45 fl oz	130	0	0	0	0	32	—	—	30	—	60	—	—
HOOD														
Natural Blenders Apple Cranberry Raspberry	1 cup (8 oz)	130	0	0	0	0	32	—	—	5	—	0	—	—
Natural Blenders Apple Grape Cherry	1 cup (8 oz)	130	0	0	0	0	32	—	—	5	—	0	—	—
Natural Blenders Apple Peach Pear	1 cup (8 oz)	120	0	0	0	0	30	—	—	5	—	0	—	—
Natural Blenders Apple Wild Blueberry Strawberry	1 cup (8 oz)	120	0	0	0	0	30	—	—	5	—	0	—	—
Natural Blenders Pineapple Orange Kiwi	1 cup (8 oz)	120	0	0	0	0	30	—	—	5	—	18	—	—
JUICY JUICE														
Apple Grape	1 box (8.45 fl oz)	120	0	0	0	1	29	—	—	10	240	60	—	—
Berry	1 box (8.45 fl oz)	130	0	0	0	1	30	—	20	15	230	60	—	—
Berry	1 bottle (6 fl oz)	90	0	0	0	1	22	—	—	10	160	60	—	—
Punch	1 box (8.45 fl oz)	140	0	0	0	1	33	—	20	10	180	60	—	—
Punch	1 bottle (6 fl oz)	100	0	0	0	1	23	—	—	10	130	60	—	—
Tropical	1 bottle (6 fl oz)	110	0	0	0	1	26	—	—	10	110	60	—	—
Tropical	1 box (8.45 fl oz)	150	0	0	0	1	36	—	20	10	160	60	—	—
KERN'S														
Apple Strawberry Nectar	6 fl oz	110	0	0	0	0	26	—	20	0	120	60	—	—
Apricot Pineapple Nectar	6 fl oz	110	0	0	0	0	27	—	20	5	190	27	—	1500
Banana Pineapple Nectar	6 fl oz	110	0	0	0	1	27	—	—	0	160	27	—	—
Coconut Pineapple Nectar	6 fl oz	140	0	0	0	1	26	—	—	25	120	27	—	—
Orange Banana Nectar	6 fl oz	110	0	0	0	1	25	—	20	0	180	60	—	—

FOOD	PORTION	CALORIES	FAT	SAT FAT	CHOL	PROTEIN	CARBO	FIBER	CALCIUM	SOD	POTAS	VIT C	FOLIC	VIT A
KERN'S (CONT.)														
Strawberry Banana Nectar	6 fl oz	110	0	0	0	0	28	—	—	0	110	27	—	—
Tropical Nectar	6 fl oz	110	0	0	0	0	27	—	—	5	90	27	—	—
KOOL-AID														
Bursts Great Bluedini	1 (7 oz)	100	0	0	0	0	24	0	0	30	15	0	—	0
Bursts Kickin' Kiwi Lime	1 (7 oz)	100	0	0	0	0	24	0	0	30	15	0	—	0
Bursts Oh Yeah Orange Pineapple	1 (7 oz)	100	0	0	0	0	24	0	0	30	15	0	—	0
Bursts Slammin' Strawberry Kiwi	1 (7 oz)	100	0	0	0	0	24	0	0	30	15	0	—	0
Bursts Tropical Punch	1 (7 oz)	100	0	0	0	0	24	0	0	30	15	0	—	0
Splash Grape Berry Punch	1 serv (8 oz)	120	0	0	0	0	31	0	0	35	15	0	—	0
Splash Kiwi Strawberry Drink	1 serv (8 oz)	110	0	0	0	0	29	0	0	35	15	0	—	0
Splash Tropical Punch	1 serv (8 oz)	120	0	0	0	0	31	0	0	35	15	0	—	0
LIBBY														
Strawberry Banana Nectar	1 can (11.5 fl oz)	220	0	0	0	tr	51	—	20	10	250	60	—	—
MAUNA LA'I														
Island Guava Hawaiian Guava Fruit Juice Drink	8 fl oz	130	0	0	0	0	32	0	—	35	30	60	—	0
Mango & Hawaiian Guava Fruit Juice Drink	8 fl oz	130	0	0	0	0	33	0	—	35	—	60	—	0
Paradise Guava Hawaiian Guava & Passion Fruit Juice Drink	8 fl oz	130	0	0	0	0	32	0	—	35	65	60	—	500
MINUTE MAID														
Berry Punch Box	8.45 fl oz	130	0	0	0	0	31	—	—	25	—	—	—	—
Berry Punch Chilled	8 fl oz	130	0	0	0	0	31	—	—	25	—	—	—	—
Citrus Punch Chilled	8 fl oz	130	0	0	0	0	31	—	—	25	—	—	—	—
Fruit Punch Box	8.45 fl oz	120	0	0	0	0	31	—	—	25	—	—	—	—
Fruit Punch Chilled	8 fl oz	120	0	0	0	0	31	—	—	25	—	—	—	—
Juices To Go Citrus Punch	1 can (11.5 fl oz)	180	0	0	0	0	45	—	—	40	—	—	—	—
Juices To Go Citrus Punch	1 bottle (10 fl oz)	160	0	0	0	0	39	—	—	35	—	—	—	—
Juices To Go Concord Punch	1 can (11.5 fl oz)	180	0	0	0	0	46	—	—	40	—	—	—	—

FOOD	PORTION	CALORIES	FAT	SAT FAT	CHOL	PROTEIN	CARBO	FIBER	CALCIUM	SOD	POTAS	VIT C	FOLIC	VIT A
MINUTE MAID (CONT.)														
Juices To Go Concord Punch	1 bottle (10 fl oz)	160	0	0	0	0	40	—	—	35	—	—	—	—
Juices To Go Concord Punch	1 bottle (16 fl oz)	130	0	0	0	0	32	—	—	25	—	—	—	—
Juices To Go Fruit Punch	1 can (11.5 fl oz)	180	0	0	0	0	44	—	—	40	—	—	—	—
Juices To Go Fruit Punch	1 bottle (10 fl oz)	160	0	0	0	0	39	—	—	35	—	—	—	—
Juices To Go Fruit Punch	1 bottle (16 fl oz)	120	0	0	0	0	31	—	—	25	—	—	—	—
Juices To Go Orange Blend	1 bottle (10 fl oz)	150	0	0	0	0	37	—	—	35	520	12	—	—
Juices To Go Orange Blend	1 can (11.5 fl oz)	170	0	0	0	0	43	—	—	40	600	42	—	—
Naturals Apple Cranberry	8 fl oz	170	0	0	0	0	42	—	—	25	—	—	—	—
Naturals Concord Medley	8 fl oz	130	0	0	0	0	32	—	—	25	—	—	—	—
Naturals Fruit Medley	8 fl oz	120	0	0	0	0	31	—	—	25	—	—	—	—
Naturals Orange Grape Medley	8 fl oz	120	0	0	—	0	30	—	—	25	420	—	—	—
Naturals Tropical Medley	8 fl oz	120	0	0	0	0	31	—	—	25	—	—	—	—
Tropical Punch Box	8.45 fl oz	130	0	0	0	0	32	—	—	25	—	—	—	—
Tropical Punch Chilled	8 fl oz	120	0	0	0	0	31	—	—	25	—	—	—	—
MOTT'S														
Apple Cranberry Blend	10 fl oz	180	0	0	0	0	44	0	0	15	80	0	—	0
Apple Cranberry From Concentrate as prep	8 fl oz	120	0	0	0	0	30	0	20	20	300	2	—	0
Apple Grape From Concentrate as prep	8 fl oz	120	0	0	0	0	30	0	0	20	240	1	—	0
Apple Raspberry Blend	10 fl oz	140	0	0	0	0	33	0	0	10	70	4	—	0
Apple Raspberry From Concentrate	8.45 fl oz	120	0	0	0	0	30	0	0	25	270	6	—	0
Fruit Basket Apple Raspberry Juice Cocktail as prep	8 fl oz	130	0	0	0	0	30	0	20	5	150	15	—	0
Fruit Basket Tropical Blend Juice Cocktail as prep	8 fl oz	120	0	0	0	0	30	0	20	5	160	15	—	0

FOOD	PORTION	CALORIES	FAT	SAT FAT	CHOL	PROTEIN	CARBO	FIBER	CALCIUM	SOD	POTAS	VIT C	FOLIC	VIT A
MOTT'S (CONT.)														
Fruit Punch From Concentrate	8.45 fl oz	120	0	0	0	0	29	0	0	20	230	2	—	0
Fruit Punch From Concentrate	10 fl oz	170	0	0	0	0	42	0	0	0	120	1	—	0
Grape Apple	10 fl oz	170	0	0	0	0	41	0	0	10	60	0	—	0
Pineapple Orange	10 fl oz	170	0	0	0	0	42	0	20	15	30	0	—	0
NANTUCKET NECTARS														
Orange Mango	8 fl oz	130	0	0	0	0	32	0	0	5	—	60	—	100
OCEAN SPRAY														
Cran*Grape	8 fl oz	170	0	0	0	0	41	0	—	35	—	60	—	0
Cran*Raspberry	8 fl oz	140	0	0	0	0	36	0	—	35	—	60	—	0
Cran*Strawberry	8 fl oz	140	0	0	0	0	36	tr	—	35	—	60	—	0
Cranapple	8 fl oz	160	0	0	0	0	41	tr	—	35	—	60	—	0
Cranapple Reduced Calorie	8 fl oz	50	0	0	0	0	13	0	—	35	125	60	—	0
Fruit Punch	8 fl oz	130	0	0	0	0	32	0	—	35	—	60	—	0
Kiwi Strawberry Cooler	8 fl oz	120	0	0	0	0	31	0	—	35	0	60	—	600
Ruby Red & Tangerine Grapefruit Juice Drink	8 fl oz	130	0	0	0	0	32	0	—	35	75	60	—	0
ODWALLA														
Boyzenberry Mango	8 fl oz	140	0	0	0	1	34	2	0	20	—	60	—	4000
C Monster	16 fl oz	300	0	0	0	4	72	4	40	110	—	1200	—	4000
Fruitshake Blackberry	8 fl oz	160	0	0	0	1	39	3	20	50	—	5	—	200
Guanaba Dabba Doo!	8 fl oz	130	0	0	0	2	29	0	20	35	—	27	—	200
Lotta Colada	8 fl oz	160	3	—	—	2	33	2	20	45	—	21	—	300
Mango Tango	8 fl oz	150	3	—	—	1	37	6	20	55	—	0	—	4000
Mo Beta	16 fl oz	280	1	—	—	3	69	3	60	290	—	480	—	50000
Raspberry Smoothie	8 fl oz	140	0	0	0	2	35	2	20	25	—	15	—	500
Strawberry Banana Smoothie	8 fl oz	100	0	0	0	1	26	2	20	10	—	15	—	100
Strawberry Go Man Go	8 fl oz	100	1	—	—	1	26	2	0	25	—	5	—	2250
Super Protein	16 fl oz	400	6	—	—	10	40	5	350	250	—	54	—	1500
PEK														
Mango Guava Ecstasy	1 bottle (20 fl oz)	110	0	0	0	0	27	0	250	20	—	60	200	2500
Passionate Peach Grapefruit	8 fl oz	110	0	0	0	0	27	0	250	20	—	60	200	2500
SHASTA PLUS														
Apple-Strawberry	1 can (11.5 oz)	160	0	0	0	0	41	0	—	45	—	60	—	—

FOOD	PORTION	CALORIES	FAT	SAT FAT	CHOL	PROTEIN	CARBO	FIBER	CALCIUM	SOD	POTAS	VIT C	FOLIC	VIT A
SHASTA PLUS (CONT.)														
Fruit Punch	1 can (11.5 oz)	160	0	0	0	0	39	0	—	45	—	60	—	—
Pineapple-Cherry	1 can (11.5 oz)	160	0	0	0	0	40	0	—	45	—	60	—	—
SNAPPLE														
Diet Kiwi Strawberry	8 fl oz	13	0	0	0	0	3	—	0	10	65	—	—	300
Fruit Punch	8 fl oz	120	0	0	0	0	29	—	0	5	10	—	—	0
Kiwi Strawberry Cocktail	8 fl oz	130	0	0	0	0	33	—	0	10	—	—	—	300
Melonberry Cocktail	8 fl oz	120	0	0	0	0	29	—	0	10	—	—	—	0
Vitamin Supreme	10 fl oz	150	0	0	0	0	38	—	40	20	—	60	—	5000
SQUEEZIT														
Berry B. Wild	1 (6.75 fl oz)	90	0	0	0	0	22	—	—	0	10	—	—	—
Chucklin' Cherry	1 (6.75 fl oz)	90	0	0	0	0	23	—	—	5	10	—	—	—
Grumpy Grape	1 (6.75 fl oz)	90	0	0	0	0	23	—	—	0	10	—	—	—
Mean Green Puncher	1 (6.75 fl oz)	90	0	0	0	0	23	—	—	0	5	—	—	—
Silly Billy Strawberry	1 (6.75 fl oz)	90	0	0	0	0	23	—	—	0	<5	—	—	—
Smarty Arty Orange	1 (6.75 fl oz)	90	0	0	0	0	23	—	—	50	5	—	—	—
TROPICANA														
Berry Punch	8 fl oz	120	0	0	0	0	29	—	—	25	—	—	—	—
Citrus Punch	8 fl oz	140	0	0	0	0	36	—	—	20	—	—	—	—
Citrus Punch	1 bottle (10 fl oz)	180	0	0	0	0	45	—	—	15	—	8	—	—
Cranberry Punch	8 fl oz	140	0	0	0	0	34	—	—	10	—	—	—	—
Cranberry Punch	1 bottle (10 fl oz)	170	0	0	0	0	43	—	—	10	—	—	—	—
Cranberry Punch	1 can (11.5 fl oz)	200	0	0	0	0	49	—	—	15	—	—	—	—
Fruit Punch	1 container (10 fl oz)	160	0	0	0	0	39	—	—	25	—	—	—	—
Fruit Punch	8 fl oz	130	0	0	0	0	31	—	—	25	—	—	—	—
Fruit Punch	1 bottle (10 fl oz)	150	0	0	0	0	39	—	—	25	—	—	—	—
Fruit Punch	1 can (11.5 fl oz)	170	0	0	0	0	42	—	—	30	—	—	—	—
Orange Pineapple	8 fl oz	110	0	0	0	tr	27	—	—	15	340	10	—	—
Orange Pineapple	1 bottle (10 fl oz)	130	0	0	0	tr	32	—	—	15	420	110	—	—
Pineapple Punch	1 bottle (10 fl oz)	160	0	0	0	0	39	—	—	20	—	20	—	—
Pineapple Punch	8 fl oz	120	0	0	0	0	31	—	—	15	—	15	—	—
Season's Best Cranberry Medley	8 fl oz	120	0	0	0	tr	29	—	—	20	260	100	—	—

FOOD	PORTION	CALORIES	FAT	SAT FAT	CHOL	PROTEIN	CARBO	FIBER	CALCIUM	SOD	POTAS	VIT C	FOLIC	VIT A
TROPICANA (CONT.)														
Tropics Apple Cranberry Kiwi	8 fl oz	120	0	0	0	tr	30	—	—	15	250	—	—	—
Tropics Orange Strawberry Banana	8 fl oz	110	0	0	0	tr	27	—	—	5	380	10	—	—
Tropics Orange Kiwi Passion	8 fl oz	100	0	0	0	tr	26	—	—	15	300	10	—	—
Tropics Orange Peach Mango	8 fl oz	110	0	0	0	tr	28	—	—	15	300	10	—	—
Tropics Orange Pineapple	8 fl oz	110	0	0	0	tr	27	—	—	15	340	10	—	—
Tropics Pineapple Passion	8 fl oz	120	0	0	0	tr	30	—	—	25	200	—	—	—
Twister Apple Raspberry Blackberry	1 can (11.5 fl oz)	180	0	0	0	0	44	—	—	25	—	—	—	—
Twister Apple Raspberry Blackberry	8 fl oz	120	0	0	0	0	31	—	—	20	—	—	—	—
Twister Apple Raspberry Blackberry	1 bottle (10 fl oz)	150	0	0	0	0	38	—	—	25	—	—	—	—
Twister Cranberry Raspberry Strawberry	8 fl oz	120	0	0	0	0	31	—	—	5	—	—	—	—
Twister Cranberry Raspberry Strawberry	1 bottle (10 fl oz)	160	0	0	0	tr	39	—	—	5	—	—	—	—
Twister Light Cranberry Raspberry Strawberry	8 fl oz	45	0	0	0	tr	11	—	—	10	—	160	—	—
Twister Light Cranberry Raspberry Strawberry	1 container (10 fl oz)	50	0	0	0	tr	13	—	—	15	—	160	—	—
Twister Light Orange Cranberry	1 container (10 fl oz)	35	0	0	0	0	9	—	—	25	—	60	—	—
Twister Light Orange Cranberry	8 fl oz	30	0	0	0	0	7	—	—	20	—	140	—	—
Twister Light Orange Cranberry	1 container (10 fl oz)	35	0	0	0	0	9	—	—	25	—	140	—	—
Twister Light Orange Raspberry	8 fl oz	35	0	0	0	0	9	—	—	20	—	140	—	—
Twister Light Orange Raspberry	1 container (10 fl oz)	45	0	0	0	0	11	—	—	25	—	140	—	—
Twister Light Orange Strawberry Banana	1 container (10 fl oz)	45	0	0	0	tr	11	—	—	25	—	120	—	—

FOOD	PORTION	CALORIES	FAT	SAT FAT	CHOL	PROTEIN	CARBO	FIBER	CALCIUM	SOD	POTAS	VIT C	FOLIC	VIT A
TROPICANA (CONT.)														
Twister Orange Cranberry	8 fl oz	120	0	0	0	tr	29	—	—	15	—	15	—	—
Twister Orange Cranberry	1 bottle (10 fl oz)	140	0	0	0	tr	36	—	—	20	—	15	—	—
Twister Orange Peach	1 can (11.5 fl oz)	160	0	0	0	tr	41	—	—	20	—	20	—	—
Twister Orange Peach	8 fl oz	120	0	0	0	tr	29	—	—	20	—	50	—	—
Twister Orange Peach	1 bottle (10 fl oz)	140	0	0	0	tr	36	—	—	25	—	50	—	—
Twister Orange Raspberry	8 fl oz	120	0	0	0	0	29	—	—	20	—	10	—	—
Twister Orange Raspberry	1 bottle (10 fl oz)	140	0	0	0	tr	36	—	—	20	—	10	—	—
Twister Orange Strawberry Banana	1 container (10 fl oz)	140	0	0	0	tr	35	—	—	20	—	10	—	—
Twister Strawberry Banana	1 bottle (10 fl oz)	140	0	0	0	tr	35	—	—	20	—	30	—	—
Twister Strawberry Banana	8 fl oz	120	0	0	0	tr	29	—	—	20	—	30	—	—
Twister Strawberry Banana	1 can (11.5 fl oz)	160	0	0	0	tr	41	—	—	30	—	40	—	—
Twister Strawberry Guava	1 bottle (10 fl oz)	140	0	0	0	tr	35	—	—	25	—	20	—	—
Twister Strawberry Guava	8 fl oz	110	0	0	0	tr	28	—	—	20	—	20	—	—
VERYFINE														
Apple Cherryberry	8 fl oz	130	0	0	0	0	33	—	—	<25	20	30	—	—
Apple Cranberry	1 bottle (10 oz)	190	0	0	0	0	48	0	0	10	—	60	—	0
Apple Quenchers Black Cherry White Grape	8 fl oz	120	0	0	0	0	30	0	0	10	—	60	—	0
Apple Quenchers Cranberry Tangerine	8 fl oz	120	0	0	0	0	31	0	0	10	—	60	—	0
Apple Quenchers Peach Kiwi	8 fl oz	130	0	0	0	0	33	0	0	25	—	60	—	0
Apple Quenchers Peach Plum	8 fl oz	130	0	0	0	0	32	0	0	25	—	60	—	0
Apple Quenchers Pear Passionfruit	8 fl oz	120	0	0	0	0	31	0	0	15	—	60	—	0
Apple Quenchers Raspberry Cherry	8 fl oz	120	0	0	0	0	31	0	0	25	—	60	—	0
Apple Quenchers Raspberry Lime	8 fl oz	120	0	0	0	0	30	0	0	25	—	60	—	0
Apple Quenchers Strawberry Banana	8 fl oz	120	0	0	0	0	30	0	0	20	—	60	—	0

FOOD	PORTION	CALORIES	FAT	SAT FAT	CHOL	PROTEIN	CARBO	FIBER	CALCIUM	SOD	POTAS	VIT C	FOLIC	VIT A
VERYFINE (CONT.)														
Chillers Artic Mango Tangerine	8 fl oz	110	0	0	0	0	27	tr	0	5	—	60	—	0
Chillers Freezing Fruit Punch	8 fl oz	130	0	0	0	0.	33	0	0	20	—	60	—	0
Chillers Lemon Lime Blizzard	8 fl oz	120	0	0	0	0	29	0	0	5	—	60	—	0
Chillers Shivering Strawberry Melon	1 can (11.5 oz)	160	0	0	0	0	41	0	0	10	—	60	—	0
Chillers Tropical Freeze	8 fl oz	120	0	0	0	0	30	0	0	10	—	60	—	0
Cranberry Raspberry	8 fl oz	160	0	0	0	0	41	0	0	10	—	60	—	0
Fruit Punch	1 bottle (10 oz)	170	0	0	0	0	42	0	0	25	—	60	—	0
Juice-Ups Berry	8 fl oz	140	0	0	0	0	34	0	0	15	—	60	—	0
Juice-Ups Fruit Punch	8 fl oz	140	0	0	0	0	34	0	0	15	—	60	—	0
Juice-Ups Orange Punch	8 fl oz	140	0	0	0	0	35	0	0	15	—	60	—	0
Orange Strawberry	8 fl oz	120	0	0	0	0	31	0	0	30	—	60	—	0
Papaya Punch	1 bottle (10 oz)	160	0	0	0	0	39	0	0	25	—	60	—	0
Pineapple Orange	1 bottle (10 oz)	160	0	0	0	0	39	0	0	20	—	60	—	0
Strawberry Banana	1 can (11.5 oz)	160	0	0	0	0	40	0	0	15	—	60	—	0
Strawberry Banana Punch	1 can (11.5 oz)	190	0	0	0	0	48	0	0	30	—	60	—	0

FRUIT MIXED

(*see also individual names*)

CANNED

FOOD	PORTION	CALORIES	FAT	SAT FAT	CHOL	PROTEIN	CARBO	FIBER	CALCIUM	SOD	POTAS	VIT C	FOLIC	VIT A
fruit cocktail in heavy syrup	½ cup	93	tr	tr	0	1	24	—	8	7	112	2	—	262
fruit cocktail juice pack	½ cup	56	tr	tr	0	1	15	—	10	4	118	3	—	378
fruit cocktail water pack	½ cup	40	tr	tr	0	1	10	—	6	5	115	3	—	305
fruit salad in heavy syrup	½ cup	94	tr	tr	0	tr	24	—	8	7	103	3	—	646
fruit salad in light syrup	½ cup	73	tr	tr	0	tr	19	—	8	7	104	3	—	541
fruit salad juice pack	½ cup	62	tr	tr	0	1	16	—	14	7	144	4	—	744
fruit salad water pack	½ cup	37	tr	tr	0	tr	10	—	8	4	95	2	—	536
mixed fruit in heavy syrup	½ cup	92	tr	tr	0	tr	24	—	1	5	108	88	—	248

FOOD	PORTION	CALORIES	FAT	SAT FAT	CHOL	PROTEIN	CARBO	FIBER	CALCIUM	SOD	POTAS	VIT C	FOLIC	VIT A
tropical fruit salad in heavy syrup	½ cup	110	tr	—	0	1	29	—	17	3	168	22	—	162
DEL MONTE														
Fruit Cocktail Fruit Naturals	½ cup (4.4 oz)	60	0	0	0	0	15	1	0	10	—	2	—	200
Fruit Cocktail In Heavy Syrup	½ cup (4.5 oz)	100	0	0	0	0	24	1	0	10	—	2	—	200
Fruit Cocktail Lite	½ cup (4.4 oz)	60	0	0	0	0	15	1	0	10	—	2	—	200
Lite Mixed Fruits Chunky	½ cup (4.4 oz)	60	0	0	0	0	15	1	0	10	—	2	—	200
Mixed Fruits Chunky Fruit Naturals	½ cup (4.4 oz)	60	0	0	0	0	15	1	0	10	—	2	—	200
Mixed Fruits Chunky In Heavy Syrup	½ cup (4.5 oz)	100	0	0	0	0	24	1	0	10	—	2	—	200
Snack Cups Mixed Fruit Fruit Naturals	1 serv (4.5 oz)	60	0	0	0	0	16	1	0	10	—	4	—	200
Snack Cups Mixed Fruit Fruit Naturals EZ-Open Lid	1 serv (4.5 oz)	60	0	0	0	0	15	1	0	10	—	4	—	200
Snack Cups Mixed Fruit In Heavy Syrup	1 serv (4.5 oz)	100	0	0	0	0	24	1	0	10	—	4	—	200
Snack Cups Mixed Fruit In Heavy Syrup EZ-Open Lid	1 serv (4.2 oz)	90	0	0	0	0	23	1	0	10	—	4	—	200
Snack Cups Mixed Fruit Lite	1 serv (4.5 oz)	60	0	0	0	0	16	1	0	10	—	4	—	200
Snack Cups Mixed Fruit Lite EZ-Open Lid	1 serv (4.5 oz)	60	0	0	0	0	15	1	0	10	—	4	—	200
DOLE														
Tropical Fruit Salad	½ cup	70	0	—	0	0	17	—	—	10	—	—	—	—
HUNT'S														
Fruit Cocktail	½ cup (4.5 oz)	90	0	0	0	0	23	1	1	15	—	2	—	20
LIBBY														
Chunky Mixed Lite	½ cup (4.3 oz)	60	0	0	0	0	14	1	0	5	85	1	—	200
Fruit Cocktail Lite	½ cup (4.3 oz)	60	0	0	0	0	15	1	0	10	120	1	—	200
DRIED														
mixed	11 oz pkg	712	1	tr	0	7	188	—	110	52	2332	11	—	7155
DEL MONTE														
Mixed	⅓ cup (1.4 oz)	110	0	0	0	0	30	5	0	50	—	1	—	1250
PLANTERS														
Fruit'n Nut Mix	1 oz	140	9	2	0	4	13	2	20	105	200	—	—	—

FOOD	PORTION	CALORIES	FAT	SAT FAT	CHOL	PROTEIN	CARBO	FIBER	CALCIUM	SOD	POTAS	VIT C	FOLIC	VIT A
SONOMA														
Diced	⅓ cup (1.4 oz)	120	0	0	0	1	31	3	0	0	—	2	—	400
Mixed Fruit	5-8 pieces (1.4 oz)	120	0	0	0	1	30	3	0	0	—	2	—	500
FROZEN														
mixed fruit sweetened	1 cup	245	tr	tr	0	4	61	—	18	8	327	188	—	806
BIG VALLEY														
Burst O' Berries	⅔ cup (4.9 oz)	70	0	0	0	1	16	3	30	0	—	42	—	150
California Tropics	⅔ cup (4.9 oz)	60	0	0	0	1	15	2	0	0	—	96	—	1000
Cup A Fruit	1 pkg (4 oz)	50	0	0	0	tr	7	2	0	0	—	168	—	500
Mixed	4.9 oz	60	0	0	0	1	14	2	13	0	—	90	—	1000
BIRDS EYE														
Mixed Fruit	½ cup (4.4 oz)	90	0	0	0	tr	23	—	—	5	—	42	—	200
DOLE														
Applesauce Strawberry	1 pkg (4 oz)	60	0	0	0	tr	15	1	0	0	—	144	—	200

FRUIT SNACKS

FOOD	PORTION	CALORIES	FAT	SAT FAT	CHOL	PROTEIN	CARBO	FIBER	CALCIUM	SOD	POTAS	VIT C	FOLIC	VIT A
fruit leather	1 bar (0.8 oz)	81	1	1	0	tr	18	—	7	18	32	16	—	27
fruit leather pieces	1 pkg (0.9 oz)	92	2	tr	0	tr	21	—	5	109	44	15	—	31
fruit leather pieces	1 oz	97	2	tr	0	tr	22	—	5	114	48	16	—	33
fruit leather rolls	1 lg (0.7 oz)	73	1	tr	0	tr	18	—	7	13	62	1	—	24
fruit leather rolls	1 sm (0.5 oz)	49	tr	tr	0	tr	12	—	4	8	41	1	—	16
BETTY CROCKER														
Fruit Roll-Ups Peel 'N Build	2 rolls (1 oz)	110	1	—	0	0	24	—	—	105	—	30	—	—
BROCK														
Beauty & The Beast	1 pkg (0.9 oz)	90	0	0	0	1	21	—	—	25	—	—	—	—
Cinderella	1 pkg (0.9 oz)	90	0	0	0	1	21	—	—	25	—	—	—	—
Dinosaurs	1 pkg (0.9 oz)	90	0	0	0	1	21	—	—	25	—	—	—	—
Ninja Trolls	1 pkg (0.9 oz)	90	0	0	0	1	21	—	—	25	—	—	—	—
Sharks	1 pkg (0.9 oz)	90	0	0	0	1	21	—	—	25	—	—	—	—
DEL MONTE														
Sierra Trail Mix	¼ cup (1.2 oz)	150	8	3	0	4	20	3	40	65	—	4	—	0
Sierra Trail Mix	1 pkg (1 oz)	120	6	2	0	3	16	2	40	50	—	2	—	0
Sierra Trail Mix	1 pkg (0.9 oz)	110	6	2	0	3	15	2	40	45	—	2	—	0
FAVORITE BRANDS														
Cherry Fruit Snack	1 pkg (0.9 oz)	80	0	0	0	1	19	—	—	15	—	15	—	1250
Creepy Crawler Fruit Snacks	1 pkg (0.9 oz)	80	0	0	0	1	19	—	—	15	—	15	—	1250
Dinosaur Fruit Snack	1 pkg (0.9 oz)	80	0	0	0	1	19	—	—	15	—	15	—	1250
Grape Fruit Snack	1 pkg (0.9 oz)	80	0	0	0	1	19	—	—	15	—	15	—	1250
Space Alien Fruit Snack	1 pkg (0.9 oz)	80	0	0	0	1	19	—	—	15	—	15	—	1250
Sports Fruit Snacks	1 pkg (0.9 oz)	80	0	0	0	1	19	—	—	15	—	15	—	1250

FOOD	PORTION	CALORIES	FAT	SAT FAT	CHOL	PROTEIN	CARBO	FIBER	CALCIUM	SOD	POTAS	VIT C	FOLIC	VIT A
FAVORITE BRANDS (CONT.)														
Strawberry Fruit Snack	1 pkg (0.9 oz)	80	0	0	0	1	19	—	—	15	—	15	—	1250
Teenage Mutant Ninja Turtle Fruit Snacks	1 pkg (0.9 oz)	80	0	0	0	1	19	—	—	15	—	15	—	1250
The Mega Roll Strawberry	1 pkg (1 oz)	110	3	2	—	0	22	2	—	15	—	15	—	1250
The Roll Cherry	1 pkg (0.75 oz)	80	2	1	—	0	16	1	—	10	—	15	—	1250
The Roll Strawberry	1 pkg (0.75 oz)	80	2	1	—	0	16	1	—	10	—	15	—	1250
Troll Fruit Snacks	1 pkg (0.9 oz)	80	0	0	0	1	19	0	—	15	—	15	—	1250
Zoo Animal Fruit Snacks	1 pkg (0.9 oz)	80	0	0	0	1	19	—	—	15	—	15	—	1250
HEALTH VALLEY														
Bakes Apple	1 bar	100	3	—	0	2	16	3	15	25	95	3	15	4
Bakes Date	1 bar	100	3	—	0	3	16	3	12	25	100	3	16	5
Bakes Raisin	1 bar	100	3	—	0	2	16	3	14	20	105	4	17	5
Fat Free Fruit Bars 100% Organic Apple	1 bar	140	tr	—	0	3	33	4	20	10	280	—	—	—
Fat Free Fruit Bars 100% Organic Apricot	1 bar	140	tr	—	0	3	33	4	20	10	280	—	—	—
Fat Free Fruit Bars 100% Organic Date	1 bar	140	tr	—	0	3	33	4	20	10	280	—	—	—
Fat Free Fruit Bars 100% Organic Raisin	1 bar	140	tr	—	0	3	33	4	20	10	280	—	—	—
Fruit & Fitness Bars	2 bars	200	5	—	0	4	35	5	39	75	290	—	14	292
Oat Bran Bakes Apricot	1 bar	100	3	—	0	2	16	2	9	15	125	1	9	1
Oat Bran Bakes Fig & Nut	1 bar	110	3	—	0	2	16	2	11	10	120	1	9	14
Oat Bran Jumbo Fruit Bar Almond & Date	1 bar	170	5	—	0	4	28	7	25	10	110	3	20	30
Oat Bran Jumbo Fruit Bars Raisin & Cinnamon	1 bar	160	2	—	0	3	32	6	58	10	125	7	20	3
Rice Bran Jumbo Fruit Bars Almond & Date	1 bar	160	5	—	0	3	27	4	45	5	280	4	4	117
SENECA														
Apple Chips	12 chips (1 oz)	140	7	1	0	0	20	2	0	15	85	18	—	0

FOOD	PORTION	CALORIES	FAT	SAT FAT	CHOL	PROTEIN	CARBO	FIBER	CALCIUM	SOD	POTAS	VIT C	FOLIC	VIT A
SENSIBLE FOODS														
Crackin' Fruit Cherry Berry	1 pkg (0.6 oz)	51	0	0	0	1	13	1	10	85	—	10	—	300
Crackin' Fruit Tropical Fruit	1 pkg (0.6 oz)	65	1	0	0	tr	16	1	10	61	—	10	—	1200
SONOMA														
Trail Mix	¼ cup (1.4 oz)	160	7	3	0	3	24	2	20	5	—	0	—	0
SOVEX														
Fruit Bites Jungle Pals	1 pkg (0.9 oz)	90	1	—	0	0	21	—	—	15	—	—	—	—
STRETCH ISLAND														
Fruit Leather Berry Blackberry	2 pieces (1 oz)	90	0	0	0	0	24	3	0	0	—	5	—	0
Fruit Leather Chunky Cherry	2 pieces (1 oz)	90	0	0	0	0	24	2	0	0	—	6	—	0
Fruit Leather Great Grape	2 pieces (1 oz)	90	0	0	0	0	24	2	20	0	—	4	—	0
Fruit Leather Organic Apple	2 pieces (1 oz)	90	0	0	0	0	24	2	0	10	—	1	—	0
Fruit Leather Organic Grape	2 pieces (1 oz)	90	0	0	0	0	24	2	0	5	—	1	—	0
Fruit Leather Organic Raspberry	2 pieces (1 oz)	90	0	0	0	0	25	2	0	10	—	1	—	0
Fruit Leather Rare Raspberry	2 pieces (1 oz)	90	0	0	0	0	24	2	0	0	—	2	—	0
Fruit Leather Snappy Apple	2 pieces (1 oz)	90	0	0	0	0	25	3	0	0	—	2	—	0
Fruit Leather Tangy Apricot	2 pieces (1 oz)	90	0	0	0	1	23	2	0	0	—	1	—	0
Fruit Leather Truly Tropical	2 pieces (1 oz)	90	0	0	0	tr	22	1	0	0	—	2	—	0
SUNBELT														
Fruit Boosters Apple	1 (1.3 oz)	130	2	0	0	1	27	0	0	60	—	0	—	0
Fruit Boosters Blueberry	1 (1.3 oz)	130	2	0	0	1	27	1	0	60	—	0	—	0
Fruit Boosters Strawberry	1 (1.3 oz)	130	2	0	0	1	27	0	0	65	—	1	—	0
Fruit Jammers	1 (1 oz)	100	1	1	0	0	23	0	0	20	—	0	—	0
WEIGHT WATCHERS														
Apple & Cinnamon	1 pkg (0.5 oz)	50	0	0	0	0	13	2	0	125	—	0	—	0
Apple Chips	1 pkg (0.75 oz)	70	0	0	0	0	18	3	0	125	—	0	—	0
Peach & Strawberry	1 pkg (0.5 oz)	50	0	0	0	0	13	2	0	125	—	0	—	0

GARBANZO

(*see* CHICKPEAS)

GARLIC

clove	1	4	tr	tr	0	tr	1	—	5	1	12	1	tr	0
powder	1 tsp	9	tr	—	0	tr	2	—	2	1	31	—	—	—

FOOD	PORTION	CALORIES	FAT	SAT FAT	CHOL	PROTEIN	CARBO	FIBER	CALCIUM	SOD	POTAS	VIT C	FOLIC	VIT A
WATKINS														
Garlic & Chive Seasoning	1 tbsp (7 g)	25	2	0	5	1	2	0	40	280	—	0	—	0
Garlic Lover's Herb Blend	¼ tsp (0.5 oz)	0	0	0	0	0	0	0	0	0	—	0	—	0
Liquid Spice	1 tbsp (0.5 oz)	120	14	2	0	0	0	0	0	0	—	0	—	0
GEFILTE FISH														
READY-TO-EAT														
sweet	1 piece (1.5 oz)	35	1	tr	12	4	3	—	10	220	38	—	1	37
GELATIN														
MIX														
low calorie	½ cup	8	0	0	0	2	0	0	tr	9	45	0	0	0
mix artifically sweetened as prep	½ cup (4.1 oz)	8	0	—	0	1	1	—	1	56	0	0	—	0
mix artifically sweetened as prep	1 pkg 4 serv (16.5 oz)	33	0	—	0	5	3	—	10	224	1	0	—	0
mix as prep	1 pkg 4 serv (19 oz)	319	0	0	0	7	76	—	12	227	6	0	—	0
mix as prep	½ cup (4.7 oz)	80	0	0	0	2	19	—	3	57	1	0	—	0
mix not prep	1 pkg (3 oz)	324	0	0	0	7	77	—	—	216	6	0	—	0
mix w/ fruit as prep	½ cup (3.7 oz)	73	tr	—	0	1	18	—	5	30	110	4	—	30
mix w/ fruit as prep	1 pkg 8 serv (19 oz)	588	2	—	0	10	144	—	40	242	887	32	—	242
powder unsweetened	1 oz	94	0	tr	—	24	0	—	15	55	4	0	—	0
powder unsweetened	1 pkg (7 g)	23	0	tr	—	6	0	—	4	14	1	0	—	0
EMES														
Kosher-Jel	½ cup (4 fl oz)	60	0	0	0	tr	15	—	tr	7	10	tr	—	—
Kosher-Jel Plain	1 tbsp (7 g)	21	0	0	0	tr	5	1	—	tr	tr	—	—	—
JELL-O														
1-2-3-Brand Strawberry as prep	⅔ cup (5.2 oz)	130	2	1	0	2	26	0	0	50	0	0	—	0
Apricot as prep	½ cup (5 oz)	80	0	0	0	2	19	0	0	80	0	0	—	0
Berry Black as prep	½ cup (5 oz)	80	0	0	0	2	19	0	0	80	0	0	—	0
Berry Blue as prep	½ cup (5 oz)	80	0	0	0	2	19	0	0	80	0	0	—	0
Black Cherry as prep	½ cup (5 oz)	80	0	0	0	2	19	0	0	80	0	0	—	0
Cherry as prep	½ cup (5 oz)	80	0	0	0	2	19	0	0	100	0	0	—	0
Cranberry Raspberry as prep	½ cup (5 oz)	80	0	0	0	2	19	0	0	75	0	0	—	0
Cranberry Strawberry as prep	½ cup (5 oz)	80	0	0	0	2	19	0	0	75	0	0	—	0
Cranberry as prep	½ cup (5 oz)	80	0	0	0	0	19	0	0	75	0	0	—	0
Grape as prep	½ cup (5 oz)	80	0	0	0	2	19	0	0	80	0	0	—	0
Lemon as prep	½ cup (5 oz)	80	0	0	0	2	19	0	0	120	0	0	—	0

FOOD	PORTION	CALORIES	FAT	SAT FAT	CHOL	PROTEIN	CARBO	FIBER	CALCIUM	SOD	POTAS	VIT C	FOLIC	VIT A
JELL-O (CONT.)														
Lime as prep	½ cup (5 oz)	80	0	0	0	2	19	0	0	90	0	0	—	0
Mango as prep	½ cup (5 oz)	80	0	0	0	2	19	0	0	80	0	0	—	0
Mixed Fruit as prep	½ cup (5 oz)	80	0	0	0	2	19	tr	0	80	0	0	—	0
Orange as prep	½ cup (5 oz)	80	0	0	0	2	19	0	0	80	0	0	—	0
Peach as prep	½ cup (5 oz)	80	0	0	0	2	19	0	0	80	0	0	—	0
Peach Passion Fruit as prep	½ cup (5 oz)	80	0	0	0	2	19	0	0	80	0	0	—	0
Pineapple as prep	½ cup (5 oz)	80	0	0	0	2	19	0	0	80	0	0	—	0
Raspberry as prep	½ cup (5 oz)	80	0	0	0	2	19	0	0	80	0	0	—	0
Sparkling White Grape as prep	½ cup (5 oz)	80	0	0	0	2	19	0	0	80	0	0	—	0
Strawberry Banana as prep	½ cup (5 oz)	80	0	0	0	2	19	0	0	80	0	0	—	0
Strawberry Kiwi as prep	½ cup (5 oz)	80	0	0	0	2	19	0	0	80	0	0	—	0
Strawberry as prep	½ cup (5 oz)	80	0	0	0	2	19	0	0	90	0	0	—	0
Sugar Free Cherry as prep	½ cup (4.2 oz)	10	0	0	0	1	0	0	0	70	0	0	—	0
Sugar Free Cranberry as prep	½ cup (4.2 oz)	10	0	0	0	1	0	0	0	80	0	0	—	0
Sugar Free Lemon	½ cup (4.2 oz)	10	0	0	0	1	0	0	0	55	0	0	—	0
Sugar Free Lime as prep	½ cup (4.2 oz)	10	0	0	0	1	0	0	0	60	0	0	—	0
Sugar Free Mixed Fruit as prep	½ cup (4.2 oz)	10	0	0	0	1	0	0	0	50	0	0	—	0
Sugar Free Orange as prep	½ cup (4.2 oz)	10	0	0	0	1	0	0	0	65	0	0	—	0
Sugar Free Raspberry as prep	½ cup (4.2 oz)	10	0	0	0	1	0	0	0	55	0	0	—	0
Sugar Free Strawberry Banana as prep	½ cup (4.2 oz)	10	0	0	0	1	0	0	0	50	0	0	—	0
Sugar Free Strawberry as prep	½ cup (4.2 oz)	10	0	0	0	1	0	0	0	55	0	0	—	0
Sugar Free Strawberry Kiwi as prep	½ cup (4.2 oz)	10	0	0	0	1	0	0	0	60	0	0	—	0
Sugar Free Watermelon as prep	½ cup (4.2 oz)	10	0	0	0	1	0	0	0	55	0	0	—	0
Watermelon as prep	½ cup (5 oz)	80	0	0	0	2	19	0	0	80	0	0	—	0
Wild Strawberry as prep	½ cup (5 oz)	80	0	0	0	2	19	0	0	120	0	0	—	0
KOJEL														
Diet	1 serv	10	tr	—	—	1	4	—	—	16	—	—	—	—

FOOD	PORTION	CALORIES	FAT	SAT FAT	CHOL	PROTEIN	CARBO	FIBER	CALCIUM	SOD	POTAS	VIT C	FOLIC	VIT A
ROYAL														
Apple	½ cup	80	0	0	0	2	19	—	—	95	0	9	—	—
Blackberry	½ cup	80	0	0	0	2	19	—	—	95	0	9	—	—
Cherry	½ cup	80	0	0	0	2	19	—	—	95	0	9	—	—
Cherry Sugar Free	½ cup	8	0	0	0	1	1	—	—	90	0	12	—	—
Concord Grape	½ cup	80	0	0	0	2	19	—	—	130	0	12	—	—
Fruit Punch	½ cup	80	0	0	0	2	19	—	—	90	0	12	—	—
Lemon	½ cup	80	0	0	0	2	19	—	—	250	0	12	—	—
Lemon-Lime	½ cup	80	0	0	0	2	19	—	—	95	0	9	—	—
Lime	½ cup	80	0	0	0	2	19	—	—	125	0	12	—	—
Lime Sugar Free	½ cup	8	0	0	0	1	1	—	—	100	0	12	—	—
Mixed Berry	½ cup	80	0	0	0	2	19	—	—	90	0	12	—	—
Orange	½ cup	80	0	0	0	2	19	—	—	95	0	9	—	—
Orange Sugar Free	½ cup	10	0	0	0	1	1	—	—	90	0	12	—	—
Peach	½ cup	80	0	0	0	2	19	—	—	95	0	4	—	—
Pineapple	½ cup	80	0	0	0	2	19	—	—	95	0	12	—	—
Raspberry	½ cup	80	0	0	0	2	19	—	—	125	0	12	—	—
Raspberry Sugar Free	½ cup	8	0	0	0	1	1	—	—	90	0	12	—	—
Strawberry	½ cup	80	0	0	0	2	19	—	—	105	0	15	—	—
Strawberry Banana Sugar Free	½ cup	8	0	0	0	1	1	—	—	85	0	12	—	—
Strawberry Orange	½ cup	80	0	0	0	2	19	—	—	110	0	12	—	—
Strawberry Sugar Free	½ cup	8	0	0	0	1	1	—	—	90	0	12	—	—
Tropical Fruit	½ cup	80	0	0	0	2	19	—	—	110	0	12	—	—
READY-TO-EAT														
DEL MONTE														
Gel Snack Cups Blue Berry	1 serv (3.5 oz)	70	0	0	0	0	19	tr	0	40	—	0	—	0
Gel Snack Cups Cherry	1 serv (3.5 oz)	70	0	0	0	0	19	tr	0	40	—	0	—	0
Gel Snack Cups Orange	1 serv (3.5 oz)	70	0	0	0	0	19	tr	0	40	—	0	—	0
Gel Snack Cups Strawberry	1 serv (3.5 oz)	70	0	0	0	0	19	tr	0	40	—	0	—	0
HANDI-SNACKS														
Gels Blue Raspberry	1 serv (4 oz)	80	0	0	0	0	20	0	0	45	30	0	—	0
Gels Cherry	1 serv (4 oz)	80	0	0	0	0	20	0	0	45	30	0	—	0
Gels Orange	1 serv (3.5 oz)	80	0	0	0	0	20	0	0	45	30	0	—	0
Gels Strawberry	1 serv (3.5 oz)	80	0	0	0	0	20	0	0	40	30	0	—	0
HUNT'S														
Snack Pack Juicy Gels Cherry	1 (4 oz)	100	0	0	0	0	25	0	15	42	—	2	—	0
Snack Pack Juicy Gels Lemon Lime	1 (4 oz)	100	0	0	0	0	25	0	15	42	—	2	—	0

FOOD	PORTION	CALORIES	FAT	SAT FAT	CHOL	PROTEIN	CARBO	FIBER	CALCIUM	SOD	POTAS	VIT C	FOLIC	VIT A
HUNT'S (CONT.)														
Snack Pack Juicy Gels Mixed Fruit	1 (4 oz)	100	0	0	0	0	25	0	15	42	—	2	—	0
Snack Pack Juicy Gels Orange	1 (4 oz)	100	0	0	0	0	25	0	15	42	—	2	—	0
Snack Pack Juicy Gels Strawberry	1 (4 oz)	100	0	0	0	0	25	0	15	42	—	2	—	0
JELL-O														
Berry Black	1 serv (3.5 oz)	70	0	0	0	1	17	0	0	40	0	0	—	0
Berry Blue	1 serv (3.5 oz)	70	0	0	0	1	17	0	0	40	0	0	—	0
Cherry	1 serv (3.5 oz)	70	0	0	0	1	17	0	0	40	0	0	—	0
Orange	1 serv (3.5 oz)	70	0	0	0	1	17	0	0	40	0	0	—	0
Orange Strawberry Banana	1 serv (3.5 oz)	70	0	0	0	1	17	0	0	40	0	0	—	0
Raspberry	1 serv (3.5 oz)	70	0	0	0	1	17	0	0	40	0	0	—	0
Rhymin' Lymon	1 serv (3.5 oz)	70	0	0	0	1	17	0	0	40	0	0	—	0
Strawberry	1 serv (3.5 oz)	70	0	0	0	1	17	0	0	40	0	0	—	0
Strawberry Kiwi	1 serv (3.5 oz)	10	0	0	0	1	0	0	0	45	0	0	—	0
Sugar Free Orange	1 serv (3.2 oz)	10	0	0	0	1	0	0	0	45	0	0	—	0
Sugar Free Raspberry	1 serv (3.2 oz)	10	0	0	0	1	0	0	0	45	0	0	—	0
Sugar Free Strawberry	1 serv (3.2 oz)	10	0	0	0	1	0	0	0	45	0	0	—	0
Tropical Berry	1 serv (3.5 oz)	10	0	0	0	1	0	0	0	45	0	0	—	0
Tropical Fruit Punch	1 serv (3.5 oz)	70	0	0	0	1	17	0	0	40	0	0	—	0
Wild Watermelon	1 serv (3.5 oz)	70	0	0	0	1	17	0	0	40	0	0	—	0
KOZY SHACK														
Gel Treat Cherry	1 pkg (4 oz)	100	0	0	0	0	25	1	20	25	—	0	—	0
Gel Treat Lemon Lime	1 pkg (4 oz)	100	0	0	0	0	25	1	20	25	—	0	—	0
Gel Treat Orange	1 pkg (4 oz)	100	0	0	0	0	25	1	20	25	—	0	—	0
Gel Treat Strawberry	1 pkg (4 oz)	100	0	0	0	0	25	1	20	25	—	0	—	0
Gel Treat Sugar Free Orange	1 pkg (4 oz)	10	0	0	0	0	2	1	20	25	—	0	—	0
Gel Treat Sugar Free Strawberry	1 pkg (4 oz)	10	0	0	0	0	2	1	20	25	—	0	—	0
GIBLETS														
capon simmered	1 cup (5 oz)	238	8	3	629	38	0	—	19	80	222	13	601	19236
chicken floured & fried	1 cup (5 oz)	402	19	6	647	47	6	—	26	164	478	13	550	17298
chicken simmered	1 cup (5 oz)	228	7	2	570	37	1	—	18	85	229	12	545	10774
turkey simmered	1 cup (5 oz)	243	7	2	606	39	3	—	18	85	291	3	501	8753
GINGER														
ground	1 tsp (1.8 g)	6	tr	tr	0	tr	1	—	2	1	24	—	—	3
root fresh	¼ cup	17	tr	tr	0	tr	4	—	4	3	100	1	—	0

FOOD	PORTION	CALORIES	FAT	SAT FAT	CHOL	PROTEIN	CARBO	FIBER	CALCIUM	SOD	POTAS	VIT C	FOLIC	VIT A
KA-ME														
Crystallized Slices	5 pieces (1 oz)	100	0	0	0	0	25	1	20	23	—	6	—	—
Sliced	20 pieces (0.5 oz)	0	0	0	0	0	0	0	0	70	—	0	—	—
GINKGO NUTS														
canned	1 oz	32	tr	tr	0	1	6	—	1	87	51	—	—	—
dried	1 oz	99	tr	tr	0	3	21	—	6	4	283	8	—	310
raw	1 oz	52	tr	tr	0	1	11	—	1	1	145	4	—	158
GIZZARDS														
chicken simmered	1 cup (5 oz)	222	5	2	281	5	2	—	14	97	259	2	77	273
turkey simmered	1 cup (5 oz)	236	6	2	336	43	1	—	22	79	306	2	75	268
SHADY BROOK														
Turkey	4 oz	130	4	1	180	22	—	—	—	90	—	—	—	—
GOAT														
roasted	3 oz	122	3	1	64	23	0	—	15	73	344	—	5	—
GOOSE														
w/ skin roasted	6.6 oz	574	41	13	172	47	0	—	25	132	618	0	4	131
w/ skin roasted	½ goose (1.7 lbs)	2362	170	53	708	195	0	—	104	543	2546	0	17	541
w/o skin roasted	5 oz	340	18	7	138	41	0	—	20	108	554	—	—	—
w/o skin roasted	½ goose (1.3 lbs)	1406	75	27	569	171	0	—	84	447	2291	—	—	—
GOOSEBERRIES														
canned in light syrup	½ cup	93	tr	tr	0	1	24	—	20	3	97	13	4	174
fresh	1 cup	67	1	tr	0	1	15	—	38	1	297	42	—	435
GRANOLA														
(*see also* CEREAL BARS, NUTRITIONAL SUPPLEMENTS)														
BARS														
almond	1 (0.8 oz)	117	6	3	0	2	15	—	7	60	64	—	—	—
almond	1 (1 oz)	140	7	4	0	2	18	—	9	73	77	—	—	—
chewy chocolate coated chocolate chip	1 (1 oz)	132	7	4	1	2	18	1	29	57	89	0	7	—
chewy chocolate coated chocolate chip	1 (1.25 oz)	165	9	5	2	2	23	1	36	71	111	0	9	—
chewy chocolate coated peanut butter	1 (1 oz)	144	9	5	3	3	15	—	31	55	96	—	—	37
chewy chocolate coated peanut butter	1 (1.3 oz)	187	11	6	4	4	20	—	40	71	124	—	—	48
chewy raisin	1 (1 oz)	127	5	3	0	2	19	1	29	80	103	0	6	0
chewy raisin	1 (1.5 oz)	191	8	4	0	3	28	2	43	120	154	0	9	0
chocolate chip	1 (1 oz)	124	5	3	0	2	20	1	22	97	71	—	—	—

FOOD	PORTION	CALORIES	FAT	SAT FAT	CHOL	PROTEIN	CARBO	FIBER	CALCIUM	SOD	POTAS	VIT C	FOLIC	VIT A
chocolate chip	1 (0.8 oz)	103	4	3	0	2	17	1	18	81	59	—	—	—
chocolate chip chewy	1 (1.5 oz)	178	7	4	1	3	29	2	39	116	145	0	9	—
chocolate chip chewy	1 (1 oz)	119	5	3	0	2	10	1	26	77	96	0	5	—
chocolate chip graham & marshmallow chewy	1 (1 oz)	121	4	3	0	2	20	1	25	90	78	0	6	—
nut & raisin chewy	1 (1 oz)	129	6	3	0	2	18	2	24	72	111	0	9	—
peanut	1 (0.8 oz)	113	5	1	0	3	15	1	9	66	72	—	—	—
peanut	1 (1 oz)	136	6	1	0	3	18	—	11	79	86	—	—	—
peanut butter	1 (0.8 oz)	114	6	1	0	2	15	—	10	67	69	—	—	—
peanut butter	1 (1 oz)	137	7	1	0	3	18	—	12	80	82	—	—	—
peanut butter chewy	1 (1 oz)	121	5	1	0	3	18	1	26	116	83	0	9	—
peanut butter & chocolate chip chewy	1 (1 oz)	122	6	2	0	3	18	1	23	93	107	0	9	—
plain	1 (1 oz)	134	7	1	0	3	18	2	17	83	95	tr	7	43
plain	1 (0.9 oz)	115	4	1	0	3	19	1	15	72	82	tr	6	37
plain chewy	1 (1 oz)	126	5	2	0	2	19	1	30	79	92	0	7	0
CARNATION														
Chocolate Chunk	1 (1.26 oz)	140	5	2	0	2	23	1	500	65	—	15	—	1250
Honey & Oats	1 (1.26 oz)	130	4	2	0	2	23	1	500	60	—	15	—	1250
FI-BAR														
Coconut	1	120	4	1	0	2	20	6	—	30	100	—	—	—
Peanut Butter	1	130	4	1	0	3	20	6	—	30	100	—	—	—
GENERAL MILLS														
Nature Valley Cinnnamon	1	120	5	1	0	2	17	1	—	70	60	—	—	—
Nature Valley Oat Bran Honey Graham	1	110	4	tr	0	2	16	1	—	90	60	—	—	—
Nature Valley Oats N'Honey	1	120	5	1	0	2	17	1	—	65	60	—	—	—
Nature Valley Peanut Butter	1	120	6	1	0	2	15	1	—	70	70	—	—	—
Nature Valley Rice Bran Cinnamon Graham	1	90	4	tr	0	1	13	1	—	75	55	—	—	—
GRIST MILL														
Chewy Apple Cinnamon	1 (1 oz)	120	4	1	0	2	21	1	—	35		—	—	—
Chewy Chocolate Chip	1 (1 oz)	130	4	1	0	2	21	1	20	30		—	—	—
Chewy Chunky Nut & Raisin	1 (1 oz)	130	6	2	0	3	18	1	—	35		—	—	—

FOOD	PORTION	CALORIES	FAT	SAT FAT	CHOL	PROTEIN	CARBO	FIBER	CALCIUM	SOD	POTAS	VIT C	FOLIC	VIT A
GRIST MILL (CONT.)														
Chewy Peanut Butter	1 (1 oz)	130	5	1	0	3	20	1	—	45	—	1	—	—
Chewy Peanut Butter Chocolate	1 (1 oz)	130	4	1	0	3	20	2	—	40	—	—	—	—
Chocolate Snack Chocolate Chip	1 (1.2 oz)	180	10	5	5	3	21	1	40	60	—	0	—	0
Chocolate Snack Nutty Fudge	1 (1.3 oz)	190	11	5	5	3	19	2	20	90	—	0	—	0
Crunchy Cinnamon	1 (0.8 oz)	110	5	1	0	3	16	1	10	60	—	0	—	0
Crunchy Oats 'N Honey	1 (0.8 oz)	110	5	1	0	3	15	1	10	60	—	0	—	0
KELLOGG'S														
Low Fat Crunchy Almond & Brown Sugar	1 (0.7 oz)	80	2	0	0	2	16	1	0	60	—	0	40	500
Low Fat Crunchy Apple Spice	1 (0.7 oz)	80	2	0	0	2	16	1	0	60	—	0	40	500
Low Fat Crunchy Cinnamon Raisin	1 (0.7 oz)	80	2	0	0	2	16	1	0	60	—	0	40	500
KUDOS														
Chocolate Chunk	1 (0.7 oz)	90	3	1	0	1	13	1	200	60	—	6	—	500
Chocolate Coated Chocolate Chip	1 (1 oz)	120	5	3	5	2	18	1	200	75	—	6	—	500
Chocolate Coated Milk & Cookies	1 (1 oz)	130	5	3	5	2	18	1	200	70	—	6	—	500
Chocolate Coated Nutty Fudge	1 (1 oz)	130	5	3	5	2	18	1	200	65	—	6	—	500
Chocolate Coated Peanut Butter	1 (1 oz)	130	5	3	5	2	18	1	200	85	—	6	—	500
Low Fat Blueberry	1 (0.7 oz)	90	2	0	0	1	15	1	200	90	—	6	—	500
Low Fat Strawberry	1 (0.7 oz)	80	2	0	0	1	15	1	200	90	—	6	—	500
NATURE'S CHOICE														
Carob Chip	1 bar (0.7 oz)	80	3	0	0	2	16	2	—	5	—	—	—	—
Cinnamon & Raisin	1 bar (0.7 oz)	80	2	0	0	2	16	3	—	5	—	—	—	—
Oats 'n Honey	1 bar (0.7 oz)	80	2	0	0	2	15	2	—	5	—	—	—	—
Peanut Butter	1 bar (0.7 oz)	80	3	0	0	2	14	2	—	5	—	—	—	—
SUNBELT														
Chewy Chocolate Chip	1 (1.25 oz)	160	7	3	0	2	23	2	20	65	—	0	—	0
Chewy Chocolate Chip	1 (1.8 oz)	220	10	4	0	3	32	2	20	95	—	0	—	0
Chewy Oats & Honey	1 (1 oz)	130	5	2	0	2	19	1	20	65	—	0	—	0
Chewy Oats & Honey	1 (1.7 oz)	210	9	4	0	3	32	2	20	105	—	0	—	0

FOOD	PORTION	CALORIES	FAT	SAT FAT	CHOL	PROTEIN	CARBO	FIBER	CALCIUM	SOD	POTAS	VIT C	FOLIC	VIT A
SUNBELT (CONT.)														
Chewy With Almonds	1 (1 oz)	130	7	2	0	2	17	2	20	60	—	0	—	0
Chewy With Almonds	1 (1.5 oz)	190	10	3	0	3	25	2	40	95	—	0	—	0
Chewy With Raisins	1 (1.2 oz)	150	6	2	0	2	25	2	20	65	—	0	—	0
Fudge Dipped Chewy Chocolate Chip	1 (1.5 oz)	190	8	4	0	3	28	2	20	80	—	0	—	0
Fudge Dipped Chewy Macaroo	1 bar (2 oz)	280	17	9	0	3	32	3	20	90	—	0	—	0
Fudge Dipped Chewy Macaroo	1 (1.4 oz)	200	13	7	0	2	22	2	20	60	—	0	—	0
Fudge Dipped Chewy With Peanuts	1 bar (1.5 oz)	210	12	3	0	3	24	2	20	65	—	0	—	0
Fudge Dipped Chewy With Peanuts	1 (2 oz)	270	15	4	0	4	32	2	20	95	—	0	—	0
CEREAL														
GOOD SHEPHERD														
Crunchy	1 oz	130	5	—	0	3	19	2	20	15	80	—	—	—
Honey Almond	1 oz	120	4	—	0	3	20	2	20	10	85	—	—	—
Organic 5 Grain Muesli	1 oz	160	3	—	0	4	27	3	10	55	55	—	—	—
Organic Brown Rice	1 oz	130	4	—	0	3	16	4	—	35	20	—	—	—
Organic Wheat Free	1 oz	90	3	—	0	3	39	2	40	3	155	—	—	—
Organic Wheat Free Apple Cinnamon	1 oz	125	4	—	0	3	20	3	—	35	30	—	—	—
Organic Wheat Free Blueberry Amaranth	1 oz	110	1	—	0	3	22	2	—	10	135	—	—	—
Organic Wheat Free Strawberry Amaranth	1 oz	110	1	—	0	3	22	2	—	12	120	—	—	—
GRIST MILL														
Low-Fat With Raisins	⅔ cup (1.9 oz)	220	3	1	0	5	42	3	0	100	40	0	100	750
KELLOGG'S														
Low Fat	½ cup (1.9 oz)	210	3	1	0	5	43	3	20	120	135	0	100	750
Low Fat With Raisins	⅔ cup (1.9 oz)	210	3	1	0	5	43	3	20	135	160	0	100	750
NATURE VALLEY														
100% Natural Oat Cinnamon & Raisin	¾ cup (1.9 oz)	240	8	1	0	5	38	3	40	90	190	0	—	0

FOOD	PORTION	CALORIES	FAT	SAT FAT	CHOL	PROTEIN	CARBO	FIBER	CALCIUM	SOD	POTAS	VIT C	FOLIC	VIT A
NATURE VALLEY (CONT.)														
100% Natural Oat Fruit & Nut	⅔ cup (1.9 oz)	250	11	2	0	6	34	3	40	75	190	0	—	0
STONE-BUHR														
Hot Apple	⅓ cup (1.6 oz)	153	1	0	0	5	31	5	20	0	—	0	—	0
SUNBELT														
Banana Nut	1.9 oz	250	9	4	1	5	37	4	80	60	—	1	—	0
Fruit & Nut	1.9 oz	230	7	3	1	6	38	4	60	100	—	0	—	0
Low Fat	1.9 oz	200	3	1	0	5	42	4	20	80	—	0	—	0
UNCLE ROY'S														
Cashew Raisin	½ cup (1.6 oz)	180	6	1	0	8	32	3	—	20	—	—	—	—
Fat Free Apple Cinnamon	½ cup (1.6 oz)	175	1	tr	0	8	38	3	—	20	—	—	—	—
Fat Free Wild Cherry	½ cup (1.6 oz)	175	1	tr	0	6	38	3	—	20	—	—	—	—
Fruit & Nut	½ cup (1.6 oz)	175	5	1	0	6	30	3	—	20	—	—	—	—
Low Fat Berries Jubilee	½ cup (1.6 oz)	175	3	1	0	6	34	3	—	20	—	—	—	—
Low Fat Crispy	½ cup (1.4 oz)	160	3	1	0	4	31	3	—	20	—	—	—	—
Low Fat Luscious Raspberry	½ cup (1.6 oz)	175	3	1	0	6	34	3	—	20	—	—	—	—
Low Fat True Blueberry	½ cup (1.6 oz)	175	3	1	0	6	34	3	—	20	—	—	—	—
Maple Date Nut	½ cup (1.6 oz)	180	6	1	0	6	29	3	—	20	—	—	—	—
Nut Butter & Almonds	½ cup (1.6 oz)	195	8	1	0	6	29	3	—	20	—	—	—	—
Organic Golden Honey	½ cup (1.6 oz)	190	6	1	0	5	30	3	—	20	—	—	—	—
Organic Maple Nut'N Rice	½ cup (1.4 oz)	170	6	1	0	4	27	3	—	20	—	—	—	—
Organic Maple Raisin	½ cup (1.6 oz)	190	6	1	0	5	30	3	—	20	—	—	—	—
GRAPE JUICE														
bottled	1 cup	155	tr	tr	0	1	38	—	22	7	334	tr	7	20
frzn sweetened as prep	1 cup	128	tr	tr	0	tr	32	—	9	5	53	60	3	19
frzn sweetened not prep	6 oz	386	1	tr	0	1	96	—	28	15	159	180	9	58
grape drink	6 oz	84	0	0	0	0	22	—	12	10	64	1	2
BAMA														
Juice	8.45 fl oz	120	0	0	0	0	29	—	—	25	20	—	30	—
BRIGHT & EARLY														
Frozen	8 fl oz	140	0	0	0	0	34	—	—	5	—	60	—	—
CAPRI SUN														
Drink	1 pkg (7 oz)	100	0	0	0	0	25	0	0	20	20	0	—	0
EVERFRESH														
Juice	1 can (8 oz)	150	0	0	0	0	38	0	—	10	—	—	—	—

FOOD	PORTION	CALORIES	FAT	SAT FAT	CHOL	PROTEIN	CARBO	FIBER	CALCIUM	SOD	POTAS	VIT C	FOLIC	VIT A
HI-C														
Box	8.45 fl oz	130	0	0	0	0	33	—	—	30	—	60	—	—
Drink	8 fl oz	130	0	0	0	0	32	—	—	30	—	60	—	—
Drink	1 can (11.5 fl oz)	180	0	0	0	0	46	—	—	45	—	84	—	—
JUICY JUICE														
Drink	1 box	130	0	0	0	1	31	—	—	10	180	60	—	—
Drink	1 bottle (6 fl oz)	90	0	0	0	1	22	—	—	5	120	60	—	—
KOOL-AID														
Bursts Grape Drink	1 (7 oz)	100	0	0	0	0	25	0	0	30	15	9	—	0
Drink as prep w/ sugar	1 serv (8 oz)	100	0	0	0	0	25	0	0	10	0	6	—	0
Drink Mix as prep	1 serv (8 oz)	60	0	0	0	0	16	0	0	0	0	6	—	0
Sugar Free Drink Mix as prep	1 serv (8 oz)	5	0	0	0	0	0	0	0	0	0	6	—	0
MINUTE MAID														
Chilled	8 fl oz	130	0	0	0	0	33	—	—	5	—	—	—	—
Grape Punch frzn	8 fl oz	130	0	0	0	0	32	—	—	5	—	—	—	—
Punch Chilled	8 fl oz	130	0	0	0	0	32	—	—	25	—	—	—	—
MOTT'S														
Drink	10 fl oz	170	0	0	0	0	42	0	0	50	40	0	—	0
Fruit Basket Cocktail as prep	8 fl oz	130	0	0	0	1	32	0	20	5	160	15	—	0
SENECA														
Blush Grape Juice frzn as prep	8 fl oz	170	0	0	0	0	39	0	0	0	105	60	—	0
Fortified With Vitamin C frzn as prep	8 fl oz	170	0	0	0	0	39	0	40	24	105	60	—	0
Sweetened frzn as prep	8 fl oz	140	0	0	0	0	39	0	40	24	105	—	—	0
White Grape Juice frzn as prep	8 fl oz	140	0	0	0	0	33	0	0	0	35	60	—	0
SHASTA PLUS														
Grape Drink	1 can (11.5 oz)	160	0	0	0	0	39	0	—	45	—	60	—	—
SIPPIN' PAK														
100% Pure	8.45 fl oz	130	0	0	0	1	32	—	20	25	150	—	—	—
SNAPPLE														
Grapeade	8 fl oz	120	0	0	0	0	30	—	0	5	0	—	—	0
TROPICANA														
Season's Best	8 fl oz	160	0	0	0	tr	39	—	—	25	—	—	—	—
VERYFINE														
100% Juice	1 bottle (10 oz)	200	0	0	0	0	47	0	0	35	—	2	—	0

FOOD	PORTION	CALORIES	FAT	SAT FAT	CHOL	PROTEIN	CARBO	FIBER	CALCIUM	SOD	POTAS	VIT C	FOLIC	VIT A
VERYFINE (CONT.)														
Chillers Glacial Grape	1 can (11.5 oz)	160	0	0	0	0	41	0	0	10	—	60	—	0
Grape Drink	1 bottle (10 oz)	160	0	0	0	0	41	0	0	10	—	36	—	0
Juice-Ups	8 fl oz	130	0	0	0	0	32	0	0	10	—	60	—	0

GRAPE LEAVES

FOOD	PORTION	CALORIES	FAT	SAT FAT	CHOL	PROTEIN	CARBO	FIBER	CALCIUM	SOD	POTAS	VIT C	FOLIC	VIT A
fresh raw	1 (3 g)	3	tr	tr	0	tr	1	tr	11	tr	8	tr	2	810
CEDAR'S														
Grape Leaves Stuffed With Rice	6 pieces (4.9 oz)	180	8	1	0	4	22	8	0	870	—	0	—	0

GRAPEFRUIT

FOOD	PORTION	CALORIES	FAT	SAT FAT	CHOL	PROTEIN	CARBO	FIBER	CALCIUM	SOD	POTAS	VIT C	FOLIC	VIT A
CANNED														
juice pack	½ cup	46	tr	tr	0	1	11	—	19	9	209	42	—	0
unsweetened	1 cup	93	tr	tr	0	1	22	—	18	3	378	72	26	18
water pack	½ cup	44	tr	tr	0	1	11	—	18	2	161	27	11	0
FRESH														
red	½	37	tr	tr	0	1	9	—	13	0	158	47	15	318
red sections	1 cup	69	tr	tr	0	1	18	—	25	1	296	88	28	595
DOLE														
Grapefruit	½	50	0	—	0	1	14	6	—	0	230	65	—	776

GRAPEFRUIT JUICE

FOOD	PORTION	CALORIES	FAT	SAT FAT	CHOL	PROTEIN	CARBO	FIBER	CALCIUM	SOD	POTAS	VIT C	FOLIC	VIT A
fresh	1 cup	96	tr	tr	0	1	23	—	22	2	400	94	—	—
frzn as prep	1 cup	102	tr	tr	0	1	24	—	19	2	337	83	9	22
frzn not prep	6 oz	302	1	tr	0	4	72	—	18	6	1002	248	26	65
sweetened	1 cup	116	tr	tr	0	1	28	—	20	4	405	67	26	0
AFTER THE FALL														
Pink	1 bottle (10 oz)	100	0	0	0	1	23	—	20	10	320	78	—	0
APPLE & EVE														
Made In The Shade Ruby Red	8 fl oz	130	0	0	0	0	32	—	—	35	—	60	—	—
CRYSTAL GEYSER														
Juice Squeeze	1 bottle (12 fl oz)	150	0	0	0	1	36	—	—	20	—	—	—	—
DEL MONTE														
Juice	8 fl oz	100	0	0	0	2	24	1	40	20	—	72	—	300
EVERFRESH														
Juice	1 can (8 oz)	90	0	0	0	0	22	0	—	0	—	—	—	—
Ruby Red Cocktail	1 can (8 oz)	130	0	0	0	0	32	0	—	0	—	—	—	—
FRESH SAMANTHA														
Juice	1 cup (8 oz)	101	0	0	0	3	24	tr	0	0	—	54	8	0
HOOD														
Select	1 cup (8 oz)	100	0	0	0	0	23	—	—	1	—	90	—	—
MINUTE MAID														
Frozen	8 fl oz	100	0	0	0	0	23	—	—	25	—	60	—	—

FOOD	PORTION	CALORIES	FAT	SAT FAT	CHOL	PROTEIN	CARBO	FIBER	CALCIUM	SOD	POTAS	VIT C	FOLIC	VIT A
MINUTE MAID (CONT.)														
Juices To Go	1 can (11.5 fl oz)	140	0	0	0	0	33	—	—	40	500	90	—	—
Juices To Go	1 bottle (10 fl oz)	120	0	0	0	0	29	—	—	35	430	60	—	—
Juices To Go	1 bottle (16 fl oz)	100	0	0	0	0	23	—	—	25	350	48	—	—
Juices To Go Pink Cocktail	1 bottle (10 fl oz)	140	0	0	0	0	34	—	—	35	—	—	—	—
Juices To Go Pink Cocktail	1 bottle (16 fl oz)	110	0	0	0	0	27	—	—	25	—	—	—	—
Juices to Go Pink Cocktail	8 fl oz	160	0	0	0	0	39	—	—	40	—	—	—	—
MOTT'S														
From Concentrate as prep	8 fl oz	120	0	0	0	2	27	0	0	10	440	78	—	0
OCEAN SPRAY														
100% Juice	8 oz	100	0	0	0	1	24	tr	—	35	240	60	—	0
Pink Juice Cocktail	8 oz	110	0	0	0	tr	28	0	—	35	140	60	—	0
Ruby Red Drink	8 oz	130	0	0	0	0	33	0	—	35	50	60	—	0
ODWALLA														
Juice	8 fl oz	90	0	0	0	2	20	—	20	5	—	78	—	300
SNAPPLE														
Juice	10 fl oz	110	0	0	0	0	25	—	20	45	340	60	—	0
Pink Grapefruit Cocktail	8 fl oz	120	0	0	0	0	31	—	20	5	0	—	—	0
TREE OF LIFE														
Juice	8 fl oz	100	0	0	0	1	26	0	0	10	280	78	—	0
TROPICANA														
Juice	1 container (6 fl oz)	80	0	0	0	tr	19	—	—	0	300	30	—	—
Juice	8 fl oz	90	0	0	0	tr	23	—	—	0	390	35	—	—
Ruby Red	1 container (10 fl oz)	120	0	0	0	tr	30	—	—	0	490	100	—	—
Ruby Red	8 fl oz	100	0	0	0	tr	25	—	—	0	400	120	—	—
Season's Best	1 bottle (7 fl oz)	80	0	0	0	tr	19	—	—	5	240	90	—	—
Season's Best	1 bottle (10 fl oz)	110	0	0	0	tr	27	—	—	5	350	120	—	—
Season's Best	8 fl oz	90	0	0	0	tr	22	—	—	5	280	100	—	—
Season's Best	1 can (11.5 fl oz)	120	0	0	0	tr	31	—	—	5	360	100	—	—
Twister Light Pink	8 fl oz	40	0	0	0	tr	10	—	—	20	—	140	—	—
Twister Light Pink	1 container (10 fl oz)	50	0	0	0	tr	12	—	—	25	—	140	—	—
Twister Pink	1 container (10 fl oz)	140	0	0	0	tr	35	—	—	25	—	40	—	—

FOOD	PORTION	CALORIES	FAT	SAT FAT	CHOL	PROTEIN	CARBO	FIBER	CALCIUM	SOD	POTAS	VIT C	FOLIC	VIT A
TROPICANA (CONT.)														
Twister Pink	1 can (11.5 fl oz)	160	0	0	0	tr	40	—	—	30	—	50	—	—
Twister Pink	8 fl oz	110	0	0	0	tr	28	—	—	20	—	40	—	—
VERYFINE														
100% Juice	1 bottle (10 oz)	110	0	0	0	0	25	0	0	20	—	60	—	0
Pink	1 bottle (10 oz)	150	0	0	0	0	38	0	0	35	—	60	—	0
Ruby Red	8 fl oz	120	0	0	0	0	29	0	0	25	—	60	—	0

GRAPES

FOOD	PORTION	CALORIES	FAT	SAT FAT	CHOL	PROTEIN	CARBO	FIBER	CALCIUM	SOD	POTAS	VIT C	FOLIC	VIT A
CANNED														
thompson seedless in heavy syrup	½ cup	94	tr	tr	0	1	25	—	13	7	132	1	—	81
thompson seedless water pack	½ cup	48	tr	tr	0	1	13	—	13	7	131	1	—	81
FRESH														
DOLE														
Grapes	1½ cup	85	0	—	0	1	24	2	—	3	—	—	—	—

GRAVY

(see also SAUCE)

FOOD	PORTION	CALORIES	FAT	SAT FAT	CHOL	PROTEIN	CARBO	FIBER	CALCIUM	SOD	POTAS	VIT C	FOLIC	VIT A
CANNED														
au jus	1 cup	38	tr	tr	1	3	6	—	10	—	—	2	—	0
chicken	1 cup	189	14	3	5	5	13	—	48	1375	260	0	—	880
mushroom	1 cup	120	6	1	0	3	13	—	17	1259	253	0	—	0
turkey	1 cup	122	5	1	5	6	12	—	10	—	—	0	—	0
FRANCO-AMERICAN														
Au Jus	2 oz	10	0	—	—	0	2	—	—	330	—	—	—	—
Beef	2 oz	25	1	—	—	0	4	—	—	340	—	—	—	—
Chicken	2 oz	45	4	—	—	0	3	—	—	240	—	—	—	200
Chicken Giblet	2 oz	30	2	—	—	1	3	—	—	310	—	—	—	—
Cream	2 oz	35	2	—	—	0	4	—	—	220	—	—	—	—
Mushroom	2 oz	25	1	—	—	0	3	—	—	290	—	—	—	—
Pork	2 oz	40	3	—	—	0	3	—	—	330	—	—	—	—
Turkey	2 oz	30	2	—	—	0	3	—	—	290	—	—	—	—
GRAVYMASTER														
Seasoning	¼ tsp	3	0	0	0	tr	1	—	tr	14	3	—	—	—
RUDY'S FARM														
Sausage Gravy	¼ cup (2 oz)	50	1	1	10	3	7	0	—	330	—	—	—	—
MIX														
chicken as prep	1 cup	83	2	1	3	3	14	—	39	1133	—	—	—	—
mushroom as prep	1 cup	70	1	1	1	2	14	—	49	1402	—	—	—	—
pork as prep	1 cup	76	2	1	3	2	13	—	32	1235	—	—	—	—
turkey as prep	1 cup	87	2	1	3	3	15	—	50	1498	—	—	—	—

FOOD	PORTION	CALORIES	FAT	SAT FAT	CHOL	PROTEIN	CARBO	FIBER	CALCIUM	SOD	POTAS	VIT C	FOLIC	VIT A
CAJUN KING														
Oil-Less Roux And Gravy Mix	3.5 oz	394	4	—	—	12	78	—	47	348	—	12	—	242
DURKEE														
Au Jus as prep	¼ cup	5	0	0	0	0	1	0	0	320	—	0	—	0
Brown as prep	¼ cup	10	1	0	0	0	3	0	0	250	—	0	—	0
Brown Herb as prep	¼ cup	15	1	0	0	1	3	0	0	350	—	0	—	0
Brown Mushroom as prep	¼ cup	15	0	0	0	1	3	0	0	300	—	0	—	0
Brown Onion as prpe	¼ cup	15	0	0	0	1	4	0	0	290	—	0	—	0
Chicken as prep	¼ cup	20	1	0	0	1	4	0	0	350	—	0	—	0
Country as prep	¼ cup	35	2	1	0	1	5	0	0	370	—	0	—	0
Homestyle as prep	¼ cup	15	1	0	0	1	3	0	40	240	—	0	—	0
Mushroom as prep	¼ cup	15	0	0	0	1	3	0	0	230	—	0	—	0
Onion as prep	¼ cup	10	0	0	0	1	3	0	0	310	—	0	—	0
Pork as prep	¼ cup	10	0	0	0	1	3	0	0	240	—	0	—	0
Sausage as prep	¼ cup	35	2	1	0	1	5	0	0	570	—	0	—	0
Swiss Steak as prep	¼ cup	15	0	0	0	0	4	0	0	370	—	0	—	0
Turkey as prep	¼ cup	20	0	0	0	1	4	0	0	270	—	0	—	0
FRENCH'S														
Au Jus as prep	¼ cup	5	0	0	0	0	1	0	0	220	—	0	—	0
Brown as prep	¼ cup	10	1	0	0	0	3	0	0	250	—	0	—	0
Chicken as prep	¼ cup	25	1	0	0	1	4	0	0	250	—	0	—	0
Country as prep	¼ cup	35	2	1	0	1	5	0	0	370	—	0	—	0
Herb Brown as prep	¼ cup	15	1	0	0	1	3	0	0	350	—	0	—	0
Homestyle as prep	¼ cup	10	1	0	0	0	3	0	0	230	—	0	—	0
Mushroom as prep	¼ cup	10	1	0	0	0	3	0	0	250	—	0	—	0
Onion	¼ cup	15	1	0	0	0	4	0	0	260	—	0	—	0
Pork as prep	¼ cup	10	1	0	0	0	3	0	0	250	—	0	—	0
Sausage as prep	¼ cup	35	2	1	0	1	5	0	0	570	—	0	—	0
Turkey as prep	¼ cup	20	0	0	0	1	4	0	0	270	—	0	—	0
HAIN														
Brown	¼ pkg	16	0	0	0	1	3	—	100	600	550	—	—	—
LOMA LINDA														
Gravy Quik Brown	1 tbsp (5 g)	20	0	0	0	tr	4	0	0	370	5	0	—	0
Gravy Quik Chicken	1 tbsp (5 g)	20	0	0	0	1	3	0	0	410	30	0	—	0
Quik Gravy Country	1 tbsp (5 g)	25	1	0	0	tr	4	0	0	250	5	0	—	0
Quik Gravy Mushroom	1 tbsp (5 g)	15	0	0	0	tr	3	tr	0	300	30	0	—	0
Quik Gravy Onion	1 tbsp (5 g)	20	0	0	0	tr	3	tr	0	230	20	0	—	0
PILLSBURY														
Brown	¼ cup	15	0	0	0	tr	3	—	0	300	5	0	—	0
Chicken	¼ cup	25	1	—	—	tr	4	—	0	230	20	0	—	0

FOOD	PORTION	CALORIES	FAT	SAT FAT	CHOL	PROTEIN	CARBO	FIBER	CALCIUM	SOD	POTAS	VIT C	FOLIC	VIT A
PILLSBURY (CONT.)														
Home Style	¼ cup	15	0	0	0	tr	3	—	0	300	5	0	—	0

GREAT NORTHERN BEANS

FOOD	PORTION	CALORIES	FAT	SAT FAT	CHOL	PROTEIN	CARBO	FIBER	CALCIUM	SOD	POTAS	VIT C	FOLIC	VIT A
CANNED														
ALLEN														
Great Northern	½ cup (4.5 oz)	100	1	0	0	6	19	7	60	310	—	1	—	0
GREEN GIANT														
Great Northern	½ cup (4.4 oz)	100	1	0	0	6	18	6	100	290	—	0	—	0
TRAPPEY														
With Sausage	½ cup (4.5 oz)	100	1	1	0	6	18	7	40	460	—	0	—	0
DRIED														
cooked	1 cup	210	1	tr	0	15	37	—	121	4	692	2	181	2
BEAN CUISINE														
Dried	½ cup	115	1	—	0	8	—	5	—	5	310	—	62	—
HURST														
HamBeens w/ Ham	3 tbsp (1.2 oz)	120	1	0	0	7	22	11	60	63	—	0	—	0

GREEN BEANS

FOOD	PORTION	CALORIES	FAT	SAT FAT	CHOL	PROTEIN	CARBO	FIBER	CALCIUM	SOD	POTAS	VIT C	FOLIC	VIT A
CANNED														
ALLEN														
Cut	½ cup (4.2 oz)	30	1	0	0	0	6	3	40	320	—	2	—	400
Cut No Added Salt	½ cup (4.2 oz)	15	0	0	0	0	3	2	40	10	—	2	—	400
French Style	½ cup (4.2 oz)	25	0	0	0	tr	4	2	40	300	—	0	—	400
Italian	½ cup (4.2 oz)	35	1	0	0	1	7	3	40	320	—	4	—	200
Shell Outs	½ cup (4.5 oz)	30	0	0	0	2	6	2	40	460	—	2	—	200
ALMA														
Cut	½ cup (4.2 oz)	30	1	0	0	0	6	3	40	320	—	2	—	400
CREST TOP														
Cut	½ cup (4.2 oz)	30	1	0	0	0	6	3	40	320	—	2	—	400
DEL MONTE														
Cut	½ cup (4.3 oz)	20	0	0	0	1	4	2	20	360	—	5	—	300
Cut 50% Less Salt	½ cup (4.3 oz)	20	0	0	0	1	4	2	20	180	—	5	—	300
Cut Italian	½ cup (4.3 oz)	30	0	0	0	1	6	3	20	360	—	9	—	200
Cut No Salt Added	½ cup (4.3 oz)	20	0	0	0	1	4	2	20	10	—	5	—	300
French Style	½ cup (4.3 oz)	20	0	0	0	1	4	2	20	360	—	5	—	300
French Style 50% Less Salt	½ cup (4.3 oz)	20	0	0	0	1	4	2	20	180	—	5	—	300
French Style No Salt Added	½ cup (4.3 oz)	20	0	0	0	1	4	2	20	10	—	5	—	300
French Style Seasoned	½ cup (4.3 oz)	20	0	0	0	1	4	2	20	360	—	5	—	300
Whole	½ cup (4.3 oz)	20	0	0	0	1	4	2	20	360	—	5	—	300
GABELLE														
Cut	½ cup (4.2 oz)	30	1	0	0	0	6	3	40	320	—	2	—	400
GREEN GIANT														
Cut	½ cup (4.2 oz)	20	0	0	0	tr	4	1	20	400	—	2	—	300

FOOD	PORTION	CALORIES	FAT	SAT FAT	CHOL	PROTEIN	CARBO	FIBER	CALCIUM	SOD	POTAS	VIT C	FOLIC	VIT A
GREEN GIANT (CONT.)														
Cut 50% Less Sodium	½ cup (4.2 oz)	20	0	0	0	tr	4	1	20	200	—	1	—	400
French Style	½ cup (4.1 oz)	20	0	0	0	tr	4	1	20	390	—	2	—	300
Kitchen Sliced	½ cup (4.2 oz)	20	0	0	0	tr	4	1	20	400	—	4	—	200
Whole	½ cup (4.1 oz)	25	0	0	0	tr	5	2	20	330	—	2	—	200
SENECA														
Cut	½ cup	20	0	0	0	1	6	2	40	360	105	5	—	200
Cuts Natural Pack	½ cup	25	0	0	0	1	6	2	20	0	105	6	—	200
French	½ cup	20	0	0	0	1	6	2	40	360	105	5	—	200
French Natural Pack	½ cup	25	0	0	0	1	6	2	20	0	105	6	—	200
Whole	½ cup	20	0	0	0	1	6	2	40	360	105	5	—	200
SUNSHINE														
Cut	½ cup (4.2 oz)	30	1	0	0	0	6	3	40	320	—	2	—	400
Italian	½ cup (4.2 oz)	35	1	0	0	1	7	3	40	320	—	4	—	200
FRESH														
cooked	½ cup	22	tr	tr	0	1	5	—	29	2	185	6	21	413
FROZEN														
cooked	½ cup	18	tr	tr	0	1	4	—	31	9	76	6	—	359
BIRDS EYE														
French w/ Toasted Almonds	¾ cup (4.1 oz)	80	4	0	0	3	7	3	60	500	—	1	—	200
FRESH LIKE														
Cut	3.5 oz	29	tr	—	—	1	7	1	41	6	149	11	—	534
French	3.5 oz	29	tr	—	—	1	7	1	46	6	174	9	—	459
Italian	3.5 oz	35	tr	—	—	2	8	1	41	6	255	16	—	440
Whole	3.5 oz	29	tr	—	—	1	6	1	39	6	181	11	—	686
GREEN GIANT														
Cut	¾ cup (2.8 oz)	25	0	0	0	1	5	2	20	0	—	6	—	200
Harvest Fresh & Almonds	⅔ cup (2.8 oz)	60	3	0	0	2	5	2	40	95	—	5	—	200
Harvest Fresh Cut	⅔ cup (2.9 oz)	25	0	0	0	tr	5	2	40	95	—	6	—	400
STOUFFER'S														
Green Bean Mushroom Casserole	1 serv (4 oz)	130	8	2	2	3	12	2	60	450	190	2	—	200
TREE OF LIFE														
Green Beans	⅔ cup (2.8 oz)	25	0	0	0	1	4	2	20	10	—	1	—	200
GREENS														
CANNED														
ALLEN														
Mixed	½ cup (4.2 oz)	30	1	0	0	1	8	4	150	10	—	6	—	5500
SUNSHINE														
Mixed	½ cup (4.2 oz)	30	1	0	0	1	8	4	150	10	—	6	—	5500

FOOD	PORTION	CALORIES	FAT	SAT FAT	CHOL	PROTEIN	CARBO	FIBER	CALCIUM	SOD	POTAS	VIT C	FOLIC	VIT A
GROUNDCHERRIES														
fresh	½ cup	37	tr	—	0	1	8	—	6	—	—	8	—	504
GROUPER														
cooked	1 fillet (7.1 oz)	238	3	1	95	50	0	—	42	107	959	—	—	—
cooked	3 oz	100	1	tr	40	21	0	—	18	45	403	—	—	—
raw	3 oz	78	1	tr	31	16	0	—	23	45	410	—	—	—
GUANABANA JUICE														
LIBBY														
Nectar	1 can (11.5 fl oz)	210	0	0	0	0	50	—	—	25	90	60	—	—
GUAVA														
fresh	1	45	1	tr	0	1	11	—	18	2	256	165	—	713
guava sauce	½ cup	43	tr	tr	0	tr	11	—	8	4	268	174	—	337
GUAVA JUICE														
KERN'S														
Nectar	6 fl oz	110	0	0	0	0	28	—	—	0	60	24	—	—
LIBBY														
Nectar	1 can (11.5 fl oz)	220	0	0	0	0	54	—	20	10	130	60	—	—
SNAPPLE														
Guava Mania	8 fl oz	110	0	0	0	0	29	—	0	0	25	—	—	0
GUINEA HEN														
w/ skin raw	½ hen (12.1 oz)	545	22	—	—	81	0	—	—	—	—	—	—	—
w/o skin raw	½ hen (9.3 oz)	292	7	—	166	55	0	—	—	—	—	—	—	—
HADDOCK														
FRESH														
cooked	1 fillet (5.3 oz)	168	1	tr	110	36	0	—	64	131	598	—	—	95
cooked	3 oz	95	1	tr	63	21	0	—	36	74	339	—	—	54
raw	3 oz	74	1	tr	49	16	0	—	28	58	264	—	—	47
roe raw	3½ oz	130	2	—	360	24	2	—	—	—	—	14	—	—
FROZEN														
GORTON'S														
Fishmarket Fresh	5 oz	110	1	—	—	25	0	—	—	120	—	—	—	—
Microwave Entree Haddock In Lemon Butter	1 pkg	360	21	10	100	23	19	—	20	730	—	—	—	200
MRS. PAUL'S														
Crunchy Batter Fillets	2 fillets	190	5	—	25	14	22	—	—	580	—	—	—	—
Light Fillets	1 fillet	220	9	—	45	17	15	—	20	350	—	—	—	—
VAN DE KAMP'S														
Battered Fillets	2 (4 oz)	260	16	3	30	13	18	0	40	530	—	0	—	0

FOOD	PORTION	CALORIES	FAT	SAT FAT	CHOL	PROTEIN	CARBO	FIBER	CALCIUM	SOD	POTAS	VIT C	FOLIC	VIT A
VAN DE KAMP'S (CONT.)														
Breaded Fillets	2 (3.5 oz)	280	17	3	25	12	19	0	0	310	—	0	—	—
Lightly Breaded Fillets	1 (4 oz)	220	10	2	30	14	19	0	20	410	—	0	—	0
SMOKED														
smoked	3 oz	99	1	tr	65	21	0	—	41	649	353	—	—	62
smoked	1 oz	33	tr	tr	21	7	0	—	14	214	116	—	—	21
HALIBUT														
FRESH														
atlantic & pacific cooked	3 oz	119	2	tr	35	23	0	—	51	59	490	—	—	152
atlantic & pacific cooked	½ fillet (5.6 oz)	223	5	1	65	42	0	—	95	110	916	—	—	284
FROZEN														
VAN DE KAMP'S														
Battered Fillets	3 (4 oz)	300	21	3	20	13	16	0	40	520	—	0	—	0
HALVA														
(*see* SESAME)														
HAM														
(*see also* HAM DISHES, PORK, TURKEY)														
boneless 11% fat roasted	3 oz	151	8	3	50	19	0	0	7	1275	—	0	3	0
canned extra lean roasted	3 oz	116	4	1	26	18	tr	0	5	965	—	0	4	0
canned extra lean roasted	1 cup	190	7	2	42	30	1	0	8	1589	—	0	7	0
center slice country style lean roasted	4 oz	220	9	3	80	31	tr	0	11	3045	—	0	6	0
patty cooked	1 patty (2 oz)	203	18	7	43	8	1	0	5	632	—	0	2	0
steak boneless extra lean	1 (2 oz)	69	2	1	26	11	0	0	2	720	—	18	2	0
ALPINE LACE														
Boneless Cooked	2 oz	60	2	1	25	9	1	0	—	440	—	—	—	—
ARMOUR														
Chopped Ham canned	2 oz	120	9	—	35	8	2	—	—	880	—	—	—	—
Deviled Ham canned	1 pkg (3 oz)	200	16	—	60	14	0	—	—	800	—	—	—	—
CARL BUDDIG														
Ham	1 oz	50	3	1	20	5	1	0	0	400	75	0	—	0
Honey Ham	1 oz	50	3	1	30	5	1	—	0	400	75	0	—	0
HEALTHY CHOICE														
Baked Cooked	3 slices (2.2 oz)	70	2	1	30	12	1	0	0	560	—	0	—	0
Cooked	3 slices (2.2 oz)	70	2	1	30	12	1	0	0	580	—	0	—	0

FOOD	PORTION	CALORIES	FAT	SAT FAT	CHOL	PROTEIN	CARBO	FIBER	CALCIUM	SOD	POTAS	VIT C	FOLIC	VIT A
HEALTHY CHOICE (CONT.)														
Deli-Thin Baked Cooked With Natural Juices	6 slices (2 oz)	60	2	1	25	10	2	0	0	500	—	0	—	0
Deli-Thin Cooked	6 slices (2 oz)	60	2	1	30	10	1	0	0	510	—	0	—	0
Deli-Thin Honey With Natural Juices	6 slices (2 oz)	60	2	1	25	10	2	0	0	540	—	0	—	0
Deli-Thin Smoked With Natural Juices	6 slices (2 oz)	60	2	1	25	10	1	0	0	530	—	0	—	0
Fresh-Trak Cooked	1 slice (1 oz)	30	1	0	10	5	1	0	0	250	—	0	—	0
Fresh-Trak Honey	1 slice (1 oz)	30	1	0	15	5	1	0	0	250	—	0	—	0
Honey Boneless	3 oz	100	3	1	40	15	5	0	0	580	—	0	—	0
Smoked	3 slices (2.2 oz)	70	2	1	30	13	1	0	0	560	—	0	—	0
Variety Pack Regular	3 slice (2.2 oz)	70	2	1	30	12	1	0	0	570	—	0	—	0
HILLSHIRE														
Brown Sugar	1 oz	40	2	—	—	4	2	—	—	440	—	—	—	—
Cooked Ham	1 oz	30	1	—	—	5	tr	—	—	470	—	—	—	—
Deli Select Baked Ham	1 slice	10	tr	—	—	2	tr	—	—	95	—	—	—	—
Deli Select Brown Sugar Baked	1 slice	10	tr	—	—	2	tr	—	—	90	—	—	—	—
Deli Select Cajun Ham	1 slice	10	tr	—	—	2	tr	—	—	120	—	—	—	—
Deli Select Honey Ham	1 slice	10	tr	—	—	2	tr	—	—	100	—	—	—	—
Deli Select Lower Salt	1 slice	10	tr	—	—	2	tr	—	—	80	—	—	—	—
Deli Select Smoked Ham	1 slice	10	tr	—	—	2	tr	—	—	95	—	—	—	—
Flavor Pack 90-99% Fat Free Brown Sugar Baked	1 slice (0.6 oz)	20	tr	—	—	3	1	—	—	170	—	—	—	—
Flavor Pack 90-99% Fat Free Honey Ham	1 slice (0.6 oz)	20	tr	—	—	3	1	—	—	180	—	—	—	—
Flavor Pack 90-99% Fat Free Smoked	1 slice (0.6 oz)	20	tr	—	—	3	tr	—	—	170	—	—	—	—
Genuine Baked	1 oz	35	1	—	—	5	1	—	—	290	—	—	—	—
Honey Ham	1 oz	40	2	—	—	4	2	—	—	440	—	—	—	—
Lower Salt	1 oz	30	1	—	—	5	1	—	—	300	—	—	—	—
Lunch 'N Munch Cooked Ham/ Swiss	1 pkg (4.5 oz)	360	22	—	—	20	19	—	—	1380	—	—	—	—

FOOD	PORTION	CALORIES	FAT	SAT FAT	CHOL	PROTEIN	CARBO	FIBER	CALCIUM	SOD	POTAS	VIT C	FOLIC	VIT A
HILLSHIRE (CONT.)														
Lunch 'N Munch Cooked Ham/ Swiss Oreo	1 pkg (4.125 oz)	370	21	—	—	16	30	—	—	1160	—	—	—	—
Lunch 'N Munch Cooked Ham/ Swiss Snickers/Hi-C	1 pkg (4.25 oz + 6 fl oz)	470	21	—	—	16	54	—	—	1180	—	—	—	—
Lunch 'N Munch Honey Ham/ Cheddar/ Snickers/Hi-C	1 pkg (4.25 oz + 6 fl oz)	500	23	—	—	17	56	—	—	1030	—	—	—	—
HORMEL														
Black Label Canned (refrigerated)	3 oz	100	5	2	40	14	1	0	0	1020	—	0	—	0
Black Label Canned (self stable)	3 oz	110	5	2	45	14	0	0	0	970	—	0	—	0
Cure 81 Half Ham	3 oz	100	5	2	45	16	0	0	0	890	—	0	—	0
Curemaster	3 oz	80	3	1	40	14	0	0	0	940	—	0	—	0
Deviled Ham	4 tbsp (2 oz)	150	12	4	40	9	2	0	0	430	—	0	—	0
Ham & Cheese Patties	1 patty (2 oz)	190	17	6	45	7	0	0	20	470	—	0	—	0
Ham Patties	1 (2 oz)	180	17	6	35	7	1	0	0	550	—	0	—	0
Light & Lean 97 Sliced	1 slice (1 oz)	25	1	0	15	4	0	0	0	340	—	0	—	0
Primissimo Proscuitti	2 oz	120	7	3	50	15	0	0	0	1080	—	0	—	0
Spiral Cure 81	3 oz	150	9	5	50	15	1	0	0	1090	—	0	—	0
JONES														
Family Ham	1 slice	40	2	—	14	6	tr	—	—	290	—	—	—	—
Ham Slices	1 slice	30	1	—	21	5	tr	—	—	200	—	—	—	—
JORDAN'S														
Healthy Trim 97% Fat Free Cooked	1 slice (1 oz)	30	1	0	10	5	2	0	0	180	—	0	—	0
Healthy Trim 97% Fat Free EZ Serve	1 slice (1 oz)	30	1	1	15	5	2	0	0	180	—	0	—	0
Healthy Trim 97% Fat Free Virginia	1 slice (1 oz)	30	1	1	15	5	2	0	0	180	—	0	—	0
KRAKUS														
Ham	1 oz	25	1	—	25	5	1	—	3	355	97	—	—	—
LOUIS RICH														
Carving Board Baked	2 slices (1.6 oz)	50	2	1	25	8	1	0	0	550	—	0	—	0
Carving Board Honey Glazed Thin	6 slices (2.1 oz)	70	2	1	30	11	2	0	0	750	—	0	—	0

FOOD	PORTION	CALORIES	FAT	SAT FAT	CHOL	PROTEIN	CARBO	FIBER	CALCIUM	SOD	POTAS	VIT C	FOLIC	VIT A
LOUIS RICH (CONT.)														
Carving Board Honey Glazed Traditional	2 slices (1.6 oz)	50	2	1	25	8	1	0	0	560	—	0	—	0
Carving Board Smoked	1 slice (1.6 oz)	45	2	1	20	8	0	0	0	570	—	0	—	0
Dinner Slices Baked	1 slice (3.3 oz)	80	2	1	40	16	1	0	0	1150	—	0	—	0
MR. TURKEY														
Deli Cuts Honey Cured	3 slices	35	1	—	20	5	1	—	—	300	—	—	—	—
OSCAR MAYER														
Baked	3 slices (2.2 oz)	70	3	1	30	11	2	0	0	790	—	0	—	0
Boiled	3 slices (2.2 oz)	60	3	1	30	10	0	0	0	820	—	0	—	0
Chopped	1 slice (1 oz)	50	3	2	15	4	1	0	0	340	—	0	—	0
Dinner Slice	3 oz	80	3	1	40	14	0	0	0	1010	—	0	—	0
Dinner Steaks	1 (2 oz)	60	2	1	30	10	0	0	0	750	—	0	—	0
Free Baked	3 slices (1.6 oz)	35	0	0	15	7	1	0	0	520	—	0	—	0
Free Honey	3 slices (1.6 oz)	35	0	0	15	7	2	0	0	580	—	0	—	0
Free Smoked	3 slices (1.6 oz)	35	0	0	15	7	1	0	0	550	—	0	—	0
Ham & Cheese Loaf	1 slice (1 oz)	70	5	3	20	4	1	0	0	350	—	0	—	0
Honey	3 slices (2.2 oz)	70	3	1	30	10	2	0	0	760	—	0	—	0
Lower Sodium	3 slices (2.2 oz)	70	3	1	30	10	2	0	0	520	—	0	—	0
Lunchables Cookies/Ham/ Swiss	1 pkg (4.2 oz)	360	19	8	50	18	29	tr	250	1420	—	0	—	300
Lunchables Dessert Chocolate Pudding/Ham/ American	1 pkg (6.2 oz)	390	20	9	55	18	34	tr	250	1540	—	0	—	200
Lunchables Ham/ Cheddar	1 pkg (4.5 oz)	340	20	11	75	21	19	0	250	1830	—	0	—	300
Smoked	3 slices (2.2 oz)	60	3	1	30	11	0	0	0	760	—	0	—	0
RUSSER														
Baked	2 oz	70	3	1	30	9	4	—	—	750	—	—	—	—
Canadian Brand Maple	2 oz	70	2	1	30	9	4	—	—	750	—	—	—	—
Chopped	2 oz	130	9	3	30	7	5	—	—	540	—	—	—	—
Cooked Ham	2 oz	60	2	1	30	9	2	—	—	650	—	—	—	—
Ham & Cheese Loaf	2 oz	120	8	2	30	8	5	—	—	600	—	—	—	—

FOOD	PORTION	CALORIES	FAT	SAT FAT	CHOL	PROTEIN	CARBO	FIBER	CALCIUM	SOD	POTAS	VIT C	FOLIC	VIT A
RUSSER (CONT.)														
Honey & Maple Cured	2 oz	70	2	1	30	9	3	—	—	550	—	—	—	—
Honey Cured	2 oz	60	3	1	30	9	2	—	—	600	—	—	—	—
Hot	2 oz	70	2	1	30	9	3	—	—	750	—	—	—	—
Light Cooked	2 oz	60	2	1	30	9	2	—	—	400	—	—	—	—
Light Smoked	2 oz	60	2	1	30	9	2	—	—	400	—	—	—	—
Smoked Virginia	2 oz	70	3	1	30	9	3	—	—	750	—	—	—	—
Spiced	2 oz	160	12	3	30	7	5	—	—	540	—	—	—	—
SARA LEE														
Bavarian Brand Baked	2 oz	80	4	1	40	9	1	—	—	610	—	9	—	—
Bavarian Brand Baked Honey	2 oz	80	4	1	40	9	2	—	—	490	—	9	—	—
Golden Cure Smoked	2 oz	80	4	2	30	9	1	—	—	650	—	9	—	—
Honey Ham	2 oz	60	2	1	25	10	2	—	—	520	—	12	—	—
Honey Roasted	2 oz	90	5	2	30	9	3	—	—	590	—	12	—	—
SPAM														
Spread	4 tbsp (2 oz)	140	12	4	40	8	1	0	0	570	—	0	—	0
UNDERWOOD														
Deviled	2.08 oz	220	19	6	50	8	tr	—	—	430	150	—	—	—
Deviled Light	2.08 oz	120	8	1	35	11	1	—	—	250	190	9	—	—
Deviled Smoked	2.08 oz	190	18	6	65	9	tr	—	—	260	140	—	—	—
WEIGHT WATCHERS														
Deli Thin Oven Roasted	5 slices (⅓ oz)	12	tr	—	5	2	tr	—	—	95	—	—	—	—
Deli Thin Oven Roasted Honey Ham	5 slices (⅓ oz)	12	tr	—	5	2	tr	—	—	95	—	—	—	—
Deli Thin Premium Smoked	5 slices (⅓ oz)	12	tr	—	5	2	tr	—	—	85	—	—	—	—
Oven Roasted Honey Ham	2 slices (¾ oz)	25	1	—	15	4	tr	—	—	220	—	—	—	—
Oven Roasted Smoked	2 slices (¾ oz)	25	1	—	15	4	tr	—	—	220	—	—	—	—
Premium Cooked	2 slices (¾ oz)	25	1	—	15	4	tr	—	—	220	—	—	—	—

HAM DISHES

FROZEN

FOOD	PORTION	CALORIES	FAT	SAT FAT	CHOL	PROTEIN	CARBO	FIBER	CALCIUM	SOD	POTAS	VIT C	FOLIC	VIT A
CROISSANT POCKET														
Stuffed Sandwich Ham & Cheddar	1 piece (4.5 oz)	360	17	7	45	13	39	5	100	710	—	15	—	500
HOT POCKET														
Stuffed Sandwich Ham & Cheese	1 (4.5 ox)	340	15	7	45	14	37	4	250	840	—	0	—	300
TAKE-OUT														
sandwich w/ cheese	1	353	15	6	58	21	33	—	130	772	290	3	71	319

HAMBURGER

(*see also* BEEF)

FROZEN

FOOD	PORTION	CALORIES	FAT	SAT FAT	CHOL	PROTEIN	CARBO	FIBER	CALCIUM	SOD	POTAS	VIT C	FOLIC	VIT A
JIMMY DEAN														
Burger	1 (2 oz)	220	21	7	40	7	0	0	—	380	—	—	—	—
Flamed Broiled Cheeseburger	1 (6.3 oz)	540	34	14	80	28	34	1	—	760	—	—	—	—
Mini Cheeseburger	2 (3 oz)	270	14	9	35	14	23	1	—	530	—	—	—	—
KID CUISINE														
Beef Patty Sandwich w/ Cheese	1 (8.5 oz)	410	15	5	15	12	58	4	150	540	—	0	—	100
RUDY'S FARM														
Mild Burger	1 (3 oz)	360	35	12	65	11	0	0	—	730	—	—	—	—
WHITE CASTLE														
Cheeseburger	2 (3.6 oz)	310	17	9	30	15	23	6	80	480	—	0	—	100
Hamburger	2 (3.2 oz)	270	14	6	20	12	23	5	20	270	—	0	—	0
TAKE-OUT														
double patty w/ bun	1 reg	544	28	10	99	30	43	—	87	554	363	0	38	0
double patty w/ cheese & bun	1 reg	457	28	13	110	28	22	—	232	635	308	0	29	332
double patty w/ cheese & double bun	1 reg	461	22	10	80	22	44	—	224	892	285	0	36	276
double patty w/ cheese ketchup mayonnaise onion pickle tomato & bun	1 reg	416	21	8	60	21	35	—	171	1051	335	2	23	398
double patty w/ ketchup mayonnaise onion pickle tomato & bun	1 reg	649	35	13	94	30	53	—	169	920	389	3	34	371
double patty w/ ketchup cheese mayonnaise mustard pickle tomato & bun	1 lg	706	44	18	141	38	40	—	240	1149	596	tr	48	348
double patty w/ ketchup mustard mayonnaise onion pickle tomato & bun	1 lg	540	27	11	122	34	40	—	102	791	569	1	27	102
double patty w/ ketchup mustard onion pickle & bun	1 reg	576	32	12	102	32	39	—	92	742	527	1	45	53

FOOD	PORTION	CALORIES	FAT	SAT FAT	CHOL	PROTEIN	CARBO	FIBER	CALCIUM	SOD	POTAS	VIT C	FOLIC	VIT A
single patty w/ bacon ketchup cheese mustard onion pickle & bun	1 lg	609	37	16	112	32	37	—	162	1044	331	2	33	406
single patty w/ bun	1 lg	400	23	8	71	23	25	—	74	474	268	0	32	0
single patty w/ bun	1 reg	275	12	4	36	12	31	—	63	387	145	0	25	0
single patty w/ cheese & bun	1 reg	320	15	6	50	15	32	—	140	500	165	0	26	153
single patty w/ ketchup cheese ham mayonnaise pickle tomato & bun	1 lg	745	48	21	122	40	38	—	301	1713	539	7	50	505
single patty w/ ketchup mustard mayonnaise onion pickle tomato & bun	1 reg	279	13	4	26	13	27	—	63	504	227	2	18	82
triple patty w/ cheese & bun	1 lg	769	51	22	161	56	27	—	282	1211	821	3	51	359
triple patty w/ ketchup mustard pickle & bun	1 lg	693	41	16	142	50	29	—	65	713	785	1	31	158

HAZELNUTS

FOOD	PORTION	CALORIES	FAT	SAT FAT	CHOL	PROTEIN	CARBO	FIBER	CALCIUM	SOD	POTAS	VIT C	FOLIC	VIT A
dried blanched	1 oz	191	19	1	0	4	5	—	55	1	131	—	—	20
dried unblanched	1 oz	179	18	1	0	4	4	—	53	1	125	tr	20	19
dry roasted unblanched	1 oz	188	19	1	0	3	5	—	55	1	131	—	—	—

CRUMPY

Chocolate Hazelnut Spread	1 tbsp (0.5 oz)	80	5	1	0	tr	8	0	0	5	—	0	—	0

HEART

FOOD	PORTION	CALORIES	FAT	SAT FAT	CHOL	PROTEIN	CARBO	FIBER	CALCIUM	SOD	POTAS	VIT C	FOLIC	VIT A
beef simmered	3 oz	148	5	1	164	24	tr	—	5	54	198	1	2	0
chicken simmered	1 cup (5 oz)	268	11	3	350	11	tr	—	27	69	192	3	116	41
lamb braised	3 oz	158	7	3	212	21	2	—	12	54	160	6	2	0
pork braised	1 cup	215	7	2	320	34	1	0	10	51	—	3	6	32
pork braised	1	191	7	2	285	30	1	0	9	45	—	3	5	28
turkey simmered	1 cup (5 oz)	257	9	3	327	39	3	—	19	79	265	3	114	40
veal braised	3 oz	158	6	2	150	25	tr	—	7	50	169	—	—	0

HEARTS OF PALM

FOOD	PORTION	CALORIES	FAT	SAT FAT	CHOL	PROTEIN	CARBO	FIBER	CALCIUM	SOD	POTAS	VIT C	FOLIC	VIT A
canned	1 cup (5.1 oz)	41	1	tr	0	4	7	—	84	622	259	12	57	0
canned	1 (1.2 oz)	9	tr	tr	0	1	2	—	19	141	58	3	13	0

HERBAL TEA

(see TEA/HERBAL TEA)

HERBS/SPICES

(see also individual names)

FOOD	PORTION	CALORIES	FAT	SAT FAT	CHOL	PROTEIN	CARBO	FIBER	CALCIUM	SOD	POTAS	VIT C	FOLIC	VIT A
curry powder	1 tsp	6	tr	—	0	tr	1	—	10	1	31	tr	—	20
poultry seasoning	1 tsp	5	tr	—	0	tr	1	—	15	tr	10	tr	—	39
pumpkin pie spice	1 tsp	6	tr	—	0	tr	1	—	12	1	11	tr	—	4
AC'CENT														
Flavor Enhancer	½ tsp	5	0	0	0	0	0	0	0	300	0	0	—	0
Herbal All Purpose Seasoning	½ tsp	0	0	0	0	0	0	0	0	0	0	0	—	0
CHI-CHI'S														
Seasoning Mix	1 tsp (3 g)	10	0	0	0	0	1	0	0	290	—	2	—	0
GOLDEN DIPT														
All Purpose Seafood	¼ tsp	2	0	0	0	0	0	—	—	85	—	—	—	—
Blackened Redfish	¼ tsp	2	0	0	0	0	0	—	—	140	—	—	—	100
Broiled Fish	¼ tsp	2	0	0	0	0	0	—	—	125	—	—	—	—
Cajun Style Shrimp & Crab	¼ tsp	2	0	0	0	0	0	—	—	200	—	—	—	—
Lemon Pepper Seafood	¼ tsp	8	0	0	0	1	1	—	—	115	—	—	—	—
KA-ME														
Five Spice Powder	¼ tsp (1 g)	0	0	0	0	0	1	0	0	0	—	—	—	—
LAWRY'S														
Seasoning Blend Sloppy Joe	1 pkg	126	tr	—	0	3	28	1	—	3442	22	—	—	—
MCILHENNY														
Crab Boil	3 oz	378	17	5	4	17	40	32	318	95	—	tr	—	495
MRS. DASH														
Extra Spicy	⅛ tsp (0.02 oz)	2	0	—	0	tr	tr	—	—	1	8	—	—	—
Garlic & Herb	⅛ tsp (0.02 oz)	2	tr	—	tr	tr	tr	—	—	tr	22	—	—	—
Lemon & Herb	⅛ tsp (0.02 oz)	2	0	—	0	tr	tr	—	—	1	6	—	—	—
Low Pepper No Garlic	⅛ tsp (0.02 oz)	2	0	—	0	tr	tr	—	—	tr	8	—	—	—
Original Blend	⅛ tsp (0.02 oz)	2	0	0	0	tr	tr	—	—	1	6	—	—	—
Table Blend	⅛ tsp (0.02 oz)	2	0	—	0	tr	tr	—	—	1	8	—	—	—
WATKINS														
Apple Bake Seasoning	¼ tsp (0.5 g)	0	0	0	0	0	0	0	0	0	—	0	—	0
Barbecue Spice	¼ tsp (0.5 g)	0	0	0	0	0	0	0	0	30	—	0	—	0
Bean Soup Seasoning	¾ tsp (2 g)	5	0	0	0	0	1	0	0	150	—	0	—	100

FOOD	PORTION	CALORIES	FAT	SAT FAT	CHOL	PROTEIN	CARBO	FIBER	CALCIUM	SOD	POTAS	VIT C	FOLIC	VIT A
WATKINS (CONT.)														
Beef Jerky Seasoning	2 tsp (6 g)	15	0	0	0	1	3	0	0	600	—	0	—	0
Chicken Seasoning	½ tsp (1 g)	0	0	0	0	0	0	0	0	110	—	0	—	0
Cole Slaw Seasoning	½ tsp (1.5 g)	5	0	0	0	0	1	0	0	190	—	0	—	0
Egg Sensations	1 tsp (3 g)	10	0	0	0	0	1	0	0	180	—	0	—	0
Fajita Seasoning	½ tsp (3 g)	10	0	0	0	0	2	0	0	0	—	0	—	500
Grill Seasoning	¼ tsp (1 g)	0	0	0	0	0	0	0	0	210	—	0	—	0
Ground Beef Seasoning	⅛ tsp (0.5 g)	0	0	0	0	0	0	0	0	70	—	0	—	0
Italian Blend	1 tsp (3 g)	1	0	0	0	0	2	0	0	120	—	0	—	0
Meat Tenderizer	⅛ tsp (0.5 g)	0	0	0	0	0	0	0	0	140	—	0	—	0
Meatloaf Seasoning	½ tsp (5 g)	15	0	0	0	1	4	0	0	270	—	0	—	100
Mexican Blend	½ tbsp (4 g)	15	0	0	0	0	3	0	0	90	—	2	—	150
Omelet & Souffle Seasoning	¾ tsp (2 g)	5	0	0	0	0	1	0	0	110	—	4	—	0
Oriental Ginger Garlic Liquid Spice Blend	1 tbsp (0.5 oz)	120	14	2	0	0	0	0	0	0	—	0	—	0
Potato Salad Seasoning	¼ tsp (1 g)	0	0	0	0	0	0	0	0	135	—	0	—	0
Pumpkin Pie Spice	¼ tsp (0.5 g)	0	0	0	0	0	0	0	0	0	—	0	—	0
Smokehouse Liquid Blend	1 tbsp (0.5 oz)	120	14	2	0	0	0	0	0	0	—	0	—	0
Soup & Vegetable Seasoning	¼ tsp (0.5 g)	0	0	0	0	0	0	0	0	70	—	0	—	0
Spanish Seasoning Blend	¼ tsp (0.5 oz)	0	0	0	0	0	0	0	0	0	—	2	—	0
HERRING														
atlantic cooked	3 oz	172	10	2	65	20	0	—	63	98	356	1	—	87
atlantic cooked	1 fillet (5 oz)	290	17	4	110	33	0	—	105	165	599	1	—	146
atlantic raw	3 oz	134	8	2	51	15	0	—	49	76	278	1	—	80
roe canned	3.5 oz	118	3	—	—	22	tr	—	15	—	—	—	—	—
roe raw	3½ oz	130	2	—	360	24	2	—	—	—	—	14	—	—
TAKE-OUT														
atlantic kippered	1 fillet (1.4 oz)	87	5	1	33	10	0	—	33	367	179	tr	—	51
atlantic pickled	½ oz	39	3	tr	2	2	1	—	12	131	10	—	tr	129
HICKORY NUTS														
dried	1 oz	187	18	2	0	4	5	—	17	0	124	—	—	—
HOMINY														
CANNED														
white	1 cup (5.6 oz)	482	1	tr	0	2	23	4	16	336	14	0	2	176
ALLEN														
Golden	½ cup (4.5 oz)	120	1	0	0	2	27	4	0	340	—	0	—	300

FOOD	PORTION	CALORIES	FAT	SAT FAT	CHOL	PROTEIN	CARBO	FIBER	CALCIUM	SOD	POTAS	VIT C	FOLIC	VIT A
ALLEN (CONT.)														
Mexican	½ cup (4.5 oz)	120	1	0	0	2	25	3	0	340	—	0	—	300
White	½ cup (4.5 oz)	100	1	0	0	2	22	4	0	340	—	0	—	200
UNCLE WILLIAM														
Golden	½ cup (4.5 oz)	120	1	0	0	2	27	4	0	340	—	0	—	300
Mexican	½ cup (4.5 oz)	120	1	0	0	2	25	3	0	340	—	0	—	300
White	½ cup (4.5 oz)	100	1	0	0	2	22	4	0	340	—	0	—	200
VAN CAMP'S														
Golden	½ cup (4.3 oz)	80	1	0	0	1	17	1	0	540	15	—	0	0
White	½ cup (4.3 oz)	80	1	0	0	1	15	1	0	530	15	—	0	0
HONEY														
honey	1 tbsp (0.7 oz)	64	0	0	0	tr	17	—	1	1	11	tr	0	0
honey	1 cup (11.9 oz)	1031	0	0	0	1	279	—	20	12	176	2	5	0
BURLESON'S														
Clover	1 tbsp	60	0	0	0	tr	16	0	1	1	21	—	—	—
Creamed	1 tbsp	60	0	0	0	tr	16	0	1	1	21	—	—	—
Natural	1 tbsp	60	0	0	0	tr	16	0	1	1	21	—	—	—
Pure	1 tbsp	60	0	0	0	tr	16	0	1	1	21	—	—	—
Raw	1 tbsp	60	0	0	0	tr	16	0	1	1	21	—	—	—
Rocky Mountain Clover	1 tbsp	60	0	0	0	tr	16	0	1	1	21	—	—	—
TREE OF LIFE														
Alfalfa	1 tbsp (0.7 oz)	60	0	0	0	0	17	—	—	0	—	—	—	—
Avocado	1 tbsp (0.7 oz)	60	0	0	0	0	17	—	—	0	—	—	—	—
Buckwheat	1 tbsp (0.7 oz)	60	0	0	0	0	17	—	—	0	—	—	—	—
Clover	1 tbsp (0.7 oz)	60	0	0	0	0	17	—	—	0	—	—	—	—
Honeybear Wildflower	1 tbsp (0.7 oz)	60	0	0	0	0	17	—	—	0	—	—	—	—
Orange	1 tbsp (0.7 oz)	60	0	0	0	0	17	—	—	0	—	—	—	—
Tupelo	1 tbsp (0.7 oz)	60	0	0	0	0	17	—	—	0	—	—	—	—
Wildflower	1 tbsp (0.7 oz)	60	0	0	0	0	17	—	—	0	—	—	—	—
HONEYDEW														
FRESH														
cubed	1 cup	60	tr	—	0	1	16	—	10	17	461	42	—	68
wedge	¹⁄₁₀	46	tr	—	0	1	12	—	8	13	350	32	—	52
CHIQUITA														
Fresh	1 cup	70	0	—	0	—	—	—	—	—	—	—	—	—
DOLE														
Honeydew	¹⁄₁₀	50	0	—	0	1	12	1	—	50	410	—	—	—
FROZEN														
BIG VALLEY														
Balls	¾ cup (4.9 oz)	45	0	0	0	1	11	1	0	16	—	30	—	0
HORSE														
roasted	3 oz	149	5	2	58	24	0	—	7	47	322	2	—	—

FOOD	PORTION	CALORIES	FAT	SAT FAT	CHOL	PROTEIN	CARBO	FIBER	CALCIUM	SOD	POTAS	VIT C	FOLIC	VIT A
HORSERADISH														
HEBREW NATIONAL														
White	1 tbsp	7	0	0	0	0	1	—	—	160	—	—	—	—
HELUVA GOOD CHEESE														
Horseradish	1 tsp (5 g)	0	0	0	0	0	0	—	—	6	—	—	—	—
KA-ME														
Wasabi Powder	¼ tsp (1 g)	0	0	0	0	0	1	0	0	0	—	—	—	—
KRAFT														
Cream Style	1 tsp (5 g)	0	0	0	0	0	0	0	0	50	10	1	—	0
Horseradish Sauce	1 tsp (5 g)	20	2	0	<5	0	tr	0	0	35	0	0	—	0
Prepared	1 tsp (5 g)	0	0	0	0	0	0	0	0	50	10	1	—	0
ROSOFF'S														
Red	1 tbsp (0.5 oz)	8	0	0	0	0	2	—	—	160	—	—	—	—
White	1 tbsp (0.5 oz)	7	0	0	0	0	1	—	—	160	—	—	—	—
SCHORR'S														
Red	1 tbsp (0.5 oz)	8	0	0	0	0	2	—	—	160	—	—	—	—
White	1 tbsp (0.5 oz)	7	0	0	0	0	1	—	—	160	—	—	—	—
HOT CAKES														
(*see* PANCAKES)														
HOT COCOA														
(*see* COCOA)														
HOT DOG														
(*see also* MEAT SUBSTITUTES, SAUSAGE, SAUSAGE SUBSTITUTES)														
beef & pork	1 (2 oz)	183	17	6	29	6	1	—	6	639	95	15	2	—
beef & pork	1 (1.5 oz)	144	13	5	22	5	1	—	6	504	75	12	2	—
chicken	1 (1.5 oz)	116	9	2	45	6	3	—	43	617	—	—	—	—
pork cheesefurter smokie	1 (1.5 oz)	141	12	5	29	6	1	—	25	465	89	8	—	—
turkey	1 (1.5 oz)	102	8	—	48	6	1	—	48	642	80	—	—	—
APPLEGATE FARMS														
Natural Turkey	1 (1.5 oz)	120	5	2	40	14	1	0	20	450	—	0	—	0
EMPIRE														
Chicken	1 (2 oz)	100	7	2	70	8	1	0	40	465	—	0	—	0
Turkey	1 (2 oz)	90	6	2	35	9	1	0	40	410	—	0	—	0
HEALTH VALLEY														
Weiners	1	96	8	—	49	5	1	0	—	90	32	—	—	—
Weiners Turkey	1	96	8	—	35	5	1	0	—	112	39	—	—	—
HEALTHY CHOICE														
Beef	1 (1.8 oz)	60	2	1	20	7	5	0	20	480	—	2	—	0
Bunsize	1 (2 oz)	70	2	1	20	8	5	0	20	590	—	4	—	0
Franks	1 (1.6 oz)	50	2	1	15	6	4	0	20	450	—	4	—	0
Jumbo	1 (2 oz)	70	2	1	20	8	5	0	20	570	—	4	—	0
HEBREW NATIONAL														
Beef	1 (1.7 oz)	150	14	—	30	6	—	—	—	370	—	—	—	—
Cocktail Beef	6 (1.8 oz)	160	15	—	35	6	—	—	—	410	—	—	—	—

FOOD	PORTION	CALORIES	FAT	SAT FAT	CHOL	PROTEIN	CARBO	FIBER	CALCIUM	SOD	POTAS	VIT C	FOLIC	VIT A
HEBREW NATIONAL (CONT.)														
Dinner Beef	1 (4 oz)	350	34	—	75	14	—	—	—	890	—	—	—	—
Reduced Fat Beef	1 (1.7 oz)	120	10	—	25	5	—	—	—	350	—	—	—	—
HILLSHIRE														
Franks Bun Size Beef	2 oz	180	16	—	—	7	2	—	—	560	—	—	—	—
Light & Mild Franks Jumbo	1 link	110	8	—	—	7	2	—	—	570	—	—	—	—
Light & Mild Wieners	1 link	90	7	—	—	6	2	—	—	580	—	—	—	—
Lit'l Franks Beef	2 oz	180	16	—	—	7	1	—	—	580	—	—	—	—
Lit'l Wieners	2 oz	180	16	—	—	8	2	—	—	560	—	—	—	—
Weiners Natural Casing	2 oz	180	17	—	—	6	2	—	—	470	—	—	—	—
Wieners Bun Size	2 oz	180	16	—	—	7	2	—	—	550	—	—	—	—
HORMEL														
Fat Free	1 (1.8 oz)	45	0	0	15	5	5	0	0	580	—	6	—	0
Fat Free Beef	1 (1.8 oz)	45	0	0	10	6	5	0	0	590	—	6	—	0
JORDAN'S														
Healthy Trim Low Fat	1 (1.8 oz)	70	3	1	25	8	3	0	0	350	—	0	—	0
Healthy Trim Low Fat Skinless	1 (1.8 oz)	70	3	1	25	8	3	0	0	350	—	0	—	0
LOUIS RICH														
Bun Length	1 (2 oz)	110	8	3	55	6	3	0	80	650	—	0	—	0
Cheese	1 (1.6 oz)	90	6	3	40	6	2	0	100	480	—	0	—	0
Franks	1 (1.6 oz)	80	6	2	40	5	2	0	60	510	—	0	—	0
MR. TURKEY														
Bun Size	1	130	11	—	50	6	2	—	—	670	—	—	—	—
Cheese	1	140	12	—	50	7	2	—	—	670	—	—	—	—
Hot Dog	1	110	9	—	40	5	2	—	—	540	—	—	—	—
OSCAR MAYER														
Beef	1 (1.6 oz)	140	13	6	30	5	1	0	0	460	—	0	—	0
Big & Juicy Franks Deli Style	1 (2.7 oz)	230	22	10	50	9	1	0	0	680	—	0	—	0
Big & Juicy Franks Original	1 (2.7 oz)	240	22	9	45	9	1	0	0	700	—	0	—	0
Big & Juicy Franks Quarter Pound	1 (4 oz)	350	32	13	65	13	2	0	20	1050	—	0	—	0
Big & Juicy Weiners Hot 'N Spicy	1 (2.7 oz)	220	20	8	45	10	1	0	0	750	—	0	—	0
Big & Juicy Weiners Smokie Links	1 (2.7 oz)	220	19	7	50	10	1	0	0	770	—	0	—	0
Big & Juicy Wieners Original	1 (2.7 oz)	240	22	9	45	9	1	0	0	690	—	0	—	0
Bun-Length Beef	1 (2 oz)	180	17	7	35	6	2	0	0	580	—	0	—	0
Cheese	1 (1.6 oz)	140	13	5	35	5	1	0	80	510	—	0	—	0

FOOD	PORTION	CALORIES	FAT	SAT FAT	CHOL	PROTEIN	CARBO	FIBER	CALCIUM	SOD	POTAS	VIT C	FOLIC	VIT A
OSCAR MAYER (CONT.)														
Free Beef	1 (1.8 oz)	40	0	0	15	7	3	0	0	460	—	0	—	0
Free Turkey & Beef	1 (1.8 oz)	35	0	0	15	6	2	0	0	490	—	0	—	0
Jumbo Beef	1 (2 oz)	180	17	7	35	6	2	0	0	580	—	0	—	0
Light Beef	1 (2 oz)	110	8	4	30	6	2	0	0	620	—	0	—	0
Wieners	1 (1.6 oz)	150	13	5	35	5	1	0	20	430	—	0	—	0
Wieners Bun-Length	1 (2 oz)	190	17	6	40	6	2	0	40	550	—	0	—	0
Wieners Light	1 (2 oz)	110	8	4	35	7	2	0	20	590	—	0	—	0
Wieners Little	6 (2 oz)	180	17	6	35	6	2	0	0	570	—	0	—	0
RUSSER														
Lil'Salt Deli Franks	1 (2.67 oz)	160	11	4	40	11	3	—	—	640	—	—	—	—
SHOFAR														
Kosher Beef	1 (1.8 oz)	150	14	5	20	6	0	0	0	370	—	0	—	0
Kosher Beef Reduced Fat Reduced Sodium	1 (1.8 oz)	120	10	4	25	7	0	0	0	360	—	0	—	100
TYSON														
Chicken Cheese	1	145	11	—	—	7	1	—	—	680	—	—	—	—
Chicken Hot Dog	1	115	10	—	—	6	1	—	—	700	—	—	—	—
WAMPLER LONGACRE														
Chicken	1 (1.6 oz)	110	9	—	50	6	0	—	—	400	—	—	—	—
Chicken	1 (2 oz)	130	11	—	65	8	0	—	—	440	—	—	—	—
Turkey	1 (1.6 oz)	110	9	—	45	6	0	—	—	400	—	—	—	—
Turkey	1 (2 oz)	130	11	—	60	8	0	—	—	440	—	—	—	—
TAKE-OUT														
corndog	1	460	19	5	79	17	56	—	101	972	262	0	60	207
w/ bun chili	1	297	13	5	51	14	31	—	19	480	166	3	50	58
w/ bun plain	1	242	15	5	44	10	18	—	24	671	143	tr	30	0

HUMMUS

FOOD	PORTION	CALORIES	FAT	SAT FAT	CHOL	PROTEIN	CARBO	FIBER	CALCIUM	SOD	POTAS	VIT C	FOLIC	VIT A
hummus	1 cup	420	21	3	0	12	50	—	124	599	427	19	146	61
ATHENOS														
Roasted Red Pepper	2 tbsp (1.1 oz)	60	4	1	0	2	6	1	0	210	—	0	—	0
CASBAH														
Mix as prep	¼ cup	120	5	0	0	5	15	1	40	180	—	1	—	—
CEDAR'S														
No Salt Added Hommus Tahini	2 tbsp (1 oz)	50	2	0	0	3	5	3	—	70	—	—	—	—
TAKE-OUT														
hummus	⅓ cup	140	7	1	0	4	17	—	41	200	142	6	49	20

HYACINTH BEANS

FOOD	PORTION	CALORIES	FAT	SAT FAT	CHOL	PROTEIN	CARBO	FIBER	CALCIUM	SOD	POTAS	VIT C	FOLIC	VIT A
dried cooked	1 cup	228	1	—	0	16	40	—	77	13	653	0	—	—

ICE CREAM AND FROZEN DESSERTS

(*see also* ICES AND ICE POPS, PUDDING POPS, SHERBET, YOGURT FROZEN)

FOOD	PORTION	CALORIES	FAT	SAT FAT	CHOL	PROTEIN	CARBO	FIBER	CALCIUM	SOD	POTAS	VIT C	FOLIC	VIT A
chocolate	½ cup (4 fl oz)	143	7	4	22	3	19	—	72	50	164	1	10	275

FOOD	PORTION	CALORIES	FAT	SAT FAT	CHOL	PROTEIN	CARBO	FIBER	CALCIUM	SOD	POTAS	VIT C	FOLIC	VIT A
dixie cup chocolate	1 (3.5 fl oz)	125	6	4	20	2	16	—	63	44	145	tr	9	241
dixie cup strawberry	1 (3.5 fl oz)	112	5	—	17	2	16	—	70	35	109	5	7	185
dixie cup vanilla	1 (3.5 fl oz)	116	6	4	25	2	14	—	74	46	115	tr	3	237
freeze dried ice cream chocolate strawberry & vanilla	1 pkg (0.75 oz)	158	5	2	1	2	24	1	20	97	—	0	—	200
french vanilla soft serve	½ gal	3014	180	108	1226	56	306	—	1886	1228	2704	7	73	6353
french vanilla soft serve	½ cup (4 fl oz)	185	11	6	78	4	19	—	113	52	152	1	7	464
strawberry	½ cup (4 fl oz)	127	6	—	19	2	18	—	79	40	124	5	8	211
vanilla	½ cup (4 fl oz)	132	7	4	29	2	16	—	85	53	131	tr	3	270
vanilla light	½ cup (2.3 oz)	92	3	2	9	3	15	—	92	56	139	1	4	109
vanilla rich	½ cup (2.6 oz)	178	12	7	45	3	17	—	87	41	118	1	4	476
vanilla soft serve	½ cup	111	2	1	10	4	19	—	138	62	194	1	6	90
vanilla 10% fat	½ gal	2153	115	71	476	38	254	—	1406	929	2052	6	22	4341
vanilla 16% fat	½ gal	2805	190	118	256	33	256	—	1213	868	1771	5	19	7199
vanilla light	½ gal	1469	45	28	146	41	232	—	1409	836	2117	6	24	1708
vanilla light	1 cup	184	6	4	18	5	29	—	176	105	265	1	3	214
vanilla light soft serve	½ gal	1787	37	23	106	64	307	—	2195	1303	3298	9	38	1400
vanilla light soft serve	1 cup	223	5	3	13	8	38	—	274	163	412	1	5	175
3 MUSKETEERS														
Single Chocolate	1 (2 fl oz)	160	10	6	20	2	16	0	60	30	60	—	—	200
Single Vanilla	1 (2 fl oz)	160	10	6	15	2	16	0	60	30	60	—	—	200
Snack Chocolate	1 (0.72 fl oz)	60	4	2	5	1	6	0	20	10	20	—	—	—
Snack Vanilla	1 (0.72 fl oz)	60	4	2	5	1	6	0	20	10	20	—	—	—
BEN & JERRY'S														
Banana Walnut	½ cup (3.9 oz)	290	21	9	75	5	26	1	—	50	—	—	—	—
Butter Pecan	½ cup (3.9 oz)	310	26	11	100	4	20	1	100	160	—	0	—	750
Cherry Garcia	½ cup (3.7 oz)	240	16	10	80	4	25	0	100	60	—	0	—	750
Cherry Vanilla	½ cup (3.9 oz)	240	15	9	85	3	26	0	—	60	—	—	—	—
Chocolate Chip Cookie Dough	½ cup (3.7 oz)	270	17	9	80	4	30	0	100	95	—	1	—	750
Chocolate Fudge Brownie	½ cup (3.7 oz)	250	14	9	50	4	31	2	100	100	—	0	—	500
Chunky Monkey	½ cup (3.7 oz)	280	19	10	70	4	29	1	100	50	—	1	—	500
Coconut Almond	½ cup (3.7 oz)	260	20	9	80	5	19	1	—	80	—	—	—	—
Coconut Almond Fudge Chip	½ cup (3.8 oz)	320	25	14	75	6	24	2	150	85	—	0	—	500
Coffee Almond Fudge	½ cup (3.7 oz)	290	20	9	75	6	24	2	150	85	—	1	—	750
Coffee Toffee Crunch	½ cup (3.7 oz)	280	19	10	80	4	28	0	100	120	—	0	—	750

FOOD	PORTION	CALORIES	FAT	SAT FAT	CHOL	PROTEIN	CARBO	FIBER	CALCIUM	SOD	POTAS	VIT C	FOLIC	VIT A
BEN & JERRY'S (CONT.)														
English Toffee Crunch	½ cup (4 oz)	310	21	12	90	4	30	0	100	130	—	0	—	750
Mint Chocolate Cookie	½ cup (3.8 oz)	260	17	10	80	4	27	1	100	120	—	0	—	750
New York Super Fudge Chunk	½ cup (3.7 oz)	290	20	11	50	5	28	2	100	55	—	0	—	500
No Fat Strawberry	½ cup (3.3 oz)	140	0	0	0	3	31	0	100	60	—	6	—	100
No Fat Vanilla Fudge Swirl	½ cup (3.1 oz)	150	0	0	0	3	32	0	100	80	—	0	—	100
Peanut Butter Cup	½ cup (4.1 oz)	370	26	12	75	8	30	2	150	140	—	0	—	500
Pop Chocolate Chip Cookie Dough	1 (4.1 oz)	450	28	15	60	6	48	1	100	150	—	1	—	750
Pop English Toffee Crunch	1 (3.7 oz)	340	23	15	75	4	35	0	100	55	—	0	—	750
Pop Vanilla	1 (3.9 oz)	360	28	15	75	5	30	0	100	75	—	1	—	500
Rain Forest Crunch	½ cup (3.7 oz)	300	23	11	85	5	24	0	100	140	—	0	—	750
Smooth Aztec Harvest Coffee	½ cup (3.8 oz)	230	16	10	90	4	22	0	100	55	—	0	—	750
Smooth Deep Dark Chocolate	½ cup (3.9 oz)	260	15	9	55	4	32	2	100	55	—	1	—	500
Smooth Double Chocolate Fudge	½ cup (4.1 oz)	280	16	9	55	5	35	3	100	60	—	1	—	750
Smooth Mocho Fudge	½ cup (4 oz)	270	18	10	85	5	30	1	150	65	—	1	—	750
Smooth Vanilla	½ cup (3.8 oz)	230	17	10	95	4	21	0	150	55	—	0	—	750
Smooth Vanilla Bean	½ cup (3.8 oz)	230	17	10	95	4	21	0	150	55	—	0	—	750
Smooth Vanilla Caramel Fudge	½ cup (4.1 oz)	280	17	10	95	4	33	1	100	75	—	1	—	750
Smooth White Russian	½ cup (3.8 oz)	240	16	10	90	4	23	0	100	55	—	0	—	750
Vanilla	½ cup (3.7 oz)	230	17	10	95	4	21	0	150	55	—	0	—	750
Wavy Gravy	½ cup (4.1 oz)	330	24	10	80	6	29	2	150	95	—	1	—	750
BON BONS														
Vanilla With Milk Chocolate Coating	8 pieces	330	23	13	20	3	27	0	80	60	—	0	—	200
Vanilla With Milk Chocolate Coating	5 pieces	200	14	8	10	2	17	0	40	35	—	0	—	100
BORDEN														
Buttered Pecan	½ cup	180	12	—	—	3	16	—	80	65	130	—	—	400
Chocolate Swirl	½ cup	130	6	—	—	2	18	—	60	65	105	—	—	200
Dutch Chocolate Olde Fashioned Recipe	½ cup	130	6	—	—	2	16	—	80	65	140	—	—	200

FOOD	PORTION	CALORIES	FAT	SAT FAT	CHOL	PROTEIN	CARBO	FIBER	CALCIUM	SOD	POTAS	VIT C	FOLIC	VIT A
BORDEN (CONT.)														
Fat Free Black Cherry	½ cup	90	tr	tr	0	2	21	—	100	40	120	0	—	0
Fat Free Chocolate	½ cup	100	tr	tr	0	3	21	—	100	50	120	0	—	0
Fat Free Peach	½ cup	90	tr	tr	0	2	21	—	100	40	120	0	—	0
Fat Free Strawberry	½ cup	90	tr	tr	0	2	21	—	100	40	120	0	—	0
Fat Free Vanilla	½ cup	90	tr	tr	0	3	20	—	100	50	130	0	—	0
Ice Milk Chocolate	½ cup	100	2	—	—	3	18	—	100	80	160	—	—	200
Ice Milk Strawberry	½ cup	90	2	—	—	2	17	—	80	65	130	—	—	—
Ice Milk Vanilla	½ cup	90	2	—	—	2	17	—	100	65	130	—	—	—
Strawberries 'N Cream Olde Fashioned Recipe	½ cup	130	5	—	—	2	19	—	60	55	85	—	—	200
Strawberry	½ cup	130	6	—	—	2	18	—	80	55	105	—	—	200
Sundae Cone	1	210	12	—	—	3	23	—	60	110	—	—	—	200
Vanilla Olde Fashioned Recipe	½ cup	130	7	—	—	2	15	—	80	55	105	—	—	300
BOUNTY														
Cherry/Dark	1 (0.84 fl oz)	70	5	3	5	1	8	0	—	20	20	—	—	—
Coconut/Dark	1 (0.84 fl oz)	70	5	3	5	1	7	0	—	20	20	—	—	—
Coconut/Milk	1 (0.84 fl oz)	70	5	3	5	1	7	0	20	20	20	—	—	—
BREYERS														
Butter Pecan	½ cup (2.4 oz)	180	12	6	35	3	14	0	80	115	—	0	—	300
Caramel Praline Crunch	½ cup (2.6 oz)	180	9	5	30	3	22	0	80	30	—	0	—	300
Cherry Vanilla	½ cup (2.4 oz)	150	8	5	30	3	17	0	80	30	—	0	—	300
Chocolate	½ cup (2.4 oz)	160	9	6	30	2	18	tr	60	20	—	0	—	300
Chocolate Chip	½ cup (2.4 oz)	170	10	7	35	3	17	0	80	35	—	0	—	300
Chocolate Chip Cookie Dough	½ cup (2.5 oz)	180	10	6	35	3	20	0	80	50	—	0	—	400
Chocolate Rainbow	½ cup (2.4 oz)	120	10	6	25	3	16	0	100	40	—	0	—	300
Coffee	½ cup (2.4 oz)	150	9	6	35	3	15	0	80	35	—	0	—	300
Cookies N Cream	½ cup (2.4 oz)	170	9	6	30	3	19	0	80	45	—	0	—	300
Creamsicle	½ cup (2.8 oz)	130	4	3	15	2	22	0	60	30	—	0	—	200
Double Chocolate Fudge	½ cup (2.6 oz)	150	9	6	40	2	23	tr	80	50	—	0	—	300
Fat Free Caramel Praline	½ cup (2.5 oz)	120	0	0	<5	3	25	0	100	90	—	0	—	300
Fat Free Chocolate	½ cup (2.4 oz)	90	0	0	0	3	19	tr	100	55	—	0	—	300
Fat Free Mint Cookies N Cream	½ cup (2.4 oz)	100	0	0	<5	3	21	0	100	75	—	0	—	300
Fat Free Strawberry	½ cup (2.4 oz)	90	0	0	0	3	19	0	100	50	—	6	—	300
Fat Free Take Two Vanilla Strawberry	½ cup (2.4 oz)	80	0	0	<5	3	19	0	100	55	—	4	—	300
Fat Free Vanilla	½ cup (2.4 oz)	90	0	0	0	3	19	tr	100	65	—	0	—	300

FOOD	PORTION	CALORIES	FAT	SAT FAT	CHOL	PROTEIN	CARBO	FIBER	CALCIUM	SOD	POTAS	VIT C	FOLIC	VIT A
BREYERS (CONT.)														
Fat Free Vanilla Chocolate Strawberry	½ cup (2.4 oz)	90	0	0	0	3	19	0	100	55	—	2	—	300
Fat Free Vanilla Fudge Twirl	½ cup (2.5 oz)	100	0	0	0	3	22	tr	100	65	—	0	—	300
French Vanilla	½ cup (2.4 oz)	160	10	6	105	4	15	0	80	40	—	0	—	400
Fruit Rainbow	½ cup (2.4 oz)	140	8	5	30	2	16	0	100	35	—	0	—	300
Hershey w/ Almonds	½ cup (2.7 oz)	190	8	5	25	3	23	tr	100	20	—	0	—	300
Light Butter Pecan	½ cup (2.3 oz)	120	4	1	<5	4	19	0	100	130	—	0	—	300
Light Caramel Praline Pecan	½ cup (3 oz)	180	5	3	15	4	30	0	150	90	—	0	—	300
Light French Chocolate	½ cup (2.4 oz)	150	5	3	30	4	22	tr	150	55	—	0	—	300
Light Mint Chocolate Chip	½ cup (2.4 oz)	140	5	3	10	3	21	0	150	50	—	1	—	300
Light Vanilla	½ cup (2.4 oz)	130	5	3	35	3	18	0	100	45	—	0	—	300
Light Vanilla Chocolate Strawberry	½ cup (2.4 oz)	120	3	2	10	4	19	0	150	50	—	1	—	300
Light Low Fat Brown Marble Fudge	½ cup (2.6 oz)	130	2	1	5	4	26	tr	100	65	—	0	—	300
Light Low Fat French Vanilla	½ cup (2.3 oz)	110	2	1	30	3	20	0	100	45	—	0	—	400
Light Low Fat Swiss Almond Fudge	½ cup (2.5 oz)	130	3	2	5	4	24	tr	100	60	—	0	—	300
Low Fat Butter Pecan	½ cup (2.6 oz)	150	7	2	15	3	21	0	80	125	—	0	—	100
Low Fat Vanilla	½ cup (2.6 oz)	120	3	2	15	3	22	0	80	40	—	0	—	100
Low Fat Vanilla Chocolate Strawberry	½ cup (2.6 oz)	120	3	2	10	3	22	0	60	40	—	4	—	100
Mint Chocolate Chip	½ cup (2.4 oz)	170	10	7	35	3	17	0	80	35	—	0	—	300
No Sugar Added Fudge Twirl	½ cup (2.6 oz)	100	5	3	25	3	14	0	100	55	—	0	—	300
No Sugar Added Mint Chocolate Chip	½ cup (2.4 oz)	100	5	4	25	3	12	0	100	50	—	0	—	300
No Sugar Added Vanilla	½ cup (2.4 oz)	90	5	3	25	3	11	0	100	50	—	0	—	300
No Sugar Added Vanilla Chocolate Strawberry	½ cup (2.4 oz)	90	5	3	25	3	11	0	100	45	—	0	—	300
Peach	½ cup (2.4 oz)	130	6	4	25	2	17	0	60	25	—	0	—	300
Peanut Butter Cup	½ cup (2.7 oz)	210	12	6	30	4	24	tr	80	90	—	0	—	300
Rocky Road	½ cup (2.5 oz)	180	9	5	25	2	24	tr	40	25	—	0	—	200

FOOD	PORTION	CALORIES	FAT	SAT FAT	CHOL	PROTEIN	CARBO	FIBER	CALCIUM	SOD	POTAS	VIT C	FOLIC	VIT A
BREYERS (CONT.)														
Soft'N Creamy Vanilla	½ cup (2.3 oz)	150	7	5	30	2	19	0	80	35	—	0	—	300
Soft'N Creamy Vanilla Chocolate Strawberry	½ cup (2.3 oz)	150	7	5	30	2	19	0	80	35	—	1	—	300
Strawberry	½ cup (2.4 oz)	130	7	5	30	2	15	0	60	30	—	12	—	300
Take Two Vanilla Chocolate	½ cup (2.5 oz)	160	9	6	35	3	17	0	80	35	—	0	—	300
Take Two Vanilla Orange Sherbet	½ cup (2.7 oz)	130	5	3	20	2	21	0	60	30	—	0	—	200
Vanilla	½ cup (2.4 oz)	150	9	6	35	3	15	0	80	35	—	0	—	300
Vanilla Chocolate Strawberry	½ cup (2.4 oz)	150	8	5	30	2	16	0	60	30	—	2	—	300
Vanilla Fudge Twirl	½ cup (2.6 oz)	160	8	5	35	3	19	tr	80	35	—	0	—	300
Viennetta Cappuccino	½ cup (2.4 oz)	190	11	7	35	3	19	0	80	35	—	0	—	400
Viennetta Chocolate	½ cup (2.4 oz)	190	12	8	25	3	18	0	100	40	—	0	—	300
Viennetta Vanilla	½ cup (2.4 oz)	190	11	7	40	3	19	0	100	40	—	0	—	300
BUTTERFINGER														
Bar	1 (2.5 oz)	170	12	7	15	2	14	0	60	40	—	0	—	100
Nuggets	8	340	24	13	20	3	29	0	100	65	—	0	—	0
CALIFORNIA JOE														
Soft Serve Chocolate	½ cup (2.5 oz)	72	0	0	0	5	11	1	150	60	—	0	—	600
Soft Serve Vanilla	½ cup (2.5 oz)	70	0	0	0	5	11	1	150	60	—	0	—	600
CARNATION														
Sundae Cup Strawberry	1 (3.3 oz)	200	8	5	30	2	29	0	40	55	—	2	—	200
COOL CREATIONS														
Cookies & Cream Sandwich	1 (3.5 oz)	240	11	4	15	2	34	1	60	250	—	0	—	400
Mini Sandwich	1 (2.3 oz)	110	5	2	10	1	16	0	20	70	—	0	—	100
DOVEBAR														
Almond	1 (3.67 fl oz)	335	22	12	35	5	30	0	100	75	150	—	—	400
Bite Size Almond Praline	1 (0.75 fl oz)	80	5	3	7	1	8	0	20	15	20	—	—	—
Bite Size Cherry Royale	1 (0.75 fl oz)	70	5	3	8	1	8	0	—	10	20	—	—	—
Bite Size Classic Vanilla	1 (0.75 fl oz)	70	5	3	8	1	7	0	—	10	20	—	—	—
Bite Size French Vanilla	1 (0.75 fl oz)	70	5	3	15	1	7	0	—	10	20	—	—	—
Bite Size Mint Supreme	1 (0.75 fl oz)	80	5	3	7	1	8	0	—	5	20	—	—	—
Caramel Pecan	1 (3.67 fl oz)	350	35	12	35	4	35	0	100	85	100	—	—	400

FOOD	PORTION	CALORIES	FAT	SAT FAT	CHOL	PROTEIN	CARBO	FIBER	CALCIUM	SOD	POTAS	VIT C	FOLIC	VIT A
DOVEBAR (CONT.)														
Chocolate Milk Chocolate	1 (3.8 fl oz)	340	21	13	40	4	35	0	100	80	100	—	—	400
Coffee Cashew	1 (3.67 fl oz)	335	22	13	35	4	31	0	80	55	100	—	—	400
Crunchy Cookie	1 (3.8 fl oz)	340	21	13	40	4	35	0	150	65	100	—	—	400
Peanut	1 (3.8 fl oz)	380	25	13	40	7	35	0	150	100	150	—	—	400
Single Vanilla/Dark	1 (2 fl oz)	200	12	7	20	2	24	0	60	50	60	—	—	200
Vanilla Dark Chocolate	1 (3.8 fl oz)	340	22	13	45	4	34	0	100	65	100	—	—	500
Vanilla Milk Chocolate	1 (3.8 fl oz)	340	21	13	40	4	34	0	150	60	100	—	—	400
DRUMSTICK														
Cone Chocolate	1 (4.6 oz)	340	19	10	25	6	37	2	100	95	—	0	—	200
Cone Chocolate Dipped	1 (4.6 oz)	340	17	10	25	5	41	1	100	95	—	0	—	200
Cone Vanilla	1 (4.6 oz)	350	20	11	20	6	36	2	100	95	—	0	—	200
Cone Vanilla Caramel	1 (4.6 oz)	360	20	12	25	6	39	6	100	100	—	0	—	200
Cone Vanilla Fudge	1 (4.6 oz)	370	21	11	20	6	40	2	100	105	—	0	—	200
EAGLE BRAND														
Vanilla	½ cup	150	9	—	—	3	16	—	100	55	150	—	—	300
EDY'S														
American Dream Chocolate	3 oz	90	1	—	0	2	20	—	—	45	—	—	—	—
American Dream Chocolate Chip	3 oz	100	1	—	0	2	22	—	—	45	—	—	—	—
American Dream Cookies'N'Cream	3 oz	100	1	—	0	2	22	—	—	45	—	—	—	—
American Dream Mocha Almond Fudge	3 oz	110	1	—	0	3	24	—	—	45	—	—	—	—
American Dream Rocky Road	3 oz	110	1	—	0	3	24	—	—	45	—	—	—	—
American Dream Strawberry	3 oz	70	tr	—	0	2	16	—	—	40	—	—	—	—
American Dream Toasted Almond	3 oz	110	1	—	0	3	24	—	—	45	—	—	—	—
American Dream Vanilla	3 oz	80	tr	—	0	2	18	—	—	45	—	—	—	—
American Dream Vanilla Chocolate Strawberry	3 oz	80	1	—	0	2	18	—	—	45	—	—	—	—
Light Almond Praline	4 oz	140	5	2-3	15	5	18	—	—	50	—	—	—	—
Light Banana-Politan	4 oz	110	4	2-3	15	3	15	—	—	50	—	—	—	—
Light Butter Pecan	4 oz	140	5	2-3	15	5	18	—	—	50	—	—	—	—
Light Cafe Au Lait	4 oz	110	4	2-3	15	3	13	—	—	50	—	—	—	—

FOOD	PORTION	CALORIES	FAT	SAT FAT	CHOL	PROTEIN	CARBO	FIBER	CALCIUM	SOD	POTAS	VIT C	FOLIC	VIT A
EDY'S (CONT.)														
Light Candy Bar	4 oz	140	5	2-3	15	4	20	—	—	50	—	—	—	—
Light Chocolate Chip	4 oz	120	4	2-3	15	4	16	—	—	50	—	—	—	—
Light Chocolate Fudge Mousse	4 oz	130	5	2-3	15	4	18	—	—	50	—	—	—	—
Light Cookies 'N' Cream	4 oz	120	5	2-3	15	3	18	—	—	50	—	—	—	—
Light Dreamy Caramel Cream	4 oz	140	4	2-3	15	4	16	—	—	50	—	—	—	—
Light Malt Ball 'N' Fudge	4 oz	140	5	2-3	15	4	20	—	—	50	—	—	—	—
Light Marble Fudge	4 oz	120	4	2-3	15	5	15	—	—	50	—	—	—	—
Light Mocha Almond Fudge	4 oz	140	5	2-3	15	6	19	—	—	50	—	—	—	—
Light Peanut Butter & Chocolate	4 oz	130	5	2-3	15	6	19	—	—	50	—	—	—	—
Light Raspberry Truffle	4 oz	110	5	2-3	15	4	19	—	—	50	—	—	—	—
Light Rocky Road	4 oz	130	5	2-3	15	4	17	—	—	50	—	—	—	—
Light Strawberry	4 oz	110	4	2-3	15	3	15	—	—	50	—	—	—	—
Light Vanilla	4 oz	100	4	2-3	15	3	13	—	—	50	—	—	—	—
Vanilla Chocolate Strawberry	4 oz	110	4	2-3	15	4	14	—	—	50	—	—	—	—
FI-BAR														
Banana Cream	1 bar	93	tr	—	—	2	21	—	—	—	—	—	—	—
Cocoa-Fudge 'N Cream	1 bar	93	tr	—	—	2	21	—	—	—	—	—	—	—
Raspberries 'N Cream	1 bar	93	tr	—	—	2	21	—	—	—	—	—	—	—
Wildberry Cream	1 bar	93	tr	—	—	2	21	—	—	—	—	—	—	—
FLINTSTONES														
Cool Cream	1 (2.75 oz)	90	2	1	5	1	18	0	40	30	—	30	—	0
Push-Up	1 (2.75 oz)	100	2	1	5	1	20	0	40	25	—	30	—	0
FRIENDLY'S														
Black Raspberry	½ cup	150	7	5	30	2	17	0	—	35	—	—	—	—
Chocolate Almond Chip	½ cup	170	10	6	35	3	18	0	—	45	—	—	—	—
Forbidden Chocolate	½ cup	150	9	5	30	3	14	0	—	40	—	—	—	—
Fudge Nut Brownie	½ cup	200	11	7	25	3	23	0	—	60	—	—	—	—
Heath English Toffee	½ cup (2.7 oz)	190	10	6	30	3	24	0	60	240	—	0	—	300
Purely Pistachio	½ cup	160	10	6	35	3	16	0	—	50	—	—	—	—
Vanilla	½ cup	150	8	5	35	2	16	0	—	40	—	—	—	—
Vanilla Chocolate Strawberry	½ cup	150	8	5	30	2	16	tr	—	35	—	—	—	—

FOOD	PORTION	CALORIES	FAT	SAT FAT	CHOL	PROTEIN	CARBO	FIBER	CALCIUM	SOD	POTAS	VIT C	FOLIC	VIT A
FRIENDLY'S (CONT.)														
Vienna Mocha Chunk	½ cup	180	11	7	30	3	19	0	—	50	—	—	—	—
FRUSEN GLADJE														
Butter Pecan	½ cup	280	21	9	60	5	16	—	150	160	220	—	—	500
Chocolate	½ cup	240	17	9	75	5	17	—	150	65	230	—	—	500
GOOD HUMOR														
Banana Bob	1 (3 fl oz)	155	7	6	5	2	22	0	80	55	—	0	—	0
Bar Classic Toasted Almond	1 (3.1 fl oz)	170	9	4	10	2	22	1	60	40	—	0	—	500
Bar Classic Vanilla	1 (3.1 fl oz)	190	10	8	15	2	22	0	80	35	—	0	—	200
Bar Classic Almond	1 (3.1 fl oz)	210	12	8	15	2	21	1	100	50	—	0	—	200
Bar Sidewalk Sundae	1	280	20	17	15	4	21	2	80	65	—	0	—	100
Bubble O'Bill	1 (3.6 fl oz)	170	10	8	15	2	20	1	100	45	—	0	—	200
Bubble Play	1	110	1	1	—	0	25	—	80	5	—	—	—	—
Chip Burrrger	1 (4.7 oz)	320	15	9	20	4	44	1	60	190	—	0	—	200
Chip Sandwich	1 (4.7 fl oz)	320	15	9	20	4	44	1	60	190	—	0	—	200
Choco Taco	1 (4.4 fl oz)	320	17	11	20	3	38	1	60	100	—	0	—	200
Chocolate Eclair Classic	1 (3.1 fl oz)	170	9	3	10	2	21	1	40	60	—	0	—	300
Classic Candy Center Crunch Vanilla	1	280	21	17	15	2	21	0	0	75	—	0	—	200
Colonel Crunch Chocolate	1 (3.1 oz)	160	7	4	10	2	21	1	40	60	—	0	—	100
Colonel Crunch Strawberry	1 (3.1 oz)	170	8	6	10	1	22	0	40	45	—	0	—	100
Combo Cup	1 (6.2 fl oz)	200	10	7	35	3	25	1	100	65	—	0	—	400
Cone Olde Nut Sundae	1 (3.9 oz)	230	9	6	5	4	32	2	80	100	—	0	—	0
Cone Sidewalk Sundae	1 (4.2 oz)	270	14	11	10	4	31	1	60	125	—	0	—	200
Creamee Burrrger	1 (4.7 oz)	310	17	12	20	0	40	1	80	150	—	0	—	200
Crunch Classic Candy Center	1 (3.1 fl oz)	260	19	14	10	2	21	1	60	60	—	0	—	100
Dinosaur Bar	1	110	2	1	—	0	25	—	80	5	—	—	—	—
Far Frog	1 (3.6 fl oz)	150	8	7	20	1	19	1	60	45	—	0	—	200
Fun Box Ice Cream Sandwich	1 (3.1 fl oz)	160	5	3	10	3	27	1	40	140	—	0	—	200
King Cone	1 (5.7 fl oz)	300	14	11	25	5	38	2	120	110	—	0	—	400
King Cone Classic Vanilla	1 (4.8 oz)	300	10	6	20	4	48	1	80	110	—	0	—	300
King Cone Strawberry	1 (5.7 oz)	250	10	7	25	3	38	1	100	105	—	4	—	300
Light Chocolate Chocolate Chip	½ cup (2.4 oz)	130	4	3	10	3	20	tr	100	40	—	0	—	200

FOOD	PORTION	CALORIES	FAT	SAT FAT	CHOL	PROTEIN	CARBO	FIBER	CALCIUM	SOD	POTAS	VIT C	FOLIC	VIT A
GOOD HUMOR (CONT.)														
Light Chocolate Chip	½ cup (2.4 oz)	130	4	3	10	3	20	0	100	45	—	0	—	200
Light Coffee	½ cup (2.4 oz)	110	3	2	15	3	18	0	100	45	—	0	—	200
Light Cookies N'Cream	½ cup (2.4 oz)	130	3	2	10	3	21	0	100	70	—	0	—	200
Light Heavenly Hash	½ cup (2.4 oz)	140	4	2	10	3	23	tr	80	45	—	0	—	200
Light Praline Almond Crunch	½ cup (2.4 oz)	130	3	2	15	3	20	0	100	65	—	0	—	200
Light Toffee Bar Crunch	½ cup (2.4 oz)	130	4	3	15	3	20	0	100	55	—	0	—	200
Light Vanilla	½ cup (2.4 oz)	110	3	2	15	3	19	0	100	50	—	0	—	200
Light Vanilla Chocolate Strawberry	½ cup (2.4 oz)	110	3	2	10	3	19	0	100	45	—	0	—	200
Light Vanilla Fudge	½ cup (2.6 oz)	120	3	2	15	2	21	0	100	50	—	0	—	200
Magmun Almond	1 (4.2 fl oz)	270	12	7	30	5	35	5	150	50	—	5	—	400
Magnum Chocolate	1 (4.2 fl oz)	260	12	8	30	1	38	2	100	60	—	0	—	400
Number One Bar	1 (4.1 fl oz)	190	11	9	15	2	22	1	60	45	—	0	—	200
Popsicle Ice Cream Bar	1 (3.1 fl oz)	160	11	9	15	2	15	1	60	35	—	0	—	200
Popsicle Ice Cream Sandwich	1 (3.6 fl oz)	190	8	4	15	3	28	1	60	120	—	0	—	200
Sandwich Classic Chip Cookie	1 (4.1 fl oz)	300	13	8	18	3	43	1	60	215	—	0	—	300
Sandwich Giant Neapolitan	1 (5.2 fl oz)	260	10	7	20	3	39	1	80	150	—	0	—	300
Sandwich Giant Vanilla	1 (5.2 fl oz)	240	10	6	20	4	35	1	80	160	—	0	—	200
Sandwich Ice Cream	1	190	8	4	15	3	28	1	60	120	—	0	—	200
Sandwich Sidewalk Sundae	1 (3.1 oz)	160	5	3	10	3	27	1	40	140	—	0	—	200
Sandwich Sprinkle	1 (3.1 fl oz)	180	6	4	10	2	28	1	40	65	—	0	—	200
Strawberry Shortcake Bar Classic	1 (3.1 fl oz)	160	8	4	10	1	20	1	40	60	—	0	—	100
Sundae Twist Cup	1	160	3	2	10	2	33	0	150	100	—	0	—	0
Toffee Taco	1 (4.4 fl oz)	300	16	10	15	3	35	1	60	120	—	0	—	200
WWF Bar	1 (3.7 fl oz)	200	10	8	15	2	24	1	60	100	—	0	—	300
X-Men Bar	1 (3 fl oz)	150	6	3	15	2	23	0	40	90	—	0	—	200
HAAGEN-DAZS														
Baileys Original Irish Cream	½ cup (3.6 oz)	280	18	11	110	4	23	0	150	100	—	0	—	500
Brownies A La Mode	½ cup (3.7 oz)	280	18	11	100	5	25	0	100	130	—	0	—	400
Butter Pecan	½ cup (3.7 oz)	320	24	11	105	5	20	tr	150	140	—	0	—	500

FOOD	PORTION	CALORIES	FAT	SAT FAT	CHOL	PROTEIN	CARBO	FIBER	CALCIUM	SOD	POTAS	VIT C	FOLIC	VIT A
HAAGEN-DAZS (CONT.)														
Cappuccino Commotion	½ cup (3.6 oz)	310	21	12	100	5	25	1	150	105	—	0	—	500
Caramel Cone Explosion	½ cup (3.6 oz)	310	20	12	95	5	27	tr	100	130	—	0	—	500
Chocolate	½ cup (3.7 oz)	270	18	11	115	5	22	1	150	75	—	0	—	500
Chocolate Chocolate Chip	½ cup (3.7 oz)	300	20	12	100	5	26	2	100	70	—	0	—	500
Coffee	½ cup (3.7 oz)	270	18	11	120	5	21	0	150	85	—	0	—	500
Cookie Dough Dynamo	½ cup (3.6 oz)	300	19	12	95	4	29	0	100	140	—	0	—	500
Cookies & Cream	½ cup (3.6 oz)	270	17	11	110	5	23	0	150	115	—	0	—	500
DiSaronno Amaretto	½ cup (3.6 oz)	260	15	9	95	4	26	0	100	80	—	0	—	500
Macadamia Brittle	½ cup (3.7 oz)	300	20	11	110	4	25	0	150	120	—	0	—	500
Multi Pack Bars Caramel Cone Explosion	1 (3.1 oz)	330	22	13	60	4	30	tr	100	150	—	0	—	300
Multi Pack Bars Chocolate & Dark Chocolate	1 (3.2 oz)	320	22	15	70	4	27	3	100	70	—	0	—	300
Multi Pack Bars Coffee & Almond Crunch	1 (3 oz)	290	21	12	80	4	22	tr	100	70	—	0	—	400
Multi Pack Bars Iced Cappuccino Explosion	1 (2.9 oz)	290	21	12	70	4	21	tr	100	60	—	0	—	400
Multi Pack Bars Triple Brownie Overload	1 (3 oz)	320	23	12	80	4	23	1	100	95	—	0	—	300
Multi Pack Bars Vanilla & Almonds	1 (3 oz)	300	22	12	70	5	21	1	150	65	—	0	—	400
Multi Pack Bars Vanilla & Dark Chocolate	1 (3.2 oz)	320	22	15	70	5	27	4	100	50	—	0	—	400
Multi Pack Bars Vanilla & Milk Chocolate	1 (3 oz)	280	20	12	75	4	20	0	100	65	—	0	—	400
Peanut Butter Burst	½ cup (3.6 oz)	330	22	11	95	6	26	1	100	150	—	0	—	500
Rum Raisin	½ cup (3.7 oz)	270	17	10	110	4	22	0	100	75	—	0	—	500
Single Pack Bars Caramel Cone Explosion	1 (3.3 oz)	350	23	14	65	4	32	tr	100	160	—	0	—	400
Single Pack Bars Chocolate & Dark Chocolate	1 (3.9 oz)	400	27	18	85	5	33	4	100	90	—	0	—	400
Single Pack Bars Coffee & Almond Crunch	1 (3.7 oz)	360	26	15	100	5	27	1	150	85	—	0	—	500

FOOD	PORTION	CALORIES	FAT	SAT FAT	CHOL	PROTEIN	CARBO	FIBER	CALCIUM	SOD	POTAS	VIT C	FOLIC	VIT A
HAAGEN-DAZS (CONT.)														
Single Pack Bars Cookie Dough Dynamo	1 (3.5 oz)	380	25	14	65	4	34	1	100	125	—	0	—	400
Single Pack Bars Iced Cappuccino	1 (3.4 oz)	330	24	14	80	5	24	tr	150	70	—	0	—	400
Single Pack Bars Triple Brownie Overload	1 (3.5 oz)	380	27	14	95	5	28	1	100	110	—	0	—	500
Single Pack Bars Vanilla & Almonds	1 (3.7 oz)	370	27	14	90	6	26	1	150	80	—	0	—	500
Single Pack Bars Vanilla & Dark Chocolate	1 (3.9 oz)	400	27	18	85	5	33	4	100	65	—	0	—	500
Single Pack Bars Vanilla & Milk Chocolate	1 (3.5 oz)	330	25	14	90	5	24	tr	150	75	—	0	—	500
Strawberry	½ cup (3.7 oz)	250	16	10	95	4	23	tr	150	80	—	9	—	500
Strawberry Cheesecake Craze	½ cup (3.7 oz)	290	18	10	100	4	28	tr	100	160	—	2	—	500
Triple Brownie Overload	½ cup (3.5 oz)	300	20	11	90	5	26	0	100	100	—	0	—	500
Vanilla	½ cup (3.7 oz)	270	18	11	120	5	21	0	150	85	—	0	—	500
Vanilla Fudge	½ cup (3.7 oz)	280	18	11	105	5	25	0	150	105	—	0	—	500
Vanilla Swiss Almond	½ cup (3.7 oz)	310	21	11	105	6	23	1	150	80	—	0	—	500
HEALTHY CHOICE														
Black Forest	½ cup (2.5 oz)	120	2	1	5	3	23	1	80	50	—	0	—	200
Bordeaux Cherry Chocolate Chip	½ cup (2.5 oz)	110	2	2	<5	3	19	tr	100	55	—	0	—	200
Butter Pecan Crunch	½ cup (2.5 oz)	120	2	1	<5	3	22	1	100	60	—	0	—	200
Cappuccino Chocolate Chunk	½ cup (2.5 oz)	120	2	1	10	3	32	1	80	60	—	0	—	200
Cookies 'N Cream	½ cup (2.5 oz)	120	2	2	<5	3	21	tr	100	90	—	0	—	200
Double Fudge Swirl	½ cup (2.5 oz)	120	2	2	<5	3	21	1	100	50	—	0	—	200
Fudge Brownie	½ cup (2.5 oz)	120	2	1	5	3	22	2	80	55	—	0	—	200
Malt Caramel Cone	½ cup (2.5 oz)	120	2	1	10	3	22	1	80	60	—	0	—	200
Mint Chocolate Chip	½ cup (2.5 oz)	120	2	1	<5	3	21	tr	100	50	—	0	—	200
Peanut Butter Cookie Dough 'N Fudge	½ cup (2.5 oz)	120	2	1	<5	3	22	tr	100	60	—	0	—	200
Praline & Caramel	½ cup (2.5 oz)	130	2	1	<5	3	25	tr	100	70	—	0	—	200
Rocky Road	½ cup (2.5 oz)	140	2	1	<5	3	28	2	100	60	—	0	—	200
Vanilla	½ cup	100	2	2	5	3	18	1	100	50	—	2	—	300
HEATH														
Bar	1 (2.5 oz)	160	12	8	15	1	13	0	40	35	—	0	—	100

FOOD	PORTION	CALORIES	FAT	SAT FAT	CHOL	PROTEIN	CARBO	FIBER	CALCIUM	SOD	POTAS	VIT C	FOLIC	VIT A
HEATH (CONT.)														
Nuggets	8	180	11	7	25	2	18	0	80	45	—	0	—	0
HOOD														
Bar Orange Cream	1 bar (1.8 oz)	90	2	1	5	1	18	0	40	30	—	0	—	0
Bar Vanilla	1 bar (1.6 oz)	160	12	9	15	1	11	0	40	45	—	0	—	100
Caramel Butterscotch Blast	½ cup (2.3 oz)	160	8	5	25	2	20	0	60	70	—	0	—	200
Chocolate	½ cup (2.3 oz)	140	7	5	30	2	17	0	60	40	—	0	—	200
Chocolate Chip	½ cup (2.3 oz)	160	9	6	30	2	18	0	60	55	—	0	—	200
Chocolate Eclair	1 bar (1.6 oz)	150	10	3	5	1	14	0	20	45	—	0	—	0
Christmas Tree	½ cup (2.3 oz)	140	7	5	30	2	18	0	60	45	—	0	—	300
Coffee	½ cup (2.3 oz)	140	7	5	30	2	16	0	60	50	—	0	—	300
Cookie Dough Delight	½ cup (2.3 oz)	160	8	5	30	2	21	0	60	70	—	2	—	200
Cookies N Cream	½ cup (2.3 oz)	160	8	5	30	2	19	0	60	75	—	0	—	200
Cooler Cups	1 (2.1 oz)	80	1	1	<5	tr	18	0	20	25	—	0	—	0
Crispy Bar	1 (1.9 oz)	180	13	10	20	2	15	0	40	40	—	0	—	200
Egg Nog	½ cup (2.3 oz)	130	6	4	25	2	17	0	60	45	—	0	—	200
Fabulous Fudge & Peanut Butter Swirled Fudge Bars	1 bar (2.1 oz)	110	4	2	10	1	17	0	40	45	—	0	—	0
Fabulous Fudgies Assorted Bars	1 bar (2.1 oz)	100	3	2	10	1	19	0	40	50	—	0	—	0
Fat Free Chocolate Passion	½ cup (2.5 oz)	100	0	0	0	3	23	0	100	50	—	0	—	0
Fat Free Classic Harlequin	½ cup (2.5 oz)	100	0	0	0	2	23	0	80	50	—	0	—	0
Fat Free Double Brownie Sundae	½ cup (2.5 oz)	120	0	0	0	2	27	0	80	60	—	0	—	0
Fat Free Heavenly Hash	½ cup (2.5 oz)	120	0	0	0	2	27	0	80	75	—	0	—	0
Fat Free Mississippi Mud Pie	½ cup (2.5 oz)	130	0	0	0	3	29	0	80	75	—	0	—	0
Fat Free Praline Pecan Delight	½ cup (2.5 oz)	120	0	0	0	2	27	0	80	55	—	0	—	0
Fat Free Raspberry Blush	½ cup (2.5 oz)	120	0	0	0	2	26	0	80	55	—	0	—	0
Fat Free Super Strawberry Swirl	½ cup (2.5 oz)	100	0	0	0	2	23	0	80	40	—	1	—	0
Fat Free Vanilla Fudge Twist	½ cup (2.5 oz)	120	0	0	0	2	26	0	80	50	—	0	—	0
Fat Free Very Vanilla	½ cup (2.5 oz)	100	0	0	0	2	23	0	100	50	—	0	—	0
Fudge Bars	1 bar (2.7 oz)	100	1	0	0	2	21	0	100	80	—	0	—	0
Grasshopper Pie	½ cup (2.3 oz)	160	7	4	25	2	22	0	60	70	—	2	—	200
Heavenly Hash	½ cup (2.3 oz)	140	6	4	20	2	21	0	60	55	—	0	—	200

FOOD	PORTION	CALORIES	FAT	SAT FAT	CHOL	PROTEIN	CARBO	FIBER	CALCIUM	SOD	POTAS	VIT C	FOLIC	VIT A
HOOD (CONT.)														
Hendrie's Cherry Chocolate Dips	1 bar (1.3 oz)	120	9	7	15	1	11	0	40	30	—	0	—	100
Hoodsie Cup Vanilla & Chocolate	1 (1.7 oz)	100	5	4	20	2	12	0	40	35	—	0	—	200
Light Almond Praline Delight	½ cup (2.4 oz)	110	5	3	15	3	23	0	80	75	—	0	—	200
Light Brownie Nut Sundae	½ cup (2.4 oz)	140	5	3	10	3	22	0	80	55	—	0	—	200
Light Caribbean Coffee Royale	½ cup (2.4 oz)	110	4	2	15	2	18	0	100	50	—	0	—	200
Light Chocolate Almond Chip Sundae	½ cup (2.4 oz)	140	5	3	10	3	22	0	80	60	—	0	—	200
Light Chocolate Chocolate Chip Cookie Dough	½ cup (2.4 oz)	140	5	3	15	3	21	0	80	70	—	0	—	200
Light Cookies N Cream	½ cup (2.4 oz)	130	4	3	15	2	21	0	100	70	—	0	—	200
Light Heath Toffee Chunk Swirl	½ cup (2.4 oz)	140	5	3	15	2	23	0	80	95	—	0	—	200
Light Heavenly Hash	½ cup (2.4 oz)	130	4	3	10	2	22	0	80	55	—	0	—	100
Light Maple Sugar Shack	⅓ cup (2.4 oz)	130	4	2	10	2	23	0	80	65	—	0	—	200
Light Massachusetts Mud Pie	½ cup (2.4 oz)	140	5	3	10	3	20	0	100	60	—	0	—	200
Light Raspberry Swirl	½ cup (2.4 oz)	120	3	2	10	2	22	0	80	55	—	0	—	200
Light Strawberry Supreme	½ cup (2.4 oz)	110	3	2	15	2	19	0	100	45	—	2	—	200
Light Triple Nut Cluster Sundae	½ cup (2.4 oz)	140	5	2	10	3	22	0	80	50	—	0	—	200
Light Vanilla	½ cup (2.4 oz)	110	4	3	15	2	18	0	100	50	—	2	—	200
Light Vanilla Chocolate Strawberry	½ cup (2.4 oz)	110	4	2	15	2	18	0	100	45	—	0	—	200
Low Fat No Sugar Added Caramel Swirl	½ cup (2.4 oz)	120	3	2	10	3	18	0	100	80	—	0	—	200
Low Fat No Sugar Added Chocolate Supreme	½ cup (2.4 oz)	120	3	2	10	4	19	0	100	60	—	0	—	200
Low Fat No Sugar Added Mocha Fudge	½ cup (2.4 oz)	110	3	2	10	3	18	0	100	45	—	0	—	200
Low Fat No Sugar Added Raspberry Swirl	½ cup (2.4 oz)	110	3	2	10	3	17	0	100	45	—	0	—	200

FOOD	PORTION	CALORIES	FAT	SAT FAT	CHOL	PROTEIN	CARBO	FIBER	CALCIUM	SOD	POTAS	VIT C	FOLIC	VIT A
HOOD (CONT.)														
Low Fat No Sugar Added Vanilla	½ cup (2.4 oz)	100	3	2	10	3	14	0	100	50	—	0	—	300
Maple Walnut	½ cup (2.3 oz)	160	9	5	30	3	16	0	60	45	—	0	—	300
Rockets	1 (2 oz)	120	5	4	20	1	18	1	60	50	—	0	—	200
Sandwich Light	1 (2.2 oz)	160	4	2	10	3	29	1	60	160	—	0	—	100
Sandwich Vanilla	1 (2.2 oz)	180	7	4	20	3	27	1	40	170	—	0	—	200
Sports Bar	1 (2.9 oz)	250	17	13	25	3	23	0	80	55	—	0	—	200
Spumoni	½ cup (2.3 oz)	140	9	5	30	2	17	0	60	45	—	0	—	200
Strawberry	½ cup (2.3 oz)	130	7	5	30	2	16	0	60	45	—	0	—	200
Super Sortment Chocolate & Banana Fudge Bar	1 bar (2.1 oz)	100	3	2	10	1	18	0	40	30	—	0	—	0
Super Sortment Root Beer Float & Orange Cream Bar	1 bar (1.5 oz)	70	3	2	10	1	12	0	20	25	—	0	—	0
Vanilla	½ cup (2.3 oz)	140	7	5	30	2	16	0	60	50	—	0	—	300
Vanilla Chocolate Patchwork	½ cup (2.3 oz)	140	7	5	30	2	17	0	60	45	—	0	—	300
Vanilla Chocolate Strawberry	½ cup (2.3 oz)	140	7	5	30	2	16	0	60	45	—	0	—	300
Vanilla Fudge	½ cup (2.3 oz)	140	6	4	25	2	20	0	60	55	—	0	—	200
KLONDIKE														
Almond Bar	1 (5.2 fl oz)	310	21	14	25	3	26	3	150	90	—	0	—	400
Caramel Crunch	1 (5.2 fl oz)	300	18	13	30	3	31	tr	150	95	—	0	—	500
Chocolate Chocolate Bar	1 (5.2 fl oz)	280	20	14	20	3	22	tr	80	60	—	0	—	400
Coffee Bar	1 (5.2 fl oz)	290	20	14	15	3	25	0	100	65	—	0	—	400
Dark Chocolate Bar	1 (5.2 fl oz)	290	20	14	30	3	24	tr	120	75	—	0	—	400
Gold Bar	1 (5.2 fl oz)	340	23	12	34	5	30	1	130	60	—	0	—	600
Krispy Bar	1 (5.2 fl oz)	300	20	13	25	3	28	0	100	85	—	0	—	400
Krunch	1 (3.1 fl oz)	200	13	9	20	3	17	1	80	160	—	0	—	250
Lite Bar	1 (2.3 fl oz)	110	6	4	5	3	14	1	100	55	—	0	—	0
Lite Bar Caramel	1 (2.4 fl oz)	120	6	5	5	3	18	1	80	65	—	0	—	0
Movie Bites Chocolate	8 pieces (4.6 fl oz)	340	26	3	25	3	22	1	80	50	—	0	—	200
Movie Bites Vanilla	8 pieces (4.6 fl oz)	320	22	18	25	3	27	1	120	60	—	0	—	300
Original Bar	1 (5.2 fl oz)	290	20	14	15	3	24	0	100	65	—	0	—	300
Sandwich Chocolate	1 (5.2 fl oz)	270	10	6	20	4	41	2	100	200	—	0	—	400
Sandwich Lite	1 (2.9 fl oz)	100	2	2	5	3	18	1	40	105	—	0	—	0
Sandwich Vanilla	1 (5.2 fl oz)	250	9	6	20	4	37	1	100	230	—	0	—	400
MARS														
Almond Bar	1 (1.85 fl oz)	210	14	6	15	4	20	0	80	45	100	—	—	200
MEADOW GOLD														
Sundae Cone	1	210	12	—	—	3	23	—	60	110	—	—	—	200

FOOD	PORTION	CALORIES	FAT	SAT FAT	CHOL	PROTEIN	CARBO	FIBER	CALCIUM	SOD	POTAS	VIT C	FOLIC	VIT A
MILKY WAY														
Single Chocolate/ Milk	1 (2 fl oz)	210	11	7	20	3	24	0	80	60	80	—	—	200
Snack Chocolate/ Milk	1 (0.72 fl oz)	70	4	3	5	1	9	0	20	25	20	—	—	—
Snack Vanilla/Dark	1 (0.72 fl oz)	70	4	3	5	1	9	0	20	25	20	—	—	—
MOCHA MIX														
Berry Berry Berry	½ cup	140	6	2	0	tr	20	0	0	60	—	1	—	0
Dutch Chocolate	½ cup (2.3 oz)	140	8	2	0	1	16	0	0	80	—	0	—	0
Mocha Almond Fudge	½ cup (2.3 oz)	150	8	2	0	1	19	0	0	65	—	0	—	0
Neapolitan	½ cup (2.3 oz)	140	7	2	0	1	18	0	0	70	—	0	—	0
Strawberry Swirl	½ cup (2.3 oz)	140	6	2	0	tr	20	0	0	55	—	0	—	0
Vanilla	½ cup (2.3 oz)	140	7	2	0	1	18	0	0	70	—	0	—	0
NESTLE CRUNCH														
Chocolate	1 bar (3 oz)	200	14	9	15	2	18	0	60	40	—	0	—	100
Cones	1 (4.6 oz)	300	16	10	25	4	36	2	100	95	—	0	—	200
Crunch King	1 (4 oz)	270	19	14	20	3	21	0	80	45	—	0	—	0
Nuggets	8 pieces	140	9	5	10	2	12	0	120	30	—	0	—	0
Reduced Fat	1 (2.5 oz)	130	7	5	5	3	14	0	40	40	—	0	—	0
Vanilla	1 bar (3 oz)	200	14	9	15	2	17	0	60	40	—	0	—	100
PERRY'S														
No Fat No Sugar Added Caramel	½ cup (2.8 oz)	90	0	0	0	4	25	1	150	90	—	1	—	500
No Fat No Sugar Added Chocolate	½ cup (2.6 oz)	80	0	0	0	5	21	2	150	80	—	1	—	500
No Fat No Sugar Added Peach	½ cup (2.9 oz)	90	0	0	0	3	24	tr	100	70	—	12	—	500
No Fat No Sugar Added Strawberry	½ cup (2.8 oz)	90	0	0	0	4	23	tr	150	75	—	1	—	500
No Fat No Sugar Added Vanilla	½ cup (2.6 oz)	80	0	0	0	4	21	tr	150	80	—	1	—	500
RICE DREAM														
Bar Chocolate	1	270	16	—	0	1	33	—	—	115	—	—	—	—
Bar Chocolate Nutty	1	330	23	—	0	5	29	—	—	110	—	—	—	—
Bar Strawberry	1	260	15	—	0	1	31	—	—	110	—	—	—	—
Bar Vanilla	1	275	16	—	0	1	33	—	—	120	—	—	—	—
Bar Vanilla Nutty	1	330	23	—	0	5	29	—	—	100	—	—	—	—
Cappuccino	½ cup	130	5	—	0	1	17	—	—	80	—	—	—	—
Carob	½ cup	130	5	—	0	1	20	—	—	80	—	—	—	—
Carob Almond	½ cup	140	6	—	0	1	20	—	—	80	—	—	—	—
Carob Chip	½ cup	140	6	—	0	1	20	—	—	80	—	—	—	—
Carob Chip Mint	½ cup	140	6	—	0	1	20	—	—	80	—	—	—	—
Cocoa Marble Fudge	½ cup	140	6	—	0	1	19	—	—	80	—	—	—	—

FOOD	PORTION	CALORIES	FAT	SAT FAT	CHOL	PROTEIN	CARBO	FIBER	CALCIUM	SOD	POTAS	VIT C	FOLIC	VIT A
RICE DREAM (CONT.)														
Dream Pie Chocolate	1	380	19	—	0	3	47	—	—	225	—	—	—	—
Dream Pie Mint	1	380	19	—	0	3	47	—	—	225	—	—	—	—
Dream Pie Mocha	1	380	19	—	0	3	47	—	—	225	—	—	—	—
Dream Pie Vanilla	1	380	19	—	0	3	47	—	—	225	—	—	—	—
Lemon	½ cup	130	5	—	0	1	17	—	—	80	—	—	—	—
Peanut Butter Fudge	½ cup	160	7	—	0	3	19	—	—	100	—	—	—	—
Strawberry	½ cup	130	5	—	0	1	17	—	—	80	—	—	—	—
Vanilla	½ cup	130	5	—	0	1	17	—	—	80	—	—	—	—
Vanilla Fudge	½ cup	140	6	—	0	1	21	—	—	80	—	—	—	—
Vanilla Swiss Almond	½ cup	140	6	—	0	1	20	—	—	80	—	—	—	—
Wildberry	½ cup	130	5	—	0	1	17	—	—	80	—	—	—	—
SEALTEST														
American Glory	½ cup (2.4 oz)	130	6	4	25	2	17	0	80	45	—	1	—	200
Butter Pecan	½ cup (2.4 oz)	160	9	5	30	3	16	0	80	115	—	0	—	200
Candy Cane Crunch	½ cup (2.4 oz)	150	6	4	25	2	21	0	60	50	—	0	—	200
Chocolate	½ cup (2.4 oz)	140	7	4	25	3	19	tr	80	50	—	0	—	200
Chocolate Butter Pecan	½ cup (2.4 oz)	150	8	5	30	3	17	0	80	85	—	0	—	200
Chocolate Chip	½ cup (2.4 oz)	150	8	5	30	3	18	0	80	50	—	0	—	200
Coconut Chocolate	½ cup (2.4 oz)	160	8	6	25	3	18	tr	80	55	—	0	—	200
Coffee	½ cup (2.4 oz)	140	7	4	30	2	16	0	80	55	—	0	—	200
Cupid's Scoops	½ cup (2.5 oz)	140	6	4	25	2	20	0	80	55	—	0	—	200
Dessert Bar Free Chocolate Fudge	1	90	0	0	0	3	19	—	60	30	170	—	—	—
Dessert Bar Free Vanilla Strawberry Swirl	1	80	0	0	0	2	17	—	60	40	100	—	—	—
Dessert Bar Free Vanilla Fudge	1	80	0	0	0	3	18	—	80	30	120	—	—	—
Free Black Cherry	½ cup	100	0	0	0	2	25	—	100	45	125	—	—	200
Free Chocolate	½ cup	100	0	0	0	3	23	—	100	50	190	—	—	200
Free Peach	½ cup	100	0	0	0	2	23	—	80	45	115	—	—	200
Free Strawberry	½ cup	100	0	0	0	2	23	—	80	40	170	—	—	200
Free Vanilla	½ cup	100	0	0	0	3	24	—	100	45	130	—	—	200
Free Vanilla Fudge Royale	½ cup	100	0	0	0	3	24	—	100	50	140	—	—	200
Free Vanilla Strawberry Royale	½ cup	100	0	0	0	3	25	—	80	35	150	—	—	200
French Vanilla	½ cup (2.4 oz)	140	8	5	60	3	16	0	80	50	—	0	—	300
Fudge Royale	½ cup (2.5 oz)	150	7	4	25	3	19	0	80	55	—	0	—	200
Heavenly Hash	½ cup (2.4 oz)	150	7	4	25	3	20	tr	80	50	—	0	—	200
Maple Walnut	½ cup (2.4 oz)	160	9	5	30	3	16	0	80	50	—	0	—	200

FOOD	PORTION	CALORIES	FAT	SAT FAT	CHOL	PROTEIN	CARBO	FIBER	CALCIUM	SOD	POTAS	VIT C	FOLIC	VIT A
SEALTEST (CONT.)														
Strawberry	½ cup (2.4 oz)	130	6	4	25	2	19	0	60	45	—	1	—	200
Triple Chocolate Passion	½ cup (2.5 oz)	160	7	5	25	3	21	tr	80	50	—	0	—	200
Vanilla	½ cup (2.4 oz)	140	7	5	30	2	16	0	80	55	—	0	—	200
Vanilla Chocolate Strawberry	½ cup (2.4 oz)	140	6	4	25	2	18	0	80	50	—	0	—	200
Vanilla With Orange Sherbet	½ cup (2.7 oz)	130	4	3	20	2	22	0	60	45	—	0	—	200
SNICKERS														
Single	1 (2 fl oz)	220	13	6	15	4	22	0	80	65	100	—	—	200
Snack	1 (1 fl oz)	110	7	3	5	2	11	0	40	35	40	—	—	—
STARBUCKS														
Biscotti Bliss	½ cup	240	12	7	55	4	30	—	100	70	—	—	—	—
Caffe Almond Fudge	½ cup	260	13	7	55	5	30	—	100	80	—	—	—	—
Caffe Almond Roast	1 bar	280	18	9	3	4	26	—	60	45	—	—	—	—
Dark Roast Expresso Swirl	½ cup	220	10	6	55	4	29	—	100	60	—	—	—	—
Frappuccino	1 bar (2.8 oz)	110	2	1	10	4	20	0	100	45	—	0	—	200
Italian Roast Coffee	½ cup	230	12	7	65	5	26	—	100	50	—	—	—	—
Javachip	½ cup	250	13	8	60	4	29	—	100	55	—	—	—	—
Low Fat Latte	½ cup	170	3	2	10	5	31	—	100	65	—	—	—	—
Low Fat Mocha Mambo	½ cup	170	3	2	10	5	32	—	100	75	—	—	—	—
Vanilla Mochachip	½ cup	270	16	10	75	5	27	—	100	60	—	—	—	—
TOFU ICE CREME														
Carob	4 fl oz	190	8	—	0	2	28	—	—	55	—	—	—	—
Vanilla	4 fl oz	190	8	—	0	2	28	—	—	55	—	—	—	—
TOFUTTI														
Frutti Vanilla Apple Orchard	4 fl oz	100	0	0	0	2	20	—	—	90	—	—	—	—
TURKEY HILL														
Black Cherry	½ cup (2.3 oz)	140	7	5	25	2	18	0	80	30	—	0	—	300
Butter Pecan	½ cup (2.3 oz)	170	11	5	30	2	16	0	80	50	—	0	—	300
Choco Mint Chip	½ cup (2.3 oz)	160	10	6	30	2	17	0	80	45	—	0	—	300
Cookies 'N Cream	½ cup (2.3 oz)	160	9	5	30	2	19	0	80	60	—	0	—	300
Lite Butter Pecan	½ cup (2.3 oz)	130	6	3	15	3	17	0	100	80	—	0	—	300
Lite Choco Mint Chip	½ cup (2.3 oz)	140	5	4	15	3	19	0	100	75	—	0	—	300
Lite Cookies 'N Cream	½ cup (2.3 oz)	130	5	3	15	3	21	0	100	90	—	0	—	300
Lite Vanilla & Chocolate	½ cup (2.3 oz)	110	3	2	15	3	18	0	100	60	—	0	—	300
Lite Vanilla Bean	½ cup (2.3 oz)	110	3	2	15	3	18	0	100	65	—	0	—	300

FOOD	PORTION	CALORIES	FAT	SAT FAT	CHOL	PROTEIN	CARBO	FIBER	CALCIUM	SOD	POTAS	VIT C	FOLIC	VIT A
TURKEY HILL (CONT.)														
Neapolitan	½ cup (2.3 oz)	150	8	5	30	2	18	0	80	30	—	0	—	300
Rocky Road	½ cup (2.3 oz)	170	8	4	30	3	23	0	80	40	—	0	—	200
Tin Roof Sundae	½ cup (2.3 oz)	160	9	5	30	2	19	0	80	70	—	0	—	200
Vanilla	½ cup (2.3 oz)	140	8	5	30	2	16	0	80	35	—	0	—	300
Vanilla & Chocolate	½ cup (2.3 oz)	150	8	5	30	2	17	0	80	35	—	0	—	300
Vanilla Bean	½ cup (2.3 oz)	140	8	5	30	2	16	0	80	35	—	0	—	300
ULTRA SLIM-FAST														
Bar Fudge	1	90	tr	—	0	2	17	2	100	50	150	6	40	500
Bar Vanilla Cookie Crunch	1	90	4	—	0	3	14	1	100	70	90	6	40	500
Chocolate	4 oz	100	tr	—	0	5	19	2	150	45	150	9	60	750
Chocolate Fudge	4 oz	120	tr	—	0	5	24	2	150	65	155	9	60	750
Peach	4 oz	100	tr	—	0	4	22	2	150	55	170	9	60	750
Pralines & Caramel	4 oz	120	tr	—	0	4	25	2	150	95	160	9	60	750
Sandwich Vanilla	1	140	2	—	0	4	28	1	100	220	130	6	40	500
Sandwich Vanilla Chocolate	1	140	2	—	0	4	28	1	100	220	120	6	40	500
Sandwich Vanilla Oatmeal	1	150	3	—	0	4	26	3	100	160	110	6	40	500
Vanilla	4 oz	90	tr	—	0	5	19	2	150	55	180	9	60	750
Vanilla Fudge Cookie	4 oz	110	tr	—	0	5	24	2	150	90	160	9	60	750
WEIGHT WATCHERS														
Chocolate Dip	1 bar	100	6	3	5	2	11	0	80	15	—	0	—	100
Chocolate Mousse	1 bar	40	1	1	5	2	9	1	80	20	—	0	—	200
Chocolate Treat	1 bar	100	1	0	0	3	20	1	100	25	—	0	—	0
English Toffee Crunch	1 bar	110	6	3	5	2	12	1	80	30	—	0	—	200
Orange Vanilla Treat	1 bar	40	1	0	5	2	10	1	60	15	—	0	—	200
Vanilla Sandwich	1 bar	150	3	1	5	3	28	1	150	150	—	0	—	200
TAKE-OUT														
cone vanilla light soft serve	1 (4.6 oz)	164	6	4	28	4	24	—	153	92	169	1	5	211
gelato chocolate hazelnut	½ cup (5.3 oz)	370	29	4	92	9	26	2	179	49	352	1	35	76
gelato vanilla	½ cup (3 oz)	211	15	8	151	3	18	0	67	78	77	tr	15	191
sundae caramel	1 (5.4 oz)	303	9	5	25	7	49	—	189	195	318	3	12	263
sundae hot fudge	1 (5.4 oz)	284	9	5	21	6	48	—	207	182	395	2	9	221
sundae strawberry	1 (5.4 oz)	269	8	4	21	6	45	—	161	92	270	2	18	222

ICE CREAM CONES AND CUPS

FOOD	PORTION	CALORIES	FAT	SAT FAT	CHOL	PROTEIN	CARBO	FIBER	CALCIUM	SOD	POTAS	VIT C	FOLIC	VIT A
sugar cone	1	40	tr	tr	0	1	8	tr	4	32	14	0	1	0
wafer cone	1	17	tr	tr	0	tr	3	tr	1	6	4	0	0	0
COMET														
Cups	1 (5 g)	20	0	—	0	0	1	tr	—	20	0	—	—	—

FOOD	PORTION	CALORIES	FAT	SAT FAT	CHOL	PROTEIN	CARBO	FIBER	CALCIUM	SOD	POTAS	VIT C	FOLIC	VIT A
COMET (CONT.)														
Sugar Cones	1 (12 g)	50	0	—	0	tr	11	tr	—	40	15	—	—	—
Waffle Cone	1 (17 g)	70	1	0	0	1	14	1	—	30	10	—	—	—
DUTCH MILL														
Chocolate Covered Wafer Cups	1 (0.5 oz)	80	5	2	0	1	8	0	0	—	—	0	—	0
KEEBLER														
Sugar Cones	1	45	tr	tr	0	1	11	—	—	35	25	—	—	—
Vanilla Cups	1	15	tr	tr	0	tr	4	—	—	20	5	—	—	—
OREO														
Chocolate Cones	1 (13 g)	50	1	0	0	1	10	tr	—	110	60	—	—	—
TEDDY GRAHAMS														
Cinnamon Cones	1 (0.5 oz)	60	1	0	0	1	13	tr	—	55	30	—	—	—

ICE CREAM TOPPINGS

(*see also* SYRUP)

FOOD	PORTION	CALORIES	FAT	SAT FAT	CHOL	PROTEIN	CARBO	FIBER	CALCIUM	SOD	POTAS	VIT C	FOLIC	VIT A
butterscotch	2 tbsp (1.4 oz)	103	tr	tr	—	1	27	—	22	143		—	—	—
caramel	2 tbsp (1.4 oz)	103	tr	tr	—	1	27	—	22	143		—	—	—
marshmallow cream	1 oz	88	tr	—	0	1	23	—	1	13	1	—	0	0
marshmallow cream	1 jar (7 oz)	615	tr	—	0	3	157	—	6	90	9	—	2	2
pineapple	2 tbsp (1.5 oz)	106	0	—	0	tr	28	—	9	26	133	25	1	9
pineapple	1 cup (11.5 oz)	861	—	—	0	1	226	—	75	214	1078	199	9	72
strawberry	2 tbsp (1.5 oz)	107	tr	—	0	tr	28	—	10	9	31	11	1	9
strawberry	1 cup (11.5 oz)	863	1	—	0	1	225	—	81	73	248	85	5	61
walnuts in syrup	2 tbsp (1.4 oz)	167	9	1	0	2	22	—	—	—	—	—	—	—
BEN & JERRY'S														
Hot Fudge	(1.3 oz)	140	7	3	10	2	19	2	40	25	—	0	—	200
CRUMPY														
Chocolate Hazelnut Spread	1 tbsp (0.5 oz)	80	5	1	0	tr	8	0	0	5	—	0	—	0
HERSHEY														
Chocolate Shoppe Candy Bar Sprinkles York	2 tbsp (1.1 oz)	170	8	5	<5	2	22	2	0	0	—	0	—	0
KRAFT														
Butterscotch	2 tbsp (1.4 oz)	130	2	1	<5	tr	28	0	0	150	40	0	—	200
Caramel	2 tbsp (1.4 oz)	120	0	0	0	2	28	0	60	90	90	0	—	0
Chocolate	2 tbsp (1.4 oz)	110	0	0	0	2	26	1	20	30	190	0	—	0
Hot Fudge	2 tbsp (1.4 oz)	140	5	2	0	1	24	tr	40	100	85	0	—	0
Pineapple	2 tbsp (1.4 oz)	110	0	0	0	0	28	0	0	15	15	5	—	0
Strawberry	2 tbsp (1.4 oz)	110	0	0	0	0	29	0	0	15	25	4	—	0
MARZETTI														
Caramel Apple	2 tbsp	60	7	2	5	1	23	0	40	95	—	0	—	100

FOOD	PORTION	CALORIES	FAT	SAT FAT	CHOL	PROTEIN	CARBO	FIBER	CALCIUM	SOD	POTAS	VIT C	FOLIC	VIT A
MARZETTI (CONT.)														
Caramel Apple Reduced Fat	2 tbsp	30	3	2	5	1	26	0	40	100	—	0	—	100
Peanut Butter Caramel	2 tbsp	60	6	1	0	3	21	1	0	135	—	0	—	0
PLANTERS														
Nut	2 tbsp (0.5 oz)	100	9	1	0	3	3	1	—	0	100	—	—	—

ICED TEA

(*see also* TEA/HERBAL TEA)

FOOD	PORTION	CALORIES	FAT	SAT FAT	CHOL	PROTEIN	CARBO	FIBER	CALCIUM	SOD	POTAS	VIT C	FOLIC	VIT A
MIX														
instant artifically sweetened lemon flavored as prep w/ water	8 oz	5	0	0	0	tr	1	—	5	24	41	0	5	0
instant sweetened lemon flavor as prep w/ water	9 oz	87	tr	tr	0	tr	22	—	6	—	50	0	10	0
instant unsweetened lemon flavor as prep w/ water	8 oz	4	0	0	0	tr	0	—	5	14	49	0	—	0
4C														
Instant	8 oz	90	0	—	—	0	22	—	—	0	15	—	—	—
BIGELOW														
Nice Over Ice	5 fl oz	1	tr	—	0	tr	tr	—	11	1	58	—	—	—
CELESTIAL SEASONINGS														
Iced Delight	8 fl oz	4	tr	—	0	tr	1	—	—	14	31	—	—	—
CRYSTAL LIGHT														
Decaffeinated as prep	1 serv (8 oz)	5	0	0	0	0	tr	0	0	0	20	0	—	0
Iced Tea as prep	1 serv (8 oz)	5	0	0	0	0	0	0	0	0	15	0	—	0
Peach Tea as prep	1 serv (8 oz)	5	0	0	0	0	0	0	0	0	15	0	—	0
Raspberry Tea as prep	1 serv (8 oz)	5	0	0	0	0	0	0	0	0	15	0	—	0
LIPTON														
100% Tea Decaffeinated as prep	1 serv	0	0	0	0	0	0	—	—	0	—	0	—	—
100% Tea Unsweetened as prep	1 serv	0	0	0	0	0	0	—	—	0	—	0	—	—
100% Tea as prep	1 serv	0	0	0	0	0	0	—	—	0	—	0	—	—
Calorie Free as prep	1 serv	0	0	0	0	0	0	—	—	0	—	0	—	—
Decaffeinated Ice Tea Brew as prep	1 serv (8 oz)	0	0	0	0	0	0	0	0	0	—	—	0	—	0
Decaffeinated Lemon as prep	1 serv	90	0	0	0	0	22	—	—	0	—	0	—	—

FOOD	PORTION	CALORIES	FAT	SAT FAT	CHOL	PROTEIN	CARBO	FIBER	CALCIUM	SOD	POTAS	VIT C	FOLIC	VIT A
LIPTON (CONT.)														
Diet Decaffeinated Lemon as prep	1 serv	5	0	0	0	0	1	—	—	0	—	0	—	—
Diet Lemon as prep	1 serv	5	0	0	0	0	1	—	—	0	—	0	—	—
Diet Peach as prep	1 serv	5	0	0	0	0	1	—	—	0	—	0	—	—
Diet Raspberry as prep	1 serv	5	0	0	0	0	1	—	—	0	—	0	—	—
Diet Tea & Lemondage as prep	1 serv	10	0	0	0	0	2	—	—	5	—	0	—	—
Herbal Iced Collection	1 tea bag	0	0	0	0	0	tr	—	—	0	—	0	—	—
Ice Tea Brew as prep	1 serv (8 oz)	0	0	0	0	0	0	0	0	0	—	0	—	0
Lemon as prep	1 serv	90	0	0	0	0	22	—	—	0	—	0	—	—
Lemon as prep	1 pkg (0.5 oz)	50	0	0	0	0	13	—	—	0	—	0	—	—
Natural Brew 100% Tea Decaffeinated as prep	1 serv	0	0	0	0	0	0	—	—	0	—	0	—	—
Natural Brew 100% Tea as prep	1 serv	0	0	0	0	0	0	—	—	0	—	0	—	—
Natural Brew Diet Lemon as prep	1 serv	5	0	0	0	0	1	—	—	0	—	0	—	—
Natural Brew Diet Peach as prep	1 serv	5	0	0	0	0	1	—	—	0	—	0	—	—
Natural Brew Diet Tropical as prep	1 serv	5	0	0	0	0	1	—	—	0	—	0	—	—
Natrual Brew Tropical as prep	1 serv	90	0	0	0	0	22	—	—	0	—	0	—	—
Natural Brew Unsweetened Lemon as prep	1 serv	0	0	0	0	0	tr	—	—	0	—	0	—	—
Peach as prep	1 serv	90	0	0	0	0	22	—	—	0	—	0	—	—
Tea & Lemonade as prep	1 serv	90	0	0	0	0	22	—	—	0	—	0	—	—
NESTEA														
Peach as prep	8 oz	88	tr	—	0	tr	22	—	4	25	93	—	—	—
Raspberry as prep	8 oz	88	tr	—	0	tr	22	—	4	25	64	—	—	—
READY-TO-DRINK														
ARIZONA														
Lemon	1 bottle (16 oz)	180	0	0	0	0	50	—	—	40	—	—	—	—
Raspberry	8 fl oz	95	0	0	0	0	25	—	—	20	—	—	—	—
CLEARLY CANADIAN														
Clearly Tea Original	8 fl oz	80	0	—	—	—	19	—	18	9	1	—	—	—
Clearly Tea Tangy Lemon	8 fl oz	80	0	—	—	—	19	—	18	9	1	—	—	—

FOOD	PORTION	CALORIES	FAT	SAT FAT	CHOL	PROTEIN	CARBO	FIBER	CALCIUM	SOD	POTAS	VIT C	FOLIC	VIT A
CRYSTAL LIGHT														
Lemon	1 serv (8 oz)	5	0	0	0	0	0	0	0	40	50	0	—	0
Peach Tea	1 serv (8 oz)	5	0	0	0	0	0	0	0	40	35	0	—	0
Raspberry Tea	1 serv (8 oz)	5	0	0	0	0	0	0	0	40	35	0	—	0
LIPTON														
Carribean Cooler	1 can (12 oz)	130	0	0	0	0	34	—	—	75	—	0	—	—
Diet Lemon	8 oz	0	0	0	0	0	0	—	—	10	—	0	—	—
Diet Lemon	1 bottle (16 oz)	10	0	0	0	0	0	—	—	10	—	0	—	—
Green Tea & Passion Fruit	1 bottle (16 oz)	160	0	0	0	0	38	—	—	10	—	0	—	—
Lemon	8 oz	80	0	0	0	0	20	—	—	15	—	15	—	—
Lemon	1 can (12 oz)	120	0	0	0	0	33	—	—	75	—	0	—	—
Lemon	1 bottle (16 oz)	180	0	0	0	0	42	—	—	10	—	0	—	—
Natural Lemon	1 box (8 oz)	100	0	0	0	0	25	—	—	10	—	60	—	—
Peach	1 bottle (16 oz)	220	0	0	0	0	52	—	—	10	—	0	—	—
Raspberry	8 oz	80	0	0	0	0	20	—	—	15	—	0	—	—
Raspberry	1 bottle (16 oz)	220	0	0	0	0	52	—	—	10	—	0	—	—
Raspberry Blast	1 can (12 oz)	130	0	0	0	0	35	—	—	75	—	0	—	—
Southern Style Extra Sweet No Lemon	1 bottle (16 oz)	240	0	0	·0	0	58	—	—	10	—	0	—	—
Southern Style Lemon	1 bottle (16 oz)	200	0	0	0	0	50	—	—	10	—	0	—	—
Southern Style Sweetened No Lemon	1 bottle (16 oz)	200	0	0	·0	0	48	—	—	10	—	0	—	—
Sweet	8 oz	80	0	0	0	0	20	—	—	15	—	0	—	—
Sweetened No Lemon	1 bottle (16 oz)	140	0	0	0	0	36	—	—	10	—	0	—	—
Sweetened Lemon	8 oz	80	0	0	0	0	20	—	—	15	—	15	—	—
Tangerine Twist	1 can (12 oz)	120	0	0	0	0	33	—	—	75	—	0	—	—
Tea & Lemonade	1 bottle (16 oz)	220	0	0	0	0	52	—	—	10	—	0	—	—
Unsweetened No Lemon	1 bottle (16 oz)	0	0	0	0	0	0	—	—	10	—	0	—	—
NESTEA														
With Sugar & Lemon	1 can (11.5 fl oz)	127	0	0	0	0	32	—	2	36	91	—	—	—
With Sugar & Lemon	1 bottle (16 fl oz)	176	0	0	0	0	44	—	3	50	126	—	—	—
ROYAL MISTIC														
Diet	12 fl oz	8	0	0	0	0	2	—	—	34	50	—	—	—
Lemon	12 fl oz	144	0	0	0	0	36	—	—	26	60	—	—	—
Orange	12 fl oz	144	0	0	0	0	36	—	—	26	62	—	—	—

FOOD	PORTION	CALORIES	FAT	SAT FAT	CHOL	PROTEIN	CARBO	FIBER	CALCIUM	SOD	POTAS	VIT C	FOLIC	VIT A
ROYAL MISTIC (CONT.)														
Wild Berry	12 fl oz	144	0	0	0	0	36	—	—	34	66	—	—	—
SCHWEPPES														
Ice Tea	8 fl oz	90	0	0	0	0	22	0	—	60	—	—	—	—
SNAPPLE														
Cranberry	8 fl oz	110	0	0	0	0	27	—	0	10	—	—	—	0
Diet	8 fl oz	0	0	0	0	0	1	—	0	10	20	—	—	0
Diet Peach	8 fl oz	0	0	0	0	0	1	—	0	10	40	—	—	0
Diet Raspberry	8 fl oz	0	0	0	0	0	1	—	0	10	55	—	—	0
Lemon	8 fl oz	110	0	0	0	0	27	—	0	10	20	0	—	0
Mango	8 fl oz	110	0	0	0	0	27	—	0	5	24	—	—	0
Mint	8 fl oz	120	0	0	0	0	29	—	0	10	—	—	—	0
Old Fashioned	8 fl oz	80	0	0	0	0	20	—	0	10	—	—	—	0
Orange	8 fl oz	110	0	0	0	0	27	—	0	10	—	—	—	0
Peach	8 fl oz	110	0	0	0	0	27	—	0	10	20	—	—	0
Raspberry	8 fl oz	120	0	0	0	0	29	—	0	10	20	—	—	0
Strawberry	8 fl oz	100	0	0	0	0	26	—	0	10	15	—	—	0
TROPICANA														
Diet Lemon Fruit	8 fl oz	15	0	0	0	0	4	—	—	25	—	—	—	—
Lemon Fruit	8 fl oz	100	0	0	0	0	25	—	—	25	—	—	—	—
Peach Fruit	1 can (11.5 fl oz)	160	0	0	0	0	41	—	—	20	—	—	—	—
Peach Fruit	1 bottle (10 fl oz)	140	0	0	0	0	35	—	—	20	—	—	—	—
Peach Fruit	8 fl oz	120	0	0	0	0	28	—	—	15	—	—	—	—
Raspberry Fruit	1 can (11.5 fl oz)	160	0	0	0	0	41	—	—	15	—	—	—	—
Raspberry Fruit	8 fl oz	120	0	0	0	0	28	—	—	15	—	—	—	—
Raspberry Fruit	1 bottle (10 fl oz)	140	0	0	0	0	34	—	—	20	—	—	—	—
Tangerine Fruit	8 fl oz	110	0	0	0	0	27	—	—	20	—	—	—	—
Tangerine Fruit	1 bottle (10 fl oz)	140	0	0	0	0	34	—	—	30	—	—	—	—
Tangerine Fruit	1 can (11.5 fl oz)	170	0	0	0	0	42	—	—	30	—	—	—	—
Twister Apple Berry	8 fl oz	100	0	0	0	0	28	—	—	15	—	100	—	—
Twister Lemon Citrus	8 fl oz	110	0	0	0	0	28	—	—	5	—	100	—	—
TURKEY HILL														
Diet Decaffeinated	1 cup (8 oz)	0	0	0	0	0	0	—	—	0	—	—	—	—
Raspberry Cooler	1 cup (8 oz)	110	0	0	0	0	28	—	—	0	—	—	—	—
Regular	1 cup (8 oz)	90	0	0	0	0	22	—	—	0	—	—	—	—

ICES AND ICE POPS

(*see also* ICE CREAM AND FROZEN DESSERTS, PUDDING POPS, SHERBET, YOGURT FROZEN)

FOOD	PORTION	CALORIES	FAT	SAT FAT	CHOL	PROTEIN	CARBO	FIBER	CALCIUM	SOD	POTAS	VIT C	FOLIC	VIT A
fruit & juice bar	1 (3 fl oz)	75	tr	—	0	1	19	—	5	3	48	1	5	27
gelatin pop	1 (1.5 oz)	31	0	0	0	1	7	—	—	20	1	—	0	0

FOOD	PORTION	CALORIES	FAT	SAT FAT	CHOL	PROTEIN	CARBO	FIBER	CALCIUM	SOD	POTAS	VIT C	FOLIC	VIT A
ice coconut pineapple	½ cup (4 fl oz)	109	3	—	0	0	23	—	0	34	—	13	—	0
ice fruit w/ Equal	1 bar (1.7 oz)	12	0	0	0	tr	3	—	1	3	13	0	0	0
ice lime	½ cup (4 fl oz)	75	0	0	0	tr	31	—	—	—	3	1	—	0
ice pop	1 (2 fl oz)	42	0	0	0	0	11	—	0	7	2	0	—	0
COOL CREATIONS														
10 Pack	1 pop (2 oz)	60	0	0	0	0	14	0	0	5	—	0	—	0
Lion King Cone	1 (4 oz)	280	14	9	15	3	36	1	60	90	—	0	—	200
Mickey Mouse Bar	1 (2.5 oz)	110	7	3	10	1	12	0	40	25	—	0	—	100
Mickey Mouse Bar	1 (4 oz)	170	11	4	15	2	17	0	60	40	—	0	—	200
Surprise Pops	1 (2 oz)	60	0	0	0	0	14	0	0	5	—	0	—	0
DOLE														
Fruit 'N Juice Coconut	1 bar (4 oz)	210	7	5	10	3	33	0	80	50	—	1	—	100
Fruit 'N Juice Lemonade	1 bar (4 oz)	120	0	0	0	1r	28	0	0	55	—	6	—	0
Fruit 'N Juice Lime	1 bar (4 oz)	110	0	0	0	0	28	0	0	55	—	1	—	0
Fruit 'N Juice Peach Passion	1 bar (2.5 oz)	70	0	0	0	0	17	0	0	5	—	6	—	0
Fruit 'N Juice Pineapple Coconut	1 bar (4 oz)	140	4	4	0	1	27	0	0	5	—	1	—	0
Fruit 'N Juice Pineapple Orange Banana	1 bar (2.5 oz)	70	0	0	0	0	16	0	20	5	—	6	—	0
Fruit 'N Juice Pineapple Orange Banana	1 bar (4 oz)	110	0	0	0	0	26	0	20	5	—	15	—	0
Fruit 'N Juice Raspberry	1 bar (2.5 oz)	70	0	0	0	0	16	0	0	5	—	1	—	0
Fruit 'N Juice Strawberry	1 bar (2.5 oz)	70	0	0	0	0	17	0	0	5	—	15	—	0
Fruit 'N Juice Strawberry	1 bar (4 oz)	110	0	0	0	0r	26	0	0	5	—	15	—	0
Fruit Juice Grape	1 bar (1.75 oz)	45	0	0	0	0	11	0	0	5	—	15	—	0
Fruit Juice No Sugar Added Grape	1 bar (1.75 oz)	25	0	0	0	0	6	0	0	5	—	15	—	0
Fruit Juice No Sugar Added Strawberry	1 bar (1.75 oz)	25	0	0	0	0	6	0	0	5	—	5	—	0
Fruit Juice Raspberry	1 bar (1.75 oz)	45	0	0	0	0	11	0	0	5	—	1	—	0
Fruit Juice Raspberry	1 bar (1.75 oz)	25	0	0	0	0	6	0	0	5	—	2	—	0
Fruit Juice Strawberry	1 bar (1.75 oz)	45	0	0	0	0	11	0	0	5	—	6	—	0

FOOD	PORTION	CALORIES	FAT	SAT FAT	CHOL	PROTEIN	CARBO	FIBER	CALCIUM	SOD	POTAS	VIT C	FOLIC	VIT A
FI-BAR														
Juice Bar Lemoney-Lime	1 bar	63	tr	—	—	tr	15	—	—	—	—	—	—	—
Juice Bar Strawberry Nectar	1 bar	63	tr	—	—	tr	15	—	—	—	—	—	—	—
Juice Bar Tropical Delight	1 bar	63	tr	—	—	tr	15	—	—	—	—	—	—	—
FLINTSTONES														
Rock Pops	1 (3.5 oz)	80	0	0	0	0	20	0	0	5	—	30	—	0
FROZFRUIT														
Banana Cream	1 bar (4 oz)	150	7	5	25	1	20	1	40	20	—	2	—	300
Cantaloupe	1 bar (4 oz)	60	0	0	0	0	35	0	0	5	—	15	—	1000
Cappuccino Cream	1 bar (3 oz)	140	6	4	25	1	18	0	40	20	—	0	—	300
Cherry	1 bar (4 oz)	70	0	0	0	1	18	1	0	0	—	2	—	300
Coconut Cream	1 bar (4 oz)	170	11	8	20	2	17	2	40	25	—	0	—	200
Kiwi Strawberry	1 bar (4 oz)	90	0	0	0	0	23	2	20	0	—	36	—	100
Lemon	1 bar (4 oz)	90	0	0	0	0	22	0	0	10	—	6	—	0
Lemon Iced Tea	1 bar (4 oz)	80	0	0	0	0	19	0	0	10	—	0	—	0
Lime	1 bar (4 oz)	90	0	0	0	0	21	0	0	10	—	2	—	0
Orange	1 bar (4 oz)	90	0	0	0	0	21	0	0	15	—	12	—	0
Pina Colada Cream	1 bar (4 oz)	170	8	6	20	2	23	1	40	20	—	4	—	200
Pineapple	1 bar (4 oz)	80	0	0	0	0	19	0	0	0	—	6	—	0
Raspberry	1 bar (4 oz)	80	0	0	0	0	20	1	0	5	—	6	—	100
Strawberry	1 bar (4 oz)	80	0	0	0	0	20	1	0	20	—	21	—	0
Strawberry Banana Cream	1 bar (4 oz)	140	6	3	20	1	22	1	40	20	—	9	—	300
Strawberry Cream	1 bar (4 oz)	130	5	3	20	1	21	1	40	20	—	15	—	300
Tropical	1 bar (4 oz)	90	0	0	0	0	23	1	0	0	—	9	—	200
Watermelon	1 bar (4 oz)	50	0	0	0	0	13	0	0	0	—	1	—	100
GOOD HUMOR														
Big Stick Cherry Pineapple	1 (3.6 fl oz)	50	0	0	0	0	12	0	0	—	5	0	—	0
Big Stick Popsicle	1 (3.6 fl oz)	50	0	0	0	0	12	—	—	5	—	—	—	—
Calippo Cherry	1 (3.8 fl oz)	100	0	0	0	0	23	—	—	5	—	—	—	—
Calippo Grape Lemon	1 (3.9 fl oz)	90	0	0	0	0	22	—	—	0	—	—	—	—
Calippo Orange	1 (3.9 fl oz)	90	0	0	0	0	23	—	—	0	—	—	—	—
Citrus Bites	1 (1.8 fl oz)	35	0	0	0	0	9	—	—	0	—	—	—	—
Creamsicle Orange	1 (2.8 fl oz)	110	3	2	10	1	20	0	40	30	—	0	—	200
Creamsicle Orange	1 (1.8 fl oz)	70	2	1	5	1	13	0	20	15	—	0	—	0
Creamsicle Orange Raspberry	1 (2.6 fl oz)	100	3	2	10	1	19	0	40	25	—	0	—	200
Creamsicle Sugar Free	1 (1.8 fl oz)	25	0	0	0	0	5	—	—	10	—	—	—	—
Flinstones Push-Up Yabba Dabba Doo Orange	1 (2.75 fl oz)	90	1	—	—	1	20	—	20	20	—	30	—	—

FOOD	PORTION	CALORIES	FAT	SAT FAT	CHOL	PROTEIN	CARBO	FIBER	CALCIUM	SOD	POTAS	VIT C	FOLIC	VIT A
GOOD HUMOR (CONT.)														
Fudgsicle Bar	1 (2.8 fl oz)	90	1	1	5	3	17	1	80	55	—	0	—	0
Fudgsicle Pop	1 (1.8 fl oz)	60	1	1	5	2	12	0	60	40	—	0	—	0
Fudgsicle Sugar Free	1 (1.8 fl oz)	40	1	1	<5	1	8	1	60	35	—	0	—	0
Fun Box Fudge Bar	1 (2.3 fl oz)	80	1	1	5	1	16	0	40	65	—	0	—	0
Fun Box Pops	1 (2 fl oz)	35	0	0	0	0	10	—	—	5	—	—	—	—
Fun Box Twin Box Cherry	1 (2.6 fl oz)	50	0	0	0	0	14	—	—	10	—	—	—	—
Fun Box Twin Pop Banana	1 (2.6 fl oz)	50	0	0	0	0	14	—	—	10	—	—	—	—
Fun Box Twin Pop Blue Raspberry	1 (2.6 fl oz)	50	0	0	0	0	14	—	—	10	—	—	—	—
Fun Box Twin Pop Cherry Lemon	1 (2.6 fl oz)	50	0	0	0	0	14	—	—	10	—	—	—	—
Fun Box Twin Pop Orange Cherry Grape	1 (2.6 fl oz)	50	0	0	0	0	14	—	—	10	—	—	—	—
Fun Box Twin Pop Root Beer	1 (2.6 fl oz)	50	0	0	0	0	14	—	—	10	—	—	—	—
Garfield Bar	1 (3.9 fl oz)	90	0	0	0	0	22	—	—	0	—	—	—	—
Great White	1 (3.1 fl oz)	70	1	—	—	0	18	—	—	0	—	—	—	—
Hyperstripe	1 (2.8 fl oz)	80	0	0	0	0	21	—	—	0	—	—	—	—
Ice Stripe Cherry Orange	1 (1.5 fl oz)	35	0	0	0	0	9	0	0	0	—	0	—	0
Jumbo Jet Star	1 (4.7 fl oz)	80	0	0	0	0	20	—	—	0	—	—	—	—
Laser Blazer	1 (2.6 fl oz)	70	0	0	0	0	16	—	—	5	—	—	—	—
Popsicle All Natural	1 (1.8 fl oz)	45	0	0	0	0	10	—	—	5	—	—	—	—
Popsicle Orange Cherry Grape	1 (1.8 fl oz)	45	0	0	0	0	11	—	—	0	—	—	—	—
Popsicle Rainbow Pops	1 (1.8 fl oz)	45	0	0	0	0	11	—	—	0	—	—	—	—
Popsicle Rootbeer Banana Lime	1 (1.8 fl oz)	45	0	0	0	0	11	—	—	0	—	—	—	—
Popsicle Strawberry Raspberry Wildberry	1 (1.8 fl oz)	45	0	0	0	0	11	—	—	0	—	—	—	—
Popsicle Supersicle Traffic Signal	1	80	0	0	0	0	20	—	—	0	—	—	—	—
Popsicle Twin Pop Cherry	1 (2.6 fl oz)	70	0	0	0	0	16	—	—	0	—	—	—	—
Popsicle Twin Pop Orange Cherry Grape Lime	1 (2.6 fl oz)	70	0	0	0	0	16	—	—	5	—	—	—	—
Snow Cone	1	60	0	—	5	0	14	—	—	5	—	2	—	—
Snowfruit Coconut Bar	1 (3.75 fl oz)	150	4	3	10	2	27	1	60	35	—	0	—	200

FOOD	PORTION	CALORIES	FAT	SAT FAT	CHOL	PROTEIN	CARBO	FIBER	CALCIUM	SOD	POTAS	VIT C	FOLIC	VIT A
GOOD HUMOR (CONT.)														
Snowfruit Orange Bar	1	140	0	0	0	tr	34	tr	—	10	—	36	—	—
Snowfruit Strawberry Bar	1	120	0	0	0	0	31	tr	—	15	—	4	—	—
Snowfruit Tropical Fruit Bar	1	110	0	0	0	0	28	—	—	10	—	—	—	—
Sugar Free Pop Orange Cherry Grape	1 (1.8 fl oz)	15	0	0	0	0	3	—	—	0	—	—	—	—
Super Mario Bar	1	120	1	1	—	0	27	—	60	10	—	—	—	—
Supersicle Cherry Banana	1 (4.7 fl oz)	80	0	0	0	0	20	—	—	0	—	—	—	—
Supersicle Cherry Cola	1 (4.7 fl oz)	80	0	0	0	0	20	—	—	0	—	—	—	—
Supersicle Double Fudge	1 (4.7 fl oz)	150	2	1	10	5	29	1	150	95	—	0	—	100
Supersicle Firecracker	1 (4.7 fl oz)	90	0	0	0	0	20	—	—	0	—	—	—	—
Supersicle Firecracker Jr.	1	72	0	0	0	0	10	—	—	0	—	—	—	—
Supersicle Sour Tower	1	80	0	0	0	0	20	—	—	0	—	—	—	—
Swirl Bubble Gum	1 (2.7 fl oz)	55	0	0	0	0	13	—	—	0	—	—	—	—
Swirl Cherry Banana	1 (2.7 fl oz)	55	0	0	0	0	13	—	—	0	—	—	—	—
Torpedo Cherry	1 (1.8 fl oz)	35	0	0	0	0	10	0	0	5	—	0	—	0
Twister Blue Raspberry Cherry Cherry Cola Cherry	1 (1.8 fl oz)	45	0	0	0	0	10	—	—	0	—	—	—	—
Twister Cherry Lemon Orange Lemon	1 (1.8 fl oz)	45	0	0	0	0	10	—	—	0	—	—	—	—
Vampire's Deadly Secret	1 (2.8 fl oz)	100	0	0	0	0	24	—	—	10	—	—	—	—
Watermelon Bar	1 (3.6 fl oz)	80	0	0	0	0	20	—	—	0	—	—	—	—
HAAGEN-DAZS														
Sorbet Banana Strawberry	½ cup (4 oz)	140	0	0	0	tr	34	tr	0	5	—	9	—	0
Sorbet Chocolate	½ cup (4 oz)	130	0	—	0	2	30	2	0	80	—	0	—	0
Sorbet Manago	½ cup (4 oz)	120	0	—	0	0	30	tr	0	0	—	12	—	1500
Sorbet Orchard Peach	½ cup (4 oz)	140	0	0	0	tr	35	tr	0	0	—	5	—	200
Sorbet Raspberry	½ cup (4 oz)	120	0	—	0	0	29	1	0	5	—	0	—	0
Sorbet Strawberry	½ cup (4 oz)	130	0	—	0	0	33	1	0	0	—	15	—	0
Sorbet Zesty Lemon	½ cup (4 oz)	130	0	—	0	0	32	tr	0	5	—	4	—	0

FOOD	PORTION	CALORIES	FAT	SAT FAT	CHOL	PROTEIN	CARBO	FIBER	CALCIUM	SOD	POTAS	VIT C	FOLIC	VIT A
HAAGEN-DAZS (CONT.)														
Sorbet & Cream Orange	½ cup (3.7 oz)	200	9	5	60	2	27	0	80	45	—	9	—	300
Sorbet & Cream Raspberry	½ cup (3.7 oz)	190	9	5	60	3	23	tr	80	45	—	5	—	300
Sorbet Bar Chocolate	1 (2.7 oz)	80	0	—	0	1	20	1	0	50	—	0	—	0
Sorbet Bar Wild Berry	1 (2.7 oz)	90	0	—	0	0	22	tr	0	5	—	2	—	0
HOOD														
Hendrie's Sizzle'N Sour Stix	1 bar (2 oz)	80	tr	0	5	0	15	0	20	15	—	0	—	0
Hoodsie Pop	1 (3.3 oz)	60	0	0	0	0	16	—	—	0	—	—	—	—
Natural Blenders Pineappple	1 bar (1 oz)	60	0	0	0	0	16	—	—	0	—	27	—	—
Natural Blenders Raspberry	1 bar (1 oz)	60	0	0	0	0	16	—	—	0	—	27	—	—
Natural Blenders Strawberry	1 bar (1 oz)	60	0	0	0	0	16	—	—	0	—	27	—	—
Pop Banana	1 (3.3 oz)	60	0	0	0	0	16	—	—	0	—	—	—	—
Pop Blue Raspberry	1 (3.3 oz)	60	0	0	0	0	16	—	—	0	—	—	—	—
Pop Cherry	1 (3.3 oz)	60	0	0	0	0	16	—	—	0	—	—	—	—
Pop Grape	1 (3.3 oz)	60	0	0	0	0	16	—	—	0	—	—	—	—
Pop Orange	1 (3.3 oz)	60	0	0	0	0	16	—	—	0	—	—	—	—
Pop Root Beer	1 (3.3 oz)	60	0	0	0	0	16	—	—	0	—	—	—	—
Super Sortment Juice Bars	1 bar (1.9 oz)	40	0	0	0	0	10	—	—	0	—	6	—	—
LIFESAVERS														
Ice Pops	1	35	0	0	0	0	9	0	—	0	0	27	—	—
Ice Pops	1 (1.75 oz)	35	0	0	0	0	9	0	—	0	0	27	—	—
MR. FREEZE														
Assorted	2 bars (3 oz)	45	0	0	0	0	11	0	0	20	0	0	—	0
Tropical	2 bars (3 oz)	45	0	0	0	0	11	0	0	20	0	0	—	0
SUNKIST														
Orange Juice Bar	1 (3.4 fl oz)	80	1	—	—	0	19	—	—	5	—	—	—	—
Wildberry	1 (3.4 fl oz)	120	1	—	—	0	27	—	—	10	—	—	—	—
TOFUTTI														
Frutti Apricot Mango	4 fl oz	100	0	0	0	2	20	—	—	90	—	—	—	—
Frutti Three Berry	4 fl oz	100	0	0	0	2	20	—	—	90	—	—	—	—

ICING

(see CAKE ICING)

INSTANT BREAKFAST

(see BREAKFAST DRINKS)

JALAPENO

(see PEPPERS)

JAM/JELLY/PRESERVES

FOOD	PORTION	CALORIES	FAT	SAT FAT	CHOL	PROTEIN	CARBO	FIBER	CALCIUM	SOD	POTAS	VIT C	FOLIC	VIT A
all flavors jam	1 tbsp (0.7 oz)	48	0	0	0	tr	13	tr	—	—	—	—	—	—

FOOD	PORTION	CALORIES	FAT	SAT FAT	CHOL	PROTEIN	CARBO	FIBER	CALCIUM	SOD	POTAS	VIT C	FOLIC	VIT A
all flavors jam	1 pkg (0.5 oz)	34	0	0	0	tr	9	tr	—	—	—	—	—	—
all flavors jelly	1 tbsp (0.7 oz)	52	0	0	0	tr	14	tr	—	—	—	—	—	—
all flavors jelly	1 pkg (0.5 oz)	38	0	0	0	tr	10	tr	—	—	—	—	—	—
all flavors preserve	1 pkg (0.5 oz)	34	0	0	0	tr	9	tr	—	—	—	—	—	—
all flavors preserve	1 tbsp (0.7 oz)	48	0	0	0	tr	13	tr	—	—	—	—	—	—
apple butter	1 tbsp (0.6 oz)	33	0	0	0	0	9	—	1	0	16	tr	—	0
apple butter	1 cup (9.9 oz)	519	1	—	0	tr	135	—	13	1	258	5	—	0
apple jelly	1 tbsp (0.7 oz)	52	0	0	0	tr	14	tr	2	7	12	tr	0	3
apple jelly	1 pkg (0.5 oz)	38	0	0	0	tr	10	tr	1	5	9	tr	0	2
linganberry jam	0.5 oz	23	tr	tr	—	tr	6	tr	—	—	—	—	—	—
orange marmalade	1 pkg (0.5 oz)	34	0	0	0	0	9	—	5	8	5	1	5	7
orange marmalade	1 tbsp (0.7 oz)	49	0	0	0	tr	13	—	8	11	7	1	7	9
strawberry jam	1 pkg (0.5 oz)	34	0	0	0	tr	9	tr	3	6	11	1	5	2
strawberry jam	1 tbsp (0.7 oz)	48	0	0	0	tr	13	tr	4	8	15	2	7	2
strawberry preserve	1 pkg (0.5 oz)	34	0	0	0	tr	9	tr	3	6	11	1	5	2
strawberry preserve	1 tbsp (0.7 oz)	48	0	0	0	tr	13	tr	4	8	15	2	7	2
BAMA														
Apple Butter	2 tsp	25	0	0	0	0	6	—	—	5	10	—	—	—
Apple Jelly	2 tsp	30	0	0	0	0	8	—	—	5	5	—	—	—
Grape Jelly	2 tsp	30	0	0	0	0	8	—	—	5	5	—	—	—
Peach Preserves	2 tsp	30	0	0	0	0	8	—	—	5	10	—	—	—
Red Plum Jam	2 tsp	30	0	0	0	0	8	—	—	5	5	—	—	—
Strawberry Preserves	2 tsp	30	0	0	0	0	8	—	—	5	10	—	—	—
ESTEE														
Apple Reduced Calorie	1 pkg (0.5 oz)	10	0	0	0	0	2	—	—	25	10	—	—	—
Apple Slice	1 tbsp (0.5 oz)	10	0	0	0	0	2	—	—	20	30	—	—	—
Apricot	1 tbsp (0.5 oz)	5	0	0	0	0	1	—	—	20	35	—	—	—
Blackberry	1 tbsp (0.5 oz)	5	0	0	0	0	1	—	—	25	25	—	—	—
Cherry	1 tbsp (0.5 oz)	5	0	0	0	0	1	—	—	20	25	—	—	—
Grape	1 tbsp (0.5 oz)	10	0	0	0	0	2	—	—	20	35	—	—	—
Orange	1 tbsp (0.5 oz)	10	0	0	0	0	2	—	—	20	35	—	—	—
Peach	1 tbsp (0.5 oz)	5	0	0	0	0	1	—	—	20	25	—	—	—
Red Raspberry	1 tbsp (0.5 oz)	5	0	0	0	0	1	—	—	25	30	—	—	—
Strawberry	1 tbsp (0.5 oz)	10	0	0	0	0	2	—	—	—	20	—	—	—
HARVEST MOON														
Apricot Fruit Spread	1 tbsp (0.6 oz)	35	0	0	0	0	9	—	—	0	—	—	—	—
Blueberry Fruit Spread	1 tbsp (0.6 oz)	35	0	0	0	0	9	—	—	0	—	—	—	—
Cherry Fruit Spread	1 tbsp (0.6 oz)	35	0	0	0	0	9	—	—	0	—	—	—	—
Grape Fruit Spread	1 tbsp (0.6 oz)	35	0	0	0	0	9	—	—	0	—	—	—	—
Peach Fruit Spread	1 tbsp (0.6 oz)	35	0	0	0	0	9	—	—	0	—	—	—	—
Raspberry Fruit Spread	1 tbsp (0.6 oz)	35	0	0	0	0	9	—	—	0	—	—	—	—

FOOD	PORTION	CALORIES	FAT	SAT FAT	CHOL	PROTEIN	CARBO	FIBER	CALCIUM	SOD	POTAS	VIT C	FOLIC	VIT A
HARVEST MOON (CONT.)														
Strawberry Fruit Spread	1 tbsp (0.6 oz)	35	0	0	0	0	9	—	—	0	—	—	—	—
RED WING														
Apple Jelly	1 tbsp (0.7 oz)	50	0	0	0	0	13	0	0	5	—	0	—	0
Apple Blackberry Jelly	1 tbsp (0.7 oz)	50	0	0	0	0	13	0	0	5	—	0	—	0
Apple Cherry Jelly	1 tbsp (0.7 oz)	50	0	0	0	0	13	0	0	10	—	0	—	0
Apple Currant Jelly	1 tbsp (0.7 oz)	50	0	0	0	0	13	0	0	15	—	0	—	0
Apple Grape Jelly	1 tbsp (0.7 oz)	50	0	0	0	0	13	0	0	10	—	0	—	0
Apple Raspberry Jelly	1 tbsp (0.7 oz)	50	0	0	0	0	13	0	0	5	—	0	—	0
Apple Strawberry Jelly	1 tbsp (0.7 oz)	50	0	0	0	0	13	0	0	5	—	0	—	0
Black Raspberry Jelly	1 tbsp (0.7 oz)	50	0	0	0	0	13	0	0	5	—	0	—	0
Blackberry Jelly	1 tbsp (0.7 oz)	50	0	0	0	0	13	0	0	5	—	0	—	0
Cherry Jelly	1 tbsp (0.7 oz)	50	0	0	0	0	13	0	0	5	—	0	—	0
Concord Grape Jelly	1 tbsp (0.7 oz)	50	0	0	0	0	13	0	0	5	—	0	—	0
Crabapple Jelly	1 tbsp (0.7 oz)	50	0	0	0	0	13	0	0	10	—	0	—	0
Cranberry Jelly	1 tbsp (0.7 oz)	50	0	0	0	0	13	0	0	10	—	0	—	0
Cranberry Grape Jelly	1 tbsp (0.7 oz)	50	0	0	0	0	13	0	0	10	—	0	—	0
Currant Jelly	1 tbsp (0.7 oz)	50	0	0	0	0	13	0	0	10	—	0	—	0
Damson Plum Jelly	1 tbsp (0.7 oz)	50	0	0	0	0	13	0	0	5	—	0	—	0
Elderberry Jelly	1 tbsp (0.7 oz)	50	0	0	0	0	13	0	0	5	—	0	—	0
Grape Jelly	1 tbsp (0.7 oz)	50	0	0	0	0	13	0	0	5	—	0	—	0
Mint Jelly	1 tbsp (0.7 oz)	50	0	0	0	0	13	0	0	5	—	0	—	0
Mint Apple Jelly	1 tbsp (0.7 oz)	50	0	0	0	0	13	0	0	5	—	0	—	0
Mixed Fruit Jelly	1 tbsp (0.7 oz)	50	0	0	0	0	13	0	0	5	—	0	—	0
Red Plum Jelly	1 tbsp (0.7 oz)	50	0	0	0	0	13	0	0	10	—	0	—	0
Red Raspberry Jelly	1 tbsp (0.7 oz)	50	0	0	0	0	13	0	0	5	—	0	—	0
Strawberry Jelly	1 tbsp (0.7 oz)	50	0	0	0	0	13	0	0	5	—	0	—	0
Strawberry Apple Jelly	1 tbsp (0.7 oz)	50	0	0	0	0	13	0	0	10	—	0	—	0
TREE OF LIFE														
Apricot Fruit Spread	1 tbsp (0.6 oz)	45	0	0	0	0	12	—	—	0	—	—	—	—
Blueberry Fruit Spread	1 tbsp (0.6 oz)	35	0	0	0	0	9	—	—	0	—	—	—	—
Cherry Fruit Spread	1 tbsp (0.6 oz)	40	0	0	0	0	10	—	—	0	—	—	—	—
Grape Fruit Spread	1 tbsp (0.6 oz)	35	0	0	0	0	8	—	—	0	—	—	—	—
Peach Fruit Spread	1 tbsp (0.6 oz)	45	0	0	0	0	12	—	—	0	—	—	—	—
Raspberry Fruit Spread	1 tbsp (0.6 oz)	30	0	0	0	0	7	—	—	0	—	—	—	—

FOOD	PORTION	CALORIES	FAT	SAT FAT	CHOL	PROTEIN	CARBO	FIBER	CALCIUM	SOD	POTAS	VIT C	FOLIC	VIT A
TREE OF LIFE (CONT.)														
Strawberry Fruit Spread	1 tbsp (0.6 oz)	35	0	0	0	0	9	—	—	0	—	12	—	—
WHISTLING WINGS														
Blueberry Jam	1 oz	50	tr	—	—	tr	12	tr	5	2	14	tr	—	—
Raspberry Jam	1 oz	60	tr	—	—	tr	14	1	7	1	29	tr	—	—

JAPANESE FOOD
(*see* ASIAN FOOD, SUSHI)

JAVA PLUM

FOOD	PORTION	CALORIES	FAT	SAT FAT	CHOL	PROTEIN	CARBO	FIBER	CALCIUM	SOD	POTAS	VIT C	FOLIC	VIT A
fresh	3	5	tr	—	0	tr	1	—	2	1	7	1	—	0
fresh	1 cup	82	tr	—	0	1	21	—	25	18	106	19	—	5

JELLY
(*see* JAM/JELLY/PRESERVE)

JERUSALEM ARTICHOKE
(*see* ARTICHOKE)

KALE

FOOD	PORTION	CALORIES	FAT	SAT FAT	CHOL	PROTEIN	CARBO	FIBER	CALCIUM	SOD	POTAS	VIT C	FOLIC	VIT A
FRESH														
chopped cooked	½ cup	21	tr	tr	0	1	4	—	47	15	148	27	9	4810
raw chopped	½ cup	21	tr	tr	0	1	3	—	46	15	152	41	10	3026
scotch chopped cooked	½ cup	18	tr	tr	0	1	4	—	86	29	178	34	9	1296
DOLE														
Chopped	½ cup	17	1	—	0	1	3	—	—	15	152	41	—	3026
FROZEN														
chopped cooked	½ cup	20	tr	tr	0	2	4	—	90	10	209	16	9	4130

KETCHUP

FOOD	PORTION	CALORIES	FAT	SAT FAT	CHOL	PROTEIN	CARBO	FIBER	CALCIUM	SOD	POTAS	VIT C	FOLIC	VIT A
DEL MONTE														
Ketchup	1 tbsp (0.5 oz)	15	0	0	0	0	4	0	0	190	—	1	—	100
ESTEE														
Imitation Sodium Free	1 pkg (0.5 oz)	15	0	—	—	0	3	—	—	0	95	—	—	—
HAIN														
Natural	1 tbsp	16	0	0	0	0	4	—	—	155	—	—	—	—
Natural No Salt Added	1 tbsp	16	0	0	0	0	4	—	—	5	—	—	—	—
HEALTHY CHOICE														
Ketchup	1 tbsp (0.5 oz)	9	0	0	0	tr	2	tr	tr	97	—	2	—	4
HEINZ														
Hot	1 tbsp	14	0	0	0	0	3	—	—	185	60	—	—	—
Lite	1 tbsp	8	0	0	0	0	2	—	—	115	65	—	—	100
HUNT'S														
Ketchup	1 tbsp (0.6 oz)	16	tr	0	0	tr	3	0	4	198	—	1	—	35
No Salt Added	1 tbsp (0.6 oz)	16	tr	0	0	tr	3	0	2	6	—	1	—	35
MCILHENNY														
Ketchup	1 tbsp (0.6 oz)	23	tr	tr	0	tr	5	tr	tr	128	—	1	—	732

FOOD	PORTION	CALORIES	FAT	SAT FAT	CHOL	PROTEIN	CARBO	FIBER	CALCIUM	SOD	POTAS	VIT C	FOLIC	VIT A
MCILHENNY (CONT.)														
Spicy	1 tbsp (0.6 oz)	23	tr	tr	tr	tr	5	tr	tr	128	—	1	—	732
MUIR GLEN														
Organic	1 tbsp (0.6 oz)	15	0	—	0	0	3	0	0	190	—	1	—	100
RED WING														
Extra Fancy	1 tbsp (0.6 oz)	20	0	0	0	0	5	0	0	190	—	0	—	0
TREE OF LIFE														
Ketchup	1 tbsp (0.5 oz)	10	0	0	0	0	3	—	0	25	—	6	—	400
Salsa Ketchup	1 tbsp (0.5 oz)	10	0	0	0	0	3	—	0	50	—	9	—	300
KIDNEY														
beef simmered	3 oz	122	3	1	329	22	0	—	15	114	152	1	83	1055
lamb braised	3 oz	117	3	1	481	20	1	—	15	128	151	10	69	387
pork cooked	1 cup	211	7	2	672	36	0	0	18	112	—	9	57	364
pork cooked	3 oz	128	4	1	408	22	0	0	11	68	—	9	35	221
veal braised	3 oz	139	5	1	672	22	0	—	25	93	135	7	18	569
KIDNEY BEANS														
CANNED														
kidney beans	1 cup	208	1	tr	0	13	38	—	69	889	658	3	126	0
red	1 cup	216	1	tr	0	13	40	—	62	873	658	3	129	0
B&M														
Red Baked Beans	½ cup (4.6 oz)	170	2	1	<5	7	32	6	60	440	—	0	—	0
EDEN														
Organic	½ cup (4.6 oz)	100	0	0	0	8	18	10	60	15	440	—	—	—
FRIEND'S														
Red Baked Beans	½ cup (4.6 oz)	160	1	0	<5	7	32	6	60	510	—	0	—	0
GOYA														
Spanish Style	7.5 oz	140	1	—	0	13	29	10	75	760	700	3	—	444
GREEN GIANT														
Dark Red	½ cup (4.5 oz)	110	0	0	0	6	18	5	40	400	—	0	—	0
Light Red	½ cup (4.5 oz)	110	0	0	0	8	20	6	60	340	—	0	—	0
HUNT'S														
Red	½ cup (4.5 oz)	94	1	0	0	6	20	5	4	484	—	tr	—	0
PROGRESSO														
Red	½ cup (4.6 oz)	110	1	0	0	7	20	8	40	280	—	0	—	0
TRAPPEY														
Dark Red	½ cup (4.5 oz)	130	1	0	0	8	22	8	60	310	—	0	—	0
Light Red	½ cup (4.5 oz)	120	1	0	0	6	22	8	40	340	—	0	—	0
Light Red New Orleans Style With Bacon	½ cup (4.5 oz)	110	1	1	0	6	20	6	40	410	—	0	—	0
Light Red With Jalapeno	½ cup (4.5 oz)	110	1	0	0	6	19	6	20	420	—	0	—	0
With Chili Gravy	½ cup (4.5 oz)	110	1	0	0	6	20	7	40	510	—	0	—	1000
VAN CAMP'S														
Dark Red	½ cup (4.6 oz)	90	0	0	0	6	20	6	40	760	280	—	0	0

FOOD	PORTION	CALORIES	FAT	SAT FAT	CHOL	PROTEIN	CARBO	FIBER	CALCIUM	SOD	POTAS	VIT C	FOLIC	VIT A
VAN CAMP'S (CONT.)														
Light Red	½ cup (4.6 oz)	90	0	0	0	6	20	6	40	390	290	—	0	0
DRIED														
california red cooked	1 cup	219	tr	tr	0	16	40	—	116	7	741	2	131	5
cooked	1 cup	225	1	tr	0	15	40	—	0	4	713	2	229	0
red cooked	1 cup	225	1	tr	0	15	40	—	50	4	713	2	229	0
royal red cooked	1 cup	218	tr	tr	0	17	39	—	78	8	669	2	130	5
ARROWHEAD														
Red	¼ cup (1.6 oz)	160	1	0	0	11	29	10	60	0	450	0	—	0
SPROUTS														
cooked	1 lb	152	3	tr	0	22	21	—	84	—	878	162	—	8
raw	½ cup	27	tr	tr	0	4	4	—	16	—	172	36	—	2

KIWI JUICE

AFTER THE FALL

FOOD	PORTION	CALORIES	FAT	SAT FAT	CHOL	PROTEIN	CARBO	FIBER	CALCIUM	SOD	POTAS	VIT C	FOLIC	VIT A
Kiwi Bear	1 cup (8 oz)	100	0	0	0	1	24	0	0	15	—	5	—	0

KIWIS

DOLE

FOOD	PORTION	CALORIES	FAT	SAT FAT	CHOL	PROTEIN	CARBO	FIBER	CALCIUM	SOD	POTAS	VIT C	FOLIC	VIT A
Fresh	2	90	1	—	0	1	18	4	—	0	450	143	—	136
SONOMA														
Dried	7-8 pieces (1 oz)	90	1	0	0	2	19	2	40	0	—	84	—	0

KNISH

JOSHUA'S

FOOD	PORTION	CALORIES	FAT	SAT FAT	CHOL	PROTEIN	CARBO	FIBER	CALCIUM	SOD	POTAS	VIT C	FOLIC	VIT A
Coney Island Potato	1 (4.6 oz)	280	8	2	0	1	52	1	100	610	—	0	—	100
TAKE-OUT														
cheese & blueberry	1 (7 oz)	378	13	—	40	24	40	—	—	—	—	—	—	—
cheese & cherry	1 (7 oz)	378	13	—	40	24	40	—	—	—	—	—	—	—
everything	1 (7 oz)	221	8	—	0	7	34	—	—	—	—	—	—	—
kashe	1 (7 oz)	270	8	—	0	7	45	—	—	—	—	—	—	—
potato	1 med (3.5 oz)	166	6	2	36	4	25	tr	27	235	179	4	17	113
potato	1 lg (7 oz)	332	12	3	72	8	49	1	54	470	358	8	35	225
potato w/ broccoli & cheese	1 (7 oz)	312	15	—	24	12	33	—	—	—	—	—	—	—
potato w/ spinach & mushroom	1 (7 oz)	214	8	—	0	6	32	—	—	—	—	—	—	—

KOHLRABI

FOOD	PORTION	CALORIES	FAT	SAT FAT	CHOL	PROTEIN	CARBO	FIBER	CALCIUM	SOD	POTAS	VIT C	FOLIC	VIT A
raw sliced	½ cup	19	tr	tr	0	1	4	—	17	14	245	43	—	25
sliced cooked	½ cup	24	tr	tr	0	1	5	—	20	17	279	44	—	29

KUMQUATS

FOOD	PORTION	CALORIES	FAT	SAT FAT	CHOL	PROTEIN	CARBO	FIBER	CALCIUM	SOD	POTAS	VIT C	FOLIC	VIT A
fresh	1	12	tr	—	0	tr	3	—	8	1	37	7	—	57

FOOD	PORTION	CALORIES	FAT	SAT FAT	CHOL	PROTEIN	CARBO	FIBER	CALCIUM	SOD	POTAS	VIT C	FOLIC	VIT A
LAMB														
(*see also* LAMB DISHES)														
FRESH														
cubed lean only braised	3 oz	190	7	3	92	29	0	—	13	60	221	—	18	—
cubed lean only broiled	3 oz	158	6	2	77	24	0	—	11	65	285	—	19	—
ground broiled	3 oz	240	17	7	82	21	0	—	19	69	288	—	16	—
leg lean & fat Choice roasted	3 oz	219	14	6	79	22	14	—	9	56	266	—	17	—
loin chop w/ bone lean & fat Choice broiled	1 chop (2.3 oz)	201	15	6	64	16	0	—	13	49	209	—	12	—
loin chop w/ bone lean only Choice broiled	1 chop (1.6 oz)	100	5	2	44	14	0	—	9	39	175	—	11	—
rib chop lean & fat Choice broiled	3 oz	307	25	11	84	19	0	—	16	64	230	—	12	—
rib chop lean only Choice broiled	3 oz	200	11	4	78	24	0	—	14	73	266	—	18	—
shank lean & fat Choice braised	3 oz	206	11	5	90	24	0	—	17	61	218	—	14	—
shank lean & fat Choice roasted	3 oz	191	11	4	77	22	0	—	8	55	277	—	19	—
shoulder chop w/ bone lean & fat Choice braised	1 chop (2.5 oz)	244	17	7	84	21	0	—	18	51	216	—	13	—
shoulder chop w/ bone lean only Choice braised	1 chop (1.9 oz)	152	8	3	66	19	0	—	14	41	185	—	12	—
sirloin lean & fat Choice roasted	3 oz	248	21	7	82	21	0	—	10	58	256	—	14	—
FROZEN														
New Zealand lean & fat cooked	3 oz	259	19	9	93	21	0	—	14	39	138	—	—	—
New Zealand lean only cooked	3 oz	175	8	3	93	25	0	—	11	43	160	—	—	—
LAMBSQUARTERS														
chopped cooked	½ cup	29	1	tr	0	3	5	—	232	—	—	33	—	8730
LECITHIN														
(*see* SOY)														
LEEKS														
chopped cooked	¼ cup	8	tr	tr	0	tr	2	—	8	3	23	1	6	12
cooked	1 (4.4 oz)	38	tr	tr	0	1	9	—	37	13	108	5	30	57
freeze dried	1 tbsp	1	0	0	0	tr	tr	—	1	0	5	tr	1	1
raw	1 (4.4 oz)	76	tr	tr	0	2	18	—	73	25	223	15	80	110
raw chopped	¼ cup	16	tr	tr	0	tr	4	—	15	5	47	3	17	25

FOOD	PORTION	CALORIES	FAT	SAT FAT	CHOL	PROTEIN	CARBO	FIBER	CALCIUM	SOD	POTAS	VIT C	FOLIC	VIT A
LEMON														
fresh	1 med	22	tr	tr	0	1	12	—	66	3	157	83	—	32
peel	1 tbsp	0	tr	tr	0	tr	1	—	8	0	10	8	—	3
wedge	1	5	tr	tr	0	tr	3	—	16	1	39	21	—	8
DOLE														
Fresh	1	18	0	—	0	0	4	0	—	0	65	—	—	—
LEMON EXTRACT														
VIRGINIA DARE														
Extract	1 tsp	22	0	—	0	—	—	—	0	—	—	—	—	—
LEMON GRASS														
fresh	1 cup (2.4 oz)	66	tr	tr	0	1	17	0	44	4	484	tr	50	7
fresh	1 tbsp (5 g)	5	tr	tr	0	tr	1	0	3	tr	35	tr	4	1
LEMON JUICE														
bottled	1 tbsp	3	tr	tr	0	tr	1	—	2	3	15	4	2	2
fresh	1 tbsp	4	0	—	0	tr	1	—	1	0	19	7	2	3
frzn	1 tbsp	3	tr	tr	0	tr	1	—	1	0	14	5	1	2
AFTER THE FALL														
Spicy Lemon	1 can (12 oz)	150	0	0	0	tr	37	0	20	35	85	1	—	0
REALEMON														
Juice	1 fl oz	6	0	0	0	0	2	—	—	5	30	9	—	—
LEMONADE														
FROZEN														
as prep w/ water	1 cup	100	tr	tr	0	tr	26	—	8	8	38	10	6	53
not prep	1 can (6 oz)	397	tr	tr	0	1	103	—	15	8	148	39	22	209
BRIGHT & EARLY														
Lemonade	8 fl oz	120	0	0	0	0	30	—	—	5	—	60	—	—
MINUTE MAID														
Country Style	8 fl oz	120	0	0	0	0	30	—	—	0	—	—	—	—
Cranberry Lemonade	8 fl oz	80	0	0	0	0	30	—	—	0	—	—	—	—
Lemonade	8 fl oz	110	0	0	0	0	29	—	—	0	—	—	—	—
Pink	8 fl oz	120	0	0	0	0	30	—	—	0	—	—	—	—
Raspberry	8 fl oz	120	0	0	0	0	30	—	—	0	—	—	—	—
SENECA														
as prep	8 fl oz	110	0	0	0	0	27	1	0	0	35	15	—	0
MIX														
powder as prep w/ water	9 fl oz	113	tr	tr	0	0	29	—	29	19	1	34	0	0
powder w/ equal	1 pitcher (67 oz)	40	0	0	0	tr	10	—	408	58	6	47	0	0
4C														
Instant as prep	8 fl oz	80	0	—	—	0	20	—	—	0	5	—	—	—
COUNTRY TIME														
Lem'n Berry Sippers Cranberry Raspberry Lemonade as prep	1 serv (8 oz)	90	0	0	0	0	21	0	0	0	0	0	—	0

FOOD	PORTION	CALORIES	FAT	SAT FAT	CHOL	PROTEIN	CARBO	FIBER	CALCIUM	SOD	POTAS	VIT C	FOLIC	VIT A
COUNTRY TIME (CONT.)														
Lem'n Berry Sippers Raspberry Lemonade as prep	1 serv (8 oz)	90	0	0	0	0	21	0	0	0	0	0	—	—
Lem'n Berry Sippers Strawberry Lemonade as prep	1 serv (8 oz)	90	0	0	0	0	21	0	0	0	0	0	—	0
Lem'n Berry Sippers Wildberry Lemonade as prep	1 serv (8 oz)	90	0	0	0	0	21	0	0	0	0	0	—	0
Lem'n Berry Sippers Sugar Free Strawberry Lemonade as prep	1 serv (8 oz)	5	0	0	0	0	0	0	0	0	0	0	—	0
Lemonade as prep	1 serv (8 oz)	70	0	0	0	0	17	0	0	15	5	6	—	0
Pink as prep	1 serv (8 oz)	70	0	0	0	0	17	0	0	15	5	6	—	0
Sugar Free Pink as prep	1 serv (8 oz)	5	0	0	0	0	0	0	0	0	40	6	—	0
Sugar Free as prep	1 serv (8 oz)	5	0	0	0	0	0	0	0	0	40	6	—	0
CRYSTAL LIGHT														
Lemonade as prep	1 serv (8 oz)	5	0	0	0	0	0	0	0	0	60	6	—	0
Pink as prep	1 serv (8 oz)	5	0	0	0	0	0	0	0	0	40	6	—	0
KOOL-AID														
Lemonade as prep	1 serv (8 oz)	70	0	0	0	0	17	0	0	0	0	6	—	0
Mix as prep w/ sugar	1 serv (8 oz)	100	0	0	0	0	25	0	0	10	0	6	—	0
Pink as prep w/ sugar	1 serv (8 oz)	100	0	0	0	0	25	0	0	10	0	6	—	0
Soarin' Strawberry Lemonade as prep	1 serv (8 oz)	70	0	0	0	0	17	0	0	15	0	6	—	0
Soarin' Strawberry Lemonade as prep w/ sugar	1 serv (8 oz)	100	0	0	0	0	25	0	0	0	0	6	—	0
Sugar Free Soarin' Strawberry Lemonade as prep	1 serv (8 oz)	5	0	0	0	0	0	0	0	0	0	6	—	0
Sugar Free Mix as prep	1 serv (8 oz)	5	0	0	0	0	0	0	0	0	0	6	—	0
READY-TO-DRINK														
AFTER THE FALL														
Apple Raspberry	1 bottle (10 oz)	120	0	0	0	1	29	—	0	15	100	9	—	0
CRYSTAL GEYSER														
Juice Squeeze Pink	1 bottle (12 fl oz)	140	0	0	0	0	34	—	—	20	—	—	160	—
CRYSTAL LIGHT														
Lemonade	1 serv (8 oz)	5	0	0	0	0	0	0	0	20	160	0	—	0
Pink	1 serv (8 oz)	5	0	0	0	0	0	0	0	20	160	0	—	0

FOOD	PORTION	CALORIES	FAT	SAT FAT	CHOL	PROTEIN	CARBO	FIBER	CALCIUM	SOD	POTAS	VIT C	FOLIC	VIT A
DIET RITE														
Salt/Sodium Free	8 fl oz	2	0	0	0	0	1	—	—	0	52	—	—	—
EVERFRESH														
Lemonade	1 can (8 oz)	120	0	0	0	0	29	0	—	0	—	—	—	—
Ruby Red	1 can (8 oz)	110	0	0	0	0	27	0	—	0	—	—	—	—
FRUITOPIA														
Lemonade	8 fl oz	120	0	0	0	0	29	—	—	25	—	—	—	—
MINUTE MAID														
Chilled	8 fl oz	110	0	0	0	0	28	—	—	25	—	—	—	—
Cranberry Chilled	8 fl oz	120	0	0	0	0	31	—	—	25	—	—	—	—
Juices To Go	1 bottle (16 fl oz)	110	0	0	0	0	28	—	—	25	—	—	—	—
Juices To Go	1 can (11.5 fl oz)	160	0	0	0	0	40	—	—	40	—	—	—	—
Juices To Go Canberry Lemonade	1 bottle (16 fl oz)	110	0	0	0	0	29	—	—	25	—	—	—	—
Juices To Go Raspberry Lemonade	1 bottle (16 fl oz)	120	0	0	0	0	29	—	—	25	—	—	—	—
Pink Chilled	8 fl oz	110	0	0	0	0	28	—	—	25	—	—	—	—
Raspberry Chilled	8 fl oz	120	0	0	0	0	30	—	—	0	—	—	—	—
MOTT'S														
Lemonade	10 fl oz	160	0	0	0	0	41	0	20	20	50	7	—	0
NEHI														
Lemonade	8 fl oz	130	0	0	0	0	35	—	—	35	20	—	—	—
NEWMAN'S OWN														
Lemonade	1 bottle (10 oz)	140	0	0	0	0	34	0	0	45	—	2	—	0
Roadside Virginia	8 fl oz	110	0	0	0	0	27	0	0	40	—	2	—	0
ODWALLA														
Honey	8 fl oz	70	0	0	0	0	26	0	0	10	—	9	—	0
Strawberry	8 fl oz	150	0	0	0	0	40	2	0	35	—	12	—	500
ROYAL MISTIC														
Lemonade Limeade	16 fl oz	230	0	0	0	0	57	—	—	19	59	—	—	—
Tropical Pink	16 fl oz	230	0	0	0	0	57	—	—	11	35	—	—	—
SANTA CRUZ														
Organic	8 oz	100	0	0	0	0	24	—	20	0	45	—	—	750
SHASTA PLUS														
Lemonade	1 can (11.5 oz)	160	0	0	0	0	40	0	—	45	—	60	—	—
SNAPPLE														
Diet Pink	8 fl oz	13	0	0	0	0	3	—	0	10	—	—	—	0
Lemonade	8 fl oz	110	0	0	0	0	29	—	0	10	15	0	—	0
Pink	8 fl oz	110	0	0	0	0	26	—	0	15	—	—	—	0
Strawberry	8 fl oz	110	0	0	0	0	26	—	0	5	10	—	—	0

FOOD	PORTION	CALORIES	FAT	SAT FAT	CHOL	PROTEIN	CARBO	FIBER	CALCIUM	SOD	POTAS	VIT C	FOLIC	VIT A
TROPICANA														
Lemonade	1 can (11.5 oz)	160	0	0	0	tr	39	—	—	20	—	—	—	—
Lemonade	8 fl oz	110	0	0	0	tr	28	—	—	20	—	—	—	—
Twister Wild Berry	8 fl oz	120	0	0	0	0	30	—	—	5	—	100	—	—
TURKEY HILL														
Lemonade	8 fl oz	110	0	0	0	0	29	—	—	0	—	—	—	—
VERYFINE														
Chillers	1 can (11.5 oz)	190	0	0	0	0	48	0	0	15	—	60	—	0
Chillers Cherry	8 fl oz	120	0	0	0	0	29	0	0	15	—	60	—	0
Chillers Peach	8 fl oz	120	0	0	0	0	31	0	0	15	—	60	—	0
Chillers Pink	1 can (11.5 oz)	180	0	0	0	0	45	0	0	15	—	60	—	0
Chillers Strawberry	1 can (11.5 oz)	170	0	0	0	0	43	0	0	20	—	60	—	0
LENTILS														
CANNED														
EDEN														
Organic w/ Sweet Onion & Bay Leaf	½ cup (4.6 oz)	90	0	0	0	8	13	4	40	210	230	—	—	—
HEALTH VALLEY														
Fast Menu Hearty Lentils Garden Vegetables	7½ oz	150	4	—	0	13	16	16	87	200	361	4	23	5000
Fast Menu Organic Lentils With Tofu Weiner	7½ oz	170	5	—	0	15	15	15	150	260	340	1	—	5000
DRIED														
cooked	1 cup	231	1	tr	0	18	40	—	37	4	731	3	358	15
FROZEN														
NATURAL TOUCH														
Lentil Rice Loaf	1 in slice (3.2 oz)	170	9	3	0	8	14	4	20	370	160	0	—	750
MIX														
CASBAH														
Pilaf as prep	1 cup	200	tr	0	0	10	38	2	60	400	—	2	—	2300
SPROUTS														
raw	½ cup	40	tr	tr	0	3	8	—	9	4	122	6	38	17
TAKE-OUT														
indian sambar	1 serv	236	5	2	10	15	37	9	—	189	—	—	—	—
LETTUCE														
(see also SALAD)														
iceberg	1 leaf	3	tr	tr	0	tr	tr	tr	4	2	32	1	11	66
looseleaf shredded	½ cup	5	tr	tr	0	tr	1	—	19	3	74	5	—	532
DOLE														
Butter	1 head	21	tr	—	0	2	4	2	—	8	8	13	—	1581

FOOD	PORTION	CALORIES	FAT	SAT FAT	CHOL	PROTEIN	CARBO	FIBER	CALCIUM	SOD	POTAS	VIT C	FOLIC	VIT A
DOLE (CONT.)														
Iceberg	⅙ med head	20	0	—	0	1	4	1	—	10	114	3	—	166
Leaf shredded	1½ cup	12	0	—	0	1	1	1	—	40	220	15	—	1596
Romaine shredded	1½ cups	18	1	—	0	1	2	1	—	40	150	20	—	2184
WESTERN EXPRESS														
Heart's Of Romaine	6 leaves (3 oz)	20	1	0	0	1	3	1	20	0	—	2	—	1000
LIMA BEANS														
CANNED														
large	1 cup	191	tr	tr	0	12	36	—	50	809	531	0	121	0
lima beans	½ cup	93	tr	tr	0	6	17	—	35	309	334	11	—	214
ALLEN														
Green	½ cup (4.5 oz)	120	1	0	0	7	23	8	40	370	—	0	—	0
Green & White	½ cup (4.5 oz)	110	1	1	0	6	20	9	40	280	—	0	—	0
DEL MONTE														
Green	½ cup (4.4 oz)	80	0	0	0	4	15	4	20	360	—	4	—	100
EAST TEXAS FAIR														
Green	½ cup (4.5 oz)	120	1	0	0	7	23	8	40	370	—	0	—	0
SENECA														
Limas	½ cup	80	0	0	0	4	15	5	60	240	315	12	—	0
TRAPPEY														
Baby Green With Bacon	½ cup (4.5 oz)	120	1	1	0	6	22	6	20	330	—	0	—	0
DRIED														
cooked	½ cup	104	tr	tr	0	6	20	—	27	14	485	9	—	315
HURST														
HamBeens Large Limas w/ Ham	1 serv	120	1	0	0	7	22	9	20	63	—	0	—	0
FROZEN														
cooked	½ cup	94	tr	tr	0	6	18	—	19	26	370	5	—	150
fordhook cooked	½ cup	85	tr	tr	0	5	16	—	19	45	347	11	—	162
BIRDS EYE														
Baby	½ cup (3.3 oz)	130	0	0	0	7	24	6	20	115	—	15	—	100
Fordhook	½ cup (3.3 oz)	100	0	0	0	6	19	5	20	10	—	15	—	100
FRESH LIKE														
Baby	3.5 oz	138	1	—	—	7	25	2	34	106	494	19	—	231
GREEN GIANT														
Butter Sauce	⅔ cup (3.6 oz)	120	3	2	<5	6	18	6	20	330	—	2	—	300
Harvest Fresh Baby	½ cup (2.7 oz)	80	0	0	0	4	15	4	20	130	—	5	—	0
LIME														
fresh	1	20	tr	tr	0	tr	7	—	22	1	68	20	6	7
LIME JUICE														
bottled	1 tbsp	3	tr	tr	0	tr	1	—	2	2	12	1	1	3
fresh	1 tbsp	4	tr	tr	0	tr	1	—	2	0	17	5	—	2

FOOD	PORTION	CALORIES	FAT	SAT FAT	CHOL	PROTEIN	CARBO	FIBER	CALCIUM	SOD	POTAS	VIT C	FOLIC	VIT A
AFTER THE FALL														
Caribbean Lime	1 can (12 oz)	170	0	0	0	2	42	0	20	25	60	2	—	0
Key West	1 cup (8 oz)	100	0	0	0	1	25	0	0	10	—	9	—	0
ODWALLA														
Summertime Lime	8 fl oz	90	0	0	0	0	23	0	0	10	—	5	—	0
REALIME														
Juice	1 oz	6	0	0	0	0	2	—	—	10	25	5	—	—

LIQUOR/LIQUEUR

(*see also* BEER AND ALE, CHAMPAGNE, DRINK MIXERS, MALT, WINE, WINE COOLERS)

FOOD	PORTION	CALORIES	FAT	SAT FAT	CHOL	PROTEIN	CARBO	FIBER	CALCIUM	SOD	POTAS	VIT C	FOLIC	VIT A
aquavit	3.5 oz	229	0	0	—	0	0	0	—	—	—	0	—	0
bloody mary	5 oz	116	tr	tr	0	1	5	—	10	332	216	20	20	508
bourbon & soda	4 oz	105	0	0	0	0	0	—	4	16	2	0	0	0
coffee liqueur	1½ oz	174	tr	tr	0	0	24	—	1	4	15	0	0	0
coffee w/ cream liqueur	1½ oz	154	7	5	—	1	10	—	7	43	15	0	0	—
cognac	3.5 oz	233	0	0	0	0	1	0	—	—	—	0	—	0
creme de menthe	1½ oz	186	tr	tr	0	0	21	—	0	3	0	—	0	0
daiquiri	2 oz	111	0	0	0	0	4	—	3	1	13	1	1	2
gin	1½ oz	110	0	0	0	0	0	—	0	1	0	0	0	0
gin & tonic	7.5 oz	171	0	0	0	0	16	—	4	10	12	1	1	2
gin ricky	4 oz	150	0	0	0	—	—	—	2	—	—	—	—	—
manhattan	2 oz	128	0	0	0	0	2	—	1	2	15	0	tr	0
martini	2½ oz	156	0	0	0	0	tr	—	1	2	13	0	tr	—
pina colada	4½ oz	262	3	1	0	1	40	—	11	9	100	7	14	3
planter's punch	3½ oz	175	0	0	0	—	—	—	4	—	—	—	—	—
rum	1½ oz	97	0	0	0	0	0	—	0	0	1	0	0	0
screwdriver	7 oz	174	tr	tr	0	1	18	—	16	2	325	67	75	133
tequila sunrise	5½ oz	189	tr	tr	0	1	15	—	10	7	178	13	—	166
tom collins	7½ oz	121	0	0	0	tr	3	—	10	39	18	4	2	2
vodka	1½ oz	97	0	0	0	0	0	—	0	0	0	0	0	0
whiskey	1½ oz	105	0	0	0	0	tr	—	0	0	1	0	0	0
whiskey sour	3 oz	123	tr	tr	0	tr	5	—	5	10	48	11	5	7
whiskey sour mix not prep	1 pkg (0.6 oz)	64	0	0	0	tr	16	—	45	46	3	1	0	5

LIVER

(*see also* PATE)

FOOD	PORTION	CALORIES	FAT	SAT FAT	CHOL	PROTEIN	CARBO	FIBER	CALCIUM	SOD	POTAS	VIT C	FOLIC	VIT A
beef braised	3 oz	137	4	2	331	21	3	—	6	59	200	19	184	30327
beef pan-fried	3 oz	184	7	2	410	23	7	—	9	90	309	19	187	30689
chicken stewed	1 cup (5 oz)	219	8	3	883	34	1	—	20	71	196	22	1077	22925
duck raw	1 (1.5 oz)	60	2	1	227	8	2	—	5	—	—	—	24	17559
goose raw	1 (3.3 oz)	125	4	1	—	15	6	—	40	132	216	—	—	29138
lamb braised	3 oz	187	7	3	426	26	2	—	7	48	188	3	62	21203
lamb fried	3 oz	202	11	4	419	22	3	—	8	105	299	11	340	22098
pork braised	3 oz	140	4	1	302	22	3	0	9	42	—	20	139	5297
turkey simmered	1 cup (5 oz)	237	8	3	876	34	5	—	15	89	272	3	932	17614

FOOD	PORTION	CALORIES	FAT	SAT FAT	CHOL	PROTEIN	CARBO	FIBER	CALCIUM	SOD	POTAS	VIT C	FOLIC	VIT A
veal braised	3 oz	140	6	2	477	18	2	—	6	45	174	26	645	22851
veal fried	3 oz	208	10	4	280	25	3	—	10	112	372	18	272	15978
SHADY BROOK														
Turkey	4 oz	160	5	2	530	23	—	—	—	110	—	—	—	—
LOBSTER														
(*see also* CRAYFISH)														
CANNED														
PROGRESSO														
Rock Lobster Sauce	½ cup (4.3 oz)	100	7	1	5	3	6	2	20	430	—	0	—	300
FRESH														
northern cooked	1 cup	142	1	tr	104	30	2	—	88	551	510	—	16	126
northern cooked	3 oz	83	1	tr	61	17	1	—	52	323	299	—	9	74
northern raw	3 oz	77	1	—	81	77	tr	—	—	—	—	—	—	—
northern raw	1 lobster (5.3 oz)	136	1	—	143	28	1	—	—	—	—	—	—	—
FROZEN														
CAJUN COOKIN'														
Crawfish Etouffee	12 oz	390	10	—	—	23	51	—	100	1110	380	—	—	500
LOGANBERRIES														
frzn	1 cup	80	tr	—	0	2	19	—	38	1	213	23	38	52
LONGANS														
fresh	1	2	0	0	0	tr	tr	—	0	0	9	3	—	—
LOQUATS														
fresh	1	5	tr	tr	0	tr	1	—	2	0	26	—	—	—
LOTUS														
root raw sliced	10 slices	45	tr	tr	0	2	14	—	36	33	450	36	—	0
root sliced cooked	10 slices	59	tr	tr	0	1	14	—	23	40	323	24	—	0
seeds dried	1 oz	94	1	tr	0	4	18	—	46	1	389	0	—	14
LOX														
(*see* SALMON)														
LUPINES														
dried cooked	1 cup	197	5	1	0	26	16	—	85	7	407	—	—	—
LYCHEES														
fresh	1	6	tr	—	0	tr	2	—	0	0	16	7	—	0
KA-ME														
Whole Pitted In Syrup	15 pieces (5 oz)	130	0	0	0	0	32	0	—	26	—	—	—	—
MACADAMIA NUTS														
dried	1 oz	199	21	3	0	2	4	—	20	1	104	—	—	0
oil roasted	1 oz	204	22	3	0	2	4	—	13	3	94	0	—	3
MACFARMS OF HAWAII														
Chocolate Covered	¼ cup (1.3 oz)	210	16	6	5	3	18	2	60	25	—	0	—	0
Dry Roasted Salted	¼ cup (1.3 oz)	220	23	4	0	3	4	3	20	65	—	0	—	0

FOOD	PORTION	CALORIES	FAT	SAT FAT	CHOL	PROTEIN	CARBO	FIBER	CALCIUM	SOD	POTAS	VIT C	FOLIC	VIT A
MACFARMS OF HAWAII (CONT.)														
Kona Coffee Dark Chocolate Covered	¼ cup (1.3 oz)	210	16	6	5	3	18	2	60	25	—	0	—	0
MAUNA LOA														
Candy Glazed	1 oz	170	14	—	5	1	11	—	—	80	—	—	—	—
Chocolate Covered	1 oz	170	13	—	0	2	12	—	40	21	—	—	—	—
Honey Roasted	1 oz	200	17	—	0	2	8	—	—	80	—	—	—	—
Macadamia Nut Brittle	1 oz	150	8	—	6	1	19	—	—	140	—	—	—	100
Roasted & Salted	1 oz	210	21	—	0	2	4	—	—	75	—	—	—	—

MACARONI

(see PASTA)

MACE

FOOD	PORTION	CALORIES	FAT	SAT FAT	CHOL	PROTEIN	CARBO	FIBER	CALCIUM	SOD	POTAS	VIT C	FOLIC	VIT A
ground	1 tsp	8	1	tr	0	tr	1	—	4	1	8	—	—	14

MACKEREL

FOOD	PORTION	CALORIES	FAT	SAT FAT	CHOL	PROTEIN	CARBO	FIBER	CALCIUM	SOD	POTAS	VIT C	FOLIC	VIT A
FRESH														
atlantic cooked	3 oz	223	15	4	64	20	0	—	13	71	341	tr	—	153
atlantic raw	3 oz	174	12	3	60	16	0	—	10	76	267	tr	—	140
spanish cooked	1 fillet (5.1 oz)	230	9	3	107	34	0	—	19	96	808	—	—	—
spanish cooked	3 oz	134	5	2	62	20	.0	—	11	56	471	—	—	—
spanish raw	3 oz	118	5	2	65	16	0	—	10	50	379	—	—	—

MALANGA

FOOD	PORTION	CALORIES	FAT	SAT FAT	CHOL	PROTEIN	CARBO	FIBER	CALCIUM	SOD	POTAS	VIT C	FOLIC	VIT A
fresh	½ cup	137	tr	—	—	2	32	—	—	—	—	8	—	0

MALT

FOOD	PORTION	CALORIES	FAT	SAT FAT	CHOL	PROTEIN	CARBO	FIBER	CALCIUM	SOD	POTAS	VIT C	FOLIC	VIT A
nonalcoholic	12 fl oz	32	0	0	0	1	5	—	25	—	—	—	—	—
BARTLES & JAYMES														
Malt Cooler Berry	12 fl oz	210	0	0	0	0	32	—	—	5	—	—	—	—
Malt Cooler Black Cherry	12 fl oz	190	0	0	0	0	30	—	—	5	—	—	—	—
Malt Cooler Light Berry	12 fl oz	140	0	0	0	0	29	—	—	0	—	—	—	—
Malt Cooler Mandarin Lemon	12 fl oz	210	0	0	0	0	34	—	—	5	—	—	—	—
Malt Cooler Margarita	12 fl oz	250	0	0	0	0	44	—	—	40	—	—	—	—
Malt Cooler Original	12 fl oz	180	0	0	0	0	27	—	—	0	—	—	—	—
Malt Cooler Peach	12 fl oz	200	0	0	0	0	31	—	—	5	—	—	—	—
Malt Cooler Pina Colada	12 fl oz	270	0	0	0	0	48	—	—	5	—	—	—	—
Malt Cooler Planter's Punch	12 fl oz	220	0	0	0	0	35	—	—	5	—	—	—	—
Malt Cooler Red Sangria	12 fl oz	190	0	0	0	0	29	—	—	5	—	—	—	—

FOOD	PORTION	CALORIES	FAT	SAT FAT	CHOL	PROTEIN	CARBO	FIBER	CALCIUM	SOD	POTAS	VIT C	FOLIC	VIT A
BARTLES & JAYMES (CONT.)														
Malt Cooler Strawberry	12 fl oz	200	0	0	0	0	31	—	—	5	—	—	—	—
Malt Cooler Strawberry Daiquiri	12 fl oz	220	0	0	0	0	35	—	—	5	—	—	—	—
Malt Cooler Tropical	12 fl oz	220	0	0	0	0	36	—	—	5	—	—	—	—

MALTED MILK
POWDER

CARNATION

Chocolate	3 tbsp (0.7 oz)	90	1	1	0	1	18	tr	0	40	115	0	—	0
Original	3 tbsp (0.7 oz)	90	2	1	5	3	15	tr	40	40	115	0	—	0

MAMMY-APPLE

fresh	1	431	4	—	0	4	106	—	93	127	398	118	—	1946

MANGO

fresh	1	135	1	tr	0	1	35	—	21	4	322	57	—	8060

CANNED

KA-ME

Mango	4 pieces (5 oz)	102	0	0	0	0	25	0	—	10	—	—	—	—

DRIED

RAINFOREST FARMS

Slices	6 slices (1.3 oz)	140	1	0	0	1	33	2	0	108	—	18	—	4000

SONOMA

Pieces	8 pieces (2 oz)	180	1	0	0	0	44	0	20	50	—	6	—	1750

MANGO JUICE

AFTER THE FALL

Hawaiian Mango	1 can (12 oz)	180	0	0	0	0	45	0	20	20	380	1	—	0
Mango Ginger	1 can (12 oz)	150	0	0	0	tr	35	0	20	25	190	1	—	0

FRESH SAMANTHA

Mango Mama	1 cup (8 oz)	125	1	0	0	2	33	2	20	0	—	54	32	2250

KERN'S

Nectar	6 fl oz	100	0	0	0	0	28	—	—	0	60	27	—	750

LIBBY

Nectar	1 can (11.5 fl oz)	210	0	0	0	0	52	—	40	10	130	60	—	1500

SNAPPLE

Diet Mango Madness	8 fl oz	13	0	0	0	0	3	—	0	10	50	—	—	0
Mango Madness Cocktail	8 fl oz	110	0	0	0	0	29	—	0	10	12	—	—	0

TANG

Drink Mix as prep	1 serv (8 oz)	100	0	0	0	0	25	0	40	0	0	60	—	500

MARGARINE

(see also BUTTER BLENDS, BUTTER SUBSTITUTES)

FOOD	PORTION	CALORIES	FAT	SAT FAT	CHOL	PROTEIN	CARBO	FIBER	CALCIUM	SOD	POTAS	VIT C	FOLIC	VIT A
squeeze soybean & cottonseed	1 tsp	34	4	1	0	tr	0	—	3	37	4	tr	tr	155
stick corn	1 tsp	34	4	1	0	0	0	—	1	44	2	tr	tr	155
stick corn	1 stick (4 oz)	815	91	15	0	1	1	—	34	1070	48	tr	1	3750
stick salted	1 stick (4 oz)	815	91	18	0	1	1	—	34	1069	48	tr	1	3750
stick salted	1 tsp	39	4	1	0	0	0	—	1	44	2	tr	tr	155
stick unsalted	1 tsp	34	4	1	0	0	0	—	1	tr	1	tr	tr	155
stick unsalted	1 stick (4 oz)	809	91	17	0	1	1	—	20	2	28	tr	1	3750
tub corn	1 cup	1626	183	32	0	2	1	—	60	2449	86	tr	2	7507
tub corn	1 tsp	34	4	1	0	0	0	—	1	51	2	tr	tr	155
tub diet	1 cup	800	90	18	0	1	1	—	41	2226	59	tr	2	7672
tub diet	1 tsp	17	2	tr	0	0	0	—	1	46	1	tr	tr	159
tub safflower	1 tsp	34	4	tr	0	0	0	—	1	51	2	tr	tr	21
tub safflower	1 cup	1626	183	21	0	2	1	—	60	2449	86	tr	2	2254
tub salted	1 tsp	34	4	1	0	0	0	—	1	51	2	tr	tr	155
tub salted	1 cup	1626	183	31	0	2	1	—	60	2449	86	tr	2	7507
tub soybean salted	1 cup	1626	183	31	0	2	1	—	60	2449	86	tr	2	7507
tub soybean salted	1 tsp	34	4	1	0	0	0	—	1	51	2	tr	tr	155
tub soybean unsalted	1 tsp	34	4	1	0	0	0	—	1	1	2	tr	tr	155
tub soybean unsalted	1 cup	1626	182	31	0	2	2	—	60	63	86	tr	2	7507
tub unsalted	1 cup	1626	182	31	0	0	0	—	60	63	86	tr	2	7507
tub unsalted	1 tsp	34	4	1	0	0	0	—	1	1	2	tr	tr	155
BLUE BONNET														
Stick	1 tbsp	100	11	2	0	0	0	—	—	95	5	—	—	500
Tub	1 tbsp	100	11	2	0	0	0	—	—	95	5	—	—	500
Whipped	1 tbsp	80	9	1	0	0	0	—	—	100	5	—	—	500
FLEISCHMANN'S														
Stick	1 tbsp	100	11	2	0	0	0	—	—	95	5	—	—	500
Stick Light Corn Oil	1 tbsp	80	8	1	0	0	0	—	—	70	10	—	—	500
Stick Sweet Unsalted	1 tbsp	100	11	2	0	0	0	—	—	0	0	—	—	500
HAIN														
Stick Safflower	1 tbsp	100	11	2	0	0	0	—	—	170	—	—	—	500
Stick Safflower Unsalted	1 tbsp	100	11	2	0	0	0	—	—	<5	—	—	—	500
Tub Safflower	1 tbsp	100	11	2	0	0	0	—	—	170	—	—	—	500
HOLLYWOOD														
Safflower	1 tbsp	100	11	2	0	0	0	—	—	130	0	—	—	500
Safflower Unsalted Sweet	1 tbsp	100	11	2	0	0	0	—	—	2	—	—	—	500
Soft Spread	1 tbsp	90	10	1	0	0	1	0	—	135	0	—	—	500

FOOD	PORTION	CALORIES	FAT	SAT FAT	CHOL	PROTEIN	CARBO	FIBER	CALCIUM	SOD	POTAS	VIT C	FOLIC	VIT A
LAND O'LAKES														
Stick	1 tbsp (0.5 oz)	90	10	2	0	0	0	—	—	95	—	—	—	500
Stick With Sweet Cream	1 tbsp (0.5 oz)	90	10	2	0	0	0	—	—	95	—	—	—	400
Stick With Sweet Cream Unsalted	1 tbsp (0.5 oz)	90	10	2	0	0	0	—	—	0	—	—	—	400
Tub	1 tbsp (0.5 oz)	80	8	2	0	0	0	—	—	90	—	—	—	500
Tub With Sweet Cream	1 tbsp (0.5 oz)	80	8	2	0	0	0	—	—	70	—	—	—	400
NUCANOLA														
Stick	1 tbsp	90	10	1	0	0	0	—	—	90	—	—	—	500
PARKAY														
Squeeze	1 tbsp (0.5 oz)	80	9	2	0	0	0	0	0	120	0	0	—	500
Stick	1 tbsp (0.5 oz)	90	10	2	0	0	0	0	0	110	5	0	—	500
Stick ⅓ Less Fat	1 tbsp (0.5 oz)	70	7	2	0	0	0	0	0	120	0	0	—	500
Tub	1 tbsp (0.5 oz)	60	7	2	0	0	0	0	0	110	0	0	—	500
Tub Light	1 tbsp (0.5 oz)	50	6	1	0	0	0	0	0	120	0	0	—	500
Tub Soft	1 tbsp (0.5 oz)	100	11	2	0	0	0	0	0	105	10	0	—	500
Tub Soft Diet	1 tbsp (0.5 oz)	50	6	1	0	0	0	0	0	110	0	0	—	500
Whipped	1 tbsp (0.3 oz)	70	7	2	0	0	0	0	0	70	5	0	—	300
PROMISE														
Spread Soft	1 tbsp	80	8	2	0	—	—	—	—	—	—	—	—	—
Spread Stick	1 tbsp	90	10	3	0	—	—	—	—	—	—	—	—	—
Spread Light Soft	1 tbsp	50	6	1	0	—	—	—	—	—	—	—	—	—
Spread Light Stick	1 tbsp	50	6	2	0	—	—	—	—	—	—	—	—	—
Ultra Soft	1 tbsp	30	4	0	0	—	—	—	—	—	—	—	—	—
Ultra Spread Fat Free	1 tbsp	5	0	0	0	—	—	—	—	—	—	—	—	—
SMART BALANCE														
No Trans Fat	1 tbsp (0.5 oz)	120	14	4	0	0	0	—	—	0	—	—	—	500
No Trans Fat Light	1 tbsp (0.5 oz)	45	5	2	0	0	0	—	—	100	—	—	—	500
No Trans Fat Spread	1 tbsp (0.5 oz)	80	9	3	0	0	0	—	—	90	—	—	—	500
SMART BEAT														
Light Unsalted	1 tbsp (0.5 oz)	25	3	0	0	0	0	—	—	0	—	—	—	500
Squeeze Fat Free	1 tbsp (0.5 oz)	5	0	0	0	0	1	—	—	100	—	—	—	500
Super Light Trans Fat Free	1 tbsp (0.5 oz)	20	2	0	0	0	0	—	—	105	—	—	—	500
Tub	1 tbsp	25	3	tr	0	0	0	—	—	110	—	—	—	500
Tub Unsalted	1 tbsp	25	3	tr	0	0	0	—	—	0	—	—	—	500
TREE OF LIFE														
Canola Soft	1 tbsp (0.5 oz)	100	11	2	0	0	0	—	—	110	—	—	—	500
Stick 100% Soy	1 tbsp (0.5 oz)	100	11	2	0	0	0	—	—	110	—	—	—	500
Stick 100% Soy Salt Free	1 tbsp (0.5 oz)	100	11	2	0	0	0	—	—	0	—	—	—	500
Stick Canola Soy	1 tbsp (0.5 oz)	100	11	2	0	0	0	—	—	110	—	—	—	500

FOOD	PORTION	CALORIES	FAT	SAT FAT	CHOL	PROTEIN	CARBO	FIBER	CALCIUM	SOD	POTAS	VIT C	FOLIC	VIT A
TREE OF LIFE (CONT.)														
Stick Canola Soy Salt Free	1 tbsp (0.5 oz)	100	11	2	0	0	0	—	—	0	—	—	—	500
WEIGHT WATCHERS														
Light	1 tbsp	45	4	1	0	0	2	0	0	70	5	0	—	500
Light Sodium Free	1 tbsp	45	4	1	0	0	2	0	0	0	—	0	—	500
MARINADE														
(*see* SAUCE)														
MARJORAM														
dried	1 tsp	2	tr	—	0	tr	tr	—	12	tr	9	—	—	48
MARSHMALLOW														
marshmallow	1 reg (0.3 oz)	23	0	0	0	tr	6	—	0	3	0	0	0	0
marshmallow	1 cup (1.6 oz)	146	tr	—	0	1	37	—	1	22	2	0	—	0
CAMPFIRE														
Large	2	40	0	0	0	0	10	—	—	10	0	—	—	—
Miniature	24	40	0	0	0	0	10	—	—	10	0	—	—	—
JOYVA														
Twists Chocolate Covered	2 (1.5 oz)	190	4	2	0	1	21	0	0	20	—	0	—	0
JUST BORN														
Peeps	5 (1.5 oz)	160	0	0	0	1	40	—	—	15	—	—	—	—
MATZO														
egg	1 (1 oz)	111	1	tr	—	4	22	1	11	6	43	—	—	12
egg & onion	1 (1 oz)	111	1	tr	—	3	22	1	10	81	24	—	3	—
plain	1 (1 oz)	112	tr	tr	0	3	24	1	4	0	32	0	4	0
whole wheat	1 (1 oz)	99	tr	tr	0	4	22	3	7	1	89	0	10	0
GOODMAN'S														
Matzo Ball Mix 50% Less Salt	2 tbsp (0.5 oz)	50	0	0	0	1	11	0	20	150	—	0	—	0
Matzo Ball Mix as prep	2 tbsp (0.5 oz)	60	0	0	0	2	12	1	20	190	—	0	—	0
HOROWITZ MARGARETEN														
Egg Milk Chocolate Coated	1 oz	97	4	3	8	3	16	1	20	7	—	—	—	—
MANISCHEWITZ														
Egg Dark Chocolate Coated	½ matzo (1 oz)	97	3	2	8	2	17	1	—	7	—	—	—	—
STREIT'S														
Dietetic	1 (1 oz)	100	0	0	0	3	23	1	0	0	—	0	—	0
Lightly Salted	1 (1 oz)	110	1	0	0	3	23	1	0	65	—	0	—	0
Matzoh Meal	¼ cup (1 oz)	110	1	0	0	3	24	1	0	0	—	0	—	0
Passover	1 (1 oz)	110	1	0	0	3	25	1	0	0	—	0	—	0
Unsalted	1 (0.9 oz)	100	1	0	0	3	22	1	0	0	—	0	—	0
Whole Wheat	1 (1 oz)	110	1	0	0	5	24	4	0	0	—	0	—	0
MAYONNAISE														
(*see also* MAYONNAISE TYPE SALAD DRESSING, RELISH)														
mayonnaise	1 cup	1577	175	26	130	2	6	—	40	1250	75	—	—	616

FOOD	PORTION	CALORIES	FAT	SAT FAT	CHOL	PROTEIN	CARBO	FIBER	CALCIUM	SOD	POTAS	VIT C	FOLIC	VIT A
mayonnaise	1 tbsp	99	11	2	8	tr	tr	—	2	78	5	—	—	39
reduced calorie	1 tbsp	34	3	1	4	0	2	—	—	75	—	—	—	—
reduced calorie	1 cup	556	46	8	58	1	38	—	—	1193	—	—	—	—
sandwich spread	1 tbsp	60	5	1	12	tr	3	—	—	—	—	—	—	—
BAMA														
Mayonnaise	1 tbsp	100	11	—	—	0	0	—	—	65	0	—	—	—
BENNETT'S														
Mayonnaise	1 tbsp	110	12	—	—	0	1	—	—	65	0	—	—	—
HAIN														
Canola	1 tbsp	60	5	0	0	0	2	—	—	160	25	—	—	—
Canola	1 tbsp	100	11	1	5	0	tr	—	—	100	5	—	—	—
Cold Processed	1 tbsp	110	12	2	5	0	0	—	—	70	0	—	—	—
Eggless No Salt Added	1 tbsp	110	12	2	0	0	0	—	—	<5	0	—	—	—
Light Low Sodium	1 tbsp	60	6	1	10	0	2	—	—	95	45	—	—	—
Real No Salt Added	1 tbsp	110	12	2	5	0	0	—	—	0	45	—	—	—
Safflower	1 tbsp	110	12	1	5	0	0	—	—	70	0	—	—	—
HOLLYWOOD														
Canola	1 tbsp	100	11	3	5	0	tr	—	—	100	5	—	—	—
Mayonnaise	1 tbsp	110	12	1	5	0	0	—	—	80	0	—	—	—
Safflower	1 tbsp	100	12	1	5	0	0	—	—	75	0	—	—	—
KRAFT														
Fat Free	1 tbsp (0.6 oz)	10	0	0	0	0	2	0	0	120	10	0	—	0
Light	1 tbsp (0.5 oz)	50	5	1	5	0	2	0	0	90	10	0	—	0
Real	1 tbsp (0.5 oz)	100	11	2	5	0	0	0	0	75	0	0	—	0
MCILHENNY														
Spicy	1 tbsp (0.5 oz)	108	12	3	8	tr	1	tr	2	94	—	tr	—	73
RED WING														
"H" Style	1 tbsp (0.5 oz)	110	11	2	10	0	1	0	0	80	—	0	—	0
SMART BEAT														
Canola Oil	1 tbsp	40	4	tr	0	0	1	—	—	110	—	—	—	—
Corn Beat	1 tbsp	40	4	tr	0	0	1	—	—	110	—	—	—	—
Fat Free	1 tbsp	10	0	0	0	0	3	—	—	135	5	—	—	—
WEIGHT WATCHERS														
Fat Free	1 tbsp	10	0	0	0	0	3	0	0	105	—	0	—	0
Light	1 tbsp	25	2	0	5	0	1	0	0	130	—	0	—	0
Light Low Sodium	1 tbsp	25	2	1	5	0	1	0	0	40	—	0	—	0

MAYONNAISE TYPE SALAD DRESSING

(*see also* MAYONNAISE, RELISH)

FOOD	PORTION	CALORIES	FAT	SAT FAT	CHOL	PROTEIN	CARBO	FIBER	CALCIUM	SOD	POTAS	VIT C	FOLIC	VIT A
home recipe	1 cup	400	24	7	—	11	38	—	214	1872	309	2	—	1048
home recipe	1 tbsp	25	2	1	—	1	2	—	13	117	19	tr	—	66
mayonnaise type salad dressing	1 cup	916	78	12	60	2	56	—	33	1670	21	—	—	517
mayonnaise type salad dressing	1 tbsp	57	5	1	4	tr	4	—	—	—	—	—	—	32

FOOD	PORTION	CALORIES	FAT	SAT FAT	CHOL	PROTEIN	CARBO	FIBER	CALCIUM	SOD	POTAS	VIT C	FOLIC	VIT A
reduced calorie w/o cholesterol	1 cup	1084	107	17	0	tr	36	—	—	794	—	—	—	—
reduced calorie w/o cholesterol	1 tbsp	68	7	1	0	7	2	—	—	49	—	—	—	—
BAMA														
Dressing	1 tbsp	50	4	—	—	0	3	—	—	105	0	—	—	—
MIRACLE WHIP														
Free	1 tbsp (0.5 oz)	15	0	0	0	0	2	0	0	125	10	0	—	0
Light	1 tbsp (0.5 oz)	35	3	0	<5	0	2	0	0	130	0	0	—	0
Salad Dressing	1 tbsp (0.6 oz)	70	7	1	5	0	2	0	0	95	0	0	—	0
NAYONAISE														
Cholesterol Free	1 tbsp (0.5 oz)	35	3	tr	0	1	1	tr	7	104	22	tr	tr	tr
Fat Free	1 tbsp (0.5 oz)	11	tr	tr	0	tr	2	tr	1	107	3	tr	0	0
SPIN BLEND														
Cholesterol Free	1 tbsp	40	4	1	0	0	2	—	—	110	—	—	—	—
Dressing	1 tbsp	60	5	1	10	0	3	—	—	110	—	—	—	—
WEIGHT WATCHERS														
Fat Free Whipped Dressing	1 tbsp	15	0	0	0	0	3	0	0	95	—	0	—	0

MEAT STICKS

FOOD	PORTION	CALORIES	FAT	SAT FAT	CHOL	PROTEIN	CARBO	FIBER	CALCIUM	SOD	POTAS	VIT C	FOLIC	VIT A
jerky beef	1 oz	96	4	1	32	11	4	—	—	815	—	—	—	—
jerky beef	1 lg piece (0.7 oz)	67	3	1	22	8	3	—	—	569	—	—	—	—
smoked	1 (0.7 oz)	109	10	4	26	4	1	—	13	293	—	—	0	—
smoked	1 oz	156	14	6	38	6	2	—	19	420	—	—	0	—
PEMMICAN														
Original Tender Kippered Beef Steak	1	110	5	3	35	12	3	0	—	1100	—	0	—	—
SLIM JIM														
Spicy	1 (0.28 oz)	45	4	2	5	2	0	0	—	110	—	2	—	0

MEAT SUBSTITUTES

(*see also* BACON SUBSTITUTES, CHICKEN SUBSTITUTES, SAUSAGE SUBSTITUTES, TURKEY SUBSTITUTES)

FOOD	PORTION	CALORIES	FAT	SAT FAT	CHOL	PROTEIN	CARBO	FIBER	CALCIUM	SOD	POTAS	VIT C	FOLIC	VIT A
simulated sausage	1 patty (38 g)	97	7	1	0	7	4	—	24	137	88	0	10	243
simulated sausage	1 link (25 g)	64	5	1	0	5	2	—	16	222	58	0	7	160
simulated meat product	1 oz	88	1	tr	0	11	11	—	57	3	—	—	—	9
BOCA BURGERS														
Chef Max's Original	1 patty (2.5 oz)	110	2	1	3	14	9	4	—	296	316	—	—	—
Hint of Garlic	1 patty (2.5 oz)	110	2	1	3	14	9	4	—	296	316	—	—	—
Vegan Original	1 patty (2.5 oz)	84	0	0	0	12	9	5	—	269	338	—	—	—
GARDENBURGER														
Classic Greek	1 (2.5 oz)	120	3	2	10	6	17	2	80	310	—	1	—	300

FOOD	PORTION	CALORIES	FAT	SAT FAT	CHOL	PROTEIN	CARBO	FIBER	CALCIUM	SOD	POTAS	VIT C	FOLIC	VIT A
GARDENBURGER (CONT.)														
Fire Roasted Vegetable	1 (2.5 oz)	120	3	2	10	7	17	2	100	270	—	6	—	300
Hamburger Style	1 (2.5 oz)	90	0	0	0	16	7	3	80	370	—	6	—	0
Hamburger Style w/ Cheese	1 (2.5 oz)	110	3	2	5	16	7	3	100	380	—	6	—	100
Savory Mushroom	1 (2.5 oz)	120	3	2	10	6	18	4	100	270	—	0	—	100
GREEN GIANT														
Southwestern Style	1 patty (3.2 oz)	140	4	2	0	18	9	5	80	370	—	0	—	0
HARVEST BURGERS														
For Recipes	⅔ cup (2.1 oz)	90	0	0	0	14	8	4	80	270	—	0	—	0
Italian Style	1 patty (3.2 oz)	140	5	2	0	17	8	5	80	370	—	0	—	0
Original	1 (3 oz)	140	4	2	0	18	8	5	80	370	—	0	—	0
HARVEST DIRECT														
TVP Beef Chunks	3.5 oz	280	1	tr	0	52	32	18	—	15	2200	—	—	—
TVP Beef Chunks Flavored	3.5 oz	250	1	tr	0	48	30	17	—	2000	2900	—	—	—
TVP Beef Strips	3.5 oz	280	1	tr	0	52	32	18	—	15	2200	—	—	—
TVP Ground Beef	3.5 oz	280	1	tr	0	52	32	18	—	15	2200	—	—	—
TVP Ground Beef Flavored	3.5 oz	250	1	tr	0	48	30	17	—	2000	2900	—	—	—
KEN & ROBERT'S														
Veggie Burger	1 (62 g)	110	2	0	0	5	19	—	—	390	215	—	—	—
KNOX MOUNTAIN FARM														
Wheat Balls Mix	1 serv (¹/₁₀ pkg)	110	1	—	—	14	9	2	60	360				
LIGHTLIFE														
American Grill	2.75 oz	110	3	1	0	13	8	—	—	325	—	—	—	—
Barbecue Grill	2.75 oz	130	6	1	0	11	10	—	—	336	—	—	—	—
Smart Deli Slices	2 slices (1.5 oz)	44	0	0	0	8	1	—	—	290	—	—	—	—
Smart Dogs	1 (1.5 oz)	40	0	0	0	8	1	—	—	290	—	—	—	—
Smart Dogs To Go	1 (5 oz)	115	0	0	0	13	19	—	—	300	—	—	—	—
Vegetarian Sloppy Joe	4.3 oz	130	6	1	0	9	11	—	—	310	—	—	—	—
LOMA LINDA														
Big Franks	1 (1.8 oz)	110	7	1	0	10	2	2	0	240	50	0	—	—
Big Franks Low Fat	1 (1.8 oz)	80	3	1	0	11	3	2	0	220	50	0	—	0
Corn Dogs	1 (2.5 oz)	200	9	2	0	10	18	3	0	500	40	0	—	0
Dinner Cuts	2 pieces (3.2 oz)	90	2	1	0	17	3	2	0	500	40	0	—	0
Nuteena	⅜ in slice (1.9 oz)	160	13	5	0	6	6	2	0	120	170	0	—	0
Patty Mix not prep	⅓ cup (0.9 oz)	90	1	0	0	14	7	5	20	480	400	0	—	0

FOOD	PORTION	CALORIES	FAT	SAT FAT	CHOL	PROTEIN	CARBO	FIBER	CALCIUM	SOD	POTAS	VIT C	FOLIC	VIT A
LOMA LINDA (CONT.)														
Redi-Burger	⅝ in slice (3 oz)	120	3	1	0	18	7	4	0	450	140	0	—	0
Sandwich Spread	¼ cup (1.9 oz)	80	5	1	0	4	7	3	20	260	140	0	—	100
Savory Dinner Loaf Mix not prep	⅓ cup (0.9 oz)	90	2	0	0	14	7	5	20	560	410	0	—	0
Swiss Stake	1 piece (3.2 oz)	120	6	1	0	9	8	4	20	430	230	0	—	0
Tender Bits	6 pieces (3 oz)	110	5	1	0	11	7	3	0	440	55	0	—	0
Tender Rounds	6 pieces (2.8 oz)	120	5	1	0	14	5	3	0	330	70	0	—	0
Vege-Burger	¼ cup (1.9 oz)	70	2	1	0	11	2	2	0	115	30	0	—	0
Vita Burger Chunks not prep	¼ cup (0.7 oz)	70	1	0	0	10	6	3	40	350	500	0	—	0
Vita Burger Granules	3 tbsp (0.7 oz)	70	1	0	0	10	6	3	40	350	500	0	—	0
MIDLAND HARVEST														
Burger n' Loaf Chili w/o Beans	0.8 oz	90	3	1	0	9	7	2	80	225	425	—	—	—
Burger n' Loaf Herbs & Spice	3.2 oz	140	5	1	0	16	7	4	100	250	450	—	—	—
Burger n' Loaf Italian	3.2 oz	140	5	1	0	16	7	4	100	375	500	—	—	—
Burger n' Loaf Original	3.2 oz	140	5	1	0	16	7	4	100	350	450	—	—	—
Burger n' Loaf Sloppy Joe w/o Sauce	0.8 oz	80	2	1	0	8	9	1	60	165	360	—	—	—
Burger n' Loaf Taco	2.7 oz	90	2	tr	0	7	7	1	50	250	350	—	—	—
MORNINGSTAR FARMS														
Better'n Burger	1 (2.7 oz)	70	0	0	0	11	6	3	60	360	390	0	—	0
Burger Style Recipe Crumbles	⅔ cup (1.9 oz)	90	3	0	0	10	4	2	20	260	100	0	—	0
Deli Franks	1 (1.6 oz)	110	7	1	0	10	3	2	0	520	50	0	—	0
Garden Grille	1 patty (2.5 oz)	120	3	1	<5	6	18	4	60	280	130	0	—	0
Garden Veggie Patties	1 patty (2.4 oz)	100	3	1	0	10	9	4	40	350	180	0	—	0
Ground Meatless	½ cup (1.9 oz)	60	0	0	0	10	4	2	20	260	100	0	—	0
Prime Patties	1 (2.7 oz)	110	2	0	0	19	5	3	60	300	170	0	—	0
Quarter Prime	1 patty (3.4 oz)	140	2	0	0	24	6	3	60	370	210	9	—	0
Southwestern Veggie Burger Kit	¼ pkg (0.9 oz)	90	0	0	0	12	9	4	60	360	300	0	—	0
Spicy Black Bean Burger	1 (2.7 oz)	110	1	0	0	11	16	5	40	470	260	0	—	0
NATURAL TOUCH														
Dinner Entree	1 patty (3 oz)	220	15	3	0	19	2	2	40	380	100	0	—	0

FOOD	PORTION	CALORIES	FAT	SAT FAT	CHOL	PROTEIN	CARBO	FIBER	CALCIUM	SOD	POTAS	VIT C	FOLIC	VIT A
NATURAL TOUCH (CONT.)														
Garden Veggie Pattie	1 (2.4 oz)	110	3	1	0	10	8	3	0	280	160	0	—	200
Loaf Mix not prep	4 tbsp (1 oz)	100	1	0	0	14	10	7	40	700	410	0	—	0
Okara Pattie	1 (2.2 oz)	110	5	1	0	11	4	3	40	360	170	0	—	0
Original Veggie Burger Kit not prep	¼ pkg (0.8 oz)	80	0	0	0	14	6	4	60	360	150	0	—	0
Southwestern Veggie Burger Kit not prep	¼ pkg (0.9 oz)	90	0	0	0	12	9	4	60	360	300	0	—	0
Spicy Black Bean Burger	1 (2.7 oz)	100	1	0	0	11	15	5	60	330	230	0	—	100
Stroganoff Mix not prep	4 tbsp (0.8 oz)	90	4	2	10	5	10	3	60	610	230	0	—	0
Taco Mix not prep	3 tbsp (0.6 oz)	90	1	0	0	8	5	3	20	590	380	1	—	400
Vegan Burger	1 (2.7 oz)	70	0	0	0	11	6	3	60	370	390	0	—	0
Vegan Burger Crumbles	½ cup (1.9 oz)	60	0	0	0	10	4	2	20	260	100	0	—	0
Vege Frank	1 (1.6 oz)	100	6	1	0	10	2	2	0	470	50	0	—	0
NEWMENU														
VegiBurger	1 patty (3 oz)	110	1	0	0	13	12	1	—	320	—	—	—	—
VegiDogs	1 (1.5 oz)	45	0	0	0	9	1	0	—	170	—	—	—	—
QUORN														
Burger	1 patty (3 oz)	100	4	2	0	11	9	4	34	420	—	—	—	—
SOVEX														
Better Than Burger?	½ cup (1.9 oz)	165	2	1	0	20	25	9	90	52	—	5	—	50
SOY IS US														
Beef Not!	½ cup (1.75 oz)	140	2	1	0	25	15	9	160	5	—	0	—	0
TRADER JOE'S														
French Village Burger Champignon No Soy No Preservatives	1 patty (3.4 oz)	190	3	1	10	11	29	6	80	120	—	0	—	200
VEGGIE PATCH														
Burgeriffics	1 (2.5 oz)	110	3	—	0	14	8	4	60	410	—	—	—	—
Perfectly Franks	1 (1.7 oz)	70	2	—	0	10	2	1	20	340	—	—	—	—
Veggie Rounds	1 (2.5 oz)	120	3	—	0	12	15	4	80	250	—	—	—	—
Veggitinos Meatballs	5 (2.8 oz)	120	4	—	0	13	10	3	60	470	—	—	—	—
WHITE WAVE														
Meatless Healthy Franks	1 (1.5 oz)	90	2	0	0	13	6	0	0	350	—	0	—	0
Meatless Jumbo Franks	1 (3 oz)	170	3	1	0	26	11	0	20	690	—	1	—	0

FOOD	PORTION	CALORIES	FAT	SAT FAT	CHOL	PROTEIN	CARBO	FIBER	CALCIUM	SOD	POTAS	VIT C	FOLIC	VIT A
WHITE WAVE (CONT.)														
Meatless Sandwich Slices Beef	2 slices (1.6 oz)	90	0	0	0	14	8	1	0	270	—	1	—	0
Meatless Sandwich Slices Bologna	2 slices (1.6 oz)	120	8	2	0	8	5	1	40	370	—	0	—	0
Meatless Sandwich Slices Pastrami	2 slices (1.6 oz)	90	0	0	0	14	8	1	0	270	—	1	—	0
Meatless Healthy Franks	1 (1.5 oz)	90	2	0	0	13	6	—	—	350	—	—	—	—
Veggie Burger	1 patty (2.5 oz)	110	3	0	0	5	16	2	60	210	—	6	—	1250
WORTHINGTON														
Beef Style Meatless	3/8 in slice (1.9 oz)	110	7	1	0	9	4	3	0	620	45	0	—	0
Bolono	3 slices (2 oz)	80	4	1	0	10	2	2	40	720	120	0	—	0
Choplets	2 slices (3.2 oz)	90	2	1	0	17	3	2	0	500	40	0	—	0
Corn Beef Meatless	4 slices (2 oz)	140	9	2	0	10	5	2	0	520	60	0	—	0
Country Stew	1 cup (8.4 oz)	210	9	2	0	13	20	5	60	830	270	0	—	2250
Dinner Roast	3/4 in slice (3 oz)	180	12	2	<5	12	5	3	40	580	55	0	—	0
FriPats	1 patty (2.2 oz)	60	6	1	0	14	4	3	60	320	125	0	—	0
Granburger not prep	3 tbsp (0.6 oz)	60	1	0	0	10	3	2	40	410	220	0	—	0
Multigrain Cutlet	2 slices (3.2 oz)	100	2	1	0	15	5	4	0	390	30	0	—	0
Numete	3/8 in slice (1.9 oz)	130	10	3	0	6	5	3	0	270	160	0	—	0
Prime Stakes	1 piece (3.2 oz)	140	9	2	0	9	4	4	0	440	80	0	—	0
Prosage Patties	1 (1.3 oz)	100	3	1	0	9	3	2	0	300	100	0	—	0
Prosage Roll	5/8 in slice (1.9 oz)	140	10	2	0	10	2	2	0	390	80	0	—	0
Protose	3/8 in slice (1.9 oz)	130	7	1	0	13	5	3	0	280	50	0	—	0
Salami Meatless	3 slices (2 oz)	130	8	1	0	12	2	2	20	930	95	0	—	0
Savory Slices	3 slices (2.9 oz)	150	9	4	0	10	6	3	0	540	40	0	—	0
Smoked Beef Meatless	6 slices (2 oz)	120	6	1	0	11	6	3	0	730	150	0	—	0
Stakelets	1 piece (2.5 oz)	140	8	2	0	12	6	2	40	480	95	0	—	0
Veelets	1 patty (2.5 oz)	180	9	2	0	14	10	5	40	390	120	0	—	0
Vegetable Skallops	1/2 cup (3 oz)	90	2	1	0	15	3	2	0	410	10	0	—	0
Vegetable Steaks	2 pieces (2.5 oz)	80	2	1	0	15	3	3	0	300	20	0	—	0

FOOD	PORTION	CALORIES	FAT	SAT FAT	CHOL	PROTEIN	CARBO	FIBER	CALCIUM	SOD	POTAS	VIT C	FOLIC	VIT A
WORTHINGTON (CONT.)														
Vegetarian Burger	¼ cup (1.9 oz)	60	2	0	0	9	2	1	0	270	25	0	—	0
Veja Links Low Fat	1 (1.1 oz)	40	2	0	0	5	1	0	0	190	20	0	—	0
Wham	2 slices (1.6 oz)	80	5	1	0	7	1	0	0	430	90	0	—	0
ZOGLO'S														
Crispy Vegetarian Cutlets	1 (3.5 oz)	200	10	2	0	20	10	2	300	300	—	18	—	1500
Savory Vegetarian Kebabs	1 serv (2.8 oz)	135	5	1	0	18	5	2	250	240	—	15	—	1250
Tender Vegetarian Burgers	1 (2.6 oz)	150	7	1	0	17	5	2	250	230	—	15	—	1250
Vegetable Patties	1 (2.6 oz)	130	5	1	0	11	10	2	250	270	—	15	—	1250
Vegetarian Franks	1 (2.6 oz)	125	5	1	0	15	5	2	250	240	—	15	—	1250

MELON

(*see also individual names*)

FROZEN

FOOD	PORTION	CALORIES	FAT	SAT FAT	CHOL	PROTEIN	CARBO	FIBER	CALCIUM	SOD	POTAS	VIT C	FOLIC	VIT A
melon balls	1 cup	55	tr	—	0	1	14	—	17	53	484	11	45	3096
BIG VALLEY														
Mixed	¾ cup (4.9 oz)	40	0	0	0	1	10	1	0	16	—	30	—	1500

MEXICAN FOOD

(*see* SALSA, SAUCE, SPANISH FOODS, TORTILLA)

MILK

(*see also* CHOCOLATE, COCOA, MILK DRINKS, MILKSHAKE)

CANNED

FOOD	PORTION	CALORIES	FAT	SAT FAT	CHOL	PROTEIN	CARBO	FIBER	CALCIUM	SOD	POTAS	VIT C	FOLIC	VIT A
condensed sweetened	1 oz	123	3	2	13	3	21	—	108	49	142	1	4	125
condensed sweetened	1 cup	982	27	17	104	24	166	—	868	389	1136	8	34	1004
evaporated	½ cup	169	10	6	37	9	13	—	329	122	382	2	10	306
evaporated skim	½ cup	99	tr	tr	5	10	14	—	369	147	423	2	11	500
CARNATION														
Evaporated	2 tbsp	40	3	2	10	2	3	—	80	35	—	—	—	—
Evaporated Lowfat	2 tbsp	25	1	—	5	2	3	—	80	35	—	—	—	100
Lite Evaporated Skimmed	½ cup (4 fl oz)	100	tr	—	5	9	14	—	300	150	—	—	—	500
Sweetened Condensed	2 tbsp	130	3	2	10	3	22	—	100	45	—	—	—	100
EAGLE														
Sweetened Condensed	⅓ cup	320	9	—	—	7	52	—	300	120	360	—	—	200
PET														
Evaporated	½ cup	170	10	—	36	8	12	—	300	140	—	—	—	200
Evaporated Filled	½ cup	150	8	1	5	8	12	—	300	140	—	2	—	500
Evaporated Light Skimmed	½ cup	100	tr	—	10	9	14	—	350	150	—	—	—	500

FOOD	PORTION	CALORIES	FAT	SAT FAT	CHOL	PROTEIN	CARBO	FIBER	CALCIUM	SOD	POTAS	VIT C	FOLIC	VIT A
DRIED														
buttermilk	1 tbsp	25	tr	tr	5	2	3	—	77	34	103	tr	3	14
nonfat instantized	1 pkg (3.2 oz)	244	tr	tr	12	32	47	—	837	499	1552	5	45	2157
CARNATION														
Nonfat	⅓ cup dry	80	0	—	<5	8	12	—	300	125	—	1	—	500
NUTRA/BALANCE														
Lactose Reduced as prep	8 oz	80	tr	—	—	8	12	—	300	125	390	1	—	500
SACO														
Cultured Buttermilk	4 tbsp (0.8 oz)	80	tr	0	4	5	13	0	220	166	—	1	—	50
SANALAC														
As Prep	8 oz	80	tr	—	4	8	12	0	300	125	380	1	—	100
REFRIGERATED														
1%	1 cup	102	3	2	10	8	12	—	300	123	381	2	12	500
1%	1 qt	409	10	6	39	32	47	—	1200	493	1524	9	50	2000
1% protein fortified	1 qt	477	12	7	39	39	54	—	1397	574	1774	11	58	2000
1% protein fortified	1 cup	119	3	2	10	10	14	—	349	143	444	3	15	500
2%	1 cup	121	5	3	18	8	12	—	297	122	377	2	12	500
2%	1 qt	485	19	12	73	33	47	—	1187	487	1507	9	50	2000
buttermilk	1 cup	99	2	1	9	8	12	—	285	257	371	2	—	81
buttermilk	1 qt	396	9	5	34	32	47	—	1141	1028	1483	10	—	323
goat	1 cup	168	10	7	28	9	11	—	326	122	499	3	1	451
goat	1 qt	672	40	26	111	35	43	—	1303	486	1995	13	6	1806
human	1 cup	171	11	5	34	3	17	—	79	42	126	12	13	593
indian buffalo	1 cup	236	17	11	46	9	13	—	412	127	434	5	14	434
low sodium	1 cup	149	8	5	33	8	11	—	246	6	617	—	—	317
nonfat	1 cup	86	tr	tr	4	8	12	—	302	125	406	2	13	500
nonfat	1 qt	342	2	1	18	33	48	—	1209	505	1623	10	51	2000
nonfat protein fortified	1 qt	400	2	2	20	39	55	—	1407	578	1786	11	59	2000
nonfat protein fortified	1 cup	100	1	tr	5	10	14	—	352	144	446	3	15	500
sheep	1 cup	264	17	11	—	15	13	—	474	108	334	10	—	360
whole	1 cup	150	8	5	33	8	11	—	291	120	370	2	12	307
BODYWISE														
Nonfat	8 fl oz	100	0	0	5	10	14	0	350	150	—	2	—	500
BORDEN														
Acidophilus 1%	8 fl oz	100	2	—	—	8	11	—	300	130	340	2	—	500
Buttermilk Lowfat Golden Churn	8 fl oz	120	4	—	—	8	11	—	300	250	360	2	—	200
Hi-Calcium	8 fl oz	150	8	—	—	8	11	—	1000	130	340	2	—	200
Hi-Protein 2%	8 fl oz	140	5	—	—	10	13	—	350	150	340	4	—	500
Milk	8 fl oz	150	8	—	—	8	11	—	300	130	340	2	—	200
Skim	8 fl oz	90	1	—	—	8	12	—	300	130	340	2	—	500
Skim-line	8 fl oz	100	1	—	—	10	13	—	350	150	340	4	—	500

FOOD	PORTION	CALORIES	FAT	SAT FAT	CHOL	PROTEIN	CARBO	FIBER	CALCIUM	SOD	POTAS	VIT C	FOLIC	VIT A
CALIMILK														
CalciMilk	8 fl oz	102	3	2	10	8	12	0	498	123	381	2	12	500
COOL COW														
Low Fat	1 cup (8 oz)	110	3	1	<5	9	12	0	300	125	—	2	—	500
FARMLAND														
1%	8 fl oz	100	3	2	10	8	12	0	300	130	—	1	—	500
2%	8 fl oz	130	5	3	20	8	12	0	300	130	—	1	—	500
Cholesterol Reduced	8 oz	150	8	—	10	8	11	—	300	125	370	2	—	200
Easylac 1%	8 fl oz	100	2	—	10	8	11	—	300	125	380	2	—	500
Easylac Nonfat	8 fl oz	90	0	—	5	8	12	—	300	125	380	2	—	500
Skim	8 fl oz	80	0	0	<5	8	12	0	300	130	—	1	—	500
Skim Plus	8 fl oz	110	0	0	<5	11	17	0	400	170	—	4	—	500
FRIENDSHIP														
Buttermilk	8 fl oz	120	4	3	15	9	12	0	300	125	—	2	—	500
HOOD														
1%	1 cup (8 oz)	110	3	2	15	8	13	0	300	125	—	2	—	500
Better Taste 2%	1 cup (8 oz)	130	5	3	20	8	13	0	300	125	—	2	—	500
Buttermilk	1 cup (8 oz)	90	0	0	<5	9	13	0	300	220	—	2	—	0
Whole	1 cup (8 oz)	150	8	5	35	8	12	0	300	125	—	2	—	300
LACTAID														
1%	8 fl oz	102	3	2	10	8	12	0	300	123	381	2	12	500
Nonfat	8 fl oz	86	tr	tr	4	8	12	0	302	126	406	2	13	500
NUFORM														
1%	1 cup (8 oz)	120	3	2	15	10	15	0	350	150	—	15	—	500
Skim	1 cup (8 oz)	100	0	0	<5	10	15	0	350	150	—	15	—	500
SILOVET														
Skim	1 cup (8 oz)	90	0	0	<5	9	13	0	300	125	—	2	—	500
VIVA														
2%	8 fl oz	120	5	—	—	8	11	—	500	125	340	2	—	500
Skim	8 fl oz	100	1	—	—	10	13	—	350	150	340	4	—	500
WEIGHT WATCHERS														
Skim	1 cup	90	0	0	5	9	13	0	300	130	280	2	—	500
SHELF-STABLE														
PARMALAT														
1%	1 cup (8 oz)	110	3	2	15	9	13	0	300	135	—	2	—	500
2%	1 cup (8 oz)	130	5	3	20	9	13	0	300	130	—	2	—	500
Skim	1 cup (8 oz)	90	1	0	5	8	13	0	300	130	—	2	—	500
Whole	1 cup (8 oz)	160	8	5	35	9	13	0	300	130	—	2	—	300

MILK DRINKS

(*see also* BREAKFAST DRINKS, CHOCOLATE, COCOA, MILKSHAKES)

FOOD	PORTION	CALORIES	FAT	SAT FAT	CHOL	PROTEIN	CARBO	FIBER	CALCIUM	SOD	POTAS	VIT C	FOLIC	VIT A
chocolate milk	1 cup	208	8	5	30	8	26	—	280	149	417	2	12	302
chocolate milk	1 qt	833	34	21	122	32	103	—	1121	596	1669	9	47	1210
chocolate milk 1%	1 cup	158	3	2	7	8	26	—	287	152	426	2	12	500
chocolate milk 1%	1 qt	630	10	6	29	32	104	—	1147	607	1702	9	48	2000

FOOD	PORTION	CALORIES	FAT	SAT FAT	CHOL	PROTEIN	CARBO	FIBER	CALCIUM	SOD	POTAS	VIT C	FOLIC	VIT A
chocolate milk 2%	1 cup	179	5	3	17	8	26	—	284	150	422	2	12	500
strawberry flavor mix as prep w/ whole milk	9 oz	234	8	5	33	8	33	—	292	128	370	2	12	308
BODY WISE														
Chocolate Nonfat Milk	1 cup (8 fl oz)	180	0	0	5	11	35	1	400	170	620	2	—	500
BORDEN														
Chocolate Lowfat Dutch Brand	8 fl oz	180	5	—	—	8	25	—	300	180	350	2	—	500
BOSCO														
Chocolate Milk	1 cup (8 fl oz)	230	8	—	—	8	33	—	200	110	370	9	—	500
HOOD														
Chocolate Lowfat	1 cup (8 oz)	150	2	1	10	8	27	0	300	240	—	2	—	500
LACTAID														
Chocolate Milk 1%	8 fl oz	158	3	2	7	8	26	tr	287	152	426	2	12	500
MEADOW GOLD														
Chocolate Milk	8 fl oz	210	8	—	—	8	25	—	300	240	—	2	—	200
PARMALAT														
Chocolate 2%	1 box (8 oz)	180	5	3	20	8	28	1	300	115	—	2	—	500
QUIK														
Banana Powder	2 tbsp (0.8 oz)	90	0	0	0	0	27	0	0	0	0	0	—	0
Cookies n Cream Powder	2 tbsp (0.8 oz)	100	1	1	0	1	21	1	0	190	0	0	—	0
Strawberry Powder	2 tbsp (0.8 oz)	90	0	0	0	0	22	0	0	0	0	0	—	0

MILK SUBSTITUTES

(see also COFFEE WHITENERS)

FOOD	PORTION	CALORIES	FAT	SAT FAT	CHOL	PROTEIN	CARBO	FIBER	CALCIUM	SOD	POTAS	VIT C	FOLIC	VIT A
imitation milk	1 cup	150	8	2	tr	4	15	—	79	191	279	0	0	0
imitation milk	1 qt	600	33	7	2	17	60	—	317	764	1116	0	0	0
BETTER THAN MILK														
Carob	8 fl oz	130	5	—	0	2	20	—	500	175	—	—	—	—
Chocolate	8 fl oz	125	5	—	0	2	17	—	500	175	—	—	—	—
Light	8 fl oz	80	tr	—	0	2	15	—	500	120	140	—	—	—
Natural	8 fl oz	90	5	—	0	2	10	—	500	120		—	—	—
EDENBLEND														
Original	8 fl oz	120	3	1	0	7	16	0	33	85	270	0	28	0
EDENSOY														
Carob	8 fl oz	150	4	1	0	6	23	0	67	105	330	0	38	0
Extra Original	8 oz	130	4	1	0	10	13	0	200	105	440	tr	40	1500
Extra Original	8 fl oz	130	5	1	0	9	12	0	195	100	450	0	44	1500
Extra Vanilla	8 fl oz	150	3	0	0	6	23	0	200	90	290	tr	40	1500
Original	8 oz	130	4	1	0	10	13	0	80	105	440	0	40	0
Vanilla	8 oz	150	3	0	0	6	32	0	60	90	290	0	40	0
HEALTH VALLEY														
Soo Moo	1 cup	120	6	—	0	6	12	0	40	55	120	—	—	95

FOOD	PORTION	CALORIES	FAT	SAT FAT	CHOL	PROTEIN	CARBO	FIBER	CALCIUM	SOD	POTAS	VIT C	FOLIC	VIT A
RICE DREAM														
Carob Lite	8 fl oz	150	3	—	0	1	32	—	20	80	—	1	—	—
Chocolate	8 fl oz	190	3	—	0	1	44	—	20	80	—	1	—	—
Chocolate	8 fl oz	190	3	—	0	1	44	—	20	80	—	1	—	—
Lite Organic Original	8 fl oz	130	2	—	0	1	28	—	20	80	—	1	—	—
Lite Vanilla	8 fl oz	130	2	—	0	1	30	—	20	80	—	1	—	—
VEGELICIOUS														
Milk	8 fl oz	100	2	—	0	2	18	—	300	125	100	6	40	500
VITAMITE														
Non-Dairy 2% Fat	1 cup (8 oz)	110	5	2	0	3	14	0	200	120	110	0	—	500
Non-Diary Nonfat	1 cup (8 oz)	90	0	0	0	1	21	0	200	70	280	0	—	500
VITASOY														
Carob Supreme	8 fl oz	210	6	1	0	8	32	1	60	160	410	—	—	—
Cocoa Light	8 fl oz	130	2	0	0	4	25	1	80	130	200	—	—	—
Original Creamy	8 fl oz	160	7	1	0	9	14	1	80	180	310	—	—	—
Original Light	8 fl oz	90	2	0	0	4	15	1	80	95	125	—	—	—
Rich Cocoa	8 fl oz	210	6	1	0	8	32	1	100	180	360	—	—	—
Vanilla Light	8 fl oz	110	2	0	0	4	20	1	80	95	110	—	—	—
Vanilla Delite	8 fl oz	190	6	1	0	7	27	1	80	130	220	—	—	—
WESTSOY														
Cocoa Lite	8 fl oz	140	2	tr	0	4	25	—	20	95	210	—	—	—
Plain Lite	8 fl oz	100	2	tr	0	4	16	—	20	100	170	—	—	—
Vanilla Lite	8 fl oz	110	2	tr	0	3	20	—	20	80	170	—	—	—
MILKSHAKE														
chocolate	10 oz	360	11	7	37	10	58	—	319	273	567	1	10	263
strawberry	10 oz	319	8	—	31	10	53	—	320	234	516	2	9	340
thick shake chocolate	10.6 oz	356	8	5	32	9	63	—	396	333	672	0	15	258
thick shake vanilla	11 oz	350	10	6	37	12	56	—	457	299	572	0	21	357
vanilla	10 oz	314	8	5	32	10	51	—	344	232	492	2	9	368
D'FROSTA SHAKE														
Vanilla	1 serv (13.5 oz)	340	9	6	40	11	57	1	394	200	510	3	—	335
FREEZE FLIP														
Fruit Shake No Fat Lactose Free Black Raspberry	1 serv (6 oz)	150	0	0	0	1	37	1	2	25	5	44	—	2
FROSTEE														
Chocolate	8 fl oz	200	8	—	—	2	30	—	—	160	220	—	—	—
Strawberry	8 fl oz	180	7	—	—	2	27	—	40	150	250	—	—	—
HOOD														
Shake Up Chocolate	1 cup (8 oz)	240	6	4	20	9	38	0	300	290	—	2	—	200
Shake Up Strawberry	1 cup (8 oz)	220	5	3	20	8	36	0	300	270	—	2	—	200

FOOD	PORTION	CALORIES	FAT	SAT FAT	CHOL	PROTEIN	CARBO	FIBER	CALCIUM	SOD	POTAS	VIT C	FOLIC	VIT A
HOOD (CONT.)														
Shake Up Vanilla	1 cup (8 oz)	220	5	3	20	8	36	0	300	270	—	2	—	200
MILKY WAY														
Shake	1 (10 fl oz)	390	16	10	60	9	54	0	250	235	250	2	—	500
PARMALAT														
Shake A Shake Chocolate	1 box (6 oz)	180	4	2	15	8	29	1	250	140	—	2	—	0
Shake A Shake Orange Vanilla	1 box (6 oz)	110	3	2	10	6	14	0	150	55	—	tr	—	200
Shake A Shake Vanilla	1 box (6 oz)	170	3	2	15	8	28	0	250	140	—	2	—	0
WEIGHT WATCHERS														
Chocolate Fudge Shake Mix as prep	1 pkg	80	1	0	0	6	12	2	250	140	—	0	—	300

MILLET
FOOD	PORTION	CALORIES	FAT	SAT FAT	CHOL	PROTEIN	CARBO	FIBER	CALCIUM	SOD	POTAS	VIT C	FOLIC	VIT A
cooked	½ cup	143	1	tr	0	4	28	—	4	2	74	0	—	—

MINERAL/BOTTLED WATER
FOOD	PORTION	CALORIES	FAT	SAT FAT	CHOL	PROTEIN	CARBO	FIBER	CALCIUM	SOD	POTAS	VIT C	FOLIC	VIT A
CANADA DRY														
Sparkling Water	8 fl oz	0	0	0	0	0	0	0	—	10	—	—	—	—
CRYSTAL GEYSER														
Sparking Natural Wild Cherry	1 bottle (12 fl oz)	0	0	0	0	0	0	—	—	70	—	—	—	—
Sparkling Lemon	1 bottle (12 fl oz)	0	0	0	0	0	0	—	—	70	—	—	—	—
Sparkling Mineral	1 bottle (12 fl oz)	0	0	0	0	0	0	—	—	70	—	—	—	—
Sparkling Natural Cola Berry	1 bottle (12 fl oz)	0	0	0	0	0	0	—	—	70	—	—	—	—
Sparkling Orange	1 bottle (12 fl oz)	0	0	0	0	0	0	—	—	70	—	—	—	—
EVIAN														
Water	1 liter	0	0	0	0	0	0	0	78	5	1	—	—	—
GLACIER SPRINGS														
Drinking Water	8 fl oz	0	0	0	0	0	0	0	—	0	—	—	—	—
LACROIX														
Sparking Berry	12 fl oz	0	0	0	0	—	—	—	—	—	—	—	—	—
Sparkling Lemon	12 fl oz	0	0	0	0	—	—	—	—	—	—	—	—	—
Sparkling Lime	12 fl oz	0	0	0	0	—	—	—	—	—	—	—	—	—
Sparkling Orange	12 fl oz	0	0	0	0	—	—	—	—	—	—	—	—	—
Sparkling Regular	12 fl oz	0	0	0	0	—	—	—	—	—	—	—	—	—
Spring	1 bottle (12 oz)	0	0	0	0	0	0	0	—	<8	—	—	—	—
MT SHASTA														
Natural Spring	1 bottle (20 oz)	0	0	0	0	0	0	0	—	<13	—	—	—	—
SAN PELLEGRINO														
Acqua Panna	8 fl oz	0	0	0	0	0	0	0	3	0	—	—	—	—

FOOD	PORTION	CALORIES	FAT	SAT FAT	CHOL	PROTEIN	CARBO	FIBER	CALCIUM	SOD	POTAS	VIT C	FOLIC	VIT A
SAN PELLEGRINO (CONT.)														
Mineral Water	1 liter (33.8 oz)	0	0	0	0	0	0	—	204	41	3	—	—	—
SARATOGA														
Sparkling	1 liter	0	0	0	0	0	0	—	67	19	2	—	—	—
WATER JOE														
Caffeine Enhanced	8 fl oz	0	0	0	0	0	0	—	—	0	—	—	—	—
MISO														
EDEN														
Genmai Miso Organic	1 tbsp (0.5 oz)	25	1	0	0	2	3	tr	9	810	80	0	—	0
Hacho Miso Organic	1 tbsp (0.5 oz)	35	2	0	0	3	2	1	0	600	160	2	—	0
Kome Miso Organic	1 tbsp (0.6 oz)	25	1	0	0	2	3	tr	0	850	55	1	—	0
Mugi Miso Organic	1 tbsp (0.6 oz)	25	1	0	0	2	3	1	9	760	75	2	—	0
Shiro Miso Organic	1 tbsp (0.6 oz)	35	1	0	0	2	5	1	0	410	25	0	—	0
MOLASSES														
blackstrap	1 tbsp (0.7 oz)	47	0	0	0	0	12	—	172	11	498	—	0	0
blackstrap	1 cup (11.5 oz)	771	tr	—	0	0	199	—	2821	180	8174	—	2	0
molasses	1 tbsp (0.7 oz)	53	0	0	0	0	14	—	41	7	293	—	0	0
molasses	1 cup (11.5 oz)	873	1	—	0	0	226	—	671	120	4802	—	1	0
BRER RABBIT														
Dark	2 tbsp	110	0	0	0	0	28	—	150	20	750	—	—	—
Light	2 tbsp	110	0	0	0	0	29	—	150	15	670	—	—	—
MCILHENNY														
Molasses	1 tbsp (0.7 oz)	66	tr	tr	0	tr	16	tr	22	9	—	tr	—	38
TREE OF LIFE														
Blackstrap	1 tbsp (0.5 oz)	45	0	0	0	0	11	—	140	15	—	—	—	—
MOOSE														
roasted	3 oz	114	1	tr	66	25	0	—	5	58	284	4	—	—
MOTH BEANS														
dried cooked	1 cup	207	1	tr	0	14	37	—	6	17	538	2	—	17
MOUSSE														
FROZEN														
PEPPERIDGE FARM														
San Francisco Chocolate Mousse	1	490	34	18	150	4	41	—	80	75	—	—	—	—
SARA LEE														
Chocolate Mint Mousse	⅕ pkg (4.3 oz)	440	28	21	30	6	40	2	—	100	—	—	—	—
WEIGHT WATCHERS														
Chocolate Mousse	1 (2.75 oz)	190	5	2	5	6	31	3	60	150	—	0	—	0

FOOD	PORTION	CALORIES	FAT	SAT FAT	CHOL	PROTEIN	CARBO	FIBER	CALCIUM	SOD	POTAS	VIT C	FOLIC	VIT A
HOME RECIPE														
chocolate	½ cup (7.1 oz)	447	33	19	299	9	33	—	202	87	296	—	—	1134
crab	¼ cup	364	20	—	136	—	—	—	272	—	—	—	—	—
orange	½ cup	87	5	—	1	3	19	—	71	24	—	—	—	—
MIX														
ROYAL														
Chocolate Mousse No-Bake	⅛ pie	130	4	0	0	3	21	—	40	190	105	—	—	—
TAKE-OUT														
chocolate	½ cup (7.1 oz)	447	33	19	299	9	33	—	202	87	296	—	—	1134

MUFFIN

FOOD	PORTION	CALORIES	FAT	SAT FAT	CHOL	PROTEIN	CARBO	FIBER	CALCIUM	SOD	POTAS	VIT C	FOLIC	VIT A
FROZEN														
HEALTH VALLEY														
Almond & Date Oat Bran Fancy Fruit	1	180	4	—	0	4	31	8	41	80	210	2	—	54
Fat Free Apple Spice	1	140	tr	—	0	4	30	5	20	110	250	1	—	—
Fat Free Banana	1	130	tr	—	0	4	29	5	20	110	530	1	—	—
Fat Free Raisin Spice	1	140	tr	—	0	4	32	5	20	100	250	1	—	—
Oat Bran Fancy Fruit Blueberry	1	140	4	—	0	4	32	8	62	100	210	5	14	36
Oat Bran Fancy Fruit Raisin	1	180	5	—	0	4	5	8	58	90	190	7	15	60
Rice Bran Fancy Fruit Raisin	1	210	7	—	0	5	7	6	47	125	400	5	8	2
PEPPERIDGE FARM														
Banana Nut	1	170	6	1	30	3	28	—	20	220	—	—	—	—
Blueberry	1	170	7	1	25	2	27	1	20	250	—	1	—	—
Cholesterol Free Multi Grain Muesli	1	200	8	1	0	4	30	—	40	230	—	—	—	—
Cholesterol Free Oatbran With Apple	1	190	7	1	0	3	29	—	40	200	—	—	—	—
Cholesterol Free Raisin Bran	1	170	6	1	0	4	30	—	60	280	—	1	—	—
Cinnamon Swirl	1	190	6	1	35	2	30	1	20	170	—	—	—	—
Corn	1	180	7	1	30	3	27	—	20	260	—	—	—	—
SARA LEE														
Blueberry	1 (2.2 oz)	220	11	2	15	3	27	tr	—	170	—	—	—	—
Corn	1 (2.2 oz)	260	14	3	25	3	30	1	—	220	—	—	—	—
Oat Bran	1	210	8	—	0	4	35	—	150	320	—	1	—	1250
WEIGHT WATCHERS														
Chocolate Chocolate Chip	1 (2.5 oz)	190	2	1	0	3	39	4	80	350	—	0	—	0

FOOD	PORTION	CALORIES	FAT	SAT FAT	CHOL	PROTEIN	CARBO	FIBER	CALCIUM	SOD	POTAS	VIT C	FOLIC	VIT A
WEIGHT WATCHERS (CONT.)														
Fat Free Banana	1 (2.5 oz)	170	0	0	0	3	41	3	80	310	—	0	—	0
Fat Free Blueberry	1 (2.5 oz)	160	0	0	0	3	38	2	60	290	—	0	—	0
HOME RECIPE														
blueberry as prep w/ 2% milk	1 (2 oz)	163	6	1	21	4	23	—	108	251	70	1	7	81
blueberry as prep w/ whole milk	1 (2 oz)	165	6	1	23	6	23	—	107	251	70	1	7	63
corn as prep w/ 2% milk	1 (2 oz)	180	7	1	24	4	25	—	148	334	83	tr	10	137
corn as prep w/ whole milk	1 (2 oz)	183	7	2	25	4	25	—	147	333	82	tr	10	118
plain as prep w/ 2% milk	1 (2 oz)	169	7	1	22	4	24	—	114	266	69	tr	7	80
plain as prep w/ whole milk	1 (2 oz)	172	7	1	24	4	24	—	113	266	68	tr	7	61
wheat bran as prep w/ 2% milk	1 (2 oz)	161	7	1	19	4	24	—	106	335	181	5	30	478
wheat bran as prep w/ whole milk	1 (2 oz)	164	7	2	20	4	24	—	106	335	181	5	30	459
MIX														
blueberry	1 (1¾ oz)	149	4	1	23	3	24	—	13	219	39	—	—	—
corn	1 (1.75 oz)	160	5	1	31	4	25	—	37	397	65	tr	6	105
wheat bran as prep	1 (1¾ oz)	138	5	1	34	5	23	—	16	233	73	0	—	51
ARROWHEAD														
Bran	⅓ cup (1.4 oz)	150	2	0	0	7	26	7	100	160	100	0	—	0
Oat Bran Wheat Free	⅓ cup (1.5 oz)	160	4	2	0	7	23	7	100	310	290	0	—	0
BETTY CROCKER														
Apple Cinnamon	1	120	4	1	25	2	18	—	20	140	40	—	—	—
Apple Cinnamon No Cholesterol Recipe	1	110	2	1	0	2	18	—	20	140	40	—	—	—
Banana Nut	1	120	5	1	25	2	17	—	20	140	65	—	—	—
Banana Nut No Cholesterol Recipe	1	110	4	1	0	2	17	—	20	140	65	—	—	—
Blueberry Streusel Bake Shop	1	210	8	—	—	3	31	—	20	230	65	—	—	—
Cinnamon Streusel	1	200	9	2	30	2	17	—	40	240	80	—	—	—
Oat Bran	1	190	8	2	35	4	25	—	60	240	150	—	—	—
Oat Bran No Cholesterol Recipe	1	180	7	2	0	4	25	—	60	240	150	—	—	—
Twice The Blueberries	1	120	4	1	20	2	18	—	20	140	35	—	—	—

FOOD	PORTION	CALORIES	FAT	SAT FAT	CHOL	PROTEIN	CARBO	FIBER	CALCIUM	SOD	POTAS	VIT C	FOLIC	VIT A
BETTY CROCKER (CONT.)														
Twice The Blueberries No Cholesterol Recipe	1	110	3	1	0	2	18	—	20	140	35	—	—	—
Wild Blueberry	1	120	4	1	25	2	18	—	40	150	65	—	—	—
Wild Blueberry Light	1	70	tr	—	20	1	16	—	—	140	25	—	—	—
Wild Blueberry Light No Cholesterol Recipe	1	70	tr	—	0	1	16	—	—	140	25	—	—	—
Wild Blueberry No Cholesterol Recipe	1	110	3	tr	0	2	18	—	40	150	65	—	—	—
DROMEDARY														
Corn Muffin	1	120	4	—	—	3	20	—	40	270	50	—	—	100
FLAKO														
Corn	⅓ cup (1.4 oz)	160	4	1	0	3	29	1	20	380	35	0	—	—
HAIN														
Oat Bran Apple Cinnamon	1	140	3	—	0	4	28	5	60	200	160	—	—	—
Oat Bran Banana Nut	1	140	4	—	0	4	26	4	60	190	170	—	—	—
Oat Bran Raspberry Spice	1	140	3	—	0	5	27	4	40	190	160	—	—	—
JIFFY														
Apple Cinnamon as prep	1	190	7	3	33	2	28	1	60	360	—	0	—	0
Banana Nut as prep	1	180	7	4	27	2	25	1	60	420	—	0	—	0
Blueberry as prep	1	190	7	4	36	2	28	1	60	288	—	0	—	0
Bran With Dates as prep	1	170	6	3	36	2	26	3	60	240	—	0	—	0
Corn as prep	1	180	4	2	0	2	28	1	80	320	—	0	—	0
Honey Date as prep	1	170	5	2	30	2	27	1	60	240	—	0	—	0
Oatmeal as prep	1	180	7	2	27	2	26	2	60	270	—	0	—	0
WANDA'S														
Blue Corn	¼ cup mix per serv (1.2 oz)	130	1	0	0	4	25	1	60	350	—	0	—	0
READY-TO-EAT														
blueberry	1 (2 oz)	158	4	1	17	3	27	2	33	255	70	1	—	—
corn	1 (2 oz)	174	5	1	—	3	29	—	42	297	39	—	—	118
oat bran wheat free	1 (2 oz)	154	4	1	0	4	28	4	36	224	289	—	10	—
toaster type blueberry	1	103	3	tr	—	2	18	—	4	158	27	0	—	105
toaster type corn	1	114	4	1	—	2	19	—	6	142	30	0	—	32
toaster type wheat bran w/ raisins	1 (1.3 oz)	106	3	1	—	2	19	—	13	178	60	0	—	64

FOOD	PORTION	CALORIES	FAT	SAT FAT	CHOL	PROTEIN	CARBO	FIBER	CALCIUM	SOD	POTAS	VIT C	FOLIC	VIT A
ARNOLD														
Bran'nola	1 (2.3 oz)	160	1	0	0	6	30	2	60	220	—	—	—	—
Raisin	1 (2.3 oz)	160	1	0	0	6	33	2	40	220	—	—	—	—
DUTCH MILL														
Apple Oat Bran	1 (2 oz)	180	5	1	0	3	31	1	60	210	—	0	—	0
Banana Walnut	1 (2 oz)	220	6	2	5	3	33	1	40	210	—	0	—	100
Carrot	1 (2 oz)	190	7	2	30	3	31	1	40	230	—	0	—	3000
Corn	1 (2 oz)	190	6	3	40	4	31	1	40	280	—	0	—	300
Cranberry Orange	1 (2 oz)	170	6	3	55	3	26	1	40	290	—	0	—	200
Raisin Bran	1 (2 oz)	230	5	3	30	2	37	3	40	330	—	0	—	200
ENTENMANN'S														
Blueberry	1 (2 oz)	200	8	—	—	3	29	—	—	250	—	—	—	—
FREIHOFER'S														
Corn Toasters	1 (1.3 oz)	130	6	1	15	2	18	0	20	210	—	0	—	0
HOSTESS														
Mini Apple Cinnamon	5 (2 oz)	260	16	3	45	3	28	3	20	180	60	—	—	—
Mini Banana Nut	5 (2 oz)	260	16	2	40	3	28	tr	20	160	90	—	—	—
Mini Blueberry	5 (2 oz)	240	13	2	40	3	30	tr	20	180	55	—	—	—
Mini Chocolate Chip	5 (2 oz)	260	15	5	35	3	29	1	—	170	85	—	—	—
Muffin Loaf Blueberry	1 (3.8 oz)	440	19	3	80	5	62	2	60	460	85	—	—	—
Oat Bran	1 (1.5 oz)	160	8	1	0	2	22	tr	—	150	45	—	—	—
Oat Bran Banana Nut	1 (1.5 oz)	150	6	1	0	2	22	1	—	160	70	—	—	—
WEIGHT WATCHERS														
Fat Free Apple Crisp	1 (2.5 oz)	160	0	0	0	3	37	1	40	290	—	0	—	0
Fat Free Cranberry Orange	1 (2.5 oz)	160	0	0	0	3	38	1	40	290	—	0	—	0
Fat Free Double Chocolate	1 (2.5 oz)	180	0	0	0	3	40	2	60	300	—	0	—	0
Fat Free Wild Blueberry	1 (2.5 oz)	160	0	0	0	3	36	1	40	280	—	0	—	0
Low Fat Apple Cinnamon	1 (2.5 oz)	170	3	2	15	4	35	2	60	200	—	0	—	200
Low Fat Blueberry	1 (2.5 oz)	180	3	0	0	4	37	2	60	200	—	0	—	100
Low Fat Carrot	1 (2.5 oz)	160	3	0	0	4	34	2	60	200	—	0	—	3000
Low Fat Chocolate Chip	1 (2.5 oz)	180	3	1	0	4	38	2	60	200	—	0	—	100
Low Fat Cranberry Orange	1 (2.5 oz)	180	3	0	0	4	38	2	60	190	—	0	—	100
Low Fat Lemon Poppy	1 (2.5 oz)	190	3	0	0	4	38	2	100	200	—	0	—	100
MULBERRIES														
fresh	1 cup	61	1	—	0	2	14	—	55	14	271	51	—	35

FOOD	PORTION	CALORIES	FAT	SAT FAT	CHOL	PROTEIN	CARBO	FIBER	CALCIUM	SOD	POTAS	VIT C	FOLIC	VIT A
MULLET														
striped cooked	3 oz	127	4	1	54	21	0	—	26	61	389	—	—	120
striped raw	3 oz	99	3	1	42	16	0	—	34	55	304	—	7	104
MUNG BEANS														
DRIED														
cooked	1 cup	213	1	tr	0	14	39	—	55	4	536	2	321	48
SPROUTS														
canned	½ cup	8	tr	tr	0	1	1	—	9	—	17	tr	6	14
cooked	½ cup	13	tr	tr	0	1	3	—	7	6	63	7	—	8
raw	½ cup	16	tr	tr	0	2	3	—	7	3	77	7	32	11
stir fried	½ cup	31	tr	tr	0	3	7	—	8	—	—	—	—	—
MUNGO BEANS														
dried cooked	1 cup	190	1	tr	1	14	33	—	95	13	416	2	170	56
MUSHROOMS														
CANNED														
pieces	½ cup	19	tr	tr	0	1	4	—	—	—	—	—	10	0
straw	1 cup (6.4 oz)	58	1	tr	0	7	8	5	18	699	699	0	69	0
whole	1 (0.4 oz)	3	tr	tr	0	tr	1	—	—	—	—	—	2	0
BINB														
Pieces & Stems	1 can (4.2 oz)	30	0	0	0	3	4	2	0	460	—	0	—	0
Sliced	1 can (4.2 oz)	30	0	0	0	3	4	2	0	460	—	0	—	0
Sliced With Garlic	1 can (4.2 oz)	35	1	0	0	3	4	1	0	410	—	0	—	0
Whole	1 can (4.2 oz)	30	0	0	0	3	4	2	0	460	—	0	—	0
GREEN GIANT														
Pieces & Stems	½ cup (4.2 oz)	30	0	0	0	3	4	2	0	440	—	0	—	0
Sliced	½ cup (4.2 oz)	30	0	0	0	2	3	2	0	440	—	0	—	0
Whole	½ cup (4.2 oz)	30	0	0	0	3	4	2	0	440	—	0	—	0
KA-ME														
Stir Fry	½ cup (4.5 oz)	20	0	0	0	2	3	2	20	380	—	1	—	—
Straw Whole Peeled	½ cup (4.5 oz)	20	0	0	0	2	3	2	20	380	—	1	—	—
SENECA														
Mushrooms	½ cup	25	0	0	0	0	3	2	0	552	210	2	—	0
DRIED														
cloud ear	1 (5 g)	13	tr	—	0	tr	3	3	7	2	34	0	2	0
cloud ears	1 cup (1 oz)	80	tr	—	0	3	20	20	45	10	211	0	11	0
shiitake	4 (½ oz)	44	tr	tr	0	1	11	—	2	2	230	—	—	0
straw	1 piece (6 g)	2	tr	0	0	tr	tr	tr	1	21	21	0	2	0
FRESH														
oyster raw	1 lg (5.2 oz)	55	1	—	0	6	9	4	9	46	764	0	70	71
oyster raw	1 sm (0.5 oz)	6	tr	—	0	1	1	tr	1	5	77	0	7	7
shitake cooked	4 (2.5 oz)	40	tr	tr	0	1	10	—	2	3	85	tr	—	0
whole cooked	1 (0.4 oz)	3	tr	tr	0	tr	1	—	1	0	43	1	2	0

FOOD	PORTION	CALORIES	FAT	SAT FAT	CHOL	PROTEIN	CARBO	FIBER	CALCIUM	SOD	POTAS	VIT C	FOLIC	VIT A
MOTHER EARTH														
Organic	4 oz	35	1	—	0	3	5	tr	—	0	280	—	—	—
FROZEN														
EMPIRE														
Breaded	7 (2.8 oz)	90	1	0	0	4	16	1	0	390	—	0	—	0
FRESH LIKE														
Mushrooms	3.5 oz	28	tr	—	—	3	4	1	6	15	414	3	—	0
MUSSELS														
blue raw	1 cup	129	3	1	42	18	6	—	39	429	479	—	—	—
blue raw	3 oz	73	2	tr	24	10	3	—	22	243	272	—	—	—
fresh blue cooked	3 oz	147	4	1	48	20	6	—	28	313	228	—	—	—
MUSTARD														
dry mustard seed yellow	1 tsp	15	1	tr	0	1	1	—	17	tr	23	—	—	2
yellow ready-to-use	1 tsp	5	tr	tr	0	tr	tr	—	4	63	7	0	—	0
BLANCHARD & BLANCHARD														
Mustard	1 tsp (5 g)	0	0	0	0	0	0	0	0	45	—	0	—	0
ESTEE														
Sodium Free	1 pkg (0.5 oz)	5	1	—	—	tr	tr	—	—	0	15	—	—	—
GREY POUPON														
Country Dijon	1 tsp	6	0	0	0	0	0	0	—	120	10	—	—	—
Dijon	1 tsp	6	0	0	0	0	0	0	—	120	10	—	—	—
Parisian	1 tsp	6	0	0	0	0	0	0	—	55	5	—	—	—
HAIN														
Stone Ground	1 tbsp	14	1	—	0	1	1	—	—	185	—	—	—	—
Stone Ground No Salt Added	1 tbsp	14	1	—	0	1	1	—	—	10	—	—	—	—
HEINZ														
Mild Yellow	1 tbsp	8	tr	0	0	1	1	—	—	175	20	—	—	—
Spicy Brown	1 tbsp	14	1	—	0	1	1	—	—	115	20	—	—	—
KA-ME														
Hot Mustard Powder Chinese Style	¼ tsp (1 g)	5	0	0	0	0	1	1	0	0	—	—	—	—
KOSCIUSZKO														
Spicy Brown	1 tsp	5	tr	—	0	tr	tr	—	—	60	—	—	—	—
KRAFT														
Horseradish Mustard	1 tsp (5 g)	0	0	0	0	0	0	0	0	55	5	0	—	0
Mustard	1 tsp (5 g)	0	0	0	0	0	0	0	0	60	5	0	—	0
MCILHENNY														
Coarse Ground	1 tsp (0.2 oz)	4	tr	tr	0	tr	tr	tr	5	39	—	tr	—	8
Spicy	1 tsp (0.2 oz)	6	tr	tr	0	tr	tr	1	30	28	—	tr	—	9
PLOCHMAN														
Dijon	1 tsp (5 g)	7	tr	—	0	tr	tr	—	—	82	—	—	—	—
Spoonable Salad	1 tsp (5 g)	4	tr	—	0	tr	tr	—	—	53	—	—	—	—

FOOD	PORTION	CALORIES	FAT	SAT FAT	CHOL	PROTEIN	CARBO	FIBER	CALCIUM	SOD	POTAS	VIT C	FOLIC	VIT A
PLOCHMAN (CONT.)														
Squeeze Salad	1 tsp (5 g)	4	tr	—	0	tr	tr	—	—	53	—	—	—	—
Stone Ground	1 tsp (5 g)	6	tr	—	0	tr	tr	—	—	60	—	—	—	—
RUSSER														
Deli	1 tsp (5 g)	4	0	0	—	0	0	—	—	65	—	—	—	—
TREE OF LIFE														
Dijon	1 tsp (5 g)	0	0	0	0	0	0	—	—	66	—	—	—	—
Dijon Imported	1 tsp (5 g)	5	0	0	0	tr	tr	—	—	120	—	—	—	—
Low Sodium	1 tsp (5 g)	3	0	0	0	tr	tr	—	—	50	—	—	—	—
Stone Ground	1 tsp (5 g)	0	0	0	0	0	0	—	—	55	—	—	—	—
Yellow	1 tsp (5 g)	0	0	0	0	0	0	—	—	55	—	—	—	—
WATKINS														
Country Mill	1 tsp (7 g)	15	1	0	—	0	2	0	0	110	—	0	—	0
Dusseldorf	1 tsp (7 g)	10	0	0	—	0	1	0	0	110	—	0	—	0
Horseradish	1 tsp (7 g)	10	0	0	—	0	1	0	0	120	—	0	—	0
Jalapeno	1 tsp (7 g)	10	0	0	—	0	1	0	0	150	—	0	—	0
Onion	1 tsp (7 g)	10	0	0	—	0	1	0	0	110	—	0	—	0
Parisienne	1 tsp (7 g)	10	0	0	—	0	1	0	0	110	—	0	—	0
MUSTARD GREENS														
fresh chopped cooked	½ cup	11	tr	tr	0	2	1	—	52	11	141	18	—	2122
fresh raw chopped	½ cup	7	tr	tr	0	1	1	—	29	7	99	20	—	1484
frozen chopped cooked	½ cup	14	tr	tr	0	2	2	—	75	19	104	10	—	3352
ALLEN														
Mustard Greens	½ cup (4.1 oz)	30	1	0	0	1	5	3	150	10	—	9	—	3500
BIRDS EYE														
Chopped	1 cup (3 oz)	30	0	0	0	2	2	2	80	20	—	15	—	2250
SUNSHINE														
Mustard Greens	½ cup (4.1 oz)	30	1	0	0	1	5	3	150	10	—	9	—	3500
NATTO														
natto	½ cup	187	10	1	0	16	13	—	191	6	642	11	—	0
NAVY BEANS														
CANNED														
navy	1 cup	296	1	tr	0	20	54	—	123	1173	755	2	163	4
ALLEN														
Navy Beans	½ cup (4.5 oz)	110	1	0	0	6	19	6	60	380	—	0	—	0
EDEN														
Organic	½ cup (4.3 oz)	100	1	0	0	6	18	7	69	15	280	0	—	0
TRAPPEY														
With Bacon	½ cup (4.5 oz)	110	2	1	0	6	17	7	40	420	—	0	—	0
With Bacon & Jalapeno	½ cup (4.5 oz)	110	2	1	0	6	17	7	40	420	—	0	—	0
DRIED														
cooked	1 cup	259	1	tr	0	16	48	—	128	2	669	2	255	3

FOOD	PORTION	CALORIES	FAT	SAT FAT	CHOL	PROTEIN	CARBO	FIBER	CALCIUM	SOD	POTAS	VIT C	FOLIC	VIT A
HURST														
HamBeens w/ Ham	3 tbsp (1.2 oz)	120	1	0	0	8	20	11	40	63	—	2	—	0
SPROUTS														
cooked	3½ oz	78	1	—	0	—	—	—	16	—	—	—	—	—
raw	½ cup	35	tr	—	0	—	—	—	8	—	—	—	—	—

NECTARINE

DOLE														
Nectarine	1	70	1	—	0	1	16	3	—	0	—	—	—	—

NEUFCHATEL

neufchatel	1 oz	74	7	4	22	3	1	—	21	113	32	0	3	321
neufchatel	1 pkg (3 oz)	221	20	13	65	8	3	—	64	339	97	0	10	964
PHILADELPHIA														
Neufchatel	1 oz	70	6	4	20	3	tr	0	20	120	30	0	—	300
WISPRIDE														
Garden Vegetable Cup	2 tbsp (1.1 oz)	60	5	3	15	3	2	0	150	180	—	2	—	100
Garlic & Herb Cup	2 tbsp (1.1 oz)	60	5	3	15	3	2	0	150	180	—	2	—	100

NON-DAIRY CREAMERS

(*see* COFFEE WHITENERS)

NON-DAIRY WHIPPED TOPPINGS

(*see* WHIPPED TOPPINGS)

NOODLE DISHES

(*see also* NOODLES and PASTA DINNERS)

FOOD	PORTION	CALORIES	FAT	SAT FAT	CHOL	PROTEIN	CARBO	FIBER	CALCIUM	SOD	POTAS	VIT C	FOLIC	VIT A
CANNED														
VAN CAMP'S														
Noodlee Weenee	1 can (8 oz)	230	8	2	20	7	34	1	0	680	240	—	8	500
FROZEN														
LUIGINO'S														
Stroganoff	1 pkg (8 oz)	310	17	5	55	14	25	2	40	920	—	0	—	400
MIX														
KRAFT														
Noodle Classics Cheddar Cheese as prep	1 cup (7.4 oz)	400	19	5	70	13	47	1	150	760	360	0	40	750
Noodle Classics Savory Chicken as prep	1 cup (8.5 oz)	340	13	3	55	10	46	2	40	1370	360	0	40	200
LA CHOY														
Ramen Noodles Beef as prep	1 cup	200	8	1	0	6	33	4	7	865	40	—	—	—
Ramen Noodles Chicken as prep	1 cup	200	7	1	0	6	29	4	7	740	40	—	—	—
LIPTON														
Noodles & Sauce Alfredo Broccoli as prep	1 cup (2.2 oz)	340	14	6	80	12	43	2	150	970	—	5	100	500

FOOD	PORTION	CALORIES	FAT	SAT FAT	CHOL	PROTEIN	CARBO	FIBER	CALCIUM	SOD	POTAS	VIT C	FOLIC	VIT A
LIPTON (CONT.)														
Noodles & Sauce Alfredo as prep	1 cup (2.2 oz)	330	14	6	80	15	42	2	150	1040	—	0	100	500
Noodles & Sauce Beef as prep	1 cup (2.1 oz)	280	10	2	60	8	43	2	0	910	—	0	100	300
Noodles & Sauce Butter as prep	1 cup (2.2 oz)	310	14	6	70	8	41	2	0	870	—	0	100	400
Noodles & Sauce Butter & Herb as prep	1 cup (2.2 oz)	300	13	5	65	9	42	2	0	780	—	0	100	200
Noodles & Sauce Chicken Broccoli as prep	1 cup (2.1 oz)	310	11	4	70	11	44	2	80	840	—	4	100	400
Noodles & Sauce Chicken Tetrazzini as prep	1 cup (2 oz)	300	12	4	70	10	41	2	80	950	—	0	100	500
Noodles & Sauce Chicken as prep	1 cup (2.1 oz)	290	11	3	65	8	42	2	0	830	—	0	100	500
Noodles & Sauce Creamy Chicken as prep	1 cup (2.1 oz)	320	13	5	75	11	42	2	80	810	—	0	100	1000
Noodles & Sauce Parmesan as prep	1 cup (2.1 oz)	330	15	6	75	14	40	2	150	850	—	2	100	500
Noodles & Sauce Sour Cream & Chives as prep	1 cup (2.2 oz)	310	14	6	70	10	41	2	20	870	—	1	100	400
Noodles & Sauce Stroganoff as prep	1 cup (2 oz)	300	11	4	70	11	40	2	80	950	—	0	100	500
NOODLES BY LEONARDO														
Macaroni & Cheese as prep	1 cup (2.5 oz)	250	1	0	0	10	49	2	60	530	—	0	—	0
ULTRA SLIM-FAST														
Noodles & Alfredo Sauce	2.3 oz	240	4	—	—	9	47	4	150	1110	240	18	—	750
Noodles & Beef	2.3 oz	230	3	—	—	8	45	4	150	1070	160	18	—	750
Noodles & Cheese	2.3 oz	230	4	—	—	9	44	4	150	770	240	18	—	750
Noodles & Chicken Sauce	2.3 oz	220	3	—	—	8	45	4	150	980	140	18	—	750
Noodles & Tomato Herb Sauce	2.3 oz	220	3	—	—	8	46	5	150	1090	260	18	—	750
SHELF-STABLE														
HORMEL														
Microcup Meals Noodles & Chicken	1 cup (7.5 oz)	200	9	3	40	8	20	1	20	1140	—	0	—	500
NOODLES														
cellophane	1 cup	492	tr	tr	0	tr	121	—	35	14	14	0	—	0
chow mein	1 cup (1.6 oz)	237	14	2	0	4	25	2	9	189	52	0	39	39
egg	1 cup (38 g)	145	2	tr	36	5	27	—	12	8	89	0	11	23

FOOD	PORTION	CALORIES	FAT	SAT FAT	CHOL	PROTEIN	CARBO	FIBER	CALCIUM	SOD	POTAS	VIT C	FOLIC	VIT A
egg cooked	1 cup (5.6 oz)	213	2	tr	53	8	40	2	19	11	45	0	102	32
japanese soba cooked	1 cup (4 oz)	113	tr	tr	0	6	24	—	5	68	40	0	8	0
japanese somen cooked	1 cup (6.2 oz)	231	tr	tr	0	7	48	—	14	283	51	0	4	0
rice cooked	1 cup (6.2 oz)	192	tr	tr	0	2	44	2	7	33	7	0	5	0
spinach/egg cooked	1 cup (5.6 oz)	211	3	1	53	8	39	4	30	19	59	0	102	165
AZUMAYA														
Chinese	4 oz	293	1	—	—	11	60	—	14	530	—	tr	—	—
Japanese	4 oz	289	1	—	—	11	59	—	15	542	—	1	—	—
CREAMETTE														
Egg	2 oz	220	3	—	—	8	40	—	20	20	135	—	—	—
HERB'S														
Egg Fine	2 oz	220	2	0	60	10	42	2	20	5	125	0	—	95
Egg Medium	2 oz	220	2	0	60	10	42	2	20	5	125	0	—	95
Kluski Medium	2 oz	220	2	0	60	10	42	2	20	5	125	0	—	95
Kluski Wide	2 oz	220	2	0	60	10	42	2	20	5	125	0	—	95
HODGSON MILL														
Veggie Egg	2 oz	200	2	1	35	9	37	2	20	25	—	0	—	0
Whole Wheat Egg	2 oz	190	2	1	30	10	34	4	20	20	—	0	—	100
Whole Wheat Spinach Egg	2 oz	190	2	1	30	10	32	5	20	45	—	0	—	100
KA-ME														
Chinese Egg	½ cup (2 oz)	210	2	1	53	7	40	2	—	3	—	—	—	—
Chinese Plain	½ cup (2 oz)	200	0	0	0	5	45	1	—	1	—	—	—	—
Chuka Soba Curly Noodles	2 oz	200	1	0	0	6	42	1	—	310	—	—	—	—
Lo Mein Wide Chinese	½ cup (2 oz)	200	0	0	0	5	45	1	—	1	—	—	—	—
Py Mai Fun Rice Sticks	2 oz	193	0	0	0	0	48	0	—	100	—	—	—	—
Sai Fun Bean Thread	1 cup (2 oz)	190	0	0	0	0	50	1	30	0	—	—	—	—
Soba Shin Shu Japanese Buckwheat	2 oz	200	1	0	0	9	40	2	20	80	—	—	—	—
Tomoshiraga Somen Noodles	2 oz	190	1	0	0	5	41	1	—	670	—	—	—	—
Udon Japanese Thick	2 oz	190	1	0	0	5	41	1	—	670	—	—	—	—
LA CHOY														
Chow Mein Narrow	½ cup	150	8	1	0	3	16	tr	6	320	35	—	—	—
Chow Mein Wide	½ cup	150	8	1	0	3	16	tr	6	300	35	—	—	—
Rice	½ cup	130	5	—	0	2	21	tr	4	420	35	—	—	—
NOODLES BY LEONARDO														
Egg Fine	2 oz	210	2	1	80	9	39	2	20	10	—	0	—	200
Egg Medium	2 oz	210	2	1	80	9	39	2	20	30	—	0	—	200

FOOD	PORTION	CALORIES	FAT	SAT FAT	CHOL	PROTEIN	CARBO	FIBER	CALCIUM	SOD	POTAS	VIT C	FOLIC	VIT A
NOODLES BY LEONARDO (CONT.)														
Egg Wide	2 oz	210	2	1	80	9	39	2	20	30	—	0	—	200
SAN GIORGIO														
Egg	2 oz	210	3	—	70	10	38	—	—	15	—	—	—	—
SHOFAR														
No Yolks	2 oz	210	0	0	0	91	41	3	0	30	—	0	—	0

NOPALES

FOOD	PORTION	CALORIES	FAT	SAT FAT	CHOL	PROTEIN	CARBO	FIBER	CALCIUM	SOD	POTAS	VIT C	FOLIC	VIT A
cooked	1 cup (5.2 oz)	23	tr	—	0	2	5	—	245	30	290	8	4	685
raw sliced	½ cup (1.5 oz)	7	tr	—	0	1	1	—	70	9	137	6	1	178
raw sliced	1 cup (3 oz)	14	tr	—	0	1	3	—	140	19	275	12	3	357

NUTMEG

FOOD	PORTION	CALORIES	FAT	SAT FAT	CHOL	PROTEIN	CARBO	FIBER	CALCIUM	SOD	POTAS	VIT C	FOLIC	VIT A
ground	1 tsp	12	1	1	0	tr	1	—	4	tr	8	—	—	2
WATKINS														
Ground	¼ tsp (0.5 g)	0	0	0	0	0	0	0	0	0	—	0	—	0

NUTRITIONAL SUPPLEMENTS

(*see also* BREAKFAST BAR, BREAKFAST DRINKS, SPORTS DRINKS)

FOOD	PORTION	CALORIES	FAT	SAT FAT	CHOL	PROTEIN	CARBO	FIBER	CALCIUM	SOD	POTAS	VIT C	FOLIC	VIT A
BENEFIT														
Chocolate	1 serv	120	2	—	—	11	15	1	300	200	460	21	120	1500
Nutrition Bar	1 (2 oz)	240	8	—	0	9	33	tr	200	190	125	21	140	1750
Vanilla	1 serv	120	2	—	—	11	15	tr	300	220	400	21	120	1500
BOOST														
Chocolate	1 can (8 oz)	240	4	1	5	10	40	0	300	130	400	60	140	1250
Vanilla	8 oz	240	4	1	5	10	40	0	300	130	400	60	140	1250
CALIFORNIA JOE														
All Natural Protein Drink Mix as prep	1 serv (8 oz)	165	4	2	0	12	21	0	240	166	21	—	—	—
CALORIE SHED														
Shake Fat Free No Sugar Caramel Ripple	½ cup (4 fl oz)	70	0	0	5	3	21	2	60	45	200	0	—	300
Shake Fat Free No Sugar Chocolate	½ cup (4 fl oz)	70	0	0	5	3	21	2	60	45	200	0	—	300
Shake Fat Free No Sugar Marshmellow Nougat	½ cup (4 fl oz)	70	0	0	5	3	21	2	60	45	200	0	—	300
DYNATRIM														
Dutch Chocolate as prep w/ 1% milk	8 oz	220	4	—	—	17	33	6	500	300	890	21	140	1750
Strawberry Royale as prep w/ 1% milk	8 oz	220	4	—	—	17	33	6	500	300	—	21	140	1750
Vanilla as prep w/ 1% milk	8 oz	220	4	—	—	17	33	6	500	300	—	21	140	1750
ENSURE														
Honey Graham Crunch	1 bar (2.23 oz)	130	3	1	<5	6	21	2	250	115	200	21	60	750

FOOD	PORTION	CALORIES	FAT	SAT FAT	CHOL	PROTEIN	CARBO	FIBER	CALCIUM	SOD	POTAS	VIT C	FOLIC	VIT A
ESSENTIAL														
Protein Powder	1 serv (0.6 oz)	70	tr	0	0	16	6	tr	98	5	750	—	100	—
FI-BAR														
Apple	1 (1 oz)	90	3	—	0	2	15	5	—	12	—	—	—	—
Cocoa Almond	1	130	4	—	0	3	21	4	—	20	—	—	—	—
Cocoa Peanut	1	130	4	—	0	3	20	4	—	20	—	—	—	—
Cranberry & Wild Berries	1 (1 oz)	100	3	—	0	2	13	4	—	20	—	—	—	—
Lemon	1 (1 oz)	90	3	—	0	2	15	5	—	12	—	—	—	—
Mandarin Orange	1 (1 oz)	99	4	—	0	2	15	5	—	12	—	—	—	—
Nuggets Almond Cappuccino Crunch	1 pkg	136	6	—	0	1	18	—	—	—	—	—	—	—
Nuggets Almond Butter Crunch	1 pkg	163	11	—	0	4	12	—	—	—	—	—	—	—
Nuggets Coconut Almond Crunch	1 pkg	136	6	—	0	1	18	—	—	—	—	—	—	—
Nuggets Peanut Butter Crunch	1 pkg	160	10	—	0	4	12	—	—	—	—	—	—	—
Raspberry	1 (1 oz)	100	3	—	0	2	13	4	—	20	—	—	—	—
Strawberry	1 (1 oz)	100	3	—	0	2	13	4	—	20	—	—	—	—
Treat Yourself Right Almond	1	152	6	—	0	3	22	5	—	38	—	—	—	—
Treat Yourself Right Peanutty Butter	1	152	5	—	0	4	18	5	—	56	—	—	—	—
Vanilla Almond	1	130	4	—	0	3	21	4	—	20	—	—	—	—
Vanilla Peanut	1	130	4	—	0	3	20	4	—	20	—	—	—	—
GATORADE														
GatorBar	1 (1.17 oz)	110	1	0	0	1	13	1	150	10	—	42	120	750
GatorLode	1 can (11.6 fl oz)	280	0	0	0	0	71	—	—	90	—	18	—	—
GatorPro	1 can (11 fl oz)	360	6	1	0	17	59	0	400	270	990	60	180	1250
ReLode	1 pkt (0.75 oz)	80	0	0	0	0	17	—	—	25	—	—	—	—
GENISOY														
Soy Protein Powder	1 scoop (0.6 oz)	60	0	0	0	14	0	—	250	180	70	15	100	1250
Soy Protein Shake Chocolate	1 scoop (1.2 oz)	120	0	0	0	14	17	2	250	170	230	15	100	1250
Soy Protein Shake Vanilla	1 scoop (1.2 oz)	130	0	0	0	14	18	0	250	180	70	15	100	1250
Soy Protein Bar Chocolate	1 bar (2.2 oz)	210	0	0	0	14	36	1	250	190	300	15	—	1250
Soy Protein Bar Chocolate Coated	1 bar (2.2 oz)	220	4	3	0	14	33	1	250	190	300	15	100	1250
NANCY GREY'S														
Shake Hi-Protein Black Raspberry	1 cup (8 fl oz)	340	16	10	65	10	40	0	300	160	—	2	—	500

FOOD	PORTION	CALORIES	FAT	SAT FAT	CHOL	PROTEIN	CARBO	FIBER	CALCIUM	SOD	POTAS	VIT C	FOLIC	VIT A
NANCY GREY'S (CONT.)														
Shake Hi-Protein Chocolate	1 cup (8 fl oz)	340	15	10	60	10	42	—	286	140	480	2	—	554
Shake Hi-Protein Vanilla	1 cup (8 fl oz)	340	16	10	65	10	40	0	298	160	370	2	—	580
NITEBITE														
Chocolate Fudge	1 bar (0.9 oz)	100	4	1	5	3	15	0	0	40	65	0	—	0
Peanut Butter	1 bar (0.9 oz)	100	4	1	5	3	15	0	0	80	45	0	—	0
NUTRA/BALANCE														
EggPro	4 oz	200	4	—	18	8	33	—	250	105	294	—	—	500
Frozen Pudding Butterscotch	4 oz	225	8	—	0	7	31	—	150	220	204	—	—	750
Frozen Pudding Chocolate	4 oz	225	8	—	0	7	31	—	150	220	204	—	—	750
Frozen Pudding Tapioca	4 oz	225	8	—	0	7	31	—	150	220	204	—	—	750
Frozen Pudding Vanilla	4 oz	225	8	—	0	7	31	—	150	220	204	—	—	750
NUTRASHAKE														
Chocolate	4 oz	200	6	—	18	6	31	—	230	55	222	—	—	150
Strawberry	4 oz	200	6	—	18	6	31	—	230	55	222	—	—	150
Vanilla	4 oz	200	6	—	18	6	31	—	230	55	222	—	—	150
With Fiber Strawberry	6 oz	300	2	—	0	11	60	—	375	110	330	—	—	300
With Fiber Vanilla	6 oz	300	2	—	0	11	60	—	375	110	330	—	—	300
POWER BAR														
Malt-Nut	1 bar (2.3 oz)	230	3	1	0	10	45	3	300	90	110	60	400	0
RESOURCE														
Fructose Sweetened	1 pkg (8 oz)	250	11	—	—	15	23	3	220	230	270	38	100	1250
Fruit Beverage	1 pkg (8 oz)	180	0	—	—	9	36	—	135	55	15	38	50	625
Liquid Food	1 pkg (8 oz)	250	9	—	—	8	34	—	125	210	380	38	50	625
Plus Liquid Food	1 pkg (8 oz)	355	13	—	—	13	47	—	167	300	490	38	75	890
SEGO														
Lite Chocolate	10 fl oz	150	3	—	5	11	20	—	500	480	690	15	—	1250
Lite Dutch Chocolate	10 fl oz	150	3	—	5	11	20	—	500	480	690	15	—	1250
Lite French Vanilla	10 fl oz	150	4	—	5	11	17	—	500	390	600	15	—	1250
Lite Strawberry	10 fl oz	150	4	—	5	11	17	—	500	390	600	15	—	1250
Lite Vanilla	10 fl oz	150	4	—	5	11	17	—	500	390	600	15	—	1250
Very Chocolate	10 fl oz	225	1	—	5	11	43	—	500	450	690	15	—	1250
Very Chocolate Malt	10 fl oz	225	1	—	5	11	43	—	500	450	690	15	—	1250
Very Strawberry	10 fl oz	225	5	—	5	11	34	—	500	360	600	15	—	1250
Very Vanilla	10 fl oz	225	5	—	5	11	34	—	500	360	600	15	—	1250

FOOD	PORTION	CALORIES	FAT	SAT FAT	CHOL	PROTEIN	CARBO	FIBER	CALCIUM	SOD	POTAS	VIT C	FOLIC	VIT A
SLIM-FAST														
Powder Chocolate as prep w/ skim milk	8 oz	190	1	—		9	14	32	2	450	210	720	21	120	1750
Powder Chocolate Malt as prep w/ skim milk	8 oz	190	tr	—		9	14	32	2	450	230	590	21	120	1750
Powder Strawberry as prep w/ skim milk	8 oz	190	1	—		9	14	32	2	450	220	720	21	120	1750
Powder Vanilla as prep w/ skim milk	8 oz	190	1	—		6	14	32	2	450	220	720	21	120	1750
SUSTACAL														
Vanilla	8 oz	240	6	1	<5	15	33	tr	240	220	490	13	90	1110
SWEET SUCCESS														
Chewy Bar Chocolate Brownie	1 (1.6 oz)	120	4	2	<5	2	28	3	150	35	—	9	60	750
Chewy Bar Chocolate Peanut Butter	1 (1.6 oz)	120	4	2	<5	2	23	3	150	35	—	9	60	750
Chewy Bar Chocolate Raspberry	1 (1.6 oz)	120	4	2	<5	2	23	3	150	35	—	9	60	750
Chewy Bar Chocolate Chip	1 (1.6 oz)	120	4	2	<5	2	23	3	150	35	—	9	60	750
Chewy Bar Oatmeal Raisin	1 (1.6 oz)	120	4	2	<5	2	23	3	150	30	—	9	60	750
Chocolate Raspberry Truffle	1 can (10 fl oz)	200	3	1	5	12	38	6	500	220	—	21	140	1750
Chocolate Raspberry as prep w/ skim milk	9 fl oz	180	1	1	6	14	30	6	500	360	—	21	140	1750
Chocolate Mocha Supreme	1 can (10 fl oz)	200	3	1	5	12	38	6	500	220	—	21	140	1750
Chocolate Mocha Supreme as prep w/ skim milk	9 fl oz	180	tr	1	6	14	30	6	500	356	—	21	140	1750
Classic Chocolate Chip as prep w/ skim milk	9 fl oz	180	1	2	6	14	30	6	500	288	—	21	140	1750
Creamy Milk Chocolate	1 carton (12 fl oz)	220	2	1	<5	14	45	6	500	300	—	0	140	1750
Creamy Milk Chocolate	1 can (10 fl oz)	200	3	1	5	12	38	6	500	240	—	21	140	1750
Creamy Milk Chocolate as prep w/ skim milk	9 fl oz	180	1	1	6	14	30	6	500	336	—	21	140	1750
Creamy Vanilla Delight as prep w/ skim milk	9 fl oz	180	tr	1	6	14	33	6	500	312	—	21	140	1750

FOOD	PORTION	CALORIES	FAT	SAT FAT	CHOL	PROTEIN	CARBO	FIBER	CALCIUM	SOD	POTAS	VIT C	FOLIC	VIT A
SWEET SUCCESS (CONT.)														
Dark Chocolate Fudge	1 can (10 fl oz)	200	3	1	5	12	38	6	500	220	—	21	140	1750
Dark Chocolate Fudge	1 carton (12 fl oz)	220	2	1	<5	14	45	6	500	310	—	0	140	1750
Dark Chocolate Fudge as prep w/ skim milk	9 fl oz	180	1	1	6	14	30	6	500	356	—	21	140	1750
Rich Chocolate Almond	1 carton (12 fl oz)	220	2	1	<5	14	45	6	500	300	—	0	140	1750
Rich Chocolate Almond	1 can (10 fl oz)	200	3	1	5	12	38	6	500	240	—	21	140	1750
Rich Chocolate Almond as prep w/ skim milk	9 fl oz	180	tr	1	6	14	30	6	500	356	—	21	140	1750
Smooth Vanilla Creme	1 can (10 fl oz)	200	3	1	5	12	38	6	500	220	—	21	140	1750
THE PUMPER														
Body Building MilkShake Chocolate	1 serv (13.5 oz)	390	2	1	5	21	80	5	468	260	1060	4	—	536
ULTRA SLIM-FAST														
Cafe Mocha as prep w/ skim milk	8 oz	200	tr	—		8	15	38	6	450	280	800	21	120	1750
Chocolate Royale as prep w/ skim milk	8 oz	200	1	—		8	14	36	5	450	230	800	21	120	1750
Crunch Bar Cocoa Almond	1	110	3	—		0	2	19	3	150	30	110	9	60	750
Crunch Bar Cocoa Raspberry	1	100	3	—		0	2	21	3	150	30	110	9	60	750
Crunch Bar Vanilla Almond	1	110	4	—		0	2	18	3	150	30	110	9	60	750
Dutch Chocolate as prep w/ water	8 oz	220	tr	—		8	14	40	5	500	260	680	21	120	1750
French Vanilla as prep w/ skim milk	8 oz	190	tr	—		8	14	36	4	450	250	730	21	120	1750
French Vanilla as prep w/ water	8 oz	220	tr	—		8	14	40	4	500	260	640	21	120	1750
Fruit Juice Mix as prep w/ fruit juice	8 oz	200	tr	—		12	11	43	6	450	80	590	21	120	1750
Nutrition Bar Dutch Chocolate	1	130	4	—		5	6	17	6	100	90	150	21	80	1750
Nutrition Bar Peanut Butter	1	140	6	—		5	7	15	7	100	100	160	21	80	1750
Pina Colada as prep w/ skim milk	8 oz	180	tr	—		8	14	36	6	450	250	730	21	120	1750
Ready-To-Drink Chocolate Royale	12 oz	250	1	—		5	11	45	5	500	240	1300	tr	120	1750

FOOD	PORTION	CALORIES	FAT	SAT FAT	CHOL	PROTEIN	CARBO	FIBER	CALCIUM	SOD	POTAS	VIT C	FOLIC	VIT A
ULTRA SLIM-FAST (CONT.)														
Ready-To-Drink Chocolate Royale	11 oz	230	3	—	5	11	42	5	500	220	1200	21	120	1750
Ready-To-Drink French Vanilla	12 oz	220	tr	—	5	13	38	5	500	240	760	tr	120	1750
Ready-To-Drink French Vanilla	11 oz	230	5	—	5	12	38	5	500	190	1160	21	120	1750
Ready-To-Drink Strawberry Supreme	12 oz	220	1	—	5	13	38	5	500	240	760	tr	120	1750
Strawberry Supreme as prep w/ water	8 oz	220	tr	—	8	14	40	4	500	260	640	21	120	1750
Strawberry as prep w/ skim milk	8 oz	190	1	—	8	14	36	4	450	250	710	21	120	1750
VITA-J														
Apple Juice	11.5 fl oz	8	0	0	0	1	2	—	—	25	—	60	400	5000
Fruit Punch	11.5 fl oz	8	0	0	0	1	2	—	—	25	—	60	400	5000
Grapefruit Cocktail w/ Raspberry	11.5 fl oz	8	0	0	0	1	2	—	—	25	—	60	400	5000
Orange Juice	11.5 fl oz	8	0	0	0	1	2	—	—	25	—	60	400	5000
NUTS MIXED														
(*see also individual names*)														
dry roasted w/ peanuts	1 oz	169	15	2	0	5	7	—	20	3	169	tr	14	4
dry roasted w/ peanuts salted	1 oz	169	15	2	0	5	7	—	20	223	169	tr	14	4
oil roasted w/ peanuts	1 oz	175	16	2	0	5	6	—	31	3	165	tr	24	6
oil roasted w/ peanuts salted	1 oz	175	16	2	0	5	6	—	31	217	165	tr	24	6
oil roasted w/o peanuts	1 oz	175	16	3	0	4	6	—	30	3	154	tr	16	6
oil roasted w/o peanuts salted	1 oz	175	16	3	0	4	6	—	30	233	154	tr	0	6
FISHER														
Mixed Deluxe Lightly Salted	1 oz	180	16	3	0	6	5	—	40	—	—	—	—	—
Mixed Deluxe Salted	1 oz	180	16	3	0	6	5	—	40	95	—	—	—	—
Mixed Oil Roasted 25% More Cashews Lightly Salted	1 oz	180	16	3	0	6	5	—	20	50	—	—	—	—
Mixed Oil Roasted 25% More Cashews Salted	1 oz	180	16	3	0	6	5	—	20	110	—	—	—	—
Nut & Fruit Pina Colada	1 oz	150	10	2	0	4	13	—	20	50	—	—	—	—

FOOD	PORTION	CALORIES	FAT	SAT FAT	CHOL	PROTEIN	CARBO	FIBER	CALCIUM	SOD	POTAS	VIT C	FOLIC	VIT A
FISHER (CONT.)														
Nut & Fruit Raisin Cranberry	1 oz	150	10	2	0	4	12	—	—	70	—	—	—	—
Nut & Fruit Tropical Fruit	1 oz	140	8	1	0	4	15	—	20	90	—	—	—	—
Nut Toppings Oil Roasted With Peanuts	1 oz	190	17	3	0	6	6	—	20	150	—	—	—	—
Peanuts Cashews	1 oz	170	13	2	0	6	8	—	—	110	—	—	—	—
GUY'S														
Mixed With Peanuts	1 oz	180	16	—	0	7	3	—	20	140	180	—	—	—
Tasty Mix	1 oz	130	7	—	0	3	14	—	20	510	55	4	—	200
PLANTERS														
Cashews & Peanuts Honey Roasted	1 oz	150	12	2	0	5	10	2	20	125	150	—	—	—
Deluxe Oil Roasted	1 oz	170	16	2	0	5	6	2	40	110	170	—	—	—
Dry Roasted	1 oz	170	14	2	0	6	7	2	40	250	180	—	—	—
Honey Roasted	1 oz	140	13	2	0	5	9	2	20	85	150	—	—	—
Lightly Salted Oil Roasted	1 oz	170	15	2	0	6	6	2	20	55	160	—	—	—
No Brazils Lightly Salted Oil Roasted	1 oz	170	15	2	0	6	6	2	40	55	180	—	—	—
No Brazils Oil Roasted	1 oz	170	15	2	0	5	6	2	40	110	180	—	—	—
Oil Roasted	1 oz	170	15	3	0	6	5	2	40	115	180	—	—	—
Select Mix Cashews Almonds & Macadamias Oil Roasted	1 oz	170	16	3	0	4	6	2	40	90	160	—	—	—
Select Mix Cashews Almonds & Pecans Oil Roasted	1 oz	170	15	2	0	4	7	2	40	95	160	—	—	—
Unsalted Oil Roasted	1 oz	170	15	2	0	6	6	3	20	0	180	—	—	—
OHELOBERRIES														
fresh	1 cup	39	tr	—	0	1	10	—	10	2	54	8	—	1162
OIL														
(*see also* FAT)														
almond	1 cup	1927	218	1	0	0	0	—	—	—	—	—	—	—
almond	1 tbsp	120	14	1	0	0	0	—	—	—	—	—	—	—
apricot kernel	1 tbsp	120	14	1	0	0	0	—	—	—	—	—	—	—
apricot kernel	1 cup	1927	218	14	0	0	0	—	—	—	—	—	—	—
butter oil	1 cup	1795	204	127	524	1	0	—	—	—	—	—	—	7688
butter oil	1 tbsp	112	13	8	33	tr	0	—	—	—	—	—	—	480
corn	1 cup	1927	218	28	0	0	0	—	—	—	—	—	—	—

FOOD	PORTION	CALORIES	FAT	SAT FAT	CHOL	PROTEIN	CARBO	FIBER	CALCIUM	SOD	POTAS	VIT C	FOLIC	VIT A
corn	1 tbsp	120	14	2	0	0	0	—	—	—	—	—	—	—
cottonseed	1 cup	1927	218	56	0	0	0	—	—	—	—	—	—	—
cottonseed	1 tbsp	120	14	4	0	0	0	—	—	—	—	—	—	—
cupu assu	1 tbsp	120	14	7	0	0	0	—	—	—	—	—	—	—
grapeseed	1 tbsp	120	14	1	0	0	0	—	—	—	—	—	—	—
hazelnut	1 cup	1927	218	1	0	0	0	—	—	—	—	—	—	—
hazelnut	1 tbsp	120	14	1	0	0	0	—	—	—	—	—	—	—
olive	1 tbsp	119	14	2	0	0	0	—	tr	0	—	—	—	—
olive	1 cup	1909	216	26	0	0	0	—	tr	tr	—	—	—	—
palm	1 tbsp	120	14	7	0	0	0	—	—	—	—	—	—	—
palm	1 cup	1927	218	107	0	0	0	—	—	—	—	—	—	—
peanut	1 tbsp	119	14	2	0	0	0	—	tr	tr	0	—	—	—
peanut	1 cup	1909	216	36	0	0	0	—	tr	tr	tr	—	—	—
poppyseed	1 tbsp	120	14	2	0	0	0	—	—	—	—	—	—	—
poppyseed	3.5 fl oz	900	100	2	0	0	0	—	—	—	—	—	—	—
rice bran	1 tbsp	120	14	3	0	0	0	—	—	—	—	—	—	—
safflower	1 tbsp	120	14	1	0	0	0	—	—	—	—	—	—	—
safflower	1 cup	1927	218	20	0	0	0	—	—	—	—	—	—	—
sesame	1 tbsp	120	14	2	0	0	0	—	—	—	—	—	—	—
sheanut	1 tbsp	120	14	6	0	0	0	—	—	—	—	—	—	—
soybean	1 tbsp	120	14	2	0	0	0	—	tr	0	—	—	—	—
soybean	1 cup	1927	218	31	0	0	0	—	tr	tr	—	—	—	—
sunflower	1 cup	1927	218	23	0	0	0	—	—	—	—	—	—	—
sunflower	1 tbsp	120	14	1	0	0	0	—	—	—	—	—	—	—
teaseed	1 tbsp	120	14	3	0	0	0	—	—	—	—	—	—	—
tomatoseed	1 tbsp	120	14	3	0	0	0	—	—	—	—	—	—	—
vegetable soybean & cottonseed	1 cup	1927	218	2	0	0	0	—	—	—	—	—	—	—
vegetable soybean & cottonseed	1 tbsp	120	14	2	0	0	0	—	—	—	—	—	—	—
walnut	1 cup	1927	218	20	0	0	0	1	—	—	—	—	—	—
walnut	1 tbsp	120	14	1	0	0	0	—	—	—	—	—	—	—
wheat germ	1 tbsp	120	14	3	0	0	0	—	—	—	—	—	—	—
ARROWHEAD														
Flax Seed	1 tbsp (0.5 fl oz)	120	14	1	—	0	0	0	—	0	—	—	—	150
Hazelnut	1 tbsp (0.5 fl oz)	120	14	1	0	0	0	0	0	0	—	0	—	0
BERTOLLI														
Extra Light	1 tbsp	120	14	—	0	—	—	—	—	—	—	—	—	—
CRISCO														
Corn Canola	1 tbsp (0.5 fl oz)	120	14	2	0	0	0	—	—	0	—	—	—	—
Oil	1 tbsp (0.5 fl oz)	120	14	2	0	0	0	—	—	0	—	—	—	—

FOOD	PORTION	CALORIES	FAT	SAT FAT	CHOL	PROTEIN	CARBO	FIBER	CALCIUM	SOD	POTAS	VIT C	FOLIC	VIT A
CRISCO (CONT.)														
Puritan Canola	1 tbsp (0.5 fl oz)	120	14	1	0	0	0	0	0	0	—	0	—	0
EDEN														
Hot Pepper Sesame	1 tbsp (0.5 oz)	130	14	2	0	0	0	0	0	0	—	0	—	0
Safflower	1 tbsp (0.5 oz)	120	14	1	0	0	0	—	—	0	—	—	—	—
Sesame	1 tbsp (0.5 oz)	140	15	2	0	0	0	—	—	0	—	—	—	—
Toasted Sesame	1 tbsp (0.5 oz)	130	14	2	0	0	0	0	0	0	—	0	—	0
HAIN														
All Blend	1 tbsp	120	14	2	0	0	0	—	—	0	0	—	—	—
Almond	1 tbsp	120	14	1	0	0	0	—	—	0	0	—	—	—
Apricot Kernel	1 tbsp	120	14	1	0	0	0	—	—	0	0	—	—	—
Avocado	1 tbsp	120	14	1	0	0	0	—	—	0	0	—	—	—
Canola	1 tbsp	120	14	1	0	0	0	—	—	0	0	—	—	—
Canola Organic	1 tbsp	120	14	1	0	0	0	—	—	0	0	—	—	—
Coconut	1 tbsp	120	14	12	0	0	0	—	—	0	0	—	—	—
Corn	1 tbsp	120	14	2	0	0	0	—	—	0	0	—	—	—
Garlic & Oil	1 tbsp	120	14	3	0	0	0	—	—	0	0	—	—	—
Olive	1 tbsp	120	14	2	0	0	0	—	—	0	0	—	—	—
Peanut	1 tbsp	120	14	2	0	0	0	—	—	0	0	—	—	—
Rice Bran	1 tbsp	120	14	3	0	0	0	—	—	0	0	—	—	—
Safflower	1 tbsp	120	14	1	0	0	0	—	—	0	0	—	—	—
Safflower Hi-Oleic	1 tbsp	120	14	1	0	0	0	—	—	0	0	—	—	—
Safflower Organic	1 tbsp	120	14	1	0	0	0	—	—	0	0	—	—	—
Sesame	1 tbsp	120	14	2	0	0	0	—	—	0	0	—	—	—
Soy	1 tbsp	120	14	2	0	0	0	—	—	0	0	—	—	—
Sunflower	1 tbsp	120	14	2	0	0	0	—	—	0	0	—	—	—
Sunflower Organic	1 tbsp	120	14	2	0	0	0	—	—	0	0	—	—	—
Walnut	1 tbsp	120	14	2	0	0	0	—	—	0	0	—	—	—
HOLLYWOOD														
Canola	1 tbsp	120	14	1	0	0	0	—	—	0	0	—	—	—
Peanut	1 tbsp	120	14	4	0	0	0	—	—	0	0	—	—	—
Safflower	1 tbsp	120	14	1	0	0	0	—	—	0	0	—	—	—
Soy	1 tbsp	120	14	3	0	0	0	—	—	0	0	—	—	—
Sunflower	1 tbsp	120	14	2	0	0	0	—	—	0	0	—	—	—
HOUSE OF TSANG														
Hot Chili Sesame	1 tsp (5 g)	45	5	1	0	0	0	0	0	0	—	0	—	0
Mongolian Fire	1 tsp (5 g)	45	5	1	0	0	0	0	0	0	—	0	—	0
Pure Sesame	1 tsp (5 g)	45	5	1	0	0	0	0	0	0	—	0	—	0
Singapore Curry	1 tsp (5 g)	45	5	1	0	0	0	0	0	0	—	0	—	0
Wok Oil	1 tbsp (0.5 oz)	130	14	3	0	0	0	0	0	0	—	0	—	0
KA-ME														
Chili Hot	1 tbsp (0.5 fl oz)	130	14	2	0	0	0	0	0	0	—	—	—	—
Sesame	1 tbsp (0.5 fl oz)	130	14	2	0	0	0	0	0	0	—	—	—	—

FOOD	PORTION	CALORIES	FAT	SAT FAT	CHOL	PROTEIN	CARBO	FIBER	CALCIUM	SOD	POTAS	VIT C	FOLIC	VIT A
KA-ME (CONT.)														
Sesame Tempura	1 tbsp (0.5 fl oz)	130	14	3	0	0	0	0	0	0	—	—	—	—
ORVILLE REDENBACHER'S														
Oil	1 tbsp	120	14	2	0	0	0	0	—	0	0	—	—	—
PAM														
Butter	⅓ sec spray (0.3 g)	0	0	0	0	0	0	—	—	0	—	—	—	—
Cooking Spray	⅓ sec spray (0.3 g)	0	0	0	0	0	0	—	—	0	—	—	—	—
Olive Oil	⅓ sec spray (0.3 g)	0	0	0	0	0	0	—	—	0	—	—	—	—
PLANTERS														
Peanut	1 tbsp (0.5 oz)	120	14	3	0	0	0	—	—	0	0	—	—	—
Popcorn	1 tbsp (0.5 oz)	120	14	3	0	0	0	—	—	0	0	—	—	—
PROGRESSO														
Olive Extra Light	1 tbsp	119	14	2	0	0	0	0	—	0	0	—	—	—
Olive Extra Mild	1 tbsp (0.5 oz)	120	14	2	0	0	0	0	0	0	—	0	—	0
Olive Extra Virgin	1 tbsp (0.5 oz)	120	14	2	0	0	0	0	0	0	—	0	—	0
Olive Riviera Blend	1 tbsp (0.5 oz)	120	14	2	0	0	0	0	0	0	—	0	—	0
SMART BEAT														
Canola	1 tbsp	120	14	1	0	0	0	—	—	0	—	—	—	—
Oil	1 tbsp	120	14	1	0	0	0	—	—	0	—	—	—	—
TREE OF LIFE														
Almond	1 tbsp (0.5 g)	130	14	1	0	0	0	—	—	0	—	—	—	—
Apricot Kernel	1 tbsp (0.5 g)	130	14	1	0	0	0	—	—	0	—	—	—	—
Avocado	1 tbsp (0.5 g)	130	14	3	0	0	0	—	—	0	—	—	—	—
Macadamia Nut	1 tbsp (0.5 g)	130	14	2	0	0	0	—	—	0	—	—	—	—
Olive Extra Virgin Organic	1 tbsp (0.5 g)	130	14	1	0	0	0	—	—	0	—	—	—	—
Sesame	1 tbsp (0.5 g)	130	14	2	0	0	0	—	—	0	—	—	—	—
Toasted Sesame	1 tbsp (0.5 oz)	130	14	2	0	0	0	0	—	0	—	—	—	—
WEIGHT WATCHERS														
Butter Spray	⅓ second spray	0	0	0	0	0	0	0	0	0	—	0	—	0
Cooking Spray	⅓ second spray	0	0	0	0	0	0	0	0	0	—	0	—	0
WESSON														
Canola	1 tbsp	120	14	1	0	0	0	0	0	0	0	0	—	0
Cooking Spray Lite	0.5 sec spray	0	0	—	0	0	0	0	0	0	—	0	—	0
Corn	1 tbsp	120	14	2	0	0	0	0	0	0	0	0	—	0
Olive	1 tbsp	120	14	2	0	0	0	0	0	0	0	0	—	0
Sunflower	1 tbsp	120	14	2	0	0	0	0	0	0	0	0	—	0
Vegetable	1 tbsp	120	14	2	0	0	0	0	0	0	0	0	—	0
FISH OIL														
HAIN														
Cod Liver	1 tbsp	120	14	—	85	0	0	—	—	0	0	—	—	35000

FOOD	PORTION	CALORIES	FAT	SAT FAT	CHOL	PROTEIN	CARBO	FIBER	CALCIUM	SOD	POTAS	VIT C	FOLIC	VIT A
HAIN (CONT.)														
Cod Liver Cherry	1 tbsp	120	14	—	75	0	0	—	—	0	0	—	—	35000
Cod Liver Mint	1 tbsp	120	14	—	85	0	0	—	—	0	0	—	—	35000

OKRA

CANNED

ALLEN

Cut	½ cup (4.4 oz)	25	0	0	0	1	6	3	80	400	—	12	—	200

MCILHENNY

Pickled	2 pieces (1 oz)	7	tr	tr	0	tr	1	1	27	18	—	tr	—	148

TRAPPEY

Cocktail Hot	2 pieces (1 oz)	8	tr	tr	0	tr	2	1	19	139	—	tr	—	113
Cocktail Mild	1 piece (1 oz)	9	tr	tr	0	1	1	1	22	207	—	1	—	34
Creole Gumbo	½ cup (4.2 oz)	35	0	0	0	2	6	3	60	290	—	9	—	750
Cut	½ cup (4.4 oz)	25	0	0	0	1	6	3	80	400	—	12	—	200

FRESH

raw	8 pods	36	tr	tr	0	2	7	—	77	8	287	20	83	627
raw sliced	½ cup	19	tr	tr	0	1	4	—	41	4	151	11	44	330
sliced cooked	½ cup	25	tr	tr	0	1	6	—	50	4	257	13	37	460
sliced cooked	8 pods	27	tr	tr	0	2	6	—	54	5	273	14	39	489

FROZEN

sliced cooked	½ cup	34	tr	tr	0	2	8	—	88	3	215	11	134	473
sliced cooked	1 pkg (10 oz)	94	1	tr	0	5	21	—	245	8	597	31	371	1311

BIRDS EYE

Cut	¾ cup (2.9 oz)	25	0	0	0	1	5	3	60	35	—	2	—	100
Whole	9 pods (3 oz)	25	0	0	0	1	5	3	60	35	—	2	—	100

FRESH LIKE

Cut	3.5 oz	26	tr	—	—	3	6	1	76	3	187	10	—	481
Whole	3.5 oz	32	tr	—	—	2	7	1	87	2	236	15	—	444

OLIVES

green	4 med	15	2	tr	0	tr	tr	tr	8	312	7	0	—	40
green	3 extra lg	15	2	tr	0	tr	tr	tr	8	312	7	0	—	40

PROGRESSO

Oil Cured	6 (0.5 oz)	80	6	1	0	0	3	1	0	330	—	0	—	0
Olive Salad (drained)	2 tbsp (0.8 oz)	25	3	0	0	0	1	1	0	360	—	0	—	0

ONION

CANNED

chopped	½ cup	21	tr	tr	0	1	5	—	51	416	124	—	—	—
whole	1 (2.2 oz)	12	tr	tr	0	1	3	—	29	234	70	—	—	—

VLASIC

Lightly Spiced Cocktail Onions	1 oz	4	0	0	0	0	1	—	—	365	—	—	—	—

WATKINS

Liquid Spice	1 tbsp (0.5 oz)	120	14	2	0	0	0	0	0	0	—	0	—	0

FOOD	PORTION	CALORIES	FAT	SAT FAT	CHOL	PROTEIN	CARBO	FIBER	CALCIUM	SOD	POTAS	VIT C	FOLIC	VIT A
DRIED														
flakes	1 tbsp	16	tr	tr	0	tr	4	—	13	1	81	4	8	0
powder	1 tsp	7	tr	—	0	tr	2	—	8	1	20	0	—	—
WATKINS														
Flakes	¼ tsp (1 g)	0	0	0	0	0	0	0	0	0	—	0	—	0
FRESH														
welsh raw	3½ oz	34	tr	tr	0	2	7	—	18	—	—	27	—	—
ANTIOCH FARMS														
Vidalia	1 med	60	0	—	0	1	14	3	40	10	200	12	tr	tr
DOLE														
Green Chopped	1 tbsp	2	tr	—	0	tr	tr	tr	—	0	15	3	—	300
Medium	1	60	0	—	0	1	14	3	—	10	208	11	—	0
FROZEN														
chopped cooked	½ cup	30	tr	tr	0	tr	7	—	17	12	114	3	14	36
chopped cooked	1 tbsp	4	tr	tr	0	tr	1	—	2	2	16	tr	0	5
rings	7 (2.5 oz)	285	19	6	0	4	27	—	21	263	90	1	9	158
rings cooked	2 (0.7 oz)	81	5	2	0	1	8	—	6	75	26	tr	3	45
whole cooked	3½ oz	28	tr	0	0	tr	7	—	27	8	101	5	13	21
BIRDS EYE														
Pearl Onions In Cream Sauce	½ cup (4.4 oz)	60	2	1	10	2	8	1	40	280	—	0	—	0
FRESH LIKE														
Diced	3.5 oz	29	0	—	—	1	7	0	18	7	125	4	—	14
Whole	3.5 oz	37	tr	—	—	1	8	1	36	10	142	7	—	16
KINERET														
Rings	6 (3 oz)	200	10	3	0	3	25	0	60	310	85	2	—	200
MRS. PAUL'S														
Crispy Onion Rings	2½ oz	190	12	—	—	2	19	—	20	230	—	—	—	—
ORE IDA														
Chopped	¾ cup (3 oz)	25	0	0	0	tr	6	1	0	20	75	4	—	0
Onion Ringers	6 pieces (3 oz)	240	14	3	0	3	26	2	20	250	135	2	—	200
TAKE-OUT														
fried	½ cup (7.5 oz)	176	11	6	—	3	17	—	57	—	—	20	—	540
rings breaded & fried	8 to 9	275	16	7	14	4	31	—	73	430	129	tr	11	8

OPOSSUM

FOOD	PORTION	CALORIES	FAT	SAT FAT	CHOL	PROTEIN	CARBO	FIBER	CALCIUM	SOD	POTAS	VIT C	FOLIC	VIT A
roasted	3 oz	188	9	—	—	26	0	—	—	—	—	—	—	—

ORANGE

FOOD	PORTION	CALORIES	FAT	SAT FAT	CHOL	PROTEIN	CARBO	FIBER	CALCIUM	SOD	POTAS	VIT C	FOLIC	VIT A
CANNED														
DEL MONTE														
Mandarin In Heavy Syrup	½ cup (4.4 oz)	80	0	0	0	0	19	tr	0	10	—	12	—	0
DOLE														
Mandarin Segments	½ cup	70	tr	—	0	0	19	—	—	10	—	—	—	—

FOOD	PORTION	CALORIES	FAT	SAT FAT	CHOL	PROTEIN	CARBO	FIBER	CALCIUM	SOD	POTAS	VIT C	FOLIC	VIT A
DOLE (CONT.)														
Pineapple Mandarin Segments	½ cup	80	tr	—	0	0	19	—	—	5	—	—	—	—
FRESH														
peel	1 tbsp	6	tr	tr	0	tr	2	—	10	0	13	8	—	25
DOLE														
Orange	1	50	0	—	0	1	13	6	—	0	270	78	—	96
ORANGE EXTRACT														
VIRGINIA DARE														
Virginia Dare	1 tsp	22	0	—	0	—	—	—	0	—	—	—	—	—
ORANGE JUICE														
canned	1 cup	104	tr	tr	0	1	25	—	21	6	436	86	—	432
chilled	1 cup	110	1	tr	0	2	25	—	24	2	473	82	45	194
fresh	1 cup	111	tr	tr	0	2	26	—	27	2	496	124	—	496
orange drink	6 oz	94	0	0	0	0	24	—	12	31	33	64	—	33
AFTER THE FALL														
Juice	1 bottle (10 oz)	110	0	0	0	2	26	—	20	10	470	96	—	200
BRIGHT & EARLY														
Chilled	8 fl oz	120	0	0	0	0	30	—	—	30	—	60	—	—
Frozen	8 fl oz	120	0	0	0	0	30	—	—	10	—	60	—	—
CAPRI SUN														
Drink	1 pkg (7 oz)	100	0	0	0	0	25	0	0	20	40	0	—	0
DEL MONTE														
Juice	8 fl oz	110	0	0	0	2	27	tr	40	25	—	72	—	200
EVERFRESH														
Juice	1 can (8 oz)	100	0	0	0	0	24	0	—	0	—	—	—	—
Ruby Red Orange Drink	1 can (8 oz)	130	0	0	0	0	33	0	—	0	—	—	—	—
FRESH SAMANTHA														
Juice	1 cup (8 oz)	109	1	0	0	4	24	1	20	0	—	84	40	200
HI-C														
Box	8.45 fl oz	130	0	0	0	0	33	—	—	30	—	60	—	—
Drink	8 fl oz	130	0	0	0	0	32	—	—	25	—	60	—	—
Drink	1 can (11.5 fl oz)	180	0	0	0	0	45	—	—	40	—	84	—	—
HOOD														
From Concentrate	1 cup (8 oz)	120	0	0	0	0	30	—	—	20	—	96	—	—
Select	1 cup (8 oz)	120	0	0	0	0	30	—	—	2	—	96	—	—
With Calcium	1 cup (8 oz)	120	0	0	0	0	30	—	300	20	—	96	—	—
KOOL-AID														
Drink Mix Orange as prep	1 serv (8 oz)	60	0	0	0	0	16	0	0	5	0	6	—	0
Orange Drink as prep w/ sugar	1 serv (8 oz)	100	0	0	0	0	25	0	0	10	0	6	—	0

FOOD	PORTION	CALORIES	FAT	SAT FAT	CHOL	PROTEIN	CARBO	FIBER	CALCIUM	SOD	POTAS	VIT C	FOLIC	VIT A
LIBBY														
Juice	6 fl oz	80	0	0	0	1	20	—	20	0	320	72	—	300
MINUTE MAID														
Box	8.45 fl oz	120	0	0	0	0	28	—	—	25	500	54	—	—
Calcium Rich Chilled	8 fl oz	120	0	0	0	0r	27	—	300	25	480	78	—	—
Calcium Rich frzn	8 fl oz	120	0	0	0	0	27	—	300	0	480	96	—	—
Chilled	8 fl oz	110	0	0	0	0	27	—	—	25	480	78	—	—
Country Style Chilled	8 fl oz	110	0	0	0	0	27	—	—	25	480	72	—	—
Country Style frzn	8 fl oz	110	0	0	0	0	27	—	—	0	480	96	—	—
Juices To Go	1 can (11.5 fl oz)	160	0	0	0	0	39	—	—	35	690	126	—	—
Juices To Go	1 bottle (16 fl oz)	110	0	0	0	0	27	—	—	25	480	72	—	—
Juices To Go	1 bottle (10 fl oz)	140	0	0	0	0	34	—	—	30	600	90	—	—
Orange Punch Box	8.45 fl oz	130	0	0	0	0	33	—	—	25	—	—	—	—
Premium Choice ·Chilled	8 fl oz	110	0	0	0	0	27	—	—	0	480	72	—	—
Pulp Free Chilled	8 fl oz	110	0	0	0	0	27	—	—	25	480	78	—	—
Pulp Free frzn	8 fl oz	110	0	0	0	0	27	—	—	0	—	96	—	—
Reduced Acid frzn	8 fl oz	110	0	0	0	0	27	—	—	0	480	96	—	—
MOTT'S														
From Concentrate	10 fl oz	130	1	0	0	2	29	0	20	20	630	84	—	400
OCEAN SPRAY														
100% Juice	8 fl oz	120	0	0	0	0	31	0	—	35	300	78	—	0
ODWALLA														
Juice	8 fl oz	110	1	—	—	2	25	1	20	25	—	150	—	500
SHASTA PLUS														
Orange Drink	1 can (11.5 oz)	160	0	0	0	0	40	0	—	45	—	60	—	—
SIPPIN' PAK														
100% Pure	8.45 fl oz	110	0	0	0	1	26	—	20	25	380	60	—	100
SNAPPLE														
Juice	10 fl oz	130	0	0	0	0	29	—	40	55	410	60	—	0
Orangeade	8 fl oz	120	0	0	0	0	31	—	0	10	—	—	—	0
TANG														
Orange Drink as prep	1 serv (8 oz)	90	0	0	0	0	23	0	80	0	50	60	—	500
Sugar Free Orange as prep	1 serv (8 oz)	5	0	0	0	0	0	0	tr	0	75	60	—	500
TREE OF LIFE														
Juice	8 fl oz	110	0	0	0	1	27	0	0	10	360	78	—	0
TROPICANA														
Double Vitamin C with Vitamin E	8 fl oz	110	0	0	0	2	26	—	20	0	450	144	60	—

FOOD	PORTION	CALORIES	FAT	SAT FAT	CHOL	PROTEIN	CARBO	FIBER	CALCIUM	SOD	POTAS	VIT C	FOLIC	VIT A
TROPICANA (CONT.)														
Frozen as prep	6 fl oz	110	0	0	0	tr	27	—	—	5	430	130	—	—
Juice	1 container (6 fl oz)	80	0	0	0	tr	20	—	—	0	320	15	—	—
Juice	1 container (8 fl oz)	110	0	0	0	tr	27	—	—	0	430	45	—	—
Juice	8 fl oz	110	0	0	0	tr	27	—	—	0	430	45	—	—
Juice	1 container (10 fl oz)	130	0	0	0	tr	33	—	—	0	530	60	—	—
Prue Premium Calcium & Extra Vitamin C	8 fl oz	110	0	0	0	2	26	—	350	0	450	108	60	—
Prue Premium Vitamins C&E	8 fl oz	110	0	0	0	2	26	—	20	0	450	144	60	—
Season's Best	1 can (11.5 fl oz)	140	0	0	0	tr	36	—	—	5	600	130	—	—
Season's Best	1 bottle (7 fl oz)	90	0	0	0	tr	23	—	—	0	370	110	—	—
Season's Best	1 bottle (10 fl oz)	130	0	0	0	tr	33	—	—	5	530	160	—	—
Season's Best Homestyle	8 fl oz	110	0	0	0	tr	27	—	—	5	430	100	—	—
VERYFINE														
100% Juice	1 bottle (10 oz)	150	0	0	0	0	37	2	0	45	—	60	—	0
Chillers Artric Orange	8 fl oz	130	0	0	0	0	33	0	0	10	—	60	—	0
Juice Blend	1 can (11.5 oz)	160	0	0	0	0	39	0	0	10	—	42	—	0
Orange Drink	1 bottle (10 oz)	160	0	0	0	0	41	0	0	90	—	36	—	0

OREGANO
ground	1 tsp	5	tr	tr	0	tr	1	—	24	tr	25	—	—	104
WATKINS														
Liquid Spice	1 tbsp (0.5 oz)	120	14	2	0	0	0	0	0	0	—	0	—	0

ORGAN MEATS
(*see* BRAINS, GIBLETS, GIZZARD, HEART, KIDNEY, LIVER, SWEETBREADS)

ORIENTAL FOOD
(*see* ASIAN FOOD, EGG ROLLS, DINNER, NOODLES, RICE, SUSHI)

OSTRICH
ostrich	3 oz	127	3	—	54	—	—	—	—	—	—	—	—	—

OYSTERS
CANNED														
eastern	1 cup	170	6	2	136	18	10	—	111	277	568	—	22	—
eastern	3 oz	58	2	1	46	6	3	—	38	95	195	—	8	—
BUMBLE BEE														
Whole	½ cup (3.5 oz)	100	4	1	55	10	6	0	20	490	260	—	—	—

FOOD	PORTION	CALORIES	FAT	SAT FAT	CHOL	PROTEIN	CARBO	FIBER	CALCIUM	SOD	POTAS	VIT C	FOLIC	VIT A
FRESH														
eastern cooked	6 med	58	2	1	46	6	3	—	38	94	192	—	8	—
eastern cooked	3 oz	117	4	1	93	12	7	—	76	190	389	—	15	—
eastern raw	1 cup	170	6	2	136	18	10	—	111	277	568	—	25	—
eastern raw	6 med	58	2	1	46	6	3	—	38	94	192	—	8	—
pacific raw	1 med	41	1	tr	—	5	2	—	4	53	84	—	—	—
pacific raw	3 oz	69	2	tr	—	8	4	—	7	90	143	—	—	—
TAKE-OUT														
battered & fried	6 (4.9 oz)	368	18	5	109	13	40	—	27	677	182	4	13	363
breaded & fried	6 (4.9 oz)	368	18	5	109	13	40	—	27	677	182	4	13	363
eastern breaded & fried	6 med (88 g)	173	11	3	72	8	10	—	54	367	215	—	12	—
eastern breaded & fried	3 oz	167	11	3	69	7	10	—	53	355	208	—	12	—
oysters rockefeller	3 oysters	66	2	—	38	7	5	—	102	80	—	—	—	—

PANCAKE/WAFFLE SYRUP

FOOD	PORTION	CALORIES	FAT	SAT FAT	CHOL	PROTEIN	CARBO	FIBER	CALCIUM	SOD	POTAS	VIT C	FOLIC	VIT A
(see also SYRUP)														
low calorie	1 tbsp	12	0	0	0	0	3	0	—	—	—	0	0	0
maple	1 cup (11.1 oz)	824	1	—	0	tr	212	—	211	27	643	0	1	—
maple	1 tbsp (0.8 oz)	52	0	—	0	0	13	—	13	2	41	0	0	—
pancake syrup	1 tbsp (0.7 oz)	57	0	0	0	0	15	—	0	17	0	0	0	0
pancake syrup	1 cup (11 oz)	903	0	0	0	0	238	—	4	290	7	0	0	0
pancake syrup light	1 oz	46	0	—	0	0	13	—	0	57	1	0	0	0
pancake syrup w/ butter	1 tbsp (0.7 oz)	59	tr	tr	1	0	15	—	0	20	1	0	0	12
pancake syrup w/ butter	1 cup (11 oz)	933	5	3	14	tr	234	—	6	307	9	0	0	193
AUNT JEMIMA														
Butter Rich	¼ cup (2.8 oz)	210	0	0	0	0	52	—	—	170	0	—	—	—
Butterlite	¼ cup (2.5 oz)	100	0	0	0	0	26	—	—	150	0	—	—	—
Lite	¼ cup (2.5 oz)	100	0	0	0	0	27	—	—	160	0	—	—	—
Syrup	¼ cup (2.8 oz)	210	0	0	0	0	53	—	—	120	10	—	—	—
BRER RABBIT														
Dark	2 tbsp	120	0	0	0	0	31	—	20	0	135	—	—	—
Light	2 tbsp	120	0	0	0	0	31	—	20	0	85	—	—	—
ESTEE														
Lite Maple	¼ cup (2.4 oz)	80	0	0	0	0	20	—	—	125	—	—	—	—
LOG CABIN														
Country Kitchen	1 oz	103	0	0	0	0	27	—	1	22	—	—	—	—
Lite	1 oz	49	0	0	0	0	13	—	—	92	1	—	—	—
MRS. RICHARDSON'S														
Lite	¼ cup (2.5 oz)	100	0	0	0	0	26	—	—	160	0	—	—	—
Original Recipe	¼ cup (2.8 oz)	210	0	0	0	0	52	—	—	115	5	—	—	—
RED WING														
Lite	¼ cup (2 oz)	100	0	0	0	0	26	0	0	115	—	0	—	0

FOOD	PORTION	CALORIES	FAT	SAT FAT	CHOL	PROTEIN	CARBO	FIBER	CALCIUM	SOD	POTAS	VIT C	FOLIC	VIT A
RED WING (CONT.)														
Syrup	¼ cup (2 oz)	210	0	0	0	0	53	0	0	30	—	0	—	0
TREE OF LIFE														
Maple	¼ cup (2.1 oz)	200	0	0	0	0	53	—	60	7	—	—	—	—

PANCAKES

FOOD	PORTION	CALORIES	FAT	SAT FAT	CHOL	PROTEIN	CARBO	FIBER	CALCIUM	SOD	POTAS	VIT C	FOLIC	VIT A
FROZEN														
buttermilk	1 4 in diam (1.3 ox)	83	1	tr	3	2	16	—	22	183	26	—	—	36
plain	1 4 in diam (1.3 oz)	83	1	tr	3	2	16	—	22	183	26	—	—	36
AUNT JEMIMA														
Blueberry	3 (3.4 oz)	210	4	1	15	6	40	2	20	670	130	0	—	0
Buttermilk	3 (3 oz)	180	3	1	15	5	34	2	40	590	150	0	—	0
Lowfat	3 (3.4 oz)	130	2	0	0	4	33	8	150	580	55	0	—	0
Original	3 (3.4 oz)	200	3	1	15	6	40	2	20	700	140	0	—	0
DOWNYFLAKE														
Blueberry	3	290	9	—	—	5	48	—	80	920	90	—	—	—
Buttermilk	3	280	9	—	—	5	45	—	60	920	115	—	—	—
Pancakes And Sausages	1 pkg (5.5 oz)	430	23	—	—	11	47	—	80	1170	210	—	—	—
Regular	3	280	9	—	—	5	45	—	60	920	115	—	—	—
GREAT STARTS														
Pancakes And Sausages	6 oz	460	22	—	—	15	52	—	80	920	—	—	—	—
Pancakes With Bacon	4½ oz	400	20	—	—	11	43	—	60	1000	—	—	—	—
Silver Dollar Pancakes And Sausage	3¾ oz	310	14	—	—	10	37	—	40	680	—	—	—	—
Whole Wheat Pancakes With Lite Links	5½ oz	350	16	—	—	15	39	—	40	600	—	—	—	—
JIMMY DEAN														
Flapstick	1 (2.5 oz)	240	14	4	20	6	22	1	—	320	—	—	—	—
Flapstick Blueberry	1 (2.5 oz)	260	15	4	15	6	23	1	—	320	—	—	—	—
QUAKER														
Lite Pancakes & Lite Links	1 pkg (6 oz)	310	10	—	48	14	43	—	300	970	80	—	—	—
Lite Pancakes & Lite Syrup	1 pkg (6 oz)	260	3	—	32	10	53	—	300	860	100	—	—	—
Pancakes & Sausages	1 pkg (6 oz)	420	16	—	62	12	57	—	250	1140	190	—	—	—
HOME RECIPE														
plain	1 (4 in diam)	86	4	1	23	2	11	—	83	157	50	tr	5	75
MIX														
buckwheat	1 (4 in diam)	62	2	1	20	2	9	—	77	160	70	tr	—	70

FOOD	PORTION	CALORIES	FAT	SAT FAT	CHOL	PROTEIN	CARBO	FIBER	CALCIUM	SOD	POTAS	VIT C	FOLIC	VIT A
buttermilk	1 4 in diam (1.3 oz)	74	1	tr	—	2	14	tr	48	239	67	—	—	12
plain	1-4 in diam (1.3 oz)	74	1	tr	—	2	14	tr	48	239	67	—	—	12
sugar free low sodium	1 (3 in diam)	44	tr	tr	0	1	9	—	13	58	85	0	1	14
whole wheat	1 (4 in diam)	92	3	1	27	4	13	—	110	252	123	tr	—	99
ARROWHEAD														
Multigrain Pancake & Waffle Mix	¼ cup (1.2 oz)	120	1	0	0	5	24	3	100	260	170	0	—	0
AUNT JEMIMA														
Buckwheat Pancake & Waffle Mix	¼ cup (1.4 oz)	120	1	0	0	5	28	4	150	560	135	—	8	—
Buttermilk Pancake & Waffle Mix	⅓ cup (1.9 oz)	190	2	1	10	6	38	2	200	480	180	—	8	—
Original Pancake & Waffle Mix	⅓ cup (1.6 oz)	150	1	0	0	4	34	1	0	620	45	—	0	—
Pancake & Waffle Mix Regular	⅓ cup (1.9 oz)	190	2	1	15	6	39	1	20	470	115	—	8	—
Pancake & Waffle Mix Whole Wheat	¼ cup (1.4 oz)	130	1	0	0	6	28	3	150	560	200	—	16	—
BETTY CROCKER														
Buttermilk	3 (4 in diam)	280	10	—	—	8	39	—	150	810	190	—	—	—
BISQUICK														
Apple Cinnamon Shake 'N Pour	3 (4 in diam)	240	3	—	0	6	47	—	100	880	110	—	—	—
Blueberry Shake 'N Pour	3 (4 in diam)	270	3	—	0	6	54	—	100	840	100	—	—	—
Buttermilk Shake 'N Pour	3 (4 in diam)	250	3	—	0	6	49	—	100	880	95	—	—	—
Original Shake 'N Pour	3 (4 in diam)	250	3	—	0	6	49	—	100	880	100	—	—	—
ESTEE														
Pancake Mix Fat Free as prep	4 (4 in diam)	180	0	0	0	4	40	1	50	255	340	0	—	0
FAST SHAKE														
Blueberry	1 serv (2.5 oz)	251	3	—	2	7	50	—		685	250	—	—	—
Buttermilk	1 serv (2.5 oz)	258	3	—	2	8	50	—		770	270	—	—	—
Original	1 serv (2.5 oz)	266	4	—	tr	6	50	—		736	250	—	—	—
HEALTH VALLEY														
Pancake Mix not prep	1 oz	100	1	—	0	4	20	3	20	170	250	1	14	3
HODGSON MILL														
Buckwheat	⅓ cup (1.8 oz)	160	1	0	0	5	35	1	20	550	—	0	—	0

FOOD	PORTION	CALORIES	FAT	SAT FAT	CHOL	PROTEIN	CARBO	FIBER	CALCIUM	SOD	POTAS	VIT C	FOLIC	VIT A
HUNGRY JACK														
Potato as prep	3 (3 in diam)	90	2	0	50	3	16	1	100	380	—	0	—	0
STONE-BUHR														
Buckwheat	¼ cup (1.4 oz)	130	1	0	0	5	29	3	200	410	—	0	—	0
Oat Bran	¼ cup (1.4 oz)	130	0	0	0	5	30	2	200	330	—	0	—	0
Whole Wheat	¼ cup (1.4 oz)	120	1	0	0	5	25	3	200	330	—	0	—	0
WANDA'S														
Blue Corn	⅓ cup mix per serv (1.7 oz)	170	2	0	0	7	32	2	100	480	—	0	—	0
TAKE-OUT														
blueberry	1 (4 in diam)	84	4	1	21	2	11	—	78	157	52	1	5	76
buckwheat	1 (4 in diam)	55	2	1	20	2	6	—	59	125	66	tr	—	60
w/ butter & syrup	3	519	14	6	57	8	91	—	128	1103	250	3	34	281
PANCREAS														
(*see* SWEETBREADS)														
PAPAYA														
fresh	1	117	tr	tr	0	2	30	—	72	8	780	188	—	6122
fresh cubed	1 cup	54	tr	tr	0	1	14	—	33	4	359	87	—	2819
KA-ME														
Papaya	¾ cup	120	0	0	0	0	29	1	20	15	—	—	—	—
SONOMA														
Dried Pieces	2 pieces (2 oz)	200	4	0	0	0	41	6	100	60	—	0	—	1750
PAPAYA JUICE														
nectar	1 cup	142	tr	tr	0	tr	36	—	24	14	78	8	5	277
EVERFRESH														
Premium Drink	1 can (8 oz)	140	0	0	0	0	35	0	—	0	—	—	—	—
GOYA														
Nectar	6 oz	110	0	—	0	1	27	—	21	10	35	15	—	400
KERN'S														
Nectar	6 fl oz	110	0	0	0	0	27	—	—	5	90	27	—	—
LIBBY														
Nectar	1 can (11.5 fl oz)	210	0	0	0	tr	51	—	40	10	180	60	—	—
PAPRIKA														
paprika	1 tsp	6	tr	tr	0	tr	1	—	4	1	49	1	—	1273
WATKINS														
Ground	¼ tsp (0.5 oz)	0	0	0	0	0	0	0	0	0	—	0	—	200
PARSLEY														
dry	1 tsp	1	tr	—	0	tr	tr	—	4	1	11	tr	—	70
dry	1 tbsp	1	tr	—	0	tr	tr	—	1	2	25	1	6	253
DOLE														
Chopped	1 tbsp	10	tr	—	0	tr	1	tr	—	4	54	9	—	520
PARSNIPS														
fresh cooked	1 (5.6 oz)	130	tr	tr	0	2	31	—	59	17	588	21	93	0

FOOD	PORTION	CALORIES	FAT	SAT FAT	CHOL	PROTEIN	CARBO	FIBER	CALCIUM	SOD	POTAS	VIT C	FOLIC	VIT A
fresh sliced cooked	½ cup	63	tr	tr	0	1	15	—	29	8	287	10	45	0
raw sliced	½ cup	50	tr	tr	0	1	12	—	24	7	251	11	45	0

PASSION FRUIT

purple fresh	1	18	tr	—	0	tr	4	—	2	5	63	5	—	126

PASSION FRUIT JUICE

purple	1 cup	126	tr	—	0	1	34	—	9	—	—	74	—	1771
yellow	1 cup	149	tr	—	0	2	36	—	9	15	687	45	—	5953
SNAPPLE														
Passion Supreme	10 fl oz	160	0	0	0	0	39	—	20	20	—	0	—	0

PASTA

(*see also* NOODLES, PASTA DINNERS, PASTA SALAD)

DRY														
corn cooked	1 cup (4.9 oz)	176	1	tr	0	4	39	7	1	0	43	0	8	80
elbows cooked	1 cup (4.9 oz)	197	1	tr	0	7	40	2	10	1	43	0	98	0
shells small cooked	1 cup (4 oz)	162	1	tr	0	5	33	2	8	1	36	0	81	0
shells small protein fortified cooked	1 cup (4 oz)	189	tr	tr	0	9	36	—	12	6	48	0	94	0
spaghetti cooked	1 cup (4.9 oz)	197	1	tr	0	7	40	2	10	1	43	0	98	0
spaghetti protein fortified cooked	1 cup (4.9 oz)	230	tr	tr	0	11	44	2	14	7	59	0	115	0
spinach spaghetti cooked	1 cup (4.9 oz)	182	1	tr	0	6	37	—	42	20	81	0	17	213
spirals cooked	1 cup (4.7 oz)	189	tr	tr	0	6	38	2	9	1	42	0	94	0
vegetable cooked	1 cup (4.7 oz)	172	tr	tr	0	6	36	6	15	8	42	0	87	71
whole wheat cooked	1 cup (4.9 oz)	174	tr	tr	0	7	37	4	21	4	62	0	7	0
whole wheat spaghetti cooked	1 cup (4.9 oz)	174	1	tr	0	7	37	6	21	4	62	0	7	0
ANTHONY														
Pasta	2 oz	210	1	0	0	7	42	tr	16	0	110	—	—	0
BARILLA														
Conchiglie Rigate	1 cup (2 oz)	200	1	0	0	6	40	2	0	0	—	0	120	0
Gemelli as prep	1 cup (2 oz)	200	1	0	0	7	42	2	0	0	—	0	—	0
Pennette Rigate	1 ⅓ cups (2 oz)	200	1	0	0	7	42	2	0	0	—	0	120	0
BELLA VIA														
Angel Hair	2 oz	200	0	0	0	8	40	—	—	0	—	—	—	—
Artichoke Angel Hair as prep	⅝ cup	200	0	0	0	8	40	—	—	0	—	—	—	—
Artichoke Spaghetti as prep	⅝ cup	200	0	0	0	8	40	—	—	0	—	—	—	—
Elbows	2 oz	200	0	0	0	8	40	—	—	0	—	—	—	—
Fettucini as prep	⅝ cup	200	0	0	0	8	40	—	—	0	—	—	—	—
Linguini	2 oz	200	0	0	0	8	40	—	—	0	—	—	—	—
Penne as prep	⅝ cup	200	0	0	0	8	40	—	—	0	—	—	—	—
Rotelli	2 oz	200	0	0	0	8	40	—	—	0	—	—	—	—

FOOD	PORTION	CALORIES	FAT	SAT FAT	CHOL	PROTEIN	CARBO	FIBER	CALCIUM	SOD	POTAS	VIT C	FOLIC	VIT A
BELLA VIA (CONT.)														
Shells	2 oz	200	0	0	0	8	40	—	—	0	—	—	—	—
Spaghetti	2 oz	200	0	0	0	8	40	—	—	0	—	—	—	—
Ziti	2 oz	200	0	0	0	8	40	—	—	0	—	—	—	—
CLASSICO														
Gnocchi Di Toscana	1 cup (2 oz)	210	1	0	0	7	42	2	0	0	—	0	—	0
CREAMETTE														
Elbow Macaroni not prep	2 oz	210	1	—	—	7	42	—	—	5	115	—	—	—
Spaghetti not prep	2 oz	210	1	—	—	7	42	—	—	5	115	—	—	—
Spinach Ribbons not prep	2 oz	210	1	—	—	7	42	—	40	70	210	—	—	—
DE BOLE'S														
Whole Wheat Organic Elbows	2 oz	210	2	0	0	7	40	5	0	0	—	0	—	0
DECECCO														
Whole Wheat Linguine cooked	2 oz	180	2	0	<5	8	33	7	20	0	—	0	—	0
DEFINO														
Lasagna No Boil	1 oz	102	tr	—	0	3	20	—	—	2	—	—	—	—
Ribbons No Boil	2 oz	204	2	—	0	6	40	—	—	3	—	—	—	—
DELVERDE														
Spaghetti Whole Wheat	2 oz	206	1	1	0	7	42	5	20	1	—	0	—	0
EDEN														
Elbows Whole Wheat Organic	2 oz	210	2	0	0	10	39	6	21	0	260	0	—	88
Elbows Whole Wheat Vegetable Organic	2 oz	210	2	0	0	10	39	6	21	0	260	0	—	88
Kudzu And Sweet Potato Pasta	2 oz	190	0	0	0	0	47	0	6	0	30	0	—	0
Kudzu Kiri Pasta	2 oz	190	0	0	0	0	47	0	6	0	30	0	—	0
Mung Bean Pasta Harusame	2 oz	190	0	0	0	0	47	0	11	5	10	0	—	0
Organic Endless Tubes	½ cup (1.9 oz)	210	1	0	0	8	41	4	20	0	150	1	—	0
Ribbons Durum Wheat Curry Organic	2 oz	220	1	0	0	8	44	3	17	0	180	0	—	90
Ribbons Durum Wheat Organic	2 oz	220	1	0	0	8	44	3	17	0	180	0	—	90
Ribbons Durum Wheat Paella Organic	2 oz	220	1	0	0	8	44	3	17	0	180	0	—	90

FOOD	PORTION	CALORIES	FAT	SAT FAT	CHOL	PROTEIN	CARBO	FIBER	CALCIUM	SOD	POTAS	VIT C	FOLIC	VIT A
EDEN (CONT.)														
Ribbons Durum Wheat Parsley Garlic Organic	2 oz	220	1	0	0	8	44	3	17	0	180	0	—	90
Ribbons Durum Wheat Pesto Organic	2 oz	220	1	0	0	8	44	3	17	0	180	0	—	90
Ribbons Whole Wheat Spinach Organic	2 oz	200	2	0	0	8	40	7	31	10	370	0	—	175
Rice Pasta Bifun	2 oz	200	1	0	0	5	44	0	13	5	10	0	—	0
Shells Durum Wheat Vegetable Organic	2 oz	210	1	0	0	7	42	2	18	10	126	0	—	127
Soba	2 oz	200	2	0	0	8	38	2	20	70	115	0	—	0
Soba 100% Buckwheat	2 oz	200	0	0	0	5	41	3	9	30	190	0	—	24
Soba Lotus Root	2 oz	190	1	0	0	9	37	4	21	470	170	0	—	0
Soba Mugwort	2 oz	190	1	0	0	8	37	2	26	550	140	0	—	0
Soba Wild Yam Jinenjo	2 oz	190	1	0	0	9	37	2	20	510	150	0	—	0
Somen	2 oz	200	2	0	0	8	38	3	20	80	115	0	—	0
Spaghetti Durum Wheat Organic	2 oz	210	1	0	0	7	42	2	18	10	125	0	—	127
Spaghetti Kamut Organic	2 oz	210	2	0	0	10	38	6	14	0	240	0	—	0
Spaghetti Pasley Garlic Organic	2 oz	210	1	0	0	7	42	2	18	10	125	0	—	127
Spaghetti Whole Wheat Organic	2 oz	210	2	0	0	10	39	6	21	0	260	0	—	88
Spirals Durum Wheat Vegetable Organic	2 oz	210	1	0	0	7	42	2	18	10	126	0	—	127
Spirals Kamut Organic	2 oz	210	2	0	0	10	38	6	14	0	240	0	—	0
Spirals Sesame Rice Organic	2 oz	200	2	0	0	10	37	6	72	0	280	0	—	0
Spirals Whole Wheat Vegetable Organic	2 oz	210	2	0	0	10	39	6	21	0	260	0	—	88
Udon	2 oz	200	2	0	0	8	38	3	20	80	115	0	—	0
Udon Brown Rice	2 oz	200	2	0	0	8	38	3	20	80	135	0	—	0
GIOIA														
Pasta	2 oz	210	1	0	0	7.	42	tr	16	0	110	—	—	0
HEALTH VALLEY														
Lasagna Whole Wheat	2 oz	170	1	—	0	9	40	7	20	10	240	3	39	5
Lasagna Spinach Whole Wheat	2 oz	170	1	—	0	9	40	7	20	15	240	4	119	2869

FOOD	PORTION	CALORIES	FAT	SAT FAT	CHOL	PROTEIN	CARBO	FIBER	CALCIUM	SOD	POTAS	VIT C	FOLIC	VIT A
HEALTH VALLEY (CONT.)														
Spagehetti Amaranth	2 oz	170	1	—	0	7	40	9	20	10	240	2	28	0
Spaghetti Oat Bran	2 oz	120	1	—	0	4	23	4	15	2	126	1	14	9
Spaghetti Spinach Whole Wheat	2 oz	170	1	—	0	9	40	7	20	15	240	4	119	2869
Spaghetti Whole Wheat	2 oz	170	1	—	0	9	40	7	20	10	240	3	39	5
HODGSON MILL														
Spaghetti Whole Wheat Spinach not prep	2 oz	190	2	1	0	9	35	5	20	25	—	0	—	0
Veggie Bows not prep	2 oz	200	1	0	0	8	41	1	0	15	—	0	—	0
Veggie Rotini not prep	2 oz	200	1	0	0	8	41	1	0	15	—	0	—	0
Veggie Wagon Wheels not prep	2 oz	200	1	0	0	8	41	1	0	15	—	0	—	0
Whole Wheat Spirals not prep	2 oz	190	1	1	0	9	34	6	20	10	—	0	—	0
LA MOLISANA														
Radiatori	2 oz	230	1	—	0	7	48	—	—	30	—	—	—	—
LUPINI														
Elbow uncooked	½ cup (2 oz)	190	2	0	0	10	37	5	40	0	200	0	—	0
Spaghetti Light uncooked	½ cup (2 oz)	190	2	0	0	10	37	5	40	0	200	0	—	0
Spaghetti With Triticale	1/7 pkg (2 oz)	190	3	1	0	9	38	6	40	5	330	0	—	0
LUXURY														
Pasta	2 oz	210	1	0	0	7	42	tr	16	0	110	—	—	0
MERLINO'S														
Pasta	2 oz	210	1	0	0	7	42	tr	16	0	110	—	—	0
NOODLES BY LEONARDO														
Capellini	2 oz	200	1	0	0	8	40	2	0	10	—	0	—	0
Elbows not prep	½ cup (2 oz)	200	1	0	0	8	40	2	0	10	—	0	—	0
Fettucini	2 oz	200	1	0	0	8	40	2	0	10	—	0	—	0
Linguine not prep	½ cup (2 oz)	200	1	0	0	8	40	2	0	10	—	0	—	0
Rigatoni	2 oz	200	1	0	0	8	40	2	0	10	—	0	—	0
Rotini	2 oz	200	1	0	0	8	40	2	0	10	—	0	—	0
Shells not prep	½ cup (2 oz)	200	1	0	0	8	40	2	0	10	—	0	—	0
Spaghetti not prep	½ cup (2 oz)	200	1	0	0	8	40	2	0	10	—	0	—	0
Spaghettini	2 oz	200	1	0	0	8	40	2	0	10	—	0	—	0
Vermicelli not prep	½ cup (2 oz)	200	1	0	0	8	40	2	0	10	—	0	—	0
PENN DUTCH														
Pasta	2 oz	210	1	0	0	7	42	tr	16	0	110	—	—	0
POMI														
Capellini	2 oz	210	1	—	0	7	41	—	—	<5	—	—	—	—

FOOD	PORTION	CALORIES	FAT	SAT FAT	CHOL	PROTEIN	CARBO	FIBER	CALCIUM	SOD	POTAS	VIT C	FOLIC	VIT A
PRINCE														
Egg	2 oz	221	3	1	70	8	40	1	19	3	75	0	—	130
Pasta	2 oz	210	1	0	0	7	42	tr	16	0	110	—	—	0
Rainbow	2 oz	210	1	0	0	8	42	1	1	5	150	0	—	0
Spinach Egg	2 oz	220	3	—	70	8	40	1	20	65	190	0	—	0
PRITIKIN														
Spaghetti Whole Wheat	⅛ box (2 oz)	190	1	0	0	—	40	—	—	0	120	—	—	—
Spiral	⅔ cup (2 oz)	190	1	0	0	—	40	—	—	10	140	—	—	—
RED CROSS														
Pasta	2 oz	210	1	0	0	7	42	tr	16	0	110	—	—	0
RONCO														
Pasta	2 oz	210	1	0	0	7	42	tr	16	0	110	—	—	0
RONZONI														
Elbows	¾ cup (2 oz)	210	1	—	0	9	40	—	—	0	—	—	—	—
Fettucini	¾ cup (2 oz)	210	1	—	0	9	40	—	—	0	—	—	—	—
Fusilli	¾ cup (2 oz)	210	1	—	0	9	40	—	—	0	—	—	—	—
Lasagne	¾ cup (2 oz)	210	1	—	0	9	40	—	—	0	—	—	—	—
Manicotti	¾ cup (2 oz)	210	1	—	0	9	40	—	—	0	—	—	—	—
Mostaccioli	¾ cup (2 oz)	210	1	—	0	9	40	—	—	0	—	—	—	—
Rigatoni	¾ cup (2 oz)	210	1	—	0	9	40	—	—	0	—	—	—	—
Rotelle uncooked	¾ cup (2 oz)	210	1	—	0	9	40	—	—	0	—	—	—	—
Rotini uncooked	¾ cup (2 oz)	210	1	—	0	9	40	—	—	0	—	—	—	—
Shells uncooked	¾ cup (2 oz)	210	1	—	0	9	40	—	—	0	—	—	—	—
Shells Jumbo	¾ cup (2 oz)	210	1	—	0	9	40	—	—	0	—	—	—	—
Spaghetti not prep	¾ cup (2 oz)	210	1	—	0	9	40	—	—	0	—	—	—	—
Tubettini	¾ cup (2 oz)	210	1	—	0	9	40	—	—	0	—	—	—	—
SAN GIORGIO														
Bowties Egg	2 oz	210	3	—	70	10	38	—	—	15	—	—	—	—
Capellini	2 oz	210	1	—	0	9	40	2	—	0	—	—	—	—
Elbow Macaroni	2 oz	210	1	—	0	9	40	2	—	0	—	—	—	—
Fettuccine Egg	2 oz	210	3	—	70	10	38	—	—	15	—	—	—	—
Fettuccini Florentine	2 oz	210	3	—	70	10	38	—	—	15	—	—	—	—
Lasagne	2 oz	210	1	—	0	9	40	2	—	0	—	—	—	—
Linguini	2 oz	210	1	—	0	9	40	2	—	0	—	—	—	—
Manicotti	2 oz	210	1	—	0	9	40	2	—	0	—	—	—	—
Rigatoni	2 oz	210	1	—	0	9	40	2	—	0	—	—	—	—
Rotini	2 oz	210	1	—	0	9	40	2	—	0	—	—	—	—
Shells	2 oz	210	1	—	0	9	40	2	—	0	—	—	—	—
Spaghetti	2 oz	210	1	—	0	9	40	2	—	0	—	—	—	—
Spaghetti Thin	2 oz	210	1	—	0	9	40	2	—	0	—	—	—	—
Vermicelli	2 oz	210	1	—	0	9	40	2	—	0	—	—	—	—
Ziti Cut	2 oz	210	1	—	0	9	40	2	—	0	—	—	—	—
TREE OF LIFE														
Cajun as prep	⅝ cup (4.9 oz)	200	1	0	0	8	40	1	40	50	—	0	—	100

FOOD	PORTION	CALORIES	FAT	SAT FAT	CHOL	PROTEIN	CARBO	FIBER	CALCIUM	SOD	POTAS	VIT C	FOLIC	VIT A
TREE OF LIFE (CONT.)														
Confetti as prep	⅝ cup (4.9 oz)	200	1	0	0	8	40	1	40	50	—	0	—	100
Garlic & Parsley as prep	⅝ cup (4.9 oz)	200	1	0	0	8	40	1	40	50	—	0	—	100
Jamaican Spice as prep	⅝ cup (4.9 oz)	200	1	0	0	8	40	1	40	50	—	0	—	100
Lemon Pepper as prep	⅝ cup (4.9 oz)	200	1	0	0	8	40	1	40	50	—	0	—	100
Spinach as prep	⅝ cup (4.9 oz)	200	1	0	0	8	40	1	40	50	—	0	—	100
Tex Mex as prep	⅝ cup (4.9 oz)	200	1	0	0	8	40	1	40	50	—	0	—	100
Thai as prep	⅝ cup (4.9 oz)	200	1	0	0	8	40	1	40	50	—	0	—	100
Tomato Basil as prep	⅝ cup (4.9 oz)	200	1	0	0	8	40	1	40	50	—	0	—	100
VIMCO														
Pasta	2 oz	210	1	0	0	7	42	tr	16	0	110	—	—	0
FRESH														
cooked	2 oz	75	1	tr	33	3	14	—	3	3	14	0	36	11
spinach cooked	2 oz	74	1	tr	19	3	14	—	10	3	21	0	36	59
CONTADINA														
Angel's Hair	1¼ cup (2.8 oz)	240	3	1	90	10	43	2	20	30	—	0	—	0
Fettuccine	1¼ cup (2.9 oz)	250	4	1	85	10	45	2	20	30	—	0	—	0
Fettuccine Cholesterol Free	1 cup (2.9 oz)	240	3	0	0	9	46	2	0	16	—	0	—	0
Light Ravioli Cheese	1 cup (3.1 oz)	240	5	2	60	13	35	2	100	340	—	0	—	0
Light Ravioli Garden Vegetable	1¼ cup (3.8 oz)	290	6	4	65	15	43	3	150	370	—	0	—	750
Light Tortellini Garlic & Cheese	1 cup (3.6 oz)	280	5	3	55	15	50	3	80	390	—	0	—	0
Linguine	1¼ cup (3 oz)	260	4	1	95	10	47	2	20	30	—	0	—	0
Linguine Cholesterol Free	1¼ cup (3.1 oz)	250	3	0	0	9	49	2	0	20	—	0	—	0
Ravioli Beef And Garlic	1¼ cup (4 oz)	350	14	5	110	17	39	3	40	350	—	0	—	100
Ravioli Cheese	1 cup (3.1 oz)	280	12	6	85	13	31	2	200	350	—	0	—	0
Ravioli Chicken And Rosemary	1¼ cup (4 oz)	330	12	4	85	13	43	3	60	420	—	0	—	0
Tagliatelli Spinach	1¼ cup (3.1 oz)	270	4	1	105	12	46	4	60	110	—	0	—	200
Tortellini Spianch Three Cheese	¾ cup (3.1 oz)	280	5	3	55	13	38	3	150	380	—	0	—	200
Tortelloni Cheese	¾ cup (3 oz)	260	6	3	45	13	39	3	150	330	—	0	—	0
Tortelloni Cheese And Basil	1 cup (4 oz)	360	11	4	65	16	49	3	200	380	—	0	—	200
Tortelloni Chicken And Prosciutto	1 cup (3.8 oz)	360	13	4	75	15	46	3	80	440	—	0	—	100

FOOD	PORTION	CALORIES	FAT	SAT FAT	CHOL	PROTEIN	CARBO	FIBER	CALCIUM	SOD	POTAS	VIT C	FOLIC	VIT A
CONTADINA (CONT.)														
Tortelloni Chicken And Vegetable	¾ cup (2.9 oz)	260	7	2	45	10	39	2	20	220	—	0	—	200
Tortelloni Spicy Italian Sausage And Bell Pepper	1 cup (3.6 oz)	330	10	4	90	13	47	3	40	280	—	0	—	100
DI GIORNO														
Angel's Hair	1 cup	160	2	0	0	6	31	2	0	115	110	0	40	0
Beef & Roasted Garlic Tortellini	1 cup	340	11	4	50	14	46	1	80	390	200	0	60	0
Fettuccine	1 cup	200	2	0	0	8	38	2	0	140	140	0	60	0
Four Cheese Raviolo	1 cup	350	15	9	70	14	40	2	250	390	200	0	60	400
Herb Linguine	1 cup	200	2	0	0	8	38	2	20	140	150	0	60	0
Italian Sausage Ravioli In Green Bell Pepper Pasta	1¼ cup	350	12	6	55	14	45	3	100	570	250	0	60	200
Lemon Chicken Tortellini In Cracked Black Pepper Pasta	1 cup	270	5	3	40	13	42	1	60	290	150	0	40	100
Light Cheese Ravioli	1 cup	280	7	4	40	15	40	2	250	400	170	0	60	400
Linguine	1 cup	200	2	0	0	8	38	2	0	140	140	0	60	0
Mozzarella Garlic Tortelloni	1 cup	300	8	5	45	15	42	1	250	400	150	0	60	200
Pesto Tortelloni	1 cup	320	8	5	45	16	46	3	250	430	230	0	60	200
Portabello Mushroom Tortelloni	1 cup	310	7	5	40	13	48	3	200	490	360	0	60	300
Red Bell Pepper Fettuccine	1 cup	200	2	0	0	8	38	2	0	140	130	2	60	300
Spinach Fettuccine	1 cup	190	2	0	0	8	38	2	40	160	220	0	60	200
Sun-Dried Tomato Ravioli	1⅓ cup	380	14	8	55	17	48	3	250	600	420	1	60	750
Three Cheese Tortellini	¾ cup	250	7	4	35	11	37	2	150	300	125	0	40	100
HERB'S														
Fettucine Bell Pepper Basil	2 oz	220	2	0	60	10	42	2	20	5	125	0	—	95
Fettucine Parsley Garlic	2 oz	220	2	0	60	10	42	2	20	5	125	0	—	95
Fettucine Spinach	2 oz	220	2	0	60	10	42	2	20	5	125	0	—	95
Ribbons Vegetable	2 oz	220	2	0	60	10	42	2	20	5	125	0	—	95
Ribbons Whole Wheat	2 oz	200	2	0	0	8	40	7	31	10	370	0	—	175
Rotini Mixed Vegetable	2 oz	210	1	0	0	7	42	2	20	10	125	0	—	181

FOOD	PORTION	CALORIES	FAT	SAT FAT	CHOL	PROTEIN	CARBO	FIBER	CALCIUM	SOD	POTAS	VIT C	FOLIC	VIT A
HERB'S (CONT.)														
Shells Mixed Vegetable	2 oz	210	1	0	0	7	42	2	20	10	125	0	—	181
TRIOS														
Ravioli Cracked Pepper Garlic Cheese	1 cup (4.3 oz)	340	9	5	50	15	48	0	200	380	—	0	—	200
HOME RECIPE														
made w/o egg cooked	2 oz	71	1	tr	0	2	14	—	3	42	11	0	25	0
plain made w/ egg cooked	2 oz	74	1	tr	23	3	13	—	6	47	12	0	25	33

PASTA DINNERS

(*see also* DINNER, PASTA SALAD)

CANNED

FOOD	PORTION	CALORIES	FAT	SAT FAT	CHOL	PROTEIN	CARBO	FIBER	CALCIUM	SOD	POTAS	VIT C	FOLIC	VIT A
CHEF BOYARDEE														
ABC's & 1,2,3's In Cheese Flavor Sauce	7.5 oz	180	1	tr	3	5	37	—	—	940	—	—	—	100
ABC's & 1,2,3's w/ Mini Meatballs	7.5 oz	260	11	4	17	7	32	2	—	1005	—	—	—	—
Beef Ravioli	7.5 oz	190	4	2	11	7	31	2	—	1160	—	—	—	400
Beef Ravioli 99% Fat Free	1 cup (8.6 oz)	210	1	0	15	9	41	3	20	1150	—	0	—	750
Beefaroni	7.5 oz	220	7	1	18	7	31	2	—	1145	—	—	—	300
Cheese Ravioli In Meat Sauce	7.5 oz	200	3	—	10	6	37	—	20	1010	—	—	—	200
Dinosaurs In Cheese Flavor Sauce	7.5 oz	180	1	tr	3	6	36	—	20	880	—	—	—	200
Dinosaurs w/ Meatballs	7.5 oz	240	9	3	17	8	32	4	—	900	—	—	—	300
Elbows In Beef Sauce	7.5 oz	210	7	—	15	8	29	—	—	1000	—	—	—	300
Lasagna	7.5 oz	230	9	—	18	7	31	—	—	1080	—	—	—	300
Lasagna In Garden Vegetable Sauce	7.5 oz	170	1	tr	3	5	34	—	20	940	—	2	—	750
Macaroni & Cheese	7.5 oz	180	5	tr	20	7	27	1	60	970	—	—	—	400
Pasta Rings & Meatballs	7.5 oz	220	8	3	25	8	33	4	20	990	—	1	—	400
Rigatoni	7.5 oz	210	6	—	17	8	31	—	20	1080	—	5	—	500
Rings & Franks	7.5 oz	190	5	2	20	7	31	3	20	980	—	4	—	300
Shells In Meat Sauce	7.5 oz	210	6	—	15	8	32	—	20	1090	—	5	—	500
Shells In Mushroom Sauce	7.5 oz	170	1	tr	2	6	35	—	20	1080	—	4	—	500
Spaghetti & Meat Balls	7.5 oz	230	7	—	20	7	29	—	—	1060	—	—	—	200

FOOD	PORTION	CALORIES	FAT	SAT FAT	CHOL	PROTEIN	CARBO	FIBER	CALCIUM	SOD	POTAS	VIT C	FOLIC	VIT A
CHEF BOYARDEE (CONT.)														
Tic Tac Toes In Cheese Flavor Sauce	7.5 oz	170	1	tr	2	5	36	3	20	930	—	—	—	200
Tic Tac Toes w/ Mini Meatballs	7.5 oz	250	10	3	16	7	32	3	—	1035	—	—	—	400
Turtles In Sauce	7.5 oz	160	1	—	3	5	33	2	—	870	—	1	—	200
Turtles w/ Meatballs	7.5 oz	210	8	3	20	7	30	2	20	990	—	1	—	300
FRANCO-AMERICAN														
Beef RavioliO's In Meat Sauce	½ can (7½ oz)	250	8	—	—	10	35	—	20	920	—	6	—	500
CircusO's Pasta In Tomato & Cheese Sauce	½ can (7⅜ oz)	170	2	—	—	5	33	—	20	860	—	—	—	500
CircusO's Pasta With Meatballs In Tomato Sauce	½ can (7⅜ oz)	210	8	—	—	9	25	—	20	950	—	4	—	500
Macaroni & Cheese	½ can (7⅜ oz)	170	6	—	—	6	24	—	80	870	—	—	—	500
Spaghetti In Tomato Sauce w/ Cheese	½ can (7⅜ oz)	180	2	—	—	5	36	—	20	840	—	—	—	400
Spaghetti w/ Meatballs In Tomato Sauce	½ can (7⅜ oz)	220	8	—	—	10	28	—	20	870	—	—	—	400
SpaghettiO's With Meatballs	½ can (7⅜ oz)	220	9	—	—	9	25	—	20	950	—	—	—	400
SpaghettiO's With Sliced Franks	½ can (7⅜ oz)	220	9	—	—	8	26	—	20	1000	—	—	—	400
SpaghettiO's In Tomato & Cheese Sauce	½ can (7⅜ oz)	170	2	—	—	5	33	—	20	860	—	—	—	500
SportyO's In Tomato & Cheese Sauce	½ can (7½ oz)	170	2	—	—	5	33	—	20	860	—	—	—	500
SportyO's Pasta With Meatballs In Tomato Sauce	½ can (7⅜ oz)	210	8	—	—	9	25	—	20	950	—	4	—	500
TeddyO's In Tomato & Cheese Sauce	½ can (7½ oz)	170	2	—	—	5	33	—	40	900	—	—	—	500
TeddyO's Pasta With Meatballs	½ can (7⅜ oz)	210	8	—	—	9	25	—	40	950	—	4	—	500
HORMEL														
Spaghetti & Meatballs	1 can (7.5 oz)	210	7	4	20	10	28	2	20	940	—	2	—	400
KID'S KITCHEN														
Microwave Meals Cheezy Mac & Beef	1 cup (7.5 oz)	260	7	3	30	15	33	1	100	910	—	1	—	400

FOOD	PORTION	CALORIES	FAT	SAT FAT	CHOL	PROTEIN	CARBO	FIBER	CALCIUM	SOD	POTAS	VIT C	FOLIC	VIT A
KID'S KITCHEN (CONT.)														
Microwave Meals Noodle Rings & Chicken	1 cup (7.5 oz)	150	4	2	30	10	17	1	40	1110	—	0	—	0
Microwave Meals Spaghetti Rings & Franks	1 cup (7.5 oz)	240	9	4	30	9	32	1	80	810	—	2	—	400
PROGRESSO														
Beef Ravioli	1 cup (9.1 oz)	260	5	2	5	9	45	4	40	940	—	4	—	1000
Cheese Ravioli	1 cup (9.1 oz)	220	2	1	<5	7	43	4	40	930	—	2	—	750
VAN CAMP'S														
Spaghetti Weenee	1 can (8 oz)	230	8	2	20	7	34	1	0	670	230	—	8	400
FROZEN														
AMY'S ORGANIC														
Macaroni & Cheese	1 pkg (9 oz)	390	14	8	40	17	50	4	—	550	—	—	—	—
Macaroni & Soy Cheese	1 pkg (9 oz)	360	14	1	0	16	42	4	—	500	—	—	—	—
Pasta Primavera	1 pkg (9.5 oz)	320	12	7	65	15	39	3	—	680	—	—	—	—
Ravioli w/ Sauce	1 pkg (9.5 oz)	340	12	3	20	15	44	6	—	580	—	—	—	—
Tofu Vegetable Lasagna	1 pkg (9.5 oz)	300	10	1	0	18	41	4	—	630	—	—	—	—
Vegetable Lasagna	1 pkg (9.5 oz)	300	10	4	15	15	39	5	—	680	—	—	—	—
Whole Meals Cannelloni	1 pkg (9 oz)	260	11	5	20	11	32	5	—	560	—	—	—	—
ARMOUR														
Classics Chicken Fettucini	1 meal (10 oz)	230	8	4	25	16	25	6	80	520	—	9	—	2500
BANQUET														
Family Entree Lasagna w/ Meat Sauce	1 serv (8 oz)	240	7	3	15	12	32	5	150	650	—	72	—	750
Family Entree Macaroni & Beef	1 serv (8 oz)	230	7	3	25	6	31	3	100	810	—	1	—	—
Family Entree Macaroni & Cheese	1 serv (8 oz)	300	10	5	25	14	39	2	250	1190	—	0	—	100
Family Entree Noodles & Chicken	1 serv (8 oz)	210	9	3	40	10	24	2	60	810	—	0	—	50
Family Entree Noodles & Beef	1 serv (7.47 oz)	140	4	2	35	11	16	2	20	1120	—	1	—	0
BIRDS EYE														
Easy Recipe Meal Starter Cheesy Cheese	1 serv	280	8	2	69	9	30	2	40	336	—	27	—	1000
Easy Recipe Meal Starter Chicken Primavera as prep	1 serv	280	8	2	69	6	30	2	40	336	—	27	—	1000

FOOD	PORTION	CALORIES	FAT	SAT FAT	CHOL	PROTEIN	CARBO	FIBER	CALCIUM	SOD	POTAS	VIT C	FOLIC	VIT A
BIRDS EYE (CONT.)														
Easy Recipe Meal Starter Chicken Alfredo as prep	1 serv	280	8	2	69	8	30	2	40	336	—	27	—	1000
Pasta Secrets Creamy Peppercorn	2 ⅓ cups (6.6 oz)	300	15	6	25	7	29	2	200	460	—	4	—	3000
Pasta Secrets Italian Pesto	2 ⅓ cups (6.4 oz)	240	9	2	5	9	32	2	100	700	—	18	—	1500
Pasta Secrets Primavera	2 ⅓ cups (6.6 oz)	230	10	3	10	9	26	3	200	430	—	30	—	2000
Pasta Secrets Three Cheese	2 cups (6.1 oz)	230	8	3	5	9	31	2	100	590	—	21	—	1750
Pasta Secrets White Cheddar	2 cups (6.3 oz)	240	10	3	10	7	30	2	200	560	—	21	—	1250
Pasta Secrets Zesty Garlic	2 cups (5.9 oz)	240	10	3	5	7	31	2	150	310	—	15	—	1750
BUDGET GOURMET														
Cheese Ravioli	1 meal (9.5 oz)	290	13	6	30	12	34	—	200	750	410	12	—	5000
Lasagna Italian Sausage	1 meal (10 oz)	430	23	—	45	20	34	—	300	830	390	12	—	5000
Lasagna Vegetable	1 meal (10.5 oz)	390	10	5	15	16	36	—	300	770	430	5	—	4000
Lasagne Three Cheese	1 meal (10 oz)	390	17	—	70	23	26	—	450	640	350	9	—	5000
Lasagne With Meat Sauce	1 meal (9.4 oz)	290	11	4	30	18	30	—	200	720	460	5	—	5000
Linguini With Shrimp & Clams	1 meal (9.5 oz)	280	10	5	45	14	34	—	100	710	320	9	—	200
Linguini With Shrimp And Clams	1 meal (10 oz)	270	9	—	50	12	35	—	80	1160	400	6	—	4500
Macaroni & Cheese	1 meal (5.75 oz)	230	12	—	35	9	22	—	200	570	120	1	—	600
Macaroni & Cheese With Cheddar & Parmesan	1 meal (10.5 oz)	330	8	4	30	19	49	—	350	760	230	1	—	300
Mainicotti Cheese	1 meal (10 oz)	440	24	—	75	20	36	—	350	740	600	6	—	9500
Pasta Alfredo With Broccoli	1 meal (5.5 oz)	210	10	—	30	8	22	—	200	630	150	5	—	400
Penne Pasta With Chunky Tomato Sauce & Italian Sausage	1 meal (10 oz)	320	9	2	5	13	34	—	80	590	390	15	—	750
Rigatoni In Cream Sauce With Broccoli & Chicken	1 meal (10.8 oz)	290	7	3	30	19	44	—	250	710	310	1	—	400

FOOD	PORTION	CALORIES	FAT	SAT FAT	CHOL	PROTEIN	CARBO	FIBER	CALCIUM	SOD	POTAS	VIT C	FOLIC	VIT A
BUDGET GOURMET (CONT.)														
Spaghetti With Chunky Tomato & Meat Sauce	1 meal (10 oz)	300	8	2	35	18	44	—	60	470	400	9	—	400
Tortellini Cheese	1 meal (5.5 oz)	200	8	—	20	8	25	—	100	530	200	5	—	4500
Ziti In Marinara Sauce	1 meal (6.25 oz)	200	9	—	10	7	23	—	80	600	220	5	—	2500
DINING LIGHT														
Cheese Cannelloni	9 oz	310	9	—	70	19	38	—	350	650	520	5	—	750
FORMAGG														
Penne Pasta Alfredo	⅔ cup (5 oz)	190	2	0	0	7	35	0	200	470	—	0	—	500
Penne Pasta Primavera	⅔ cup (5 oz)	190	2	0	0	7	35	0	200	470	—	0	—	500
Vegetable Pasta & Caesar Italian Garden	⅔ cup (5 oz)	190	2	0	0	7	35	0	200	470	—	0	—	500
GREEN GIANT														
Create A Meal Creamy Alfredo as prep	1¼ cups (10 oz)	380	12	5	75	34	33	4	250	990	—	27	—	2250
Create A Meal Creamy Cheddar as prep	1½ cups (10 oz)	290	10	6	45	20	29	4	200	1470	—	36	—	3000
Create A Meal Creamy Chicken Noodle as prep	1¼ cups (10 oz)	350	11	5	65	28	34	3	150	970	—	5	—	3000
Pasta Accents Alfredo	2 cups (5.6 oz)	210	5	3	15	9	25	4	150	480	—	12	—	300
Pasta Accents Creamy Cheddar	2 ⅓ cups (6.7 oz)	250	8	3	15	9	36	5	150	700	—	6	—	4000
Pasta Accents Florentine	2 cups (7.3 oz)	310	9	3	20	13	44	5	300	910	—	5	—	6000
Pasta Accents Garden Herb Seasoning	2 cups (6.8 oz)	230	7	4	15	9	32	7	80	750	—	9	—	1750
Pasta Accents Garlic Seasoning	2 cups (6.6 oz)	260	10	5	15	7	36	5	60	640	—	5	—	2500
Pasta Accents Primavera	2¼ cups (7 oz)	320	12	5	20	13	40	7	150	500	—	15	—	750
Pasta Accents White Cheddar Sauce	1¾ cups (5.6 oz)	300	12	4	20	10	38	4	200	570	—	12	—	500
HEALTHY CHOICE														
Beef Macaroni Casserole	1 meal (8.5 oz)	200	1	1	15	14	34	5	40	450	—	54	—	500
Cheese Ravioli Parmigiana	1 meal (9 oz)	250	4	2	20	11	44	6	150	290	—	0	—	750

FOOD	PORTION	CALORIES	FAT	SAT FAT	CHOL	PROTEIN	CARBO	FIBER	CALCIUM	SOD	POTAS	VIT C	FOLIC	VIT A
HEALTHY CHOICE (CONT.)														
Chicken Broccoli Alfredo	1 meal (12.1 oz)	370	8	3	45	23	53	6	100	470	—	12	—	1500
Chicken Fettucini Alfredo	1 meal (8.5 oz)	250	3	1	30	20	34	3	80	370	—	0	—	0
Classics Pasta Shells Marinara	1 meal (12 oz)	360	3	2	25	25	59	5	400	390	—	0	—	500
Classics Turkey Fettuccine Alla Crema	1 meal (12.5 oz)	350	4	2	30	28	50	5	100	370	—	5	—	1000
Fettucini Alfredo	1 meal (8 oz)	240	5	2	10	9	39	3	100	430	—	0	—	0
Lasagna Roma	1 meal (13.5 oz)	390	5	2	15	26	60	9	150	580	—	0	—	500
Macaroni & Cheese	1 meal (9 oz)	290	5	2	15	15	45	4	300	580	—	0	—	0
Spaghetti Bolognese	1 meal (10 oz)	260	3	1	15	14	43	5	40	470	—	15	—	500
Three Cheese Manicotti	1 meal (11 oz)	310	9	5	20	16	41	7	300	450	—	1	—	750
Vegetable Pasta Italiano	1 meal (10 oz)	220	1	0	0	8	44	6	40	340	—	0	—	1750
Zucchini Lasagna	1 meal (14 oz)	330	2	1	10	20	58	11	200	310	—	6	—	1250
KID CUISINE														
Macaroni & Cheese	1 pkg (10.6 oz)	420	12	5	25	10	68	3	150	920	—	0	—	400
Mini Cheese Ravioli	1 pkg (9.82 oz)	320	5	2	10	7	63	6	60	780	—	0	—	200
LE MENU														
Entree LightStyle Garden Vegetables Lasagna	10½ oz	260	8	—	25	11	35	—	150	500	—	48	—	1250
Entree LightStyle Lasagna With Meat Sauce	10 oz	290	8	—	30	19	36	—	150	510	—	18	—	1250
Entree LightStyle Meat Sauce & Cheese Tortellini	8 oz	250	8	—	15	11	34	—	80	480	—	42	—	500
Entree LightStyle Spaghetti With Beef Sauce And Mushrooms	9 oz	280	6	—	15	12	45	—	40	450	—	36	—	750
LightStyle 3-Cheese Stuffed Shells	10 oz	280	8	—	25	17	34	—	250	690	—	30	—	1250
LightStyle Cheese Tortellini	10 oz	230	6	—	15	10	35	—	100	460	—	42	—	4200
Manicotto With Three Cheeses	11¾ oz	390	15	—	—	19	44	—	500	870	—	15	—	1000
LEAN CUISINE														
Alfredo Pasta Primavera	1 pkg (10 oz)	290	7	3	10	11	46	3	150	570	300	12	—	400

FOOD	PORTION	CALORIES	FAT	SAT FAT	CHOL	PROTEIN	CARBO	FIBER	CALCIUM	SOD	POTAS	VIT C	FOLIC	VIT A
LEAN CUISINE (CONT.)														
Angel Hair Pasta	1 pkg (10 oz)	220	3	1	0	8	41	6	80	420	560	12	—	1250
Bow Tie Pasta & Creamy Tomato Sauce	1 pkg (9.5 oz)	260	6	2	35	9	43	6	100	550	450	27	—	1500
Cafe Classics Bow Tie Pasta & Chicken	1 pkg (9.5 oz)	250	5	1	45	16	34	3	80	530	710	21	—	1750
Cafe Classics Cheese Lasagna w/ Chicken Scaloppini	1 pkg (10 oz)	290	8	2	30	21	33	3	150	590	560	9	—	500
Cheddar Bake With Pasta	1 pkg (9 oz)	220	6	3	15	11	30	3	250	590	320	6	—	1750
Cheese Cannelloni	1 pkg (9.1 oz)	230	4	2	15	20	28	3	350	570	490	6	—	500
Cheese Lasagna Casserole	1 pkg (10 oz)	270	6	3	10	6	40	5	200	590	420	9	—	1750
Cheese Ravioli	1 pkg (8.5 oz)	270	7	3	45	11	40	5	150	580	470	4	—	500
Cheese Stuffed Shells	1 serv (8.9 oz)	230	5	3	15	11	34	3	250	590	450	6	—	400
Chicken Fettucini	1 pkg (9.25 oz)	280	6	2	35	21	36	4	150	590	380	0	—	400
Chicken Lasagna	1 pkg (10 oz)	270	8	3	35	19	30	5	250	590	390	2	—	2500
Classic Cheese Lasagna	1 pkg (11.5 oz)	270	5	3	25	16	41	6	400	590	560	6	—	750
Fettucini Alfredo	1 pkg (9 oz)	300	7	3	15	12	47	2	200	550	230	0	—	0
Fettucini Primavera	1 pkg (10 oz)	270	7	3	15	13	38	4	250	580	370	0	—	2000
Five Cheese Lasagna	1 serv (8 oz)	210	4	2	25	13	31	4	300	590	440	6	—	500
Lasagne With Meat Sauce	1 pkg (10.5 oz)	290	6	4	25	21	37	4	300	560	580	12	—	750
Macaroni & Beef	1 pkg (10 oz)	270	4	2	25	15	43	4	60	590	520	0	—	400
Macaroni & Cheese	1 pkg (10 oz)	290	7	4	20	13	43	4	250	590	200	0	—	0
Penne Pasta Bolognese	1 pkg (9.5 oz)	270	6	3	25	15	39	4	60	570	450	12	—	2500
Penne Pasta w/ Tomato Basil Sauce	1 pkg (10 oz)	270	4	1	0	8	52	5	60	350	560	15	—	750
Spaghetti w/ Meat Sauce	1 pkg (11.5 oz)	290	5	2	20	11	50	7	60	570	550	9	—	500
Spaghetti w/ Meatballs	1 pkg (9.5 oz)	280	6	2	20	16	40	4	80	570	510	6	—	500
Vegetable Lasagna	1 pkg (10.5 oz)	260	7	3	20	15	35	5	350	590	530	9	—	2500
LIFE CHOICE														
Linguini Roma	1 meal (13.2 oz)	230	1	0	0	8	48	6	60	580	—	15	—	750
Sun Dried Tomato Manicotti	1 meal (11.65 oz)	220	3	1	5	11	39	7	100	540	—	5	—	3500

FOOD	PORTION	CALORIES	FAT	SAT FAT	CHOL	PROTEIN	CARBO	FIBER	CALCIUM	SOD	POTAS	VIT C	FOLIC	VIT A
LIFE CHOICE (CONT.)														
Vegetable Lasagna Primavera	1 meal (11.2 oz)	170	1	1	5	10	30	8	200	600	—	0	—	2250
LUIGINO'S														
& Pomodoro Sauc With Meatballs	1 pkg (9 oz)	320	11	4	15	12	43	2	60	890	—	2	—	0
& Pomodoro Sauce With Meatballs	1 cup (6.3 oz)	270	9	3	10	10	36	2	60	740	—	2	—	0
Cheese Ravioli & Alfredo With Broccoli Sauce	1 pkg (8.5 oz)	420	25	13	70	18	30	2	500	890	—	0	—	1250
Cheese Tortellini & Alfredo Sauce With Broccoli	1 pkg (8 oz)	390	24	12	65	17	28	2	450	840	—	0	—	1250
Fettuccine Alfredo	1 cup (7.5 oz)	330	11	4	20	13	36	3	40	510	—	0	—	200
Fettuccine Alfredo	1 pkg (9.4 oz)	390	14	5	30	16	45	4	100	630	—	0	—	300
Fettuccine Alfredo With Broccoli	1 pkg (9.2 oz)	360	16	8	25	14	39	4	200	500	—	0	—	750
Fettuccine Carbonara	1 pkg (9 oz)	360	13	4	35	15	47	3	200	760	—	0	—	750
Lasagna Alfredo	1 pkg (9 oz)	360	20	6	30	16	30	2	100	660	—	0	—	400
Lasagna Alfredo	1 cup (6.3 oz)	300	17	5	25	13	25	2	40	550	—	0	—	0
Lasagna Pollo	1 pkg (9 oz)	320	14	5	30	16	33	3	150	610	—	0	—	500
Lasagna With Meat Sauce	1 pkg (9 oz)	290	10	4	20	15	36	2	0	820	—	2	—	200
Lasagna With Meat Sauce	1 cup (7.2 oz)	240	8	3	15	12	30	2	0	680	—	2	—	200
Lasagna With Vegetables	1 pkg (9 oz)	290	10	3	20	14	35	2	0	630	—	2	—	200
Linguini With Clams & Sauce	1 pkg (9 oz)	270	6	2	10	12	42	2	40	650	—	0	—	200
Linguini With Red Sauce &	1 pkg (9 oz)	260	6	1	0	11	41	3	150	540	—	0	—	400
Linguini With Seafood	1 pkg (9 oz)	290	8	2	0	10	45	4	100	740	—	0	—	400
Macaroni & Cheese	1 pkg (9 oz)	370	15	6	20	13	45	3	250	750	—	0	—	750
Macaroni & Cheese	1 cup (7.2 oz)	310	12	7	15	11	37	2	250	620	—	0	—	750
Marinara Sauce Penne Pasta Italian Sausage & Peppers	1 pkg (9 oz)	350	17	4	35	18	32	2	0	880	—	4	—	200
Marinara Sauce Penne Pasta Italian Sausage & Peppers	1 cup (7.4 oz)	290	14	3	30	15	27	2	0	730	—	4	—	400
Meat Ravioli & Pomodoro Sauce	1 pkg (8.5 oz)	320	13	5	50	15	37	3	250	1060	—	0	—	1250
Minestrone With Penne Pasta	1 cup (6.3 oz)	180	6	1	5	10	21	1	0	640	—	0	—	400

FOOD	PORTION	CALORIES	FAT	SAT FAT	CHOL	PROTEIN	CARBO	FIBER	CALCIUM	SOD	POTAS	VIT C	FOLIC	VIT A
LUIGINO'S (CONT.)														
Penne Pollo	1 pkg (9 oz)	330	14	5	20	15	36	3	100	530	—	0	—	400
Penne Primavera	1 pkg (9 oz)	350	10	4	25	15	50	3	60	330	—	0	—	200
Rigatoni Pomodoro Italiano	1 pkg (9 oz)	290	8	2	0	15	40	4	80	710	—	0	—	1500
Shells & Cheese With Jalapenos	1 pkg (8.5 oz)	360	15	6	30	14	41	2	250	700	—	0	—	750
Spaghetti Bolognese	1 pkg (9 oz)	270	8	3	20	13	38	4	0	820	—	2	—	200
Spaghetti Marinara	1 pkg (10 oz)	250	2	1	0	11	49	3	40	680	—	1	—	200
Spinach Ravioli & Primavera Sauce	1 pkg (8.5 oz)	360	17	8	45	15	36	2	300	800	—	0	—	200
MORTON														
Macaroni & Cheese	1 serv (8 oz)	220	6	3	15	9	34	2	100	960	—	1	—	200
MRS. PAUL'S														
Entrees Light Seafood Lasagne	9½ oz	290	8	—	57	14	39	—	250	750	—	2	—	100
Entrees Light Seafood Rotini	9 oz	240	6	—	25	12	34	—	200	570	—	1	—	—
PALMAZONE														
Macaroni 'n Cheese	½ pkg (6 oz)	260	7	—	20	13	36	—	150	320	—	—	—	400
PASTA FAVORITES														
Chicken Pasta Primavera	1 pkg (10.5 oz)	330	13	5	25	13	40	6	80	930	—	12	—	2500
Fettuccini Alfredo	1 pkg (10.5 oz)	370	18	8	30	12	39	4	150	940	—	18	—	300
Italian Sausage & Peppers	1 pkg (10.5 oz)	340	13	4	10	11	43	7	60	840	—	60	—	500
Lasagna	1 pkg (10.5 oz)	290	9	2	10	14	39	6	150	900	—	60	—	750
Macaroni & Cheese	1 pkg (10.5 oz)	350	12	4	20	13	47	5	150	1070	—	24	—	1250
Pasta Primavera	1 pkg (10.5 oz)	320	14	6	20	10	40	7	80	920	—	9	—	2500
Spaghetti w/ Meatballs	1 pkg (10.5 oz)	370	16	5	35	14	40	6	80	1040	—	60	—	1250
Vegetable Lasagna	1 pkg (10.5 oz)	260	6	2	10	11	41	7	150	850	—	60	—	750
White Cheddar & Rotini	1 pkg (10.5 oz)	350	12	5	15	12	48	6	200	900	—	6	—	5000
SENOR FELIX'S														
Lasagna Southwestern	1 serv (6 oz)	160	7	4	15	8	15	2	200	380	—	21	—	500
STOUFFER'S														
Cheddar Pasta w/ Beef & Tomatoes	1 pkg (11 oz)	450	19	10	51	25	45	3	350	1130	380	5	—	400
Cheese Manicotti	1 pkg (9 oz)	380	17	9	45	18	38	4	450	880	450	2	—	500

FOOD	PORTION	CALORIES	FAT	SAT FAT	CHOL	PROTEIN	CARBO	FIBER	CALCIUM	SOD	POTAS	VIT C	FOLIC	VIT A
STOUFFER'S (CONT.)														
Cheese Ravioli	1 pkg (10.6 oz)	380	13	6	100	15	51	6	250	700	450	12	—	750
Chicken Lasagna	1 serv (7.8 oz)	320	17	5	30	13	29	4	200	750	325	5	—	2000
Fettucini Alfredo	1 pkg (10 oz)	520	28	16	100	16	17	4	300	1060	190	0	—	100
Fettucini Primavera	1 pkg (10 oz)	430	20	12	50	13	49	5	250	1100	250	0	—	2500
Five Cheese Lasagna	1 pkg (10.75 oz)	360	13	7	35	21	40	6	350	960	470	6	—	500
Grilled Chicken & Angel Hair Pasta	1 pkg (10.9 oz)	380	13	4	40	25	40	5	250	750	320	0	—	1500
Homestyle Chicken Fettucini	1 pkg (10.5 oz)	390	15	4	65	31	32	3	300	1250	520	1	—	200
Homestyle Chicken Parmigiana w/ Spaghetti	1 pkg (12 oz)	460	16	4	45	24	54	5	150	1060	670	12	—	750
Homestyle Veal Parmigiana w/ Spaghetti	1 pkg (11.9 oz)	430	17	5	80	21	49	6	150	1120	680	12	—	750
Lasagna Bake	1 pkg (10.25 oz)	370	12	5	30	18	47	6	150	900	440	9	—	500
Lasagna w/ Meat Sauce	1 pkg (10.5 oz)	370	14	7	45	23	39	4	250	1050	550	12	—	750
Macaroni & Cheese	1 cup (6 oz)	320	16	7	30	13	31	3	300	990	210	0	—	100
Macaroni & Cheese w/ Broccoli	1 pkg (10.5 oz)	360	17	8	25	15	37	5	300	1050	400	9	—	750
Macaroni & Beef	1 pkg (11.5 oz)	420	20	8	50	20	40	5	60	1530	630	9	—	750
Noodles Romanoff	1 pkg (12 oz)	490	25	6	60	18	48	4	150	1400	280	0	—	250
Pasta Shells w/ American Cheese	1 cup (6 oz)	260	10	4	20	11	31	2	250	1190	280	0	—	100
Salisbury Steak w/ Macaroni & Cheese	1 serv (11.3 oz)	410	19	8	70	26	34	2	250	1230	360	2	—	100
Spaghetti w/ Meat Sauce	1 pkg (10 oz)	350	12	4	35	15	46	5	60	570	430	9	—	500
Spaghetti w/ Meatballs	1 pkg (12.6 oz)	440	15	5	50	19	56	5	60	830	500	5	—	500
Tuna Noodle Casserole	1 pkg (10 oz)	320	10	4	40	20	37	0	200	1130	390	0	—	100
Turkey Tettrazini	1 pkg (10 oz)	360	17	7	55	19	33	1	100	1060	380	2	—	100
Vegetable Lasagna	1 pkg (10.5 oz)	440	20	8	35	21	43	5	500	1110	470	0	—	3000
SWANSON														
Homestyle Lasagne With Meat Sauce	10½ oz	400	15	—	—	26	39	—	500	1070	—	6	—	750
Homestyle Macaroni & Cheese	10 oz	390	19	—	—	17	37	—	450	1150	—	1	—	100

FOOD	PORTION	CALORIES	FAT	SAT FAT	CHOL	PROTEIN	CARBO	FIBER	CALCIUM	SOD	POTAS	VIT C	FOLIC	VIT A
SWANSON (CONT.)														
Homestyle Spaghetti With Italian Style Meatballs	13 oz	490	18	—	—	23	60	—	100	940	—	12	—	1250
Macaroni & Cheese	7 oz	200	8	—	—	7	24	—	150	740	—	—	—	400
Macaroni & Cheese	12¼ oz	370	15	—	—	13	48	—	250	1070	—	6	—	3500
Spaghetti & Meatballs	12½ oz	390	17	—	—	14	46	—	100	1100	—	12	—	750
TABATCHNICK														
Macaroni & Cheese	7.5 oz	280	12	6	26	14	30	2	250	840	—	tr	—	0
TYSON														
Parmigiana	1 pkg (11.25 oz)	380	17	—	36	19	37	—	—	1100				
ULTRA SLIM-FAST														
Pasta Primavera	12 oz	340	9	—	25	18	52	5	350	730	440	15	40	4000
Spaghetti With Beef & Mushroom Sauce	12 oz	370	10	—	25	20	49	0	100	990	610	5	80	500
WEIGHT WATCHERS														
Smart Ones Angel Hair Pasta	1 pkg (9 oz)	170	2	0	0	8	29	4	100	520	—	9	—	500
Smart Ones Bowtie Pasta & Mushrooms Marsala	1 pkg (9.65 oz)	280	9	4	10	13	36	5	200	560	—	2	—	100
Smart Ones Chicken Fettucini	1 pkg (10 oz)	290	7	2	50	19	39	4	100	590	—	6	—	500
Smart Ones Creamy Rigatoni w/ Broccoli & Chicken	1 pkg (9 oz)	230	2	1	20	14	40	4	150	670	—	5	—	750
Smart Ones Fettucini Alfredo w/ Broccoli	1 pkg (8.5 oz)	230	6	3	20	10	34	3	250	450	—	1	—	300
Smart Ones Lasagna Florentine	1 pkg (10 oz)	200	2	0	10	10	34	5	200	500	—	9	—	1500
Smart Ones Lasagna Alfredo	1 pkg (9 oz)	300	7	4	25	15	45	2	250	650	—	6	—	200
Smart Ones Lasagna w/ Meat Sauce	1 pkg (10.25 oz)	270	7	3	35	14	38	6	400	570	—	2	—	1500
Smart Ones Lasagna w/ Meat Sauce	1 pkg (9 oz)	240	2	1	10	13	43	4	150	520	—	5	—	500
Smart Ones Macaroni & Cheese	1 pkg (9 oz)	220	2	1	5	9	42	4	100	640	—	0	—	300

FOOD	PORTION	CALORIES	FAT	SAT FAT	CHOL	PROTEIN	CARBO	FIBER	CALCIUM	SOD	POTAS	VIT C	FOLIC	VIT A
WEIGHT WATCHERS (CONT.)														
Smart Ones Pasta & Spinach Romano	1 pkg (10.4 oz)	240	8	4	5	11	32	4	250	510	—	9	—	1500
Smart Ones Pasta w/ Tomato Basil Sauce	1 pkg (9.6 oz)	260	9	4	10	12	33	5	200	360	—	4	—	200
Smart Ones Penne Pasta w/ Sun-Dried Tomatoes	1 pkg (10 oz)	290	9	3	15	12	41	4	200	560	—	15	—	500
Smart Ones Penne Pollo	1 pkg (10 oz)	290	5	2	35	22	40	3	150	620	—	4	—	300
Smart Ones Ravioli Florentine	1 pkg (8.5 oz)	220	2	1	5	9	43	4	100	490	—	9	—	2000
Smart Ones Spaghetti Marinara	1 pkg (9 oz)	280	7	2	5	9	46	5	80	690	—	12	—	750
Smart Ones Spaghetti w/ Meat Sauce	1 pkg (10 oz)	290	6	2	15	17	41	4	0	560	—	9	—	500
Smart Ones Spicy Penne & Ricotta	1 pkg (10.2 oz)	280	6	2	5	12	45	5	150	370	—	4	—	300
Smart Ones Tuna Noodle Casserole	1 pkg (9.5 oz)	270	7	4	40	13	39	4	200	670	—	6	—	500
Smart Ones Zita Mozzarella	1 pkg (9 oz)	280	6	2	5	11	45	4	100	430	—	5	—	300
HOME RECIPE														
macaroni & cheese	1 cup	430	22	10	44	17	40	—	362	1086	240	1	—	860
spaghetti w/ meatballs & tomato sauce	1 cup	330	12	4	89	19	39	—	124	1009	665	22	—	1590
MIX														
CASBAH														
Pasta Fasul	1 pkg (1.6 oz)	150	1	0	0	11	10	2	80	490	—	9	—	350
HAIN														
Pasta & Sauce Creamy Parmesan	¼ pkg	150	3	—	10	8	22	—	100	400	190	—	—	300
Pasta & Sauce Creamy Swiss	¼ pkg	170	4	—	—	6	26	—	80	360	5	—	—	—
Pasta & Sauce Fettuccine Alfredo	¼ pkg	180	4	—	—	5	27	—	60	420	50	—	—	—
Pasta & Sauce Italian Herb	¼ pkg	110	2	—	—	4	17	—	40	160	5	—	—	—
Pasta & Sauce Primavera	¼ pkg	140	4	—	10	7	20	—	100	430	180	2	—	2250
Pasta & Sauce Tangy Cheddar	¼ pkg	180	6	—	3	6	24	—	80	350	120	—	—	100

FOOD	PORTION	CALORIES	FAT	SAT FAT	CHOL	PROTEIN	CARBO	FIBER	CALCIUM	SOD	POTAS	VIT C	FOLIC	VIT A
KRAFT														
Deluxe Macaroni & Cheese Four Cheese Blend as prep	1 cup (6.2 oz)	320	10	7	25	14	44	1	200	910	170	0	60	500
Deluxe Macaroni & Cheese Original as prep	1 cup (6.1 oz)	320	10	6	25	14	44	1	200	730	190	0	60	500
Light Deluxe Macaroni & Cheese as prep	1 cup (6.5 oz)	290	5	3	15	14	48	1	200	810	310	0	60	200
Macaroni & Cheese All Shapes as prep	1 cup (6.9 oz)	410	18	5	10	12	49	1	100	750	340	0	60	750
Macaroni & Cheese Original as prep	1 cup (6.9 oz)	410	18	5	10	12	49	1	100	750	340	0	60	750
Macaroni & Cheese Original as prep light recipe	1 cup (6.4 oz)	290	6	2	10	12	48	2	150	580	310	0	60	200
Premium Macaroni & Cheese Cheesy Alfredo as prep	1 cup (6.9 oz)	410	19	5	10	11	49	2	150	810	330	0	60	750
Premium Macaroni & Cheese Mild White Cheddar as prep	1 cup (6.8 oz)	410	19	4	10	12	49	1	150	740	330	0	60	1000
Premium Macaroni & Cheese Thick 'N Creamy as prep	1 cup (7.6 oz)	420	19	5	15	13	50	2	150	760	360	0	60	750
Premium Macaroni & Cheese Three Cheese as prep	1 cup (6.9 oz)	410	18	4	10	12	49	2	150	790	330	0	60	750
Spaghetti Classics Mild Italian as prep	1 cup (9.1 oz)	240	3	1	<5	11	46	3	60	850	590	9	40	500
Spaghetti Classics Tangy Italian as prep	1 cup (8.9 oz)	240	2	1	0	11	46	3	60	830	590	9	40	500
Spaghetti Classics Zesty Cheese as prep	1 cup (8.6 oz)	240	2	1	5	11	46	3	60	800	630	9	40	500
Spaghetti Classics w/ Meat Sauce as prep	1 cup (8.2 oz)	330	10	4	15	11	47	3	60	810	410	4	40	750
LIPTON														
Pasta & Sauce Angel Hair Chicken Broccoli as prep	1 cup	260	8	1	0	8	43	2	0	810	—	4	100	300

FOOD	PORTION	CALORIES	FAT	SAT FAT	CHOL	PROTEIN	CARBO	FIBER	CALCIUM	SOD	POTAS	VIT C	FOLIC	VIT A
LIPTON (CONT.)														
Pasta & Sauce Angel Hair Parmesan as prep	1 cup	280	11	3	10	8	41	2	40	960	—	0	100	400
Pasta & Sauce Bow Tie Chicken Primavera as prep	1 cup	290	10	4	10	9	43	2	100	820	—	1	100	1000
Pasta & Sauce Bow Tie Italian Cheese as prep	1 cup	300	12	5	15	10	41	tr	150	900	—	0	100	400
Pasta & Sauce Butter & Herbs as prep	1 cup	270	10	3	5	7	40	2	0	830	—	0	100	0
Pasta & Sauce Cheddar Broccoli as prep	1 cup	340	11	4	15	11	49	1	150	970	—	4	120	500
Pasta & Sauce Chicken Herb Parmesan as prep	1 cup	80	9	2	5	8	43	2	40	910	—	0	100	400
Pasta & Sauce Chicken Stir-Fry as prep	1 cup	270	8	1	0	8	43	2	20	900	—	1	100	750
Pasta & Sauce Creamy Garlic as prep	1 cup	350	13	5	15	10	50	1	100	980	—	0	100	500
Pasta & Sauce Creamy Mushroom as prep	1 cup	320	11	4	15	10	46	0	100	870	—	0	100	400
Pasta & Sauce Mild Cheddar Cheese as prep	1 cup	290	10	4	10	10	41	tr	150	930	—	0	100	400
Pasta & Sauce Roasted Garlic Chicken as prep	1 cup	290	10	3	10	9	43	tr	400	880	—	0	100	400
Pasta & Sauce Roasted Garlic & Olive Oil w/ Tomato as prep	1 cup	270	9	2	0	8	42	2	0	880	—	2	100	500
Pasta & Sauce Rotini Primavera as prep	1 cup	320	12	5	15	10	45	2	100	980	—	4	100	750
Pasta & Sauce Savory Herb w/ Garlic as prep	1 cup	280	9	3	5	8	52	2	20	890	—	0	100	300
Pasta & Sauce Three Cheese Rotini as prep	1 cup	320	12	5	15	11	44	tr	150	970	—	0	100	400
MELTING POT														
Terrazza Black Beans & Penne	1 cup	180	1	0	0	8	36	2	20	480	—	1	—	100

FOOD	PORTION	CALORIES	FAT	SAT FAT	CHOL	PROTEIN	CARBO	FIBER	CALCIUM	SOD	POTAS	VIT C	FOLIC	VIT A
MELTING POT (CONT.)														
Terrazza Florentine Red Beans & Fusilli	1 cup	220	1	0	<5	10	43	2	40	350	—	0	—	500
Terrazza Red Lentils & Bow Ties	1 cup	240	2	1	40	13	42	5	20	390	—	0	—	200
Terrazza Tuscan White Beans & Gemell	1 cup	220	1	0	<5	10	44	3	40	450	—	1	—	100
NILE SPICE														
Pasta'n Sauce Mediterranean	1 pkg	210	5	3	10	9	33	2	100	640	—	2	—	0
Pasta'n Sauce Parmesan	1 pkg	200	3	2	10	8	36	1	80	470	—	2	—	200
Pasta'n Sauce Primavera	1 pkg	200	4	3	10	9	34	2	150	610	—	9	—	750
ULTRA SLIM-FAST														
Macaroni & Cheese	2.3 oz	230	3	—	—	9	46	4	150	770	200	18	—	750
UNCLE BEN														
Country Inn Pasta & Sauce Angel Hair Parmesan	1 serv (2.2 oz)	245	5	—	13	10	39	3	65	926	134	2	—	271
Country Inn Pasta & Sauce Broccoli & White Cheddar	1 serv (2.2 oz)	240	5	—	8	9	40	2	57	799	54	1	—	0
Country Inn Pasta & Sauce Butter & Herb	1 serv (2 oz)	230	6	—	10	7	36	1	31	885	53	14	—	34
Country Inn Pasta & Sauce Creamy Garlic	1 serv (2.4 oz)	261	5	—	8	9	45	2	32	599	55	0	—	31
Country Inn Pasta & Sauce Fettuccine Alfredo	1 serv (2.2 oz)	310	6	—	12	9	41	2	42	656	53	tr	—	0
Country Inn Pasta & Sauce Herb Linguine	1 serv (2.2 oz)	240	3	—	5	9	43	2	29	654	55	4	—	27
Country Inn Pasta & Sauce Mushroom Fettuccine	1 serv (2.2 oz)	250	6	—	12	9	41	2	32	638	53	0	—	42
Country Inn Pasta & Sauce Vegetable Alfredo	1 serv (2.2 oz)	240	5	—	11	9	42	2	36	548	53	3	—	48
VELVEETA														
Rotini & Cheese w/ Broccoli as prep	1 cup (7.2 oz)	400	16	10	50	18	47	2	300	1230	270	4	60	750

FOOD	PORTION	CALORIES	FAT	SAT FAT	CHOL	PROTEIN	CARBO	FIBER	CALCIUM	SOD	POTAS	VIT C	FOLIC	VIT A
VELVEETA (CONT.)														
Shells & Cheese Bacon as prep	1 cup (6.8 oz)	360	14	8	40	17	43	1	250	1140	230	0	60	500
Shells & Cheese Original as prep	1 cup (6.6 oz)	360	13	8	40	16	44	1	250	1030	210	0	60	500
Shells & Cheese Salsa as prep	1 cup (7.5 oz)	380	14	9	40	17	47	2	250	1180	300	0	60	750
SHELF-STABLE														
CHEF BOYARDEE														
Microwave Main Meal Beans & Pasta	10.5 oz	200	1	tr	10	14	44	10	100	1030	—	1	—	300
Microwave Main Meal Beef Ravioli Suprema	10.5 oz	290	4	—	10	12	52	5	20	1390	—	4	—	750
Microwave Main Meal Cheese Ravioli Suprema	10.5 oz	290	4	—	10	12	52	5	60	1360	—	4	—	500
Microwave Main Meal Fettuccine	10.5 oz	290	9	4	25	13	46	6	20	1010	—	6	—	750
Microwave Main Meal Lasagna	10.5 oz	290	8	—	20	13	41	5	40	1000	—	4	—	500
Microwave Main Meal Meat Tortellini	10.5 oz	220	4	2	30	12	53	6	20	980	—	6	—	500
Microwave Main Meal Noodles w/ Chicken	10.5 oz	170	1	—	20	13	27	3	20	1120	—	—	—	200
Microwave Main Meal Peas & Pasta	10.5 oz	190	2	tr	0	9	39	6	40	1020	—	4	—	750
Microwave Main Meal Spaghetti Suprema	10.5 oz	200	7	—	20	11	37	7	40	1000	—	2	—	500
Microwave Main Meal Zesty Macaroni	10.5 oz	290	8	—	25	14	40	5	20	1300	—	—	—	1000
Microwave Main Meal Ziti In Sauce	10.5 oz	210	tr	tr	0	8	52	7	20	1030	—	4	—	750
HORMEL														
Microcup Meals Lasagna	1 cup (7.5 oz)	250	14	7	25	8	24	1	40	950	—	0	—	300
Microcup Meals Macaroni & Cheese	1 cup (7.5 oz)	260	11	6	35	11	30	1	100	690	—	0	—	300
Microcup Meals Ravioli w/ Tomato Sauce	1 cup (7.5 oz)	220	6	2	15	8	34	2	60	840	—	2	—	200
Microcup Meals Spaghetti & Meatballs	1 cup (7.5 oz)	220	7	4	25	11	28	1	60	930	—	0	—	500

FOOD	PORTION	CALORIES	FAT	SAT FAT	CHOL	PROTEIN	CARBO	FIBER	CALCIUM	SOD	POTAS	VIT C	FOLIC	VIT A
KID'S KITCHEN														
Microwave Meals Beefy Macaroni	1 cup (7.5 oz)	190	6	3	30	11	23	2	40	790	—	0	—	750
Microwave Meals Macaroni & Cheese	1 cup (7.5 oz)	260	11	6	35	11	30	1	100	690	—	0	—	300
Microwave Meals Mini Ravioli	1 cup (7.5 oz)	240	7	3	20	10	34	1	40	950	—	1	—	500
Microwave Meals Spaghetti & Meatballs	1 cup (7.5 oz)	220	7	4	25	11	28	1	60	950	—	0	—	500
Microwave Meals Spaghetti Ring & Meatballs	1 cup (7.5 oz)	250	7	3	20	11	35	3	60	1200	—	1	—	400
LUNCH BUCKET														
Elbows In Tomato Sauce	1 pkg (7.5 oz)	190	2	—	—	4	38	—	—	860	—	—	—	—
Lasagna With Meatsauce	1 pkg (7.5 oz)	220	4	—	30	8	38	—	—	870	—	—	—	—
Light'n Healthy Italian Style Pasta	1 pkg (7.5 oz)	130	1	—	10	7	23	—	—	630	—	—	—	—
Light'n Healthy Pasta In Wine Sauce	1 pkg (7.5 oz)	130	3	—	10	5	21	—	—	600	—	—	—	—
Light'n Healthy Pasta'n Garden Vegetables	1 pkg (7.5 oz)	150	1	—	0	4	30	—	—	630	—	—	—	—
Macaroni'n Cheese	1 pkg (7.5 oz)	210	9	—	—	9	24	—	—	990	—	—	—	—
Pasta'n Chicken	1 pkg (7.5 oz)	180	6	—	45	9	22	—	—	860	—	—	—	—
Spaghetti'n Meatsauce	1 pkg (7.5 oz)	240	5	—	30	9	39	—	—	870	—	—	—	—
MY OWN MEAL														
Cheese Tortellini	1 pkg (10 oz)	340	10	3	15	15	49	6	350	1000	—	15	—	1000
TAKE-OUT														
macaroni & cheese	1 cup	230	10	5	24	9	26	—	199	730	139	tr	—	260
PASTA MACHINE MIX														
WANDA'S														
Dried Tomato	⅓ cup mix per serv (1.9 oz)	202	1	0	0	7	42	1	10	0	—	0	—	0
Durum & Semolina	⅓ cup mix per serv (1.9 oz)	199	1	0	0	7	42	1	10	0	—	0	—	0
Semolina Blend	⅓ cup mix per serv (1.9 oz)	202	1	0	0	7	42	1	10	0	—	0	—	0
Spinach	⅓ cup mix per serv (1.9 oz)	202	1	0	0	7	42	1	10	0	—	0	—	0
Whole Wheat & Semolina	⅓ cup mix per serv (1.9 oz)	198	1	0	0	7	41	4	10	2	—	0	—	0

PASTA SALAD

MIX

KRAFT

FOOD	PORTION	CALORIES	FAT	SAT FAT	CHOL	PROTEIN	CARBO	FIBER	CALCIUM	SOD	POTAS	VIT C	FOLIC	VIT A
Herb & Garlic as prep	¾ cup (4.9 oz)	280	14	2	0	6	34	2	2	670	170	2	40	500
Pasta Salad Classic Ranch w/ Bacon as prep	¾ cup (4.7 oz)	350	22	4	10	7	32	2	0	480	150	0	40	400
Pasta Salad Creamy Ceasar as prep	¾ cup (4.8 oz)	340	21	4	15	7	31	2	60	630	320	4	40	200
Pasta Salad Garden Primavera as prep	¾ cup (5 oz)	240	8	2	<5	8	35	2	60	710	190	4	40	300
Pasta Salad Italian 97% Fat Free as prep	¾ cup (4.9 oz)	190	2	1	<5	8	3534	2	100	740	220	4	40	300
Pasta Salad Parmesan Peppercorn as prep	¾ cup (4.9 oz)	360	23	4	15	7	29	2	60	570	150	1	40	500

SUDDENLY SALAD

FOOD	PORTION	CALORIES	FAT	SAT FAT	CHOL	PROTEIN	CARBO	FIBER	CALCIUM	SOD	POTAS	VIT C	FOLIC	VIT A
Classic Pasta Low Fat Recipe as prep	¾ cup	180	3	1	0	5	34	1	0	830	150	0	—	0
Classic Pasta as prep	¾ cup	220	7	1	0	5	34	1	0	830	150	0	—	0
Garden Italian 98% Fat Free as prep	¾ cup	140	1	0	0	5	29	2	20	540	130	0	—	750

TAKE-OUT

FOOD	PORTION	CALORIES	FAT	SAT FAT	CHOL	PROTEIN	CARBO	FIBER	CALCIUM	SOD	POTAS	VIT C	FOLIC	VIT A
elbow macaroni salad	3.5 oz	160	5	2	0	3	26	—	—	590	—	1	—	—
italian style pasta salad	3.5 oz	140	7	1	0	3	15	—	20	480	—	9	—	300
mustard macaroni salad	3.5 oz	190	10	1	0	4	23	—	—	560	—	4	—	—
pasta salad w/ vegetables	3.5 oz	140	4	3	0	4	21	—	40	210	—	4	—	—

PASTRY

(*see* BROWNIE, CAKE, DANISH PASTRY)

PATE

CANNED

FOOD	PORTION	CALORIES	FAT	SAT FAT	CHOL	PROTEIN	CARBO	FIBER	CALCIUM	SOD	POTAS	VIT C	FOLIC	VIT A
chicken liver	1 tbsp (13 g)	109	2	—	—	2	1	—	1	—	—	—	—	94
chicken liver	1 oz	238	4	—	—	4	2	—	3	—	—	—	—	205
goose liver smoked	1 oz	131	12	—	43	3	1	—	—	—	—	—	—	—
goose liver smoked	1 tbsp (13 g)	60	6	—	20	1	1	—	—	—	—	—	—	—
liver	1 oz	90	8	—	—	4	tr	—	20	198	39	0	17	936
liver	1 tbsp (13 g)	41	4	—	—	5	tr	—	9	91	18	0	8	429

FOOD	PORTION	CALORIES	FAT	SAT FAT	CHOL	PROTEIN	CARBO	FIBER	CALCIUM	SOD	POTAS	VIT C	FOLIC	VIT A
SELLS														
Liver	2.08 oz	190	16	—	90	8	4	—	—	470	170	—	—	650
PEACH														
CANNED														
halves in heavy syrup	1 half	60	tr	tr	0	tr	16	—	8	5	74	2	3	269
halves in light syrup	1 half	44	tr	tr	0	tr	12	—	3	4	79	2	3	286
halves juice pack	1 half	34	tr	tr	0	tr	9	—	15	3	98	3	—	294
halves water pack	1 half	18	tr	tr	0	tr	5	—	2	3	76	2	3	410
spiced in heavy syrup	1 cup	180	tr	tr	0	1	49	—	15	9	206	13	—	768
spiced in heavy syrup	1 fruit	66	tr	tr	0	tr	18	—	5	3	75	5	—	279
DEL MONTE														
Halves Cling In Heavy Syrup	½ cup (4.5 oz)	100	0	0	0	0	24	1	0	10	—	5	—	300
Halves Cling Lite	½ cup (4.4 oz)	60	0	0	0	0	15	1	0	10	—	5	—	300
Halves Cling Melba In Heavy Syrup	½ cup (4.5 oz)	100	0	0	0	0	24	1	0	10	—	5	—	300
Halves Freestone In Heavy Syrup	½ cup (4.5 oz)	100	0	0	0	0	24	1	0	10	—	1	—	100
Sliced Cling Fruit Naturals	½ cup (4.4 oz)	60	0	0	0	0	15	1	0	10	—	5	—	300
Sliced Cling In Heavy Syrup	½ cup (4.5 oz)	100	0	0	0	0	24	1	0	10	—	5	—	300
Sliced Cling Lite	½ cup (4.4 oz)	60	0	0	0	0	15	1	0	10	—	5	—	300
Sliced Freestone In Heavy Syrup	½ cup (4.5 oz)	100	0	0	0	0	24	1	0	10	—	1	—	100
Sliced Freestone Lite	½ cup (4.4 oz)	60	0	0	0	0	14	1	0	10	—	1	—	100
Snack Cups Diced Fruit Naturals	1 serv (4.5 oz)	60	0	0	0	0	16	1	0	10	—	5	—	300
Snack Cups Diced Fruit Naturals EZ-Open Lid	1 serv (4.2 oz)	60	0	0	0	0	15	1	0	10	—	5	—	300
Snack Cups Diced In Heavy Syrup	1 serv (4.5 oz)	100	0	0	0	0	24	1	0	10	—	5	—	300
Snack Cups Diced In Heavy Syrup EZ-Open Lid	1 serv (4.2 oz)	90	0	0	0	0	23	1	0	10	—	5	—	300
Snack Cups Diced Lite	1 serv (4.5 oz)	60	0	0	0	0	16	1	0	10	—	5	—	300
Snack Cups Diced Lite EZ-Open Lid	1 serv (4.2 oz)	60	0	0	0	0	15	1	0	10	—	5	—	300
Whole Cling In Heavy Syrup	½ cup (4.2 oz)	100	0	0	0	0	24	tr	0	10	—	5	—	300
HUNT'S														
Halves	½ cup (4.5 oz)	100	0	0	0	1	24	1	1	10	—	2	—	30

FOOD	PORTION	CALORIES	FAT	SAT FAT	CHOL	PROTEIN	CARBO	FIBER	CALCIUM	SOD	POTAS	VIT C	FOLIC	VIT A
HUNT'S (CONT.)														
Slices	½ cup (4.5 oz)	100	0	0	0	1	24	1	1	10	—	2	—	30
LIBBY														
Halves Yellow Cling Lite	½ cup (4.4 oz)	60	0	0	0	1	13	1	0	10	105	1	—	300
Sliced Yellow Cling Lite	½ cup (4.4 oz)	60	0	0	0	1	13	1	0	10	105	1	—	300
DRIED														
halves cooked w/ sugar	½ cup	139	tr	tr	0	1	36	—	11	3	395	5	tr	243
halves cooked w/o sugar	½ cup	99	tr	tr	0	1	25	—	12	3	413	5	tr	254
DEL MONTE														
Sun Dried	⅓ cup (1.4 oz)	90	0	0	0	1	28	5	0	0	—	6	—	600
SONOMA														
Pieces	3-5 pieces (1.4 oz)	120	0	0	0	1	31	1	0	0	—	2	—	1000
FRESH														
sliced	1 cup	73	tr	tr	0	1	19	—	9	1	334	11	6	910
DOLE														
Peach	2	70	0	—	0	1	19	1	—	0	—	—	—	—
FROZEN														
slices sweetened	1 cup	235	tr	tr	0	2	60	—	6	16	325	235	—	709
BIG VALLEY														
Freestone	⅔ cup (4.9 oz)	50	0	0	0	1	13	1	0	0	—	168	—	1250
PEACH JUICE														
nectar	1 cup	134	tr	tr	0	1	35	—	13	17	101	13	—	643
GOYA														
Nectar	6 oz	110	0	—	0	tr	27	—	22	30	95	1	—	414
KERN'S														
Nectar	6 fl oz	110	0	0	0	1	26	—	—	0	120	24	—	200
LIBBY														
Nectar	1 can (11.5 fl oz)	210	0	0	0	1	52	—	20	5	190	60	—	200
MOTT'S														
Fruit Basket Orchard Peach Juice Cocktail as prep	8 fl oz	130	0	0	0	0	32	0	0	0	200	15	—	300
SNAPPLE														
Dixie Peach	10 fl oz	140	0	0	0	0	39	—	40	20	—	0	—	750
PEANUT BUTTER														
ARROWHEAD														
Creamy	2 tbsp (1.1 oz)	200	15	3	0	9	6	1	20	0	—	0	—	0
Crunchy	2 tbsp (1.1 oz)	200	15	3	0	9	6	1	20	0	—	0	—	0

FOOD	PORTION	CALORIES	FAT	SAT FAT	CHOL	PROTEIN	CARBO	FIBER	CALCIUM	SOD	POTAS	VIT C	FOLIC	VIT A
BAMA														
Creamy	2 tbsp	200	17	—	0	7	6	—	—	140	130	—	—	—
Crunchy	2 tbsp	200	17	—	0	7	6	—	—	115	130	—	—	—
Jelly & Peanut Butter	2 tbsp	150	7	—	0	3	20	—	—	75	95	—	—	—
CRAZY RICHARD'S														
Natural Creamy	2 tbsp (1.1 oz)	190	16	2	0	9	6	2	20	0	—	0	—	0
ESTEE														
Chunky Sodium Free	2 tbsp (1 oz)	190	15	3	0	7	7	2	0	0	200	0	—	0
Chunky Sodium Free Sorbitol Sweetened	2 tbsp (1 oz)	190	15	3	0	7	7	2	0	0	200	0	—	0
Creamy Sodium Free	2 tbsp (1 oz)	190	15	3	0	7	7	2	0	0	200	0	—	0
Creamy Sodium Free Sorbitol Sweetened	2 tbsp (1 oz)	190	15	3	0	7	7	2	0	0	200	0	—	0
HEALTH VALLEY														
Chunky No Salt	2 tbsp	170	14	—	0	8	6	2	10	2	190	tr	26	0
Creamy No Salt	2 tbsp	170	14	—	0	8	6	3	10	2	190	tr	26	0
HOLLYWOOD														
Creamy	1 tbsp	35	3	0	0	2	1	1	—	25	45	—	—	—
Crunchy	1 tbsp	35	3	0	0	2	1	1	—	25	45	—	—	—
Unsalted	1 tbsp	35	3	0	0	2	1	1	—	0	45	—	—	—
JIF														
Creamy	2 tbsp (1.1 oz)	190	16	3	0	8	7	2	—	150	207	—	—	—
Extra Crunchy	2 tbsp (1.1 oz)	190	16	3	0	8	7	2	—	130	207	—	—	—
Reduced Fat	2 tbsp (1.3 oz)	190	12	3	0	8	15	2	—	250	—	—	24	—
Simply Creamy	2 tbsp (1.1 oz)	190	16	3	0	8	6	2	—	65	209	—	—	—
Simply Extra Crunchy	2 tbsp (1.1 oz)	190	16	3	0	8	6	2	—	50	209	—	—	—
PETER PAN														
Creamy	2 tbsp	190	16	2	0	9	6	2	—	150	230	—	—	—
Creamy Salt Free	2 tbsp	190	17	2	0	9	5	2	20	0	230	—	—	—
Crunchy	2 tbsp	190	16	2	0	9	6	2	—	150	230	—	—	—
Crunchy Salt Free	2 tbsp	190	17	2	0	9	5	2	20	0	230	—	—	—
RED WING														
Creamy	2 tbsp (1.1 oz)	200	16	3	0	7	6	2	0	140	—	0	—	0
Crunchy	2 tbsp (1.1 oz)	200	16	3	0	7	6	2	0	120	—	0	—	0
SKIPPY														
Reduced Fat Creamy	2 tbsp	190	12	3	0	9	13	1	0	200	—	0	24	0
TREE OF LIFE														
Creamy	2 tbsp (1 oz)	190	15	4	0	9	7	1	20	150	—	—	—	—
Creamy No Salt	2 tbsp (1 oz)	190	15	4	0	9	7	1	20	0	—	—	—	—
Creamy Organic	2 tbsp (1 oz)	190	16	4	0	8	7	1	20	45	—	—	—	—

FOOD	PORTION	CALORIES	FAT	SAT FAT	CHOL	PROTEIN	CARBO	FIBER	CALCIUM	SOD	POTAS	VIT C	FOLIC	VIT A
TREE OF LIFE (CONT.)														
Creamy Organic No Salt	2 tbsp (1 oz)	190	16	4	0	8	7	1	20	0	—	—	—	—
Crunchy	2 tbsp (1 oz)	190	15	4	0	9	7	1	20	150	—	—	—	—
Crunchy No Salt	2 tbsp (1 oz)	190	15	4	0	9	7	1	20	0	—	—	—	—
Crunchy Organic	2 tbsp (1 oz)	190	16	4	0	8	7	1	20	45	—	—	—	—
Crunchy Organic No Salt	2 tbsp (1 oz)	190	16	4	0	8	7	1	20	0	—	—	—	—
Peanut Wonder 78% Less Fat	2 tbsp (1 oz)	100	4	1	0	3	11	1	20	250	—	9	—	0
PEANUTS														
chocolate coated	10 (1.4 oz)	208	13	6	4	5	20	—	42	16	201	0	3	0
chocolate coated	1 cup (5.2 oz)	773	50	22	13	19	74	—	155	61	748	0	12	0
virginia oil roasted	1 oz	161	14	2	0	8	5	—	24	121	183	0	35	0
virginia oil roasted	1 cup	826	70	9	0	37	28	—	123	619	933	0	179	0
BEER NUTS														
Peanuts	1 pkg (1 oz)	180	14	—	0	7	7	—	2	60	—	—	—	—
FISHER														
Salted-In-Shell shelled	1 oz	170	14	2	0	7	6	—	—	170	—	—	—	—
Spanish Roasted	1 oz	180	16	3	0	5	6	—	—	130	—	—	—	—
FRITO LAY														
Dry Roasted	1.2 oz	190	16	—	0	7	7	—	—	300	—	—	—	—
Salted	1 oz	170	15	—	0	6	6	—	—	170	—	—	—	—
GUY'S														
Dry Roasted	1 oz	170	14	—	0	8	3	—	—	310	200	—	—	—
Spanish Salted	1 oz	170	14	—	0	8	3	—	—	170	200	—	—	—
LANCE														
Honey Toasted	1 pkg (39 g)	230	17	3	0	9	11	—	—	240	150	—	—	—
Roasted w/ Shell	1 pkg (50 g)	190	15	3	0	9	8	—	20	0	—	—	—	—
Salted	1 pkg (32 g)	190	15	3	0	9	7	—	20	105	15	—	—	—
Salted Tube	1 pkg (42 g)	240	20	4	0	12	9	—	20	120	120	—	—	—
LITTLE DEBBIE														
Salted	1 pkg (1.2 oz)	230	21	3	0	8	3	2	20	45	—	0	—	0
PENNANT														
Oil Roasted	1 oz	170	14	2	0	7	6	3	—	115	200	—	—	—
PLANTERS														
Cocktail Lightly Salted Oil Roasted	1 oz	170	15	2	0	7	5	2	—	55	190	—	—	—
Cocktail Oil Roasted	1 oz	170	14	2	0	7	6	3	—	115	200	—	—	—
Cocktail Unsalted Oil Roasted	1 oz	170	14	2	0	7	6	2	—	0	190	—	—	—
Dry Roasted	1 oz	160	13	2	0	7	6	3	20	250	180	—	—	—
Fun Size! Oil Roasted	2 pkg (1 oz)	170	15	2	0	7	6	2	—	140	190	—	—	—

FOOD	PORTION	CALORIES	FAT	SAT FAT	CHOL	PROTEIN	CARBO	FIBER	CALCIUM	SOD	POTAS	VIT C	FOLIC	VIT A
PLANTERS (CONT.)														
Heat Hot Spicy Oil Roasted	1 pkg (1.7 oz)	290	25	4	0	12	9	4	40	370	340	4	—	—
Heat Hot Spicy Oil Roasted	1 oz	160	14	2	0	7	5	2	—	190	200	—	—	—
Heat Hot Spicy Oil Roasted	1 pkg (2 oz)	330	29	4	0	14	10	5	60	390	400	4	—	100
Heat Mild Spicy Oil Roasted	1 oz	160	14	2	0	7	5	2	20	130	200	—	—	—
Honey Roasted	1 oz	160	13	2	0	6	8	2	—	90	180	—	—	—
Honey Roasted Dry Roasted	1 pkg (1.7 oz)	260	19	3	0	10	17	3	40	260	270	—	—	—
Lightly Salted Dry Roasted	1 oz	160	14	2	0	8	5	3	20	110	200	—	—	—
Lightly Salted Dry Roasted	1 pkg (1.75 oz)	290	25	3	0	13	9	4	20	190	370	—	—	—
Lightly Salted Oil Roasted	1 pkg (1.8 oz)	300	27	4	0	13	8	4	20	95	340	—	—	—
Munch'N Go Singles Heat Hot Spicy Oil Roasted	1 pkg (2.5 oz)	410	36	5	0	18	13	6	60	480	500	1	—	—
Reduced Fat Honey Roasted	⅓ cup (1 oz)	130	7	1	0	6	12	2	20	150	160	0	60	0
Salted Oil Roasted	1 pkg (1 oz)	170	15	2	0	7	5	2	20	110	190	—	—	—
Spanish Oil Roasted	1 oz	170	14	3	0	7	5	2	20	105	180	—	—	—
Spanish Raw	1 oz	150	13	3	0	7	6	3	20	5	180	—	—	—
Sweet N Crunchy	1 oz	140	7	1	0	4	16	2	—	20	115	—	—	—
Unsalted Dry Roasted	1 oz	160	14	2	0	8	6	3	—	0	200	—	—	—
WEIGHT WATCHERS														
Honey Roasted	1 pkg (0.7 oz)	100	5	1	0	7	7	2	0	100	—	0	—	0
PEAR														
CANNED														
halves in heavy syrup	1 cup	188	tr	tr	0	1	49	—	12	13	165	3	3	0
halves in heavy syrup	1 half	68	tr	tr	0	tr	15	—	4	4	51	1	1	0
halves in light syrup	1 half	45	tr	tr	0	tr	12	—	4	4	52	1	1	0
halves juice pack	1 cup	123	tr	tr	0	1	32	—	21	10	238	4	—	14
halves water pack	1 half	22	tr	tr	0	tr	6	—	—	41	5	1	1	0
DEL MONTE														
Halves Fruit Naturals	½ cup (4.4 oz)	60	0	0	0	0	15	1	0	10	—	2	—	0
Halves In Heavy Syrup	½ cup (4.5 oz)	100	0	0	0	0	24	1	0	10	—	2	—	0
Halves Lite	½ cup (4.4 oz)	60	0	0	0	0	15	1	0	10	—	2	—	0

FOOD	PORTION	CALORIES	FAT	SAT FAT	CHOL	PROTEIN	CARBO	FIBER	CALCIUM	SOD	POTAS	VIT C	FOLIC	VIT A
DEL MONTE (CONT.)														
Sliced In Heavy Syrup	½ cup (4.5 oz)	100	0	0	0	0	24	1	0	10	—	2	—	0
Sliced Lite	½ cup (4.4 oz)	60	0	0	0	0	15	1	0	10	—	2	—	0
Snack Cups Diced In Heavy Syrup	1 serv (4.5 oz)	100	0	0	0	0	24	1	0	10	—	2	—	0
Snack Cups Diced In Heavy Syrup EZ-Open Lid	1 serv (4.2 oz)	90	0	0	0	0	23	1	0	10	—	2	—	0
Snack Cups Diced Lite	1 serv (4.5 oz)	60	0	0	0	0	15	1	0	10	—	2	—	0
Snack Cups Diced Lite EZ-Open Lid	1 serv (4.2 oz)	60	0	0	0	0	15	1	0	10	—	2	—	0
LIBBY														
Halves Lite	½ cup (4.3 oz)	60	0	0	0	0	13	1	0	10	80	0	—	0
Sliced Lite	½ cup (4.3 oz)	60	0	0	0	0	13	1	0	10	80	0	—	0
DRIED														
halves	10	459	1	tr	0	3	122	—	59	10	932	12	—	6
halves	1 cup	472	1	tr	0	3	125	—	60	10	959	13	—	6
halves cooked w/ sugar	½ cup	196	tr	tr	0	1	52	—	22	4	344	5	0	56
halves cooked w/o sugar	½ cup	163	tr	tr	0	tr	43	—	21	4	331	5	0	54
MARIANI														
Pears	¼ cup	150	0	—	0	—	—	—	20	—	—	—	—	—
SONOMA														
Pieces	3-4 pieces (1.4 oz)	120	0	0	0	1	33	3	0	0	—	4	—	0
FRESH														
DOLE														
Pear	1	100	1	—	0	1	25	4	—	1	—	—	—	—
PEAR JUICE														
nectar	1 cup	149	tr	tr	0	tr	39	—	11	9	33	3	—	1
GOYA														
Nectar	6 oz	120	0	—	0	0	29	—	21	15	30	19	—	<100
KERN'S														
Nectar	6 fl oz	120	0	0	0	0	28	—	—	0	90	27	—	—
LIBBY														
Nectar	1 can (11.5 fl oz)	220	0	0	0	0	54	3	20	5	130	60	—	—
PEAS														
CANNED														
green	½ cup	59	tr	tr	0	4	11	—	17	186	147	8	38	653
ALLEN														
Crowder	½ cup (4.5 oz)	110	1	1	0	6	19	8	40	460	—	0	—	0
Purple Hull	½ cup (4.4 oz)	120	1	1	0	7	21	6	40	350	—	0	—	0

FOOD	PORTION	CALORIES	FAT	SAT FAT	CHOL	PROTEIN	CARBO	FIBER	CALCIUM	SOD	POTAS	VIT C	FOLIC	VIT A
CREST TOP														
Early June	½ cup (4.5 oz)	100	1	0	0	5	20	6	20	300	—	0	—	100
DEL MONTE														
Sweet	½ cup (4.4 oz)	60	0	0	0	3	11	4	20	360	—	18	—	200
Sweet 50% Less Salt	½ cup (4.4 oz)	60	0	0	0	3	11	4	20	180	—	18	—	200
Sweet No Salt Added	½ cup (4.4 oz)	60	0	0	0	3	11	4	20	10	—	18	—	200
Sweet Very Young	½ cup (4.4 oz)	60	0	0	0	3	10	4	0	360	—	24	—	300
EAST TEXAS FAIR														
Cream Peas	½ cup (4.4 oz)	120	1	1	0	8	20	5	40	420	—	0	—	0
Crowder	½ cup (4.5 oz)	110	1	1	0	6	19	8	40	460	—	0	—	0
Lady Peas With Snaps	½ cup (4.3 oz)	100	1	1	0	7	17	4	20	420	—	0	—	0
Peas 'n Pork	½ cup (4.5 oz)	110	2	1	0	6	19	5	40	540	—	0	—	0
Pepper Peas	½ cup (4.5 oz)	120	1	1	0	6	22	6	40	580	—	1	—	0
Purple Hull	½ cup (4.4 oz)	120	1	1	0	7	21	6	40	350	—	0	—	0
White Acre	½ cup (4.3 oz)	100	1	1	0	6	17	5	40	460	—	0	—	0
GREEN GIANT														
Sweet	½ cup (4.3 oz)	60	0	0	0	4	11	4	20	390	—	6	—	300
Sweet 50% Less Sodium	½ cup (4.3 oz)	60	0	0	0	4	11	3	20	195	—	6	—	300
HOMEFOLKS														
Crowder	½ cup (4.5 oz)	110	1	1	0	6	19	8	40	460	—	0	—	0
Purple Hull	½ cup (4.4 oz)	120	1	1	0	7	21	6	40	350	—	0	—	0
LESUEUR														
Early Peas	½ cup (4.2 oz)	60	0	0	0	4	12	3	20	380	—	6	—	300
Early Peas 50% Less Sodium	½ cup (4.2 oz)	60	0	0	0	4	11	4	20	190	—	6	—	400
Sweet	½ cup (4.2 oz)	60	0	0	0	4	12	3	20	380	—	6	—	300
Sweet 50% Less Sodium	½ cup (4.2 oz)	60	0	0	0	4	11	4	20	190	—	6	—	400
SENECA														
Natural Pack	½ cup	60	0	0	0	4	9	4	20	0	140	15	—	300
Peas	½ cup	50	0	0	0	4	9	5	20	360	140	15	—	300
SUNSHINE														
Field Peas	½ cup (4.4 oz)	120	1	1	0	7	21	6	40	350	—	0	—	0
Lady Peas	½ cup (4.3 oz)	100	1	1	0	6	17	5	40	460	—	0	—	0
TRAPPEY														
Field Peas With Bacon	½ cup (4.5 oz)	90	1	1	0	6	15	5	0	380	—	0	—	0
Field Peas With Snaps And Bacon	½ cup (4.5 oz)	110	1	1	0	6	19	4	40	380	—	0	—	0
DRIED														
split cooked	1 cup	231	1	tr	0	16	41	—	26	4	710	1	127	14
BASCOM'S														
Yellow Split as prep	½ cup	110	0	0	0	8	20	—	—	0	—	—	—	—

FOOD	PORTION	CALORIES	FAT	SAT FAT	CHOL	PROTEIN	CARBO	FIBER	CALCIUM	SOD	POTAS	VIT C	FOLIC	VIT A
HURST														
HamBeens Green Split Peas w/ Ham	1 serv	120	1	0	0	8	21	4	20	63	—	0	—	0
FRESH														
DOLE														
Sugar Peas	½ cup	30	tr	—	0	2	5	2	—	3	144	43	—	105
FROZEN														
green cooked	½ cup	63	tr	tr	0	4	11	—	19	70	134	8	47	534
snap peas cooked	½ cup	42	tr	tr	0	3	7	—	48	4	173	18	—	133
snap peas cooked	1 pkg (10 oz)	132	1	tr	0	9	23	—	150	12	549	56	—	421
BIRDS EYE														
Baby Pea Blend	¾ cup (2.6 oz)	40	0	0	0	2	7	2	0	40	—	5	—	1500
Baby Sweet	⅔ cup (3.1 oz)	70	1	0	0	5	12	4	0	105	—	9	—	300
Field Peas w/ Snaps	⅔ cup (3.4 oz)	130	1	0	0	9	24	4	40	15	—	2	—	0
Purple Hull Peas	½ cup (2.8 oz)	110	1	0	0	7	21	4	20	10	—	1	—	0
CHUN KING														
Snow Pea Pods	½ pkg (3 oz)	35	2	0	0	2	4	2	20	0	—	15	—	200
FRESH LIKE														
Green	3.5 oz	85	1	—	—	5	14	2	23	79	149	20	—	698
Tiny Green	3.5 oz	63	tr	—	—	4	12	1	26	79	149	21	—	861
GREEN GIANT														
Butter Sauce	¾ cup (4 oz)	100	2	2	<5	4	16	5	0	400	—	5	—	500
Butter Sauce LeSueur Baby Peas	¾ cup (4 oz)	100	2	2	<5	5	16	4	40	370	—	6	—	500
Harvest Fresh LeSueur Baby	⅔ cup (3.2 oz)	70	0	0	0	4	13	4	20	220	—	6	—	400
Harvest Fresh Sugar Snap	⅔ cup (3.2 oz)	50	0	0	0	3	10	3	60	95	—	6	—	0
Harvest Fresh Sweet	⅔ cup (3.3 oz)	60	0	0	0	4	12	4	0	200	—	6	—	300
LaSueur Baby Sweet	⅔ cup (2.8 oz)	60	0	0	0	5	11	5	20	150	—	6	—	400
LaSueur Early June	⅔ cup (2.8 oz)	80	0	0	0	5	11	5	20	150	—	6	—	400
LaSueur Early June w/ Mushrooms	¾ cup (3 oz)	60	0	0	0	4	10	4	0	105	—	5	—	400
Select Sugar Snap	¾ cup (2.8 oz)	35	0	0	0	2	7	3	60	0	—	6	—	300
Sweet	⅔ cup (3.1 oz)	70	0	0	0	4	13	4	20	135	—	12	—	400
TREE OF LIFE														
Peas	⅔ cup (3.1 oz)	70	0	0	0	5	12	4	0	100	—	9	—	300
SPROUTS														
raw	½ cup	77	tr	tr	0	5	17	—	21	12	229	6	87	100
PECANS														
dry roasted	1 oz	187	18	1	0	2	6	—	10	0	105	—	12	—
dry roasted salted	1 oz	187	18	1	0	2	6	—	10	260	105	—	12	—

FOOD	PORTION	CALORIES	FAT	SAT FAT	CHOL	PROTEIN	CARBO	FIBER	CALCIUM	SOD	POTAS	VIT C	FOLIC	VIT A
oil roasted	1 oz	195	20	2	0	2	5	—	10	0	102	—	—	—
oil roasted salted	1 oz	195	20	2	0	2	5	—	10	252	102	—	—	—
PLANTERS														
Chips	1 pkg (2 oz)	390	40	3	0	5	9	7	40	5	230	1	—	200
Gold Measure Halves	1 pkg (2 oz)	390	40	3	0	5	9	3	40	5	230	1	—	200
Halves	1 oz	190	20	2	0	3	4	2	20	0	115	—	—	100
Honey Roasted	1 oz	180	16	2	0	2	9	2	—	75	95	—	—	100
Pieces	1 oz	190	20	2	0	3	4	2	20	0	115	—	—	100
Pieces	1 pkg (2 oz)	390	40	3	0	5	9	3	40	5	230	1	—	200
PECTIN														
powder	1 pkg (1.75 oz)	163	tr	—	0	tr	45	—	4	100	4	—	0	1
powder	¼ pkg (0.4 oz)	39	0	0	0	0	11	—	1	24	1	—	0	0
SURE JELL														
For Lower Sugar Recipes	¼ tsp (0.7 g)	5	0	0	0	0	1	0	0	10	0	0	—	0
Pectin	¼ tsp (0.9 g)	5	0	0	0	0	1	0	0	0	0	0	—	0
PEPEAO														
pepeao dried	½ cup	36	tr	—	0	1	10	—	14	8	85	tr	—	0
pepeao raw sliced	1 cup	25	tr	—	0	tr	7	—	16	9	42	1	—	0
PEPPER														
black	1 tsp	5	tr	tr	0	tr	1	—	9	1	26	—	—	4
cayenne	1 tsp	6	tr	tr	0	tr	1	—	3	1	36	1	—	749
red	1 tsp	6	tr	tr	0	tr	1	—	3	1	36	1	—	749
white	1 tsp	7	tr	—	0	tr	2	—	6	tr	2	—	—	—
AC'CENT														
Lemon	½ tsp	0	0	0	0	0	0	0	0	0	0	0	—	0
Seasoned	½ tsp	0	0	0	0	0	0	0	0	0	0	0	—	0
LAWRY'S														
Lemon	1 tsp	6	tr	—	0	tr	1	tr	—	340	11	—	—	—
WATKINS														
Black	¼ tbsp (0.5 g)	0	0	0	0	0	0	0	0	0	—	0	—	0
Cajun	¼ tbsp (0.5 g)	0	0	0	0	0	0	0	0	25	—	0	—	0
Cracked Black	¼ tbsp (0.5 g)	0	0	0	0	0	0	0	0	0	—	0	—	0
Dijon	¼ tbsp (0.5 g)	0	0	0	0	0	0	0	0	15	—	0	—	0
Garlic Peppercorn Blend	¼ tbsp (1 g)	0	0	0	0	0	0	0	0	0	—	0	—	0
Herb	¼ tbsp (0.5 g)	0	0	0	0	0	0	0	0	0	—	0	—	0
Italian	¼ tbsp (0.5 g)	0	0	0	0	0	0	0	0	0	—	0	—	0
Lemon	¼ tbsp (1 g)	0	0	0	0	0	0	0	0	55	—	0	—	0
Mexican	¼ tbsp (0.5 g)	0	0	0	0	0	0	0	0	0	—	0	—	0
Red Pepper Flakes	¼ tsp (0.5 oz)	0	0	0	0	0	0	0	0	0	—	0	—	200

FOOD	PORTION	CALORIES	FAT	SAT FAT	CHOL	PROTEIN	CARBO	FIBER	CALCIUM	SOD	POTAS	VIT C	FOLIC	VIT A
WATKINS (CONT.)														
Royal Pepper Blend	¼ tbsp (0.5 g)	0	0	0	0	0	0	0	0	0	—	0	—	0
PEPPERS														
CANNED														
chili green	1 cup (5.5 oz)	29	tr	tr	0	1	6	2	50	552	157	0	75	175
chili green hot chopped	½ cup	17	tr	tr	0	1	4	—	5	—	—	46	—	415
chili red hot	1 (2.6 oz)	18	tr	tr	0	1	4	—	5	—	—	50	—	8681
chili red hot chopped	½ cup	17	tr	tr	0	1	4	—	5	—	—	46	—	8087
green halves	½ cup	13	tr	tr	0	1	3	—	28	958	102	33	—	109
jalapeno chopped	½ cup	17	tr	tr	0	1	3	—	18	995	92	9	—	1156
red halves	½ cup	13	tr	tr	0	1	3	—	28	958	102	33	—	364
CHI-CHI'S														
Chilies Diced Green	2 tbsp (1.2 oz)	10	0	0	0	0	1	0	0	20	—	6	—	0
Chilies Green Whole	¾ pepper (1 oz)	10	0	0	0	0	1	0	0	15	—	6	—	0
DEL MONTE														
Chilpotle In Spice Sauce	2 tbsp (1.1 oz)	20	1	0	0	tr	4	1	0	430	—	4	—	1000
Hot Chili	4 (1 oz)	10	0	0	0	0	3	tr	0	610	—	27	—	0
Jalapeno Nacho Pickled Sliced	2 tbsp (1 oz)	5	0	0	0	0	1	tr	0	340	—	6	—	100
Jalapeno Pickled Sliced	2 tbsp (1.1 oz)	5	0	0	0	0	1	tr	0	530	—	6	—	100
Jalapeno Pickled Whole	2 tbsp (1.1 oz)	5	0	0	0	0	1	tr	0	560	—	6	—	100
Jalapeno Whole	1 (0.7 oz)	3	0	0	0	0	tr	tr	0	230	—	4	—	0
HEBREW NATIONAL														
Filet	¼ pepper (1 oz)	9	0	0	0	0	2	—	—	310	—	—	—	—
Hot Cherry	⅓ pepper (1 oz)	11	0	0	0	0	2	—	—	270	—	—	—	—
Red Filet	¼ pepper (1 oz)	9	0	0	0	0	2	—	—	310	—	—	—	—
MCILHENNY														
Jalapeno Nacho Slices	12 slices (1.1 oz)	7	tr	tr	0	tr	1	1	5	70	—	tr	—	155
OLD EL PASO														
Green Chilies Chopped	2 tbsp (1 oz)	5	0	0	0	0	1	1	40	110	—	6	—	0
Green Chilies Whole	1 (1.2 oz)	10	0	0	0	0	2	1	0	230	—	9	—	200
Jalapenos Peeled	3 (1 oz)	10	0	0	0	0	1	1	40	200	—	4	—	0
Jalapenos Pickled	2 (0.9 oz)	5	0	0	0	0	1	0	0	380	—	0	—	0
Jalapenos Slices	2 tbsp (1.1 oz)	15	0	0	0	0	3	1	60	400	—	2	—	100

FOOD	PORTION	CALORIES	FAT	SAT FAT	CHOL	PROTEIN	CARBO	FIBER	CALCIUM	SOD	POTAS	VIT C	FOLIC	VIT A
PROGRESSO														
Cherry (drained)	2 tbsp (0.9 oz)	30	2	0	0	0	2	1	0	30	—	18	—	500
Fried (drained)	2 tbsp (0.9 oz)	60	5	1	0	0	3	1	0	60	—	15	—	0
Hot Cherry	1 (1 oz)	15	0	0	0	0	0	0	0	250	—	0	—	2500
Pepper Salad (drained)	2 tbsp (0.9 oz)	25	2	0	0	0	1	1	0	80	—	18	—	300
Roasted	½ piece (1 oz)	10	0	0	0	0	1	0	0	60	—	21	—	1000
Tuscan (drained)	3 (1 oz)	10	0	0	0	0	1	1	0	330	—	0	—	0
ROSOFF'S														
Sweet	¼ pepper (1 oz)	9	0	0	0	0	2	—	—	310	—	—	—	—
SCHORR'S														
Filet Peppers	1 oz	9	0	0	0	0	2	—	—	310	—	—	—	—
TRAPPEY														
Banana Mild	3 peppers (1 oz)	6	tr	tr	0	tr	1	1	3	100	—	tr	—	15
Banana Sliced Rings	21 slices (1 oz)	6	tr	tr	0	tr	1	1	10	529	—	2	—	35
Cherry Hot	2 peppers (1 oz)	7	tr	tr	0	tr	1	1	7	373	—	tr	—	691
Cherry Mild	2 peppers (1 oz)	10	tr	tr	0	tr	2	1	7	225	—	6	—	252
Dulcito Italian Pepperoncini	4 peppers (1 oz)	8	tr	tr	0	tr	2	1	6	178	—	1	—	195
In Vinegar Hot	15 peppers (1 oz)	9	tr	tr	0	tr	2	tr	8	573	—	2	—	47
Jalapeno Hot Sliced	21 slices (1 oz)	4	tr	tr	tr	tr	1	1	7	296	—	tr	—	132
Jalapeno Whole	2 peppers (1 oz)	11	0	tr	tr	tr	2	1	13	658	—	tr	—	124
Serano	7 peppers (1 oz)	7	tr	tr	0	tr	1	tr	72	37	—	tr	—	125
Tempero Golden Greek Pepperoncini	4 peppers (1 oz)	7	tr	tr	0	tr	1	1	9	470	—	tr	—	86
Torrido Santa Fe Grande	3 peppers (1 oz)	10	tr	tr	0	tr	2	tr	8	492	—	1	—	39
VLASIC														
Hot Banana Pepper Rings	1 oz	4	0	0	0	0	1	—	—	465	—	9	—	—
Hot Cherry	1 oz	10	0	0	0	0	2	—	—	425	—	15	—	100
Jalapeno Mexican Hot	1 oz	8	0	0	0	0	2	—	—	380	—	—	—	100
Mexican Tiny Hot	1 oz	6	0	0	0	0	2	—	—	430	—	1	—	—
Mild Cherry	1 oz	8	0	0	0	0	2	—	—	410	—	6	—	100
Mild Greek Pepperoncini Salad Peppers	1 oz	4	0	0	0	0	1	—	—	450	—	—	—	—

FOOD	PORTION	CALORIES	FAT	SAT FAT	CHOL	PROTEIN	CARBO	FIBER	CALCIUM	SOD	POTAS	VIT C	FOLIC	VIT A
DRIED														
ancho	1 (0.6 oz)	48	1	tr	0	2	9	4	10	7	410	0	12	3474
green	1 tbsp	1	tr	tr	0	tr	tr	—	1	1	13	8	1	25
pasilla	1 (7 g)	24	1	—	0	1	4	2	7	6	156	0	12	2503
red	1 tbsp	1	tr	tr	0	tr	tr	—	1	1	13	8	1	309
FRESH														
banana raw	1 (4 in) (1.2 oz)	9	tr	tr	0	1	2	1	5	4	84	27	10	112
banana raw	1 cup (4.4 oz)	33	1	tr	0	2	7	4	17	16	317	27	36	422
chili green hot raw	1	18	tr	tr	0	1	4	—	8	3	153	109	11	346
chili green hot raw chopped	½ cup	30	tr	tr	0	2	7	—	13	5	255	182	18	578
chili red hot raw	1 (1.6 oz)	18	tr	tr	0	1	4	—	8	3	153	109	11	4838
chili red raw chopped	½ cup	30	tr	tr	0	2	7	—	13	5	255	182	18	8063
hungarian raw	1 (0.9 oz)	8	tr	tr	0	tr	2	0	3	tr	55	0	14	38
jalapeno raw	1 (0.5 oz)	4	tr	tr	0	tr	1	tr	1	tr	30	6	7	30
jalapeno raw sliced	1 cup (3.2 oz)	27	1	tr	0	1	5	3	9	1	197	6	42	194
serrano raw	1 (6 g)	2	tr	0	0	tr	tr	tr	1	1	19	3	1	57
serrano raw chopped	1 cup (3.7 oz)	34	tr	tr	0	2	7	4	12	11	320	3	24	984
DOLE														
Medium	1	25	1	—	0	1	5	2	—	0	281	117	—	415
FROZEN														
green chopped not prep	1 oz	6	tr	tr	0	tr	1	—	3	1	26	16	4	103
red chopped	1 oz	6	tr	tr	0	tr	1	—	3	1	26	16	4	1333
BIRDS EYE														
Diced Green	¾ cup (2.9 oz)	20	0	0	0	1	4	2	0	10	—	18	—	100
PERCH														
FRESH														
cooked	3 oz	99	1	tr	98	21	0	—	87	67	293	—	—	—
cooked	1 fillet (1.6 oz)	54	1	tr	53	11	0	—	47	36	158	—	—	—
ocean perch atlantic cooked	3 oz	103	2	tr	46	20	0	—	117	82	298	—	—	39
ocean perch atlantic cooked	1 fillet (1.8 oz)	60	1	tr	27	12	0	—	69	48	175	—	—	23
ocean perch atlantic raw	3 oz	80	1	tr	36	16	0	—	91	64	232	—	—	34
raw	3 oz	77	1	tr	76	16	0	—	68	52	228	—	—	—
FROZEN														
GORTON'S														
Fishmarket Fresh Ocean Perch	5 oz	140	3	—	—	25	2	—	20	100	—	—	—	—
VAN DE KAMP'S														
Battered Fillets	2 (4 oz)	300	20	3	25	12	19	0	20	480	—	0	—	0

FOOD	PORTION	CALORIES	FAT	SAT FAT	CHOL	PROTEIN	CARBO	FIBER	CALCIUM	SOD	POTAS	VIT C	FOLIC	VIT A
PERSIMMONS														
dried japanese	1	93	tr	—	0	tr	25	—	8	1	273	0	—	190
fresh	1	32	tr	—	0	tr	8	—	7	0	78	17	—	—
fresh japanese	1	118	tr	—	0	1	31	—	13	3	270	13	13	3640
SONOMA														
Dried	6-8 pieces (1.4 oz)	140	0	0	0	1	35	3	20	10	—	72	—	500
PHEASANT														
breast w/o skin raw	½ breast (6.4 oz)	243	6	2	—	44	0	—	6	60	440	11	—	268
leg w/o skin raw	1 (3.6 oz)	143	5	2	—	24	0	—	31	48	316	—	—	209
w/ skin raw	½ pheasant (14 oz)	723	37	11	—	91	0	—	50	161	971	21	—	706
w/o skin raw	½ pheasant (12.4 oz)	470	13	4	—	83	0	—	45	131	921	21	—	181
PHYLLO DOUGH														
phyllo dough	1 oz	85	2	tr	0	2	15	—	3	137	21	0	5	0
sheet	1	57	1	tr	0	1	10	—	2	92	14	0	3	0
EKIZIAN														
Sheets	½ lb	865	17	7	123	23	151	—	47	573	233	0	61	520
PICANTE														
(*see* SALSA)														
PICKLES														
sweet gherkin	1 sm (½ oz)	20	tr	tr	0	tr	5	—	2	107	30	1	—	10
DEL MONTE														
Dill Halves	¼ pickle (1 oz)	5	0	0	0	0	tr	tr	40	370	—	0	—	0
Dill Hamburger Chips	5 pieces (1 oz)	5	0	0	0	0	1	0	60	310	—	0	—	0
Dill Sweet Chips	5 pieces (1 oz)	40	0	0	0	0	10	tr	0	210	—	0	—	0
Dill Sweet Gherkin	2 pickles (1 oz)	40	0	0	0	0	10	tr	0	210	—	0	—	0
Dill Sweet Midgets	3 pickles (1 oz)	40	0	0	0	0	10	tr	0	210	—	0	—	0
Dill Sweet Whole	2 pickles (1 oz)	40	0	0	0	0	10	tr	0	210	—	0	—	0
Dill Tiny Kosher	1½ pickle (1 oz)	5	0	0	0	0	1	tr	20	240	—	0	—	0
Dill Whole Pickles	1½ pickle (1 oz)	5	0	0	0	0	tr	tr	40	370	—	0	—	0
HEBREW NATIONAL														
Half Sour	½ pickle (1 oz)	4	0	0	0	0	1	—	—	210	—	—	—	—
Kosher	⅓ pickle (1 oz)	4	0	0	0	0	1	—	—	260	—	—	—	—
Kosher Barrel Cured Dill	1 pkg	23	0	0	0	1	4	—	—	1570	—	—	—	—

FOOD	PORTION	CALORIES	FAT	SAT FAT	CHOL	PROTEIN	CARBO	FIBER	CALCIUM	SOD	POTAS	VIT C	FOLIC	VIT A
HEBREW NATIONAL (CONT.)														
Kosher Barrel Cured Hot Dill	1 pkg	23	0	0	0	1	4	—	—	1570	—	—	—	—
Kosher Chips	3 slices (1 oz)	4	0	0	0	0	1	—	—	300	—	—	—	—
Kosher Halves	⅓ pickle (1 oz)	4	0	0	0	0	1	—	—	290	—	—	—	—
Kosher Large	⅕ pickle (1 oz)	4	0	0	0	0	1	—	—	300	—	—	—	—
Kosher Spears	½ spear (1 oz)	4	0	0	0	0	1	—	—	260	—	—	—	—
Sour Garlic	⅓ pickle (1 oz)	3	0	0	0	0	1	—	—	250	—	—	—	—
MCILHENNY														
Hot N' Sweet	4 (1 oz)	42	tr	tr	0	tr	10	tr	8	28	—	tr	—	2
ROSOFF'S														
Half Sour	⅓ pickle (1 oz)	4	0	0	0	0	1	—	—	210	—	—	—	—
Half Sour Spears	½ spear (1 oz)	4	0	0	0	0	1	—	—	200	—	—	—	—
Kosher	⅓ pickle (1 oz)	4	0	0	0	0	1	—	—	260	—	—	—	—
Kosher Halves	⅓ pickle (1 oz)	4	0	0	0	0	1	—	—	290	—	—	—	—
SCHORR'S														
Garlic	⅓ pickle (1 oz)	3	0	0	0	0	1	—	—	250	—	—	—	—
Half Sour	½ spear (1 oz)	4	0	0	0	0	1	—	—	200	—	—	—	—
Half Sour	⅓ pickle (1 oz)	4	0	0	0	0	1	—	—	210	—	—	—	—
Kosher Deli	½ pickle (1 oz)	4	0	0	0	0	1	—	—	160	—	—	—	—
Kosher Halves	⅓ pickle (1 oz)	4	0	0	0	0	1	—	—	290	—	—	—	—
Kosher Spears	½ spear (1 oz)	4	0	0	0	0	1	—	—	260	—	—	—	—
Kosher Whole	⅓ pickle (1 oz)	4	0	0	0	0	1	—	—	260	—	—	—	—
VLASIC														
Bread & Butter Chips	1 oz	30	0	0	0	0	7	—	—	160	—	—	—	—
Bread & Butter Chunks	1 oz	25	0	0	0	0	6	—	—	120	—	—	—	—
Bread & Butter Stixs	1 oz	18	0	0	0	0	5	—	—	110	—	—	—	—
Deli Bread & Butter	1 oz	25	0	0	0	0	6	—	—	120	—	—	—	—
Deli Dill Halves	1 oz	4	0	0	0	0	1	—	—	290	—	—	—	—
Half-The-Salt Hamburger Dill Chips	1 oz	2	0	0	0	0	1	—	—	175	—	—	—	—

FOOD	PORTION	CALORIES	FAT	SAT FAT	CHOL	PROTEIN	CARBO	FIBER	CALCIUM	SOD	POTAS	VIT C	FOLIC	VIT A
VLASIC (CONT.)														
Half-The-Salt Kosher Crunchy Dills	1 oz	4	0	0	0	0	1	—	—	125	—	—	—	—
Half-The-Salt Kosher Dill Spears	1 oz	4	0	0	0	0	1	—	—	120	—	—	—	—
Half-The-Salt Sweet Butter Chips	1 oz	30	0	0	0	0	7	—	—	80	—	—	—	—
Hot & Spicy Garden Mix	1 oz	4	0	0	0	0	1	—	—	380	—	4	—	100
Kosher Baby Dills	1 oz	4	0	0	0	0	1	—	—	210	—	—	—	—
Kosher Crunchy Dills	1 oz	4	0	0	0	0	1	—	—	210	—	—	—	—
Kosher Dill Gherkins	1 oz	4	0	0	0	0	1	—	—	210	—	—	—	—
Kosher Dill Spears	1 oz	4	0	0	0	0	1	—	—	175	—	—	—	—
Kosher Snack Chunks	1 oz	4	0	0	0	0	1	—	—	220	—	—	—	—
No Garlic Dill Spears	1 oz	4	0	0	0	0	1	—	—	210	—	—	—	—
Original Dills	1 oz	2	0	0	0	0	1	—	—	375	—	—	—	—
Polish Snack Chunk Dills	1 oz	4	0	0	0	0	1	—	—	300	—	1	—	—
Zesty Crunchy Dills	1 oz	4	0	0	0	0	1	—	—	250	—	—	—	—
Zesty Dill Snack Chunks	1 oz	4	0	0	0	0	1	—	—	290	—	—	—	—
Zesty Dill Spears	1 oz	4	0	0	0	0	1	—	—	230	—	—	—	—
PIE														
(*see also* PIE CRUST)														
CANNED FILLING														
apple	⅛ can (2.6 oz)	74	tr	tr	0	tr	19	1	3	32	33	—	0	—
apple	1 can (21 oz)	599	1	tr	0	1	156	6	27	259	268	—	0	—
cherry	⅛ can (2.6 oz)	85	tr	tr	0	tr	22	—	8	7	78	—	3	152
cherry	1 can (21 oz)	683	1	tr	0	3	175	—	65	54	625	—	24	1220
pumpkin pie mix	1 cup	282	tr	tr	0	3	71	—	99	561	372	10	—	22405
LIBBY														
Pumpkin Pie Mix	½ cup	100	0	—	0	<1	25	2	20	150	—	1	—	8000
NONE SUCH														
Mincemeat Condensed	¼ pkg	220	2	—	—	1	50	—	40	310	240	—	—	—
Mincemeat Ready-to-Use	⅓ cup	200	1	—	—	1	48	—	40	360	210	—	—	—
Mincemeat Ready-to-Use With Brandy & Rum	⅓ cup	220	2	—	—	1	48	—	40	260	210	—	—	—

FOOD	PORTION	CALORIES	FAT	SAT FAT	CHOL	PROTEIN	CARBO	FIBER	CALCIUM	SOD	POTAS	VIT C	FOLIC	VIT A
FROZEN														
apple	⅛ of 9 in pie (4.4 oz)	297	14	3	0	2	43	2	13	333	826	4	5	154
blueberry	⅛ of 9 in pie (4.4 oz)	289	13	2	0	2	44	—	10	406	63	—	—	175
cherry	⅛ of 9 in pie (4.4 oz)	325	14	3	0	3	50	1	15	308	102	—	10	—
chocolate creme	⅙ of 8 in pie (4 oz)	344	22	6	6	3	38	—	41	153	144	—	8	—
coconut creme	⅙ of 7 in pie (2.2 oz)	191	11	5	0	1	24	1	19	163	42	0	—	58
lemon meringue	⅙ of 8 in pie (4.5 oz)	303	10	2	51	2	53	1	63	165	100	4	10	198
peach	⅙ of 8 in pie (4.1 oz)	261	12	2	0	2	39	—	9	316	146	—	—	123
AMY'S ORGANIC														
Apple	1 serv (8 oz)	280	12	—	—	4	42	—	—	180	—	—	—	—
BANQUET														
Apple	⅕ pie (4 oz)	300	13	6	5	3	41	2	0	370	—	0	—	0
Banana Cream	⅓ pie (4.7 oz)	350	21	5	<5	3	39	1	20	290	—	0	—	0
Cherry	⅕ pie (4 oz)	290	14	6	5	3	39	2	0	310	—	0	—	0
Chocolate Cream	⅓ pie (4.7 oz)	360	20	5	<5	3	43	3	40	240	—	0	—	0
Coconut Cream	⅓ pie (4.7 oz)	350	20	6	<5	3	39	2	40	250	—	0	—	0
Lemon Cream	⅓ pie (4.7 oz)	360	20	5	<5	3	43	2	40	240	—	0	—	0
Mincemeat	⅕ pie (4 oz)	310	13	6	10	3	46	2	20	430	—	0	—	0
Peach	⅕ pie (4 oz)	260	12	5	5	3	36	2	0	340	—	6	—	0
Pumpkin	⅙ pie (4 oz)	250	8	3	20	4	40	3	60	340	—	0	—	3500
KINERET														
Apple Homestyle	⅙ pie (4 oz)	313	16	4	0	2	41	1	<10	175	—	2	—	<50
MCMILLIN'S														
Apple	4 oz	430	23	—	—	4	51	—	100	340	65	—	—	—
Berry	4 oz	430	23	—	—	3	52	—	100	410	55	—	—	—
Cherry	4 oz	430	24	—	—	3	51	—	100	350	70	—	—	100
Chocolate Pudding	4 oz	420	21	—	—	3	54	—	80	350	95	—	—	—
Coconut Pudding	4 oz	450	26	—	—	4	50	—	100	420	60	—	—	—
Lemon	4 oz	450	25	—	—	4	52	—	80	330	50	—	—	—
Peach	4 oz	430	24	—	—	4	52	—	80	370	70	—	—	—
Strawberry	4 oz	400	20	—	—	3	50	—	80	370	70	—	—	—
MRS. SMITH'S														
Apple	⅙ of 8 in pie (4.3 oz)	270	11	2	0	2	41	1	—	300	65	—	—	—
Apple	¹⁄₁₀ of 10 in pie (4.6 oz)	280	12	3	0	2	43	1	—	310	70	—	—	—
Apple	⅛ of 9 in pie (4.6 oz)	370	18	4	0	2	50	2	—	430	80	—	—	—
Apple Cranberry	⅙ of 8 in pie (4.3 oz)	280	11	2	0	2	43	1	—	290	60	—	—	—

FOOD	PORTION	CALORIES	FAT	SAT FAT	CHOL	PROTEIN	CARBO	FIBER	CALCIUM	SOD	POTAS	VIT C	FOLIC	VIT A
MRS. SMITH'S (CONT.)														
Apple Lattice Ready To Serve	1/5 of 8 in pie (4.6 oz)	310	13	3	0	2	45	2	—	350	100	—	—	—
Banana Cream	1/4 of 8 in pie (3.4 oz)	250	9	3	0	2	40	1	—	170	100	—	—	—
Berry	1/6 of 8 in pie (4.3 oz)	280	11	2	0	2	44	0	—	340	75	—	—	—
Blackberry	1/6 of 8 in pie (4.3 oz)	280	11	2	0	2	43	1	—	320	65	—	—	—
Blueberry	1/6 of 8 in pie	260	11	2	0	2	39	1	—	320	50	—	—	—
Boston Cream	1/8 of 8 in pie (2.4 oz)	170	5	2	25	2	29	0	—	140	35	—	—	—
Cherry	1/6 of 8 in pie	270	11	2	0	2	41	1	—	320	110	—	—	—
Cherry	1/8 of 9 in pie (4.6 oz)	320	13	3	0	3	48	1	—	350	140	—	—	—
Cherry Lattice Ready To Serve	1/5 of 8 in pie (4.6 oz)	320	13	3	0	3	47	1	—	340	130	—	—	—
Chocolate Cream	1/4 of 8 in pie (3.4 oz)	290	14	4	0	2	37	1	—	180	135	—	—	—
Coconut Cream	1/4 of 8 in pie (3.4 oz)	280	14	4	0	2	36	0	—	160	65	—	—	—
Coconut Custard	1/5 of 8 in pie (5 oz)	280	12	5	75	7	35	0	—	350	230	—	—	—
Dutch Apple	1/6 of 8 in pie	310	13	3	0	3	48	1	—	270	70	—	—	—
Dutch Apple	1/10 of 10 in pie (4.6 oz)	320	12	3	0	3	50	1	—	270	75	—	—	—
Dutch Apple	1/8 of 9 in pie (4.5 oz)	300	12	3	0	2	48	2	—	240	95	—	—	—
French Silk Cream	1/5 of 8 in pie (4.8 oz)	410	21	6	5	3	55	1	—	250	45	—	—	—
Hearty Pumpkin	1/5 of 8 in pie (5.2 oz)	280	10	3	60	5	46	2	—	350	300	—	—	—
Lemon Cream	1/4 of 8 in pie (3.4 oz)	270	13	3	0	2	36	0	—	150	75	—	—	—
Lemon Meringue	1/5 of 8 in pie (4.8 oz)	300	8	2	65	3	54	0	—	220	45	—	—	—
Mince	1/6 of 8 in pie (4.3 oz)	300	11	2	0	2	48	2	—	400	130	—	—	—
Peach	1/6 of 8 in pie	260	11	2	0	2	38	1	—	310	115	—	—	—
Peach	1/8 of 9 in pie (4.6 oz)	310	13	3	0	3	46	1	—	350	150	—	—	—
Pecan	1/8 of 10 in pie (4.5 oz)	500	23	4	60	5	68	1	—	460	90	—	—	—
Pumpkin	1/9 of 10 in pie (5.1 oz)	250	8	2	50	5	42	1	—	330	230	—	—	—
Pumpkin	1/5 of 8 in pie (5.2 oz)	270	8	2	45	5	44	1	—	350	230	—	—	—
Red Raspberry	1/6 of 8 in pie (4.3 oz)	280	11	2	0	2	43	0	—	310	70	—	—	—

FOOD	PORTION	CALORIES	FAT	SAT FAT	CHOL	PROTEIN	CARBO	FIBER	CALCIUM	SOD	POTAS	VIT C	FOLIC	VIT A
MRS. SMITH'S (CONT.)														
Strawberry Rhubarb	⅙ of 8 in pie (4.3 oz)	280	11	2	0	2	44	0	—	380	135	—	—	—
Strawberry Rhubarb	⅕ of 8 in pie (4.8 oz)	520	23	4	70	5	73	1	—	450	90	—	—	—
PEPPERIDGE FARM														
Hyannis Boston Cream Pie	1	230	10	4	70	4	34	2	60	125	—	—	—	200
Mississippi Mud	1	310	23	12	60	3	23	—	40	45	—	—	—	400
PET-RITZ														
Apple	⅙ pie (4.33 oz)	330	12	—	—	2	53	—	20	385	130	4	—	—
Banana Cream	⅙ pie (2.33 oz)	170	9	—	—	2	22	—	20	155	60	—	—	—
Blueberry	⅙ pie (4.33 oz)	370	12	—	—	3	50	—	20	330	105	3	—	—
Cherry	⅙ pie (4.33 oz)	300	12	—	—	3	48	—	20	330	145	2	—	400
Chocolate Cream	⅙ pie (2.33 oz)	190	8	—	—	1	27	—	20	145	80	—	—	—
Coconut Cream	⅙ pie (2.33 oz)	190	8	—	—	2	27	—	20	145	45	—	—	—
Egg Custard	⅙ pie (4.0 oz)	200	8	—	—	5	28	—	80	—	—	—	—	200
Lemon Cream	⅙ pie (2.33 oz)	190	9	—	—	2	26	—	20	150	50	—	—	—
Mince	⅙ pie (4.33 oz)	280	9	—	—	2	48	—	60	—	—	1	—	1400
Neapolitan Cream	⅙ pie (2.33 oz)	180	10	—	—	1	17	—	—	185	58	—	—	—
Peach	⅙ pie (4.33 oz)	320	12	—	—	2	51	—	—	320	150	21	—	350
Pumpkin Custard	⅙ pie (4.33 oz)	250	9	—	—	4	39	—	20	—	—	10	—	—
Strawberry Cream	⅙ pie (2.33 oz)	170	9	—	—	2	20	—	20	145	58	—	—	—
Sweet Potato	⅙ pie (3.33 oz)	150	7	—	—	2	21	—	—	110	60	2	—	1750
SARA LEE														
Chocolate Silk	⅕ pie (4.8 oz)	500	32	16	<5	4	49	2	—	440	—	—	—	—
Coconut Cream	⅕ pie (4.8 oz)	480	31	14	0	4	47	2	—	430	—	—	—	—
Fruit's Of The Forest	⅛ pie (4.6 oz)	340	19	5	0	3	40	3	—	420	—	—	—	—
Homestyle Apple	⅛ pie (4.6 oz)	340	16	4	0	3	46	1	—	310	—	—	—	—
Homestyle Blueberry	⅛ pie (4.6 oz)	360	15	4	0	3	54	2	—	340	—	—	—	—
Homestyle Cherry	⅛ pie (4.6 oz)	330	15	4	0	3	46	2	—	290	—	—	—	—
Homestyle Dutch Apple	⅛ pie (4.6 oz)	350	15	3	0	3	53	2	—	320	—	—	—	—

FOOD	PORTION	CALORIES	FAT	SAT FAT	CHOL	PROTEIN	CARBO	FIBER	CALCIUM	SOD	POTAS	VIT C	FOLIC	VIT A
SARA LEE (CONT.)														
Homestyle Mince	⅛ pie (4.6 oz)	390	17	4	0	3	56	3	—	450	—	—	—	—
Homestyle Peach	⅛ pie (4.6 oz)	330	13	3	0	3	50	2	—	250	—	—	—	—
Homestyle Pecan	⅛ pie (4.2 oz)	520	24	5	45	5	70	3	—	480	—	—	—	—
Homestyle Pumpkin	⅛ pie (4.6 oz)	260	11	3	30	4	37	2	—	460	—	—	—	—
Homestyle Raspberry	⅛ pie (4.6 oz)	380	19	5	5	3	48	2	—	330	—	—	—	—
Lemon Meringue	⅙ pie (5 oz)	350	11	3	0	2	59	5	—	460	—	—	—	—
Slice Lemon Icebox	1 (3.5 oz)	260	9	2	<5	5	41	2	—	180	—	—	—	—
Slice Southern Pecan	1 (4 oz)	470	23	4	25	4	62	2	—	420	—	—	—	—
WEIGHT WATCHERS														
Mississippi Mud	1 piece (2.45 oz)	160	5	0	45	4	24	5	80	120	—	0	—	100
HOME RECIPE														
apple	⅛ of 9 in pie (5.4 oz)	411	19	5	0	4	58	3	11	327	123	3	7	90
banana cream	⅛ of 9 in pie (5.2 oz)	398	20	6	75	7	49	—	110	355	245	2	17	386
blueberry	⅛ of 9 in pie (5.2 oz)	360	18	4	0	4	49	—	10	272	74	1	7	61
butterscotch	⅛ of 9 in pie (4.5 oz)	355	18	5	78	6	42	—	128	335	221	1	14	383
cherry	⅛ of 9 in pie (6.3 oz)	486	22	5	0	5	69	—	18	343	138	2	12	737
coconut creme	⅛ of 9 in pie (4.7 oz)	396	21	8	77	6	46	—	113	356	183	1	14	379
custard	⅛ of 9 in pie (4.5 oz)	262	11	4	87	7	34	2	107	256	159	1	13	281
lemon meringue	⅛ of 9 in pie (4.5 oz)	362	16	4	68	5	50	2	15	307	83	4	11	204
mince	⅛ of 9 in pie (5.8 oz)	477	18	4	0	18	79	—	37	419	335	10	9	36
pecan	⅛ of 9 in pie (4.3 oz)	502	27	5	106	6	64	4	39	320	163	tr	17	410
pumpkin	⅛ of 9 in pie (5.4 oz)	316	14	5	65	7	41	4	145	349	289	3	16	11833
vanilla cream	⅛ of 9 in pie (4.4 oz)	350	18	5	78	6	41	—	113	327	158	1	14	385
MIX														
banana cream no-bake	⅛ of 9 in pie (3.2 oz)	231	12	6	—	3	29	—	67	267	104	1	6	375
chocolate mousse no-bake	⅛ of 9 in pie (3.3 oz)	247	15	8	0	3	28	—	74	437	270	1	3	392
coconut creme no-bake	⅛ of 9 in pie (3.3 oz)	259	17	10	—	3	27	—	67	309	132	1	4	381

FOOD	PORTION	CALORIES	FAT	SAT FAT	CHOL	PROTEIN	CARBO	FIBER	CALCIUM	SOD	POTAS	VIT C	FOLIC	VIT A
BETTY CROCKER														
Boston Cream Classic Dessert	⅛ pie	270	6	—	—	4	50	—	150	390	110	—	—	100
JELL-O														
No Bake Chocolate Silk as prep	⅙ pie (4.4 oz)	320	16	6	5	5	37	tr	150	490	260	0	—	500
ROYAL														
Key Lime Pie Filling	mix for 1 serv	50	0	0	0	0	13	—	—	120	40	—	—	—
Lemon Pie Filling	mix for 1 serv	50	0	0	0	0	13	0	—	120	40	—	—	—
Lemon Meringue No-Bake	⅛ pie	210	5	—	—	3	38	—	—	170	45	—	—	—
READY-TO-EAT														
ENTENMANN'S														
Apple Homestyle	1 serv (2.1 oz)	140	7	—	—	1	21	—	—	150	—	—	—	—
Coconut Custard	1 serv (1.8 oz)	140	8	—	—	3	16	—	—	160	—	—	—	—
SNACK														
apple	1 (3 oz)	266	14	7	13	2	33	—	127	325	51	1	4	148
apple fried	1 (6.4 oz)	404	21	3	—	4	55	3	28	479	83	2	4	35
blueberry fried	1 (6.4 oz)	404	21	3	—	4	55	3	28	479	83	2	4	35
cherry	1 (3 oz)	266	14	7	13	2	33	—	127	325	51	1	4	148
cherry fried	1 (6.4 oz)	404	21	3	—	4	55	3	28	479	83	2	4	220
lemon	1 (3 oz)	266	14	7	13	2	33	—	127	325	51	1	4	148
lemon fried	1 (6.4 oz)	404	21	3	—	4	55	3	28	479	83	0	4	41
peach fried	1 (6.4 oz)	404	21	3	—	4	55	3	28	479	83	2	4	35
strawberry fried	1 (6.4 oz)	404	21	3	—	4	55	3	28	479	83	2	4	35
LANCE														
Pecan	1 (38 g)	350	15	3	40	4	51	—	—	70	50	—	—	200
LITTLE DEBBIE														
Marshmallow Banana	1 pkg (1.4 oz)	160	5	3	0	1	27	0	0	95	—	0	—	0
Marshmallow Banana	1 pkg (2.7 oz)	320	11	7	0	3	54	0	20	190	—	0	—	0
Marshmallow Banana	1 pkg (2 oz)	240	8	5	0	2	40	0	0	140	—	0	—	0
Marshmallow Chocolate	1 pkg (1.4 oz)	160	5	3	0	1	27	1	0	95	—	0	—	0
Marshmallow Chocolate	1 pkg (2 oz)	240	9	5	0	2	40	1	20	135	—	0	—	0
Marshmallow Chocolate	1 pkg (2.7 oz)	320	11	7	0	3	53	1	20	190	—	0	—	0
Oatmeal Creme	1 pkg (1.3 oz)	170	8	2	0	2	25	1	0	200	—	0	—	0
Oatmeal Creme	1 pkg (3 oz)	360	14	3	0	3	58	2	20	400	—	0	—	0
Oatmeal Creme	1 pkg (2.5 oz)	300	11	2	0	3	48	1	20	330	—	0	—	0
Raisin Creme	1 pkg (1.2 oz)	140	5	1	0	0	23	1	0	120	—	0	—	0
Raisin Creme	1 pkg (2.5 oz)	290	12	3	0	2	47	0	0	240	—	0	—	0

FOOD	PORTION	CALORIES	FAT	SAT FAT	CHOL	PROTEIN	CARBO	FIBER	CALCIUM	SOD	POTAS	VIT C	FOLIC	VIT A
TASTYKAKE														
Apple	1 pkg (113 g)	300	12	3	0	3	46	2	60	340	—	—	—	—
Banana Creme	1 pkg (120 g)	380	16	6	25	5	54	2	—	430	—	2	—	—
Blueberry	1 pkg (113 g)	310	9	2	0	3	55	2	—	410	—	6	—	0.2
Cherry	1 pkg (113 g)	300	10	2	0	3	49	2	20	310	—	—	—	—
Coconut Creme	1 pkg (113 g)	380	20	5	65	5	46	2	60	420	—	—	—	—
French Apple	1 pkg (120 g)	350	11	2	0	3	63	2	40	220	—	—	—	—
Lemon	1 pkg (113 g)	320	13	3	40	4	48	2	60	380	—	—	—	—
Lemon Lime	1 pkg (113 g)	320	13	3	45	4	49	1	—	310	—	—	—	—
Peach	1 pkg (113 g)	300	12	3	0	3	47	—	60	360	—	—	—	100
Pineapple Cheese	1 pkg (120 g)	340	13	3	20	5	54	2	—	410	—	—	—	—
Pumpkin	1 pkg (4 oz)	320	14	4	30	5	46	2	20	520	—	—	—	100
Strawberry	1 pkg (113 g)	340	11	3	0	3	57	1	—	300	—	—	—	—
Tasty Klair	1 pkg (113 g)	400	20	4	55	6	51	2	80	320	—	—	—	200
TAKE-OUT														
coconut custard	⅙ of 8 in pie (3.6 oz)	271	14	6	36	6	32	—	84	348	182	—	—	114
custard	⅙ pie 9 in	330	17	6	169	9	36	—	146	436	208	0	—	350
pecan	⅙ of 8 in pie (4 oz)	452	21	4	36	5	65	4	19	480	84	1	7	198
pumpkin	⅙ of 8 in pie (3.8 oz)	229	10	2	22	4	30	3	66	308	168	—	17	—

PIE CRUST

(*see also* PIE)

FOOD	PORTION	CALORIES	FAT	SAT FAT	CHOL	PROTEIN	CARBO	FIBER	CALCIUM	SOD	POTAS	VIT C	FOLIC	VIT A
FROZEN														
baked	⅛ of 9 in pie (0.6 oz)	82	5	2	—	1	8	—	3	104	18	—	—	—
baked	9 in shell (4.4 oz)	647	41	13	—	6	63	—	26	815	138	—	—	—
puff pastry baked	1 shell (1.4 oz)	223	15	2	0	3	18	—	4	101	25	0	4	0
ORONOQUE														
Deep Dish	⅙ pie (1.41 oz)	200	13	—	—	3	16	—	—	200	30	—	—	—
Pie Crust	⅙ pie (1.23 oz)	170	12	—	—	3	14	—	—	170	25	—	—	—
PEPPERIDGE FARM														
Patty Shells	1	210	15	—	—	3	16	—	—	180	—	—	—	—
Puff Pastry Sheets	¼ sheet	260	17	—	—	4	22	—	—	290	—	—	—	—
PET-RITZ														
Deep Dish	⅙ pie (1 oz)	130	8	—	7	1	12	—	—	120	30	—	—	—
Graham Cracker	⅙ pie (0.83 oz)	110	6	—	7	1	8	—	—	80	40	—	—	—
Regular	⅙ pie (0.83 oz)	110	7	—	7	1	11	—	—	110	25	—	—	—
Tart Shells	1	150	10	—	7	3	12	—	—	150	20	—	—	—

FOOD	PORTION	CALORIES	FAT	SAT FAT	CHOL	PROTEIN	CARBO	FIBER	CALCIUM	SOD	POTAS	VIT C	FOLIC	VIT A
HOME RECIPE														
9-inch crust	1	900	60	15	0	11	79	—	25	1100	90	0	—	0
baked	9 in shell (6.3 oz)	949	62	15	0	12	86	—	18	975	120	0	21	0
baked	⅛ of 9 in crust (0.8 oz)	119	8	2	0	1	11	—	2	122	15	0	3	0
MIX														
as prep	9 in crust (5.6 oz)	801	49	12	0	11	81	—	96	1167	99	0	—	0
as prep	⅛ of 9 in pie (0.7 oz)	100	6	2	0	1	10	—	12	146	12	0	—	0
BETTY CROCKER														
Pie Crust	1/16 pkg	120	8	2	0	1	10	—	—	140	15	—	—	—
Sticks	1/16 pkg	120	8	2	0	1	10	—	—	140	15	—	—	—
FLAKO														
Mix	¼ cup (0.9 oz)	130	8	3	5	2	13	1	0	170	20	—	0	—
JIFFY														
As prep	1/7 crust	180	10	4	5	2	19	tr	0	250	—	0	—	0
READY-TO-EAT														
chocolate cookie crumb baked	⅛ of 9 in pie (1 oz)	139	9	2	0	1	15	—	8	185	48	0	1	231
chocolate cookie crumb baked	9 in crust (7.7 oz)	1130	69	15	3	12	122	—	68	1502	375	tr	1	1876
chocolate cookie crumb chilled	9 in crust (7.8 oz)	1127	69	15	3	12	121	—	68	1499	374	tr	1	1872
chocolate cookie crumb chilled	⅛ of 9 in pie (1 oz)	142	9	2	0	1	15	—	9	188	47	0	tr	235
graham cracker baked	9 in crust (8.4 oz)	1181	60	12	0	10	156	—	50	1365	210	tr	17	1876
graham cracker baked	⅛ of 9 in pie (1 oz)	148	8	2	0	1	20	—	6	171	26	0	2	238
graham cracker chilled	⅛ of 9 in pie (1 oz)	150	8	2	0	1	20	—	6	173	27	0	2	239
graham cracker chilled	9 in crust (8.6 oz)	1182	60	12	0	10	155	—	50	1365	211	tr	17	1877
vanilla wafer cracker crumbs baked	9 in crust (6.1 oz)	937	64	13	69	7	89	—	74	909	140	tr	11	1950
vanilla wafer cracker crumbs baked	⅛ of 9 in pie (0.8 oz)	119	8	2	9	1	11	—	9	116	18	0	1	248
vanilla wafer cracker crumbs chilled	9 in crust (6.2 oz)	934	64	13	69	7	88	—	74	906	140	tr	11	1944
vanilla wafer cracker crumbs chilled	⅛ of 9 in pie (0.8 oz)	117	8	2	9	1	11	—	9	113	17	0	1	243

FOOD	PORTION	CALORIES	FAT	SAT FAT	CHOL	PROTEIN	CARBO	FIBER	CALCIUM	SOD	POTAS	VIT C	FOLIC	VIT A
GENERIC LABEL														
Graham	⅛ pie (0.7 oz)	110	5	3	0	1	14	1	20	110	—	0	—	0
HONEY MAID														
Graham	⅙ crust (1 oz)	140	7	2	0	1	18	tr	—	125	20	—	—	—
NABISCO														
Nilla	⅙ crust (1 oz)	140	8	2	<5	1	18	0	—	65	20	—	—	—
OREO														
Crumb Crust	⅙ crust (1 oz)	140	11	2	0	1	18	tr	—	180	55	—	—	500
READY CRUST														
Chocolate	⅛ pie 9 in	100	5	1	0	1	14	—	—	120	60	—	—	—
Chocolate	1 (3 in diam)	110	5	1	0	1	15	—	—	135	60	—	—	—
Graham	1 (3 in diam)	110	5	1	0	1	15	—	—	145	30	—	—	—
Graham	⅛ pie 9 in	100	5	1	0	1	13	—	—	130	30	—	—	—

PIEROGI

FROZEN

FOOD	PORTION	CALORIES	FAT	SAT FAT	CHOL	PROTEIN	CARBO	FIBER	CALCIUM	SOD	POTAS	VIT C	FOLIC	VIT A
EMPIRE														
Potato Cheese	3 (4.6 oz)	260	6	3	5	11	40	5	60	200	—	0	—	0
Potato Onion	3 (4.6 oz)	250	5	1	0	10	43	4	20	210	—	0	—	0
GOLDEN														
Potato Cheese	3 (4 oz)	250	8	2	35	8	38	—	56	260	320	tr	—	300
Potato Onion	3 (4 oz)	210	6	2	—	6	36	—	13	220	260	tr	—	144
MRS. T'S														
Potato And Cheddar Cheese	1 (1.3 oz)	60	tr	—	<2	2	11	—	—	170	—	—	—	—
Potato And Onion	1 (1.3 oz)	50	tr	—	<2	2	10	—	—	140	—	—	—	—

PIG'S EARS AND FEET

FOOD	PORTION	CALORIES	FAT	SAT FAT	CHOL	PROTEIN	CARBO	FIBER	CALCIUM	SOD	POTAS	VIT C	FOLIC	VIT A
ear simmered	1	184	12	4	100	18	tr	0	20	185	—	0	0	0
feet pickled	1 oz	58	5	2	26	4	tr	0	9	262	—	0	1	0
feet pickled	1 lb	921	73	25	417	61	tr	0	145	4187	—	0	18	0
feet simmered	3 oz	165	11	4	85	16	0	0	38	26	—	0	1	0
HORMEL														
Pickled Feet	2 oz	80	6	2	45	7	0	0	20	530	—	0	—	0
Pickled Hocks	2 oz	110	8	3	45	9	0	0	0	530	—	0	—	0

PIGEON

FOOD	PORTION	CALORIES	FAT	SAT FAT	CHOL	PROTEIN	CARBO	FIBER	CALCIUM	SOD	POTAS	VIT C	FOLIC	VIT A
w/ skin & bone	3.5 oz	169	10	—	110	21	0	—	45	90	330	—	—	—

PIGEON PEAS

FOOD	PORTION	CALORIES	FAT	SAT FAT	CHOL	PROTEIN	CARBO	FIBER	CALCIUM	SOD	POTAS	VIT C	FOLIC	VIT A
dried cooked	½ cup	102	tr	tr	0	6	20	—	36	5	322	0	93	2
dried cooked	1 cup	204	1	tr	0	11	39	—	72	9	644	0	186	4

PIGNOLIA

(*see* PINE NUTS)

PIKE

FOOD	PORTION	CALORIES	FAT	SAT FAT	CHOL	PROTEIN	CARBO	FIBER	CALCIUM	SOD	POTAS	VIT C	FOLIC	VIT A
northern cooked	½ fillet (5.4 oz)	176	1	tr	78	38	0	—	113	76	514	6	—	125
northern cooked	3 oz	96	1	tr	43	21	0	—	62	42	282	—	3	69

FOOD	PORTION	CALORIES	FAT	SAT FAT	CHOL	PROTEIN	CARBO	FIBER	CALCIUM	SOD	POTAS	VIT C	FOLIC	VIT A
northern raw	3 oz	75	1	tr	33	16	0	—	48	33	220	3	—	60
roe raw	3½ oz	130	2	—	360	24	2	—	—	—	—	14	—	—

PILLNUTS
canarytree dried	1 oz	204	23	9	0	3	1	—	41	1	144	—	—	12

PIMIENTOS
DROMEDARY
Pimientos	1 oz	10	0	0	0	0	2	—	—	5	45	9	—	500

PINE NUTS
pignolia dried	1 tbsp	51	5	1	0	2	1	—	3	0	60	—	—	—
pignolia dried	1 oz	146	14	2	0	7	4	—	7	1	170	—	—	—
pinyon dried	1 oz	161	17	3	0	3	5	—	2	20	178	1	—	8

PROGRESSO
Pignoli	1 jar (1 oz)	170	13	1	0	10	2	0	0	0	—	0	—	0

PINEAPPLE
CANNED
chunks in heavy syrup	1 cup	199	tr	tr	0	1	52	—	35	3	264	19	12	37
chunks juice pack	1 cup	150	tr	tr	0	1	39	—	34	4	304	24	—	95
crushed in heavy syrup	1 cup	199	tr	tr	0	1	52	—	35	3	264	19	12	37
slices in heavy syrup	1 slice	45	tr	tr	0	tr	12	—	8	1	60	4	3	8
slices in light syrup	1 slice	30	tr	tr	0	tr	8	—	8	1	61	4	3	9
slices juice pack	1 slice	35	tr	tr	0	tr	9	—	8	1	70	6	—	22
slices water pack	1 slice	19	tr	tr	0	tr	5	—	9	1	74	5	3	9
tidbits in heavy syrup	1 cup	199	tr	tr	0	1	52	—	35	3	264	19	12	37
tidbits in juice	1 cup	150	tr	tr	0	1	19	—	34	4	304	24	—	95
tidbits in water	1 cup	79	tr	tr	0	1	20	—	37	3	313	19	12	37

DEL MONTE
Chunks In Heavy Syrup	½ cup (4.3 oz)	90	0	0	0	0	24	1	0	10	—	12	—	0
Chunks In Its Own Juice	½ cup (4.4 oz)	70	0	0	0	0	17	1	0	5	—	12	—	0
Crushed In Heavy Syrup	½ cup (4.4 oz)	90	0	0	0	0	24	1	0	10	—	12	—	0
Crushed In Its Own Juice	½ cup (4.3 oz)	70	0	0	0	0	17	1	0	10	—	12	—	0
Sliced In Heavy Syrup	½ cup (4.1 oz)	90	0	0	0	0	23	1	0	10	—	12	—	0
Sliced In Its Own Juice	½ cup (4 oz)	60	0	0	0	0	16	1	0	10	—	12	—	0
Snack Cups Tidbits In Juice	1 serv (4.5 oz)	70	0	0	0	1	18	1	0	10	—	12	—	0
Snack Cups Tidbits In Juice EZ-Open Lid	1 serv (4.2 oz)	60	0	0	0	0	17	1	0	10	—	12	—	0

FOOD	PORTION	CALORIES	FAT	SAT FAT	CHOL	PROTEIN	CARBO	FIBER	CALCIUM	SOD	POTAS	VIT C	FOLIC	VIT A
DEL MONTE (CONT.)														
Spears In Its Own Juice	½ cup (4.3 oz)	70	0	0	0	0	17	1	0	5	—	12	—	0
Tidbits In Its Own Juice	½ cup (4.3 oz)	70	0	0	0	0	17	1	0	5	—	12	—	0
Wedges In Its Own Juice	½ cup (4.3 oz)	70	0	0	0	0	17	1	0	5	—	12	—	0
DOLE														
All Cuts Juice Pack	½ cup	70	tr	—	0	0	18	—	10	—	—	—	—	—
All Cuts Syrup Pack	½ cup	90	0	0	0	0	23	—	10	—	—	—	—	—
LIBBY														
Crushed	1 cup with juice	140	0	0	0	1	35	—	20	10	—	6	—	—
Sliced In Unsweetened Juice	1 cup with juice	140	0	0	0	1	35	—	20	<10	—	6	—	—
DRIED														
SONOMA														
Pieces	2 pieces (1.4 oz)	140	2	0	0	0	30	2	40	30	—	0	—	500
FRESH														
DOLE														
Pineapple	2 slices	90	1	—	0	1	21	2	—	10	165	16	—	46
FROZEN														
chunks sweetened	½ cup	104	tr	tr	0	tr	27	—	11	2	122	10	—	37
PINEAPPLE JUICE														
canned	1 cup	139	tr	tr	0	1	34	—	42	2	334	27	58	12
frzn as prep	1 cup	129	tr	tr	0	1	32	—	28	3	340	30	—	25
frzn not prep	6 oz	387	tr	tr	0	3	96	—	84	6	1020	91	—	108
AFTER THE FALL														
Mandarin Pineapple	1 can (12 oz)	150	0	0	0	1	37	0	20	25	35	2	—	0
BRIGHT & EARLY														
Frozen	8 fl oz	120	0	0	0	0	30	—	—	10	—	60	—	—
DEL MONTE														
Juice	1 serv (11.5 oz)	190	0	0	0	1	45	1	40	15	—	60	—	0
Juice	6 fl oz	80	0	0	0	tr	20	0	20	5	—	60	—	0
Juice	8 fl oz	110	0	0	0	tr	26	0	20	10	—	60	—	0
DOLE														
100% frzn as prep	8 fl oz	130	0	0	0	1	30	0	40	20	290	60	—	0
Chilled	6 fl oz	90	0	0	0	0	22	—	—	5	—	—	—	—
MINUTE MAID														
Box	8.45 fl oz	130	0	0	0	0	33	—	—	25	—	—	—	—
Frozen	8 fl oz	110	0	0	0	0	28	—	—	5	—	—	—	—
PINK BEANS														
CANNED														
GOYA														
Spanish Style	7.5 oz	140	tr	—	0	10	32	10	86	800	690	2	—	1140

FOOD	PORTION	CALORIES	FAT	SAT FAT	CHOL	PROTEIN	CARBO	FIBER	CALCIUM	SOD	POTAS	VIT C	FOLIC	VIT A
DRIED														
cooked	1 cup	252	1	tr	0	15	47	—	88	3	858	0	284	0

PINTO BEANS

FOOD	PORTION	CALORIES	FAT	SAT FAT	CHOL	PROTEIN	CARBO	FIBER	CALCIUM	SOD	POTAS	VIT C	FOLIC	VIT A
CANNED														
pinto	1 cup	186	1	tr	0	11	35	—	89	998	723	2	145	3
ALLEN														
Pinto Beans	½ cup (4.5 oz)	110	1	0	0	5	20	7	60	290	—	0	—	0
BROWN BEAUTY														
Pinto Beans	½ cup (4.5 oz)	110	1	0	0	5	20	7	60	290	—	0	—	0
CHI-CHI'S														
Pinto Beans	½ cup (4.3 oz)	100	1	0	0	6	18	3	20	540	—	0	—	0
EAST TEXAS FAIR														
Pinto Beans	½ cup (4.5 oz)	110	1	0	0	5	20	7	60	290	—	0	—	0
EDEN														
Organic	½ cup (4.6 oz)	100	0	0	0	6	18	6	60	15	350	—	—	—
Organic Spicy w/ Jalapeno & Red Peppers	½ cup (4.6 oz)	125	0	0	0	6	24	7	80	195	380	—	—	200
GEBHARDT														
Pinto Beans	4 oz	100	tr	—	0	6	19	5	37	600	400	2	—	—
GOYA														
Spanish Style	7.5 oz	140	1	—	0	11	31	10	91	860	730	2	—	1160
GREEN GIANT														
Pinto Beans	½ cup (4.4 oz)	110	1	0	0	6	20	5	80	280	—	0	—	0
OLD EL PASO														
Pinto Beans	½ cup (4.6 oz)	110	1	0	0	6	19	7	40	420	—	0	—	0
PROGRESSO														
Pinto Beans	½ cup (4.6 oz)	110	1	0	0	7	18	7	40	250	—	0	—	0
TRAPPEY														
Jalapinto With Bacon	½ cup (4.5 oz)	120	1	1	0	6	22	8	60	540	—	0	—	0
With Bacon	½ cup (4.5 oz)	120	1	1	0	6	20	7	40	270	—	0	—	0
DRIED														
cooked	1 cup	235	1	tr	0	14	44	—	82	3	800	4	294	3
ARROWHEAD														
Dried	¼ cup (1.5 oz)	150	1	0	0	10	27	8	60	0	420	0	—	0
BEAN CUISINE														
Dried	½ cup	115	1	—	0	8	—	5	—	5	310	—	62	—
HURST														
HamBeens w/ Ham	3 tbsp (1.2 oz)	120	1	0	0	7	20	6	40	63	—	1	—	0
FROZEN														
cooked	3 oz	152	tr	tr	0	9	29	—	49	—	—	1	—	0
SPROUTS														
cooked	3½ oz	22	tr	—	0	—	4	—	15	—	—	—	—	—
raw	3½ oz	62	1	—	0	—	12	—	43	—	—	—	—	—

FOOD	PORTION	CALORIES	FAT	SAT FAT	CHOL	PROTEIN	CARBO	FIBER	CALCIUM	SOD	POTAS	VIT C	FOLIC	VIT A
PINYON														
(*see* PINE NUTS)														
PISTACHIOS														
dry roasted	1 oz	172	15	2	0	4	8	—	20	2	275	—	—	—
dry roasted salted	1 cup	776	68	9	0	19	35	—	90	1040	1242	—	—	—
dry roasted salted	1 oz	172	15	2	0	4	8	—	20	260	275	—	—	—
DOLE														
Shelled	1 oz	163	14	—	0	6	7	—	—	—	—	—	—	—
Shells On	1 oz	90	7	—	0	3	3	—	—	250	140	—	—	—
FISHER														
Red Tint	1 oz	170	15	3	0	5	6	—	40	220	—	—	—	—
LANCE														
Pistachios	1 pkg (32 g)	100	8	1	0	3	4	—	20	100	160	—	—	—
PLANTERS														
Munch'N Go Singles Shelled Dry Roasted	1 pkg (2 oz)	330	29	4	0	11	14	6	60	450	510	—	—	100
Red Salted Dry Roasted	1 pkg	160	14	2	0	5	7	3	20	250	260	2	—	—
Uncolored Dry Roasted	½ cup	160	14	2	0	5	7	3	20	180	250	2	—	—
SONOMA														
Salted Shelled	¼ cup (1 oz)	190	14	2	0	6	9	3	40	220	—	0	—	0
PITANGA														
fresh	1	2	tr	—	0	tr	1	—	1	0	7	2	—	105
fresh	1 cup	57	1	—	0	1	13	—	16	5	178	46	—	2595
PIZZA														
(*see also individual restaurants in Part Two*)														
DOUGH														
BOBOLI														
Shell + Sauce	⅛ lg shell (2.6 oz)	170	3	1	5	7	28	1	80	460	—	2	—	200
Shell + Sauce	⅙ sm shell (2.6 oz)	170	3	1	5	7	29	1	80	540	—	4	—	200
HOUSE OF PASTA														
Frozen	⅛ of 14 in pie (1.9 oz)	140	1	0	0	4	27	1	0	140	—	0	—	0
JIFFY														
As prep	¼ crust	180	3	3	0	4	33	2	0	264	—	0	—	0
SASSAFRAS														
Cornmeal Pizza Crust	1 slice (1.4 oz)	140	0	0	0	4	30	1	0	240	—	0	—	0
Italian Pizza Crust Mix	1 slice (1.4 oz)	140	0	0	0	4	30	1	0	135	—	0	—	0
WANDA'S														
Crust Mix Oregano & Basil	⅒ pie (1.4 oz)	149	0	0	0	4	32	1	10	227	—	0	—	0

FOOD	PORTION	CALORIES	FAT	SAT FAT	CHOL	PROTEIN	CARBO	FIBER	CALCIUM	SOD	POTAS	VIT C	FOLIC	VIT A
WANDA'S (CONT.)														
Crust Mix Oregano & Basil Whole Wheat	1/10 pie (1.4 oz)	141	1	0	0	6	30	5	10	227	—	0	—	0
WATKINS														
Crust Mix	1/8 pkg (1.8 oz)	180	1	0	0	6	36	2	0	60	—	0	—	0
FROZEN														
AMY'S ORGANIC														
Cheese	1 (13 oz)	310	11	4	15	13	39	2	—	490	—	—	—	—
Pocket Sandwich Cheese Pizza	1 (4.5 oz)	290	9	4	20	14	38	3	—	390	—	—	—	—
Pocket Sandwich Veggie Pepperoni Pizza	1 (4.5 oz)	220	7	3	15	12	28	3	—	490	—	—	—	—
Roasted Vegetable	1 (12 oz)	270	8	1	0	6	43	3	—	470	—	—	—	—
Spinach	1 (14 oz)	320	11	4	15	13	40	2	—	490	—	—	—	—
CELESTE														
Italian Bread Deluxe	1 (5.1 oz)	290	11	3	15	16	36	3	250	1000	280	4	—	750
Italian Bread Garlic & Herb Zesty Chicken	1 (5 oz)	260	8	2	20	17	34	3	250	960	280	0	—	1000
Italian Bread Pepperoni	1 (5 oz)	320	13	4	20	17	37	3	300	1140	300	0	—	1000
Italian Bread Zesty Four Cheese	1 (4.6 oz)	300	12	6	25	15	32	3	250	820	260	5	—	750
Large Cheese	1/4 pie (4.4 oz)	320	16	8	25	14	32	3	300	590	250	0	—	1250
Large Deluxe	1/4 pie (5.5 oz)	350	18	6	20	14	35	4	200	880	360	4	—	1500
Large Pepperoni	1/4 pie (4.7 oz)	350	20	7	20	13	33	3	200	990	310	0	—	1500
Large Suprema With Meat	1/5 pie (4.6 oz)	290	16	5	15	13	27	3	200	770	280	0	—	1500
Large Zesty Four Cheese	1/4 pie (4.4 oz)	330	16	8	30	14	34	3	300	610	250	0	—	1250
Small Cheese	1 (7.5 oz)	540	25	13	45	23	60	4	500	1090	440	0	—	2250
Small Deluxe	1 (8.2 oz)	540	29	10	25	21	53	6	350	1320	530	0	—	2500
Small Hot & Zesty Four Cheese	1 (7 oz)	530	27	13	50	24	50	4	500	1090	410	0	—	1750
Small Original Four Cheese	1 (7 oz)	540	30	12	50	25	47	4	500	1040	410	0	—	2000
Small Pepperoni	1 (6.7 oz)	520	27	10	25	19	53	4	300	1280	430	0	—	2250
Small Sausage	1 (7.5 oz)	530	27	9	25	23	52	5	400	1400	460	0	—	2250
Small Suprema Vegetable	1 (7.5 oz)	480	23	8	5	20	52	5	450	1270	400	0	—	2500
Small Suprema With Meat	1 (9 oz)	580	31	10	30	25	56	7	450	1480	550	6	—	2500
Small Zesty Four Cheese	1 (7 oz)	530	27	13	50	24	50	4	500	1090	410	0	—	1750

FOOD	PORTION	CALORIES	FAT	SAT FAT	CHOL	PROTEIN	CARBO	FIBER	CALCIUM	SOD	POTAS	VIT C	FOLIC	VIT A
CROISSANT POCKET														
Stuffed Sandwich Pepperoni Pizza	1 piece (4.5 oz)	350	15	5	30	16	39	3	200	870	—	1	—	500
DI GIORNO														
Rising Crust 12 inch Four Cheese	1/6 pie (4.9 oz)	320	11	6	25	16	39	3	300	870	250	0	—	750
Rising Crust 12 inch Italian Sausage	1/6 pie (5.3 oz)	360	14	7	35	18	40	3	250	1000	300	0	—	750
Rising Crust 12 inch Pepperoni	1/6 pie (5.2 oz)	370	16	8	35	18	40	3	250	1080	320	0	—	750
Rising Crust 12 inch Supreme	1/6 pie (5.8 oz)	380	17	8	40	18	40	3	250	1100	340	1	—	750
Rising Crust 12 inch Three Meat	1/6 pie (5.4 oz)	380	16	8	40	19	40	3	250	1100	330	0	—	750
Rising Crust 12 inch Vegetable	1/6 pie (5.6 oz)	310	10	5	20	15	41	3	250	830	290	4	—	750
Rising Crust 8 inch Chicken Supreme	1/3 pie (4.8 oz)	270	9	5	30	16	33	2	200	740	230	1	—	500
Rising Crust 8 inch Four Cheese	1/3 pie (4 oz)	260	9	5	20	14	33	2	250	720	200	0	—	500
Rising Crust 8 inch Italian Sausage	1/3 pie (4.4 oz)	300	12	6	25	15	33	2	200	830	240	0	—	500
Rising Crust 8 inch Pepperoni	1/3 pie (4.2 oz)	300	13	6	30	15	33	2	200	880	253	0	—	500
Rising Crust 8 inch Spinach	1/3 pie (4.3 oz)	250	8	4	15	15	33	3	200	670	240	0	—	750
Rising Crust 8 inch Supreme	1/3 pie (4.7 oz)	310	14	6	30	15	34	2	200	900	270	1	—	500
Rising Crust 8 inch Three Meat	1/3 pie (4.4 oz)	310	13	6	30	15	34	2	200	900	260	0	—	500
Rising Crust 8 inch Vegetable	1/3 pie (4.6 oz)	250	8	4	15	13	33	2	200	680	230	2	—	500
EMPIRE														
3 Pack	1 (3 oz)	210	9	4	20	10	23	7	250	630	—	2	—	400
Bagel	1 (2 oz)	150	5	3	15	7	15	0	100	390	—	1	—	200
English Muffin	1 (2 oz)	130	5	3	15	7	15	1	200	390	—	1	—	200
Pizza	1/2 pie (5 oz)	340	13	7	30	18	38	2	350	970	—	4	—	500
HEALTHY CHOICE														
French Bread Cheese	1 (5.6 oz)	310	4	2	10	20	49	6	300	470	—	0	—	200
French Bread Pepperoni	1 (6 oz)	360	9	4	25	22	48	5	250	580	—	0	—	500
French Bread Sausage	1 (6 oz)	330	4	2	20	20	52	6	200	470	—	0	—	300
French Bread Supreme	1 (6.35 oz)	340	6	2	25	22	49	5	200	510	—	0	—	300

FOOD	PORTION	CALORIES	FAT	SAT FAT	CHOL	PROTEIN	CARBO	FIBER	CALCIUM	SOD	POTAS	VIT C	FOLIC	VIT A
HOT POCKET														
Stuffed Sandwich Pepperoni & Sausage Pizza	1 (4.5 oz)	340	16	6	30	12	38	3	250	630	—	0	—	500
Stuffed Sandwich Pepperoni Pizza	1 (4.5 oz)	350	17	8	30	13	38	2	250	780	—	0	—	500
JACK'S														
Great Combinations 12 inch Bacon Cheeseburger	¼ pie (4.7 oz)	360	18	9	45	20	31	2	250	770	350	0	—	750
Great Combinations 12 inch Double Cheese	¼ pie (4.9 oz)	380	19	11	50	21	32	2	450	670	290	0	—	1000
Great Combinations 12 inch Pepperoni	¼ pie (5.2 oz)	410	19	9	40	19	42	3	300	830	280	0	—	750
Great Combinations 12 inch Pepperoni & Mushrooms	¼ pie (4.8 oz)	340	16	7	35	17	32	2	250	740	280	0	—	750
Great Combinations 12 inch Sausage	¼ pie (5.4 oz)	390	18	8	40	18	40	3	300	700	360	0	—	750
Great Combinations 12 inch Sausage & Mushroom	¼ pie (4.9 oz)	310	15	7	30	16	29	3	250	610	340	0	—	750
Great Combinations 12 inch Sausage & Pepperoni	¼ pie (4.8 oz)	350	19	8	40	17	29	2	250	770	300	0	—	750
Great Combinations 12 inch Supreme	¼ pie (5.2 oz)	350	18	8	40	17	30	5	250	750	320	1	—	750
Great Combinations 9 inch Double Cheese	½ pie (5.5 oz)	430	21	12	55	23	38	3	500	740	300	0	—	1000
Great Combinations 9 inch Pepperoni & Sausage	½ pie (5.1 oz)	380	18	8	40	18	36	3	300	790	300	0	—	750
Naturally Rising 12 inch Bacon Cheeseburger	⅙ pie (5 oz)	350	15	7	40	18	35	2	250	680	310	0	—	500
Naturally Rising 12 inch Canadian Bacon	⅙ pie (4.9 oz)	280	9	5	30	16	34	2	250	590	280	0	—	500

FOOD	PORTION	CALORIES	FAT	SAT FAT	CHOL	PROTEIN	CARBO	FIBER	CALCIUM	SOD	POTAS	VIT C	FOLIC	VIT A
JACK'S (CONT.)														
Naturally Rising 12 inch Cheese	⅙ pie (4.5 oz)	290	10	6	25	15	35	2	250	500	260	0	—	500
Naturally Rising 12 inch Combination w/ Sausage & Pepperoni	⅙ pie (5.2 oz)	360	17	8	40	17	34	2	250	680	310	0	—	500
Naturally Rising 12 inch Pepperoni	⅙ pie (4.9 oz)	350	16	8	40	17	35	2	250	710	260	0	—	500
Naturally Rising 12 inch Pepperoni Supreme	⅙ pie (5.1 oz)	340	16	8	35	16	34	2	250	670	300	0	—	750
Naturally Rising 12 inch Sausage	⅙ pie (5.1 oz)	340	15	7	35	17	34	2	250	600	330	0	—	500
Naturally Rising 12 inch Spicy Italian Sausage	⅙ pie (5.1 oz)	330	14	7	40	17	34	2	250	680	240	0	—	500
Naturally Rising 12 inch The Works	⅙ pie (5.3 oz)	330	14	7	35	16	34	2	250	580	340	0	—	500
Naturally Rising 9 inch Cheese	⅓ pie (4.7 oz)	300	10	6	25	15	38	2	250	500	270	0	—	500
Naturally Rising 9 inch Combination w/ Sausage & Pepperoni	¼ pie (4.2 oz)	300	14	7	35	14	29	2	200	560	260	0	—	400
Naturally Rising 9 inch Pepperoni	⅓ pie (5.2 oz)	360	16	8	40	17	38	2	250	720	300	0	—	500
Naturally Rising 9 inch Sausage	⅓ pie (5.4 oz)	360	16	7	35	17	38	2	250	620	340	0	—	500
Naturally Rising 9 inch The Works	¼ pie (4.5 oz)	280	12	6	30	13	29	2	250	480	280	0	—	400
Original 12 inch Canadian Bacon	¼ pie (4.4 oz)	280	10	5	30	16	31	2	250	620	270	0	—	500
Original 12 inch Cheese	⅓ pie (5 oz)	360	13	7	30	19	41	3	350	650	290	0	—	750
Original 12 inch Hamburger	¼ pie (4.4 oz)	300	14	7	35	16	28	2	250	580	270	0	—	500
Original 12 inch Pepperoni	¼ pie (4.3 oz)	330	15	7	35	16	31	2	250	720	240	0	—	500
Original 12 inch Sausage	¼ pie (4.3 oz)	300	14	7	30	15	28	2	250	580	290	0	—	500
Original 12 inch Spicy Italian Sausage	¼ pie (4.3 oz)	290	13	6	35	15	29	2	250	650	280	0	—	500
Original 9 inch Pepperoni	½ pie (5 oz)	380	18	8	40	18	37	3	300	820	270	0	—	750
Original 9 inch Sausage	½ pie (5.1 oz)	360	16	7	35	17	36	3	300	660	340	0	—	750

FOOD	PORTION	CALORIES	FAT	SAT FAT	CHOL	PROTEIN	CARBO	FIBER	CALCIUM	SOD	POTAS	VIT C	FOLIC	VIT A
JACK'S (CONT.)														
Pizza Bursts Combination Sausage & Pepperoni	6 pieces (3 oz)	250	12	4	20	8	26	2	60	500	230	0	—	400
Pizza Bursts Pepperoni	6 pieces (3 oz)	260	14	5	20	9	25	2	100	560	200	0	—	500
Pizza Bursts Sausage	6 pieces (3 oz)	250	12	4	20	8	25	2	60	490	200	0	—	400
Pizza Bursts Supercheese	6 pieces (3 oz)	250	12	5	20	9	25	2	150	460	190	0	—	500
Pizza Bursts Supreme	6 pieces (3 oz)	250	13	4	20	8	26	2	60	520	200	0	—	400
KID CUISINE														
Cheese	1 (8 oz)	430	11	3	20	12	71	5	150	440	—	0	—	100
Hamburger	1 (8.30 oz)	400	11	4	25	14	61	6	100	530	—	6	—	200
KINERET														
Bagel Pizza	2 (4 oz)	300	10	6	30	15	39	1	200	700	—	9	—	750
Slice	1 (4.9 oz)	490	9	4	20	14	93	2	150	510	—	1	—	0
LEAN CUISINE														
French Bread Cheese	1 pkg (6 oz)	300	5	3	10	15	49	4	300	580	480	4	—	300
French Bread Deluxe	1 pkg (6.1 oz)	300	6	3	25	16	46	4	150	590	480	6	—	400
French Bread Pepperoni	1 pkg (5.25 oz)	310	7	3	20	15	46	3	250	590	420	2	—	400
LEAN POCKETS														
Stuffed Sandwich Pizza Deluxe	1 (4.5 oz)	270	8	3	25	12	37	2	200	680	—	0	—	750
OLD EL PASO														
Pizza Burrito Cheese	1 (3.5 oz)	320	9	4	20	13	27	0	250	430	—	0	—	0
Pizza Burrito Pepperoni	1 (3.5 oz)	260	10	5	20	12	31	0	150	510	—	0	—	0
Pizza Burrito Sausage	1 (3.5 oz)	260	9	4	15	11	32	0	150	420	—	0	—	0
PEPPERIDGE FARM														
Croissant Pastry Cheese	1	430	23	—	—	15	41	—	350	640	—	2	—	300
Croissant Pastry Deluxe	1	440	23	—	—	16	43	—	350	790	—	1	—	200
Croissant Pastry Pepperoni	1	420	22	—	—	14	43	—	250	690	—	4	—	300
SMALL WORLD														
Four Cheese	1 (4 oz)	240	6	3	13	10	38	1	250	350	—	0	—	100
SPECIAL DELIVERY														
Organic	⅓ pizza (5.3 oz)	320	9	5	20	13	46	1	300	500	—	0	—	100

FOOD	PORTION	CALORIES	FAT	SAT FAT	CHOL	PROTEIN	CARBO	FIBER	CALCIUM	SOD	POTAS	VIT C	FOLIC	VIT A
SPECIAL DELIVERY (CONT.)														
Organic Soy Kaas	⅓ pizza (5.3 oz)	320	7	2	0	16	47	1	40	600	—	0	—	0
STOUFFER'S														
French Bread Bacon Cheddar	1 piece (5.7 oz)	430	21	7	25	15	46	4	200	880	310	4	—	300
French Bread Cheese	1 piece (5.2 oz)	370	16	6	15	14	43	3	200	880	240	0	—	300
French Bread Cheeseburger	1 piece (6 oz)	420	20	6	30	17	44	3	200	800	320	2	—	500
French Bread Deluxe	1 piece (6.2 oz)	430	21	7	20	17	49	3	150	990	320	2	—	400
French Bread Double Cheese	1 piece (5.9 oz)	400	16	7	25	16	49	4	250	950	240	2	—	300
French Bread Pepperoni	1 piece (5.6 oz)	430	20	8	15	16	46	3	150	990	290	1	—	500
French Bread Pepperoni & Mushroom	1 piece (6.1 oz)	440	20	7	30	15	49	5	100	910	310	2	—	300
French Bread Sausage	1 piece (6 oz)	420	18	7	20	17	48	3	200	1260	330	2	—	300
French Bread Sausage & Pepperoni	1 piece (6.25 oz)	470	23	8	25	18	47	3	200	1340	350	5	—	200
French Bread Three Meat	1 piece (6.25 oz)	460	21	8	35	20	48	5	200	1200	370	4	—	500
French Bread Vegetable Deluxe	1 piece (6.4 oz)	380	16	6	20	14	46	4	300	780	230	0	—	2000
French Bread White Pizza	1 piece (5.1 oz)	460	23	7	20	18	45	5	350	700	130	0	—	200
TOMBSTONE														
Double Top Pepperoni	⅙ pie (4.5 oz)	340	19	9	45	18	24	2	350	810	300	1	—	750
Double Top Sausage	⅙ pie (4.6 oz)	320	17	9	40	18	25	2	350	760	320	2	—	750
Double Top Sausage & Pepperoni	⅙ pie (4.6 oz)	340	19	9	45	19	25	2	350	820	320	1	—	750
Double Top Supreme	⅙ pie (4.7 oz)	330	18	9	40	18	25	2	300	780	310	2	—	1000
Double Top Two Cheese	⅙ pie (5.2 oz)	380	19	11	50	22	29	2	500	760	320	2	—	1250
For One ½ Less Fat Cheese	1 pie (6.5 oz)	460	10	5	20	23	43	3	400	940	450	2	—	750
For One ½ Less Fat Vegetable	1 pie (7.2 oz)	360	9	4	10	21	48	5	350	860	500	1	—	1250
For One Extra Cheese	1 pie (6.9 oz)	520	28	13	50	26	47	3	500	940	450	1	—	1250
For One Pepperoni	1 pie (6.9 oz)	550	32	14	55	25	41	3	400	1160	500	1	—	1250

FOOD	PORTION	CALORIES	FAT	SAT FAT	CHOL	PROTEIN	CARBO	FIBER	CALCIUM	SOD	POTAS	VIT C	FOLIC	VIT A
TOMBSTONE (CONT.)														
For One Supreme	1 pie (7.5 oz)	550	32	14	55	24	42	3	350	1090	500	4	—	1250
Light Supreme	⅕ pie (4.8 oz)	270	9	4	20	17	30	3	200	720	370	1	—	750
Light Vegetable	⅕ pie (4.6 oz)	240	7	3	10	14	31	3	200	500	310	2	—	750
Original 12 inch Canadian Bacon	¼ pie (5.5 oz)	350	14	7	35	20	36	3	250	890	400	1	—	1000
Original 12 inch Deluxe	⅕ pie (4.8 oz)	310	14	6	30	15	29	3	250	690	350	4	—	750
Original 12 inch Extra Cheese	¼ pie (5.1 oz)	350	15	8	30	18	35	3	350	680	350	1	—	1000
Original 12 inch Hamburger	⅕ pie (4.4 oz)	310	15	7	30	15	29	2	200	670	320	2	—	750
Original 12 inch Pepperoni	¼ pie (5.3 oz)	400	21	9	40	19	35	3	300	930	400	1	—	1000
Original 12 inch Sausage	⅕ pie (4.4 oz)	300	14	6	30	15	29	2	200	680	340	1	—	750
Original 12 inch Sausage & Mushroom	⅕ pie (4.6 oz)	300	14	6	30	15	29	3	200	680	350	1	—	750
Original 12 inch Sausage & Pepperoni	⅕ pie (4.4 oz)	320	16	7	30	15	29	2	250	740	330	1	—	750
Original 12 inch Supreme	⅕ pie (5.1 oz)	320	16	7	30	15	29	2	250	730	330	4	—	750
Original 9 inch Deluxe	⅓ pie (4.4 oz)	280	13	6	25	14	27	2	200	630	310	1	—	750
Original 9 inch Extra Cheese	½ pie (5.6 oz)	380	19	8	30	19	40	3	350	740	390	1	—	1250
Original 9 inch Hamburger	⅓ pie (4 oz)	280	13	6	25	14	27	2	200	600	280	1	—	750
Original 9 inch Pepperoni	⅓ pie (4 oz)	300	15	7	30	14	27	2	200	680	290	1	—	750
Original 9 inch Pepperoni & Sausage	⅓ pie (4.1 oz)	300	15	7	30	14	27	2	200	710	320	1	—	750
Original 9 inch Sausage	⅓ pie (4 oz)	280	13	6	25	14	27	2	200	610	310	1	—	750
Original 9 inch Supreme	⅓ pie (4.4 oz)	310	16	7	30	15	27	2	200	720	300	2	—	750
Oven Rising Italian Sausage	⅙ pie (5.1 oz)	320	13	6	30	16	35	2	250	700	320	1	—	750
Oven Rising Pepperoni	⅙ pie (4.9 oz)	340	15	7	35	17	34	2	250	750	340	1	—	750
Oven Rising Supreme	⅙ pie (5.1 oz)	320	14	6	30	16	34	2	200	720	350	2	—	750
Oven Rising Three Cheese	⅙ pie (4.8 oz)	320	13	8	35	16	34	2	300	580	310	1	—	750
Oven Rising Three Meat	⅙ pie (5.1 oz)	340	15	7	35	17	34	2	250	750	350	1	—	750

FOOD	PORTION	CALORIES	FAT	SAT FAT	CHOL	PROTEIN	CARBO	FIBER	CALCIUM	SOD	POTAS	VIT C	FOLIC	VIT A
TOMBSTONE (CONT.)														
Thin Crust Four Meat Combo	¼ pie (5 oz)	380	23	10	45	19	26	2	300	890	360	1	—	750
Thin Crust Italian Sausage	¼ pie (5 oz)	370	22	10	45	18	26	2	300	840	360	1	—	750
Thin Crust Pepperoni	¼ pie (4.8 oz)	400	25	11	50	18	25	2	300	920	350	1	—	750
Thin Crust Supreme	¼ pie (5 oz)	380	22	10	45	18	26	2	300	840	360	2	—	750
Thin Crust Supreme Taco	¼ pie (5.1 oz)	370	23	11	50	16	27	2	250	740	370	2	—	1000
Thin Crust Three Cheese	¼ pie (4.7 oz)	360	21	11	45	19	25	2	400	690	290	1	—	1000
WEIGHT WATCHERS														
Smart Ones Deluxe Combo	1 (6.57 oz)	380	11	4	40	23	47	6	500	550	—	5	—	750
Smart Ones Pepperoni	1 (5.56 oz)	390	12	4	45	23	46	4	450	650	—	5	—	400
SAUCE														
BOBOLI														
Sauce	¼ cup (2.5 oz)	40	0	0	0	1	9	1	20	410	—	9	—	500
Sauce	1 pkg (1.2 oz)	20	0	0	0	1	4	1	0	200	—	5	—	400
CONTADINA														
Flavored With Pepperoni	¼ cup	40	2	1	—	1	6	1	20	420	—	5	—	400
Pizza Sauce	¼ cup	35	2	—	—	1	6	1	20	350	—	5	—	400
Squeeze	¼ cup	35	2	—	—	1	6	1	20	350	—	5	—	400
With Italian Cheeses	¼ cup	40	2	—	—	1	6	1	20	420	—	5	—	400
EDEN														
Pizza Pasta Sauce	½ cup (4.4 oz)	80	3	0	0	3	12	3	31	320	530	11	—	2350
MUIR GLEN														
Organic	¼ cup (2.2 oz)	40	1	—	0	1	6	2	0	230	—	1	—	100
PROGRESSO														
Pizza Sauce	¼ cup (2.2 oz)	35	1	0	0	1	5	1	20	140	—	6	—	400
RAGU														
Quick Traditional	3 tbsp (1.7 oz)	35	2	—	0	1	3	—	—	330	—	4	—	300
TREE OF LIFE														
Sauce	¼ cup (1.9 oz)	30	1	—	0	1	5	—	20	120	—	9	—	300
TAKE-OUT														
cheese deep dish individual	1 (5.5 oz)	460	24	9	20	15	47	2	250	750	—	1	—	400
PLANTAINS														
fresh uncooked	1 (6.3 oz)	218	1	—	0	2	57	—	5	7	893	33	39	2017
sliced cooked	½ cup	89	tr	—	0	1	24	—	2	4	358	8	20	700

FOOD	PORTION	CALORIES	FAT	SAT FAT	CHOL	PROTEIN	CARBO	FIBER	CALCIUM	SOD	POTAS	VIT C	FOLIC	VIT A
CHIFLES														
Plantain Chips	1 pkg (2 oz)	170	11	2	0	tr	17	2	20	14	—	4	—	400
PLUMS														
CANNED														
purple in heavy syrup	3	119	tr	tr	0	tr	31	—	12	26	121	1	3	344
purple in heavy syrup	1 cup	320	tr	tr	0	1	60	—	24	50	234	1	7	668
purple in light syrup	3	83	tr	tr	0	tr	22	—	13	26	123	1	3	352
purple in light syrup	1 cup	158	tr	tr	0	1	41	—	24	50	233	1	6	666
purple juice pack	3	55	tr	tr	0	tr	14	—	9	1	147	3	—	958
purple juice pack	1 cup	146	tr	tr	0	1	38	—	25	3	389	7	—	2542
purple water pack	1 cup	102	tr	tr	0	1	27	—	17	2	314	8	7	2276
purple water pack	3	39	tr	tr	0	tr	10	—	6	1	120	3	3	868
FRESH														
plum	1	36	tr	tr	0	1	9	—	2	0	113	6	1	213
sliced	1 cup	91	1	tr	0	1	21	—	6	1	284	16	4	533
DOLE														
Plums	2	70	1	—	0	1	17	1	—	0	—	—	—	—
POI														
poi	½ cup	134	tr	tr	0	tr	33	—	19	14	220	5	—	24
POKEBERRY SHOOTS														
cooked	½ cup	16	tr	—	0	2	3	—	43	—	—	67	—	7134
raw	½ cup	18	tr	—	0	2	3	—	42	—	—	109	—	6960
ALLEN														
Pokeberry Shoots	½ cup (4.1 oz)	35	1	0	0	2	5	3	80	5	—	36	—	9000
POLENTA														
(*see* CORNMEAL)														
POMEGRANATES														
pomegranate	1	104	tr	—	0	1	26	—	5	5	399	9	—	—
POMPANO														
florida cooked	3 oz	179	10	4	54	20	0	—	36	65	541	—	—	—
florida raw	3 oz	140	8	3	43	16	0	—	19	55	324	—	—	—
POPCORN														
(*see also* CHIPS, POPCORN CAKES, PRETZELS, SNACKS)														
air-popped	1 cup (0.3 oz)	31	tr	tr	0	1	6	2	1	0	24	0	2	16
air-popped	1 oz	108	1	tr	0	3	22	4	3	1	85	0	6	56
caramel coated	1 oz	122	4	1	—	1	22	1	12	58	31	0	—	14
caramel coated	1 cup (1.2 oz)	152	5	1	—	1	28	2	15	72	38	0	—	18
carmel coated w/ peanuts	⅔ cup (1 oz)	114	2	tr	0	2	23	1	19	84	101	0	—	18
cheese	1 cup (0.4 oz)	58	4	1	1	1	6	1	12	98	29	tr	—	27
cheese	1 oz	149	9	2	3	3	15	3	32	252	74	tr	—	69

FOOD	PORTION	CALORIES	FAT	SAT FAT	CHOL	PROTEIN	CARBO	FIBER	CALCIUM	SOD	POTAS	VIT C	FOLIC	VIT A
oil popped	1 oz	142	8	1	0	3	16	3	3	251	64	tr	5	44
oil popped	1 cup (0.4 oz)	55	3	1	0	1	6	1	1	97	25	0	2	17
BARREL O' FUN														
Baked Curl	1 oz	150	9	2	0	2	17	0	20	260	—	—	—	—
Caramel Corn	1 oz	115	1	0	0	1	25	1	—	170	—	4	—	—
Corn Pop	1 oz	190	16	1	0	0	10	0	—	230	—	—	—	—
Popcorn	1 oz	160	12	1	0	2	13	1	—	240	—	—	—	—
White Cheddar Pops	1 oz	170	13	1	0	2	11	0	110	370	—	—	—	—
CHEETOS														
Cheddar Cheese	0.5 oz	80	6	—	0	1	6	—	—	160	50	—	—	—
CHESTERS														
Microwave	3 cups	110	7	—	0	1	13	—	—	170	50	—	—	—
Microwave Butter	3 cups	120	7	—	0	2	13	—	—	180	60	—	—	—
Microwave Cheese	3 cups	110	8	—	0	2	11	—	—	230	70	—	—	—
Popcorn	0.5 oz	70	3	—	0	1	9	—	—	200	40	—	—	—
CRACKER JACK														
Original	1 oz	120	3	—	—	2	22	—	—	85	115	—	—	—
ESTEE														
No Sugar Added Caramel	1 cup (1 oz)	120	2	0	0	1	26	1	0	90	—	0	—	0
GREENFIELD														
Caramel	1 cup (1 oz)	120	2	tr	0	2	22	—	—	100	50	—	—	—
HERR'S														
Regular	3 cups (1 oz)	140	11	2	0	2	11	3	0	250	—	0	—	0
JIFFY POP														
Bag Butter	3 cups	90	5	1	0	2	11	2	—	140	—	—	—	—
Bag Lite	3 cups	70	3	tr	0	2	11	2	—	110	—	—	—	—
Bag Regular	3 cups	100	6	1	0	2	11	2	—	140	—	—	—	—
Glazed Popcorn Clusters	1 oz	120	2	tr	5	0	25	1	—	120	—	—	—	200
Microwave Butter	4 cup	140	7	—	0	3	17	3	—	270	—	—	—	—
Microwave Regular	4 cup	140	7	—	0	3	17	3	—	270	—	—	—	—
Pan Butter	4 cup	130	6	—	0	3	16	2	—	270	—	—	—	—
Pan Regular	4 cup	130	6	—	0	3	16	2	—	270	—	—	—	—
LANCE														
Cheese	1 pkg (25 g)	130	8	1	5	2	13	—	40	280	40	—	—	—
Plain	1 pkg (25 g)	140	9	2	0	2	13	—	—	210	10	—	—	—
White Cheddar Cheese	1 pkg (25 g)	140	9	3	5	2	12	—	—	170	90	—	—	—
LOUISE'S														
Fat-Free Apple Cinnamon	1 oz	100	0	0	0	1	24	1	—	80	—	—	—	—
Fat-Free Buttery Toffee	1 oz	100	0	0	0	1	24	1	—	80	—	—	—	—
Fat-Free Caramel	1 oz	100	0	0	0	1	24	1	—	80	—	—	—	—

FOOD	PORTION	CALORIES	FAT	SAT FAT	CHOL	PROTEIN	CARBO	FIBER	CALCIUM	SOD	POTAS	VIT C	FOLIC	VIT A
NEWMAN'S OWN														
Microwave Butter Flavor	3½ cups	170	11	2	0	2	16	3	0	180	—	0	—	0
Microwave Light Butter	3½ cups	110	3	1	0	2	20	3	0	90	—	0	—	0
Microwave Light Natural	3½ cups	110	3	1	0	2	20	3	0	90	—	0	—	0
Microwave Natural	3½ cups	170	11	2	0	2	16	3	0	180	—	0	—	0
Popcorn unpopped	3 tbsp	110	2	0	0	4	27	7	0	0	—	0	—	0
ORVILLE REDENBACHER'S														
Gourmet Hot Air	3 cups	40	tr	—	0	1	10	3	—	0	60	—	—	—
Gourmet Original	3 cups	80	4	—	0	1	10	3	—	0	60	—	—	—
Gourmet White	3 cups	80	4	—	0	1	10	3	—	0	60	—	—	—
Microwave Gourmet	3 cups	100	6	1	0	2	11	3	—	200	60	—	—	—
Microwave Gourmet Butter	3 cups	100	6	1	0	2	11	3	—	240	60	—	—	—
Microwave Gourmet Butter Toffee	2½ cups	210	12	3	tr	2	26	2	—	85	100	—	—	80
Microwave Gourmet Caramel	2½ cups	240	14	3	tr	2	29	2	20	90	125	—	—	40
Microwave Gourmet Cheddar Cheese	3 cups	130	8	2	2	2	14	3	—	280	70	—	—	—
Microwave Gourmet Frozen	3 cups	100	6	1	0	2	11	3	—	200	60	—	—	—
Microwave Gourmet Frozen Butter	3 cups	100	6	1	0	2	11	3	—	240	60	—	—	—
Microwave Gourmet Light	3 cups	70	3	1	0	2	8	3	—	115	60	—	—	—
Microwave Gourmet Light Butter	3 cups	70	3	1	0	2	8	3	—	110	60	—	—	—
Microwave Gourmet Salt Free	3 cups	100	6	1	0	2	11	3	—	0	60	—	—	—
Microwave Gourmet Salt Free Butter	3 cups	100	6	1	0	2	11	3	—	0	60	—	—	—
Microwave Gourmet Sour Cream 'n Onion	3 cups	160	12	3	0	2	12	3	24	270	100	2	—	—
PLANTERS														
Fiddle Faddle Caramel Fat Free	1 cup (1 oz)	110	0	0	0	tr	28	1	0	210	—	0	—	0
POP SECRET														
Microwave 94% Fat Free Butter	6 cups	110	2	0	0	4	23	4	—	230	—	—	—	—

FOOD	PORTION	CALORIES	FAT	SAT FAT	CHOL	PROTEIN	CARBO	FIBER	CALCIUM	SOD	POTAS	VIT C	FOLIC	VIT A
POP SECRET (CONT.)														
Microwave Light Butter	6 cups	120	5	1	0	3	20	4	—	260	—	—	—	—
Pop Chips	1½ cups (1 oz)	130	4	1	0	2	23	1	—	400	—	—	—	—
SMARTFOOD														
Cheddar Cheese	0.5 oz	80	5	—	6	1	7	—	20	130	50	—	—	—
Lowfat Toffee Crunch	¾ cup	110	2	tr	0	1	24	1	0	200	10	0	—	500
Reduced Fat White Cheddar	¾ cup	130	6	2	<5	3	17	3	20	260	80	0	—	0
SNYDER'S														
Butter	1 oz	140	9	—	0	2	13	3	—	140	—	—	—	2000
ULTRA SLIM-FAST														
Lite N' Tasty	½ oz	60	2	—	0	2	10	2	100	150	30	6	40	500
WEIGHT WATCHERS														
Butter	1 pkg (0.66 oz)	90	3	0	0	2	14	3	0	100	—	0	—	0
Butter Toffee	1 pkg (0.9 oz)	110	3	1	0	1	21	1	0	90	—	1	—	0
Caramel	1 pkg (0.9 oz)	100	1	0	0	1	22	1	0	45	—	0	—	0
Microwave	1 pkg (1 oz)	100	1	0	0	3	22	7	0	0	—	0	—	0
White Cheddar Cheese	1 pkg (0.66 oz)	90	4	1	0	2	12	2	0	125	—	0	—	0
WISE														
Tender Eating	0.5 oz	70	6	—	—	1	4	—	—	120	25	—	—	—
With Real Premium White Cheddar Cheese	0.5 oz	70	5	—	—	1	4	—	20	170	40	—	—	—

POPCORN CAKES

FOOD	PORTION	CALORIES	FAT	SAT FAT	CHOL	PROTEIN	CARBO	FIBER	CALCIUM	SOD	POTAS	VIT C	FOLIC	VIT A
popcorn cake	1 (0.3 oz)	38	tr	tr	0	1	8	—	1	29	33	0	—	7
GENERAL MILLS														
Popcorn Bars Caramel	1 (0.6 oz)	70	1	1	0	0	16	0	—	55	—	—	—	—
LUNDBERG														
Organic Lightly Salted	1	60	1	—	—	1	12	—	<20	140	40	tr	—	<100
Organic Unsalted	1	60	1	—	—	1	12	—	<20	3	40	tr	—	<100
Rye With Caraway Lightly Salted	1	59	0	0	—	1	14	—	<20	5	46	tr	—	<100
MOTHER'S														
Butter Flavor	1 (0.3 oz)	35	0	0	0	1	7	0	—	0	15	—	0	—
Unsalted	1 (0.3 oz)	35	0	0	0	1	7	0	—	0	20	—	0	—
ORVILLE REDENBACHER'S														
Chocolate Peanut Crunch Mini	6 pieces (0.5 oz)	60	1	0	0	2	12	1	—	20	—	—	—	—
Peanut Caramel Crunch	6 (0.5 oz)	60	1	0	0	2	13	1	—	30	—	—	—	—

FOOD	PORTION	CALORIES	FAT	SAT FAT	CHOL	PROTEIN	CARBO	FIBER	CALCIUM	SOD	POTAS	VIT C	FOLIC	VIT A
QUAKER														
Blueberry Crunch	1 (0.5 oz)	50	0	0	0	1	11	—	—	0	—	—	—	—
Butter Mini	6 (0.5 oz)	50	1	—	0	2	11	2	—	140	—	—	—	—
Butter Popped	1 (0.3 oz)	35	0	0	0	1	7	—	—	45	—	—	—	—
Caramel	1 (0.5 oz)	50	0	0	0	1	12	—	—	30	—	—	—	—
Caramel Mini	5 (0.5 oz)	50	1	—	0	1	12	1	—	70	—	—	—	—
Cheddar Cheese Mini	6 (0.5 oz)	50	1	—	0	2	11	1	—	200	—	—	—	—
Lightly Salted Mini	7 (0.5 oz)	50	1	—	0	2	12	2	—	120	—	—	—	—
Monterey Jack	1 (0.4 oz)	40	0	0	0	1	8	—	—	80	—	—	—	—
Strawberry Crunch	1 (0.5 oz)	50	0	0	0	1	11	—	—	0	—	—	—	—
White Cheddar	1 (0.4 oz)	40	0	0	0	1	8	—	—	90	—	—	—	—
POPOVER														
home recipe as prep w/ 2% milk	1 (1.4 oz)	87	3	1	46	4	11	—	38	82	65	tr	7	117
home recipe as prep w/ whole milk	1 (1.4 oz)	90	3	1	47	4	11	—	37	82	64	tr	7	97
mix as prep	1 (1.2 oz)	67	2	tr	—	3	10	—	9	143	25	—	—	—
POPPY SEEDS														
poppy seeds	1 tsp	15	1	tr	0	1	1	—	41	1	20	—	—	0
PORK														

(*see also* BACON, BACON SUBSTITUTES, CANADIAN BACON, DELI MEATS/COLD CUTS, HAM, PORK DISHES, SAUSAGE)
CANNED

FOOD	PORTION	CALORIES	FAT	SAT FAT	CHOL	PROTEIN	CARBO	FIBER	CALCIUM	SOD	POTAS	VIT C	FOLIC	VIT A
HORMEL														
Pickled Tidbits	2 oz	100	8	3	45	8	0	0	20	530	—	0	—	0
FRESH														
boston blade roast lean & fat cooked	3 oz	229	16	6	73	20	0	0	24	57	—	1	4	6
boston blade steak lean & fat cooked	3 oz	220	14	5	81	22	0	0	31	59	—	1	3	8
center loin roast lean bone in cooked	3 oz	169	8	3	67	23	0	0	21	56	—	1	3	6
center loin chop lean bone in cooked	3 oz	172	7	3	72	25	0	0	20	53	—	1	3	6
center rib chop lean & fat bone in cooked	3 oz	213	13	5	62	23	0	0	21	34	—	tr	2	6
center rib roast lean & fat bone in cooked	3 oz	217	13	5	62	23	0	0	24	39	—	tr	3	5
fresh ham rump lean roasted	3 oz	175	7	2	82	26	0	0	6	55	—	tr	3	8
fresh ham rump lean & fat roasted	3 oz	214	12	4	82	25	0	0	10	53	—	tr	3	8

FOOD	PORTION	CALORIES	FAT	SAT FAT	CHOL	PROTEIN	CARBO	FIBER	CALCIUM	SOD	POTAS	VIT C	FOLIC	VIT A
fresh ham shank lean roasted	3 oz	183	9	3	78	24	0	0	6	54	—	tr	5	7
fresh ham shank lean & fat roasted	3 oz	246	17	6	78	22	0	0	13	50	—	tr	4	8
fresh ham whole lean roasted	3 oz	179	8	3	80	25	0	0	6	54	—	tr	10	8
fresh ham whole lean roasted diced	1 cup	285	13	4	127	40	0	0	9	86	—	tr	16	12
fresh ham whole lean & fat roasted	3 oz	232	15	6	80	23	0	0	12	51	—	tr	9	9
fresh ham whole lean & fat roasted diced	1 cup	369	24	9	127	36	0	0	19	81	—	tr	14	14
ground cooked	3 oz	252	18	7	80	22	0	0	19	62	—	1	5	7
loin chop lean bone in braised	3 oz	191	11	4	71	21	0	0	20	53	—	1	3	6
loin chop lean bone in broiled	3 oz	199	12	4	71	22	0	0	20	68	—	1	3	6
loin roast lean bone in roasted	3 oz	210	13	5	79	23	0	0	25	25	—	tr	4	7
loin whole lean & fat braised	3 oz	203	12	4	68	23	0	0	18	41	—	1	3	6
loin whole lean & fat broiled	3 oz	206	12	4	68	23	0	0	16	53	—	1	4	6
loin whole lean & fat roasted	3 oz	211	12	5	70	23	0	0	16	50	—	1	5	8
lungs braised	3 oz	84	3	1	329	14	0	0	7	69	—	7	2	0
pancreas cooked	3 oz	186	9	3	268	24	0	0	14	36	—	5	4	0
ribs country style lean & fat braised	3 oz	252	18	7	74	20	0	0	25	50	—	1	3	7
shoulder arm picnic lean & fat roasted	3 oz	269	20	7	80	20	0	0	16	60	—	tr	3	7
shoulder whole lean & fat roasted	3 oz	248	18	7	77	20	0	0	20	58	—	tr	4	7
shoulder whole lean & fat roasted diced	1 cup	394	29	11	122	31	0	0	32	92	—	tr	7	11
shoulder whole lean roasted	3 oz	196	12	4	77	22	0	0	15	64	—	1	4	6
shoulder whole lean roasted doced	1 cup	311	18	6	122	34	0	0	24	101	—	1	7	9
sirloin chop lean & fat bone in braised	3 oz	208	13	5	70	22	0	0	15	43	—	1	3	6
sirloin roast lean & fat bone in cooked	3 oz	222	14	5	74	23	0	0	20	51	—	tr	5	7
spareribs braised	3 oz	338	26	10	103	25	0	0	40	79	—	0	3	9
spleen braised	3 oz	127	3	1	428	24	0	0	11	91	—	10	3	0
tail simmered	3 oz	336	30	11	110	15	0	0	11	21	—	0	3	0

FOOD	PORTION	CALORIES	FAT	SAT FAT	CHOL	PROTEIN	CARBO	FIBER	CALCIUM	SOD	POTAS	VIT C	FOLIC	VIT A
tenderloin lean roasted	3 oz	139	4	1	67	24	0	0	5	48	—	tr	5	6
top loin chop boneless lean & fat cooked	3 oz	198	11	4	64	24	0	0	18	36	—	tr	3	6
top loin roast boneless lean & fat cooked	3 oz	192	10	4	66	24	0	0	4	37	—	tr	7	7
OSCAR MAYER														
Sweet Morsel Smoked Boneless Pork Shoulder Butt	3 oz	180	15	5	50	11	0	0	0	990	—	0	—	0

PORK DISHES

JIMMY DEAN

FOOD	PORTION	CALORIES	FAT	SAT FAT	CHOL	PROTEIN	CARBO	FIBER	CALCIUM	SOD	POTAS	VIT C	FOLIC	VIT A
BBQ Pork Rib Sandwich	1 (5.4 oz)	440	23	7	55	24	36	1	—	970	—	—	—	—
TAKE-OUT														
pork roast	2 oz	70	3	1	40	10	0	—	—	390	—	1	—	—
tourtiere	1 piece (4.9 oz)	451	34	10	—	15	21	—	18	—	—	—	—	10

POSOLE

(*see* HOMINY)

POT PIE

AMY'S ORGANIC

FOOD	PORTION	CALORIES	FAT	SAT FAT	CHOL	PROTEIN	CARBO	FIBER	CALCIUM	SOD	POTAS	VIT C	FOLIC	VIT A
Broccoli	1 (7.5 oz)	430	22	10	45	11	46	4	—	630	—	—	—	—
Country Vegetable	1 (7.5 oz)	370	16	9	40	12	47	4	—	580	—	—	—	—
Shepard's	1 (8 oz)	160	4	0	0	5	27	5	—	490	—	—	—	—
Vegetable	1 (7.5 oz)	360	18	11	45	7	44	4	—	540	—	—	—	—
Vegetable Non-Dairy	1 (7.5 oz)	320	9	1	0	9	50	4	—	590	—	—	—	—
AWARD BRAND														
Beef	1 (7 oz)	350	18	8	20	7	37	3	0	1130	—	0	—	750
Chicken	1 (7 oz)	350	19	8	30	9	39	3	40	1140	—	0	—	500
BANQUET														
Family Entree Chicken Pie	1 serv (8 oz)	450	30	12	35	14	39	6	40	1010	—	—	—	750
Macaroni & Cheese	1 pkg (6.5 oz)	200	3	2	10	7	35	2	100	600	—	0	—	0
Vegetable & Cheese	1 (7 oz)	390	18	8	15	8	49	3	80	1000	—	0	—	1250
Vegetable Pie w/ Beef	1 (7 oz)	330	15	7	25	9	38	3	20	1000	—	0	—	750
Vegetable Pie w/ Chicken	1 (7 oz)	350	18	7	40	10	36	3	20	950	—	0	—	1000
Vegetable Pie w/ Turkey	1 (7 oz)	370	20	8	45	10	38	3	40	850	—	0	—	750
EMPIRE														
Chicken	1 (8.1 oz)	440	21	5	30	23	41	11	20	960	—	0	—	1000

FOOD	PORTION	CALORIES	FAT	SAT FAT	CHOL	PROTEIN	CARBO	FIBER	CALCIUM	SOD	POTAS	VIT C	FOLIC	VIT A
EMPIRE (CONT.)														
Turkey	1 (8.1 oz)	470	23	5	25	21	46	11	40	820	—	0	—	750
GREAT VALUE														
Beef	1 (7 oz)	390	19	8	35	15	38	3	20	940	—	0	—	0
Chicken	1 (7 oz)	380	20	8	35	10	39	2	20	900	—	0	—	500
Turkey	1 (7 oz)	400	22	8	35	9	42	3	20	910	—	0	—	500
LEAN CUISINE														
Chicken Pie	1 pkg (9.5 oz)	290	9	3	30	18	35	5	100	570	560	0	—	3000
Turkey & Country Vegetable	1 pkg (9.5 oz)	320	9	3	45	19	40	4	40	590	340	0	—	1250
MORTON														
Beef	1 (7 oz)	310	17	8	15	7	34	2	20	1380	—	0	—	500
Chicken	1 (7 oz)	320	18	7	25	8	32	3	40	1020	—	0	—	500
Macaroni & Cheese	1 (6 oz)	160	3	2	10	6	30	3	80	640	—	0	—	500
Turkey	1 (7 oz)	300	18	9	25	8	29	2	40	1060	—	0	—	500
OZARK VALLEY														
Chicken	1 (7 oz)	330	19	7	35	8	32	2	40	1010	—	0	—	100
Macaroni & Cheese	1 (6.5 oz)	160	3	2	<5	6	29	0	0	780	—	0	—	0
Turkey	1 (7 oz)	280	16	6	30	6	29	2	20	1030	—	0	—	100
STOUFFER'S														
Beef Pie	1 pkg (10 oz)	450	26	9	65	19	36	3	40	1140	260	1	—	2000
Chicken Pie	1 pkg (10 oz)	540	33	10	25	23	38	4	80	1080	410	5	—	5000
Turkey	1 pkg (10 oz)	530	33	9	65	21	36	3	100	1040	320	2	—	1500
SWANSON														
Beef	7 oz	370	19	—	—	12	36	—	20	730	—	—	—	1250
Beef Hungry Man	16 oz	610	31	—	—	24	58	—	40	1360	—	4	—	2250
Chicken	7 oz	380	22	—	—	11	35	—	20	760	—	—	—	2000
Chicken Homestyle	8 oz	410	21	—	—	15	41	—	40	1030	—	2	—	1500
Hungry Man Chicken	16 oz	630	35	—	—	22	57	—	60	1600	—	—	—	3000
Hungry Man Turkey	16 oz	650	36	—	—	24	57	—	60	1470	—	—	—	3000
Turkey	7 oz	380	21	—	—	11	36	—	20	720	—	—	—	1750
TAKE-OUT														
beef	⅓ of 9 in pie (7.4 oz)	515	30	8	42	21	39	—	29	596	334	6	—	4220
chicken	⅓ of 9 in pie (8.1 oz)	545	31	10	56	23	42	—	70	594	343	5	—	7220

POTATO

(*see also* CHIPS, KNISH, PANCAKES)

FOOD	PORTION	CALORIES	FAT	SAT FAT	CHOL	PROTEIN	CARBO	FIBER	CALCIUM	SOD	POTAS	VIT C	FOLIC	VIT A
CANNED														
potatoes	½ cup	54	tr	tr	0	1	12	—	5	—	206	5	6	—
ALLEN														
Refried Potatoes	½ cup (4.5 oz)	150	3	1	0	7	24	11	40	360	—	0	—	0
BUTTERFIELD														
Diced	⅔ cup (5.7 oz)	100	0	0	0	2	22	3	60	350	—	18	—	0
Sliced	½ cup (5.7 oz)	100	0	0	0	2	22	4	40	390	—	9	—	0

FOOD	PORTION	CALORIES	FAT	SAT FAT	CHOL	PROTEIN	CARBO	FIBER	CALCIUM	SOD	POTAS	VIT C	FOLIC	VIT A
BUTTERFIELD (CONT.)														
Whole	2½ pieces (5.6 oz)	90	0	0	0	2	20	2	60	330	—	15	—	0
DEL MONTE														
New Sliced	⅔ cup (5.4 oz)	60	0	0	0	1	13	2	20	360	—	12	—	0
New Whole	⅔ cup (5.5 oz)	60	0	0	0	1	13	2	20	360	—	12	—	0
HORMEL														
Au Gratin & Bacon	1 can (7.5 oz)	250	14	5	25	8	23	2	100	840	—	0	—	0
SENECA														
Potatoes	½ cup	80	0	0	0	3	15	2	0	264	385	6	—	0
SUNSHINE														
Whole	2½ pieces (5.6 oz)	90	0	0	0	2	20	2	60	330	—	15	—	0
FRESH														
baked w/ skin	1 (6.5 oz)	220	tr	tr	0	5	51	—	20	16	844	26	22	0
microwaved	1 (7 oz)	212	tr	tr	0	5	49	—	22	16	903	31	24	—
microwaved w/o skin	½ cup	78	tr	tr	0	2	18	—	4	5	321	12	10	—
raw w/o skin	1 (3.9 oz)	88	tr	tr	0	2	20	—	8	7	608	22	14	0
YUKON GOLD														
Fresh	1 (5.3 oz)	110	0	—	0	—	—	—	—	—	—	—	—	—
FROZEN														
french fries thick cut	10 strips	109	4	2	0	2	17	—	5	23	240	5	9	—
hashed brown	½ cup	170	9	4	—	2	22	—	12	27	340	5	—	—
potato puffs	½ cup	138	7	3	0	2	19	—	19	462	236	4	10	10
potato puffs as prep	1	16	1	tr	0	tr	2	—	2	52	27	1	1	1
BIRDS EYE														
Whole	3 (2.6 oz)	50	0	0	0	1	13	1	0	25	—	2	—	0
BUDGET GOURMET														
Baked With Broccoli And Cheese	1 pkg (10.5 oz)	300	10	4	30	13	40	—	300	740	890	18	—	1000
Cheddared Potatoes	1 pkg (5.5 oz)	260	16	—	35	7	22	—	150	600	330	6	—	300
Cheddared Potatoes With Broccoli	1 pkg (5 oz)	150	7	—	20	6	14	—	150	410	250	15	—	500
Three Cheese Potatoes	1 pkg (5.75 oz)	220	11	—	30	7	23	—	150	470	370	6	—	300
EMPIRE														
Crinkle Cut French Fries	½ cup (3 oz)	90	2	1	0	1	18	7	0	20	—	0	—	0
Latkes Potato Pancakes	1 (2 oz)	80	2	2	0	1	15	8	0	200	—	0	—	0
Latkes Mini Potato Pancakes	2 (2 oz)	90	3	1	0	1	16	6	0	160	—	0	—	0

FOOD	PORTION	CALORIES	FAT	SAT FAT	CHOL	PROTEIN	CARBO	FIBER	CALCIUM	SOD	POTAS	VIT C	FOLIC	VIT A
GOLDEN														
Potato Pancakes	1 (1.33 oz)	71	3	0	4	2	10	—	4	187	125	tr	—	100
HEALTHY CHOICE														
Cheddar Broccoli Potatoes	1 meal (10.5 oz)	310	5	2	10	13	53	8	200	550	—	27	—	300
Garden Potato Casserole	1 meal (9.25 oz)	200	4	2	10	11	30	6	100	520	—	21	—	1250
KINERET														
Crinkle Cut	18 pieces (3 oz)	120	4	1	0	2	20	2	—	260	—	4	—	—
Kugel	1 piece (2.5 oz)	150	10	2	30	2	13	1	0	160	—	12	—	0
Latkes	1 (1.5 oz)	90	5	—	0	2	9	2	—	150	—	—	—	—
Latkes Mini	10 (3 oz)	160	9	1	0	1	18	2	—	240	—	—	—	—
LEAN CUISINE														
Deluxe Cheddar	1 pkg (10.4 oz)	270	7	4	20	12	40	6	250	590	950	9	—	400
Roasted Potatoes w/ Broccoli & Cheddar Cheese Sauce	1 pkg (10.25 oz)	260	6	4	15	12	39	7	250	590	920	12	—	750
MICROMAGIC														
French Fries Low Fat	1 pkg (3 oz)	130	3	1	0	3	23	3	20	35	—	2	—	0
OH BOY!														
Stuffed With Cheddar Cheese	1 (6 oz)	130	4	—	0	4	20	4	60	310	510	1	—	200
Stuffed With Real Bacon	1 (6 oz)	120	3	—	5	4	20	4	20	300	550	—	—	400
ORE IDA														
Cheddar Browns	1 patty (3 oz)	90	3	1	<5	3	14	1	20	350	300	2	—	100
Cottage Fries	14 pieces (3 oz)	130	4	1	0	2	21	1	0	20	370	1	—	0
Crispers!	17 pieces (3 oz)	220	13	2	0	2	24	2	0	510	210	0	—	0
Crispers! Nacho	10 pieces (3 oz)	170	9	3	0	2	21	2	0	360	250	12	—	100
Crispers! Texas	3 oz	170	10	3	0	3	19	2	0	270	310	15	—	200
Crispy Crowns!	12 pieces (3 oz)	100	11	2	0	2	21	2	0	450	250	0	—	0
Crispy Crunchies	12 pieces (3 oz)	160	9	2	0	2	18	2	0	370	270	2	—	0
Deep Fries Crinkle Cuts	18 pieces (3 oz)	160	7	1	0	2	23	2	0	15	260	1	—	0
Deep Fries French Fries	22 pieces (3 oz)	160	7	1	0	2	22	2	0	20	250	2	—	0
Dinner Fries Country Style	8 pieces (3 oz)	110	3	1	0	2	19	1	0	20	280	5	—	0

FOOD	PORTION	CALORIES	FAT	SAT FAT	CHOL	PROTEIN	CARBO	FIBER	CALCIUM	SOD	POTAS	VIT C	FOLIC	VIT A
ORE IDA (CONT.)														
Fast Fries	23 pieces (3 oz)	140	6	2	0	2	20	2	0	230	240	12	—	0
Fast Fries Ranch	22 pieces (3 oz)	150	7	2	0	2	21	1	0	430	210	4	—	0
Golden Crinkles	16 pieces (3 oz)	120	4	1	0	2	20	2	0	25	260	1	—	0
Golden Fries	16 pieces (3 oz)	120	4	1	0	2	20	1	0	25	260	0	—	0
Golden Patties	1 (2.5 oz)	140	7	2	0	1	16	1	0	280	120	0	—	0
Golden Twirls	28 pieces (3 oz)	160	7	1	0	2	22	2	0	25	380	1	—	0
Hash Browns Country Style	1 cup (2.6 oz)	60	0	0	0	2	13	1	0	10	240	4	—	0
Hash Browns Shredded	1 patty (3 oz)	70	0	0	0	2	15	1	0	25	280	4	—	0
Hash Browns Southern Style	¾ cup (3 oz)	70	0	0	0	2	17	2	0	25	150	1	—	0
Hot Tots	9 pieces (3 oz)	150	6	1	0	2	21	2	0	380	250	4	—	0
Mashed Natural Butter	½ cup (2.1 oz)	80	2	1	<5	2	14	tr	0	140	210	4	—	100
Microwave Crinkle Cuts	1 pkg (3.5 oz)	180	8	2	0	3	26	2	0	10	460	4	—	0
Microwave Hash Browns	1 patty (2 oz)	110	6	2	0	1	13	tr	0	150	140	0	—	0
Microwave Tater Tots	1 pkg (3.75 oz)	190	10	3	0	2	26	2	0	420	160	4	—	0
O'Brien Potatoes	¾ cup (3 oz)	60	0	0	0	1	13	2	0	15	160	5	—	0
Pixie Crinkles	33 pieces (3 oz)	140	5	1	0	2	21	3	0	25	340	1	—	0
Shoestrings	38 pieces (3 oz)	150	5	1	0	2	22	2	0	20	240	0	—	0
Snackin' Fries	1 pkg (5 oz)	180	20	4	0	4	36	3	0	590	410	9	—	0
Snackin' Fries Extra Zesty	1 pkg (5 oz)	180	20	4	0	4	35	4	0	510	520	12	—	0
Tater ABC's	10 pieces (3 oz)	190	11	5	0	2	20	2	0	310	210	5	—	0
Tater Tots	9 pieces (3 oz)	160	8	2	0	2	21	2	0	340	220	1	—	0
Tater Tots Bacon	9 pieces (3 oz)	150	7	2	0	2	20	1	0	490	220	0	—	0
Tater Tots Onion	9 pieces (3 oz)	150	7	2	0	2	20	2	0	370	250	0	—	0
Toaster Hash Browns	2 patties (3.5 oz)	190	12	2	0	2	21	1	0	550	180	0	—	0
Topped Broccoli & Cheese	½ (6 oz)	150	4	2	10	5	24	4	150	410	560	12	—	200
Topped Salsa & Cheese	½ (5.5 oz)	160	5	2	10	5	25	3	150	430	580	21	—	400
Topped Vegetable Primavera	1 (6.13 oz)	160	5	2	<5	6	23	—	150	390	510	15	—	750

FOOD	PORTION	CALORIES	FAT	SAT FAT	CHOL	PROTEIN	CARBO	FIBER	CALCIUM	SOD	POTAS	VIT C	FOLIC	VIT A
ORE IDA (CONT.)														
Twice Baked Butter	1 (5 oz)	200	9	3	0	4	27	4	40	350	590	15	—	300
Twice Baked Cheddar Cheese	1 (5 oz)	190	8	3	0	4	27	3	40	460	630	2	—	0
Twice Baked Ranch	1 (5 oz)	180	6	2	0	5	27	3	60	400	420	12	—	200
Twice Baked Sour Cream & Chives	1 (5 oz)	180	6	2	0	4	28	3	40	370	620	4	—	0
Waffle Fries	15 pieces (3 oz)	140	5	2	0	2	22	2	0	35	290	2	—	0
Wedges With Skin	9 pieces (3 oz)	110	3	1	0	2	19	2	0	15	380	1	—	0
Zesties!	12 pieces (3 oz)	160	9	2	0	2	21	1	0	370	210	4	—	100
STOUFFER'S														
Au Gratin	½ cup (5.75 oz)	130	6	3	15	4	15	1	100	590	250	4		0
Scalloped	½ cup (5.75 oz)	140	6	1	<5	4	17	2	100	450	230	5		0
WEIGHT WATCHERS														
Smart Ones Baked Broccoli & Cheese	1 pkg (10 oz)	250	7	2	15	12	35	6	250	590	—	9	—	1000
HOME RECIPE														
au gratin	½ cup	160	9	6	29	6	14	—	146	528	483	12	10	322
mashed w/ whole milk & margarine	⅓ cup	66	tr	tr	2	2	13	—	17	182	236	tr	7	33
scalloped	½ cup	105	5	3	14	4	13	—	70	409	461	13	10	165
MIX														
au gratin as prep	4½ oz	127	6	4	—	3	18	—	114	601	300	4	—	—
instant mashed flakes as prep w/ whole milk & butter	½ cup	118	6	4	15	2	16	—	52	349	245	10	8	189
instant mashed flakes not prep	½ cup	78	tr	tr	0	2	18	—	5	24	239	18	9	—
scalloped as prep	4½ oz	127	6	4	—	3	18	—	49	467	278	5	2	—
BARBARA'S														
Mashed not prep	⅓ cup (0.8 oz)	70	0	0	0	2	17	1	—	10	—	—	—	—
BETTY CROCKER														
Au Gratin as prep	½ cup	110	3	1	0	2	22	1	20	610	260	0	—	0
Cheddar & Bacon as prep	½ cup	120	3	1	<5	3	21	1	40	630	280	0	—	0
Cheddar & Sour Cream as prep	½ cup	130	3	1	5	3	25	1	60	580	280	0	—	0
Chicken & Vegetable as prep	⅔ cup	130	3	1	<5	4	24	1	60	520	310	0	—	400
Chicken & Vegetable as prep	⅔ cup	140	4	1	<5	4	24	1	60	540	310	0	—	400
Creamy Garlic as prep	⅔ cup	150	5	2	<5	3	24	1	60	490	300	0	—	100

FOOD	PORTION	CALORIES	FAT	SAT FAT	CHOL	PROTEIN	CARBO	FIBER	CALCIUM	SOD	POTAS	VIT C	FOLIC	VIT A
BETTY CROCKER (CONT.)														
Hash Browns as prep	½ cup	200	8	2	0	3	31	2	20	590	550	0	—	300
Homestyle Broccoli Au Gratin as prep	½ cup	110	3	1	<5	3	21	2	40	510	310	0	—	100
Homestyle Broccoli Au Gratin Stove Top Recipe as prep	½ cup	130	4	1	<5	3	21	2	40	560	310	0	—	100
Homestyle Cheddar Cheese Stove Top Recipe as prep	½ cup	140	5	2	5	3	21	1	60	680	310	0	—	100
Homestyle Cheddar Cheese as prep	½ cup	120	3	1	<5	3	21	1	60	600	310	0	—	100
Homestyle Cheesy Scalloped Stove Top Recipe as prep	½ cup	130	5	2	5	3	20	1	60	590	310	0	—	100
Homestyle Cheesy Scalloped as prep	½ cup	120	3	1	<5	3	20	1	60	520	310	0	—	100
Julienne as prep	½ cup	110	3	1	5	3	20	1	60	600	250	0	—	100
Mashed Butter & Herb Reduced Fat Recipe as prep	½ cup	130	5	2	5	3	20	1	40	480	370	0	—	200
Mashed Butter & Herb as prep	½ cup	160	8	3	5	3	20	1	60	510	370	0	—	300
Mashed Potato Buds Reduced Fat Recipe as prep	⅔ cup	120	4	1	0	3	19	1	20	420	370	0	—	300
Mashed Potato Buds Sour Cream 'N Chive as prep	⅔ cup	190	11	3	<5	3	23	1	40	560	400	0	—	300
Mashed Potato Buds Sour Cream 'N Chive Reduced Fat as prep	⅔ cup	160	7	2	<5	3	23	1	40	520	400	0	—	300
Mashed Potato Buds as prep	⅔ cup	160	8	2	<5	3	19	1	20	460	370	0	—	300
Mashed Roasted Garlic Reduced Fat Recipe as prep	½ cup	130	5	1	0	3	19	1	40	380	370	0	—	100
Mashed Roasted Garlic as prep	½ cup	160	8	2	<5	3	19	1	40	410	370	0	—	300
Mashed Sour Cream & Chives Reduced Fat Recipe as prep	½ cup	130	4	1	<5	3	21	1	60	440	380	0	—	100
Mashed Sour Cream & Chives as prep	½ cup	160	7	2	5	3	21	1	60	470	380	0	—	300
Potato Shakers Original Low Fat Recipe as prep	⅔ cup	120	2	0	<5	3	23	2	20	560	550	0	—	100

FOOD	PORTION	CALORIES	FAT	SAT FAT	CHOL	PROTEIN	CARBO	FIBER	CALCIUM	SOD	POTAS	VIT C	FOLIC	VIT A
BETTY CROCKER (CONT.)														
Potato Shakers Original as prep	⅔ cup	140	4	1	<5	3	23	2	20	560	550	0	—	100
Potato Shakers Parmesan & Herb Low Fat Recipe as prep	⅔ cup	120	2	0	<5	3	23	2	20	490	560	0	—	0
Potato Shakers Parmesan & Herb as prep	⅔ cup	140	4	1	<5	3	23	2	20	490	560	0	—	0
Potato Shakers Zesty Cheddar Low Fat Recipe as prep	⅔ cup	120	2	1	<5	3	22	2	20	490	550	0	—	0
Potato Shakers Zesty Cheddar as prep	⅔ cup	140	5	1	<5	3	22	2	20	490	550	0	—	0
Ranch as prep	½ cup	130	2	1	<5	3	25	1	60	600	300	0	—	100
Scalloped Potatoes & Ham as prep	½ cup	120	3	1	<5	3	21	1	40	540	280	0	—	100
Scalloped as prep	½ cup	130	3	1	<5	3	23	1	60	600	320	0	—	100
Smokey Cheddar as prep	½ cup	120	3	1	<5	3	22	1	80	570	310	0	—	0
Sour Cream 'n Chive as prep	½ cup	120	3	1	5	3	22	1	60	530	310	0	—	100
Three Cheese as prep	½ cup	120	3	1	<5	3	23	1	40	580	300	0	—	0
Twice Baked Cheddar & Bacon Low Fat Recipe as prep	⅔ cup	130	3	1	<5	6	22	1	80	540	410	0	—	400
Twice Baked Cheddar & Bacon as prep	⅔ cup	210	11	3	85	6	22	1	80	610	410	0	—	400
White Cheddar as prep	½ cup	120	3	1	<5	3	22	1	40	540	270	0	—	0
COUNTRY STORE														
Mashed not prep	⅓ cup	70	0	0	0	2	15	—	—	10	180	—	—	—
HUNGRY JACK														
Au Gratin as prep	½ cup	150	5	3	10	3	24	1	80	620	—	1	—	200
Cheddar & Bacon as prep	½ cup	150	5	3	10	4	24	2	80	540	—	1	—	200
Chessy Scalloped as prep	½ cup	150	5	3	10	3	24	1	60	570	—	1	—	200
Creamy Scalloped as prep	½ cup	150	5	3	10	3	24	2	60	460	—	1	—	200
Mashed Butter Flavored as prep	½ cup	150	7	2	<5	3	19	1	60	350	—	0	—	300

FOOD	PORTION	CALORIES	FAT	SAT FAT	CHOL	PROTEIN	CARBO	FIBER	CALCIUM	SOD	POTAS	VIT C	FOLIC	VIT A
HUNGRY JACK (CONT.)														
Mashed Flakes as prep	½ cup	160	7	2	<5	3	20	1	60	240	—	0	—	300
Mashed Garlic Flavored as prep	½ cup	150	7	2	<5	3	19	1	60	360	—	0	—	300
Mashed Parsley Butter as prep	½ cup	150	7	2	<5	3	19	1	60	380	—	0	—	300
Mashed Sour Cream 'n Chives as prep	½ cup	150	7	2	<5	3	19	1	60	380	—	0	—	300
Sour Cream & Chives as prep	½ cup	160	6	4	15	3	23	1	60	510	—	2	—	300
IDAHO														
Mashed Potato Flakes as prep	½ cup	150	6	2	<5	3	20	1	60	240	—	0	—	300
Mashed Potato Granules as prep	½ cup	160	7	2	<5	3	22	2	60	300	—	0	—	300
SHAKE 'N BAKE														
Perfect Potatoes Crispy Cheddar	⅙ pkg (7 g)	30	2	2	5	2	2	0	40	380	45	0	—	0
Perfect Potatoes Herb & Garlic	⅙ pkg (7 g)	20	0	0	0	0	5	0	0	380	15	0	—	0
Perfect Potatoes Home Fries	⅙ pkg (7 g)	20	0	0	0	0	5	0	0	410	45	2	—	200
Perfect Potatoes Parmesan Peppercorn	⅙ pkg (7 g)	25	1	1	<5	1	3	0	40	300	40	0	—	0
Perfect Potatoes Savory Onion	⅙ pkg (7 g)	20	0	0	0	0	5	0	0	280	20	0	—	0
REFRIGERATED														
SIMPLY POTATOES														
Au Gratin	¼ pkg (3 oz)	130	8	—	21	3	13	—	80	370	430	4	—	250
Hash Browns	⅕ pkg (4 oz)	100	tr	—	0	3	23	—	—	410	530	5	—	100
Hash Browns Onion	⅕ pkg (4 oz)	120	tr	—	0	3	26	—	—	380	510	1	—	100
Hash Browns Southwest Style	⅕ pkg (4 oz)	100	tr	—	0	3	23	—	—	410	530	5	—	100
Mashed	⅕ pkg (4 oz)	90	2	—	0	2	15	—	—	150	290	4	—	100
Scalloped	¼ pkg (3 oz)	100	5	—	17	2	11	—	40	390	320	2	—	200
SHELF-STABLE														
LUNCH BUCKET														
Scalloped	1 pkg (7.5 oz)	160	7	—	35	4	20	—	—	770	—	—	—	—
MICRO CUP MEALS														
Microcup Meals Scalloped Potatoes w/ Ham	1 cup (7.5 oz)	240	14	6	35	7	20	2	20	920	—	0	—	0
TAKE-OUT														
baked topped w/ cheese sauce	1	475	29	11	19	15	47	—	310	381	1167	26	28	834

FOOD	PORTION	CALORIES	FAT	SAT FAT	CHOL	PROTEIN	CARBO	FIBER	CALCIUM	SOD	POTAS	VIT C	FOLIC	VIT A
baked topped w/ cheese sauce & bacon	1	451	26	10	30	18	44	—	309	973	1179	29	28	627
baked topped w/ cheese sauce & broccoli	1	402	14	9	20	14	47	—	334	484	1440	49	61	1695
baked topped w/ cheese sauce & chili	1	481	22	13	31	23	56	—	409	701	1570	32	50	768
baked topped w/ sour cream & chives	1	394	22	10	23	7	50	—	105	182	1383	34	32	1346
french fried in vegetable oil	1 reg	235	12	4	0	3	29	—	12	124	541	4	25	22
french fried in vegetable oil	1 lg	355	19	6	0	5	44	—	18	187	819	6	38	33
indian yogurt potatoes	1 serv	315	9	4	18	7	52	0	—	216	—	—	—	—
mashed	½ cup	111	4	1	2	2	18	—	27	309	303	6	0	177
mustard potato salad	3.5 oz	120	6	0	0	1	16	—	—	393	—	12	—	500
o'brien	1 cup	157	3	2	7	5	30	—	70	421	516	32	16	934
potato pancakes	1 (1.3 oz)	101	7	1	35	2	11	—	9	188	291	8	9	53
potato salad	½ cup	179	10	2	86	3	14	—	24	661	317	13	8	261
potato salad	⅓ cup	108	6	tr	57	1	13	—	13	312	256	1	24	95
potato salad w/ vegetables	3.5 oz	120	3	1	0	2	20	—	—	390	—	4	—	—

PRESERVE

(*see* JAM/JELLY/PRESERVE)

PRETZELS

(*see also* CHIPS, POPCORN, SNACKS)

FOOD	PORTION	CALORIES	FAT	SAT FAT	CHOL	PROTEIN	CARBO	FIBER	CALCIUM	SOD	POTAS	VIT C	FOLIC	VIT A
chocolate covered	1 oz	130	5	2	—	2	20	—	21	—	—	tr	—	—
chocolate covered	1 (0.4 oz)	50	2	1	—	1	8	—	8	—	—	tr	—	—
dutch twist	4 (2.1 oz)	229	2	tr	0	6	48	2	21	1029	68	0	—	0
pretzels	1 oz	108	1	tr	0	3	23	1	10	486	42	0	—	0
rods	4 (2 oz)	229	2	tr	0	6	48	2	21	1029	68	0	—	0
sticks	10	10	tr	tr	tr	tr	2	—	1	48	3	0	—	0
sticks	120 (2 oz)	229	2	tr	0	6	48	2	21	1029	68	0	—	0
twist	1 (½ oz)	65	1	tr	tr	2	13	—	4	258	16	0	—	0
twists	10 (2.1 oz)	229	2	tr	0	6	48	2	21	1029	68	0	—	0
whole wheat	2 med (2 oz)	205	2	tr	0	6	46	—	16	115	244	—	—	—
whole wheat	2 sm (1 oz)	103	1	tr	0	3	23	—	8	58	122	—	—	—
BARREL O' FUN														
Mini	1 oz	110	1	0	0	3	23	1	—	100	—	—	—	—
Sticks	1 oz	110	1	0	0	3	23	1	—	100	—	—	—	—
Twists	1 oz	110	1	0	0	3	23	1	—	100	—	—	—	—

FOOD	PORTION	CALORIES	FAT	SAT FAT	CHOL	PROTEIN	CARBO	FIBER	CALCIUM	SOD	POTAS	VIT C	FOLIC	VIT A
ESTEE														
Dutch Unsalted	2 (1.1 oz)	130	1	0	0	3	26	1	0	40	40	0	—	0
Nuggets Ranch Reduced Sodium	23 (1 oz)	130	2	1	0	3	24	tr	0	240	—	0	—	0
Nuggets Reduced Sodium	30 (1 oz)	120	2	0	0	3	24	1	0	180	—	0	—	0
Unsalted	23 (1 oz)	120	1	0	0	3	25	1	0	30	120	0	—	0
FORMAGG														
Pretzel Nuts	1 oz	120	4	1	0	2	21	tr	100	390	—	0	—	0
HERR'S														
Hard Sourdough	1 (1 oz)	100	0	0	0	3	23	2	0	450	—	0	—	0
LANCE														
Twist	1 pkg (42 g)	150	1	0	0	4	30	—	—	700	50	—	—	—
MANISCHEWITZ														
Bagel Pretzels Original	4 (1 oz)	110	0	0	0	0	22	1	40	260	—	0	—	0
MISTER SALTY														
Chips	16 (1 oz)	110	3	0	0	2	21	tr	40	620	30	—	—	—
Dutch	2 (1.1 oz)	120	1	0	0	3	25	1	—	580	50	—	—	—
Fat Free Chips	16 (1 oz)	100	0	0	0	2	22	1	80	620	30	—	—	—
Mini	22 (1 oz)	110	1	0	0	3	22	1	—	440	45	—	—	—
Sticks Fat Free	47 (1 oz)	110	0	0	0	3	23	1	—	370	30	—	—	—
Twist Fat Free	9 (1 oz)	110	0	0	0	3	23	1	—	380	35	—	—	—
MR. PHIPPS														
Chips Lower Sodium	16 (1 oz)	120	3	0	0	2	21	tr	40	410	30	—	—	—
Chips Original	16 (1 oz)	120	3	0	0	2	21	tr	40	630	30	—	—	—
Chips Original Fat Free	16 (1 oz)	100	0	0	0	2	22	tr	80	630	30	—	—	—
NESTLE														
Flipz Milk Chocolate Covered	9 pieces (1 oz)	130	5	4	<5	2	19	tr	0	135	—	0	—	0
Flipz White Fudge Covered	9 pieces (1 oz)	130	6	5	0	2	19	0	40	130	—	0	—	0
NEWMAN'S OWN														
Salted Rounds Organic	1 pkg (1.4 oz)	150	2	0	0	3	31	1	0	530	—	0	—	0
PLANTERS														
Twists	1 oz	100	1	0	0	3	23	1	—	420	30	—	—	—
Twists	1 pkg (1.5 oz)	160	1	0	0	4	35	1	—	640	45	—	—	—
QUINLAN														
Beers	1 oz	110	2	1	0	2	22	1	0	550	—	0	—	0
Hard Sourdough	1 oz	110	2	1	0	2	22	1	0	550	—	0	—	0
Logs	1 oz	110	2	1	0	2	22	1	0	550	—	0	—	0
Nuggets	1 oz	110	2	1	0	2	22	1	0	550	—	0	—	0
Rods	1 oz	110	2	1	0	2	22	1	0	550	—	0	—	0

FOOD	PORTION	CALORIES	FAT	SAT FAT	CHOL	PROTEIN	CARBO	FIBER	CALCIUM	SOD	POTAS	VIT C	FOLIC	VIT A
QUINLAN (CONT.)														
Sticks	1 oz	110	2	1	0	2	22	1	0	550	—	0	—	0
Thins	1 oz	110	2	1	0	2	22	1	0	550	—	0	—	0
ROLD GOLD														
Bavarian	3 pieces (1 oz)	120	2	—	0	3	22	—	—	430	50	—	—	—
Fat Free Hard Sour Dough	1	80	0	0	0	2	19	1	0	270	40	0	—	0
Fat Free Thins	12 pieces (1 oz)	110	0	0	0	2	23	1	0	460	30	0	—	0
Fat Free Tiny Twists	18 pieces (1 oz)	110	0	0	0	3	23	1	0	430	30	0	—	0
Pretzel Chips	1 oz	110	1	—	0	3	22	—	—	310	35	—	—	—
Pretzel Chips Cheese	1 oz	120	3	—	0	3	22	—	—	240	45	—	—	—
Rods	3 pieces (1 oz)	110	2	—	0	3	23	—	—	410	50	—	—	—
Snack Mix	½ cup (1 oz)	140	6	—	0	3	18	—	20	330	45	—	—	—
Sticks	50 pieces (1 oz)	110	2	.	0	3	23	—	—	490	50	—	—	—
SEYFART'S														
Butter Rods	1 oz	110	1	—	—	3	21	—	—	530	40	—	—	—
SNYDER'S														
Logs	1 oz	310	0	0	0	3	22	—	—	360	—	—	—	—
Minis	1 oz	310	0	0	0	3	22	—	—	460	—	—	—	—
Minis Unsalted	1 oz	310	0	0	0	3	22	—	—	70	—	tr	—	—
Nibblers	1 oz	310	0	0	0	3	22	—	—	460	—	—	—	—
Oat Bran	1 oz	120	1	—	0	2	14	—	—	300	—	—	—	—
Old Fashioned Hard	1 oz	111	0	0	0	3	23	—	—	655	—	—	—	—
Old Fashioned Hard Unsalted	1 oz	100	0	0	0	3	23	—	—	89	—	—	—	—
Old Tyme	1 oz	310	0	0	0	3	22	—	—	310	—	—	—	—
Old Tyme Unsalted	1 oz	110	0	0	0	3	22	—	—	70	—	—	—	—
Rods	1 oz	310	0	0	0	3	22	—	—	320	—	—	—	—
Sourdough Hard Buttermilk Ranch	1 oz	130	5	1	0	2	19	0	—	250	—	—	—	—
Sourdough Hard Cheddar Cheese	1 oz	160	7	1	0	4	13	0	—	320	—	—	—	—
Sourdough Hard Honey Mustard & Onion	1 oz	130	5	1	0	2	19	0	—	250	—	—	—	—
Stix	1 oz	310	0	0	0	3	22	—	—	900	—	—	—	—
Very Thins	1 oz	310	0	0	0	3	22	—	—	720	—	—	—	—
SUNSHINE														
California Pretzels	1 oz	110	2	0	0	3	22	1	—	350	—	—	—	—
ULTRA SLIM-FAST														
Lite N' Tasty	1 oz	100	tr	—	0	2	21	4	100	460	85	6	40	500

FOOD	PORTION	CALORIES	FAT	SAT FAT	CHOL	PROTEIN	CARBO	FIBER	CALCIUM	SOD	POTAS	VIT C	FOLIC	VIT A
WEIGHT WATCHERS														
Oat Bran Nuggets	1 pkg (1.5 oz)	170	3	0	0	4	33	3	0	250	—	0	—	0
PRICKLYPEAR														
fresh	1	42	1	—	0	1	10	—	58	6	226	14	—	53
PRUNE JUICE														
DEL MONTE														
Juice	8 fl oz	170	0	0	0	1	43	1	20	20	—	18	—	0
OCEAN SPRAY														
100% Juice	8 fl oz	180	0	0	0	2	44	0	—	8	480	5	—	0
PRUNES														
CANNED														
in heavy syrup	5	90	tr	tr	0	1	24	—	15	2	194	2	—	686
in heavy syrup	1 cup	245	tr	tr	0	2	65	—	40	6	528	7	—	1866
DRIED														
DEL MONTE														
Pitted	¼ cup (1.4 oz)	120	0	0	0	1	29	3	0	5	—	2	—	500
Unpitted	⅓ cup (1.4 oz)	110	0	0	0	1	12	1	0	5	—	2	—	500
SONOMA														
Pitted	¼ cup (1.4 oz)	120	0	0	0	1	29	3	0	5	—	2	—	500
SUNSWEET														
Orange Essence Pitted Prunes	6 (1.4 oz)	100	0	0	0	1	26	3	20	5	—	0	—	500
PUDDING														
(*see also* CUSTARD, PUDDING POPS)														
HOME RECIPE														
bread pudding	1 recipe 6 serv (26.4 oz)	1266	44	17	434	40	185	—	855	1741	1684	1	94	1816
chocolate as prep w/ whole milk	½ cup (5.5 oz)	221	6	3	17	5	40	—	152	137	252	1	7	193
cornstarch	½ cup (4.4 oz)	137	5	3	—	5	20	—	145	—	—	1	—	195
rice	½ cup (5.3 oz)	217	4	3	17	6	40	—	155	85	268	1	6	154
MIX														
banana as prep w/ 2% milk	½ cup (4.9 oz)	142	2	1	9	4	26	—	154	232	193	1	5	251
banana as prep w/ whole milk	½ cup (4.9 oz)	157	4	3	17	4	25	—	151	231	189	1	5	155
chocolate as prep w/ 2% milk	½ cup (5 oz)	150	3	2	9	5	28	—	161	148	240	1	—	252
chocolate as prep w/ whole milk	½ cup (5 oz)	158	5	3	17	5	26	—	158	147	232	1	—	157
coconut cream as prep w/ 2% milk	½ cup (4.9 oz)	148	4	3	9	4	25	—	154	226	223	1	—	251
coconut cream as prep w/ whole milk	½ cup (4.9 oz)	160	4	3	17	4	25	—	155	227	219	1	—	155
instant banana as prep w/ 2% milk	½ cup (5.2 oz)	152	3	1	9	4	29	—	150	435	192	1	6	250

FOOD	PORTION	CALORIES	FAT	SAT FAT	CHOL	PROTEIN	CARBO	FIBER	CALCIUM	SOD	POTAS	VIT C	FOLIC	VIT A
instant banana as prep w/ whole milk	½ cup (5.2 oz)	167	4	3	17	4	27	—	147	434	189	1	6	154
instant chocolate as prep w/ 2% milk	½ cup (5.2 oz)	149	3	2	9	3	28	—	153	418	247	1	6	254
instant chocolate as prep w/ whole milk	½ cup (5.2 oz)	164	5	3	17	5	28	—	151	417	244	1	6	157
instant coconut cream as prep w/ 2% milk	½ cup (5.2 oz)	157	3	2	0	4	28	—	150	362	194	1	7	250
instant coconut cream as prep w/ whole milk	½ cup (5.2 oz)	172	5	3	17	4	28	—	148	360	190	1	6	154
instant lemon as prep w/ 2% milk	½ cup (5.2 oz)	155	4	1	9	4	30	—	149	394	190	1	6	250
instant lemon as prep w/ whole milk	½ cup (5.2 oz)	169	4	3	17	4	30	—	146	393	187	1	6	154
instant vanilla as prep w/ 2% milk	½ cup (5 oz)	147	2	1	9	2	28	—	146	407	185	1	6	242
instant vanilla as prep w/ whole milk	½ cup (5 oz)	181	4	2	16	4	28	—	144	406	182	1	—	149
lemon	½ cup (5.1 oz)	163	2	1	77	1	36	—	11	94	7	0	—	117
rice as prep w/ 2% milk	½ cup (5.1 oz)	161	2	1	9	5	30	—	152	159	189	1	6	250
rice as prep w/ whole milk	½ cup (5.1 oz)	175	4	3	17	5	30	—	149	158	186	1	5	153
tapioca as prep w/ 2% milk	½ cup (5 oz)	147	2	1	9	4	28	—	149	172	190	1	—	250
tapioca as prep w/ whole milk	½ cup (5 oz)	161	4	3	17	4	28	—	147	171	186	1	—	154
vanilla as prep w/ 2% milk	½ cup (4.9 oz)	141	2	1	9	4	26	—	153	224	194	1	—	251
vanilla as prep w/ whole milk	½ cup (4.9 oz)	155	4	3	17	2	26	—	150	223	190	1	—	155
EMES														
Dietetic as prep w/ skim milk	½ cup (4 fl oz)	71	1	—	0	5r	13	—	—	110	—	tr	—	—
JELL-O														
Americana Rice as prep w/ skim milk	½ cup (5.2 oz)	140	0	0	<5	5	29	0	150	160	210	0	—	200
Americana Tapioca as prep w/ skim milk	½ cup (5.1 oz)	130	0	0	<5	4	28	0	150	180	200	0	—	200
Banana Cream as prep w/ 2% milk	½ cup (5.1 oz)	140	3	2	10	4	26	0	150	240	190	0	—	200
Butterscotch as prep w/ 2% milk	½ cup (5.2 oz)	160	3	2	10	4	30	0	150	190	190	0	—	200
Chocolate as prep w/ 2% milk	½ cup (5.2 oz)	150	3	2	10	5	28	tr	150	170	340	0	—	200

FOOD	PORTION	CALORIES	FAT	SAT FAT	CHOL	PROTEIN	CARBO	FIBER	CALCIUM	SOD	POTAS	VIT C	FOLIC	VIT A
JELL-O (CONT.)														
Chocolate Fudge as prep w/ 2% milk	½ cup (5.2 oz)	150	3	2	10	5	28	1	150	170	330	0	—	200
Coconut Cream as prep w/ 2% milk	½ cup (5.1 oz)	150	5	4	10	4	24	tr	150	210	220	0	—	200
Fat Free Chocolate as prep w/ skim milk	½ cup (5.2 oz)	130	0	0	<5	5	29	0	150	170	310	0	—	200
Fat Free Vanilla as prep w/ skim milk	½ cup (5.1 oz)	130	0	0	<5	4	28	0	150	200	210	0	—	200
Instant Banana Cream as prep w/ 2% milk	½ cup (5.2 oz)	150	3	2	10	4	29	0	150	410	190	0	—	200
Instant Butterscotch as prep w/ 2% milk	½ cup (5.2 oz)	150	3	2	10	4	29	0	150	450	190	0	—	200
Instant Chocolate as prep w/ 2% milk	½ cup (5.2 oz)	160	3	2	10	4	31	tr	150	470	270	0	—	200
Instant Chocolate Fudge as prep w/ 2% milk	½ cup (4.2 oz)	160	3	2	10	5	31	tr	150	440	330	0	—	200
Instant Coconut Cream as prep w/ 2% milk	½ cup (4.2 oz)	160	5	4	10	4	27	tr	150	320	220	0	—	200
Instant French Vanilla as prep w/ 2% milk	½ cup (4.2 oz)	150	3	2	10	4	29	0	150	410	190	0	—	200
Instant Lemon as prep w/ 2% milk	½ cup (4.2 oz)	150	3	2	10	4	29	0	150	370	190	0	—	200
Instant Pistachio as prep w/ 2% milk	½ cup (4.2 oz)	160	3	2	10	4	29	0	150	410	200	0	—	200
Instant Vanilla as prep w/ 2% milk	½ cup (4.2 oz)	150	3	2	10	4	29	0	150	410	190	0	—	200
Instant Fat Free Chocolate as prep w/ skim milk	½ cup (5.3 oz)	140	0	0	<5	5	31	tr	150	410	280	0	—	200
Instant Fat Free Devil's Food as prep w/ skim milk	½ cup (5.3 oz)	140	0	0	<5	5	31	tr	150	420	280	0	—	200
Instant Fat Free Sugar Free Banana as prep w/ skim milk	½ cup (4.6 oz)	70	0	0	<5	4	12	0	150	410	210	0	—	200
Instant Fat Free Sugar Free Butterscotch as prep w/ skim milk	½ cup (4.6 oz)	70	0	0	<5	4	12	0	150	400	210	0	—	200
Instant Fat Free Sugar Free Chocolate Fudge as prep w/ skim milk	½ cup (4.7 oz)	80	0	0	<5	5	14	tr	150	390	320	0	—	200

FOOD	PORTION	CALORIES	FAT	SAT FAT	CHOL	PROTEIN	CARBO	FIBER	CALCIUM	SOD	POTAS	VIT C	FOLIC	VIT A
JELL-O (CONT.)														
Instant Fat Free Sugar Free Chocolate as prep w/ skim milk	½ cup (4.6 oz)	80	0	0	<5	5	14	tr	150	390	320	0	—	200
Instant Fat Free Sugar Free Vanilla as prep w/ skim milk	½ cup (4.6 oz)	70	0	0	<5	4	12	0	150	400	210	0	—	200
Instant Fat Free Sugar Free White Chocolate as prep w/ skim milk	½ cup (4.6 oz)	70	0	0	<5	4	12	0	150	400	210	0	—	200
Instant Fat Free Vanilla as prep w/ skim milk	½ cup (5.2 oz)	140	0	0	<5	4	29	0	150	410	200	0	—	200
Instant Fat Free White Chocolate as prep w/ skim milk	½ cup (5.2 oz)	140	0	0	<5	4	29	0	150	410	200	0	—	200
Lemon as prep	½ cup (4.4 oz)	140	2	1	75	tr	29	0	0	75	75	0	—	100
Milk Chocolate as prep w/ 2% milk	½ cup (5.2 oz)	150	3	2	10	4	28	tr	150	170	260	0	—	200
Sugar Free Chocolate as prep w/ 2% milk	½ cup (4.6 oz)	90	3	2	10	5	13	tr	150	170	330	0	—	200
Sugar Free Vanilla as prep w/ 2% milk	½ cup (4.5 oz)	80	3	2	10	4	11	0	150	170	190	0	—	200
Vanilla as prep w/ 2% milk	½ cup (5.1 oz)	140	3	2	10	4	26	0	150	200	190	0	—	200
MY*T*FINE														
Butterscotch	mix for 1 serv	90	0	0	0	0	22	—	—	190	0	—	—	—
Chocolate	mix for 1 serv	100	0	0	0	1	23	0	—	135	15	—	—	—
Chocolate Almond	mix for 1 serv	100	1	0	0	1	23	—	—	135	20	—	—	—
Chocolate Fudge	mix for 1 serv	100	0	0	0	1	24	1	—	140	15	—	—	—
Lemon	mix for 1 serv	90	0	0	0	0	22	—	—	170	15	—	—	—
Vanilla	mix for 1 serv	90	0	0	0	0	22	0	—	120	0	—	—	—
Vanilla Tapioca	mix for 1 serv	80	0	0	0	0	19	—	—	160	5	—	—	—
ROYAL														
Banana Cream	mix for 1 serv	80	0	0	0	0	20	0	—	110	0	—	—	—
Banana Cream Instant	mix for 1 serv	90	0	0	0	0	22	—	—	390	25	—	—	—
Butterscotch	mix for 1 serv	90	0	0	0	0	25	0	—	180	5	—	—	—
Butterscotch Instant	mix for 1 serv	90	0	0	0	0	22	—	—	400	25	—	—	—
Cherry Vanilla Instant	mix for 1 serv	90	0	0	0	0	23	0	—	300	35	—	—	—
Chocolate	mix for 1 serv	90	0	0	0	1	22	0	—	90	40	—	—	—

FOOD	PORTION	CALORIES	FAT	SAT FAT	CHOL	PROTEIN	CARBO	FIBER	CALCIUM	SOD	POTAS	VIT C	FOLIC	VIT A
ROYAL (CONT.)														
Chocolate Almond Instant	mix for 1 serv	120	1	—	—	0	26	—	—	440	—	—	—	—
Chocolate Chocolate Chip Instant	mix for 1 serv	110	1	0	0	1	26	0	20	590	45	—	—	—
Chocolate Instant	mix for 1 serv	110	0	0	0	1	23	0	20	450	75	—	—	—
Chocolate Peanut Butter Instant	mix for 1 serv	110	1	0	0	1	26	0	20	480	45	—	—	—
Chocolate Sugar Free Instant	mix for 1 serv	50	0	—	—	0	11	—	—	420	130	—	—	—
Dark'N Sweet Chocolate	mix for 1 serv	90	0	0	0	1	22	1	—	95	30	—	—	—
Dark'N Sweet Instant	mix for 1 serv	110	0	0	0	1	25	0	20	460	40	—	—	—
Lemon Instant	mix for 1 serv	90	0	0	0	0	23	—	—	320	0	—	—	—
Pistachio Instant	mix for 1 serv	90	1	0	0	0	22	0	—	360	35	—	—	—
Strawberry Instant	mix for 1 serv	100	0	0	0	0	24	—	—	330	25	—	—	—
Toasted Coconut Instant	mix for 1 serv	100	2	—	—	0	22	—	—	450	—	—	—	—
Vanilla	mix for 1 serv	80	0	0	0	0	20	0	—	160	0	—	—	—
Vanilla Chocolate Chip Instant	mix for 1 serv	90	1	0	0	0	22	0	—	350	30	—	—	—
Vanilla Instant	mix for 1 serv	90	0	0	0	0	23	—	—	325	5	—	—	—
READY-TO-EAT														
banana	1 pkg (5 oz)	180	5	1	—	3	30	—	120	278	156	—	—	—
chocolate	1 pkg (5 oz)	189	6	1	5	4	32	—	128	183	256	3	4	51
lemon	1 pkg (5 oz)	177	4	1	0	tr	36	—	3	199	1	—	—	—
rice	1 pkg (5 oz)	231	11	2	—	3	31	—	—	121	65	—	—	—
tapioca	1 pkg (5 oz)	169	5	1	—	3	28	—	119	168	148	—	—	0
vanilla	1 pkg (4 oz)	146	4	1	8	3	25	—	99	153	128	0	0	23
DEL MONTE														
Snack Cups Banana	1 serv (4 oz)	140	4	1	0	1	25	0	60	190	—	0	—	0
Snack Cups Butterscotch	1 serv (4 oz)	140	4	1	0	1	25	0	60	170	—	0	—	0
Snack Cups Chocolate	1 serv (4 oz)	160	4	1	0	2	27	0	60	130	—	0	—	0
Snack Cups Chocolate Fudge	1 serv (4 oz)	150	4	1	0	2	25	0	60	190	—	0	—	0
Snack Cups Chocolate Peanut Butter	1 serv (4 oz)	160	4	1	0	2	28	0	60	270	—	0	—	0
Snack Cups Lite Chocolate	1 serv (4 oz)	100	1	0	0	2	19	0	60	140	—	0	—	0
Snack Cups Lite Vanilla	1 serv (4 oz)	90	1	0	0	1	18	0	60	190	—	0	—	0
Snack Cups Tapioca	1 serv (4 oz)	140	4	1	0	1	23	0	60	110	—	0	—	0

FOOD	PORTION	CALORIES	FAT	SAT FAT	CHOL	PROTEIN	CARBO	FIBER	CALCIUM	SOD	POTAS	VIT C	FOLIC	VIT A
DEL MONTE (CONT.)														
Snack Cups Vanilla	1 serv (4 oz)	150	4	1	0	1	26	0	60	150	—	0	—	0
HANDI-SNACKS														
Banana	1 serv (3.5 oz)	120	4	1	0	1	22	0	40	150	70	0	—	0
Butterscotch	1 serv (3.5 oz)	120	4	1	0	1	22	0	60	150	70	0	—	0
Chocolate	1 serv (3.5 oz)	130	4	1	0	2	23	tr	60	125	140	0	—	0
Chocolate Fudge	1 serv (3.5 oz)	130	4	1	0	2	23	tr	60	130	160	0	—	0
Fat Free Chocolate	1 serv (3.5 oz)	90	0	0	0	2	21	0	60	170	140	0	—	0
Fat Free Vanilla	1 serv (3.5 oz)	90	0	0	0	1	21	0	60	180	70	0	—	0
Tapioca	1 serv (3.5 oz)	120	4	1	0	2	21	0	60	120	75	0	—	0
Vanilla	1 serv (3.5 oz)	120	4	1	0	1	21	0	40	150	70	0	—	0
HUNT'S														
Snack Pack Banana	1 (4 oz)	158	6	2	tr	2	25	0	5	163	—	0	—	0
Snack Pack Butterscotch	1 (4 oz)	153	6	2	1	2	24	0	5	211	—	0	—	0
Snack Pack Chocolate	1 (4 oz)	167	6	2	1	2	25	0	62	173	—	0	—	0
Snack Pack Chocolate Fudge	1 (4 oz)	167	6	1	1	2	26	0	62	191	—	0	—	0
Snack Pack Chocolate Marshmallow	1 (4 oz)	155	6	2	tr	2	23	0	5	124	—	0	—	0
Snack Pack Fat Free Chocolate	1 (4 oz)	96	tr	0	tr	2	21	0	5	212	188	0	—	0
Snack Pack Fat Free Tapioca	1 (4 oz)	95	tr	0	tr	2	21	0	6	185	69	0	—	0
Snack Pack Fat Free Vanilla	1 (4 oz)	93	tr	0	1	2	21	0	5	167	72	0	—	0
Snack Pack Lemon	1 (4 oz)	162	3	1	0	tr	33	0	4	100	—	0	—	0
Snack Pack Swirl Chocolate Caramel	1 (4 oz)	168	6	1	1	2	26	0	64	176	—	0	—	0
Snack Pack Swirl Chocolate Peanut Butter	1 (4 oz)	166	6	2	1	3	25	0	64	165	—	0	—	0
Snack Pack Swirl Milk Chocolate	1 (4 oz)	164	6	2	1	2	26	0	62	175	—	0	—	0
Snack Pack Swirl Smores	1 (4 oz)	154	6	2	1	1	25	0	5	129	—	0	—	0
Snack Pack Tapioca	1 (4 oz)	151	6	1	1	2	23	0	6	134	69	0	—	0
Snack Pack Vanilla	1 (4 oz)	163	6	1	1	2	25	0	65	176	—	0	—	0
IMAGINE FOODS														
Lemon Dream	1 (4 oz)	120	0	0	0	1	30	—	—	5	—	—	—	—
JELL-O														
Chocolate	1 serv (4 oz)	160	5	2	0	3	28	0	100	190	260	0	—	100
Chocolate Marshmallow	1 serv (4 oz)	160	5	2	0	3	27	0	80	180	210	0	—	200

FOOD	PORTION	CALORIES	FAT	SAT FAT	CHOL	PROTEIN	CARBO	FIBER	CALCIUM	SOD	POTAS	VIT C	FOLIC	VIT A
JELL-O (CONT.)														
Chocolate Vanilla Swirls	1 serv (4 oz)	160	5	2	0	3	27	0	80	180	210	0	—	100
Free Chocolate	1 serv (4 oz)	100	0	0	0	3	23	tr	80	190	240	0	—	100
Free Chocolate Vanilla Swirl	1 serv (4 oz)	100	0	0	0	3	23	tr	80	210	200	0	—	100
Free Devil's Food	1 serv (4 oz)	100	0	0	0	3	23	tr	80	210	220	0	—	100
Free Rocky Road	1 serv (4 oz)	100	0	0	0	3	23	tr	80	210	200	0	—	100
Free Vanilla	1 serv (4 oz)	100	0	0	0	2	23	0	80	240	125	0	—	100
Tapioca	1 serv (4 oz)	140	4	2	0	2	26	0	80	160	125	0	—	200
Tapioca	1 serv (4 oz)	100	0	0	0	2	23	0	80	240	125	0	—	200
Vanilla	1 serv (4 oz)	160	5	2	0	2	25	0	80	170	125	0	—	100
KOZY SHACK														
Banana	1 pkg (4 oz)	130	3	2	10	3	22	1	250	150	—	2	—	100
Chocolate	1 pkg (4 oz)	140	4	2	5	3	24	1	100	150	—	0	—	100
Light Chocolate	1 pkg (4 oz)	110	1	1	5	4	22	1	150	150	—	0	—	0
Light Vanilla	1 pkg (4 oz)	110	1	0	10	4	22	0	150	160	—	0	—	0
Rice	1 pkg (4 oz)	130	3	2	17	4	23	1	100	140	—	0	—	100
Tapioca	1 pkg (4 oz)	140	3	2	5	3	25	0	150	160	—	0	—	100
Vanilla	1 pkg (4 oz)	130	3	2	10	3	22	1	150	150	—	0	—	100
MATTHEW WALKER														
Plum	3.5 oz	290	7	—	—	3	60	1	150	100	400	2	—	0
SNACK PACK														
Banana	4.25 oz	145	6	1	1	2	22	0	63	180	85	—	—	31
Butterscotch	4.25 oz	170	6	1	1	2	27	0	69	210	90	—	—	33
Chocolate	4.25 oz	170	6	1	1	2	26	0	55	120	145	—	—	27
Chocolate Marshmallow	4.25 oz	165	6	1	1	2	26	0	55	125	95	—	—	27
Chocolate Fudge	4.25 oz	165	6	1	1	2	27	0	55	125	150	—	—	27
Lemon	4.25 oz	150	4	1	0	tr	30	tr	7	75	10	—	—	—
Light Chocolate	4.25 oz	100	2	tr	1	3	20	0	95	120	210	—	—	38
Light Tapioca	4.25 oz	100	2	tr	1	2	18	0	64	105	85	—	—	30
Tapioca	4.25 oz	150	5	1	1	2	23	0	87	125	150	—	—	42
Vanilla	4.25 oz	170	6	1	1	2	27	0	63	150	85	—	—	31
SWISS MISS														
Butterscotch	4 oz	180	6	1	5	2	29	0	98	135	130	—	—	—
Chocolate	4 oz	180	6	1	5	2	29	0	100	160	250	—	—	—
Chocolate Fudge	4 oz	220	6	2	5	3	38	0	100	180	240	—	—	—
Chocolate Sundae	4 oz	220	7	2	5	2	36	0	77	140	200	—	—	—
Light Chocolate	4 oz	100	1	tr	0	3	20	0	80	120	210	—	—	20
Light Chocolate Fudge	4 oz	100	1	tr	0	3	20	0	80	120	180	—	—	20
Light Vanilla	4 oz	100	1	tr	0	2	20	0	60	105	90	—	—	—
Light Vanilla Chocolate Parfait	4 oz	100	1	tr	0	2	20	0	80	110	140	—	—	20
Tapioca	4 oz	160	5	1	5	2	27	0	99	170	130	—	—	—

FOOD	PORTION	CALORIES	FAT	SAT FAT	CHOL	PROTEIN	CARBO	FIBER	CALCIUM	SOD	POTAS	VIT C	FOLIC	VIT A
SWISS MISS (CONT.)														
Vanilla	4 oz	190	7	1	5	2	30	0	98	140	130	—	—	—
Vanilla Parfait	4 oz	180	6	1	1	2	29	0	100	150	190	—	—	—
Vanilla Sundae	4 oz	200	7	2	5	2	36	0	74	180	140	—	—	—
ULTRA SLIM-FAST														
Butterscotch	4 oz	100	tr	—	0	2	21	2	100	230	70	—	40	500
Chocolate	4 oz	100	tr	—	0	2	21	2	100	240	130	—	40	500
Vanilla	4 oz	100	tr	—	0	2	21	2	100	230	70	—	40	500
TAKE-OUT														
bread pudding	½ cup (4.4 oz)	212	7	3	83	7	31	—	143	291	282	1	16	304
chocolate	½ cup (5.5 oz)	206	4	2	9	5	41	—	155	157	256	1	7	290
tapioca	½ cup (5.3 oz)	189	7	—	124	7	26	—	159	288	216	1	14	314
vanilla	½ cup (4.3 oz)	130	4	3	17	4	20	—	145	113	185	1	5	153

PUDDING POPS

(*see also* ICE CREAM AND FROZEN DESSERTS, PUDDING)

FOOD	PORTION	CALORIES	FAT	SAT FAT	CHOL	PROTEIN	CARBO	FIBER	CALCIUM	SOD	POTAS	VIT C	FOLIC	VIT A
chocolate	1 (1.6 oz)	72	2	—	1	2	12	—	66	77	105	tr	1	52
vanilla	1 (1.6 oz)	75	2	—	1	2	13	—	61	50	65	tr	2	81

PUMMELO

FOOD	PORTION	CALORIES	FAT	SAT FAT	CHOL	PROTEIN	CARBO	FIBER	CALCIUM	SOD	POTAS	VIT C	FOLIC	VIT A
fresh	1	228	tr	—	0	5	59	—	23	7	1317	372	—	0
sections	1 cup	71	tr	—	0	1	18	—	7	2	411	116	—	0

PUMPKIN

FOOD	PORTION	CALORIES	FAT	SAT FAT	CHOL	PROTEIN	CARBO	FIBER	CALCIUM	SOD	POTAS	VIT C	FOLIC	VIT A
CANNED														
pumpkin	½ cup	41	tr	tr	0	1	10	—	32	6	251	5	15	26908
LIBBY														
Solid Pack	½ cup	60	1	—	0	2	15	4	20	5	—	5	—	17500
FRESH														
cooked mashed	½ cup	24	tr	tr	0	1	6	—	18	2	281	6	—	1320
flowers cooked	½ cup	10	tr	tr	0	1	2	—	25	4	71	3	—	1162
flowers raw	1	0	0	0	0	tr	tr	—	1	0	3	1	—	39
leaves cooked	½ cup	7	tr	tr	0	1	1	—	15	3	153	tr	—	866
leaves raw	½ cup	4	tr	tr	0	1	tr	—	8	2	87	2	—	388
raw cubed	½ cup	15	tr	tr	0	1	4	—	12	1	197	5	—	928
SEEDS														
dried	1 oz	154	13	2	0	7	5	—	12	5	229	—	—	108
roasted	1 cup	1184	96	18	0	75	31	—	97	40	1829	—	—	—
roasted	1 oz	148	12	2	0	9	4	—	12	5	229	—	—	—
salted & roasted	1 cup	1184	96	18	0	75	31	—	97	1294	1829	—	—	—
salted & roasted	1 oz	148	12	2	0	9	4	—	12	144	229	—	—	—
whole roasted	1 oz	127	6	1	0	5	15	—	16	5	261	—	—	—
whole roasted	1 cup	285	12	2	0	12	34	—	35	12	588	—	—	—
whole salted roasted	1 oz	127	6	1	0	5	15	—	16	191	261	—	—	—
whole salted roasted	1 cup	285	12	2	0	12	34	—	35	268	588	—	—	—

FOOD	PORTION	CALORIES	FAT	SAT FAT	CHOL	PROTEIN	CARBO	FIBER	CALCIUM	SOD	POTAS	VIT C	FOLIC	VIT A
PURSLANE														
cooked	1 cup	21	tr	—	0	2	4	—	90	51	561	12	—	2130
raw	1 cup	7	tr	—	0	1	1	—	28	20	213	9	—	568
QUAHOGS														
(*see* CLAM)														
QUAIL														
breast w/o skin raw	1 (2 oz)	69	2	tr	—	13	0	—	5	31	146	3	—	21
w/ skin raw	1 quail (3.8 oz)	210	13	4	—	21	0	—	14	58	235	7	8	265
w/o skin raw	1 quail (3.2 oz)	123	4	1	—	20	0	—	12	47	218	—	—	52
QUICHE														
TAKE-OUT														
lorraine	⅛ of 8 in pie	600	48	23	285	13	29	—	211	653	283	tr	—	1640
QUINCE														
fresh	1	53	tr	tr	0	tr	14	—	10	4	181	14	—	37
QUINOA														
quinoa	½ cup	318	5	tr	0	11	59	—	51	—	629	—	—	—
ARROWHEAD														
Quinoa	¼ cup (1.4 oz)	140	2	0	0	5	25	4	40	0	250	0	—	0
EDEN														
Not Prep	¼ cup (1.6 oz)	170	3	0	0	6	31	3	0	0	210	0	—	0
RABBIT														
wild w/o bone stewed	3 oz	147	3	1	104	28	0	—	15	38	292	—	—	—
RACCOON														
roasted	3 oz	217	12	—	—	25	0	—	—	—	—	—	—	—
RADICCHIO														
leaf	3.5 oz	18	tr	tr	—	1	3	1	—	—	—	—	—	—
RADISHES														
DRIED														
chinese	½ cup	157	tr	tr	0	5	37	—	165	161	2027	0	—	0
daikon	½ cup	157	tr	tr	0	5	37	—	365	161	2027	0	—	0
FRESH														
chinese raw	1 (12 oz)	62	tr	tr	0	2	14	—	91	71	767	74	—	0
chinese raw sliced	½ cup	8	tr	tr	0	tr	2	—	12	9	100	10	—	0
chinese sliced cooked	½ cup	13	tr	tr	0	tr	3	—	12	10	211	11	—	0
daikon raw	1 (12 oz)	62	tr	tr	0	2	14	—	91	71	767	74	—	0
daikon raw sliced	½ cup	8	tr	tr	0	tr	2	—	12	9	100	10	—	0
daikon sliced cooked	½ cup	13	tr	tr	0	tr	3	—	12	10	211	11	—	0
red raw	10	7	tr	tr	0	tr	2	—	9	11	104	10	12	3
red sliced	½ cup	10	tr	tr	0	tr	2	—	12	14	134	13	16	4

FOOD	PORTION	CALORIES	FAT	SAT FAT	CHOL	PROTEIN	CARBO	FIBER	CALCIUM	SOD	POTAS	VIT C	FOLIC	VIT A
DOLE														
Radishes	7	20	0	—	0	0	3	0	—	35	200	19	—	—
SPROUTS														
raw	½ cup	8	tr	tr	0	1	1	—	10	1	16	6	18	74
RAISINS														
chocolate coated	10 (0.4 oz)	39	2	1	0	tr	7	—	9	4	51	0	—	4
chocolate coated	1 cup (6.7 oz)	741	28	17	5	8	130	—	163	68	976	tr	—	71
seedless	1 tbsp	27	tr	tr	0	tr	7	—	—	—	—	—	—	—
CINDERELLA														
Seedless	½ cup	250	0	—	0	—	—	—	46	—	—	—	—	—
DEL MONTE														
Golden	¼ cup (1.4 oz)	130	0	0	0	0	31	2	0	10	—	0	—	0
Raisins	1 box (1.5 oz)	140	0	0	0	0	33	3	0	10	—	0	—	0
Raisins	1 box (1 oz)	90	0	0	0	0	22	2	0	5	—	0	—	0
Raisins	1 box (0.5 oz)	45	0	0	0	0	11	tr	0	0	—	0	—	0
Raisins	¼ cup (1.4 oz)	130	0	0	0	0	31	2	0	10	—	0	—	0
Yogurt Raisins Strawberry	1 pkg (0.9 oz)	110	3	3	0	2	20	tr	40	25	—	0	—	0
Yogurt Raisins Vanilla	1 pkg (0.9 oz)	110	3	3	0	2	20	tr	40	25	—	0	—	0
Yogurt Raisins Vanilla	1 pkg (1 oz)	120	3	3	0	2	22	tr	40	25	—	0	—	0
Yogurt Raisins Vanilla	3 tbsp (1 oz)	130	3	3	0	2	23	1	60	30	—	0	—	0
DOLE														
Golden	½ cup	250	0	0	0	3	66	—	—	25	630	—	—	—
Seedless	½ cup	250	0	0	0	3	66	—	—	15	670	—	—	—
SONOMA														
Monukka Thompson	¼ cup (1.4 oz)	130	0	0	0	1	31	2	0	10	—	0	—	0
TREE OF LIFE														
Organic	¼ cup (1.4 oz)	130	0	0	0	1	31	2	20	10	310	9	—	0
RASPBERRIES														
CANNED														
in heavy syrup	½ cup	117	tr	tr	0	1	30	—	14	4	120	11	13	43
FRESH														
raspberries	1 cup	61	1	tr	0	1	14	—	27	0	187	31	—	160
raspberries	1 pint	154	2	tr	0	3	36	—	69	0	474	78	—	406
DOLE														
Raspberries	1 cup	45	0	—	0	1	10	9	—	0	190	29	—	—
FROZEN														
sweetened	1 cup	256	tr	tr	0	2	65	—	38	1	285	41	65	149
sweetened	1 pkg (10 oz)	291	tr	tr	0	2	74	—	43	1	324	47	74	169
BIG VALLEY														
Raspberries	⅔ cup (4.9 oz)	80	0	0	0	1	18	3	30	0	—	30	—	150

FOOD	PORTION	CALORIES	FAT	SAT FAT	CHOL	PROTEIN	CARBO	FIBER	CALCIUM	SOD	POTAS	VIT C	FOLIC	VIT A
BIRDS EYE														
Red	½ cup (4.4 oz)	90	0	0	0	tr	22	5	—	5	—	18	—	—

RASPBERRY JUICE

FOOD	PORTION	CALORIES	FAT	SAT FAT	CHOL	PROTEIN	CARBO	FIBER	CALCIUM	SOD	POTAS	VIT C	FOLIC	VIT A
CRYSTAL GEYSER														
Juice Squeeze Mountain Raspberry	1 bottle (12 fl oz)	135	0	0	0	1	32	—			20	—	—	160	—
CRYSTAL LIGHT														
Raspberry Ice Drink	1 serv (8 oz)	5	0	0	0	0	0	0	0	20	60	0		0
Raspberry Ice Drink Mix as prep	1 serv (8 oz)	5	0	0	0	0	0	0	0	0	0	6	—	0
FRESH SAMANTHA														
Raspberry Dream	1 cup (8 oz)	120	1	0	0	2	30	2	20	0	—	66	40	300
KOOL-AID														
Drink Mix as prep	1 serv (8 oz)	60	0	0	0	0	17	0	0	0	0	6	—	0
Raspberry Drink as prep w/ sugar	1 serv (8 oz)	100	0	0	0	0	25	0	0	30	0	6	—	0
Splash Blue Raspberry Drink	1 serv (8 oz)	120	0	0	0	0	30	0	0	35	15	0	—	0

RED BEANS

FOOD	PORTION	CALORIES	FAT	SAT FAT	CHOL	PROTEIN	CARBO	FIBER	CALCIUM	SOD	POTAS	VIT C	FOLIC	VIT A
CANNED														
ALLEN														
Red Beans	½ cup (4.5 oz)	160	1	0	0	6	19	9	40	310	—	0	—	0
GREEN GIANT														
Red Beans	½ cup (4.5 oz)	100	1	0	0	6	19	6	40	350	—	0	—	0
HUNT'S														
Small	½ cup (4.5 oz)	89	1	0	0	6	19	6	3	713	—	1	—	0
VAN CAMP'S														
Red Beans	½ cup (4.6 oz)	90	0	0	0	6	20	5	20	560	410	—	100	0
DRIED														
BEAN CUISINE														
Dried	½ cup	115	1	—	0	8	—	5	—	5	310	—	62	—
MIX														
BEAN CUISINE														
Pasta & Beans Barcelona Red With Radiatore	½ cup	170	4	1	tr	60	170	—	—	379	—	—	—	—
MAHATMA														
Red Beans & Rice	1 cup	190	1	0	0	8	40	7	40	790	—	6	—	500

RED KIDNEY BEANS

FOOD	PORTION	CALORIES	FAT	SAT FAT	CHOL	PROTEIN	CARBO	FIBER	CALCIUM	SOD	POTAS	VIT C	FOLIC	VIT A
DRIED														
HURST														
HamBeens w/ Ham	1 serv	120	1	0	0	8	20	10	40	63	—	1	—	0

RELISH

FOOD	PORTION	CALORIES	FAT	SAT FAT	CHOL	PROTEIN	CARBO	FIBER	CALCIUM	SOD	POTAS	VIT C	FOLIC	VIT A
cranberry orange	½ cup	246	tr	—	0	tr	64	—	15	44	53	25	—	97

FOOD	PORTION	CALORIES	FAT	SAT FAT	CHOL	PROTEIN	CARBO	FIBER	CALCIUM	SOD	POTAS	VIT C	FOLIC	VIT A
DEL MONTE														
Hamburger	1 tbsp (0.5 oz)	20	0	0	0	0	6	tr	0	220	—	0	—	200
Hot Dog	1 tbsp (0.5 oz)	15	0	0	0	0	4	tr	0	140	—	0	—	0
Sweet Pickle	1 tbsp (0.5 oz)	20	0	0	0	0	5	0	0	125	—	0	—	0
GREEN GIANT														
Corn	1 tbsp (0.6 oz)	20	0	0	0	0	5	0	0	40	—	0	—	0
OLD EL PASO														
Jalapeno	1 tbsp (0.5 oz)	5	0	0	0	0	1	0	0	110	—	0	—	0
VLASIC														
Dill	1 oz	2	0	0	0	0	1	—	—	415	—	—	—	—
Hamburger	1 oz	40	0	0	0	0	9	—	—	255	—	—	—	100
Hot Dog	1 oz	40	1	—	—	0	8	—	—	255	—	1	—	—
Hot Piccalilli	1 oz	35	0	0	0	0	8	—	—	165	—	—	—	100
India	1 oz	30	0	0	0	0	8	—	—	205	—	—	—	—
Sweet	1 oz	30	0	0	0	0	8	—	—	220	—	—	—	—
RENNIN														
tablet	1 (0.9 g)	1	0	—	—	0	tr	—	34	234	3	0	—	0
RHUBARB														
fresh	½ cup	13	tr	—	0	1	3	—	52	2	175	5	4	61
frzn	½ cup	60	tr	—	0	tr	3	—	132	1	73	3	6	73
frzn as prep w/ sugar	½ cup	139	tr	—	0	tr	37	—	174	2	115	4	6	83
RICE														
(*see also* BRAN, CEREAL, FLOUR, RICE CAKES, WILD RICE)														
brown long grain cooked	½ cup	109	tr	tr	0	3	23	2	10	5	42	0	4	—
brown medium grain cooked	½ cup	109	tr	tr	0	2	23	—	10	1	77	0	4	—
glutinous cooked	½ cup	116	tr	tr	0	2	25	—	2	6	12	0	1	—
white long grain cooked	½ cup	131	tr	tr	0	3	28	tr	12	2	40	0	3	—
white long grain instant cooked	½ cup	80	tr	tr	0	2	17	tr	6	2	3	0	3	—
white medium grain cooked	½ cup	132	tr	tr	0	2	29	—	3	0	30	0	2	—
white short grain cooked	½ cup	133	tr	tr	0	2	29	—	1	0	27	0	2	—
ARROWHEAD														
Basmati Brown	¼ cup (1.5 oz)	150	1	0	0	3	33	2	20	0	90	0	—	0
Basmati White	¼ cup (1.5 oz)	150	0	0	0	4	34	tr	0	0	—	0	—	0
Brown Quick Regular	⅓ cup (1.5 oz)	150	1	0	0	3	32	2	20	0	85	0	—	0
Brown Quick Spanish Style	¼ pkg (1.4 oz)	150	1	0	0	4	30	2	20	250	85	0	—	0
Brown Quick Vegetable Herb	¼ pkg (1.4 oz)	150	1	0	0	4	30	3	20	160	80	0	—	0

FOOD	PORTION	CALORIES	FAT	SAT FAT	CHOL	PROTEIN	CARBO	FIBER	CALCIUM	SOD	POTAS	VIT C	FOLIC	VIT A
ARROWHEAD (CONT.)														
Brown Quick Wild Rice & Herb	¼ pkg (1.3 oz)	140	1	0	0	4	28	3	20	220	80	0	—	0
BIRDS EYE														
Rice & Broccoli In Cheese Sauce	1 pkg (10 oz)	290	9	3	15	8	44	2	100	1110	—	21	—	300
White & Wild	1 cup (6.6 oz)	180	4	2	10	4	31	2	40	480	—	1	—	0
BUDGET GOURMET														
Oriental Rice With Vegetables	1 pkg (5.75 oz)	230	12	—	20	4	28	—	20	420	150	9	—	1000
Rice Pilaf With Green Beans	1 pkg (5.5 oz)	230	11	—	10	4	30	—	40	510	80	9	—	400
CAROLINA														
Red Beans & Rice as prep	¼ pkg	190	1	0	0	6	40	6	40	790	—	6	—	500
CASBAH														
Basmati as prep	1 cup	158	tr	—	—	3	36	—	—	—	—	—	—	—
Jambalaya	1 pkg (1.4 oz)	130	0	0	0	4	27	1	350	500	—	24	—	1400
La Fiesta	1 pkg (1.59 oz)	170	1	0	0	6	34	0	40	400	—	—	—	100
Nutted Pilaf as prep	1 cup	220	3	0	0	6	40	1	40	460	—	0	—	0
Pilaf as prep	1 cup	200	tr	0	0	6	44	tr	40	430	—	0	—	0
Spanish Pilaf as prep	1 cup	200	1	0	0	6	44	1	140	430	—	34	—	1600
Thai Yum	1 pkg (1.7 oz)	180	3	0	0	5	33	1	50	500	—	2	—	1700
CHUN KING														
Fried Rice	1 pkg (8 oz)	290	6	2	25	11	48	5	20	1310	—	0	—	750
Fried Rice With Chicken	1 pkg (8 oz)	270	6	2	25	9	44	4	20	1330	—	0	—	100
GOODMAN'S														
Rice & Vermicelli For Beef	¾ cup	160	1	0	5	4	33	0	0	860	—	0	—	0
Rice & Vermicelli For Chicken	¾ cup	160	1	0	0	4	33	1	0	920	—	0	—	0
GOYA														
Arroz Amarillo	¼ cup (1.6 oz)	170	0	0	0	4	37	1	0	546	—	0	—	0
GREEN GIANT														
Rice & Broccoli	1 pkg (10 oz)	320	12	4	15	8	44	2	150	1000	—	18	—	4500
Rice Medley	1 pkg (10 oz)	240	3	2	5	6	46	2	40	880	—	6	—	300
Rice Pilaf	1 pkg (10 oz)	230	3	2	5	6	44	3	40	1020	—	5	—	4000
White & Wild	1 pkg (10 oz)	250	5	1	0	6	45	3	60	1000	—	5	—	300
HAIN														
Almondine	½ cup	130	5	—	0	3	17	—	—	260	100	—	—	—
Oriental 3-Grain Goodness	½ cup	120	5	—	—	4	15	—	20	300	100	—	—	750

FOOD	PORTION	CALORIES	FAT	SAT FAT	CHOL	PROTEIN	CARBO	FIBER	CALCIUM	SOD	POTAS	VIT C	FOLIC	VIT A
KITCHEN DEL SOL														
Mediterranean Paella Costa Brave as prep	½ cup (1.2 oz)	130	2	tr	0	3	23	1	40	312	—	15	—	100
Mediterranean Sunny Lemon Pilaf as prep	½ cup (1.2 oz)	110	1	0	0	3	22	1	20	210	—	42	—	750
Mediterranean Tomato & Basil With Pine Nuts	½ cup (1 oz)	110	4	1	0	2	18	1	0	270	—	27	—	200
LA CHOY														
Chinese Fried Rice	¾ cup	190	1	tr	0	4	41	tr	14	820	30	—	—	—
LIPTON														
Golden Saute Onion Mushroom	½ cup (2.1 oz)	240	4	2	0	6	45	2	0	850	—	0	—	0
Oriental Stir Fry as prep	1 cup	270	8	1	0	5	47	1	0	860	—	2	80	750
Rice & Sauce Alfredo Broccoli as prep	1 cup	320	12	5	15	9	46	1	150	990	—	6	100	500
Rice & Sauce Beef as prep	1 cup	270	8	1	0	6	47	1	0	1010	—	0	80	200
Rice & Sauce Cajun Style as prep	1 cup	270	7	1	0	7	46	1	0	910	—	4	80	500
Rice & Sauce Cajun Style w/ Beans as prep	1 cup	310	8	1	0	10	52	7	0	530	—	1	100	500
Rice & Sauce Cheddar Broccoli as prep	1 cup	280	9	3	5	7	46	1	40	1010	—	5	100	400
Rice & Sauce Chicken & Parmesan Risotto as prep	1 cup	270	9	2	0	6	43	tr	0	830	—	0	100	200
Rice & Sauce Chicken Broccoli as prep	1 cup	280	9	2	0	7	46	2	20	910	—	6	100	500
Rice & Sauce Chicken Flavor as prep	1 cup	280	9	2	5	7	45	1	0	960	—	0	60	300
Rice & Sauce Creamy Chicken as prep	1 cup	290	11	3	0	6	45	1	0	830	—	0	80	750
Rice & Sauce Herb & Butter as prep	1 cup	280	11	4	10	6	43	tr	0	880	—	0	80	300
Rice & Sauce Medley as prep	1 cup	270	9	2	5	7	44	2	0	870	—	0	80	500

FOOD	PORTION	CALORIES	FAT	SAT FAT	CHOL	PROTEIN	CARBO	FIBER	CALCIUM	SOD	POTAS	VIT C	FOLIC	VIT A
LIPTON (CONT.)														
Rice & Sauce Mushroom as prep	1 cup	270	8	1	0	6	45	1	20	960	—	0	80	0
Rice & Sauce Mushroom & Herb as prep	1 cup	290	8	2	0	6	49	1	20	620	—	1	80	300
Rice & Sauce Oriental as prep	1 cup	280	8	1	0	7	48	2	20	940	—	2	60	750
Rice & Sauce Pilaf as prep	1 cup	260	11	1	0	6	44	1	20	930	—	0	80	400
Rice & Sauce Scampi Style as prep	1 cup	270	9	2	5	6	44	1	0	900	—	0	80	200
Rice & Sauce Spanish as prep	1 cup	270	8	1	0	6	47	2	0	900	—	5	80	500
Rice & Sauce Teriyaki as prep	1 cup	270	8	1	0	5	45	1	0	910	—	0	80	300
Roasted Chicken as prep	1 cup	260	8	1	0	4	46	1	0	880	—	0	80	500
Salsa Style as prep	1 cup	220	7	1	0	4	37	2	0	540	—	4	60	400
Southwestern Chicken Flavor as prep	1 cup	260	11	1	0	5	47	1	0	840	—	2	80	750
LUIGINO'S														
Fried Rice Chicken	1 pkg (8 oz)	250	5	2	55	11	38	2	60	640	—	0	—	100
Fried Rice Pork	1 pkg (8 oz)	250	7	3	60	11	37	2	60	830	—	0	—	100
Fried Rice Pork & Shrimp	1 pkg (8 oz)	250	5	2	55	10	39	2	60	890	—	0	—	0
Fried Rice Shrimp	1 pkg (8 oz)	220	4	2	60	9	38	2	80	730	—	0	—	200
Risotto Parmesano	1 pkg (8 oz)	360	20	6	50	14	30	2	350	740	—	0	—	500
MAHATMA														
Broccoli & Cheese	1 cup	200	2	1	5	5	41	2	80	620	—	2	—	100
Jambalaya	1 cup (2 oz)	190	1	0	0	4	43	tr	20	700	—	1	—	500
Long Grain & Wild	1 cup (2 oz)	190	1	0	0	5	41	2	20	1240	—	0	—	0
Pilaf	1 cup (2 oz)	190	0	0	0	5	43	tr	0	820	—	0	—	0
Spanish	1 cup (2 oz)	180	1	0	0	4	42	2	20	760	—	4	—	0
Yellow Rice Mix	1 cup	190	0	0	0	4	43	tr	40	970	—	4	—	0
MELTING POT														
Risotto Melanese w/ Saffron	1 cup	210	0	0	0	4	48	0	0	70	—	5	—	0
Risotto Primavera	1 cup	200	1	0	0	5	44	1	0	85	—	1	—	300
Risotto Sun-Dried Tomatoes & Peas	1 cup	200	1	0	0	5	45	1	0	75	—	0	—	100
Risotto Three Cheese	1 cup	200	2	1	5	5	44	0	20	410	—	0	—	200
Risotto Wild Mushroom	1 cup	200	1	0	0	5	44	2	0	50	—	0	—	750

FOOD	PORTION	CALORIES	FAT	SAT FAT	CHOL	PROTEIN	CARBO	FIBER	CALCIUM	SOD	POTAS	VIT C	FOLIC	VIT A
MINUTE														
Boil-In-Bag White as prep	1 cup (5.7 oz)	190	0	0	0	4	42	tr	0	10	15	0	80	0
Instant Brown as prep	1 cup (5.2 oz)	170	2	0	0	4	34	2	0	10	40	0	0	0
Instant White as prep	1 cup (5.7 oz)	160	0	0	0	3	36	tr	0	5	10	0	60	0
Long Grain & Wild Seasoned w/ Herbs as prep	1 cup (7.8 oz)	230	1	0	0	6	50	1	20	950	95	0	80	0
NEAR EAST														
Barley Pilaf as prep	1 cup	220	4	1	0	6	41	5	—	620	200	—	8	500
Beef Pilaf as prep	1 cup	220	5	1	0	5	42	1	—	850	150	—	8	750
Curry Rice as prep	1 cup	220	4	1	0	5	42	1	—	660	160	—	8	1250
Lentil Pilaf as prep	1 cup	210	4	1	0	10	37	0	—	650	460	—	120	1500
Long Grain & Wild as prep	1 cup	220	5	1	0	6	42	2	—	810	170	—	8	400
Pilaf Brown Rice as prep	1 cup	220	5	1	0	6	41	2	—	710	180	—	8	1000
Pilaf Chicken as prep	1 cup	220	5	1	0	5	42	1	—	940	130	—	8	200
Pilaf Kosher as prep	1 cup	220	5	1	0	6	42	1	—	870	110	—	8	200
Spanish Pilaf as prep	1 cup	230	6	1	0	5	42	1	—	990	170	—	8	1000
OLD EL PASO														
Mexican	½ cup (4 oz)	410	2	1	0	8	90	3	150	1350	—	48	—	300
Spanish	1 cup (8.6 oz)	130	1	—	0	3	28	2	0	1340	—	0	—	0
PRITIKIN														
Mexican	⅓ cup (2 oz)	200	2	0	0	—	43	—	—	105	270	—	—	—
Oriental	⅓ cup (2 oz)	190	2	0	0	—	43	—	—	260	360	—	—	—
SUCCESS														
Beef Oriental	½ cup	190	1	0	0	5	43	2	40	920	—	9	—	0
Broccoli & Cheese	½ cup	200	2	1	10	6	41	2	80	690	—	2	—	0
Brown & Wild	½ cup	190	1	0	0	6	40	3	20	830	—	0	—	40
Classic Chicken	½ cup	150	1	0	0	4	32	1	20	720	—	2	—	100
Long Grain & Wild	½ cup	190	0	0	0	5	42	1	20	890	—	6	—	100
Pilaf	½ cup	200	0	0	0	5	44	2	20	630	—	1	—	300
Spanish	½ cup	190	1	0	0	5	43	1	80	780	—	5	—	750
ULTRA SLIM-FAST														
Oriental Style	2.3 oz	240	1	—	—	5	58	4	150	900	110	18	—	750
Rice & Chicken Sauce	2.3 oz	240	1	—	—	5	56	4	150	1080	100	18	—	750
UNCLE BEN														
Boil-In-Bag	1 serv (0.9 oz)	94	tr	—	0	2	22	tr	4	9	5	0	—	0
Brown	1 serv (1.6 oz)	158	1	—	0	4	34	1	4	1	107	0	—	0
Brown & Wild Fast Cooking	1 serv (1.3 oz)	120	1	—	tr	4	26	1	12	383	182	2	—	0

FOOD	PORTION	CALORIES	FAT	SAT FAT	CHOL	PROTEIN	CARBO	FIBER	CALCIUM	SOD	POTAS	VIT C	FOLIC	VIT A
UNCLE BEN (CONT.)														
Country Inn Broccoli Almondine	1 serv (1.2 oz)	124	2	—	tr	4	25	1	24	367	0	2	—	0
Country Inn Broccoli & White Cheddar	1 serv (1.2 oz)	131	3	—	3	4	24	1	44	288	0	1	—	32
Country Inn Broccoli Au Gratin	1 serv (1.1 oz)	116	2	—	2	4	22	1	42	342	0	3	—	29
Country Inn Chicken Stock	1 serv (1.2 oz)	123	1	—	3	4	24	1	17	269	85	1	—	20
Country Inn Chicken With Wild Rice	1 serv (1.1 oz)	108	1	—	1	3	23	1	13	359	0	0	—	5
Country Inn Creamy Chicken & Mushroom	1 serv (1.3 oz)	138	3	—	2	4	24	1	25	380	0	tr	—	63
Country Inn Creamy Chicken & Wild Rice	1 serv (1.3 oz)	135	1	—	4	4	27	1	45	340	0	tr	—	32
Country Inn Green Bean Almondine	1 serv (1.2 oz)	128	2	—	2	4	25	1	26	280	0	1	—	13
Country Inn Herbed Au Gratin	1 serv (1.2 oz)	119	2	—	3	3	24	1	38	361	0	tr	—	18
Country Inn Homestyle Chicken & Vegetables	1 serv (1.3 oz)	139	3	—	7	4	24	1	23	298	83	tr	—	53
Country Inn Rice Florentine	1 serv (1.2 oz)	212	2	—	3	4	24	1	34	354	137	1	—	26
Country Inn Vegetable Pilaf	1 serv (1.2 oz)	115	1	—	1	3	25	1	15	357	0	2	—	0
In An Instant	1 serv (1.1 oz)	111	tr	—	0	2	25	tr	0	10	7	0	—	0
Long Grain & Wild Chicken Stock Sauce	1 serv (1.3 oz)	133	2	—	5	4	25	1	19	601	80	6	—	0
Long Grain & Wild Fast Cooking	1 serv (1 oz)	101	tr	—	1	3	22	1	8	450	47	1	—	0
Long Grain & Wild Garden Vegetable Blend	1 serv (1.3 oz)	128	1	—	1	4	26	1	19	601	133	1	—	0
Long Grain & Wild Original	1 serv (1 oz)	96	tr	—	tr	3	21	1	16	363	90	2	—	0
White Converted	1 serv (1.2 oz)	123	tr	—	0	3	27	tr	12	1	48	0	—	0
VAN CAMP'S														
Spanish	1 cup (9 oz)	180	3	1	0	3	37	3	20	1290	250	—	0	1000
WATKINS														
Brown & Wild	¼ cup (1.6 oz)	160	0	0	0	4	34	3	0	10	—	0	—	0

FOOD	PORTION	CALORIES	FAT	SAT FAT	CHOL	PROTEIN	CARBO	FIBER	CALCIUM	SOD	POTAS	VIT C	FOLIC	VIT A
WATKINS (CONT.)														
Calico Medley	¼ cup (1.6 oz)	160	0	0	0	4	37	4	40	30	—	0	—	0
East/West Medley	¼ cup (1.6 oz)	160	0	0	0	6	33	5	20	0	—	0	—	0
Heartland Medley	¼ cup (1.6 oz)	160	0	0	0	5	35	4	20	10	—	0	—	0
Minnesota Medley	¼ cup (1.6 oz)	160	0	0	0	5	34	2	100	10	—	0	—	0
White & Wild	¼ cup (1.6 oz)	160	0	0	0	4	34	1	40	5	—	0	—	0
TAKE-OUT														
nasi goreng indonesian rice & vegetables	1 cup (4.9 oz)	130	0	0	0	4	28	1	20	530	—	5	—	2250

RICE CAKES

(see also POPCORN CAKES)

FOOD	PORTION	CALORIES	FAT	SAT FAT	CHOL	PROTEIN	CARBO	FIBER	CALCIUM	SOD	POTAS	VIT C	FOLIC	VIT A
brown rice	1 (0.3 oz)	35	tr	tr	0	1	7	tr	1	29	26	0	2	0
brown rice & buckwheat	1 (0.3 oz)	34	tr	tr	0	1	7	tr	1	10	27	0	2	0
brown rice & buckwheat unsalted	1 (0.3 oz)	34	tr	tr	0	1	7	tr	1	tr	27	0	2	0
brown rice & corn	1 (0.3 oz)	35	tr	tr	0	1	7	—	1	26	25	0	2	0
brown rice & rye	1 (0.3 oz)	35	tr	tr	0	1	7	tr	2	10	28	0	0	—
brown rice & sesame seed	1 (0.3 oz)	35	tr	tr	0	1	7	—	1	20	26	—	2	0
brown rice multigrain	1 (0.3 oz)	35	tr	tr	0	1	7	—	2	23	26	0	2	0
brown rice multigrain unsalted	1 (0.3 oz)	35	tr	tr	0	1	7	—	2	tr	26	0	2	0
brown rice unsalted	1 (0.3 oz)	35	tr	tr	0	1	7	tr	1	3	26	0	2	0
HAIN														
5-Grain	1	40	tr	—	—	tr	8	—	—	10	20	—	—	—
Mini Apple Cinnamon	½ oz	60	tr	—	0	1	12	0	—	10	60	—	—	—
Mini Barbeque	½ oz	70	3	—	0	1	10	0	—	50	40	—	—	—
Mini Cheese	½ oz	60	2	—	<5	1	10	0	—	100	50	—	—	—
Mini Honey Nut	½ oz	60	tr	—	0	1	11	0	—	30	40	—	—	—
Mini Nacho Cheese	½ oz	70	2	—	<5	1	10	—	—	90	95	—	—	—
Mini Plain	½ oz	60	tr	—	0	1	12	0	—	20	40	—	—	—
Mini Plain No Salt Added	½ oz	60	tr	—	0	1	12	0	—	5	40	—	—	—
Mini Ranch	½ oz	70	3	—	0	1	9	—	—	90	40	—	—	—
Mini Teriyaki	½ oz	50	tr	—	0	1	12	0	—	75	40	—	—	—
Plain	1	40	tr	—	—	tr	8	—	—	10	20	—	—	—
Plain No Salt Added	1	40	tr	—	—	tr	8	—	—	<5	35	—	—	—
Sesame	1	40	tr	—	—	tr	8	—	—	10	25	—	—	—
Sesame No Salt	1	40	tr	—	—	tr	8	—	—	<5	30	—	—	—

FOOD	PORTION	CALORIES	FAT	SAT FAT	CHOL	PROTEIN	CARBO	FIBER	CALCIUM	SOD	POTAS	VIT C	FOLIC	VIT A
KA-ME														
Cheese	16 pieces (1 oz)	120	2	0	0	3	24	0	—	180	—	—	—	—
Onion	16 pieces (1 oz)	120	1	0	0	3	25	0	—	75	—	—	—	—
Plain	16 pieces (1 oz)	120	2	0	0	3	25	0	—	15	—	—	—	—
Seaweed	16 pieces (1 oz)	120	2	0	0	3	25	0	—	100	—	—	—	—
Sesame	16 pieces (1 oz)	120	2	0	0	3	24	0	—	85	—	—	—	—
Unsalted	16 pieces (1 oz)	120	1	0	0	3	26	0	—	0	—	—	—	—
LUNDBERG														
Organic Lightly Salted	1	60	1	—	—	1	14	—	<20	120	46	tr	—	<100
Organic Unsalted	1	60	1	—	—	1	14	—	<20	3	46	tr	—	<100
Premium Lightly Salted	1	60	1	—	—	1	14	—	<20	120	46	tr	—	<100
Premium Unsalted	1	60	1	—	—	1	14	—	<20	3	46	tr	—	<100
Sesame Lightly Salted	1	59	0	0	—	1	16	—	<20	6	46	tr	—	<100
MOTHER'S														
Mini Apple	5 (0.5 oz)	50	0	0	0	1	12	0	—	40	40	—	0	—
Mini Caramel	5 (0.5 oz)	50	0	0	0	1	12	0	—	40	40	—	0	—
Mini Cinnamon	5 (0.5 oz)	50	0	0	0	1	12	0	—	40	40	—	0	—
Mini Plain Unsalted	7 (0.5 oz)	60	0	0	0	1	12	0	—	0	40	—	0	—
Multigrain Lightly Salted	1 (0.3 oz)	35	0	0	0	1	7	0	—	30	30	—	0	—
Rye Unsalted	1 (0.3 oz)	35	0	0	0	1	7	1	—	0	45	—	0	—
Wheat Unsalted	1 (0.3 oz)	35	0	0	0	1	7	1	—	0	30	—	0	—
PRITIKIN														
Mini Apple Crisp	5 (0.5 oz)	50	0	0	0	—	12	—	—	20	30	—	—	—
Multigrain	1 (0.3 oz)	35	0	0	0	—	7	—	—	20	30	—	—	—
Multigrain Unsalted	1 (0.3 oz)	35	0	0	0	—	7	—	—	0	25	—	—	—
Plain	1 (0.3 oz)	35	0	0	0	—	7	—	—	20	25	—	—	—
Plain Unsalted	1 (0.3 oz)	35	0	0	0	—	7	—	—	0	25	—	—	—
Sesame Low Sodium	1 (0.3 oz)	35	0	0	0	—	7	—	—	20	25	—	—	—
Sesame Unsalted	1 (0.3 oz)	35	0	0	0	—	7	—	—	0	25	—	—	—
QUAKER														
Apple Cinnamon	1 (0.5 oz)	50	0	0	0	1	11	—	—	0	—	—	—	—
Banana Crunch	1 (0.5 oz)	50	0	0	0	1	11	—	—	45	—	—	—	—
Cinnamon Crunch	1 (0.5 oz)	50	0	0	0	1	11	—	—	25	—	—	—	—
Mini Apple Cinnamon	5 (0.5 oz)	50	0	0	0	1	12	—	—	0	—	—	—	—

FOOD	PORTION	CALORIES	FAT	SAT FAT	CHOL	PROTEIN	CARBO	FIBER	CALCIUM	SOD	POTAS	VIT C	FOLIC	VIT A
QUAKER (CONT.)														
Mini Banana Nut	5 (0.5 oz)	50	0	0	0	1	12	—	—	40	—	—	—	—
Mini Butter Popped Corn	6 (0.5 oz)	50	0	0	0	1	12	—	—	120	—	—	—	—
Mini Caramel Corn	5 (0.5 oz)	50	0	0	0	1	12	—	—	25	—	—	—	—
Mini Chocolate Crunch	5 (0.5 oz)	50	0	0	0	1	12	—	—	10	—	—	—	—
Mini Cinnamon Crunch	5 (0.5 oz)	50	0	0	0	1	12	—	—	25	—	—	—	—
Mini Honey Nut	5 (0.5 oz)	50	0	0	0	1	12	—	—	25	—	—	—	—
Mini Monterey Jack	6 (0.5 oz)	50	0	0	0	1	11	—	—	100	—	—	—	—
Mini White Cheddar	6 (0.5 oz)	50	0	0	0	1	11	—	—	120	—	—	—	—
Salt-Free	1 (0.3 oz)	35	0	0	0	1	7	—	—	0	—	—	—	—
Salted	1 (0.3 oz)	35	0	0	0	1	7	—	—	15	—	—	—	—
TREE OF LIFE														
Fat Free Mini Apple Cinnamon	15	60	0	0	0	1	13	0	—	5	—	—	—	—
Fat Free Mini Caramel	15	60	0	0	0	1	13	0	—	10	—	—	—	—
Fat Free Mini Honey Nut	15	60	0	0	0	1	13	0	—	0	—	—	—	—
Fat Free Mini Jalapeno	15	60	0	0	0	1	13	0	—	25	—	—	—	—
Fat Free Mini Plain	15	50	0	0	0	1	12	0	—	45	—	—	—	—
ROCKFISH														
pacific cooked	3 oz	103	2	tr	38	20	0	—	10	65	442	—	—	186
pacific cooked	1 fillet (5.2 oz)	180	3	1	66	36	0	—	18	114	774	—	—	327
pacific raw	3 oz	80	1	tr	29	16	0	—	8	51	344	—	—	162
ROE														
(*see also individual fish names*)														
fish	3.5 oz	39	2	tr	105	6	tr	—	—	—	—	—	—	—
ROLL														
(*see also* BISCUIT, CROISSANT, ENGLISH MUFFIN, MUFFIN, POPOVER, SCONE)														
FROZEN														
NEW YORK														
Garlic	1 (2 oz)	210	10	2	0	3	26	1	0	370	—	0	—	200
PEPPERIDGE FARM														
Cinnamon Roll	1 (2¼ oz)	220	14	—	—	4	34	—	20	190	—	—	—	—
SARA LEE														
Deluxe Cinnamon Rolls	1 (2.7 oz)	320	15	9	40	5	41	1	—	300	—	—	—	—
Deluxe Cinnamon Rolls w/ Icing	1	370	15	9	40	5	53	1	—	300	—	—	—	—

FOOD	PORTION	CALORIES	FAT	SAT FAT	CHOL	PROTEIN	CARBO	FIBER	CALCIUM	SOD	POTAS	VIT C	FOLIC	VIT A
HOME RECIPE														
dinner as prep w/ 2% milk	1 (2½ in)	111	3	1	12	3	19	—	21	145	53	tr	15	118
dinner as prep w/ whole milk	1 (2½ in)	112	3	1	13	3	19	—	21	145	53	tr	15	108
raisin & nut	1 (2 oz)	196	7	1	13	4	30	—	36	185	123	tr	18	233
MIX														
DROMEDARY														
Hot Roll Mix	2	239	5	—	—	6	41	—	20	410	—	—	—	250
NATURAL OVENS														
German Hard	1 (2.1 oz)	138	1	0	0	5	36	1	50	140	—	—	20	—
Gourmet Dinner	1 (1 oz)	50	1	0	0	3	15	2	100	140	—	—	—	—
Hearty Sandwich	1 (1.8 oz)	110	1	0	0	5	30	2	150	140	—	—	80	—
READY-TO-EAT														
brown & serve	1 (1 oz)	85	2	tr	0	2	14	—	34	148	38	—	8	—
cheese	1 (2.3 oz)	238	12	4	—	5	29	—	78	236	—	—	—	—
cinnamon raisin	1 (2¾ in)	223	10	3	40	4	31	1	43	229	67	1	14	129
dinner	1 (1 oz)	85	2	tr	0	2	14	—	34	148	38	—	8	—
egg	1 (2½ in)	107	2	1	—	3	18	1	21	191	—	0	—	—
french	1 (1.3 oz)	105	2	tr	0	3	19	—	35	232	43	0	—	—
hamburger	1 (1½ oz)	123	2	1	—	4	22	—	60	241	60	—	—	—
hamburger multi-grain	1 (1½ oz)	113	2	1	0	4	19	2	41	197	—	0	—	—
hamburger reduced calorie	1 (1½ oz)	84	1	tr	0	4	18	3	26	190	34	—	—	—
hard	1 (3½ in)	167	2	tr	0	6	30	—	54	310	61	0	8	0
hotdog	1 (1½ oz)	123	2	1	—	4	22	—	60	241	60	—	—	—
hotdog multi-grain	1 (1½ oz)	113	2	1	0	4	19	2	41	197	—	0	—	—
hotdog reduced calorie	1 (1½ oz)	84	1	tr	0	4	18	3	26	190	34	—	—	—
kaiser	1 (3½ in)	167	2	tr	0	6	30	—	54	310	61	0	8	0
oat bran	1 (1.2 oz)	78	2	tr	0	3	13	1	28	136	—	0	—	—
rye	1 (1 oz)	81	1	tr	0	3	15	—	9	253	51	0	—	—
submarine	1 (4.7 oz)	155	2	tr	tr	5	30	—	24	313	49	0	—	0
wheat	1 (1 oz)	77	2	tr	0	2	13	—	50	96	—	0	—	0
whole wheat	1 (1 oz)	75	1	tr	0	3	15	—	30	135	77	0	8	0
ALVARADO ST. BAKERY														
Burger Buns	1 (2.2 oz)	140	2	0	0	7	27	3	—	290	—	—	—	—
Hot Dog Buns	1 (2.2 oz)	140	2	0	0	7	28	3	—	290	—	—	—	—
ARNOLD														
8-inch Francisco	1 (2.5 oz)	210	3	—	—	7	39	—	80	260	—	—	—	—
Augusto Pan Cubano	1	230	3	—	0	7	43	2	80	500	—	—	—	—
Bakery Light	1 (1.5 oz)	80	<2	0	0	4	21	4	20	190	—	—	—	—
Bran'nola Buns	1 (1.5 oz)	100	1	0	0	5	20	3	20	160	—	—	—	—
Deli Kaiser	1	170	2	—	—	5	34	—	40	—	—	—	—	—

FOOD	PORTION	CALORIES	FAT	SAT FAT	CHOL	PROTEIN	CARBO	FIBER	CALCIUM	SOD	POTAS	VIT C	FOLIC	VIT A
ARNOLD (CONT.)														
Deli Onion	1	170	2	—	—	5	34	—	40	—	—	—	—	—
Dinner Plain	1 (0.7 oz)	50	1	0	tr	2	9	1	—	80	—	—	—	—
Dinner Sesame	1 (0.7 oz)	50	1	0	tr	2	9	1	—	80	—	—	—	—
Dutch Egg	1	130	3	tr	0	4	21	2	40	180	—	—	—	—
French Francisco	1 (2.5 oz)	210	3	—	—	7	39	—	80	260	—	—	—	—
French Mini Francisco	1	130	2	—	—	4	24	—	20	140	—	—	—	—
Hamburger	1	120	2	—	0	4	20	2	20	190	—	—	—	—
Hot Dog	1 (1.5 oz)	110	2	tr	0	4	21	1	20	160	—	—	—	—
Hot Dog Bran'nola	1 (1.5 oz)	110	2	tr	0	4	18	1	20	170	—	—	—	—
Hot Dog New England Style	1	110	2	—	0	4	20	1	20	160	—	—	—	—
Italian 8-inch Savoni	1	210	3	tr	0	8	38	3	40	—	—	—	—	—
Kaiser Francisco	1 (2 oz)	180	—	—	—	6	34	—	80	230	—	—	—	—
Onion Premium	1 (2.6 oz)	180	1	—	0	7	38	2	20	340	—	—	—	—
Onion Soft	1	140	—	—	0	5	28	2	40	200	—	—	—	—
Party Petite	2	70	2	tr	—	2	10	1	—	70	—	—	—	—
Potato	1	140	2	—	0	5	25	2	40	210	—	—	—	—
Sandwich Soft Sesame	1	130	3	—	0	4	23	2	40	220	—	—	—	—
Sourdough Brown N' Serve	1 (1 oz)	100	1	—	—	3	19	—	40	120	—	—	—	—
Sourdough Francisco	1 (1 oz)	100	1	—	—	3	19	—	40	120	—	—	—	—
Wheat Old Fashioned	2	80	3	—	—	2	11	—	20	98	—	—	—	—
AUGUST BROS.														
Dinner	1	90	1	—	—	6	18	—	20	170	—	—	—	—
Kaiser	1	170	1	—	0	6	35	2	40	310	—	—	—	—
Onion	1	160	1	—	0	6	33	2	40	310	—	—	—	—
Sesame Cubano	1	170	1	—	0	6	35	2	40	310	—	—	—	—
BREAD DU JOUR														
Bavarian Cracked Wheat	1 (1.2 oz)	90	1	0	0	3	17	1	60	190	60	—	—	—
Crusty Italian	1 (1.2 oz)	80	1	0	0	4	16	tr	60	190	60	—	—	—
French Petite	1 (3.5 oz)	230	2	0	0	10	47	2	150	530	120	—	—	—
Rye	1 (1.2 oz)	90	2	0	0	3	16	1	—	230	40	—	—	—
Sourdough	1 (2.2 oz)	140	2	0	0	6	29	2	80	230	60	—	—	—
DICARLO'S														
Extra Sourdough	1 (1.6 oz)	100	1	0	0	3	20	1	—	230	—	—	—	—
French	1 (1 oz)	70	1	0	0	3	14	tr	40	150	—	—	—	—
HOME PRIDE														
Dinner Wheat	1 (1.9 oz)	160	4	1	0	5	26	2	100	270	75	—	—	—
Hamburger Potato Bun	1 (1.9 oz)	130	2	0	0	5	27	2	60	270	90	—	—	—

FOOD	PORTION	CALORIES	FAT	SAT FAT	CHOL	PROTEIN	CARBO	FIBER	CALCIUM	SOD	POTAS	VIT C	FOLIC	VIT A
HOME PRIDE (CONT.)														
Hot Dog Potato Bun	1 (1.9 oz)	130	2	0	0	5	27	2	60	270	90	—	—	—
Sandwich Roll Wheat	1 (1.9 oz)	160	4	1	0	5	26	2	100	270	75	—	—	—
White	2 (1.6 oz)	130	4	1	0	4	22	1	80	230	65	—	—	—
LEVY														
Sub Old Country	1	180	2	—	—	6	34	—	40	230				
MARTIN'S														
Big Marty Poppy	1	170	2	—	0	11	31	3	—	320	—	—	—	—
Big Marty Sesame	1	170	2	—	0	11	31	3	—	320	—	—	—	—
Hoagie	1	240	3	—	0	16	41	3	—	430	—	—	—	—
Hoagie Sesame	1	240	3	—	0	16	41	4	—	430	—	—	—	—
Potato Dinner	1	100	1	—	0	5	18	1	—	135	—	—	—	—
Potato Long	1	140	1	—	0	8	27	2	—	200	—	—	—	—
Potato Party	1	50	1	—	0	3	10	1	—	70	—	—	—	—
Potato Sandwich	1	140	1	—	0	8	26	2	—	200	—	—	—	—
Sandwich Whole Wheat 100% Stoneground	1	160	2	—	0	11	28	5	—	290	—	—	—	—
MATTHEW'S														
Salad Roll	1	110	2	—	0	5	19	2	40	190	—	—	—	—
Sandwich	1	110	2	—	0	5	19	2	40	180	—	—	—	—
PEPPERIDGE FARM														
Brown 'N Serve Club	1	100	1	—	0	3	19	1	40	190	—	—	—	—
Brown 'N Serve French	½ roll	180	2	1	0	6	36	1	60	380	—	—	—	—
Brown 'N Serve Hearth	1	50	1	—	0	2	10	tr	20	100	—	—	—	—
Dinner	1	60	2	0	<5	2	8	tr	20	95	—	—	—	—
Dinner Country Style Classic	1	50	1	0	0	2	9	0	—	90	—	—	—	—
Finger Poppy Seed	1	50	2	0	<5	2	8	tr	20	80	—	—	—	—
Finger Sesame Seed	1	60	2	0	<5	2	9	tr	20	85	—	—	—	—
Frankfurter Dijon	1	160	5	1	0	5	23	2	60	230	—	—	—	—
Frankfurter Side Sliced	1	140	3	1	0	5	24	1	60	270	—	—	—	—
Frankfurter Top Sliced	1	140	3	1	0	5.	24	1	60	270	—	—	—	—
Frankfurter w/ Poppy Seeds	1	130	2	1	0	6	23	1	60	280	—	—	—	—
French Style	1	100	1	—	0	4	20	1	40	230	—	—	—	—
Hamburger	1	130	2	1	0	5	22	1	40	240	—	—	—	—
Hamburger	1	130	2	1	0	5	22	1	40	240	—	—	—	—

FOOD	PORTION	CALORIES	FAT	SAT FAT	CHOL	PROTEIN	CARBO	FIBER	CALCIUM	SOD	POTAS	VIT C	FOLIC	VIT A
PEPPERIDGE FARM (CONT.)														
Heat & Serve Butter Crescent	1	110	6	3	15	2	13	tr	20	150	—	—	—	—
Heat & Serve Golden Twist	1	110	5	2	5	2	14	tr	20	150	—	—	—	—
Hoagie Soft	1	210	5	1	0	8	34	1	60	320	—	—	—	—
Old Fashioned	1	50	2	1	5	2	7	tr	20	85	—	—	—	—
Parker House	1	60	1	0	5	2	9	tr	20	80	—	—	—	—
Party	1	30	1	—	0	1	5	tr	—	50	—	—	—	—
Potato Sandwich	1	160	4	1	0	4	28	1	—	260	—	—	—	—
Sandwich Onion w/ Poppy Seeds	1	150	3	1	0	5	26	1	40	260	—	—	—	—
Sandwich Salad	1	110	4	—	10	4	16	—	40	150	—	—	—	—
Sandwich w/ Sesame Seeds	1	140	3	1	0	5	23	1	40	230	—	—	—	—
Soft Family	1	100	2	1	0	4	18	1	40	190	—	—	—	—
Sourdough French	1	100	1	—	0	4	19	1	40	240	—	—	—	—
ROMAN MEAL														
Brown & Serve	2 (2 oz)	140	3	tr	0	5	24	2	63	275	67	0	—	0
Dinner	2 (2 oz)	136	2	tr	0	6	24	2	64	282	68	0	—	0
Hamburger	1 (1.6 oz)	111	2	tr	0	5	19	2	52	229	55	0	—	0
Hotdog	1 (1.5 oz)	103	2	tr	0	4	18	2	48	214	52	0	—	0
Sandwich	1 (2.7 oz)	181	3	tr	0	7	31	3	88	392	96	0	—	0
Sandwich	1 (2.7 oz)	181	3	tr	0	7	31	3	88	392	96	0	—	0
SAN FRANCISCO														
Sourdough	1 (1.8 oz)	180	0	0	0	6	37	3	0	300	—	0	—	0
THE BAKER														
Honey Cinnamon Raisin	1 (2 oz)	150	2	0	0	4	31	4	20	115	—	1	—	0
WONDER														
Brown 'N Serve Buttermilk	1 (1 oz)	70	1	0	0	3	13	tr	60	160	45	—	—	—
Brown 'N Serve Wheat	1 (1 oz)	70	1	0	0	2	14	tr	40	135	25	—	—	—
Brown 'N Serve White	1 (1 oz)	70	1	0	0	2	14	tr	40	135	25	—	—	—
Dinner White Light	1 (1 oz)	60	1	0	0	3	9	4	80	150	40	—	—	—
Hamburger	1 (1.5 oz)	110	2	0	0	4	21	tr	80	250	45	—	—	—
Hamburger Light	1 (1.5 oz)	80	2	0	0	5	13	5	80	210	40	—	—	—
Hamburger Wheat	1 (2.2 oz)	170	3	0	0	6	31	1	100	370	65	—	—	—
Hot Dog	1 (1.5 oz)	110	2	0	0	4	21	tr	80	250	45	—	—	—
Hot Dog Light	1 (1.5 oz)	80	2	0	0	5	13	5	80	210	40	—	—	—
Tea Dinner Rolls	1 (1.5 oz)	80	1	0	0	4	19	5	80	210	—	—	—	—

FOOD	PORTION	CALORIES	FAT	SAT FAT	CHOL	PROTEIN	CARBO	FIBER	CALCIUM	SOD	POTAS	VIT C	FOLIC	VIT A
REFRIGERATED														
cinnamon w/ frosting	1	109	4	1	—	2	17	—	10	250	19	—	—	—
crescent	1 (1 oz)	98	4	1	0	2	14	—	6	341	45	0	—	0
ROSELLE														
fresh	1 cup	28	tr	—	0	1	6	—	123	3	118	7	—	163
ROSEMARY														
dried	1 tsp	4	tr	—	0	tr	1	—	15	1	11	1	—	38
RUTABAGA														
CANNED														
SUNSHINE														
Diced	½ cup (4.2 oz)	30	0	0	0	tr	7	3	40	220	—	1	—	0
FRESH														
cooked mashed	½ cup	41	tr	tr	0	1	9	—	50	22	344	26	19	0
raw cubed	½ cup	25	tr	tr	0	1	6	—	33	14	236	18	14	0
SABLEFISH														
smoked	1 oz	72	6	1	18	5	0	—	—	206	132	—	—	—
smoked	3 oz	218	17	4	55	15	0	—	—	626	401	—	—	—
SAFFLOWER														
seeds dried	1 oz	147	11	1	0	5	10	—	22	—	—	—	—	—
SAFFRON														
saffron	1 tsp	2	tr	—	0	tr	tr	—	1	1	12	—	—	—
SAGE														
ground	1 tsp	2	tr	tr	0	tr	tr	—	12	tr	7	tr	—	41
WATKINS														
Sage	¼ tsp (0.5 g)	0	0	0	0	0	0	0	0	0	—	0	—	0
SALAD														
(*see also* LETTUCE, PASTA SALAD)														
MIX														
DOLE														
Caesar Salad	⅓ pkg (3.5 oz)	170	14	2	5	3	9	1	40	480	110	4	32	400
Classic Blend	3.5 oz	25	1	0	0	1	4	1	0	20	170	6	0	2250
Coleslaw Blend	3.5 oz	30	1	0	0	1	5	2	40	35	230	48	8	2250
French Blend	3.5 oz	25	1	0	0	1	4	1	20	15	230	12	32	3500
Italian Blend	3.5 oz	25	1	0	0	1	3	1	40	45	200	6	60	1000
Salad-In-A-Minute Oriental	3.5 oz	110	7	1	0	2	12	2	0	290	140	18	8	1750
Salad-In-A-Minute Spinach	3.5 oz	180	9	2	0	5	19	3	40	660	85	9	<8	1000
FRESH EXPRESS														
American Salad	1½ cups (3 oz)	20	0	0	0	1	3	1	20	10	—	5	—	1000
Caesar Salad	1½ cups (3 oz)	140	11	1	10	3	8	1	40	320	—	1	—	750

FOOD	PORTION	CALORIES	FAT	SAT FAT	CHOL	PROTEIN	CARBO	FIBER	CALCIUM	SOD	POTAS	VIT C	FOLIC	VIT A
FRESH EXPRESS (CONT.)														
European Salad	1½ cups (3 oz)	20	0	0	0	1	3	1	20	10	—	4	—	750
Garden Salad	1½ cups (3 oz)	20	0	0	0	1	3	1	20	10	—	4	—	500
Italian Salad	1½ cups (3 oz)	20	0	0	0	1	3	1	20	0	—	4	—	1000
Oriental Salad	1½ cups (3 oz)	120	8	1	0	3	11	1	40	330	—	18	—	1500
Riviera Salad	1½ cups (3 oz)	10	0	0	0	1	2	1	20	0	—	9	—	750
Spinach Salad	1½ cups (3 oz)	130	3	0	0	3	23	3	40	430	—	9	—	2000
SUDDENLY SALAD														
Caesar Low Fat Recipe as prep	¾ cup	170	3	0	0	5	30	1	20	580	130	0	—	0
Caesar as prep	¾ cup	220	9	2	0	5	30	1	20	580	130	0	—	0
Italian Pepperoni Low Fat Recipe as prep	1 cup	180	2	0	0	6	35	2	20	700	190	0	—	1750
Italian Pepperoni as prep	1 cup	200	4	1	0	6	35	1	20	700	200	0	—	1750
Ranch & Bacon Low Fat Recipe as prep	¾ cup	180	2	0	<5	7	31	1	20	530	210	0	—	750
Ranch & Bacon as prep	¾ cup	320	19	3	15	7	31	1	20	490	210	0	—	750
WEIGHT WATCHERS														
Caesar Salad	1 serv (3.5 oz)	60	0	0	0	2	11	1	40	600	—	9	—	400
Caesar Salad w/ Cookies	1 pkg (4.3 oz)	160	3	1	0	4	29	3	40	670	—	9	—	400
European Salad	1 serv (3.5 oz)	60	0	0	0	2	13	2	40	530	—	9	—	750
European Salad w/ Cookies	1 pkg (4.3 oz)	160	3	1	0	3	31	2	40	620	—	9	—	750
Garden Salad	1 serv (3.5 oz)	60	0	0	0	2	12	1	20	270	—	9	—	750
Garden Salad w/ Cookies	1 pkg (4 oz)	120	2	1	0	3	24	2	20	340	—	9	—	750
TAKE-OUT														
caesar	2 cups (5 oz)	235	20	2	10	5	11	1	40	440	—	24	—	2500
tossed w/o dressing	¾ cup	16	0	0	0	1	3	—	13	27	179	24	39	1182
tossed w/o dressing	1½ cups	32	tr	0	0	3	7	—	26	53	356	48	77	2352
tossed w/o dressing w/ cheese & egg	1½ cups	102	6	3	98	9	5	—	100	119	371	10	85	822
tossed w/o dressing w/ chicken	1½ cups	105	2	tr	72	17	4	—	37	209	447	17	67	935
tossed w/o dressing w/ pasta & seafood	1½ cups (14.6 oz)	380	21	3	50	16	32	—	73	1572	600	38	100	6245

FOOD	PORTION	CALORIES	FAT	SAT FAT	CHOL	PROTEIN	CARBO	FIBER	CALCIUM	SOD	POTAS	VIT C	FOLIC	VIT A
tossed w/o dressing w/ shrimp	1½ cups	107	2	tr	180	15	7	—	60	487	404	9	87	791

SALAD DRESSING

HOME RECIPE

french	1 tbsp	88	10	2	—	0	1	—	1	92	3	tr	—	72
vinegar & oil	1 tbsp	72	8	2	0	0	tr	—	—	tr	1	—	—	—

MIX

GOOD SEASONS

Cheese Garlic as prep	2 tbsp (1 oz)	140	16	3	0	0	1	0	0	330	15	0	—	0
Fat Free Honey Mustard as prep	2 tbsp (1.2 oz)	20	0	0	0	0	5	0	0	280	30	0	—	0
Fat Free Italian as prep	2 tbsp (1.1 oz)	10	0	0	0	0	2	0	0	290	110	0	—	0
Fat Free Ranch as prep	2 tbsp (1.2 oz)	20	0	0	0	0	5	0	0	250	30	0	—	100
Fat Free Zesty Herb as prep	2 tbsp (1.1 oz)	10	0	0	0	0	2	0	0	260	70	0	—	0
Garlic & Herbs as prep	2 tbsp (1 oz)	140	15	2	0	0	1	0	0	340	10	0	—	0
Gourmet Caesar as prep	2 tbsp (1.1 oz)	150	16	3	0	0	3	0	0	300	110	0	—	0
Gourmet Parmesan Italian as prep	2 tbsp (1.1 oz)	150	16	3	0	0	2	0	0	330	25	0	—	0
Honey French as prep	2 tbsp (1.2 oz)	160	15	2	0	0	5	0	0	250	30	0	—	100
Honey Mustard as prep	2 tbsp (1.1 oz)	150	15	2	0	0	3	0	0	240	15	0	—	0
Italian as prep	2 tbsp (1 oz)	140	15	2	0	0	1	0	0	320	15	0	—	0
Mexican Spice as prep	2 tbsp (1.1 oz)	140	15	3	0	0	2	0	0	310	65	0	—	0
Mild Italian as prep	2 tbsp (1.1 oz)	150	15	3	0	0	2	0	0	370	10	0	—	0
Oriental Sesame as prep	2 tbsp (1.1 oz)	150	16	3	0	0	3	0	0	360	15	0	—	0
Reduced Calorie Italian as prep	2 tbsp (1 oz)	50	5	1	0	0	2	0	0	280	15	—	0	0
Reduced Calorie Zesty Italian as prep	2 tbsp (1 oz)	50	5	1	0	0	2	0	0	260	30	0	—	0
Roasted Garlic as prep	2 tbsp (1.1 oz)	150	15	2	0	0	2	0	0	340	15	0	—	0
Zesty Italian as prep	2 tbsp (1 oz)	140	15	2	0	0	1	0	0	220	15	0	—	0

HAIN

No Oil 1000 Island	1 tbsp	12	0	—	tr	0	3	—	—	150	60	—	—	—
No Oil Bleu Cheese	1 tbsp	14	1	—	<5	1	1	—	—	190	40	—	—	—
No Oil Buttermilk	1 tbsp	11	tr	—	0	1	1	—	—	150	40	—	—	—
No Oil Caesar	1 tbsp	6	tr	—	0	0	1	—	—	200	15	—	—	—

FOOD	PORTION	CALORIES	FAT	SAT FAT	CHOL	PROTEIN	CARBO	FIBER	CALCIUM	SOD	POTAS	VIT C	FOLIC	VIT A
HAIN (CONT.)														
No Oil French	1 tbsp	12	0	—	0	0	3	—	—	340	45	—	—	—
No Oil Garlic & Cheese	1 tbsp	6	tr	—	0	tr	1	—	—	180	15	—	—	—
No Oil Herb	1 tbsp	2	0	—	0	0	1	—	—	140	10	—	—	—
No Oil Italian	1 tbsp	2	0	—	0	0	1	—	—	170	10	—	—	—
READY-TO-EAT														
blue cheese	1 tbsp	77	8	2	—	1	1	—	12	—	—	tr	—	32
french	1 tbsp	67	6	2	—	tr	3	—	2	214	12	—	—	—
french reduced calorie	1 tbsp	22	1	tr	1	0	4	—	2	128	13	—	—	—
italian	1 tbsp	69	7	1	—	tr	2	—	1	116	2	—	—	—
italian reduced calorie	1 tbsp	16	2	tr	1	tr	1	—	0	118	2	—	—	—
russian	1 tbsp	76	8	1	—	tr	2	—	3	133	24	1	—	106
russian reduced calorie	1 tbsp	23	1	tr	1	tr	5	—	3	141	26	—	—	—
sesame seed	1 tbsp	68	7	1	0	1	1	—	—	153	—	—	—	—
thousand island	1 tbsp	59	6	1	—	tr	2	—	2	109	18	—	—	50
thousand island reduced calorie	1 tbsp	24	2	tr	2	tr	3	—	2	153	17	—	—	49
ESTEE														
Blue Cheese	2 tbsp (1 oz)	15	1	—	—	tr	1	—	—	80	—	—	—	—
Creamy French	2 tbsp (1 oz)	10	0	0	—	0	2	—	—	80	—	—	—	—
Creamy French Fat Free	1 pkg (0.5 oz)	5	0	0	0	0	1	—	—	40	15	—	—	—
Creamy Garlic	2 tbsp (1 oz)	60	0	0	—	0	2	—	—	80	—	—	—	—
Creamy Garlic Fat Free	1 pkg (0.5 oz)	5	0	0	0	0	1	—	—	40	10	—	—	—
Creamy Italian	2 tbsp (1 oz)	15	1	—	—	0	2	—	—	80	—	—	—	—
Fat Free Thousand Island	1 pkg (0.5 oz)	5	0	0	0	0	1	—	—	40	15	—	—	—
Italian	2 tbsp (1 oz)	5	0	0	—	0	1	—	—	80	—	—	—	—
Italian Fat Free	1 pkg (0.5 oz)	0	0	0	—	0	tr	—	—	40	5	—	—	—
Low Fat Blue Cheese	1 pkg (0.5 oz)	5	0	—	—	0	tr	—	—	40	10	—	—	—
Thousand Island	2 tbsp (1 oz)	10	0	0	—	0	2	—	—	80	—	—	—	—
HAIN														
1000 Island	1 tbsp	50	5	—	0	0	0	—	—	85	30	—	—	—
Canola Garden Tomato	1 tbsp	60	6	—	0	0	1	—	—	150	15	—	—	—
Canola Italian	1 tbsp	50	5	—	0	0	1	—	—	150	5	—	—	—
Canola Spicy French Mustard	1 tbsp	50	5	—	5	1	1	—	—	190	35	—	—	—
Canola Tangy Citrus	1 tbsp	50	5	—	0	0	1	—	—	75	10	—	—	—
Creamy Caesar	1 tbsp	60	6	—	<5	0	1	—	—	220	10	—	—	—

FOOD	PORTION	CALORIES	FAT	SAT FAT	CHOL	PROTEIN	CARBO	FIBER	CALCIUM	SOD	POTAS	VIT C	FOLIC	VIT A
HAIN (CONT.)														
Creamy Caesar Low Salt	1 tbsp	60	6	—	<5	0	1	—	—	15	10	—	—	—
Creamy French	1 tbsp	60	6	—	0	0	1	—	—	80	20	—	—	—
Creamy Italian	1 tbsp	80	8	—	0	0	0	—	—	100	10	—	—	—
Creamy Italian No Salt Added	1 tbsp	80	8	—	0	0	1	—	—	25	50	—	—	—
Cucumber Dill	1 tbsp	80	8	—	5	0	0	—	—	210	20	—	—	—
Dijon Vinaigrette	1 tbsp	50	5	—	<5	0	0	—	—	180	10	—	—	—
Garlic & Sour Cream	1 tbsp	70	7	—	0	0	0	—	—	100	20	—	—	—
Honey & Sesame	1 tbsp	60	5	—	0	0	2	—	—	210	25	—	—	—
Italian Cheese Vinaigrette	1 tbsp	55	6	—	<5	0	0	—	—	130	10	—	—	—
Old Fashioned Buttermilk	1 tbsp	70	7	—	0	0	0	—	—	100	20	—	—	—
Poppyseed Rancher's	1 tbsp	60	7	—	<5	0	0	—	—	105	15	—	—	—
Savory Herb No Salt Added	1 tbsp	90	10	—	0	0	0	—	—	45	25	—	—	—
Swiss Cheese Vinaigrette	1 tbsp	60	7	—	<5	0	0	—	—	160	15	—	—	—
Traditional Italian	1 tbsp	80	8	—	0	0	0	—	—	330	10	—	—	—
Traditional Italian No Salt Added	1 tbsp	60	6	—	0	0	1	—	—	20	25	—	—	—
HOLLYWOOD														
Caesar	1 tbsp	70	7	1	0	1	2	0	20	65	15	—	—	—
Creamy French	1 tbsp	70	7	1	0	0	2	0	—	45	15	—	—	—
Creamy Italian	1 tbsp	90	9	1	0	0	2	0	—	140	10	—	—	—
Dijon Vinaigrette	1 tbsp	60	6	1	0	0	2	0	—	40	25	—	—	—
Italian	1 tbsp	90	9	1	0	0	1	0	—	300	5	—	—	—
Italian Cheese	1 tbsp	80	8	1	0	0	2	0	—	60	20	—	—	—
Old Fashion Buttermilk	1 tbsp	75	8	1	0	0	1	0	—	40	15	—	—	—
Poppy Seed Rancher's	1 tbsp	75	8	1	0	0	1	0	—	35	10	—	—	—
Thousand Island	1 tbsp	60	6	1	5	0	3	0	—	15	15	—	—	—
KRAFT														
1/3 Less Fat Catalina	2 tbsp (1.2 oz)	80	5	1	0	0	9	0	0	400	70	0	—	500
1/3 Less Fat Cucumber Ranch	2 tbsp (1.1 oz)	60	5	1	0	0	2	0	0	480	20	0	—	0
1/3 Less Fat Italian	2 tbsp (1.1 oz)	70	7	1	0	0	3	0	20	240	25	0	—	0
1/3 Less Fat Ranch	2 tbsp (1.1 oz)	110	11	2	10	0	1	0	0	310	40	0	—	0
1/3 Less Fat Thousand Island	2 tbsp (1.2 oz)	70	5	1	10	0	7	0	0	340	60	0	—	0
Bacon & Tomato	2 tbsp (1.1 oz)	140	14	3	<5	tr	2	0	0	280	35	0	—	0
Buttermilk Ranch	2 tbsp (1.1 oz)	150	16	3	<5	0	1	0	0	240	20	0	—	0

FOOD	PORTION	CALORIES	FAT	SAT FAT	CHOL	PROTEIN	CARBO	FIBER	CALCIUM	SOD	POTAS	VIT C	FOLIC	VIT A
KRAFT (CONT.)														
Caesar Italian	2 tbsp (1.1 oz)	100	10	2	0	tr	2	0	20	480	25	0	—	0
Caesar Ranch	2 tbsp (1.1 oz)	110	11	2	10	1	1	0	20	290	30	0	—	0
Catalina	2 tbsp (1.1 oz)	120	10	2	0	0	7	0	0	390	35	0	—	500
Catalina With Honey	2 tbsp (1.1 oz)	130	11	2	0	0	7	0	0	320	70	0	—	0
Classic Caesar	2 tbsp (1.1 oz)	110	11	2	10	1	1	0	20	290	30	0	—	0
Coleslaw	2 tbsp (1.1 oz)	130	11	2	15	0	7	0	0	410	5	0	—	0
Creamy French	2 tbsp (1.1 oz)	160	15	3	0	0	5	0	0	270	20	0	—	1250
Creamy Garlic	2 tbsp (1.1 oz)	110	11	2	0	0	2	0	0	360	25	0	—	0
Creamy Italian	2 tbsp (1.1 oz)	110	11	2	0	0	2	0	0	250	15	0	—	0
Cucumber Ranch	2 tbsp (1.1 oz)	140	15	2	0	0	2	0	0	220	20	0	—	0
Free Blue Cheese	2 tbsp (1.2 oz)	45	0	0	0	0	11	1	0	360	30	0	—	0
Free Caesar Italian	2 tbsp (1.2 oz)	25	0	0	0	tr	4	0	20	480	50	0	—	0
Free Catalina	2 tbsp (1.2 oz)	35	0	0	0	0	8	tr	0	320	40	0	—	500
Free Classic Caesar	2 tbsp (1.2 oz)	45	0	0	0	tr	11	tr	0	360	50	0	—	0
Free Creamy Italian	2 tbsp (1.2 oz)	50	0	0	0	0	12	tr	0	330	25	0	—	0
Free French	2 tbsp (1.2 oz)	45	0	0	0	0	11	tr	0	300	25	0	—	500
Free Garlic Ranch	2 tbsp (1.2 oz)	45	0	0	0	0	11	1	0	320	30	0	—	0
Free Honey Dijon	2 tbsp (1.2 oz)	45	0	0	0	0	10	1	0	330	35	0	—	0
Free Italian	2 tbsp (1.2 oz)	20	0	0	0	0	4	0	0	430	40	0	—	0
Free Peppercorn Ranch	2 tbsp (1.2 oz)	45	0	0	0	0	11	tr	0	330	35	0	—	0
Free Ranch	1 tbsp (1.2 oz)	50	0	0	0	0	11	1	0	350	30	0	—	0
Free Red Wine Vinegar	2 tbsp (1.1 oz)	15	0	0	0	0	3	0	0	410	10	0	—	0
Free Thousand Island	2 tbsp (1.2 oz)	40	0	0	0	0	9	1	0	280	40	0	—	0
Garlic Ranch	2 tbsp (1.1 oz)	180	19	3	10	0	1	0	0	270	15	0	—	0
Herb Vinaigrette	2 tbsp (1.1 oz)	140	15	2	0	0	tr	0	0	250	10	0	—	0
Honey Dijon	2 tbsp (1.1 oz)	110	10	2	0	0	6	0	0	210	35	0	—	0
Honey Mustard	2 tbsp (1.1 oz)	110	10	2	0	0	6	0	0	210	35	0	—	0
House Italian w/ Olive Oil Blend	2 tbsp (1.1 oz)	120	12	2	<5	0	2	0	0	240	20	0	—	0
Peppercorn Ranch	2 tbsp (1 oz)	170	18	3	10	tr	1	0	20	270	15	0	—	0
Pesto Italian	2 tbsp (1.1 oz)	90	9	2	0	0	2	0	0	310	15	0	—	0
Ranch	2 tbsp (1 oz)	170	18	3	10	0	1	0	0	280	10	0	—	0
Roka Blue Cheese	2 tbsp (1.1 oz)	130	13	3	<5	tr	2	tr	0	310	35	0	—	0
Russian	2 tbsp (1.2 oz)	130	10	2	0	0	10	0	0	310	40	0	—	400
Sour Cream & Onion Ranch	2 tbsp (1 oz)	170	18	3	10	0	1	0	0	250	45	0	—	0
Thousand Island	2 tbsp (1.1 oz)	110	10	2	10	0	5	0	0	310	40	0	—	0
Thousand Island With Bacon	2 tbsp (1.1 oz)	130	12	2	0	0	5	0	0	200	35	0	—	0
Tomato & Herb Italian	2 tbsp (1.1 oz)	100	9	1	0	0	3	0	0	340	80	0	—	0

FOOD	PORTION	CALORIES	FAT	SAT FAT	CHOL	PROTEIN	CARBO	FIBER	CALCIUM	SOD	POTAS	VIT C	FOLIC	VIT A
KRAFT (CONT.)														
Zesty Italian	2 tbsp (1.1 oz)	110	11	1	0	0	2	0	0	540	10	0	—	0
MARZETTI														
Bacon Spinach Salad	2 tbsp	80	15	2	1	0	16	15	0	260	—	0	—	0
Blue Cheese	2 tbsp	160	17	3	20	1	0	0	0	230	—	1	—	0
Buttermilk & Herb	2 tbsp	180	20	3	3	0	1	0	0	260	—	0	—	0
Buttermilk Bacon Ranch	2 tbsp	180	19	3	10	0	1	0	—	270	—	0	—	0
Buttermilk Blue Cheese	2 tbsp	160	18	3	10	1	1	0	—	220	—	0	—	0
Buttermilk Parmesan Pepper	2 tbsp	170	18	3	10	0	1	0	0	310	—	0	—	0
Buttermilk Parmesan Ranch	2 tbsp	160	17	3	10	0	1	0	0	240	—	0	—	0
Buttermilk Ranch	2 tbsp	180	20	3	4	0	1	0	—	250	—	0	—	0
Buttermilk Veggie Dip	2 tbsp	170	18	3	3	0	1	0	0	240	—	0	—	0
Caesar	2 tbsp	150	16	3	0	0	1	0	0	390	—	0	—	0
Caesar Ranch	2 tbsp	190	20	3	5	0	2	0	0	300	—	0	—	0
California French	2 tbsp	160	13	2	0	0	11	0	0	240	—	0	—	0
Celery Seed	2 tbsp	160	13	2	0	0	10	0	0	180	—	0	—	0
Chunky Blue Cheese	2 tbsp	150	16	3	25	1	1	0	—	300	—	0	—	0
Classic Caesar Ranch	2 tbsp	190	20	3	5	0	2	0	0	300	—	0	—	0
Country French	2 tbsp	150	13	2	10	0	7	0	0	220	—	0	—	0
Cracked Peppercorn	2 tbsp	140	14	3	30	1	1	0	—	280	—	0	—	0
Creamy Garlic Italian	2 tbsp	160	17	3	15	0	1	0	—	140	—	1	—	0
Creamy Italian	2 tbsp	150	16	3	15	0	1	0	0	170	—	1	—	0
Crispy Celery Seed	2 tbsp	160	13	2	0	0	11	0	—	190	—	0	—	0
Dijon Honey Mustard	2 tbsp	140	13	2	20	0	6	0	—	180	—	0	—	0
Dijon Ranch	2 tbsp	170	18	3	25	0	2	0	0	190	—	0	—	0
Dutch Sweet'N Sour	2 tbsp	160	13	2	0	0	10	0	—	200	—	0	—	0
Fat Free California French	2 tbsp	45	0	0	0	0	11	0	0	330	—	0	—	0
Fat Free Honey Dijon	2 tbsp	60	0	0	0	0	14	1	0	190	—	0	—	0
Fat Free Honey French	2 tbsp	45	0	0	0	0	11	0	0	330	—	0	—	0
Fat Free Italian	2 tbsp	15	0	0	0	0	3	0	—	450	—	0	—	0
Fat Free Peppercorn Ranch	2 tbsp	30	0	0	0	0	7	1	—	420	—	0	—	0
Fat Free Ranch	2 tbsp	30	0	0	0	0	7	1	0	430	—	0	—	0

FOOD	PORTION	CALORIES	FAT	SAT FAT	CHOL	PROTEIN	CARBO	FIBER	CALCIUM	SOD	POTAS	VIT C	FOLIC	VIT A
MARZETTI (CONT.)														
Fat Free Raspberry	2 tbsp	70	0	0	0	0	18	0	0	150	—	0	—	0
Fat Free Slaw	2 tbsp	45	0	0	15	0	11	0	0	390	—	0	—	0
Fat Free Sweet & Sour	2 tbsp	45	0	0	0	0	14	0	0	290	—	0	—	0
Fat Free Thousand Island	2 tbsp	35	0	0	0	0	9	0	—	370	—	0	—	0
Garden Ranch	2 tbsp	180	19	3	3	0	1	0	0	250	—	1	—	200
Gusto Italian	2 tbsp	120	13	2	0	0	1	0	—	740	—	2	—	0
Honey Dijon	2 tbsp	140	13	2	15	0	6	0	0	170	—	0	—	0
Honey Dijon Ranch	2 tbsp	150	15	3	25	0	2	0	0	200	—	0	—	0
Honey French	2 tbsp	160	14	2	0	0	11	0	—	230	—	0	—	0
Honey French Blue Cheese	2 tbsp	160	13	2	0	1	11	0	—	260	—	0	—	0
House Caesar	2 tbsp	150	16	3	5	0	1	0	20	340	—	0	—	0
Italian With Olive Oil	2 tbsp	120	13	2	0	0	1	0	0	480	—	0	—	0
Light Blue Cheese	2 tbsp	60	6	2	15	2	4	0	20	650	—	0	—	0
Light Buttermilk Ranch	2 tbsp	90	9	2	10	0	3	0	0	280	—	0	—	0
Light California French	2 tbsp	80	6	1	0	0	8	0	0	360	—	0	—	0
Light Chunky Blue Cheese	2 tbsp	80	7	2	15	1	4	0	20	330	—	0	—	0
Light French	2 tbsp	40	2	0	0	0	6	0	0	320	—	0	—	0
Light French	2 tbsp	40	2	0	0	0	6	0	0	320	—	0	—	0
Light Honey French	2 tbsp	80	4	1	0	1	12	0	0	250	—	0	—	0
Light Italian	2 tbsp	60	5	1	0	0	3	0	0	570	—	0	—	0
Light Ranch	2 tbsp	90	8	2	5	0	7	0	0	430	—	0	—	0
Light Red Wine Vinegar & Oil	2 tbsp	20	1	0	0	0	3	0	0	490	—	0	—	0
Light Slaw	2 tbsp	60	7	1	30	0	10	0	0	380	—	0	—	0
Light Sweet & Sour	2 tbsp	100	6	1	0	0	11	0	0	260	—	0	—	0
Light Thousand Island	2 tbsp	70	5	1	20	0	6	0	0	350	—	0	—	0
Old Fashioned Poppyseed	2 tbsp	140	11	2	10	0	10	0	—	220	—	0	—	0
Olde Venice Italian	2 tbsp	130	13	2	0	0	2	0	0	490	—	0	—	0
Olde World Caesar	2 tbsp	150	16	3	5	0	1	0	0	340	—	0	—	0
Parmesan Pepper	2 tbsp	160	17	3	10	0	1	0	0	260	—	0	—	0
Peppercorn Ranch	2 tbsp	180	19	3	10	0	1	0	0	220	—	0	—	0
Poppyseed	2 tbsp	160	13	2	15	0	10	0	0	310	—	0	—	0
Potato Salad Dressing	2 tbsp	120	13	2	35	0	7	0	0	300	—	1	—	0
Ranch	2 tbsp	180	20	3	3	0	1	0	0	260	—	0	—	0

FOOD	PORTION	CALORIES	FAT	SAT FAT	CHOL	PROTEIN	CARBO	FIBER	CALCIUM	SOD	POTAS	VIT C	FOLIC	VIT A
MARZETTI (CONT.)														
Red Wine Vinegar & Oil	2 tbsp	130	14	2	0	0	2	0	0	460	—	0	—	0
Romano Cheese Caesar	2 tbsp	150	16	3	15	0	1	0	0	370	—	0	—	0
Romano Italian	2 tbsp	160	17	3	0	0	1	0	0	390	—	0	—	0
Savory Italian	2 tbsp	110	12	2	0	0	3	0	0	520	—	1	—	0
Slaw	2 tbsp	170	16	3	30	0	6	0	0	370	—	0	—	0
Southern Slaw	2 tbsp	100	11	2	20	0	14	0	0	210	—	0	—	0
Sweet & Saucy	2 tbsp	140	12	2	0	0	9	0	0	290	—	0	—	0
Sweet & Sour	2 tbsp	160	13	2	0	0	10	0	0	210	—	1	—	0
Thousand Island	2 tbsp	150	15	2	25	0	5	0	—	230	—	0	—	0
Vintage Champagne	2 tbsp	150	16	2	0	0	2	0	0	460	—	0	—	0
Wilde Raspberry	2 tbsp	150	12	2	0	0	12	0	0	65	—	0	—	0
NASOYA														
Creamy Dill	2 tbsp (1 oz)	63	5	tr	0	1	3	tr	11	145	32	tr	tr	tr
Creamy Italian	2 tbsp (1 oz)	60	5	0	0	0	3	tr	10	187	33	1	tr	39
Garden Herb	2 tbsp (1 oz)	61	5	tr	0	1	3	tr	10	148	30	tr	tr	6
Sesame Garlic	2 tbsp (1 oz)	63	5	tr	0	1	3	tr	10	137	32	tr	1	1
Thousand Island	2 tbsp (1 oz)	62	4	tr	0	1	6	tr	7	146	32	1	tr	35
NEWMAN'S OWN														
Balsamic Vinaigrette	2 tbsp (1.1 oz)	90	9	1	0	0	3	0	0	350	—	0	—	0
Caesar	2 tbsp (1.1 oz)	150	16	2	<5	1	1	0	0	450	—	0	—	0
Light Italian	2 tbsp (1.1 oz)	20	1	0	0	0	3	0	0	380	—	0	—	0
Olive Oil & Vinegar	2 tbsp (1 oz)	150	16	3	0	0	1	0	0	150	—	0	—	0
Ranch	2 tbsp (1 oz)	180	19	3	<5	1	2	0	0	170	—	0	—	0
PFEIFFER														
1000 Island	2 tbsp	140	14	2	20	0	4	0	0	220	—	0	—	0
California French	2 tbsp	140	12	2	0	0	9	0	0	290	—	0	—	0
French	2 tbsp	150	13	2	10	0	7	0	0	220	—	0	—	0
Honey Dijon	2 tbsp	140	13	2	15	0	6	0	0	170	—	0	—	0
Lite Italian	2 tbsp	50	5	1	0	0	3	0	0	410	—	0	—	0
Ranch	2 tbsp	180	20	3	3	0	1	0	0	260	—	0	—	0
Savory Italian	2 tbsp	110	12	2	0	0	3	0	0	520	—	1	—	0
PRITIKIN														
Dijon Balsamic Vinaigrette	2 tbsp (1 oz)	3	0	0	0	—	6	—	—	125	0	—	—	—
French	2 tbsp (1 oz)	35	0	0	0	—	8	—	—	130	—	—	—	—
Honey Dijon	2 tbsp (1 oz)	45	0	0	0	—	11	—	—	130	0	—	—	—
Honey French	2 tbsp (1 oz)	40	0	0	0	—	11	—	—	135	—	—	—	—
Italian	2 tbsp (1 oz)	20	0	0	0	—	5	—	—	115	—	—	—	—
Raspberry Vinaigrette	2 tbsp (1 oz)	45	0	0	0	—	11	—	—	70	—	—	—	—

FOOD	PORTION	CALORIES	FAT	SAT FAT	CHOL	PROTEIN	CARBO	FIBER	CALCIUM	SOD	POTAS	VIT C	FOLIC	VIT A
RED WING														
"K" Dressing	1 tbsp (0.5 oz)	70	7	1	5	0	4	0	0	90	—	0	—	0
Chunky Blue Cheese	2 tbsp (1 oz)	130	13	2	0	0	3	0	0	290	—	0	—	0
Creamy Ranch	2 tbsp (1 oz)	150	15	2	15	0	2	0	0	280	—	0	—	0
French Traditional	2 tbsp (1 oz)	130	11	2	0	0	8	0	0	250	—	0	—	0
Italian Traditional	2 tbsp (1 oz)	100	9	2	0	0	4	0	0	550	—	0	—	0
Spicy Sweet French	2 tbsp (1 oz)	130	11	2	0	0	8	0	0	370	—	0	—	0
Thousand Island Thick & Rich	2 tbsp (1 oz)	110	9	2	15	0	8	0	0	270	—	0	—	0
SEVEN SEAS														
⅓ Less Fat Creamy Italian	2 tbsp (1.1 oz)	60	5	1	0	0	2	0	0	500	0	0	—	0
⅓ Less Fat Italian w/ Olive Oil Blend	2 tbsp (1.1 oz)	45	4	0	0	0	2	0	0	460	10	0	—	0
⅓ Less Fat Ranch	2 tbsp (1.1 oz)	100	9	2	0	0	5	0	0	320	10	0	—	0
⅓ Less Fat Red Wine Vinegar & Oil	2 tbsp (1.1 oz)	45	4	0	0	0	3	0	0	320	10	0	—	0
⅓ Less Fat Viva Italian	2 tbsp (1.1 oz)	45	4	0	0	0	2	0	0	320	10	0	—	0
2 Cheese Italian	2 tbsp (1.1 oz)	70	7	1	0	0	3	0	0	240	25	0	—	0
Chunky Blue Cheese	2 tbsp (1.1 oz)	130	13	3	<5	tr	2	tr	0	310	35	0	—	0
Classic Caesar	2 tbsp (1.1 oz)	100	10	2	0	tr	2	0	20	480	25	0	—	0
Creamy Italian	2 tbsp (1.1 oz)	120	12	2	0	0	1	0	0	510	10	0	—	0
Free Ranch	2 tbsp (1.2 oz)	45	0	0	0	0	11	1	0	330	35	0	—	0
Free Red Wine Vinegar	2 tbsp (1.1 oz)	15	0	0	0	0	3	0	0	410	10	0	—	0
Free Sour Cream & Onion Ranch	2 tbsp (1.2 oz)	50	0	0	0	0	11	1	0	300	35	0	—	0
Free Viva Italian	2 tbsp (1.1 oz)	10	0	0	0	0	2	1	0	480	30	0	—	0
Green Goddess	2 tbsp (1.1 oz)	130	13	2	0	0	1	0	0	260	15	0	—	0
Herbs & Spices	2 tbsp (1.1 oz)	90	9	1	0	0	1	0	0	290	5	0	—	0
Ranch	2 tbsp (1.1 oz)	160	17	3	<5	0	2	0	0	260	20	0	—	0
Red Wine Vinegar & Oil	2 tbsp (1.1 oz)	90	9	1	0	0	2	0	0	500	10	0	—	0
Viva Italian	2 tbsp (1.1 oz)	90	9	1	0	0	2	0	0	370	10	0	—	0
Viva Russian	2 tbsp (1.1 oz)	150	16	3	0	0	3	0	0	210	50	0	—	0
TREE OF LIFE														
Cafe Venice	2 tbsp (1 oz)	100	12	1	0	0	2	0	0	170	—	0	—	0
Fat Free Blue Cheese	2 tbsp (1 oz)	15	1	—	—	0	2	—	40	260	—	—	—	—
Fat Free Honey French	2 tbsp (1 oz)	35	0	0	0	0	8	—	—	150	—	—	—	—
Fat Free Italian Garlic	2 tbsp (1 oz)	20	0	0	0	0	4	—	—	260	—	2	—	—

FOOD	PORTION	CALORIES	FAT	SAT FAT	CHOL	PROTEIN	CARBO	FIBER	CALCIUM	SOD	POTAS	VIT C	FOLIC	VIT A
TREE OF LIFE (CONT.)														
Fat Free Oriental Ginger	2 tbsp (1 oz)	15	0	0	0	0	3	—	—	310	—	—	—	—
Frisco's Raspberry	2 tbsp (1 oz)	120	11	1	0	0	5	0	0	80	—	2	—	0
Maison Caesar	2 tbsp (1 oz)	70	6	1	5	2	1	0	40	115	—	0	—	0
Shanghai Palace	2 tbsp (1 oz)	80	7	0	0	1	3	0	0	310	—	0	—	0
ULTRA SLIM-FAST														
French	1 tbsp	20	tr	—	0	0	4	0	100	150	—	6	—	500
Italian	1 tbsp	6	tr	—	0	0	1	0	100	170	—	6	—	500
W.J. CLARK														
Ginger Orange Vinaigrette	1 tbsp	73	7	1	0	0	tr	0	10	134	—	1	—	<50
Herbs & Romano	1 tbsp	67	6	tr	0	0	2	0	tr	111	—	tr	—	tr
Lemon Peppercorn	1 tbsp	72	7	1	0	0	tr	0	<10	135	—	2	—	0
Lime Cilantro Vinaigrette	1 tbsp	73	8	1	0	0	tr	0	<10	147	—	3	—	300
Poppy Seed	1 tbsp	75	6	tr	0	0	3	0	tr	106	—	tr	—	tr
Sweet Pepper Basil	1 tbsp	69	7	tr	0	0	2	0	tr	127	—	7	—	1500
Tarragon Honey Mustard	1 tbsp	66	6	tr	0	0	2	0	tr	139	—	tr	—	tr
WALDEN FARMS														
Fat Free Balsamic Vinaigrette	2 tbsp (1 oz)	15	0	0	0	0	3	0	0	360	—	0	—	0
Fat Free Bleu Cheese	2 tbsp (1 oz)	25	0	0	8	0	4	0	0	240	—	0	—	0
Fat Free Caesar	2 tbsp (1 oz)	25	0	0	0	1	4	0	0	360	—	0	—	0
Fat Free Creamy Italian With Parmesan	1 tbsp (1 oz)	25	0	0	0	1	4	0	0	360	—	0	—	0
Fat Free French Style	2 tbsp (1 oz)	25	0	0	0	1	4	0	0	360	—	0	—	0
Fat Free Honey Dijon	2 tbsp (1 oz)	25	0	0	0	0	6	0	0	240	—	0	—	0
Fat Free Italian	2 tbsp (1 oz)	10	0	0	0	0	2	0	0	290	—	0	—	0
Fat Free Ranch	2 tbsp (1 oz)	25	0	0	0	1	4	0	0	290	—	0	—	0
Fat Free Raspberry Vinaigrette	2 tbsp (1 oz)	20	0	0	0	0	4	0	0	290	—	0	—	0
Fat Free Russian	2 tbsp (1 oz)	30	0	0	5	0	6	0	0	240	—	0	—	0
Fat Free Sodium Free Italian	2 tbsp (1 oz)	10	0	0	0	0	2	0	0	0	—	0	—	0
Fat Free Sugar Free Italian	2 tbsp (1 oz)	0	0	0	0	0	0	0	0	290	—	0	—	0
Fat Free Thousand Island	2 tbsp (1 oz)	35	0	0	5	0	7	0	0	240	—	0	—	0
Italian With Sun Dried Tomato	2 tbsp (1 oz)	15	0	0	0	0	3	0	0	290	—	0	—	0
Ranch With Sun Dried Tomato	2 tbsp (1 oz)	25	0	0	0	1	4	0	0	290	—	0	—	0

FOOD	PORTION	CALORIES	FAT	SAT FAT	CHOL	PROTEIN	CARBO	FIBER	CALCIUM	SOD	POTAS	VIT C	FOLIC	VIT A
WEIGHT WATCHERS														
Fat Free Caesar	2 tbsp	10	0	0	0	0	1	0	0	390	—	0	—	0
Fat Free Caesar	1 pkg (0.75 oz)	5	0	0	0	0	1	0	0	290	—	0	—	0
Fat Free Creamy Italian	2 tbsp	30	0	0	0	0	7	0	0	360	—	0	—	0
Fat Free French Style	2 tbsp	40	0	0	0	0	9	0	0	200	—	0	—	0
Fat Free Honey Dijon	2 tbsp	45	0	0	0	0	11	0	0	150	—	0	—	0
Fat Free Italian	2 tbsp	10	0	0	0	0	2	0	0	360	—	0	—	0
Fat Free Ranch	2 tbsp	35	0	0	0	0	7	0	0	270	—	0	—	0
Fat Free Ranch	1 pkg (0.75 oz)	25	0	0	0	0	6	0	0	200	—	0	—	0
WISHBONE														
Caesar	2 tbsp (1 oz)	90	10	2	5	1	2	0	0	300	—	0	—	0
Chunky Blue Cheese	2 tbsp (1 oz)	150	17	3	0	1	3	0	20	290	—	0	—	0
Classic House Italian	2 tbsp (1 oz)	140	14	2	5	0	2	0	0	360	—	0	—	0
Classic Olive Oil Italian	2 tbsp (1 oz)	60	5	1	0	0	4	0	0	350	—	0	—	0
Creamy Caesar	2 tbsp (1 oz)	180	18	3	10	1	1	0	20	290	—	0	—	0
Creamy Italian	2 tbsp (1 oz)	110	10	2	0	1	4	0	20	240	—	0	—	0
Creamy Roasted Garlic	2 tbsp (1 oz)	110	10	2	0	1	3	0	0	240	—	0	—	0
Deluxe French	2 tbsp (1 oz)	120	11	2	0	0	5	0	0	170	—	0	—	0
Fat Free Chunky Blue Cheese	2 tbsp (1 oz)	35	0	0	0	0	7	tr	20	290	—	0	—	0
Fat Free Creamy Italian	2 tbsp (1 oz)	35	0	0	0	0	9	tr	0	250	—	0	—	0
Fat Free Creamy Roasted Garlic	2 tbsp (1 oz)	40	0	0	0	0	9	0	20	280	—	0	—	0
Fat Free Deluxe French	2 tbsp (1 oz)	30	0	0	0	0	7	tr	0	230	—	0	—	0
Fat Free Honey Dijon	2 tbsp (1 oz)	45	0	0	0	1	10	0	20	270	—	0	—	0
Fat Free Italian	2 tbsp (1 oz)	10	0	0	0	0	2	0	0	280	—	0	—	0
Fat Free Parmesan & Onion	2 tbsp (1 oz)	45	0	0	0	1	9	tr	20	320	—	0	—	0
Fat Free Ranch	2 tbsp (1 oz)	40	0	0	0	0	9	tr	20	280	—	0	—	0
Fat Free Red Wine Vinaigrette	2 tbsp (1 oz)	35	0	0	0	0	7	0	0	230	—	0	—	0
Fat Free Sweet N' Spicy French	2 tbsp (1 oz)	30	0	0	0	0	7	0	0	220	—	0	—	0

FOOD	PORTION	CALORIES	FAT	SAT FAT	CHOL	PROTEIN	CARBO	FIBER	CALCIUM	SOD	POTAS	VIT C	FOLIC	VIT A
WISHBONE (CONT.)														
Fat Free Thousand Island	2 tbsp (1 oz)	35	0	0	0	0	9	tr	0	290	—	0	—	100
Italian	2 tbsp (1 oz)	80	8	1	0	0	3	0	0	490	—	0	—	0
Lite French	2 tbsp (1 oz)	50	2	1	5	0	8	0	0	240	—	0	—	0
Lite Italian	2 tbsp (1 oz)	15	1	0	0	0	2	0	0	500	—	0	—	0
Lite Ranch	2 tbsp (1 oz)	100	8	1	5	0	5	0	0	300	—	0	—	0
Olive Oil Vinaigrette	2 tbsp (1 oz)	60	5	1	0	0	4	0	0	250	—	0	—	0
Oriental	2 tbsp (1 oz)	70	5	1	0	0	5	0	0	440	—	0	—	0
Parmesan & Onion	2 tbsp (1 oz)	110	10	2	5	1	5	0	20	260	—	0	—	0
Ranch	2 tbsp (1 oz)	160	17	3	10	0	1	0	20	200	—	0	—	0
Red Wine Vinaigrette	2 tbsp (1 oz)	80	5	1	0	0	9	0	0	230	—	0	—	0
Robusto Italian	2 tbsp (1 oz)	90	8	1	0	0	4	0	0	550	—	2	—	0
Russian	2 tbsp (1 oz)	110	6	1	0	0	15	0	0	350	—	0	—	0
Sweet N' Spicy French	2 tbsp (1 oz)	140	12	2	0	0	6	0	0	330	—	0	—	0
Thousand Island	2 tbsp (1 oz)	140	12	2	10	0	7	0	0	340	—	0	—	0
SALMON														
CANNED														
chum w/ bone	3 oz	120	5	1	33	18	0	—	212	414	—	—	—	51
chum w/ bone	1 can (13.9 oz)	521	20	5	144	79	0	—	920	1797	—	—	—	5483
pink w/ bone	1 can (15.9 oz)	631	27	7	—	90	0	—	969	2514	1982	0	70	250
pink w/ bone	3 oz	118	5	1	—	17	0	—	181	471	277	0	13	47
sockeye w/ bone	1 can (12.9 oz)	566	27	6	161	76	0	—	883	1987	1392	0	36	648
sockeye w/ bone	3 oz	130	6	1	37	17	0	—	203	458	321	0	8	149
BUMBLE BEE														
Keta	3.5 oz	160	8	2	60	20	0	—	150	490	340	0	—	0
Pink	3.5 oz	160	8	2	50	20	0	—	200	490	320	0	—	0
Pink Skinless & Boneless	3.25 oz	120	5	1	25	17	0	—	0	420	300	0	—	0
Red	3.5 oz	180	10	2	60	20	0	—	150	490	370	0	—	100
Red Skinless & Boneless	3.25 oz	130	6	1	30	17	0	—	0	420	310	0	—	0
FRESH														
coho cooked	3 oz	157	6	1	42	23	0	—	—	50	454	1	—	—
coho cooked	½ fillet (5.4 oz)	286	12	2	76	42	0	—	—	91	828	2	—	—
coho raw	3 oz	124	5	1	33	18	0	—	—	39	359	1	—	—
roe raw	3.5 oz	207	10	—	—	25	1	—	—	—	—	18	—	—
sockeye cooked	½ fillet (5.4 oz)	334	17	3	135	42	0	—	11	102	582	—	—	324

FOOD	PORTION	CALORIES	FAT	SAT FAT	CHOL	PROTEIN	CARBO	FIBER	CALCIUM	SOD	POTAS	VIT C	FOLIC	VIT A
sockeye cooked	3 oz	183	9	2	74	23	0	—	6	102	582	—	—	178
sockeye raw	3 oz	143	7	1	53	18	0	—	5	40	332	—	—	163
SMOKED														
chinook	1 oz	33	1	tr	7	5	0	—	3	220	49	—	1	25
chinook	3 oz	99	4	1	20	16	0	—	9	666	149	—	2	75
NATHAN'S														
Nova	2 oz	80	3	1	30	13	1	0	0	1150	—	0	—	0

SALSA

(*see also* KETCHUP, SAUCE, SPANISH FOODS)

FOOD	PORTION	CALORIES	FAT	SAT FAT	CHOL	PROTEIN	CARBO	FIBER	CALCIUM	SOD	POTAS	VIT C	FOLIC	VIT A
CASA FIESTA														
Chili Salsa	1 oz	9	tr	—	—	tr	2	—	3	117	—	tr	—	67
Picante Mild	1 oz	9	tr	—	—	tr	2	—	3	117	—	tr	—	67
CHI-CHI'S														
Con Queso	2 tbsp (1.1 oz)	90	7	3	15	3	4	0	80	480	—	0	—	0
Hot	2 tbsp (1 oz)	10	0	0	0	0	2	0	0	160	—	0	—	0
Medium	2 tbsp (1 oz)	10	0	0	0	0	2	0	0	140	—	0	—	0
Mild	2 tbsp (1 oz)	10	0	0	0	0	1	0	0	140	—	0	—	0
Picante Hot	2 tbsp (1 oz)	10	0	0	0	0	2	0	0	270	—	0	—	0
Picante Medium	2 tbsp (1 oz)	10	0	0	0	0	2	0	0	200	—	0	—	0
Picante Mild	2 tbsp (1 oz)	10	0	0	0	0	2	0	0	210	—	0	—	0
Verde Medium	2 tbsp (1.2 oz)	15	0	0	0	0	3	0	0	180	—	2	—	0
Verde Mild	2 tbsp (1.2 oz)	15	0	0	0	0	3	0	0	180	—	2	—	0
DEL MONTE														
Mexicana	2 tbsp (1.1 oz)	5	0	0	0	0	2	1	0	200	—	1	—	300
Taquera	2 tbsp (1.1 oz)	5	0	0	0	0	2	1	0	220	—	1	—	400
Verde	2 tbsp (1.1 oz)	10	0	0	0	0	2	tr	0	280	—	2	—	0
GUILTLESS GOURMET														
Picante Hot	1 oz	6	0	0	0	0	1	tr	—	133	—	—	—	—
Picante Medium	1 oz	6	0	0	0	0	1	tr	—	133	—	—	—	—
HAIN														
Hot	¼ cup	22	0	0	0	1	4	—	20	480	140	9	—	300
Mild	¼ cup	20	0	0	—	1	4	—	40	410	150	5	—	300
HELUVA GOOD CHEESE														
Cheese & Salsa	2 tbsp (1.1 oz)	80	6	5	10	3	3	0	100	210	—	1	—	200
Thick & Chunky Hot	2 tbsp (1.2 oz)	10	0	0	0	0	2	0	20	180	—	4	—	200
Thick & Chunky Mild	2 tbsp (1.2 oz)	10	0	0	0	0	2	0	20	180	—	4	—	200
HOT CHA CHA														
Medium	2 tbsp (1 oz)	5	0	0	0	0	2	—	—	0	—	—	—	—
HUNT'S														
Alfresco Medium	2 tbsp (1.1 oz)	10	tr	tr	0	tr	2	tr	9	199	—	6	—	28
Alfresco Mild	2 tbsp (1.1 oz)	10	tr	tr	0	tr	2	tr	9	199	—	6	—	28
Hot	2 tbsp (1.1 oz)	27	tr	0	0	1	6	1	10	236	—	5	—	98
Medium	2 tbsp (1.1 oz)	27	tr	0	0	1	6	1	10	236	—	5	—	98

FOOD	PORTION	CALORIES	FAT	SAT FAT	CHOL	PROTEIN	CARBO	FIBER	CALCIUM	SOD	POTAS	VIT C	FOLIC	VIT A
HUNT'S (CONT.)														
Mild	2 tbsp (1.1 oz)	27	tr	0	0	1	6	1	10	236	—	5	—	98
Picante Medium	2 tbsp (1.1 oz)	11	tr	0	0	1	2	tr	5	256	—	2	—	62
Picante Mild	2 tbsp (1.1 oz)	11	tr	0	0	1	2	tr	5	256	—	2	—	62
LOUISE'S														
Fat Free BBQ Black Bean	1 oz	10	0	0	0	0	2	0	—	110	—	—	—	—
Fat Free Black Bean	1 oz	10	0	0	0	0	2	0	—	110	—	—	—	—
Fat Free Medium	1 oz	10	0	0	0	0	3	1	—	80	—	—	—	—
Fat Free Mild	1 oz	10	0	0	0	0	3	1	—	80	—	—	—	—
Fat Free Nacho Queso	1 oz	15	0	0	0	1	3	0	—	45	—	—	—	—
MUIR GLEN														
Organic Fat Free Hot	2 tbsp (1.1 oz)	10	0	—	0	tr	2	0	0	160	—	1	—	100
Organic Fat Free Medium	2 tbsp (1.1 oz)	10	0	—	0	tr	2	0	0	160	—	1	—	100
Organic Fat Free Mild	2 tbsp (1.1 oz)	10	0	—	0	tr	2	0	0	160	—	1	—	100
NEWMAN'S OWN														
Bandito Hot	2 tbsp (1.1 oz)	10	0	0	0	0	2	tr	0	150	—	0	—	200
Bandito Medium	2 tbsp (1.1 oz)	10	0	0	0	0	2	tr	0	105	—	0	—	200
Bandito Mild	2 tbsp (1.1 oz)	10	0	0	0	0	2	tr	0	105	—	0	—	200
Peach	2 tbsp (1.1 oz)	25	0	0	0	0	6	1	0	90	—	0	—	750
Pineapple	2 tbsp (1.1 oz)	15	0	0	0	0	3	1	0	90	—	0	—	750
Roasted Garlic	2 tbsp (1.1 oz)	10	0	0	0	1	2	1	0	150	—	0	—	500
OLD EL PASO														
Green Chili Medium	2 tbsp (1 oz)	10	0	0	0	0	2	tr	20	110	—	2	—	0
Homestyle	2 tbsp (1 oz)	5	0	0	0	0	1	0	40	110	—	4	—	200
Homestyle Mild	2 tbsp (1 oz)	5	0	0	0	0	1	0	40	110	—	4	—	200
Picante Hot	2 tbsp (1 oz)	10	0	0	0	0	2	0	0	230	—	2	—	0
Picante Medium	2 tbsp (1 oz)	10	0	0	0	0	2	0	0	230	—	2	—	0
Picante Mild	2 tbsp (1 oz)	10	0	0	0	0	2	0	0	230	—	2	—	100
Picante Thick'n Chunky Hot	2 tbsp (1 oz)	10	0	0	0	0	2	0	0	160	—	2	—	100
Picante Thick'n Chunky Medium	2 tbsp (1 oz)	10	0	0	0	0	2	0	0	140	—	2	—	0
Picante Thick'n Chunky Mild	2 tbsp (1 oz)	10	0	0	0	0	2	0	0	130	—	2	—	0
Pico De Gallo Hot	2 tbsp (1 oz)	5	0	0	0	0	2	tr	0	260	—	0	—	0
Pico De Gallo Medium	1 tbsp (1 oz)	5	0	0	0	0	2	tr	0	260	—	0	—	0
Salsa Verde	2 tbsp (1 oz)	10	0	0	0	0	2	0	0	95	—	0	—	0
Thick'n Chunky Hot	2 tbsp (1 oz)	10	0	0	0	0	2	0	0	130	—	4	—	100

FOOD	PORTION	CALORIES	FAT	SAT FAT	CHOL	PROTEIN	CARBO	FIBER	CALCIUM	SOD	POTAS	VIT C	FOLIC	VIT A
OLD EL PASO (CONT.)														
Thick'n Chunky Medium	2 tbsp (1 oz)	10	0	0	0	0	2	0	0	140	—	5	—	100
Thick'n Chunky Mild	2 tbsp (1 oz)	10	0	0	0	0	2	0	0	140	—	5	—	100
ORTEGA														
Hot Green Chili	1 tbsp	6	0	0	0	0	2	—	—	190	65	4	—	—
Medium Green Chili	1 tbsp	6	0	0	0	0	1	—	—	190	55	1	—	—
Mild Green Chili	1 tbsp	8	0	0	0	0	2	—	—	190	70	1	—	—
PACE														
Picante	2 tbsp (1 fl oz)	7	0	0	0	tr	2	tr	6	294	78	2	—	60
Thick & Chunky	2 tbsp (1 fl oz)	12	0	0	0	tr	2	1	10	321	86	7	—	62
PROGRESSO														
Italian Hot	2 tbsp (1 oz)	30	0	0	0	0	2	tr	0	170	—	4	—	100
Italian Medium	2 tbsp (1 oz)	10	0	0	0	0	2	tr	0	170	—	4	—	100
Italian Mild	2 tbsp (1 oz)	10	0	0	0	0	2	tr	0	170	—	4	—	100
ROSARITA														
Chunky Hot	3 tbsp (1.5 oz)	25	tr	—	0	1	6	tr	20	300	100	17	—	92
Chunky Medium	3 tbsp (1.5 oz)	25	tr	—	0	1	6	tr	35	350	130	17	—	94
Chunky Mild	3 tbsp (1.5 oz)	25	tr	—	0	1	6	tr	50	340	130	17	—	91
Taco Salsa Chunky Medium	3 tbsp (1.5 oz)	25	tr	—	0	1	6	tr	20	310	100	16	—	87
Taco Salsa Chunky Mild	3 tbsp (1.5 oz)	25	tr	—	0	1	6	tr	19	300	90	16	—	80
TABASCO														
Picante	2 tbsp (1.5 oz)	17	tr	tr	0	1	3	1	8	313	—	tr	—	441
TACO BELL														
Smooth 'N Zesty Picante Medium	2 tbsp (1.1 oz)	15	0	0	0	0	3	tr	0	190	—	0	—	100
Smooth 'N Zesty Picante Mild	2 tbsp (1.1 oz)	15	0	0	0	0	3	tr	0	190	—	0	—	100
Thick 'N Chunky Salsa Hot	2 tbsp (1.1 oz)	15	0	0	0	0	2	tr	0	240	—	0	—	100
Thick 'N Chunky Salsa Medium	2 tbsp (1.1 oz)	15	0	0	0	0	2	tr	0	240	—	0	—	100
Thick 'N Chunky Salsa Mild	2 tbsp (1.1 oz)	15	0	0	0	tr	3	tr	0	240	—	0	—	100
TOSTITOS														
Hot	2 tbsp (1 oz)	12	0	0	0	1	3	1	0	205	50	4	—	480
Medium	2 tbsp (1 oz)	12	0	0	0	1	3	1	0	205	50	4	—	480
Mild	2 tbsp (1 oz)	12	0	0	0	1	3	1	0	205	50	4	—	480
TREE OF LIFE														
Hot	2 tbsp (1 oz)	10	0	0	0	0	2	—	20	30	—	4	—	200
Medium	2 tbsp (1 oz)	10	0	0	0	0	2	—	20	30	—	4	—	200
Mild	2 tbsp (1 oz)	10	0	0	0	0	2	—	20	30	—	4	—	200
No Salt	2 tbsp (1 oz)	10	0	0	0	0	2	—	20	20	—	4	—	200

FOOD	PORTION	CALORIES	FAT	SAT FAT	CHOL	PROTEIN	CARBO	FIBER	CALCIUM	SOD	POTAS	VIT C	FOLIC	VIT A
WATKINS														
Salsa Seasoning Blend	⅛ tsp (0.5 g)	0	0	0	0	0	0	0	0	5	—	0	—	150
Tropical	2 tbsp (1 oz)	60	0	0	0	0	13	0	0	430	—	0	—	0
WISE														
Picante	2 tbsp	12	0	0	0	0	3	—	—	130	65	—	—	750
SALSIFY														
fresh sliced cooked	½ cup	46	tr	—	0	2	10	—	32	11	192	3	—	0
raw sliced	½ cup	55	tr	—	0	2	12	—	40	13	255	5	—	0
SALT/SEASONED SALT														
(*see also* SALT SUBSTITUTES)														
salt	1 tbsp (18 g)	0	0	0	0	0	0	—	4	6976	1	—	—	—
salt	1 tsp (6 g)	0	0	0	0	0	0	—	1	2325	0	—	—	—
HAIN														
Sea Salt	1 tsp	0	0	0	0	0	0	—	—	2255	—	—	—	—
Sea Salt Iodized	1 tsp	0	0	0	0	0	0	—	—	2255	—	—	—	—
WATKINS														
Bacon Cheese Salt	¼ tbsp (1 g)	0	0	0	0	0	0	0	0	280	—	0	—	0
Butter Salt	¼ tbsp (1 g)	0	0	0	0	0	0	0	0	330	—	0	—	0
Cheese Salt	¼ tbsp (1 g)	0	0	0	0	0	0	0	0	290	—	0	—	0
Garlic Salt	¼ tsp (1 g)	0	0	0	0	0	0	0	0	270	—	0	—	0
Salt & Vinegar Seasoning	¼ tsp (1 g)	0	0	0	0	0	0	0	0	105	—	0	—	0
Seasoning Salt	¼ tsp (1 g)	0	0	0	0	0	0	0	0	270	—	0	—	0
Sour Cream & Onion Salt	¼ tbsp (1 g)	0	0	0	0	0	0	0	0	270	—	0	—	0
SALT SUBSTITUTES														
CARDIA														
Salt Alternative	1 pkg (0.6 g)	0	0	0	0	0	0	—	—	135	90	—	—	—
MRS. DASH														
Onion & Herb	⅛ tsp (0.02 oz)	2	0	—	0	tr	tr	—	—	1	5	—	—	—
NOSALT														
Salt Alternative	1 pkg (0.75 g)	0	0	0	0	2	0	—	—	0	375	—	—	—
PAPA DASH														
Lite Salt	½ tsp (1 g)	0	0	0	0	0	1	—	—	170	—	—	—	—
SANDWICH														
TAKE-OUT														
submarine w/ salami ham cheese lettuce tomato onion & oil	1	456	19	7	35	22	51	—	189	1650	394	12	—	425
SAPODILLA														
fresh	1	140	2	—	0	1	34	—	36	20	328	25	—	102
fresh cut up	1 cup	199	3	—	0	1	48	—	51	29	465	35	—	145

FOOD	PORTION	CALORIES	FAT	SAT FAT	CHOL	PROTEIN	CARBO	FIBER	CALCIUM	SOD	POTAS	VIT C	FOLIC	VIT A
SAPOTES														
fresh	1	301	1	—	0	5	76	—	88	21	773	45	—	923
SARDINES														
CANNED														
atlantic in oil w/ bone	2	50	3	tr	34	6	0	—	92	121	95	—	3	54
atlantic in oil w/ bone	1 can (3.2 oz)	192	11	1	131	23	0	—	351	465	365	—	11	206
pacific in tomato sauce w/ bone	1	68	5	1	23	6	0	—	91	157	130	tr	9	139
pacific in tomato sauce w/ bone	1 can (13 oz)	658	44	11	225	61	0	—	887	1532	1262	4	89	1351
DEL MONTE														
In Tomato Sauce	1 fish (1.4 oz)	50	3	1	25	5	1	tr	80	130	—	9	—	0
PORT CLYDE														
In Louisiana Hot Sauce	1 can (3.75 oz)	170	9	2	105	19	1	0	200	760	—	0	—	400
In Mustard Sauce	1 can (3.75 oz)	150	9	2	110	18	1	1	250	450	—	0	—	200
In Soybean Oil Select Small	1 can (3.3 oz)	220	17	4	115	19	0	0	300	360	—	0	—	100
In Soybean Oil With Hot Chilies	1 can (3.3 oz)	155	9	2	80	21	0	0	350	310	—	0	—	100
In Soybean Oil drained	1 can (3.3 oz)	220	17	4	115	19	0	0	300	360	—	0	—	100
In Spring Water	1 can (3.3 oz)	170	10	4	140	18	0	0	300	240	—	0	—	100
In Tomato Sauce	1 can (3.75 oz)	150	9	2	100	17	0	0	250	480	—	0	—	200
UNDERWOOD														
Brisling In Olive Oil	3.75 oz	260	20	—	—	19	1	—	300	450	—	—	—	200
In Mustard Sauce	3.75 oz	220	16	—	—	16	2	—	250	560	250	—	—	300
In Sild Oil drained	3.75 oz	460	42	—	—	19	1	—	300	120	—	—	—	—
In Soya Oil drained	3 oz	230	18	—	—	16	1	—	250	400	220	—	—	200
In Tomato Sauce	3.75 oz	220	16	—	—	16	2	—	250	500	270	—	—	300
With Tabasco Pepper Sauce drained	3 oz	220	16	—	—	16	1	—	250	400	180	—	—	100
VIKING'S DELIGHT														
Brisling In Olive Oil	1 can (3.75 oz)	460	42	—	—	19	1	—	300	450	—	0	—	200
Brisling In Olive Oil drained	1 can (3.75 oz)	260	20	—	—	19	1	—	300	450	—	0	—	200
SAUCE														
(*see also* BARBECUE SAUCE, GRAVY, PIZZA, SALSA, SPAGHETTI SAUCE, TOMATO)														
JARRED														
teriyaki	1 oz	30	0	0	0	2	6	—	9	1380	81	0	7	0
teriyaki	1 tbsp	15	0	0	0	1	3	—	4	690	41	0	4	0

FOOD	PORTION	CALORIES	FAT	SAT FAT	CHOL	PROTEIN	CARBO	FIBER	CALCIUM	SOD	POTAS	VIT C	FOLIC	VIT A
ARMOUR														
Chili Hot Dog	¼ cup (2.2 oz)	120	9	—	20	4	6	—	—	310	—	—	—	—
Meatless Sloppy Joe Sauce	¼ cup (2.2 oz)	30	0	0	0	0	7	—	—	430	—	—	—	—
CASA FIESTA														
Taco Mild	1 oz	9	tr	—	—	tr	2	—	3	117	—	tr	—	67
CHEEZ WHIZ														
Cheese	2 tbsp (1.2 oz)	90	7	5	20	4	3	0	100	540	105	0	—	300
Cheese Jalapeno Pepper	2 tbsp (1.2 oz)	90	7	5	25	4	3	0	100	510	90	0	—	300
Cheese Mild Salsa	2 tbsp (1.2 oz)	100	7	5	25	4	3	0	100	530	85	0	—	300
CHI-CHI'S														
Enchilada	¼ cup (2.1 oz)	30	2	1	0	0	3	0	0	210	—	0	—	500
Taco	1 tbsp (0.5 oz)	10	0	0	0	0	1	0	0	75	—	0	—	0
CONTADINA														
Sweet 'n Sour	2 tbsp	40	1	—	—	0	8	—	—	110	—	—	—	—
DEL MONTE														
Cocktail	¼ cup (2.7 oz)	100	0	0	0	1	24	0	0	910	—	2	—	1000
Sloppy Joe Hickory Flavor	¼ cup (2.4 oz)	70	0	0	0	1	18	0	40	700	—	15	—	2500
Sloppy Joe Italian Style	¼ cup (2.4 oz)	70	0	0	0	1	16	0	20	700	—	12	—	1750
Sloppy Joe Original	¼ cup (2.4 oz)	70	0	0	0	1	16	0	0	680	—	12	—	2500
EL MOLINO														
Taco Red Mild	2 tbsp	10	0	0	0	0	2	—	—	170	65	—	—	500
ESCOFFIER														
Diable	1 tbsp	20	0	0	—	0	4	—	—	160	45	—	—	—
GEBHARDT														
Enchilada Sauce	3 tbsp (1.5 oz)	25	1	1	tr	tr	2	tr	90	170	20	1	—	45
Hot Dog Chili Sauce	2 tbsp	30	1	tr	3	1	4	tr	8	180	80	—	—	2
Hot Sauce	½ tsp	tr	tr	—	0	tr	tr	tr	—	55	2	—	—	—
GOLDEN DIPT														
Cajun Style	1 oz	90	8	—	0	0	5	—	—	360	—	4	—	100
Creole	1 oz	20	1	—	0	0	2	—	—	190	—	—	—	—
Dijonaisse	1 oz	52	4	—	0	0	2	—	—	130	—	—	—	—
French White	1 oz	55	4	—	0	0	3	—	—	210	—	—	—	—
Ginger Teriyaki Marinade	1 oz	120	7	—	0	1	12	—	—	920	—	—	—	—
Lemon Butter Dill	1 oz	100	9	—	0	0	4	—	—	190	—	4	—	—
Lemon Herb Marinade	1 oz	130	14	—	0	0	2	—	—	210	—	4	—	—
Seafood Cocktail	1 tbsp	20	0	0	0	0	5	—	—	210	—	4	—	100
Seafood Cocktail Extra Hot	1 tbsp	20	0	0	0	0	5	—	—	210	—	4	—	200
Tartar	1 tbsp	70	7	—	10	0	2	—	—	100	—	6	—	—

FOOD	PORTION	CALORIES	FAT	SAT FAT	CHOL	PROTEIN	CARBO	FIBER	CALCIUM	SOD	POTAS	VIT C	FOLIC	VIT A
GOLDEN DIPT (CONT.)														
Tartar Lite	1 tbsp	50	4	—	5	0	4	—	—	40	—	—	—	—
GREEN GIANT														
Sloppy Joe	¼ cup (2.6 oz)	50	0	0	0	2	11	2	0	420	—	0	—	750
Sloppy Joe as prep w/ meat	1 serv (4.4 oz)	200	11	4	45	14	11	2	20	470	—	0	—	750
HEINZ														
Worcestershire	1 tbsp	6	0	0	0	0	1	—	—	170	50	1	—	—
HELUVA GOOD CHEESE														
Cocktail	¼ cup (1.6 oz)	40	0	0	0	0	10	—	—	410	—	—	—	—
HORMEL														
Not-So-Sloppy-Joe Sauce	¼ cup (2.2 oz)	70	0	0	0	1	15	1	20	720	—	1	—	100
HOUSE OF TSANG														
Bangkok Padang	1 tbsp (0.6 oz)	45	3	1	0	1	4	0	0	240	—	0	—	0
Hoisin	1 tsp (6 g)	15	0	0	0	0	4	0	0	120	—	0	—	0
Mandarin Marinade	1 tbsp (0.6 oz)	25	0	0	0	0	6	0	0	680	—	0	—	0
Saigon Sizzle	1 tbsp (0.6 oz)	40	1	0	0	0	8	0	0	350	—	0	—	0
Spicy Brown Bean	1 tsp (6 g)	15	0	0	0	0	3	0	0	130	—	0	—	0
Stir Fry Classic	1 tbsp (0.6 oz)	25	1	0	0	0	4	0	0	570	—	0	—	0
Stir Fry Sweet & Sour	1 tbsp (0.6 oz)	30	0	0	0	0	7	0	0	45	—	0	—	0
Stir Fry Szechuan Spicy	1 tbsp (0.6 oz)	20	1	0	0	0	4	0	0	490	—	0	—	0
Sweet & Sour Concentrate	1 tsp (6 g)	10	0	0	0	0	3	0	0	15	—	0	—	0
Teriyaki Korean	1 tbsp (0.6 oz)	30	1	0	0	0	6	0	0	430	—	0	—	0
HUNT'S														
Chicken Sensations Barbecue Flavor	1 tbsp (0.5 oz)	35	3	tr	0	tr	3	tr	7	308	—	2	—	38
Chicken Sensations Italian Garlic	1 tbsp (0.5 oz)	30	3	tr	0	tr	1	1	8	326	—	2	—	25
Chicken Sensations Lemon Herb	1 tbsp (0.5 oz)	31	3	tr	0	tr	2	tr	6	378	—	1	—	30
Chicken Sensations South Western	1 tbsp (0.5 oz)	27	3	tr	0	tr	1	tr	8	281	—	2	—	20
Pepper Sauce Original	1 tsp (5.2 g)	1	tr	0	0	tr	tr	0	1	205	—	tr	—	5
Steak	1 tbsp (0.6 oz)	10	tr	0	0	tr	2	tr	1	256	—	2	—	4
JUST RITE														
Hot Dog	2 oz	60	3	1	7	2	6	tr	14	220	170	2	—	5
KA-ME														
Black Bean Sauce	1 tbsp (0.5 oz)	10	0	0	0	1	2	1	—	550	—	—	—	—
Chili Sauce Hot Garlic	1 tbsp (0.5 oz)	15	0	0	0	0	4	1	—	115	—	—	—	—
Duck Sauce	2 tbsp (1 oz)	80	0	0	0	0	20	0	—	480	—	—	—	—

FOOD	PORTION	CALORIES	FAT	SAT FAT	CHOL	PROTEIN	CARBO	FIBER	CALCIUM	SOD	POTAS	VIT C	FOLIC	VIT A
KA-ME (CONT.)														
Fish Sauce	1 tbsp (0.5 fl oz)	10	0	0	0	1	1	0	—	1300	—	—	—	—
Hoisin Sauce	2 tbsp (1 oz)	45	0	0	0	1	10	1	—	620	—	—	—	—
Hot Sauce	1 tsp (5 g)	0	0	0	0	0	1	0	—	80	—	—	—	—
Lemon Sauce	1 tbsp (0.5 oz)	45	0	0	0	0	11	0	—	125	—	—	—	—
Mandarin Orange Sauce	2 tbsp (1 oz)	80	0	0	0	0	21	0	—	430	—	—	—	—
Oyster Sauce	1 tbsp (0.5 fl oz)	10	0	0	0	0	3	0	—	460	—	—	—	—
Plum	2 tbsp (1 fl oz)	80	0	0	0	0	19	0	—	420	—	—	—	—
Stir Fry Sauce	1 tbsp	10	0	0	0	1	1	0	—	570	—	—	—	—
Sweet & Sour	2 tbsp (1 fl oz)	50	0	0	0	0	13	0	—	270	—	—	—	—
Szechuan	1 tbsp (0.5 oz)	20	1	0	0	1	2	2	—	410	—	—	—	—
Tamari	1 tbsp (0.5 fl oz)	10	1	0	0	2	1	0	—	930	—	—	—	—
Tempura Sauce	2 tbsp (1 fl oz)	15	0	0	0	1	3	0	—	1790	—	—	—	—
Teriyaki Sauce	1 tbsp (0.5 fl oz)	10	0	0	0	0	2	0	—	480	—	—	—	—
KRAFT														
Cocktail	¼ cup (2.3 oz)	60	1	0	0	1	13	1	0	800	270	6	—	500
Fat Free Tartar Sauce	2 tbsp (1.1 oz)	25	0	0	0	0	5	0	0	200	20	0	—	0
Lemon & Herb Tartar Sauce	2 tbsp (1 oz)	150	16	3	15	0	tr	0	0	170	10	0	—	0
Reduced Fat Sandwich Spread	1 tbsp (0.5 oz)	35	3	0	0	0	3	0	0	130	5	0	—	0
Sandwich Spread	1 tbsp (0.5 oz)	50	4	1	<5	0	3	0	0	105	0	0	—	0
Sweet'n Sour	2 tbsp (1.2 oz)	60	0	0	0	0	14	0	0	125	20	0	—	0
Tartar	2 tbsp (1.1 oz)	90	9	2	10	0	4	2	0	170	15	0	—	0
LA CHOY														
Duck Sauce Sweet & Sour	1 tbsp	25	tr	—	0	tr	7	tr	—	40	10	—	—	—
Sweet & Sour	1 tbsp	25	tr	—	0	tr	7	tr	—	40	10	—	—	—
LAWRY'S														
Marinade Lemon Pepper	1 tbsp (0.5 oz)	10	1	—	—	0	1	—	—	380	—	—	—	—
Teriyaki Marinade	2 tbsp	72	tr	tr	0	6	11	tr	—	7100	520	—	—	—
LEA & PERRINS														
Steak	1 oz	40	tr	—	—	tr	10	—	—	220	—	—	—	—
MANWICH														
Bold	¼ cup (2.2 oz)	62	1	0	0	1	13	1	3	802	—	8	—	46
Burrito	¼ cup (2.2 oz)	25	tr	0	0	1	6	4	15	559	—	7	—	107
Mexican	¼ cup (2.2 oz)	27	tr	0	0	1	5	1	2	552	—	7	—	77
Original	¼ cup (2.2 oz)	32	tr	0	0	1	6	1	1	365	—	7	—	77
Taco	¼ cup (2.2 oz)	31	tr	0	0	1	7	1	9	587	—	33	—	443
Thick & Chunky	¼ cup (2.3 oz)	44	tr	0	0	1	9	1	2	737	—	7	—	79

FOOD	PORTION	CALORIES	FAT	SAT FAT	CHOL	PROTEIN	CARBO	FIBER	CALCIUM	SOD	POTAS	VIT C	FOLIC	VIT A
MARZETTI														
Teriyaki Stir-Fry	2 tbsp	80	2	0	0	2	14	0	0	820	—	0	—	0
MCILHENNY														
7 Spice Chili	2 tbsp (1.1 fl oz)	16	tr	tr	tr	1	3	1	25	191	—	tr	—	874
Sauce	2 tbsp (1.1 oz)	48	2	tr	tr	1	7	tr	9	201	—	2	—	401
Tabasco	1 tsp	1	tr	tr	tr	tr	tr	tr	1	30	—	tr	—	209
MRS. DASH														
Steak	1 tbsp (0.4 oz)	17	tr	—	0	tr	4	—	—	10	70	—	—	—
NEWMAN'S OWN														
Spicy Simmer Sauce Diavolo	½ cup (4.4 oz)	70	3	0	0	0	10	3	60	510	—	0	—	750
OLD EL PASO														
Enchilada Hot	¼ cup (2 oz)	30	2	—	0	0	4	0	0	190	—	0	—	750
Enchilada Mild	¼ cup (2 oz)	25	1	—	0	0	4	0	0	160	—	6	—	500
Green Chili Enchilada Sauce	¼ cup (2.1 oz)	30	2	—	0	tr	3	0	0	330	—	6	—	0
Taco Hot	1 tbsp (0.5 oz)	5	0	0	0	0	1	0	0	90	—	0	—	0
Taco Medium	1 tbsp (0.5 oz)	5	0	0	0	0	1	0	0	70	—	0	—	0
Taco Mild	1 tbsp (0.5 oz)	5	0	0	0	0	1	0	0	85	—	0	—	0
Taco Sauce	1 tbsp (0.5 oz)	5	0	0	0	0	1	0	0	85	—	0	—	0
Taco Sauce Extra Chunky Medium	1 tbsp (0.5 oz)	5	0	0	0	0	1	0	0	80	—	0	—	0
Taco Sauce Extra Chunky Mild	1 tbsp (0.5 oz)	5	0	0	0	0	1	0	0	80	—	0	—	0
ORTEGA														
Taco Thick & Smooth Hot	1 tbsp	8	0	0	0	0	2	0	—	105	40	2	—	200
Taco Thick & Smooth Mild	1 tbsp	8	0	0	0	0	2	0	—	115	35	2	—	100
PROGRESSO														
Alfredo	½ cup (4.4 oz)	310	27	15	75	10	5	0	300	670	—	0	—	750
RED WING														
Chili Sauce	1 tbsp (0.6 oz)	20	0	0	0	0	5	0	0	220	—	0	—	0
Seafood Cocktail	¼ cup (2 oz)	90	1	0	0	0	22	0	0	830	—	2	—	300
SAUCE ARTURO														
Original	¼ cup (2.2 fl oz)	50	1	0	0	1	8	0	0	680	—	6	—	200
SIMMER CHEF														
Golden Honey Mustard	½ cup (4 fl oz)	150	2	0	0	1	30	1	20	400	—	1	—	0
Hearty Onion & Mushroom	½ cup (4 fl oz)	50	1	0	0	1	9	1	20	670	—	0	—	0
SNOW'S														
Newburg With Sherry	⅓ cup	120	8	—	—	3	10	—	80	520	110	—	—	100

FOOD	PORTION	CALORIES	FAT	SAT FAT	CHOL	PROTEIN	CARBO	FIBER	CALCIUM	SOD	POTAS	VIT C	FOLIC	VIT A
SNOW'S (CONT.)														
Welsh Rarebit Cheese	½ cup	170	11	—	—	9	10	—	250	460	25	—	—	500
TACO BELL														
Taco Sauce Medium	2 tbsp (1.1 oz)	15	0	0	0	0	3	tr	0	160	—	0	—	200
Taco Sauce Mild	2 tbsp (1.1 oz)	15	0	0	0	0	3	tr	0	160	—	0	—	200
The Restaurant Hot Sauce	1 tsp (5 g)	0	0	0	0	0	0	0	0	50	—	0	—	0
TRAPPEY														
Indi-Pep West Indian Style Pepper Sauce	1 tsp (0.1 oz)	1	tr	0	0	tr	tr	tr	tr	41	—	tr	—	33
Mexi Pep Louisiana Hot Sauce	1 tsp (0.1 oz)	tr	tr	0	0	tr	tr	tr	1	59	—	tr	—	30
Pepper Sauce	1 tsp (0.2 oz)	1	tr	0	0	tr	tr	tr	1	85	—	tr	—	47
Red Devil Buffalo Style Hot Sauce	1 tsp (0.1 oz)	1	tr	0	0	tr	tr	tr	1	59	—	1	—	148
Red Devil Cayenne Pepper Sauce	1 tsp (0.1 oz)	1	tr	0	0	tr	tr	tr	tr	44	—	1	—	55
Worcestershire Chef Magic	1 tsp (0.1 oz)	3	tr	tr	0	tr	1	tr	1	39	—	tr	—	<5
WATKINS														
Inferno Hot Pepper Sauce	2 tbsp (1 oz)	35	0	0	0	0	8	1	0	930	—	0	—	100
Steak Sauce	1 tbsp (0.5 oz)	20	0	0	0	0	4	0	0	220	—	0	—	150
MIX														
bearnaise as prep w/ milk & butter	1 cup	701	68	42	189	8	18	—	—	1265	—	—	—	—
cheese as prep w/ milk	1 cup	307	17	9	53	16	23	—	570	1566	554	2	—	—
curry as prep w/ milk	1 cup	270	15	6	35	11	26	—	485	1276	—	—	—	—
mushroom as prep w/ milk	1 cup	228	10	5	34	11	24	—	—	1533	—	—	—	—
sourcream as prep w/ milk	1 cup	509	30	16	91	19	45	—	546	1007	733	—	—	—
stroganoff as prep	1 cup	271	11	7	38	12	34	—	521	1829	672	—	—	—
sweet & sour as prep	1 cup	294	tr	tr	0	1	73	—	41	779	66	—	—	—
teriyaki as prep	1 cup	131	1	tr	0	4	28	—	112	4791	216	—	—	—
white as prep w/ milk	1 cup	241	13	6	34	10	21	—	424	796	443	—	—	—
CAJUN KING														
Etoufee Seasoning Mix	3.5 oz	383	6	—	—	12	70	—	64	1087	—	20	—	4660
Jambalaya Seasoning Mix	3.5 oz	375	9	—	—	12	61	—	114	2855	—	16	—	2150

FOOD	PORTION	CALORIES	FAT	SAT FAT	CHOL	PROTEIN	CARBO	FIBER	CALCIUM	SOD	POTAS	VIT C	FOLIC	VIT A
DURKEE														
A La King as prep	1 cup	60	4	1	0	1	8	0	80	800	—	9	—	100
Cheese as prep	¼ cup	25	2	1	2	1	4	0	40	260	—	0	—	0
Hollandaise as prep	2 tbsp	10	0	0	0	0	2	0	0	70	—	0	—	100
Nacho Cheese as prep	2 tbsp	25	2	0	0	1	2	0	0	180	—	5	—	200
White as prep	¼ cup	20	1	0	0	0	5	0	0	330	—	0	—	0
FRENCH'S														
Cheese as prep	¼ cup	25	1	0	0	1	4	0	0	250	—	0	—	0
Hollandaise as prep	2 tbsp	10	0	0	0	0	2	0	0	75	—	0	—	0
WATKINS														
Beef Marinade	¼ tbsp (2 g)	5	0	0	0	0	1	0	0	160	—	0	—	0
Calypso Hot Pepper Sauce	1 tsp (5 g)	10	0	0	0	0	3	0	0	25	—	0	—	0
Caribbean Red Pepper Sauce	1 tsp (5 g)	10	0	0	0	0	3	0	0	25	—	0	—	0
Chicken & Pork Marinade	¼ tbsp (2 g)	5	0	0	0	0	2	0	0	280	—	0	—	0
Fish & Seafood Marinade	¼ tbsp (2 g)	10	0	0	0	0	1	0	0	100	—	0	—	0
Meat Magic	1 tsp (6 g)	10	0	0	0	0	2	0	0	190	—	0	—	0
SHELF-STABLE														
CHEEZ WHIZ														
Cheese Sqeezable	2 tbsp (1.2 oz)	100	8	4	15	2	4	0	60	470	30	0	—	200
FRESH GOURMET														
Stir 'n Sauce Italian	1 tbsp (0.5 oz)	30	1	—	—	0	5	—	—	230	—	—	—	—
SAUERKRAUT														
canned	½ cup	22	tr	tr	0	1	5	—	36	780	201	17	—	21
CLAUSSEN														
Canned	½ cup	17	tr	—	0	—	—	—	26	—	—	—	—	—
DEL MONTE														
Canned	½ cup (4.2 oz)	15	0	0	0	1	4	2	0	700	—	18	—	0
HEBREW NATIONAL														
Gallon Kraut	½ cup	25	0	0	0	0	4	—	—	800	—	—	—	—
New Kraut	½ cup (3.1 oz)	50	1	—	—	1	11	—	—	550	—	—	—	—
ROSOFF'S														
Sauerkraut	½ cup (3.2 oz)	50	1	—	—	1	11	—	—	550	—	—	—	—
SCHORR'S														
New Kraut	½ cup (3.2 oz)	50	1	—	—	1	11	—	—	550	—	—	—	—
SENECA														
Canned	2 tbsp	5	0	0	0	0	0	1	0	192	70	5	—	0
VLASIC														
Old Fashioned	1 oz	4	0	0	0	0	1	—	—	280	—	2	—	—
SAUSAGE														
(*see also* HOT DOG, SAUSAGE SUBSTITUTES)														
bierschinken	3.5 oz	174	11	—	—	18	tr	—	15	753	261	—	—	—

FOOD	PORTION	CALORIES	FAT	SAT FAT	CHOL	PROTEIN	CARBO	FIBER	CALCIUM	SOD	POTAS	VIT C	FOLIC	VIT A
bierwurst	3.5 oz	258	21	—	—	16	0	—	—	—	—	—	—	—
bockwurst	3.5 oz	276	25	—	—	12	0	—	—	700	—	—	—	—
bockwurst pork & veal raw	1 link (2.3 oz)	200	18	7	—	9	tr	—	—	—	—	—	—	—
bratwurst pork cooked	1 link (3 oz)	256	22	8	51	12	2	—	38	473	180	1	—	—
brotwurst pork	1 oz	92	8	3	18	4	1	—	14	315	80	8	—	—
brotwurst pork & beef	1 link (2.5 oz)	226	19	7	44	10	2	—	34	778	197	20	—	—
fleischwurst	3.5 oz	305	29	—	—	12	0	—	14	829	199	—	—	—
jagdwurst	3.5 oz	211	16	—	—	16	0	—	14	818	260	—	—	—
knockwurst pork & beef	1 (2.4 oz)	209	19	7	39	8	1	—	7	687	136	18	—	—
pork & beef cooked	1 link (½ oz)	52	5	2	—	2	tr	—	—	105	—	—	—	—
smoked beef cooked	1 sausage (1.4 oz)	134	12	—	29	—	—	—	4	—	—	—	—	—
smoked pork & beef	1 link (2.4 oz)	229	21	7	48	9	1	—	7	151	30	3	—	—
smoked pork & beef	1 sm link (½ oz)	54	5	2	11	2	tr	—	2	151	30	3	—	—
vienna canned	1 (½ oz)	45	4	1	8	2	tr	—	2	152	16	0	—	—
vienna canned	7 (4 oz)	315	28	10	59	12	2	—	12	1077	114	0	—	—
zungenwurst (tongue)	3.5 oz	285	24	—	—	17	0	—	—	—	—	—	—	—
AIDELLS														
Andouille Cajun Cooked	1 (3.5 oz)	220	17	8	40	16	1	—	—	770	—	—	—	—
Burmese Curry Cooked	1 (3.5 oz)	220	15	5	20	18	3	—	—	730	—	—	—	—
Chicken & Apple Fresh	1 (1.9 oz)	110	8	2	20	9	1	—	—	250	—	—	—	—
Chicken & Apple Smoked	1 (3.5 oz)	220	16	5	30	16	0	0	—	730	—	—	—	—
Chicken & Turkey New Mexico Smoked	1 (3.5 oz)	220	16	5	40	15	2	—	—	600	—	—	—	—
Chicken & Turkey Thai Fresh	1 (3.5 oz)	200	16	5	35	15	0	—	—	600	—	—	—	—
Chicken & Turkey Thai Smoked	1 (3.5 oz)	220	16	5	30	18	0	—	—	770	—	—	—	—
Chicken & Turkey With Sun-Dried Tomatoes & Basil Fresh	1 (3.5 oz)	200	15	6	35	15	1	—	—	550	—	—	—	—
Chicken & Turkey With Sun-Dried Tomatoes & Basil Smoked	1 (3.5 oz)	200	14	5	30	19	0	—	—	730	—	—	—	—
Creole Hot Cooked	1 (3.5 oz)	220	16	7	30	17	2	—	—	600	—	—	—	—

FOOD	PORTION	CALORIES	FAT	SAT FAT	CHOL	PROTEIN	CARBO	FIBER	CALCIUM	SOD	POTAS	VIT C	FOLIC	VIT A
AIDELLS (CONT.)														
Duck & Turkey Smoked	1 (3.5 oz)	220	16	4	60	17	1	—	—	700	—	—	—	—
Hunter's Cooked	1 (3.5 oz)	240	19	5	35	17	0	—	—	720	—	—	—	—
Italian Hot Fresh	1 (3.5 oz)	230	18	6	40	16	0	—	—	550	—	—	—	—
Italian Mild Fresh	1 (3.5 oz)	230	18	6	40	16	0	—	—	550	—	—	—	—
Lamb & Beef With Rosemary Fresh	1 (3.5 oz)	220	16	6	35	16	2	—	—	600	—	—	—	—
Lemon Chicken Cooked	1 (3.5 oz)	220	16	5	35	15	1	—	—	700	—	—	—	—
Mexican Chorizo Beef Fresh	1 (3.5 oz)	400	37	14	70	13	3	—	—	550	—	—	—	—
Whiskey Fennel Cooked	1 (3.5 oz)	230	18	7	65	17	1	—	—	730	—	—	—	—
ARMOUR														
Vienna Sausage 25% Less Fat	3 (1.9 oz)	130	11	—	50	6	1	—	—	420	—	—	—	—
Vienna Sausage In BBQ Sauce	3 (2.1 oz)	160	14	—	45	5	4	—	—	550	—	—	—	—
Vienna Sausage In Beef Stock	3 (1.9 oz)	170	16	—	50	5	1	—	—	420	—	—	—	—
Vienna Sausage In Hot Sauce	3 (2.1 oz)	170	15	—	50	5	3	—	—	630	—	—	—	—
Vienna Sausage Smoked	3 (1.9 oz)	170	16	—	50	5	1	—	—	420	—	—	—	—
BANNER														
Sausage Tripe	2 oz	90	5	—	85	9	2	—	—	430	—	—	—	—
BILINSKI'S														
Chicken & Vegetable	1 (3 oz)	80	2	1	40	14	2	tr	20	530	—	6	—	100
Chicken Italian With Peppers & Onions	1 (3 oz)	120	4	1	80	19	1	—	20	800	—	5	—	200
GOLDEN BROWN														
Beef	1	80	7	—	18	4	tr	—	—	160	—	—	—	—
Mild	1	100	10	—	18	3	tr	—	—	150	—	—	—	—
Spicy	1	100	9	—	18	3	tr	—	—	150	—	—	—	—
HEALTHY CHOICE														
Low Fat Smoked	2 oz	70	2	1	25	8	4	1	0	590	—	2	—	0
Low Fat Smoked Polska Kielbasa	2 oz	70	2	1	25	8	4	1	0	590	—	2	—	0
HEBREW NATIONAL														
Beef Knocks	1 (3 oz)	260	25	—	55	10	—	—	—	670	—	—	—	—
Polish Beef	1 link	240	22	—	50	12	—	—	—	680	—	—	—	—
HILLSHIRE														
Beer Bratwurst	1 (2 oz)	190	17	—	—	7	2	—	—	500	—	—	—	—
Bratwurst Fresh	1 (2 oz)	190	17	—	—	7	1	—	—	410	—	—	—	—

FOOD	PORTION	CALORIES	FAT	SAT FAT	CHOL	PROTEIN	CARBO	FIBER	CALCIUM	SOD	POTAS	VIT C	FOLIC	VIT A
HILLSHIRE (CONT.)														
Bratwurst Light Fresh	1 (2 oz)	150	11	—	—	9	2	—	—	620	—	—	—	—
Bratwurst Spicy	1 (2 oz)	180	17	—	—	8	1	—	—	490	—	—	—	—
Flavorseal Kielbasa Polska	2 oz	190	17	—	—	8	2	—	—	540	—	—	—	—
Flavorseal Kielbasa Polska Beef	2 oz	190	17	—	—	7	2	—	—	550	—	—	—	—
Flavorseal Kielbasa Polska Lite	2 oz	130	11	—	—	8	1	—	—	512	—	—	—	—
Flavorseal Kielbasa Polska Mild	2 oz	190	17	—	—	7	2	—	—	530	—	—	—	—
Flavorseal Kielbasa Polska Turkey	2 oz	90	5	—	—	9	2	—	—	500	—	—	—	—
Flavorseal Smoked	2 oz	190	17	—	—	71	2	—	—	500	—	—	—	—
Flavorseal Smoked Beef	2 oz	180	16	—	—	7	2	—	—	490	—	—	—	—
Flavorseal Smoked Beef & Cheddar	2 oz	190	15	—	—	8	1	—	—	500	—	.	—	—
Flavorseal Smoked Country Recipe	2 oz	180	16	—	—	7	2	—	—	490	—	—	—	—
Flavorseal Smoked Hot	2 oz	180	16	—	—	7	2	—	—	510	—	—	—	—
Flavorseal Smoked Lite	2 oz	130	11	—	—	8	1	—	—	512	—	—	—	—
Flavorseal Smoked Turkey	2 oz	90	5	—	—	9	2	—	—	500	—	—	—	—
Flavorseal Smoked w/ Italian Seasoning	2 oz	200	18	—	—	7	1	—	—	500	—	—	—	—
Italian Mild	1 (2 oz)	190	17	—	—	7	1	—	—	490	—	—	—	—
Italian Mild Light	1 (2 oz)	150	11	—	—	9	2	—	—	620	—	—	—	—
Italian Hot	1 (2 oz)	180	17	—	—	7	1	—	—	500	—	—	—	—
Italian Hot Light	1 (2 oz)	150	11	—	—	9	2	—	—	620	—	—	—	—
Kielbasa Fresh Polska	1 (2 oz)	190	17	—	—	7	1	—	—	410	—	—	—	—
Kielbasa Fresh Polska Lower Fat	1 (2 oz)	150	11	—	—	9	2	—	—	620	—	—	—	—
Links 80% Fat Free Cheddar Hots	2 oz	150	12	—	—	9	1	—	—	640	—	—	—	—
Links 80% Fat Free Kielbasa	2 oz	130	10	—	—	8	2	—	—	630	—	—	—	—
Links 80% Fat Free Smokies	2 oz	130	10	—	—	8	2	—	—	640	—	—	—	—
Links Brats Fully Cooked	2 oz	170	16	—	—	7	1	—	—	380	—	—	—	—
Links Bratwurst Smoked	2 oz	190	17	—	—	8	1	—	—	540	—	—	—	—

FOOD	PORTION	CALORIES	FAT	SAT FAT	CHOL	PROTEIN	CARBO	FIBER	CALCIUM	SOD	POTAS	VIT C	FOLIC	VIT A
HILLSHIRE (CONT.)														
Links Bun Size Cheddarwurst	2 oz	200	18	—	—	8	1	—	—	480	—	—	—	—
Links Bun Size Kielbasa	2 oz	180	16	—	—	8	2	—	—	570	—	—	—	—
Links Bun Size Smoked	2 oz	180	16	—	—	8	2	—	—	570	—	—	—	—
Links Bun Size Smoked Beef	2 oz	180	16	—	—	8	2	—	—	570	—	—	—	—
Links Cheddarwurst	2 oz	190	17	—	—	8	1	—	—	480	—	—	—	—
Links Cheddarwurst Lite	1 link (2.7 oz)	190	15	—	—	12	2	—	—	680	—	—	—	—
Links Hot	2 oz	190	16	—	—	8	2	—	—	530	—	—	—	—
Links Hot Beef	2 oz	190	17	—	—	8	1	—	—	560	—	—	—	—
Links Hot Lite	1 link (2.7 oz)	190	15	—	—	11	2	—	—	690	—	—	—	—
Links Keilbasa Polska	2 oz	190	17	—	—	7	2	—	—	530	—	—	—	—
Links Keilbasa Polska Lite	1 link (2.7 oz)	190	15	—	—	11	2	—	—	610	—	—	—	—
Links Knockwurst Lite	2 oz	180	16	—	—	7	1	—	—	460	—	—	—	—
Links Lit'l Polskas	2 oz	180	16	—	—	6	2	—	—	600	—	—	—	—
Links Lit'l Smokies	2 oz	180	16	—	—	8	2	—	—	600	—	—	—	—
Links Lit'l Smokies Beef	2 oz	180	16	—	—	8	2	—	—	600	—	—	—	—
Links Lit'l Smokies Cheddar	2 oz	180	16	—	—	8	2	—	—	600	—	—	—	—
Links Lit'l Smokies Light	2 oz	120	8	—	—	8	1	—	—	600	—	—	—	—
Links Polish	2 oz	190	17	—	—	7	2	—	—	520	—	—	—	—
Links Smoked	2 oz	190	18	—	—	8	1	—	—	520	—	—	—	—
Mexican Style	1 (2 oz)	190	17	—	—	7	1	—	—	410	—	—	—	—
Mexican Style Lower Fat	1 (2 oz)	150	11	—	—	9	2	—	—	620	—	—	—	—
HORMEL														
Kielbasa	2 oz	150	13	5	40	8	—	—	0	530	—	0	—	0
Light & Lean 97 Dinner Smoked	2 oz	60	2	1	20	8	2	0	0	640	—	6	—	0
Pickled Hot	6 (2 oz)	140	11	5	40	8	1	0	0	380	—	9	—	0
Pickled Smoked	6 (2 oz)	140	11	5	40	8	1	0	0	380	—	9	—	0
Smoked Summer	2 oz	200	18	8	55	8	2	0	—	970	—	—	—	—
Vienna	2 oz	140	14	5	45	5	0	0	40	420	—	0	—	0
Vienna Chicken	2 oz	110	9	3	55	6	1	0	40	400	—	0	—	0
JIMMY DEAN														
Brick Sausage	2.5 oz	270	25	9	55	10	0	0	—	550	—	—	—	—
Bulk	2.5 oz	300	28	10	55	9	0	0	—	490	—	—	—	—

FOOD	PORTION	CALORIES	FAT	SAT FAT	CHOL	PROTEIN	CARBO	FIBER	CALCIUM	SOD	POTAS	VIT C	FOLIC	VIT A
JIMMY DEAN (CONT.)														
Hickory Smoked Dinner Sausage	2 oz	170	14	5	35	7	2	0	—	500	—	—	—	—
Pattie Pre-Cooked	1 (1.9 oz)	230	22	8	45	7	0	0	—	520	—	—	—	—
Polska Kielbaska	2 oz	170	15	5	35	7	1	0	—	500	—	—	—	—
Sage Pattie	1 (2 oz)	200	19	7	45	7	0	0	—	340	—	—	—	—
Sausage Pattie Raw	1 (2 oz)	200	19	6	40	7	0	0	—	400	—	—	—	—
Skinless Link	2 (2 oz)	200	19	7	45	7	0	0	—	440	—	—	—	—
Skinless Link	4 (2 oz)	200	19	7	45	6	0	0	—	440	—	—	—	—
JONES														
Brown & Serve Bacon	1	90	8	—	19	3	tr	—	—	140	—	—	—	—
Brown & Serve Beef	1	90	9	—	18	3	tr	—	—	190	—	—	—	—
Brown & Serve Light	1	60	5	—	16	3	1	—	—	140	—	—	—	—
Brown & Serve Regular	1	100	10	—	19	3	tr	—	—	150	—	—	—	—
Cello Beef	1 slice (1 oz)	130	13	—	25	3	tr	—	—	160	—	—	—	—
Cello Hot Country	1 slice (1 oz)	110	10	—	24	4	tr	—	—	170	—	—	—	—
Cello Original	1 slice (1 oz)	100	10	—	24	4	tr	—	—	180	—	—	—	—
Dinner Link	1	280	28	—	48	6	tr	—	—	310	—	—	—	—
Golden Brown Light Links	1	60	5	—	16	3	1	—	—	130	—	—	—	—
Golden Brown Mild Pattie	1	150	14	—	29	5	tr	—	—	220	—	—	—	—
Italian	1	160	14	—	44	8	tr	—	—	420	—	—	—	—
Light Link	1	70	6	—	21	4	1	—	—	210	—	—	—	—
Little Link	1	140	14	—	24	3	tr	—	—	170	—	—	—	—
Patties	1	150	14	—	36	6	tr	—	—	270	—	—	—	—
Scrapple	1 slice	90	6	—	24	4	5	—	—	230	—	—	—	—
Scrapple	1 slice (1.5 oz)	90	6	—	24	4	5	—	—	230	—	—	—	—
LITTLE SIZZLERS														
Brown & Serve	3 links (2.1 oz)	190	22	8	45	8	1	0	0	670	—	0	—	0
Brown & Serve	2 patties (1.8 oz)	190	18	6	40	7	1	0	0	560	—	0	—	0
Cooked	2 patties (1.8 oz)	230	22	8	45	8	0	0	0	610	—	0	—	0
Cooked	3 links (1.8 oz)	230	22	8	45	8	0	0	0	610	—	0	—	0
Heat & Serve Pork cooked	3 links (1.8 oz)	230	22	8	45	8	0	0	0	610	—	0	—	0
LOUIS RICH														
Polska Kielbasa	2 oz	90	5	2	35	8	2	0	0	490	—	0	—	0
Turkey Hot	2.5 oz	120	8	3	55	12	1	0	40	430	—	0	—	0
Turkey Original	2.5 oz	120	8	3	55	12	1	0	40	430	—	0	—	0
Turkey Smoked	2 oz	90	5	2	30	8	2	0	0	490	—	0	—	0

FOOD	PORTION	CALORIES	FAT	SAT FAT	CHOL	PROTEIN	CARBO	FIBER	CALCIUM	SOD	POTAS	VIT C	FOLIC	VIT A
MR. TURKEY														
Breakfast	2.5 oz	130	9	—	65	12	0	—	—	460	—	—	—	—
Hearty Blend Polish Kielbasa	1 oz	70	6	—	23	4	1	—	—	260	—	—	—	—
Hearty Blend Smoked	1 oz	70	6	—	23	4	1	—	—	260	—	—	—	—
Hot Smoked	1 oz	45	3	—	15	4	2	—	—	250	—	—	—	—
Italian Smoked	1 oz	45	3	—	15	4	2	—	—	250	—	—	—	—
Polish Kielbasa	1 oz	45	3	—	15	4	2	—	—	250	—	—	—	—
Smoked	1 oz	45	3	—	15	4	2	—	—	250	—	—	—	—
OLD SMOKEHOUSE														
Summer Sausage	2 oz	200	18	8	55	8	2	0	0	970	—	6	—	0
OSCAR MAYER														
Pork cooked	2 links (1.7 oz)	170	15	5	40	9	1	0	0	410	—	0	—	0
Smokies Beef	1 (1.5 oz)	120	11	5	30	5	1	0	0	420	—	0	—	0
Smokies Cheese	1 (1.5 oz)	130	12	5	30	6	1	0	0	450	—	0	—	0
Smokies Link	1 (1.5 oz)	130	12	4	25	5	1	0	0	430	—	0	—	0
Smokies Little	6 (2 oz)	170	15	6	35	7	1	0	40	570	—	0	—	0
Smokies Little Cheese	6 (2 oz)	180	16	6	40	7	1	0	40	590	—	0	—	0
PERDUE														
Breakfast Links Turkey Cooked	2 links (2 oz)	100	6	2	45	9	0	—	40	430	—	—	—	—
Hot Italian Turkey Cooked	1 link (2.4 oz)	110	6	2	60	13	1	—	80	500	—	—	—	—
Sweet Italian Turkey Cooked	1 link (2.4 oz)	110	6	2	60	13	1	—	1	500	—	—	—	—
RUDY'S FARM														
Italian Hot	2.5 oz	240	22	7	50	10	0	0	—	570	—	—	—	—
Italian Mild	2.5 oz	240	22	7	50	10	0	0	—	500	—	—	—	—
Italian Mild Natural Casing	1 (2 oz)	190	17	6	40	8	0	0	—	410	—	—	—	—
Morning Right Link	3 (2.9 oz)	150	10	4	40	15	0	0	—	260	—	—	—	—
Morning Right Pattie	2 (2.9 oz)	150	10	4	40	15	0	0	—	260	—	—	—	—
Pattie Pre-Cooked	1 (1.4 oz)	100	6	2	35	13	0	1	—	200	—	—	—	—
Smoked	4 (2.1 oz)	200	18	6	40	7	1	0	—	590	—	—	—	—
Sweet Link	1 (3.9 oz)	380	35	12	80	16	1	0	—	820	—	—	—	—
SHADY BROOK														
Turkey Breakfast	2 oz	80	4	2	35	10	—	—	—	480	—	—	—	—
Turkey Hot Italian	2 oz	100	5	2	40	12	—	—	—	460	—	—	—	—
Turkey Old World Style	4 oz	190	11	3	65	20	—	—	—	850	—	—	—	—
Turkey Sweet Italian	2 oz	100	5	2	40	12	—	—	—	420	—	—	—	—

FOOD	PORTION	CALORIES	FAT	SAT FAT	CHOL	PROTEIN	CARBO	FIBER	CALCIUM	SOD	POTAS	VIT C	FOLIC	VIT A
SHOFAR														
Knockwurst Beef	1 (3 oz)	260	23	9	50	11	tr	0	0	620	—	0	—	200
TYSON														
Country Pork	3.5 oz	320	29	—	49	13	1	—	—	905	—	—	—	—
WAMPLER LONGACRE														
Breakfast Links	1 (2.8 oz)	170	12	—	20	15	2	—	—	525	—	—	—	—
Italian Links	1 (2.8 oz)	170	12	—	20	15	2	—	—	520	—	—	—	—
Tinderlings Garlic & Pepper	1 (3.5 oz)	143	5	—	55	23	3	—	—	500	—	—	—	—
Turkey	1 link (1 oz)	60	4	—	30	5	1	—	—	190	—	—	—	—
Turkey	1 pattie (2 oz)	120	8	—	60	10	4	—	—	380	—	—	—	—
TAKE-OUT														
pork	1 link (0.5 oz)	48	4	1	11	3	tr	—	4	168	47	0	—	tr
pork	1 patty (1 oz)	100	8	3	22	5	tr	—	9	349	97	0	—	tr

SAUSAGE DISHES

FOOD	PORTION	CALORIES	FAT	SAT FAT	CHOL	PROTEIN	CARBO	FIBER	CALCIUM	SOD	POTAS	VIT C	FOLIC	VIT A
JIMMY DEAN														
Italian Sausage & Mozzarella Sandwich	1 (4.5 oz)	380	22	9	40	17	28	2	—	1030	—	—	—	—

SAUSAGE SUBSTITUTES

FOOD	PORTION	CALORIES	FAT	SAT FAT	CHOL	PROTEIN	CARBO	FIBER	CALCIUM	SOD	POTAS	VIT C	FOLIC	VIT A
GARDENSAUSAGE														
Patty	1 (2.5 oz)	140	3	2	5	7	20	5	350	460	—	0	—	0
KNOX MOUNTAIN FARM														
No-So-Sausage	1 serv (1/10 pkg)	120	1	—	—	14	6	2	60	696	—	—	—	—
LIGHTLIFE														
Lean Links Breakfast	1.25 oz	69	3	tr	0	4	4	—	—	250	—	—	—	—
Lean Links Italian	1.5 oz	83	3	tr	0	5	5	—	—	300	—	—	—	—
LOMA LINDA														
Linketts	1 (1.2 oz)	70	5	1	0	7	1	1	0	160	15	0	—	0
Little Links	2 (1.6 oz)	90	6	1	0	8	2	2	0	230	25	0	—	0
MORNINGSTAR FARMS														
Breakfast Links	2 (1.6 oz)	60	3	1	0	8	2	2	0	340	60	0	—	0
Breakfast Patties	1 (1.3 oz)	70	3	1	0	8	2	2	0	170	110	0	—	0
Grillers	1 patty (2.2 oz)	140	7	2	0	14	5	3	40	260	130	0	—	0
Sausage Style Recipe Crumbles	2/3 cup (1.9 oz)	90	3	0	0	11	5	3	20	370	65	0	—	0
NATURAL TOUCH														
Vegan Sausage Crumbles	1/2 cup (1.9 oz)	60	0	0	0	10	4	2	40	300	80	0	—	0
WHITE WAVE														
Meatless Healthy Links	2 (1.6 oz)	140	10	2	0	8	5	3	40	450	—	0	—	0

FOOD	PORTION	CALORIES	FAT	SAT FAT	CHOL	PROTEIN	CARBO	FIBER	CALCIUM	SOD	POTAS	VIT C	FOLIC	VIT A
WORTHINGTON														
Leanies	1 link (1.4 oz)	110	8	2	0	7	2	1	20	430	40	0	—	0
Prosage Links	2 (1.6 oz)	60	3	1	0	8	2	2	0	340	60	0	—	0
Saucettes	1 link (1.3 oz)	90	6	1	0	6	1	1	0	200	25	0	—	0
Super Links	1 (1.7 oz)	110	8	1	0	7	2	1	0	350	30	0	—	0
Veja Links	1 (1.1 oz)	50	3	1	0	5	1	0	0	190	20	0	—	0
SAVORY														
ground	1 tsp	4	tr	—	0	tr	1	—	30	tr	15	—	—	72
SCALLOP														
FRESH														
raw	3 oz	75	1	tr	28	14	2	—	21	137	274	—	—	—
FROZEN														
MRS. PAUL'S														
Fried	2 oz	160	7	—	10	8	18	—	20	320	—	—	—	—
HOME RECIPE														
breaded & fried	2 lg	67	3	1	19	6	3	—	13	144	103	—	—	—
TAKE-OUT														
breaded & fried	6 (5 oz)	386	19	5	107	16	38	—	18	919	294	0	40	139
SCONE														
FINNEGAN'S														
Cranberry	1 (2.7 oz)	90	2	0	0	2	20	1	60	176	—	0	—	0
Irish Raisin	1 (2.7 oz)	90	2	0	0	2	20	1	60	176	—	0	—	0
TAKE-OUT														
raisin	1 (3 oz)	270	6	4	25	6	50	2	60	400	—	0	—	200
orange poppy	1 (3 oz)	260	6	4	30	6	47	2	80	400	—	0	—	300
SCROD														
GORTON'S														
Microwave Entree Baked	1 pkg	320	18	4	80	17	18	—	—	420	—	—	—	—
SEA BASS														
(*see* BASS)														
SEATROUT														
(*see* TROUT)														
SEAWEED														
agar dried	1 oz	87	tr	tr	0	2	23	—	78	29	321	0	—	0
agar fresh	1 oz	tr	tr	tr	0	tr	2	—	15	3	64	0	—	0
irishmoss fresh	1 oz	14	tr	tr	0	tr	4	—	21	19	18	—	—	—
kelp fresh	1 oz	12	tr	tr	0	tr	3	—	48	66	25	—	51	33
kombu fresh	1 oz	12	tr	tr	0	tr	3	—	48	66	25	—	51	33
laver fresh	1 oz	10	tr	tr	0	2	1	—	20	14	101	11	—	1483
nori fresh	1 oz	10	tr	tr	0	2	1	—	20	14	101	11	—	1483
spirulina dried	1 oz	83	2	1	0	16	7	—	—	309	388	13	—	—
spirulina fresh	1 oz	7	tr	tr	0	2	1	—	—	28	36	tr	—	—

FOOD	PORTION	CALORIES	FAT	SAT FAT	CHOL	PROTEIN	CARBO	FIBER	CALCIUM	SOD	POTAS	VIT C	FOLIC	VIT A
tangle fresh	1 oz	12	tr	tr	0	tr	3	—	48	66	25	—	51	33
wakame fresh	1 oz	13	tr	tr	0	1	3	—	43	249	14	1	—	103
EDEN														
Agar Agar Bars	1 tbsp (2.5 oz)	10	0	0	0	0	2	2	16	10	10	0	—	0
Agar Agar Flakes	1 tbsp (2.5 oz)	10	0	0	0	0	2	2	16	10	10	0	—	0
Arame	½ cup (0.3 oz)	30	0	0	0	1	7	7	110	120	180	0	—	536
Hiziki	½ cup (0.3 oz)	30	0	0	0	tr	6	6	110	160	480	0	—	0
Kombu	3.5 in piece (3.3 g)	10	0	0	0	0	2	1	23	90	170	0	—	0
Nori	1 sheet (2.5 g)	10	0	0	0	1	1	1	7	5	90	6	—	403
Sushi Nori	1 sheet (2.5 g)	10	0	0	0	1	1	1	7	5	90	6	—	403
Wakame	½ cup (0.3 oz)	25	0	0	0	2	4	4	76	660	480	0	—	427
Wakame Flakes	½ cup (0.3 oz)	25	0	0	0	2	4	4	89	720	35	0	—	296
MAINE COAST														
Alaria	⅓ cup (7 g)	18	0	0	0	1	3	2	90	301	522	0	—	1000
Dulse	⅓ cup (7 g)	18	0	0	0	2	3	2	10	122	547	0	—	50
Dulse Flakes	1 oz	75	1	—	—	6	13	9	60	493	2217	2	—	188
Kelp	⅓ cup (7 g)	17	0	0	0	1	3	3	70	312	784	0	—	56
Kelp Crunch	1 bar (1 oz)	129	6	1	0	3	14	2	170	109	344	0	—	0
Kelp Crunch Peanut-Raisin	1 bar (1 oz)	129	6	1	0	3	14	2	170	109	344	0	—	0
Laver	⅓ cup (7 g)	22	0	0	0	2	3	3	10	113	188	1	—	500
Sea Seasoning Dulse	1 g	3	0	0	0	0	1	—	2	17	78	—	—	6
Sea Seasoning Dulse With Celery	1 g	3	0	0	0	0	1	—	3	17	73	—	—	6
Sea Seasoning Dulse With Garlic	1 g	3	0	0	0	0	1	—	2	13	61	—	—	5
Sea Seasoning Dulse With Sesame	1 g	3	0	0	0	0	1	—	7	6	29	—	—	2
Sea Seasoning Kelp	1 g	3	0	0	0	0	1	—	20	35	111	—	—	0
Sea Seasoning Kelp With Cayenne	1 g	3	0	0	0	0	1	—	20	35	111	—	—	0
Sea Seasoning Nori	1 g	3	0	0	0	0	1	—	4	8	24	—	—	240
Sea Seasoning Nori With Ginger	1 g	3	0	0	0	0	1	—	1	3	30	—	—	160

SEITAN

(*see* WHEAT)

SEMOLINA

FOOD	PORTION	CALORIES	FAT	SAT FAT	CHOL	PROTEIN	CARBO	FIBER	CALCIUM	SOD	POTAS	VIT C	FOLIC	VIT A
dry	½ cup	303	tr	tr	0	11	61	3	14	1	157	0	61	—

SESAME

FOOD	PORTION	CALORIES	FAT	SAT FAT	CHOL	PROTEIN	CARBO	FIBER	CALCIUM	SOD	POTAS	VIT C	FOLIC	VIT A
seeds	1 tsp	16	2	—	0	1	tr	—	4	1	11	—	—	1
seeds dried	1 tbsp	52	5	1	0	2	2	—	88	1	42	0	9	1
seeds dried	1 cup	825	72	10	0	26	34	—	1404	16	674	0	139	13

FOOD	PORTION	CALORIES	FAT	SAT FAT	CHOL	PROTEIN	CARBO	FIBER	CALCIUM	SOD	POTAS	VIT C	FOLIC	VIT A
seeds roasted & toasted	1 oz	161	14	2	0	14	7	—	281	3	135	—	—	—
sesame crunch candy	20 pieces (1.2 oz)	181	12	2	0	4	18	—	—	—	—	—	—	—
sesame crunch candy	1 oz	146	9	1	0	3	14	—	—	—	—	—	—	—
sesame sticks	1 oz	153	10	2	0	3	13	—	48	422	—	0	2	25
sesame sticks unsalted	1 oz	153	10	2	0	3	13	—	48	8	—	0	2	25
tahini from roasted & toasted kernels	1 tbsp	89	8	1	0	3	3	—	64	17	62	0	—	—
tahini from stone ground kernels	1 tbsp	86	7	1	0	3	4	—	63	11	62	0	—	—
tahini from unroasted kernels	1 tbsp	85	8	1	0	3	3	—	20	0	64	—	—	—
ARROWHEAD														
Sesame Tahini	1 oz	170	17	—	0	6	4	—	40	5	105	—	—	—
CASBAH														
Tahini Sauce Mix as prep	¼ cup	160	13	0	0	4	10	tr	30	160	—	0	—	0
EDEN														
Sesame Shake	½ tsp (1.5 g)	10	1	0	0	0	0	tr	0	40	—	0	—	0
Sesame Shake Garlic	½ tsp (1.5 g)	10	1	0	0	0	0	tr	0	35	—	0	—	0
Sesame Shake Organic Seaweed	½ tsp (1.5 g)	10	1	0	0	0	0	tr	0	35	—	0	—	0
JOYVA														
Tahini	2 tbsp (1 oz)	200	18	3	0	5	3	1	0	25	—	0	—	0
PLANTERS														
Nut Mix	1 oz	150	12	2	0	5	9	2	40	240	130	—	—	—
STONE-BUHR														
Seeds Raw	4 tsp (1 oz)	180	16	3	0	8	3	1	40	10	—	0	—	0
SESBANIA														
flower	1	1	0	0	0	tr	tr	—	1	0	5	2	—	0
flowers	1 cup	5	tr	—	0	tr	1	—	4	3	37	15	—	0
flowers cooked	1 cup	23	tr	—	0	1	5	—	23	11	111	39	—	0
SHAD														
roe baked w/ butter & lemon	3.5 oz	126	3	—	—	22	2	—	13	73	132	—	—	—
roe raw	3½ oz	130	2	—	360	24	2	—	—	—	—	14	—	—
SHALLOTS														
dried	1 tbsp	3	0	0	0	tr	1	—	2	1	15	tr	1	—
raw chopped	1 tbsp	7	tr	tr	0	tr	2	—	4	1	33	1	—	—
SHARK														
batter-dipped & fried	3 oz	194	12	3	50	16	5	—	52	103	132	—	—	153
raw	3 oz	111	4	1	43	18	0	—	29	67	136	—	—	198

FOOD	PORTION	CALORIES	FAT	SAT FAT	CHOL	PROTEIN	CARBO	FIBER	CALCIUM	SOD	POTAS	VIT C	FOLIC	VIT A
SHEEPSHEAD FISH														
cooked	3 oz	107	1	tr	—	22	0	—	32	62	435	—	—	—
cooked	1 fillet (6.5 oz)	234	3	1	—	48	0	—	70	136	952	—	—	—
raw	3 oz	92	2	1	—	17	0	—	18	61	344	—	—	—
SHELLFISH														
(see individual names, SHELLFISH SUBSTITUTES)														
SHELLFISH SUBSTITUTES														
crab imitation	3 oz	87	1	—	17	10	1	—	11	715	77	—	—	—
scallop imitation	3 oz	84	tr	—	18	11	9	—	7	676	88	—	—	—
shrimp imitation	3 oz	86	1	—	31	11	8	—	16	599	76	—	—	—
surimi	3 oz	84	1	—	25	13	6	—	7	122	95	—	—	—
surimi	1 oz	28	tr	—	8	4	2	—	2	40	31	—	—	—
LOUIS KEMP														
Crab Delights Chunk Style	2 oz	54	tr	—		10	6	5	—	—	320	—	—	—
Lobster Delights	2 oz	60	tr	—		10	8	6	—	—	470	—	—	—
Maryland Style Cakes	2.5 oz	154	9	—		26	8	10	—	—	780	—	—	—
OCEAN MAGIC														
Imitation King Crab	3 oz	80	tr	—		15	8	11	—	—	740	—	—	—
SHELLIE BEANS														
canned	½ cup	37	tr	tr	0	2	8	—	36	408	133	4	—	278
SHERBET														
(see also ICES AND ICE POPS)														
orange	½ cup (4 fl oz)	132	2	1	5	1	29	—	52	44	92	4	4	73
orange	½ gal	2158	31	19	113	17	469	—	827	706	1585	31	111	1480
orange	1 bar (2.75 fl oz)	91	1	1	3	1	20	—	36	30	63	3	3	50
orange home recipe	½ cup	120	2	—	9	2	24	—	—	30	—	—	—	—
BORDEN														
Orange	½ cup	110	1	—	—	1	25	—	40	40	65	—	—	—
BREYERS														
Fat Free Orange	½ cup (3 oz)	110	0	0	0	2	27	0	60	25	—	1	—	0
Fat Free Rainbow	½ cup (3 oz)	110	0	0	0	1	28	0	60	25	—	0	—	0
Fat Free Raspberry	½ cup (3 oz)	120	0	0	0	2	28	0	60	20	—	1	—	0
Fat Free Tropical	½ cup (3 oz)	110	0	0	0	1	27	0	60	25	—	0	—	0
Orange	½ cup (3 oz)	120	1	1	5	1	26	0	40	25	—	1	—	100
Rainbow	½ cup (3 oz)	120	2	1	5	1	27	0	40	15	—	1	—	0
Raspberry	½ cup (3 oz)	120	2	1	5	1	28	0	40	15	—	0	—	0
Tropical	½ cup (3 oz)	120	1	1	5	1	27	0	40	15	—	0	—	100
HOOD														
Lime Orange Lemon	½ cup (3.1 oz)	120	1	1	<5	1	26	0	40	35	—	0	—	0

FOOD	PORTION	CALORIES	FAT	SAT FAT	CHOL	PROTEIN	CARBO	FIBER	CALCIUM	SOD	POTAS	VIT C	FOLIC	VIT A
HOOD (CONT.)														
Orange	½ cup (3.1 oz)	120	1	1	<5	1	26	0	40	35	—	0	—	0
Rainbow Swirl	½ cup (3.1 oz)	120	1	1	<5	1	26	0	40	30	—	0	—	0
Raspberry Orange Lime	½ cup (3.1 oz)	120	1	1	<5	1	26	0	40	30	—	0	—	0
SEALTEST														
Lime	½ cup (3 oz)	130	1	0	5	1	28	0	40	30	—	1	—	0
Orange	½ cup (3 oz)	130	1	1	5	1	28	0	40	30	—	1	—	0
Rainbow Orange Red Raspberry Lime	½ cup (3 oz)	130	1	1	5	1	28	0	40	25	—	1	—	0
Red Raspberry	½ cup (3 oz)	130	1	1	5	1	28	0	40	25	—	1	—	0
SHRIMP														
CANNED														
canned	1 cup	154	3	tr	222	30	1	—	75	216	269	—	2	—
canned	3 oz	102	2	tr	147	20	1	—	50	143	179	—	2	—
ROBINSON														
Canned Shrimp	2 oz	58	1	—	—	—	—	—	40	—	—	—	—	—
FRESH														
cooked	3 oz	84	1	tr	166	18	0	—	33	190	154	—	3	—
cooked	4 large	22	tr	tr	43	5	0	—	9	49	40	—	1	—
raw	3 oz	90	1	tr	130	17	1	—	44	126	157	—	3	—
raw	4 large	30	tr	tr	43	6	tr	—	15	42	52	—	1	—
FROZEN														
CAJUN COOKIN'														
Shrimp Creole	12 oz	390	11	—	—	17	55	—	80	1130	350	4	—	750
Shrimp Etouffee	17 oz	360	9	—	—	19	52	—	100	1170	240	—	—	750
Shrimp Jambalaya	12 oz	450	20	—	—	20	43	—	100	800	550	4	—	750
GORTON'S														
Butterfly Shrimp	4 oz	160	tr	—	—	19	16	—	150	540	—	—	—	—
Microwave Crunchy Shrimp	5 oz	380	20	3	65	14	35	—	60	870	—	—	—	—
Microwave Entree Shrimp Scampi	1 pkg	390	30	—	—	10	21	—	60	470	—	—	—	500
Shrimp Crisps	4 oz	280	15	—	—	9	26	—	40	740	—	—	—	—
MRS. PAUL'S														
Entrees Light Seafood & Clams With Linguini	10 oz	240	5	2	40	12	36	—	40	750	—	1	—	—
VAN DE KAMP'S														
Breaded Butterfly	7 (4 oz)	280	14	3	55	12	28	2	20	580	—	0	—	0
Breaded Popcorn	20 (4 oz)	270	13	2	35	11	28	1	40	610	—	0	—	0
Breaded Whole	7 (4 oz)	240	10	2	50	13	26	2	20	520	—	0	—	0
TAKE-OUT														
breaded & fried	3 oz	206	10	2	150	18	10	—	57	292	191	—	7	—
breaded & fried	6 to 8 (6 oz)	454	25	5	201	19	40	—	84	1447	184	0	48	119

FOOD	PORTION	CALORIES	FAT	SAT FAT	CHOL	PROTEIN	CARBO	FIBER	CALCIUM	SOD	POTAS	VIT C	FOLIC	VIT A
SMELT														
rainbow cooked	3 oz	106	3	tr	76	19	0	—	65	65	316	—	—	—
rainbow raw	3 oz	83	2	tr	60	15	0	—	51	51	247	—	—	—
SNACKS														
(*see also* CHIPS, FRUIT SNACKS, NUTS MIXED, POPCORN, PRETZELS)														
oriental mix	1 oz	155	12	—	0	6	9	—	22	235	147	tr	25	15
pork skins	1 oz	154	9	3	27	17	0	—	8	521	36	tr	—	37
pork skins barbecue	1 oz	152	9	3	33	16	1	—	12	756	51	tr	—	427
trail mix	1 oz	131	8	2	0	4	13	—	22	65	194	tr	20	5
trail mix	1 cup (5.3 oz)	693	44	8	0	21	67	—	117	343	1028	2	107	27
trail mix tropical	1 oz	115	5	2	0	2	19	—	16	3	201	2	12	14
trail mix w/ chocolate chips	1 oz	137	9	2	—	4	13	—	31	34	184	tr	18	12
trail mix w/ chocolate chips	1 cup (5.1 oz)	707	47	9	—	21	66	—	159	177	946	2	95	64
BAKEM-ETS														
Hot'N Spicy	21 pieces (1 oz)	150	9	—	25	17	1	—	—	750	55	—	—	—
Snacks	21 pieces (1 oz)	160	10	—	25	12	2	—	—	850	55	—	—	—
BARBARA'S														
Cheese Puffs Bakes	1½ cups (1 oz)	160	11	2	0	2	13	0	—	190	—	—	—	—
Cheese Puffs Jalapeno	¾ cup (1 oz)	150	9	2	0	2	15	0	—	250	—	—	—	—
Cheese Puffs Original	¾ cup (1 oz)	150	10	2	0	2	16	0	—	130	—	—	—	—
BIG DIPPER														
Bagel Chips Lowfat Barbeque	12 (1 oz)	110	2	0	0	4	21	1	40	190	—	0	40	0
Bagel Chips Lowfat Garlic	12 (1 oz)	120	2	0	0	4	21	1	0	295	—	0	40	0
Bagel Chips Lowfat Original	12 (1 oz)	110	2	0	0	4	21	1	20	150	—	0	40	0
BUGLES														
Baked Cheddar Cheese	1½ cups (1 oz)	130	4	1	0	2	22	tr	—	440	—	—	—	—
Baked Original	1½ cups (1 oz)	130	4	1	0	2	23	tr	—	380	—	—	—	—
CHEETOS														
Cheddar Valley	26 pieces (1 oz)	160	9	—	0	2	16	1	—	240	45	—	—	—
Crunchy	26 pieces (1 oz)	150	9	—	0	1	17	1	—	310	40	—	—	—
Curls	15 pieces (1 oz)	150	9	—	0	1	17	1	—	270	40	—	—	—
Flamin' Hot	26 pieces (1 oz)	150	9	—	0	2	16	1	—	240	50	—	—	—

FOOD	PORTION	CALORIES	FAT	SAT FAT	CHOL	PROTEIN	CARBO	FIBER	CALCIUM	SOD	POTAS	VIT C	FOLIC	VIT A
CHEETOS (CONT.)														
Light	38 pieces (1 oz)	140	6	—	0	2	19	1	20	280	75	—	—	—
Paws	16 pieces (1 oz)	160	10	—	0	1	15	1	—	310	45	—	—	—
Puffed Ball	38 pieces (1 oz)	160	10	—	0	2	16	1	—	360	50	—	—	—
Puffs	33 pieces (1 oz)	160	9	—	0	1	16	1	—	330	50	—	—	—
CHEEZ DOODLES														
Crunchy	1 oz	160	10	—	—	2	16	—	20	230	50	—	—	—
Puffed	1 oz	150	9	—	—	2	16	—	20	360	70	—	—	—
CHEEZ WAFFIES														
Snacks	1 oz	140	8	—	—	3	14	—	60	420	180	—	—	—
CHEX MIX														
Bold 'n Zesty	½ cup (1 oz)	140	6	1	0	3	20	2	—	370	—	—	40	—
Cheddar Cheese	½ cup (1 oz)	130	5	1	0	3	20	1	—	330	—	—	40	—
Hot 'n Spicy	⅔ cup (1 oz)	130	5	1	0	3	21	2	—	410	—	—	40	—
Traditional	⅔ cup (1 oz)	130	4	1	0	3	21	1	—	410	—	—	40	—
COMBOS														
Cheddar Cheese Cracker	1 pkg (1.7 oz)	250	13	3	5	5	28	1	60	520	—	—	—	—
Cheddar Cheese Cracker	1 oz	140	8	2	5	3	16	0	20	300	—	—	—	—
Cheddar Cheese Pretzel	1 oz	130	5	1	0	3	18	0	40	310	—	—	—	—
Cheddar Cheese Pretzel	1 pkg (1.8 oz)	240	9	2	5	5	33	1	100	560	—	—	—	—
Chili Cheese w/ Corn Shell	1 oz	140	6	1	0	2	17	1	20	420	—	—	—	100
Chili Cheese w/ Corn Shell	1 pkg (1.7 oz)	230	11	2	5	4	29	2	40	710	—	—	—	200
Mustard Pretzel	1 pkg (1.8 oz)	230	8	1	0	4	35	1	60	500	—	—	—	—
Mustard Pretzel	1 oz	130	4	1	0	2	19	1	20	270	—	—	—	—
Nacho Cheese Pretzel	1 pkg (1.7 oz)	230	8	2	0	5	34	1	80	580	—	—	—	—
Nacho Cheese Pretzel	1 oz	130	5	1	0	3	19	1	40	320	—	—	—	—
Nacho Cheese w/ Tortilla Shell	1 oz	140	6	1	0	2	17	1	20	380	—	—	—	—
Nacho Cheese w/ Tortilla Shell	1 pkg (1.7 oz)	230	11	2	0	4	30	1	40	640	—	—	—	—
Peanut Butter Cracker	1 oz	140	8	2	0	4	15	1	—	260	—	—	—	—
Pepperoni & Cheese Pizza	1 oz	140	7	1	5	2	17	0	40	280	—	—	—	—
Pepperoni & Cheese Pizza	1 pkg (1.7 oz)	240	11	2	5	4	30	1	60	480	—	—	—	—

FOOD	PORTION	CALORIES	FAT	SAT FAT	CHOL	PROTEIN	CARBO	FIBER	CALCIUM	SOD	POTAS	VIT C	FOLIC	VIT A
COMBOS (CONT.)														
Pizzeria Pretzel	1 pkg (1.8 oz)	230	8	2	0	5	35	1	80	520	—	—	—	—
Pizzeria Pretzel	1 oz	130	5	1	0	3	19	1	40	290	—	—	—	—
Tortilla Ranch	1 bag (1.7 oz)	240	12	3	5	4	29	1	20	610	—	—	—	—
Tortilla Ranch	1 oz	140	7	2	5	2	17	1	20	350	—	—	—	—
CORNNUTS														
Barbecue	1 oz	120	4	tr	0	2	22	2	—	270	70	—	tr	—
Nacho Cheese	1 oz	120	4	tr	0	2	22	2	—	180	70	—	—	—
Original	1 oz	120	4	tr	0	2	22	2	—	170	70	—	—	—
Original	1 pkg (2 oz)	260	8	2	0	5	40	4	0	340	—	0	—	0
Picante	1 oz	120	4	tr	0	2	22	2	—	260	70	—	—	—
Ranch	1 oz	120	4	tr	0	2	20	2	—	190	80	—	—	—
DOO DADS														
Snacks	1 oz	130	6	1	0	3	17	—	20	360	80	—	—	—
ENERGY FOOD FACTORY														
Poprice Cheddar Cheese	½ oz	60	3	—	0	2	8	—	—	110	—	—	—	—
Poprice Herb & Garlic	½ oz	50	2	—	0	1	10	—	—	70	—	—	—	—
Poprice Lite	½ oz	50	2	—	0	1	9	—	—	70	—	—	—	—
Poprice Original No Salt	½ oz	45	0	0	0	1	11	—	—	1	—	—	—	—
ESTEE														
Snack Crisps Apple Cinnamon	1 pkg (0.66 oz)	90	2	0	0	1	16	tr	0	70	80	0	—	0
Snack Crisps Apple Cinnamon	27 crisps (1 oz)	130	3	0	0	2	24	1	0	110	120	0	—	0
Snack Crisps Chocolate	1 pkg (0.66 oz)	90	2	0	0	2	15	1	0	70	150	0	—	0
Snack Crisps Chocolate	30 crisps (1 oz)	130	3	1	0	2	23	2	0	110	230	0	—	0
Snack Crisps Lemon	30 (1 oz)	130	3	1	5	2	23	tr	0	110	100	0	—	0
Snack Crisps Lemon	1 pkg (0.66 oz)	90	2	0	0	1	16	tr	0	70	70	0	—	0
Snack Crisps Ranch	1 pkg (0.6 oz)	90	2	0	0	2	15	0	20	135	80	0	—	0
Snack Crisps Ranch	30 (1 oz)	130	3	1	5	3	22	tr	40	200	120	0	—	0
Snack Crisps White Cheddar	1 pkg (0.6 oz)	90	2	1	5	2	14	tr	20	135	70	0	—	0
Snack Crisps With Cheddar	27 crisps (1 oz)	130	3	1	5	3	22	tr	40	200	100	0	—	0
FRITO LAY														
Corn Nuggets Toasted	1.38 oz	170	5	—	0	3	29	—	—	265	—	1	—	—
FUNYUMS														
Onion Rings	11 pieces (1 oz)	140	7	—	0	2	18	1	—	265	40	—	—	—

FOOD	PORTION	CALORIES	FAT	SAT FAT	CHOL	PROTEIN	CARBO	FIBER	CALCIUM	SOD	POTAS	VIT C	FOLIC	VIT A
HAPI														
Chili Bits	½ cup (1 oz)	110	0	0	0	3	25	1	80	180	—	0	—	0
HEALTH VALLEY														
Cheddar Lites	0.75 oz	40	2	—	tr	1	4	tr	4	35	45	tr	1	29
Cheddar Lites With Green Onion	0.75 oz	40	2	—	0	1	4	tr	—	35	45	—	—	tr
INNOVATIVE FOODS														
Roasted Sweet Corn	1 pkg (0.8 oz)	76	0	0	0	3	17	2	0	5	—	2	—	150
LANCE														
Cheese Balls	1 pkg (32 g)	190	13	3	5	2	16	—	40	420	70	—	—	—
Crunchy Cheese Twists	1 pkg (42 g)	260	16	4	0	3	25	—	20	290	30	—	—	—
Gold-N-Chees	1 pkg (39 g)	180	9	2	5	4	23	—	20	410	40	—	—	—
Pork Skins	1 pkg (14 g)	80	5	2	20	9	0	—	—	270	20	—	—	—
Pork Skins BBQ	1 pkg (14 g)	80	5	2	20	9	0	—	—	400	10	—	—	—
MR. PEANUT														
Peanut Butter Crisps Graham	12 pieces (1.1 oz)	150	8	2	0	4	18	2	—	100	90	—	—	—
MUNCHOS														
Snack	16 pieces (1 oz)	160	10	—	0	1	15	—	tr	230	180	—	—	—
PITA PUFFS														
Barbeque	35 (1 oz)	120	3	0	0	4	20	1	0	150	—	0	16	0
Lowfat Garlic	35 (1 oz)	110	1	0	0	3	22	1	0	125	—	0	40	0
Lowfat Original	35 (1 oz)	110	1	0	0	3	22	1	0	170	—	0	32	0
Lowfat Salsa	35 (1 oz)	110	1	0	0	3	21	1	0	290	—	0	40	0
Pizza	35 (1 oz)	120	2	0	0	4	21	1	0	230	—	0	16	0
Ranch	35 (1 oz)	120	2	0	0	4	21	1	0	195	—	0	24	0
PLANTERS														
Cheez Balls	1 oz	150	10	2	2	2	15	1	20	300	45	—	—	100
Cheez Balls	1 pkg (1 oz)	150	10	2	2	2	15	1	20	330	45	—	—	100
Cheez Curls	1 pkg (1.2 oz)	190	12	3	2	2	19	1	20	380	60	—	—	100
Cheez Curls	1 oz	150	10	2	2	2	15	1	20	310	45	—	—	—
Heat Snack Mix	1 oz	140	8	1	0	5	13	2	20	230	125	1	—	100
SNYDER'S														
Cheddar Cheese Twists	1 oz	150	8	—	0	2	17	—	20	200	—	—	—	1500
Kruncheez	1 oz	160	10	—	0	2	15	—	20	170	—	—	—	500
Onion Toasters	1 oz	150	8	—	0	2	17	3	60	280	—	—	—	—
Snack Mix	1 oz	170	8	1	0	2	11	tr	—	410	45	—	—	300
Sopaipillas Apple & Cinnamon	1 oz	150	8	1	0	2	18	1	—	15	—	—	—	—
SPLURGE														
Snack Mix Fat Free Original	⅔ cup (1 oz)	100	0	0	0	3	25	tr	20	340	—	0	—	0

FOOD	PORTION	CALORIES	FAT	SAT FAT	CHOL	PROTEIN	CARBO	FIBER	CALCIUM	SOD	POTAS	VIT C	FOLIC	VIT A
ULTRA SLIM-FAST														
Lite N' Tasty Cheese Curls	1 oz	110	3	—	0	2	20	3	100	360	80	6	40	500
WEIGHT WATCHERS														
Cheese Curls	1 pkg (0.5 oz)	70	3	1	0	1	10	0	0	85	—	0	—	0
SNAIL														
cooked	3 oz	233	1	tr	110	41	13	—	96	350	590	—	10	137
raw	3 oz	117	tr	tr	55	20	7	—	48	175	295	—	5	—
SNAPPER														
cooked	1 fillet (6 oz)	217	3	1	80	45	0	—	69	96	887	—	—	—
cooked	3 oz	109	1	tr	40	22	0	—	34	48	444	—	—	—
raw	3 oz	85	1	tr	31	17	0	—	27	54	355	—	—	—
SODA														
(*see also* DRINK MIXERS, MINERAL/BOTTLED WATER, SPORTS DRINKS)														
club	12 oz	0	0	0	0	0	0	—	17	75	6	0	0	0
cola	12 oz	151	tr	—	0	tr	39	—	9	14	4	0	0	0
cream	12 oz	191	0	0	0	0	49	—	19	43	4	0	0	0
diet cola	12 oz	2	0	0	0	tr	tr	—	12	21	0	0	0	0
diet cola w/ equal	12 oz	2	0	0	0	tr	tr	—	12	21	0	0	0	0
diet cola w/ saccharin	12 oz	2	0	0	0	tr	tr	—	14	57	7	0	0	0
ginger ale	12 oz can	124	0	—	0	tr	32	—	12	25	5	0	0	0
grape	12 oz	161	0	0	0	0	42	—	12	57	3	0	0	0
lemon lime	12 oz	149	0	0	0	0	38	—	9	41	4	0	0	0
orange	12 oz	177	0	0	0	0	46	—	19	49	9	0	0	0
pepper type	12 oz	151	tr	—	0	0	38	—	12	38	2	0	0	0
quinine	12 oz	125	0	0	0	0	32	—	5	15	1	0	0	0
root beer	12 oz	152	0	0	0	tr	39	—	19	49	3	0	0	0
tonic water	12 oz	125	0	0	0	0	32	—	5	15	1	0	0	0
7 UP														
Cherry	1 oz	13	0	—	0	—	—	—	0	—	—	—	—	—
Diet	1 oz	tr	0	—	0	—	—	—	0	—	—	—	—	—
Original	1 oz	12	0	—	0	—	—	—	0	—	—	—	—	—
AFTER THE FALL														
Raspberry Ginger Ale	1 can (12 oz)	150	0	0	0	1	36	0	20	25	100	1	—	0
BARRELHEAD														
Root Beer	8 fl oz	110	0	0	0	0	27	0	—	25	—	—	—	—
BURST														
Cola Strawberry	8 fl oz	117	0	0	0	tr	31	—	—	0	7	0	—	—
CANADA DRY														
Birch Beer Brown	8 fl oz	110	0	0	0	0	27	0	—	40	—	—	—	—
Birch Beer Clear	8 fl oz	110	0	0	0	0	27	0	—	40	—	—	—	—
Black Cherry Wishniak	8 fl oz	130	0	0	0	0	32	0	—	40	—	—	—	—

FOOD	PORTION	CALORIES	FAT	SAT FAT	CHOL	PROTEIN	CARBO	FIBER	CALCIUM	SOD	POTAS	VIT C	FOLIC	VIT A
CANADA DRY (CONT.)														
Cactus Cooler	8 fl oz	110	0	0	0	0	27	0	—	40	—	—	—	—
California Strawberry	8 fl oz	110	0	0	0	0	27	0	—	45	—	—	—	—
Club	8 fl oz	0	0	0	0	0	0	0	—	60	—	—	—	—
Club Sodium Free	8 fl oz	0	0	0	0	0	0	0	—	0	—	—	—	—
Concord Grape	8 fl oz	120	0	0	0	0	29	0	—	45	—	—	—	—
Diet Ginger Ale	8 fl oz	0	0	0	0	0	0	0	—	60	—	—	—	—
Diet Ginger Ale Cherry	8 fl oz	0	0	0	0	0	0	0	—	60	—	—	—	—
Diet Ginger Ale Cranberry	8 fl oz	0	0	0	0	0	tr	0	—	50	—	—	—	—
Diet Ginger Ale Lemon	8 fl oz	5	0	0	0	0	0	0	—	60	—	—	—	—
Diet Tonic Water	8 fl oz	0	0	0	0	0	0	0	—	35	—	—	—	—
Diet Tonic Water Twist Of Lime	8 fl oz	0	0	0	0	0	0	0	—	45	—	—	—	—
Ginger Ale	8 fl oz	100	0	0	0	0	25	0	—	20	—	—	—	—
Ginger Ale Cherry	8 fl oz	110	0	0	0	0	27	0	—	25	—	—	—	—
Ginger Ale Cranberry	8 fl oz	100	0	0	0	0	25	0	—	15	—	—	—	—
Ginger Ale Golden	8 fl oz	100	0	0	0	0	24	0	—	10	—	—	—	—
Ginger Ale Lemon	8 fl oz	100	0	0	0	0	25	0	—	20	—	—	—	—
Half & Half	8 fl oz	110	0	0	0	0	27	0	—	25	—	—	—	—
Hi-Spot	8 fl oz	110	0	0	0	0	28	0	—	50	—	—	—	—
Island Lime	8 fl oz	140	0	0	0	0	33	0	—	15	—	—	—	—
Jamaica Cola	8 fl oz	110	0	0	0	0	27	0	—	10	—	—	—	—
Lemon Sour	8 fl oz	100	0	0	0	0	21	0	—	15	—	—	—	—
Peach	8 fl oz	120	0	0	0	0	30	0	—	40	—	—	—	—
Pina Pineapple	8 fl oz	110	0	0	0	0	26	0	—	40	—	—	—	—
Seltzer	8 fl oz	0	0	0	0	0	0	0	—	10	—	—	—	—
Seltzer Cherry	8 fl oz	0	0	0	0	0	0	0	—	10	—	—	—	—
Seltzer Cranberry Lime	8 fl oz	0	0	0	0	0	0	0	—	10	—	—	—	—
Seltzer Grapefruit	8 fl oz	0	0	0	0	0	0	0	—	10	—	—	—	—
Seltzer Lemon Lime	8 fl oz	0	0	0	0	0	0	0	—	10	—	—	—	—
Seltzer Mandarin Orange	8 fl oz	0	0	0	0	0	0	0	—	10	—	—	—	—
Seltzer Peach	8 fl oz	0	0	0	0	0	0	0	—	10	—	—	—	—
Seltzer Raspberry	8 fl oz	0	0	0	0	0	0	0	—	10	—	—	—	—
Seltzer Strawberry	8 fl oz	0	0	0	0	0	0	0	—	10	—	—	—	—
Seltzer Tropical	8 fl oz	0	0	0	0	0	0	0	—	10	—	—	—	—
Sunripe Orange	8 fl oz	140	0	0	0	0	35	0	—	45	—	—	—	—
Tahitian Treat	8 fl oz	150	0	0	0	0	36	0	—	45	—	—	—	—
Tonic Water	8 fl oz	100	0	0	0	0	24	0	—	15	—	—	—	—

FOOD	PORTION	CALORIES	FAT	SAT FAT	CHOL	PROTEIN	CARBO	FIBER	CALCIUM	SOD	POTAS	VIT C	FOLIC	VIT A
CANADA DRY (CONT.)														
Tonic Water Twist Of Lime	8 fl oz	100	0	0	0	0	24	0	—	20	—	—	—	—
Vanilla Cream	8 fl oz	120	0	0	0	0	30	0	—	40	—	—	—	—
Vichy Water	8 fl oz	0	0	0	0	0	0	0	—	490	—	—	—	—
Wild Cherry	8 fl oz	110	0	0	0	0	28	0	—	40	—	—	—	—
CLEARLY 2														
Black Cherry	8 fl oz	2	0	—	—	—	0	—	18	9	1	—	—	—
Key Lime	8 fl oz	2	0	—	—	—	0	—	18	9	1	—	—	—
CLEARLY CANADIAN														
Alpine Fruit & Berries	8 fl oz	90	0	—	—	—	23	—	18	9	1	—	—	—
Boysenberry Mist	8 fl oz	2	0	—	—	—	0	—	18	9	1	—	—	—
Coastal Cranberry	8 fl oz	90	0	—	—	—	22	—	18	9	1	—	—	—
Country Raspberry	8 fl oz	80	0	—	—	—	19	—	18	9	1	—	—	—
Green Apple	8 fl oz	80	0	—	—	—	19	—	18	9	1	—	—	—
Mountain Blackberry	8 fl oz	100	0	—	—	—	24	—	18	9	1	—	—	—
Orchard Peach Strawberry	8 fl oz	90	0	—	—	—	22	—	18	9	1	—	—	—
Soda	8 fl oz	0	0	0	0	—	0	—	25	5	1	—	—	—
Summer Strawberry	8 fl oz	80	0	—	—	—	19	—	18	9	1	—	—	—
Western Longanberry	8 fl oz	80	0	—	—	—	19	—	18	9	1	—	—	—
Wild Cherry	8 fl oz	90	0	—	—	—	23	—	18	9	1	—	—	—
COCA-COLA														
Cherry	8 fl oz	104	0	0	0	0	28	—	—	4	0	—	—	—
Classic	8 fl oz	97	0	0	0	0	27	—	—	9	0	—	—	—
Classic Caffeine-Free	8 fl oz	97	0	0	0	0	27	—	—	9	0	—	—	—
Coke II	8 fl oz	105	0	0	0	0	29	—	—	4	0	—	—	—
Diet	8 fl oz	1	0	0	0	0	tr	—	—	4	12	—	—	—
Diet Cherry	8 fl oz	1	0	0	0	0	tr	—	—	4	12	—	—	—
Diet Coke Caffeine-Free	8 fl oz	1	0	0	0	0	tr	—	—	4	12	—	—	—
COTT														
Cola	8 fl oz	110	0	0	0	0	27	0	—	10	—	—	—	—
Ginger Ale	8 fl oz	90	0	0	0	0	20	0	—	20	—	—	—	—
Grape	8 fl oz	130	0	0	0	0	30	0	—	25	—	—	—	—
Orange	8 fl oz	140	0	0	0	0	33	0	—	25	—	—	—	—
Pineapple	8 fl oz	130	0	0	0	0	32	0	—	25	—	—	—	—
Punch	8 fl oz	130	0	0	0	0	32	0	—	25	—	—	—	—
Seltzer	8 fl oz	0	0	0	0	0	0	0	—	0	—	—	—	—
CRUSH														
Cherry	8 fl oz	140	0	0	0	0	35	0	—	30	—	—	—	—
Grape	8 fl oz	110	0	0	0	0	—	0	—	—	—	—	—	—

FOOD	PORTION	CALORIES	FAT	SAT FAT	CHOL	PROTEIN	CARBO	FIBER	CALCIUM	SOD	POTAS	VIT C	FOLIC	VIT A
CRUSH (CONT.)														
Orange	8 fl oz	140	0	0	0	0	—	0	—	—	—	—	—	—
Orange Diet	8 fl oz	0	0	0	0	0	0	0	—	—	—	—	—	—
Pineapple	8 fl oz	140	0	0	0	0	35	0	—	30	—	—	—	—
Strawberry	8 fl oz	130	0	0	0	0	—	0	—	—	—	—	—	—
Tropical Fruit Punch	1 bottle (10 fl oz)	180	0	0	0	0	44	0	0	20	33	2	—	0
Tropical Fruit Punch	1 can (11.5 fl oz)	200	0	0	0	—	—	—	16	—	—	—	—	—
DIET RITE														
Black Cherry Salt/Sodium Free	8 fl oz	2	0	0	0	0	1	—	—	0	55	—	—	—
Cola	8 fl oz	1	0	0	0	0	tr	—	—	0	43	—	—	—
Cola Caffeine/Sugar Free	8 fl oz	1	0	0	0	0	tr	—	—	7	40	—	—	—
Cola Salt/Sodium Free	8 fl oz	1	0	0	0	0	tr	—	—	tr	40	—	—	—
Fruit Punch Salt/Sodium Free	8 fl oz	2	0	0	0	0	tr	—	—	0	37	—	—	—
Golden Peach Salt/Sodium Free	8 fl oz	2	0	0	0	0	tr	—	—	0	33	—	—	—
Key Lime Salt/Sodium Free	8 fl oz	7	0	0	0	0	2	—	—	0	31	—	—	—
Pink Grapefruit Salt/Sodium Free	8 fl oz	2	0	0	0	0	1	—	—	0	43	—	—	—
Red Raspberry Salt/Sodium Free	8 fl oz	3	0	0	0	0	1	—	—	tr	81	—	—	—
Tangerine Salt/Sodium Free	8 fl oz	2	0	0	0	0	tr	—	—	0	37	—	—	—
White Grape Salt/Sodium Free	8 fl oz	1	0	0	0	0	tr	—	—	0	35	—	—	—
DR PEPPER														
Diet	1 oz	tr	0	—	0	—	—	—	0	—	—	—	—	—
Original	1 oz	13	0	—	0	—	—	—	0	—	—	—	—	—
DR. NEHI														
Soda	8 fl oz	100	0	0	0	0	26	—	—	35	28	—	—	—
FANTA														
Ginger Ale	8 fl oz	86	0	0	0	0	23	—	—	4	11	—	—	—
Grape	8 fl oz	117	0	0	0	0	31	—	—	9	0	—	—	—
Orange	8 fl oz	118	0	0	0	0	32	—	—	9	0	—	—	—
Root Beer	8 fl oz	111	0	0	0	0	29	—	—	4	13	—	—	—
FRESCA														
Soda	8 fl oz	3	0	0	0	0	tr	—	—	1	55	—	—	—
HEALTH VALLEY														
Ginger Ale	12 oz	153	1	—	0	1	35	0	—	30	10	—	—	—
Rootbeer Old Fashioned	12 oz	120	1	—	0	1	26	—	—	12	22	—	—	—

FOOD	PORTION	CALORIES	FAT	SAT FAT	CHOL	PROTEIN	CARBO	FIBER	CALCIUM	SOD	POTAS	VIT C	FOLIC	VIT A
HEALTH VALLEY (CONT.)														
Sarsaparilla Rootbeer	12 oz	153	1	—	0	1	35	—	—	27	16	—	—	—
Wild Berry	12 oz	142	1	—	0	1	33	—	—	27	5	—	—	—
HIRES														
Cream	8 fl oz	130	0	0	0	0	0	0	—	30	—	—	—	—
Cream Soda Diet	8 fl oz	0	0	0	0	0	0	0	—	35	—	—	—	—
Original Mocha	8 fl oz	100	0	0	0	0	24	0	—	45	—	—	—	—
Original Mocha Diet	8 fl oz	5	0	0	0	0	0	0	—	45	—	—	—	—
Root Beer	8 fl oz	130	0	0	0	0	31	0	—	45	—	—	—	—
Root Beer Diet	8 fl oz	0	0	0	0	0	0	0	—	70	—	—	—	—
IBC														
Root Beer	8 oz	110	0	0	0	0	29	—	—	40	—	—	—	—
KICK														
Soda	8 fl oz	120	0	0	0	0	32	—	—	35	49	—	—	—
MELLO YELLOW														
Diet	8 fl oz	4	0	0	0	0	tr	—	—	tr	37	—	—	—
Soda	8 fl oz	119	0	0	0	0	32	—	—	9	22	—	—	—
MINUTE MAID														
Berry	8 fl oz	111	0	0	0	0	30	—	—	9	0	—	—	—
Diet Orange	8 fl oz	2	0	0	0	0	0	—	—	0	43	—	—	—
Fruit Punch	8 fl oz	117	0	0	0	0	32	—	—	10	13	—	—	—
Grape	8 fl oz	121	0	0	0	0	32	—	—	9	0	—	—	—
Grapefruit	8 fl oz	108	0	0	0	0	29	—	—	9	tr	—	—	—
Orange	8 fl oz	118	0	0	0	0	32	—	—	0	14	—	—	—
Peach	8 fl oz	110	0	0	0	0	29	—	—	9	0	—	—	—
Pineapple	8 fl oz	109	0	0	0	0	30	—	—	9	0	—	—	—
Raspberry	8 fl oz	111	0	0	0	0	30	—	—	9	0	—	—	—
Soda	8 fl oz	110	0	0	0	0	29	—	—	11	0	—	—	—
Strawberry	8 fl oz	122	0	0	0	0	33	—	—	9	0	—	—	—
MOUNTAIN DEW														
Diet	8 fl oz	2	0	0	0	tr	tr	—	—	0	49	—	—	—
Soda	8 fl oz	118	0	0	0	tr	30	—	—	21	4	—	—	—
MR. PIBB														
Diet	8 fl oz	1	0	0	0	0	tr	—	—	2	20	—	—	—
Soda	6 oz	97	0	0	0	0	26	—	—	7	14	—	—	—
MUG														
Cream	8 fl oz	122	0	0	0	tr	32	—	—	21	2	—	—	—
Diet Cream	8 fl oz	2	0	0	0	tr	0	—	—	29	2	—	—	—
Diet Root Beer	8 fl oz	1	0	0	0	tr	tr	—	—	26	0	—	—	—
Root Beer	8 fl oz	141	0	0	0	tr	29	—	—	26	0	—	—	—
NEHI														
Cream	8 fl oz	120	0	0	0	0	32	—	—	0	0	—	—	—
Fruit Punch	8 fl oz	120	0	0	0	0	34	—	—	35	32	—	—	—

FOOD	PORTION	CALORIES	FAT	SAT FAT	CHOL	PROTEIN	CARBO	FIBER	CALCIUM	SOD	POTAS	VIT C	FOLIC	VIT A
NEHI (CONT.)														
Ginger Ale	8 fl oz	90	0	0	0	0	24	—	—	35	2	—	—	—
Grape	8 fl oz	120	0	0	0	0	32	—	—	35	16	—	—	—
Orange	8 fl oz	130	0	0	0	0	35	—	—	35	20	—	—	—
Peach	8 fl oz	130	0	0	0	0	34	—	—	35	32	—	—	—
Pineapple	8 fl oz	130	0	0	0	0	36	—	—	0	18	—	—	—
Quinine Water	8 fl oz	90	0	0	0	0	23	—	—	35	0	—	—	—
Root Beer	8 fl oz	120	0	0	0	0	32	—	—	35	27	—	—	—
Strawberry	8 fl oz	120	0	0	0	0	32	—	—	35	0	—	—	—
Wild Red	8 fl oz	120	0	0	0	0	32	—	—	33	15	—	—	—
OLD COLONY														
Grape	8 fl oz	140	0	0	0	0	32	0		40	—	—	—	—
ORANGINA														
Sparkling Citrus	6 fl oz	80	0	0	0	0	19	—	—	0	35	6	—	—
PEPSI														
Caffeine Free	8 fl oz	105	0	0	0	tr	27	—	—	0	7	—	—	—
Diet	8 fl oz	1	0	0	0	tr	tr	—	—	tr	21	—	—	—
Diet Caffeine Free	8 fl oz	1	0	0	0	tr	tr	—	—	tr	21	—	—	—
Regular	8 fl oz	105	0	0	0	tr	27	—	—	0	7	—	—	—
RAMBLIN' ROOT BEER														
Ramblin' Root Beer	8 fl oz	120	0	0	0	0	33	—	—	4	27	—	—	—
RAZING RAZBERRY														
Cola	8 fl oz	117	0	0	0	tr	31	—	—	0	7	0	—	—
ROYAL CROWN														
Caffeine Free Cola	8 fl oz	110	0	0	0	0	29	—	—	35	10	—	—	—
Cherry	8 fl oz	110	0	0	0	0	29	—	—	35	10	—	—	—
Cola	8 fl oz	100	0	0	0	0	28	—	—	35	10	—	—	—
Diet	8 fl oz	1	0	0	0	0	tr	—	—	tr	40	—	—	—
Diet Caffeine Free	8 fl oz	1	0	0	0	0	tr	—	—	tr	40	—	—	—
Diet Cranberry Apple Salt/ Sodium Free	8 fl oz	2	0	0	0	0	tr	—	—	1	81	—	—	—
Diet Cranberry Salt/Sodium Free	8 fl oz	2	0	0	0	0	tr	—	—	1	81	—	—	—
ROYAL MISTIC														
'N Juice Black Cherry	12 fl oz	146	0	0	0	0	36	—	—	26	14	—	—	—
'N Juice Peach Vanilla	12 fl oz	146	0	0	0	0	36	—	—	18	8	—	—	—
'N Juice Tangerine Orange	12 fl oz	146	0	0	0	0	36	—	—	30	18	—	—	—
'N Juice Tropical Supreme	12 fl oz	152	0	0	0	0	38	—	—	14	18	—	—	—
'N Juice Wild Berry	12 fl oz	156	0	0	0	0	38	—	—	30	14	—	—	—
Caribbean Fruit Punch	16 fl oz	230	0	0	0	0	57	—	—	5	11	—	—	—

FOOD	PORTION	CALORIES	FAT	SAT FAT	CHOL	PROTEIN	CARBO	FIBER	CALCIUM	SOD	POTAS	VIT C	FOLIC	VIT A
ROYAL MISTIC (CONT.)														
Grape Strawberry	16 fl oz	230	0	0	0	0	57	—	—	5	11	—	—	—
Sparkling Diet With Lime Kiwi	11.1 fl oz	0	0	0	0	0	0	—	—	<90	52	—	—	—
Sparkling Diet With Raspberry Boysenberry	11.1 fl oz	0	0	0	0	0	0	—	—	<90	52	—	—	—
Sparkling Diet With Royal Peach	11.1 fl oz	0	0	0	0	0	0	—	—	<90	52	—	—	—
Sparkling Diet With Wild Cherry	11.1 fl oz	0	0	0	0	0	0	—	—	<90	52	—	—	—
Sparkling With Lime Kiwi	11.1 fl oz	112	0	0	0	0	28	—	—	38	4	—	—	—
Sparkling With Mandarin Orange Pineappple	11.1 fl oz	120	0	0	0	0	30	—	—	18	4	—	—	—
Sparkling With Mango Passion	11.1 fl oz	112	0	0	0	0	28	—	—	34	4	—	—	—
Sparkling With Raspberry Boysenberry	11.1 fl oz	112	0	0	0	0	28	—	—	24	4	—	—	—
Sparkling With Royal Peach	11.1 fl oz	112	0	0	0	0	28	—	—	30	4	—	—	—
Sparkling With Wild Cherry	11.1 fl oz	112	0	0	0	0	28	—	—	28	4	—	—	—
SCHWEPPES														
Bitter Lemon	8 fl oz	110	0	0	0	0	28	0	—	45	—	—	—	—
Club	8 fl oz	0	0	0	0	0	0	0	—	70	—	—	—	—
Club Sodium Free	8 fl oz	0	0	0	0	0	0	0	—	0	—	—	—	—
Diet Ginger Ale	8 fl oz	0	0	0	0	0	0	0	—	75	—	—	—	—
Diet Ginger Ale Dry Grape	8 fl oz	2	0	0	0	0	0	0	—	90	—	—	—	—
Diet Ginger Ale Raspberry	8 fl oz	0	0	0	0	0	0	0	—	75	—	—	—	—
Ginger Ale	8 fl oz	90	0	0	0	0	22	0	—	50	—	—	—	—
Ginger Ale Dry Grape	8 fl oz	100	0	0	0	0	26	0	—	50	—	—	—	—
Ginger Ale Raspberry	8 fl oz	100	0	0	0	0	26	0	—	50	—	—	—	—
Ginger Beer	8 fl oz	100	0	0	0	0	25	0	—	90	—	—	—	—
Grape	8 fl oz	130	0	0	0	0	33	0	—	55	—	—	—	—
Grapefruit	8 fl oz	110	0	0	0	0	27	0	—	75	—	—	—	—
Lemon Sour	8 fl oz	110	0	0	0	0	26	0	—	25	—	—	—	—
Lemon-Lime	8 fl oz	100	0	0	0	0	25	0	—	75	—	—	—	—
Seltzer Black Berry	8 fl oz	0	0	0	0	0	0	0	—	10	—	—	—	—
Seltzer Lemon	8 fl oz	0	0	0	0	0	0	0	—	10	—	—	—	—
Seltzer Lemon Lime	8 fl oz	0	0	0	0	0	0	0	—	10	—	—	—	—

FOOD	PORTION	CALORIES	FAT	SAT FAT	CHOL	PROTEIN	CARBO	FIBER	CALCIUM	SOD	POTAS	VIT C	FOLIC	VIT A
SCHWEPPES (CONT.)														
Seltzer Lime	8 fl oz	0	0	0	0	0	0	0	—	10	—	—	—	—
Seltzer Orange	8 fl oz	0	0	0	0	0	0	0	—	10	—	—	—	—
Seltzer Peaches & Cream	8 fl oz	0	0	0	0	0	0	0	—	10	—	—	—	—
Seltzer Raspberry	8 fl oz	0	0	0	0	0	0	0		0	—	—	—	—
Tonic Citrus	8 fl oz	90	0	0	0	0	20	0	—	25	—	—	—	—
Tonic Cranberry	8 fl oz	90	0	0	0	0	20	0	—	25	—	—	—	—
Tonic Raspberry	8 fl oz	90	0	0	0	0	20	0	—	25	—	—	—	—
Tonic Water Diet	8 fl oz	0	0	0	0	0	0	0	—	85	—	—	—	—
SHASTA														
Black Cherry	1 can (12 oz)	170	0	0	0	0	41	0	—	54	—	—	—	—
Caffeine Free Cola	1 can (12 oz)	160	0	0	0	0	41	—	—	45	—	—	—	—
Cherry Cola	1 can (12 oz)	160	0	0	0	0	39	—	—	45	—	—	—	—
Club Soda	1 can (12 oz)	0	0	0	0	0	0	—	—	90	—	—	—	—
Cola	1 can (12 oz)	170	0	0	0	0	42	0	—	45	—	—	—	—
Creme	1 can (12 oz)	190	0	0	0	0	47	0	—	45	—	—	—	—
Diet Birch Beer	12 oz	4	0	—	0	—	—	—	0	—	—	—	—	—
Diet Black Cherry	1 can (12 oz)	0	0	0	0	0	0	0	—	55	—	—	—	—
Diet Caffeine Free Cola	1 can (12 oz)	0	0	0	0	0	0	0	—	55	—	—	—	—
Diet Cherry Cola	1 can (12 oz)	0	0	0	0	0	0	0	—	55	—	—	—	—
Diet Cola	1 can (12 oz)	0	0	0	0	0	0	0	—	45	—	—	—	—
Diet Creme	1 can (12 oz)	0	0	0	0	0	0	0	—	55	—	—	—	—
Diet Doc Shasta	1 can (12 oz)	0	0	0	0	0	0	0	—	45	—	—	—	—
Diet Ginger Ale	1 can (12 oz)	0	0	0	0	0	0	0	—	55	—	—	—	—
Diet Grape	1 can (12 oz)	0	0	0	0	0	0	0	—	55	—	—	—	—
Diet Grapefruit	1 can (12 oz)	0	0	0	0	0	0	0	—	45	—	—	—	—
Diet Grapefruit	1 can (12 oz)	0	0	0	0	0	0	0	—	55	—	—	—	—
Diet Kiwi-Strawberry	1 can (12 oz)	0	0	0	0	0	0	0	—	45	—	—	—	—
Diet Lemon-Lime Twist	1 can (12 oz)	0	0	0	0	0	0	0	—	55	—	—	—	—
Diet Orange	1 can (12 oz)	0	0	0	0	0	0	0	—	55	—	—	—	—
Diet Pineapple-Orange	1 can (12 oz)	0	0	0	0	0	0	0	—	55	—	—	—	—
Diet Raspberry Creme	1 can (12 oz)	0	0	0	0	0	0	0	—	45	—	—	—	—
Diet Red Pop	1 can (12 oz)	0	0	0	0	0	0	0	—	55	—	—	—	—
Diet Root Beer	1 can (12 oz)	0	0	0	0	0	0	0	—	55	—	—	—	—
Diet Strawberry	1 can (12 oz)	0	0	0	0	0	0	0	—	55	—	—	—	—
Diet Strawberry-Peach	1 can (12 oz)	0	0	0	0	0	0	0	—	55	—	—	—	—
Doc Shasta	1 can (12 oz)	160	0	0	0	0	39	0	—	45	—	—	—	—
Fruit Punch	1 can (12 oz)	200	0	0	0	0	50	0	—	45	—	—	—	—
Ginger Ale	1 can (12 oz)	130	0	0	0	0	32	0	—	45	—	—	—	—

FOOD	PORTION	CALORIES	FAT	SAT FAT	CHOL	PROTEIN	CARBO	FIBER	CALCIUM	SOD	POTAS	VIT C	FOLIC	VIT A
SHASTA (CONT.)														
Grape	1 can (12 oz)	190	0	0	0	0	48	0	—	45	—	—	—	—
Kiwi-Strawberry	1 can (12 oz)	170	0	0	0	0	43	0	—	45	—	—	—	—
Lemon-Lime Twist	1 can (12 oz)	150	0	0	0	0	38	0	—	45	—	—	—	—
Moon Mist	1 can (12 oz)	180	0	0	0	0	46	0	—	45	—	—	—	—
Orange	1 can (12 oz)	200	0	0	0	0	49	0	—	45	—	—	—	—
Peach	1 can (12 oz)	170	0	0	0	0	43	0	—	45	—	—	—	—
Pineapple	1 can (12 oz)	200	0	0	0	0	51	0	—	45	—	—	—	—
Pineapple-Orange	1 can (12 oz)	180	0	0	0	0	46	0	—	45	—	—	—	—
Quinine/Tonic	1 can (12 oz)	130	0	0	0	0	32	0	—	45	—	—	—	—
Raspberry Creme	1 can (12 oz)	170	0	0	0	0	44	0	—	45	—	—	—	—
Red Pop	1 can (12 oz)	170	0	0	0	0	43	0	—	45	—	—	—	—
Root Beer	1 can (12 oz)	170	0	0	0	0	42	0	—	45	—	—	—	—
Strawberry	1 can (12 oz)	190	0	0	0	0	46	0	—	45	—	—	—	—
Strawberry-Peach	1 can (12 oz)	170	0	0	0	0	42	0	—	45	—	—	—	—
SLICE														
Diet Lemon Lime	8 fl oz	5	0	0	0	tr	tr	—	—	1	56	—	—	—
Diet Mandarin	8 fl oz	5	0	0	0	tr	tr	—	—	10	62	—	—	—
Lemon Lime	8 fl oz	100	0	0	0	tr	26	—	—	10	55	—	—	—
Mandarin Orange	8 fl oz	128	0	0	0	tr	33	—	—	10	73	—	—	—
Red	8 fl oz	128	0	0	0	tr	33	—	—	10	27	0	—	—
SNAPPLE														
Amazin' Grape	8 fl oz	120	0	0	0	0	28	—	0	5	0	—	—	0
Cherry Lime Ricky	8 fl oz	110	0	0	0	0	27	—	0	0	—	—	—	0
Creme D'Vanilla	8 fl oz	130	0	0	0	0	33	—	0	0	0	—	—	0
French Cherry	8 fl oz	120	0	0	0	0	29	—	0	0	—	—	—	0
Kiwi Peach	8 fl oz	120	0	0	0	0	29	—	0	0	—	—	—	0
Kiwi Strawberry	8 fl oz	130	0	0	0	0	33	—	0	5	0	—	—	0
Mango Madness	8 fl oz	130	0	0	0	0	33	—	0	5	0	—	—	0
Passion Supreme	8 fl oz	120	0	0	0	0	29	—	0	0	0	—	—	0
Peach Melba	8 fl oz	120	0	0	0	0	31	—	0	0	—	—	—	0
Raspberry	8 fl oz	120	0	0	0	0	31	—	0	0	—	—	—	0
Seltzer Black Cherry	8 fl oz	0	0	0	0	0	0	—	0	0	—	—	—	0
Seltzer Lemon Lime	8 fl oz	0	0	0	0	0	0	—	0	0	—	—	—	0
Seltzer Original	8 fl oz	0	0	0	0	0	0	—	0	0	—	—	—	0
Seltzer Tangerine	8 fl oz	0	0	0	0	0	0	—	0	0	—	—	—	0
Tru Root Beer	8 fl oz	110	0	0	0	0	29	—	0	0	—	—	—	0
SPRITE														
Diet	8 fl oz	3	0	0	0	0	0	—	—	0	67	—	—	—
Soda	8 fl oz	100	0	0	0	0	26	—	—	31	0	—	—	—
SUNDROP														
Cherry	8 fl oz	130	0	0	0	0	21	0	—	15	—	—	—	—
Diet	8 fl oz	5	0	0	0	0	0	0	—	65	—	—	—	—

FOOD	PORTION	CALORIES	FAT	SAT FAT	CHOL	PROTEIN	CARBO	FIBER	CALCIUM	SOD	POTAS	VIT C	FOLIC	VIT A
SUNDROP (CONT.)														
Soda	8 fl oz	140	0	0	0	0	34	0	—	20	—	—	—	—
SUNKIST														
Cactus Cooler	8 fl oz	110	0	0	0	0	27	0	—	40	—	—	—	—
Cherry	8 fl oz	140	0	0	0	0	35	0	—	35	—	—	—	—
Diet Citrus	8 fl oz	0	0	0	0	0	0	0	—	90	—	—	—	—
Diet Orange	8 fl oz	5	0	0	0	0	0	0	—	75	—	—	—	—
Fruit Punch	8 fl oz	130	0	0	0	0	33	0	—	35	—	—	—	—
Orange	8 fl oz	140	0	0	0	0	35	0	—	40	—	—	—	—
Peach	8 fl oz	120	0	0	0	0	30	0	—	40	—	—	—	—
Pineapple	8 fl oz	140	0	0	0	0	35	0	—	35	—	—	—	—
Strawberry	8 fl oz	140	0	0	0	0	34	0	—	35	—	—	—	—
TAB														
Soda	8 fl oz	1	0	0	0	0	tr	—	—	4	12	—	—	—
TROPICAL CHILL														
Cola	8 fl oz	117	0	0	0	tr	31	—	—	0	7	0	—	—
Diet	8 fl oz	1	0	0	0	tr	tr	—	—	0	7	0	—	—
UPPER 10														
Diet	8 fl oz	3	0	0	0	0	1	—	—	0	55	—	—	—
Diet Salt/Sodium Free	8 fl oz	3	0	0	0	0	1	—	—	0	55	—	—	—
Salt Free	8 fl oz	100	0	0	0	0	29	—	—	0	17	—	—	—
Soda	8 fl oz	100	0	0	0	0	28	—	—	35	39	—	—	—
WINK														
Diet	8 fl oz	5	0	0	0	0	1	0	—	95	—	—	—	—
Soda	8 fl oz	130	0	0	0	0	31	0	—	35	—	—	—	—
YOO-HOO														
Original	9 fl oz	150	tr	tr	0	3	31	tr	100	200	250	6	8	500
SOLDIER BEANS														
BEAN CUISINE														
Dried	½ cup	115	1	—	0	8	—	5	—	5	310	—	62	—
SOLE														
FRESH														
cooked	1 fillet (4.5 oz)	148	2	tr	86	31	0	—	23	133	436	—	—	48
cooked	3 oz	99	1	tr	58	21	0	—	16	89	292	—	—	32
FROZEN														
GORTON'S														
Fishmarket Fresh	5 oz	110	1	—	—	24	1	—	—	140	—	—	—	—
Microwave Entree In Lemon Butter	1 pkg	380	24	11	120	25	17	—	20	560	—	—	—	200
Microwave Entree In Wine Sauce	1 pkg	180	8	3	90	25	3	—	60	770	—	—	—	—
MRS. PAUL'S														
Light Fillets	1 fillet	240	10	—	50	16	20	—	40	450	—	—	—	100

FOOD	PORTION	CALORIES	FAT	SAT FAT	CHOL	PROTEIN	CARBO	FIBER	CALCIUM	SOD	POTAS	VIT C	FOLIC	VIT A
VAN DE KAMP'S														
Lightly Breaded Fillets	1 (4 oz)	220	11	2	40	14	17	0	20	410	—	0	—	0
Natural Fillets	1 (4 oz)	110	2	0	50	23	0	0	20	125	—	0	—	0
TAKE-OUT														
battered & fried	3.2 oz	211	11	3	31	13	15	—	17	484	292	0	51	35
breaded & fried	3.2 oz	211	11	3	31	13	15	—	17	484	292	0	51	35

SORBET

(*see* ICES AND ICE POPS)

SORGHUM

FOOD	PORTION	CALORIES	FAT	SAT FAT	CHOL	PROTEIN	CARBO	FIBER	CALCIUM	SOD	POTAS	VIT C	FOLIC	VIT A
sorghum	½ cup	325	3	tr	0	11	72	—	27	—	336	0	—	—

SOUFFLE

FOOD	PORTION	CALORIES	FAT	SAT FAT	CHOL	PROTEIN	CARBO	FIBER	CALCIUM	SOD	POTAS	VIT C	FOLIC	VIT A
lemon chilled	1 cup	176	tr	—	2	9	34	—	175	108	—	—	—	—
raspberry chilled	1 cup	173	tr	—	3	10	34	—	190	108	—	—	—	—
spinach	1 cup	218	18	7	184	11	3	—	230	763	202	3	62	3461

SOUP

CANNED

FOOD	PORTION	CALORIES	FAT	SAT FAT	CHOL	PROTEIN	CARBO	FIBER	CALCIUM	SOD	POTAS	VIT C	FOLIC	VIT A
asparagus cream of as prep w/ milk	1 cup	161	8	3	22	6	16	—	175	1041	359	4	—	599
asparagus cream of as prep w/ water	1 cup	87	4	1	5	1	11	—	29	981	173	3	—	445
beef broth ready-to-serve	1 cup	16	1	tr	tr	3	tr	—	15	782	130	0	—	0
beef broth ready-to-serve	1 can (14 oz)	27	1	tr	1	5	tr	—	25	1294	214	0	—	0
beef noodle as prep w/water	1 cup	84	3	1	5	5	9	—	15	952	99	tr	4	629
black bean turtle soup	1 cup	218	1	tr	0	14	40	—	84	922	739	6	146	10
black bean as prep w/water	1 cup	116	2	tr	0	6	20	—	45	1198	273	1	25	506
celery cream of as prep w/ milk	1 cup	165	10	4	32	6	15	—	186	1010	309	1	9	461
celery cream of as prep w/ water	1 cup	90	6	1	15	2	9	—	40	949	123	tr	2	306
celery cream of not prep	1 can (10¾ oz)	219	14	3	34	4	21	—	98	2308	299	1	6	746
cheese as prep w/ milk	1 cup	230	15	9	48	9	16	—	288	1020	340	1	—	1243
cheese as prep w/ water	1 cup	155	10	7	30	5	11	—	142	959	154	0	—	1088
cheese not prep	1 can (11 oz)	377	25	16	72	13	26	—	345	2331	374	0	—	2643
chicken broth as prep w/ water	1 cup	39	1	tr	1	5	1	—	9	776	210	0	—	0
chicken cream of as prep w/ milk	1 cup	191	11	5	27	7	15	—	180	1046	273	1	8	715

FOOD	PORTION	CALORIES	FAT	SAT FAT	CHOL	PROTEIN	CARBO	FIBER	CALCIUM	SOD	POTAS	VIT C	FOLIC	VIT A
chicken cream of as prep w/ water	1 cup	116	7	2	10	3	9	—	34	986	87	tr	2	560
chicken gumbo as prep w/water	1 cup	56	1	tr	5	3	8	—	24	955	75	5	—	136
chicken noodle as prep w/ water	1 cup	75	2	1	7	4	9	—	17	1107	55	tr	2	711
chicken rice as prep w/ water	1 cup	251	2	tr	7	4	7	—	17	814	100	tr	1	660
clam chowder new england as prep w/ water	1 cup	95	3	tr	5	5	12	—	43	914	146	2	4	8
clam chowder new england as prep w/ milk	1 cup	163	7	3	22	9	17	—	187	992	300	4	10	164
consomme w/ gelatin not prep	1 can (10½ oz)	71	0	0	0	13	4	—	21	1550	373	2	7	0
consomme w/ gelatin as prep w/ water	1 cup	29	0	0	0	5	2	—	8	637	153	1	3	0
escarole ready-to-serve	1 cup	27	2	1	2	2	2	—	32	3865	—	—	—	2170
french onion as prep w/ water	1 cup	57	2	tr	0	4	8	—	26	1053	69	1	15	0
gazpacho ready-to-serve	1 cup	57	2	tr	0	9	1	—	24	1183	224	3	—	200
minestrone as prep w/water	1 cup	83	3	1	2	4	11	—	34	911	312	1	16	2337
mushroom cream of as prep w/ milk	1 cup	203	14	5	20	6	15	—	178	1076	270	2	—	154
mushroom cream of as prep w/ water	1 cup	129	9	2	2	2	9	—	46	1031	101	1	—	0
oyster stew as prep w/ milk	1 cup	134	8	5	32	6	10	—	167	1040	235	4	—	225
oyster stew as prep w/ water	1 cup	59	4	3	14	2	4	—	22	980	49	3	—	71
pepperpot as prep w/ water	1 cup	103	5	2	10	6	9	—	23	970	152	1	tr	856
potato cream of as prep w/ milk	1 cup	148	6	4	22	6	17	—	166	1060	323	1	9	443
potato cream of as prep w/ water	1 cup	73	2	1	5	2	11	—	20	1000	137	0	3	288
scotch broth as prep w/ water	1 cup	80	3	1	5	5	9	—	15	1012	159	1	—	2180
split pea w/ ham as prep w/ water	1 cup	189	4	2	8	10	28	—	22	1008	399	1	3	444
tomato as prep w/ milk	1 cup	160	6	3	17	6	22	—	159	932	450	68	21	849
tomato as prep w/ water	1 cup	86	2	tr	0	2	17	—	13	872	263	67	15	688

FOOD	PORTION	CALORIES	FAT	SAT FAT	CHOL	PROTEIN	CARBO	FIBER	CALCIUM	SOD	POTAS	VIT C	FOLIC	VIT A
vegetarian vegetable as prep w/ water	1 cup	72	2	tr	0	2	12	—	21	823	209	1	11	3005
vichyssoise	1 cup	148	6	4	22	6	17	—	166	1060	323	1	9	443
CAMPBELL														
Asparagus Cream Of as prep	8 oz	80	4	—	—	2	10	—	20	820	—	1	—	200
Bean Homestyle as prep	8 oz	130	1	—	—	6	25	—	60	700	—	2	—	750
Bean With Bacon as prep	8 oz	140	4	—	—	6	21	—	60	840	—	—	—	750
Beef as prep	8 oz	80	2	—	—	5	10	—	—	830	—	1	—	1000
Beef Broth as prep	8 oz	16	0	—	—	3	1	—	—	820	—	—	—	—
Beef Noodle Homestyle as prep	8 oz	80	4	—	—	5	7	—	—	810	—	1	—	—
Beef Noodle as prep	8 oz	70	3	—	—	4	7	—	—	830	—	—	—	200
Beefy Mushroom as prep	8 oz	60	3	—	—	4	5	—	—	960	—	—	—	—
Broccoli Cream Of as prep	8 oz	80	5	—	—	1	8	—	20	790	—	6	—	100
Broccoli Cream Of as prep w/ 2% milk	8 oz	140	7	—	—	5	14	—	150	850	—	6	—	300
Celery Cream Of as prep	8 oz	100	7	—	—	2	8	—	20	820	—	—	—	300
Cheddar Cheese as prep	8 oz	110	6	—	—	4	10	—	100	810	—	—	—	750
Chicken Alphabet as prep	8 oz	80	3	—	—	3	10	—	—	800	—	—	—	750
Chicken Noodle-O's as prep	8 oz	70	2	—	—	3	9	—	—	820	—	—	—	400
Chicken Vegetable as prep	8 oz	70	3	—	—	3	8	—	—	850	—	—	—	2500
Chicken & Pasta With Garden Vegetables	1 cup (8.4 oz)	90	1	0	5	6	14	1	40	850	—	1	—	2500
Chicken & Stars as prep	8 oz	60	2	—	—	3	7	—	—	870	—	—	—	400
Chicken 'n Dumplings as prep	8 oz	80	3	—	—	4	9	—	—	960	—	—	—	400
Chicken Barley as prep	8 oz	70	2	—	—	3	10	—	—	850	—	—	—	1000
Chicken Broth as prep	8 oz	30	2	—	—	1	2	—	—	710	—	—	—	—
Chicken Broth & Noodles as prep	8 oz	45	1	—	—	1	8	—	—	860	—	—	—	400
Chicken Cream Of as prep	8 oz	110	7	—	—	2	9	—	20	810	—	—	—	500
Chicken Gumbo as prep	8 oz	60	2	—	—	2	8	—	20	900	—	—	—	100

FOOD	PORTION	CALORIES	FAT	SAT FAT	CHOL	PROTEIN	CARBO	FIBER	CALCIUM	SOD	POTAS	VIT C	FOLIC	VIT A
CAMPBELL (CONT.)														
Chicken Mushroom Creamy as prep	8 oz	120	8	—	—	3	8	—	20	920	—	—	—	750
Chicken Noodle Homestyle as prep	8 oz	70	3	—	—	3	8	—	—	880	—	1	—	750
Chicken Noodle as prep	8 oz	60	2	—	—	3	8	—	—	900	—	—	—	300
Chicken With Rice as prep	8 oz	60	3	—	—	2	7	—	—	790	—	—	—	400
Chili Beef as prep	8 oz	140	5	—	—	5	20	—	20	840	—	2	—	500
Chunky Chicken Nuggets w/ Vegetables & Noodles	10¾ oz	190	6	—	—	11	24	—	40	1060	—	9	—	2500
Clam Chowder Manhattan Style as prep	8 oz	70	2	—	—	2	10	—	20	820	—	5	—	1500
Clam Chowder New England as prep	8 oz	80	3	—	—	3	12	—	20	870	—	1	—	—
Clam Chowder New England as prep w/ whole milk	8 oz	150	7	—	—	7	17	—	100	930	—	2	—	100
Consomme as prep	8 oz	25	0	—	—	4	2	—	—	750	—	—	—	—
Curly Noodle With Chicken as prep	8 oz	80	3	—	—	3	11	—	—	800	—	—	—	750
French Onion as prep	8 oz	60	2	—	—	2	9	—	20	900	—	2	—	—
Green Pea as prep	8 oz	160	3	—	—	8	25	—	—	820	—	—	—	—
Healthy Request Bean With Bacon as prep	8 oz	140	4	—	5	6	22	—	60	470	500	—	—	500
Healthy Request Chicken Noodle as prep	8 oz	60	2	—	15	3	8	—	—	460	270	—	—	300
Healthy Request Chicken With Rice as prep	8 oz	60	3	—	10	2	7	—	—	480	180	—	—	400
Healthy Request Cream Of Mushroom as prep	8 oz	60	2	—	<5	1	9	—	—	460	440	—	—	300
Healthy Request Cream Of Chicken	8 oz	70	2	—	10	2	11	—	0	490	310	—	—	400
Healthy Request Hearty Chicken Vegetable	8 oz	120	2	—	20	7	16	—	—	460	430	1	—	500
Healthy Request Ready-To-Serve Chicken Broth	8 oz	10	0	—	0	1	1	—	—	400	50	9	—	—

FOOD	PORTION	CALORIES	FAT	SAT FAT	CHOL	PROTEIN	CARBO	FIBER	CALCIUM	SOD	POTAS	VIT C	FOLIC	VIT A
CAMPBELL (CONT.)														
Healthy Request Ready-To-Serve Hearty Minestrone	8 oz	90	3	—	<2	4	13	—	40	430	540	—	—	4500
Healthy Request Ready-To-Serve Hearty Chicken Noodle	8 oz	80	2	—	25	9	7	—	20	470	400	—	—	2250
Healthy Request Ready-To-Serve Hearty Chicken Rice	8 oz	110	2	—	20	7	15	—	—	400	360	—	—	500
Healthy Request Ready-To-Serve Hearty Vegetable	8 oz	110	3	—	0	3	17	—	40	480	550	—	—	5500
Healthy Request Ready-To-Serve Hearty Vegetable Beef	8 oz	120	3	—	15	9	15	—	20	490	620	—	—	2500
Healthy Request Tomato as prep	8 oz	90	2	—	0	1	17	—	—	430	220	27	—	400
Healthy Request Tomato as prep w/ skim milk	8 oz	130	2	—	<5	5	22	—	150	490	400	27	—	750
Healthy Request Vegetable as prep	8 oz	90	2	—	<5	3	14	—	20	500	410	2	—	2000
Healthy Request Vegetable Beef as prep	8 oz	70	2	—	5	5	9	—	20	490	360	—	—	750
Home Cookin' Bean & Ham	10¾ oz	210	4	—	—	14	29	—	60	1000	—	—	—	1500
Home Cookin' Beef With Vegetables & Pasta	10¾ oz	140	2	—	—	12	18	—	20	1060	—	4	—	200
Home Cookin' Chicken Minestrone	10¾ oz	180	6	—	—	15	17	—	60	950	—	2	—	2000
Home Cookin' Chicken Gumbo With Sausages	10¾ oz	140	4	—	—	11	15	—	60	1090	—	—	—	3000
Home Cookin' Chicken Rice	10¾ oz	150	6	—	—	14	10	—	20	1090	—	—	—	1500
Home Cookin' Chicken With Noodles	10¾ oz	140	4	—	—	13	12	—	20	1150	—	—	—	3500
Home Cookin' Country Vegetable	10¾ oz	120	2	—	—	4	20	—	60	1070	—	4	—	4500
Home Cookin' Garden Tomato	10¾ oz	150	3	—	—	2	29	—	80	930	—	12	—	2750

FOOD	PORTION	CALORIES	FAT	SAT FAT	CHOL	PROTEIN	CARBO	FIBER	CALCIUM	SOD	POTAS	VIT C	FOLIC	VIT A
CAMPBELL (CONT.)														
Home Cookin' Hearty Lentil	10¾ oz	170	2	—	—	11	28	—	60	930	—	4	—	4000
Home Cookin' Minestrone	10¾ oz	140	3	—	—	4	22	—	80	1220	—	5	—	4500
Home Cookin' Split Pea With Ham	10¾ oz	230	1	—	—	16	38	—	40	1310	—	6	—	2500
Home Cookin' Vegetable Beef	10¾ oz	140	3	—	—	13	17	—	40	1160	—	9	—	5000
Minestrone as prep	8 oz	80	2	—	—	3	13	—	20	900	—	4	—	2250
Mushroom Cream Of as prep	8 oz	100	7	—	—	2	8	—	20	820	—	—	—	—
Mushroom Golden as prep	8 oz	70	3	—	—	2	9	—	—	870	—	—	—	750
Nacho Cheese as prep	8 oz	110	8	—	—	4	8	—	40	740	—	6	—	1250
Nacho Cheese as prep w/ milk	8 oz	180	12	—	—	8	13	—	200	800	—	6	—	1500
Noodles & Ground Beef as prep	8 oz	90	4	—	—	4	10	—	—	820	—	—	—	750
Onion Cream Of as prep	8 oz	100	5	—	—	2	12	—	20	830	—	—	—	300
Onion Cream Of as prep w/ whole milk & water	8 oz	140	7	—	—	4	15	—	80	860	—	—	—	400
Oyster Stew as prep	8 oz	70	5	—	—	2	5	—	—	840	—	5	—	—
Oyster Stew as prep w/ whole milk	8 oz	140	9	—	—	6	10	—	100	890	—	6	—	100
Pepper Pot as prep	8 oz	90	4	—	—	5	9	—	20	970	—	—	—	1000
Potato Cream Of as prep	8 oz	80	3	—	—	1	12	—	—	870	—	—	—	200
Potato Cream Of as prep w/ whole milk & water	8 oz	120	4	—	—	3	15	—	80	900	—	—	—	200
Ready-To-Serve Chunky Chili Beef	11 oz	290	7	—	—	21	37	—	60	1120	—	6	—	1250
Ready-To-Serve Chunky Mediterranean Vegetable	9½ oz	170	6	—	—	4	24	—	60	1010	—	6	—	5500
Ready-To-Serve Chunky Minestrone	9½ oz	160	4	—	—	6	24	—	80	870	—	6	—	4500
Ready-To-Serve Chunky Beef	10¾ oz	200	5	—	—	15	24	—	20	1100	—	6	—	5000
Ready-To-Serve Chunky Beef Stroganoff	10¾ oz	320	16	—	—	15	28	—	60	1230	—	—	—	2500

FOOD	PORTION	CALORIES	FAT	SAT FAT	CHOL	PROTEIN	CARBO	FIBER	CALCIUM	SOD	POTAS	VIT C	FOLIC	VIT A
CAMPBELL (CONT.)														
Ready-To-Serve Chunky Chicken Corn Chowder	10¾ oz	340	21	—	—	14	23	—	20	1200	—	—	—	2250
Ready-To-Serve Chunky Chicken Noodle	10¾ oz	200	7	—	—	14	20	—	20	1140	—	—	—	1000
Ready-To-Serve Chunky Chicken Vegetable	9½ oz	170	6	—	—	10	19	—	20	1080	—	5	—	6500
Ready-To-Serve Chunky Chicken With Rice	9½ oz	140	4	—	—	10	16	—	40	1060	—	4	—	6000
Ready-To-Serve Chunky Creamy Chicken Mushroom	10½ oz	270	19	—	—	12	13	—	20	1280	—	—	—	1000
Ready-To-Serve Chunky Creole Style	10¾ oz	240	8	—	—	11	31	—	60	910	—	—	—	300
Ready-To-Serve Chunky Ham 'n Butter Bean	10¾ oz	280	10	—	—	12	34	—	40	1180	—	6	—	3000
Ready-To-Serve Chunky Manhattan Style Clam Chowder	10¾ oz	160	4	—	—	7	24	—	60	1110	—	12	—	5500
Ready-To-Serve Chunky New England Clam Chowder	10¾ oz	290	17	—	—	9	26	—	60	1200	—	—	—	—
Ready-To-Serve Chunky Old Fashioned Chicken	10¾ oz	180	5	—	—	12	21	—	40	1220	—	6	—	6000
Ready-To-Serve Chunky Old Fashioned Vegetable Beef	10¾ oz	190	6	—	—	13	20	—	40	1100	—	6	—	5500
Ready-To-Serve Chunky Old Fashioned Bean w/ Ham	11 oz	290	9	—	—	14	38	—	100	1110	—	6	—	4500
Ready-To-Serve Chunky Pepper Steak	10¾ oz	180	3	—	—	14	24	—	20	1050	—	9	—	2500
Ready-To-Serve Chunky Sirloin Burger	10¾ oz	220	9	—	—	12	23	—	40	1240	—	6	—	4500
Ready-To-Serve Chunky Split Pea w/ Ham	10¾ oz	230	6	—	—	12	33	—	20	1080	—	6	—	3500

FOOD	PORTION	CALORIES	FAT	SAT FAT	CHOL	PROTEIN	CARBO	FIBER	CALCIUM	SOD	POTAS	VIT C	FOLIC	VIT A
CAMPBELL (CONT.)														
Ready-To-Serve Chunky Steak & Potato	10¾ oz	200	5	—	—	14	24	—	20	1140	—	5	—	—
Ready-To-Serve Chunky Turkey Vegetable	9⅜ oz	150	6	—	—	9	16	—	40	1060	—	6	—	6500
Ready-To-Serve Low Sodium Chicken Vegetable Beef	10¾ oz	180	5	—	—	14	19	—	40	90	—	9	—	5000
Ready-To-Serve Low Sodium Chicken Broth	10½ oz	30	1	—	—	3	2	—	20	85	—	—	—	—
Ready-To-Serve Low Sodium Chicken With Noodles	10¾ oz	170	5	—	—	13	17	—	20	90	—	2	—	1750
Ready-To-Serve Low Sodium Mushroom Cream Of	10½ oz	210	14	—	—	3	18	—	60	55	—	—	—	—
Ready-To-Serve Low Sodium Split Pea	10¾ oz	230	4	—	—	12	37	—	40	30	—	5	—	1500
Ready-To-Serve Low Sodium Tomato With Tomato Pieces	10½ oz	190	6	—	—	4	30	—	40	45	—	35	—	1500
Scotch Broth as prep	8 oz	80	3	—	—	4	9	—	—	870	—	—	—	2250
Shrimp Cream Of as prep	8 oz	90	6	—	—	2	8	—	—	810	—	—	—	—
Shrimp Cream Of as prep w/ whole milk	8 oz	160	10	—	—	5	13	—	150	860	—	1	—	200
Split Pea With Bacon as prep	8 oz	160	4	—	—	9	24	—	—	780	—	—	—	400
Teddy Bear as prep	8 oz	70	2	—	—	3	11	—	—	790	—	—	—	750
Tomato as prep	8 oz	90	2	—	—	1	17	—	—	680	—	27	—	500
Tomato as prep w/ 2% milk	8 oz	150	4	—	—	5	22	—	150	740	—	27	—	750
Tomato Bisque as prep	8 oz	120	3	—	—	2	22	—	40	820	—	18	—	500
Tomato Homestyle Cream Of as prep	8 oz	110	3	—	—	1	20	—	—	810	—	24	—	500
Tomato Homestyle Cream Of as prep w/ whole milk	8 oz	180	7	—	—	5	25	—	100	860	—	24	—	750

FOOD	PORTION	CALORIES	FAT	SAT FAT	CHOL	PROTEIN	CARBO	FIBER	CALCIUM	SOD	POTAS	VIT C	FOLIC	VIT A
CAMPBELL (CONT.)														
Tomato Rice Old Fashioned as prep	8 oz	110	2	—	—	1	22	—	—	730	—	12	—	400
Tomato Zesty as prep	8 oz	100	2	—	—	1	20	—	20	760	—	18	—	1250
Turkey Vegetable as prep	8 oz	70	3	—	—	2	8	—	—	710	—	—	—	2500
Turkey Noodle as prep	8 oz	70	2	—	—	3	9	—	—	880	—	—	—	500
Vegetable Homestyle as prep	8 oz	60	2	—	—	2	9	—	20	880	—	4	—	2250
Vegetable as prep	8 oz	90	2	—	—	3	14	—	20	830	—	4	—	2000
Vegetable Beef as prep	8 oz	70	2	—	—	4	10	—	—	780	—	2	—	2000
Vegetable Old Fashioned as prep	8 oz	60	2	—	—	2	9	—	—	880	—	1	—	2500
Vegetarian Vegetable as prep	8 oz	80	2	—	—	2	13	—	—	790	—	4	—	2000
Won Ton as prep	8 oz	40	1	—	—	2	5	—	—	850	—	—	—	—
COLLEGE INN														
Beef Broth	½ can (7 oz)	16	0	0	0	3	1	—	—	960	25	—	—	—
Chicken Broth	½ can (7 oz)	35	3	1	5	1	0	0	—	990	25	—	—	100
Chicken Broth Lower Salt	½ can (7 oz)	20	2	1	5	1	0	0	—	550	25	—	—	100
GORTON'S														
New England Clam Chowder as prep w/ whole milk	¼ can	140	5	—	15	7	17	—	150	740	—	—	—	100
GOYA														
Black Bean	7.5 oz	160	4	—	0	11	29	9	67	720	690	2	—	<100
HAIN														
Chicken Broth	8.75 fl oz	70	6	—	5	2	0	—	—	870	190	—	—	200
Chicken Broth No Salt Added	8.75 fl oz	60	5	—	5	3	0	—	—	75	150	—	—	500
Chicken Noodle	9.5 fl oz	120	4	—	20	9	11	—	20	980	190	—	—	750
Chicken Noodle No Salt Added	9.5 fl oz	120	4	—	25	9	12	—	—	90	170	—	—	1250
Creamy Mushroom	9.25 fl oz	110	4	—	15	4	16	—	20	740	230	—	—	1250
Italian Vegetable Pasta	9.5 fl oz	160	5	—	20	4	25	—	40	910	490	1	—	1250
Italian Vegetable Pasta Low Sodium	9.5 fl oz	140	6	—	20	4	22	—	40	90	310	4	—	1000
Minestrone	9.5 fl oz	170	2	—	0	8	27	—	60	1060	450	4	—	3000
Minestrone No Salt Added	9.5 fl oz	160	4	—	0	7	28	—	60	35	390	2	—	3000
Mushroom Barley	9.5 fl oz	100	2	—	10	4	17	—	20	600	180	—	—	1250
New England Clam Chowder	9.5 fl oz	180	4	—	25	8	26	—	20	780	350	9	—	1000

FOOD	PORTION	CALORIES	FAT	SAT FAT	CHOL	PROTEIN	CARBO	FIBER	CALCIUM	SOD	POTAS	VIT C	FOLIC	VIT A
HAIN (CONT.)														
Split Pea	9.5 fl oz	170	1	—	0	11	28	—	20	970	450	2	—	2250
Split Pea No Salt Added	9.5 fl oz	170	1	—	0	11	29	—	40	40	400	2	—	2500
Turkey Rice	9.5 fl oz	100	3	—	20	8	10	—	—	970	160	—	—	1000
Turkey Rice No Salt Added	9.5 fl oz	120	4	—	15	7	13	—	—	85	160	—	—	2000
Vegetable Chicken	9.5 fl oz	120	4	—	15	8	14	—	40	930	400	2	—	4500
Vegetable Chicken No Salt Added	9.5 fl oz	130	4	—	20	8	14	—	40	100	400	1	—	3000
Vegetable Broth	9.5 fl oz	45	0	—	0	1	10	—	—	1180	180	—	—	500
Vegetable Broth Low Sodium	9.5 fl oz	40	tr	—	0	1	8	—	—	85	120	—	—	400
Vegetable Split Pea	9.5 fl oz	170	1	—	0	11	28	—	20	970	450	1	—	2250
Vegetable Split Pea No Salt Added	9.5 fl oz	170	1	—	0	13	27	—	40	70	370	—	—	1250
Vegetarian Lentil	9.5 fl oz	160	3	—	5	9	25	—	40	690	500	1	—	1500
Vegetarian Lentil No Salt Added	9.5 fl oz	160	3	—	5	9	24	—	40	65	480	—	—	1250
Vegetarian Vegetable	9.5 fl oz	140	4	—	0	4	22	—	40	920	350	4	—	7500
Vegetarian Vegetable No Salt Added	9.5 fl oz	150	5	—	0	5	23	—	40	45	390	4	—	6000
HEALTH VALLEY														
Beef Broth	7.5 oz	10	tr	—	1	1	2	0	3	420	80	0	4	1
Beef Broth No Salt Added	7.5 oz	10	tr	—	1	1	2	0	3	5	80	0	4	1
Black Bean	7.5 oz	150	2	—	0	7	24	16	57	280	310	2	991	5112
Black Bean No Salt Added	7.5 oz	150	2	—	0	7	24	16	57	20	310	2	991	5112
Chicken Broth	7.5 oz	35	2	—	2	4	1	0	7	410	120	tr	3	tr
Chicken Broth No Salt Added	7.5 oz	35	2	—	2	4	1	0	7	0	120	tr	3	tr
Chunky Chicken Vegetable	7.5 oz	125	2	—	12	7	20	4	36	290	383	1	16	3283
Chunky Five Bean Vegetable	7.5 oz	110	2	—	0	4	21	11	43	290	300	3	16	5000
Chunky Five Bean Vegetable No Salt Added	7.5 oz	110	2	—	0	4	21	11	43	60	300	3	16	5000
Chunky Vegetable Chicken No Salt Added	7.5 oz	125	2	—	12	7	20	4	36	60	383	1	16	3283
Green Split Pea	7.5 oz	180	tr	—	0	11	34	15	53	290	400	1	60	5122
Green Split Pea No Salt Added	7.5 oz	180	tr	—	0	11	34	15	53	25	400	1	60	5122
Lentil	7.5 oz	220	4	—	0	13	33	10	78	290	360	1	16	5132

FOOD	PORTION	CALORIES	FAT	SAT FAT	CHOL	PROTEIN	CARBO	FIBER	CALCIUM	SOD	POTAS	VIT C	FOLIC	VIT A
HEALTH VALLEY (CONT.)														
Lentil No Salt Added	7.5 oz	220	4	—	0	13	4	10	78	25	360	1	16	5132
Manhattan Clam Chowder	7.5 oz	110	2	—	15	6	15	2	53	290	290	3	16	5106
Manhattan Clam Chowder No Salt Added	7.5 oz	110	2	—	15	6	15	2	53	60	590	3	16	5106
Minestrone	7.5 oz	130	3	—	0	6	19	13	53	290	260	1	tr	5010
Minestrone No Salt Added	7.5 oz	130	3	—	0	6	19	13	53	90	260	1	tr	5010
Mushroom Barley	7.5 oz	100	2	—	0	5	2	9	21	290	330	3	37	5325
Mushroom Barley No Salt Added	7.5 oz	100	2	—	0	5	16	9	21	20	330	3	37	5325
Potato Leek	7.5 oz	130	2	—	0	4	23	7	38	290	280	tr	8	4985
Potato Leek No Salt Added	7.5 oz	130	2	—	0	4	23	7	38	20	280	tr	8	4985
Tomato	7.5 oz	130	3	—	0	3	21	1	26	290	660	21	7	4952
Tomato No Salt Added	7.5 oz	130	3	—	0	3	21	1	26	40	660	21	7	4952
Vegetable	7.5 oz	110	1	—	0	4	20	8	33	300	300	3	38	5000
Vegetable No Salt Added	7.5 oz	110	1	—	0	4	20	8	33	40	300	3	38	5000
HEALTHY CHOICE														
Bean & Ham	1 cup (8.7 oz)	184	—	1	5	10	34	10	94	465	393	3	—	—
Beef & Potato	1 cup (8.5 oz)	119	2	1	8	9	18	3	21	635	372	5	—	176
Chicken Corn Chowder	1 cup (8.8 oz)	176	3	1	8	8	30	2	23	466	—	9	—	140
Chicken Pasta	1 cup (8.6 oz)	118	3	1	6	7	18	1	37	493	—	3	—	191
Chicken With Rice	1 cup (8.4 oz)	108	3	1	6	7	15	1	23	426	—	6	—	253
Chili Beef	1 cup (9.1 oz)	166	1	1	10	14	30	5	84	384	—	10	—	201
Clam Chowder	1 cup (8.8 oz)	123	1	1	12	6	23	2	32	481	—	2	—	0
Country Vegetable	1 cup (8.6 oz)	104	1	tr	tr	4	23	2	45	431	—	8	—	530
Cream Of Mushroom	1 cup (8.8 oz)	77	1	tr	tr	4	14	1	36	450	—	1	—	0
Cream Of Chicken With Mushrooms	1 cup (8.9 oz)	127	2	1	8	7	20	1	37	421	—	1	—	14
Cream Of Chicken With Vegetables	1 cup (8.9 oz)	127	2	1	10	7	21	1	36	384	—	1	—	99
Garden Vegetable	1 cup (8.6 oz)	118	1	tr	tr	5	26	3	43	405	—	8	—	600
Hearty Chicken	1 cup (8.7 oz)	132	3	1	19	8	20	1	40	461	—	11	—	540
Lentil	1 cup (8.7 oz)	146	1	tr	2	9	28	5	47	419	—	11	—	605
Minestrone	1 cup (8.6 oz)	112	1	tr	2	6	23	3	76	392	—	8	—	600
Old Fashion Chicken Noodle	1 cup (8.8 oz)	137	3	1	9	9	19	1	32	402	—	11	—	264
Split Pea & Ham	1 cup (8.8 oz)	155	2	1	9	11	26	2	43	399	—	6	—	361
Tomato Garden	1 cup (8.6 oz)	106	2	1	1	5	21	3	83	424	—	7	—	555

FOOD	PORTION	CALORIES	FAT	SAT FAT	CHOL	PROTEIN	CARBO	FIBER	CALCIUM	SOD	POTAS	VIT C	FOLIC	VIT A
HEALTHY CHOICE (CONT.)														
Turkey With Wild Rice	1 cup (8.4 oz)	92	2	1	2	6	13	1	30	355	—	8	—	253
Vegetable Beef	1 cup (8.8 oz)	130	1	tr	3	11	22	2	42	422	—	11	—	280
HERB-OX														
Beef Liquid	2 tsp (0.4 oz)	20	0	0	0	2	2	0	0	570	—	0	—	0
Chicken Liquid	2 tsp (0.4 oz)	15	0	0	0	1	1	0	0	620	—	0	—	0
OLD EL PASO														
Black Bean With Bacon	1 cup (8.6 oz)	160	2	1	5	11	26	7	60	960	—	0	—	0
Chicken Vegetable	1 cup (8.4 oz)	110	3	1	15	9	13	0	60	620	—	5	—	3000
Chicken With Rice	1 cup (8.4 oz)	90	3	1	15	8	10	0	40	680	—	16	—	3500
Garden Vegetable	1 cup (8.4 oz)	110	3	1	<5	5	17	0	60	710	—	5	—	3500
Hearty Beef	1 cup (8.4 oz)	120	3	2	25	10	14	0	40	690	—	9	—	2000
Hearty Chicken Noodle	1 cup (8.4 oz)	110	3	1	25	9	10	0	40	720	—	5	—	3500
PRITIKIN														
Chicken & Rice	1 cup (8.8 oz)	80	1	0	5	—	13	—	—	250	280	—	—	—
Chicken Broth	1 cup (8.5 oz)	15	0	0	0	—	1	—	—	290	60	—	—	—
Chicken Pasta	1 cup (8.6 oz)	100	1	0	5	—	18	—	—	290	160	—	—	—
Hearty Vegetable	1 cup (8.8 oz)	90	1	0	0	—	20	—	—	290	340	—	—	—
Lentil	1 cup (8.4 oz)	130	1	0	0	—	24	—	—	280	490	—	—	—
Minestrone	1 cup (8.8 oz)	90	1	0	0	—	19	—	—	290	330	—	—	—
Split Pea	1 cup (9.2 oz)	140	1	0	0	—	29	—	—	290	530	—	—	—
Three Bean Chili	½ cup (4.5 oz)	90	1	0	0	—	19	—	—	170	600	—	—	—
Vegetable Broth	1 cup (8.3 oz)	20	0	0	0	—	3	—	—	250	70	—	—	—
Vegetarian Vegetables	1 cup (9 oz)	100	0	0	0	—	23	—	—	290	290	—	—	—
PROGRESSO														
Bean And Ham	1 cup (8.4 oz)	160	2	1	10	10	25	8	80	870	—	0	—	1500
Beef	1 can (10.5 fl oz)	180	6	—	35	15	17	—	40	840	330	4	—	1250
Beef Barley	1 cup (8.5 oz)	130	4	2	25	10	13	3	40	780	—	0	—	1500
Beef Minestrone	1 cup (8.5 oz)	140	4	2	25	12	14	3	40	850	—	2	—	2000
Beef Noodle	1 cup (8.5 oz)	140	4	2	30	13	15	1	20	950	—	0	—	750
Beef Vegetable & Rotini	1 cup (8 oz)	120	4	2	20	11	10	3	20	830	—	2	—	1250
Broccoli & Shells	1 cup (8.5 oz)	70	1	0	<5	3	14	3	40	720	—	6	—	3000
Chickarina	1 cup (8.3 oz)	120	5	2	20	8	10	1	20	710	—	0	—	400
Chicken Minestrone	1 cup (8.4 oz)	120	4	1	20	10	12	2	40	790	—	0	—	2500
Chicken Vegetables & Penne	1 cup (8.4 oz)	100	3	1	10	7	11	3	20	780	—	4	—	2000
Chicken & Wild Rice	1 cup (8.4 oz)	100	2	1	20	6	15	2	20	820	—	0	—	1500
Chicken Barley	1 cup (8.5 oz)	110	3	1	15	10	14	3	20	720	—	0	—	1750

FOOD	PORTION	CALORIES	FAT	SAT FAT	CHOL	PROTEIN	CARBO	FIBER	CALCIUM	SOD	POTAS	VIT C	FOLIC	VIT A
PROGRESSO (CONT.)														
Chicken Broth	1 cup ((8.2 oz)	20	1	—	5	2	1	0	0	860	—	0	—	0
Chicken Noodle	1 can (10.5 oz)	110	3	1	25	11	10	1	20	910	—	0	—	4000
Chicken Noodle	1 cup (8.4 oz)	80	2	1	20	9	8	1	20	730	—	0	—	3000
Chicken Rice Vegetable	1 can (10.5 oz)	130	4	1	20	9	15	tr	40	940	—	0	—	1500
Chicken Rice Vegetable	1 cup (8.4 oz)	110	3	1	15	7	12	tr	20	750	—	0	—	1250
Clam & Rotini Chowder	1 cup (8.8 oz)	200	9	2	10	7	21	0	80	800	—	0	—	0
Corn Chowder	1 cup (8.6 oz)	180	10	4	10	5	20	2	0	780	—	6	—	300
Cream Of Chicken	1 cup (8.4 oz)	170	10	4	35	8	11	0	20	880	—	0	—	300
Cream Of Mushroom	1 cup (8.4 oz)	140	8	4	20	3	12	1	20	920	—	0	—	0
Creamy Tortellini	1 cup (8.4 oz)	210	15	8	30	5	15	0	150	830	—	0	—	1000
Escarole In Chicken Broth	1 cup (8.1 oz)	25	1	0	<5	2	2	0	20	980	—	0	—	750
Green Split Pea	1 cup (8.6 oz)	170	3	1	5	10	25	5	0	870	—	0	—	100
Healthy Classics Beef Barley	1 cup (8.5 oz)	140	2	1	20	11	20	3	20	490	—	4	—	2250
Healthy Classics Beef Vegetable	1 cup (8.5 oz)	150	2	1	15	10	25	6	0	410	—	5	—	2000
Healthy Classics Chicken Noodle	1 cup (8.3 oz)	80	2	1	20	7	10	1	0	480	—	0	—	3000
Healthy Classics Chicken Rice With Vegetables	1 cup (8.4 oz)	90	2	0	10	7	12	1	20	450	—	0	—	1750
Healthy Classics Cream Of Broccoli	1 cup (8.6 oz)	90	3	1	<5	2	13	2	40	580	—	6	—	300
Healthy Classics Garlic & Pasta	1 cup (8.5 oz)	100	2	0	<5	4	18	3	60	450	—	0	—	3000
Healthy Classics Lentil	1 cup (8.5 oz)	120	3	0	0	5	20	1	40	510	—	0	—	1250
Healthy Classics Minestrone	1 cup (8.5 oz)	120	3	0	0	5	20	1	40	510	—	0	—	1250
Healthy Classics New England Clam Chowder	1 cup (8.6 oz)	120	2	1	5	5	20	1	0	530	—	5	—	200
Healthy Classics Split Pea	1 cup (8.9 oz)	180	3	1	<5	10	30	5	40	420	—	0	—	1750
Healthy Classics Tomato Garden Vegetable	1 cup (8.6 oz)	100	1	0	0	3	19	4	60	480	—	5	—	1250
Healthy Classics Vegetable	1 cup (8.4 oz)	80	2	0	5	4	13	1	40	470	—	1	—	3000
Hearty Minestrone With Shells	1 cup (8.4 oz)	120	2	0	0	5	20	4	20	700	—	5	—	2000

FOOD	PORTION	CALORIES	FAT	SAT FAT	CHOL	PROTEIN	CARBO	FIBER	CALCIUM	SOD	POTAS	VIT C	FOLIC	VIT A
PROGRESSO (CONT.)														
Hearty Black Bean	1 cup (8.5 oz)	170	2	0	<5	8	30	10	60	730	—	0	—	200
Hearty Chicken	1 can (10.5 fl oz)	120	3	1	25	13	10	0	20	1070	—	4	—	2500
Hearty Chicken & Rotini	1 cup (8.4 oz)	90	2	1	20	10	8	0	0	860	—	4	—	2250
Hearty Penne In Chicken Broth	1 cup (8.4 oz)	70	1	0	<5	5	12	0	0	930	—	0	—	1750
Hearty Tomato & Rotini	1 cup (8.4 oz)	90	1	0	5	4	16	3	60	820	—	4	—	500
Hearty Vegetable With Rotini	1 cup (8.4 oz)	110	1	0	0	4	20	3	40	720	—	0	—	3000
Homestyle Chicken Vegetable	1 cup (8.4 oz)	100	3	1	15	9	10	1	0	680	—	0	—	1750
Lentil	1 can (10.5 fl oz)	170	3	0	0	11	27	8	60	930	—	0	—	1000
Lentil	1 cup (8.5 oz)	140	2	0	0	9	22	7	40	750	—	0	—	750
Lentil & Shells	1 cup (8.5 oz)	130	2	0	0	7	22	4	20	840	—	0	—	200
Lentil With Sausage	1 cup (8.5 oz)	170	7	2	15	8	19	5	20	780	—	4	—	2000
Macaroni & Bean	1 cup (8.6 oz)	160	4	1	<5	7	23	6	40	800	—	0	—	200
Manhattan Clam Chowder	1 cup (8.4 oz)	110	2	0	10	12	11	3	40	710	—	4	—	2250
Meatballs & Pasta Pearls	1 cup (8.3 oz)	140	7	3	15	7	13	0	40	700	—	0	—	750
Minestrone	1 can (10.5 fl oz)	170	4	1	0	7	27	6	80	1190	—	0	—	2500
Minestrone	1 cup (8.4 oz)	130	3	1	0	5	22	5	60	960	—	0	—	2000
New England Clam Chowder	1 can (10.5 fl oz)	220	12	4	20	7	21	2	60	1050	—	9	—	0
New England Clam Chowder	1 cup (8.4 oz)	180	10	3	15	6	17	2	40	850	—	9	—	0
Spicy Chicken & Penne	1 cup (8.5 oz)	120	4	1	20	8	13	0	20	680	—	0	—	2000
Split Pea With Ham	1 cup (8.5 oz)	160	4	2	15	9	20	5	40	830	—	2	—	1250
Tomato	1 cup (8.5 oz)	90	2	0	0	3	15	4	20	990	—	1	—	1500
Tomato Tortellini	1 cup (8.4 oz)	120	5	2	10	5	13	2	60	910	—	1	—	1500
Tomato Beef & Rotini	1 cup (8.5 oz)	140	5	2	25	11	15	2	40	750	—	0	—	200
Tortellini In Chicken Broth	1 cup (8.3 oz)	80	2	1	5	4	10	2	40	750	—	0	—	3000
Vegetable	1 cup (8.4 oz)	90	2	1	<5	4	15	3	40	850	—	1	—	3500
Zesty Minestrone	1 cup (8.3 oz)	150	6	3	10	6	17	4	60	790	—	1	—	1750
SNOW'S														
Manhattan Clam Chowder as prep w/ water	7.5 fl oz	70	2	—	—	3	9	—	40	630	210	1	—	2000

FOOD	PORTION	CALORIES	FAT	SAT FAT	CHOL	PROTEIN	CARBO	FIBER	CALCIUM	SOD	POTAS	VIT C	FOLIC	VIT A
SNOW'S (CONT.)														
New England Clam Chowder as prep w/ milk	7.5 fl oz	140	6	—	—	8	13	—	150	670	280	—	—	100
New England Corn Chowder as prep w/ milk	7.5 fl oz	150	6	—	—	5	18	—	150	640	280	—	—	200
New England Fish Chowder as prep w/ milk	7.5 fl oz	130	6	—	—	9	11	—	150	620	300	—	—	100
New England Seafood Chowder as prep w/ milk	7.5 fl oz	130	6	—	—	8	11	—	150	690	280	—	—	100
SWANSON														
Beef Broth	7¼ oz	18	1	—	—	2	1	—	—	750	—	—	—	—
Chicken Broth	7.25 oz	30	2	—	—	2	2	—	—	900	—	—	—	—
Natural Goodness Clear Chicken Broth	7¼ oz	20	1	—	—	2	1	—	—	580	—	—	—	—
Vegetable Broth	7.25 fl oz	20	1	—	—	0	3	—	—	920	—	—	—	300
WEIGHT WATCHERS														
Chicken & Rice	1 can (10.5 oz)	110	2	0	10	6	17	4	60	720	—	0	—	1000
Chicken Noodle	1 can (10.5 oz)	150	2	1	30	9	25	4	60	740	—	0	—	1000
Minestrone	1 can (10.5 oz)	130	2	1	5	5	23	6	100	760	—	1	—	3000
Vegetable	1 can (10.5 oz)	130	1	0	0	4	27	6	80	680	—	2	—	3500
FROZEN														
TABATCHNICK														
Barley Mushroom	1 serv (7.5 oz)	70	0	0	0	2	13	3	40	540	—	2	—	2500
Barley Mushroom No Salt Added	1 serv (7.5 oz)	70	0	0	0	2	13	3	40	98	—	2	—	500
Broccoli Cream Of	1 serv (7.5 oz)	90	4	2	5	3	12	3	100	740	—	2	—	8000
Cabbage	1 serv (7.5 oz)	60	0	0	0	1	14	2	80	160	—	2	—	2500
Chicken With Dumplings	1 serv (7.5 oz)	70	2	0	20	1	13	1	40	830	—	0	—	0
Corn Chowder	1 serv (7.5 oz)	150	6	2	5	3	22	1	60	650	—	2	—	0
Minestrone	1 serv (7.5 oz)	150	1	0	0	9	27	10	100	550	—	6	—	2250
New England Potato	1 serv (7.5 oz)	150	6	3	9	4	21	2	80	540	—	0	—	0
New York Chicken	1 serv (7.5 oz)	35	0	0	0	2	6	0	40	850	—	0	—	200
Old Fashion Potato	1 serv (7.5 oz)	70	0	0	0	2	16	2	20	540	—	0	—	200
Pea	1 serv (7.5 oz)	180	2	0	0	12	31	11	40	520	—	2	—	1500
Pea No Salt Added	1 serv (7.5 oz)	180	2	0	0	12	31	11	40	79	—	2	—	1500
Spinach Cream Of	1 serv (7.5 oz)	90	4	2	5	3	11	2	200	630	—	2	—	13500
Vegetable	1 serv (7.5 oz)	110	1	0	0	5	20	4	60	580	—	6	—	5000

FOOD	PORTION	CALORIES	FAT	SAT FAT	CHOL	PROTEIN	CARBO	FIBER	CALCIUM	SOD	POTAS	VIT C	FOLIC	VIT A
TABATCHNICK (CONT.)														
Vegetable No Salt Added	1 serv (7.5 oz)	110	1	0	0	5	20	4	60	77	—	6	—	5000
Wisconsin Cheddar Vegetable	1 serv (7.5 oz)	140	9	3	13	4	12	1	100	930	—	2	—	0
Yankee Bean	1 serv (7.5 oz)	160	2	0	0	10	27	11	80	570	—	0	—	500
MIX														
asparagus cream of as prep w/ water	1 cup	59	2	tr	tr	2	9	—	—	801	—	—	—	—
beef broth cube	1 cube (3.6 g)	6	tr	tr	tr	1	1	—	—	864	15	—	—	—
beef broth cube as prep w/ water	1 cup	8	tr	tr	tr	1	1	—	—	1152	20	—	—	—
celery cream of as prep w/ water	1 cup	63	2	tr	1	3	10	—	—	839	—	—	—	—
chicken broth	1 pkg (0.2 oz)	16	1	tr	1	1	1	—	11	1116	19	tr	—	30
chicken broth as prep w/ water	1 cup	21	1	tr	1	1	1	—	15	1484	25	tr	—	40
chicken broth cube	1 cube (4.8 g)	9	tr	tr	1	1	1	—	—	1152	18	—	—	—
chicken broth cube as prep w/ water	1 cup	13	tr	tr	1	1	2	—	—	792	24	—	—	—
chicken cream of as prep w/ water	1 cup	107	5	3	3	2	13	—	76	1184	215	—	—	—
chicken noodle as prep w/ water	1 cup	53	1	tr	3	3	7	—	32	1284	31	tr	1	63
french onion not prep	1 pkg (1.4 oz)	115	2	1	2	5	21	—	55	3493	260	1	6	8
leek as prep w/ water	1 cup	71	2	1	3	2	11	—	—	966	—	—	—	—
onion as prep w/ water	1 cup	28	1	tr	0	1	5	—	13	848	63	tr	2	2
tomato as prep w/ water	1 cup	102	2	1	1	2	19	—	54	943	295	5	7	832
4C														
Noodle	8 oz	50	2	—	—	2	7	—	—	960	60	—	—	—
Onion Reduced Salt	8 oz	30	1	—	—	1	5	—	60	760	60	1	—	—
ARMOUR														
Bouillon Cubes Beef	1 (4 g)	5	0	0	0	0	1	—	—	920	—	—	—	—
Bouillon Cubes Chicken	1 (4 g)	5	0	0	0	0	1	—	—	910	—	—	—	—
ARROWHEAD														
Bean & Barley	¼ cup (1.9 oz)	170	0	0	0	12	35	7	40	0	610	0	—	0
BEAN CUISINE														
Bean Bouillabisse	1 cup (7.5 fl oz)	174	tr	tr	0	6	18	5	80	5	—	10	—	1650
Island Black Bean	1 cup (8.7 fl oz)	210	4	1	0	9	33	10	150	504	—	27	—	1000

FOOD	PORTION	CALORIES	FAT	SAT FAT	CHOL	PROTEIN	CARBO	FIBER	CALCIUM	SOD	POTAS	VIT C	FOLIC	VIT A
BEAN CUISINE (CONT.)														
Lots of Lentil	1 cup (7.7 oz)	166	tr	tr	0	6	19	6	90	7	—	9	—	150
Mesa Maize	1 cup (9.2 fl oz)	179	tr	tr	0	6	21	6	90	9	—	32	—	250
Rocky Mountain Red Bean	1 cup (8.6 oz)	202	tr	tr	0	7	24	8	130	7	—	17	—	<50
Sante Fe Corn Chowder	1 cup (9.2 oz)	179	tr	tr	0	6	21	6	90	9	—	32	—	250
Thick As Fog Split Pea	1 cup (8.6 fl oz)	189	tr	tr	0	8	21	1	40	13	—	7	—	3150
Ultima Pasta E Fagioli	1 cup (8.6 fl oz)	179	tr	0	0	7	22	4	90	8	—	5	—	2350
White Bean Provencal	1 cup (7.7 fl oz)	166	tr	tr	0	6	19	6	90	7	—	9	—	150
CAMPBELL														
Bean With Bacon 'n Ham Microwave	7½ oz	230	5	—	—	8	38	—	60	830	—	1	—	750
Chicken Noodle Microwave	7½ oz	100	4	—	—	5	11	—	—	870	—	—	—	1250
Chicken Noodle as prep	8 oz	100	2	—	—	5	16	—	20	710	—	—	—	—
Chicken With Rice Microwave	7½ oz	100	4	—	—	3	14	—	—	820	—	—	—	1500
Chili Beef Microwave	7½ oz	190	4	—	—	7	32	—	40	870	—	1	—	1000
Hearty Noodle as prep	8 oz	90	1	—	—	4	15	—	20	840	—	—	—	1000
Noodle as prep	8 oz	110	2	—	—	5	19	—	20	700	—	—	—	—
Onion as prep	8 oz	30	0	—	—	1	7	—	—	700	—	—	—	—
Vegetable as prep	8 oz	40	0	—	—	1	8	—	20	710	—	—	—	500
Vegetable Beef Microwave	7½ oz	100	2	—	—	5	16	—	20	830	—	2	—	1250
CAMPBELL'S CUP														
Beef Noodle	1 (1.35 oz)	130	2	—	—	6	23	—	20	1270	—	1	—	1250
Chicken Noodle	1 (1.35 oz)	140	3	—	—	7	22	—	—	1340	—	1	—	—
Chicken Noodle w/ White Meat as prep	6 oz	90	2	—	—	6	12	—	—	770	—	—	—	—
Creamy Chicken w/ White Meat as prep	6 oz	90	4	—	—	3	12	—	20	1020	—	—	—	—
Hearty Noodles With Vegetables	1 (1.7 oz)	180	2	—	—	7	32	—	20	1320	—	1	—	750
Noodle With Chicken Broth as prep	6 oz	90	2	—	—	4	15	—	20	910	—	—	—	500
CASBAH														
Black Bean	1 pkg (1.7 oz)	170	2	0	0	9	30	9	80	530	—	15	—	1100

FOOD	PORTION	CALORIES	FAT	SAT FAT	CHOL	PROTEIN	CARBO	FIBER	CALCIUM	SOD	POTAS	VIT C	FOLIC	VIT A
CASBAH (CONT.)														
Split Pea	1 pkg (2.3 oz)	230	1	0	0	15	40	10	50	500	—	1	—	450
Sweet Corn Chowder	1 pkg (1.2 oz)	125	1	0	0	4	26	2	20	440	—	15	—	200
Vegetarian Chili	1 pkg (1.8 oz)	170	2	0	0	10	31	7	70	430	—	24	—	2500
CUP-A-RAMEN														
Beef With Vegetables Low Fat as prep	8 oz	220	2	—	—	7	44	—	20	1600	—	1	—	2000
Beef With Vegetables as prep	8 oz	270	10	—	—	6	38	—	20	1530	—	—	—	1000
Chicken With Vegetables Low Fat as prep	8 oz	220	2	—	—	7	44	—	20	1500	—	1	—	2000
Chicken With Vegetables as prep	8 oz	270	10	—	—	6	38	—	20	1470	—	1	—	1000
Oriental With Vegetables Low Fat as prep	8 oz	220	2	—	—	7	44	—	20	1400	—	1	—	2000
Oriental With Vegetables as prep	8 oz	270	10	—	—	6	38	—	20	1210	—	1	—	750
Shrimp With Vegetables Low Fat as prep	8 oz	230	2	—	—	7	45	—	20	1290	—	1	—	1250
Shrimp With Vegetables as prep	8 oz	280	10	—	—	6	40	—	20	1190	—	2	—	1500
CUP-A-SOUP														
Broccoli & Cheese as prep	1 serv (6 oz)	70	3	1	5	2	9	tr	40	550	—	4	—	0
Chicken Vegetable as prep	1 serv (6 oz)	50	1	0	10	1	10	0	0	520	—	0	16	0
Chicken Broth as prep	1 serv (6 oz)	20	0	0	0	1	3	0	0	440	—	0	—	0
Chicken Broth w/ Pasta Fat Free as prep	1 serv (6 oz)	45	0	0	0	2	8	0	0	450	—	0	16	0
Chicken Noodle as prep	1 serv (6 oz)	50	1	0	10	2	8	0	0	540	—	0	16	0
Cream Of Chicken as prep	1 serv (6 oz)	70	2	0	0	1	12	tr	0	640	—	0	—	0
Creamy Chicken Vegetable as prep	1 serv (6 oz)	80	5	2	0	2	10	tr	20	590	—	0	—	200
Creamy Mushroom as prep	1 serv (6 oz)	60	2	0	0	1	10	0	0	610	—	0	—	0
Green Pea as prep	1 serv (6 oz)	80	1	0	0	4	12	3	0	520	—	0	—	0
Hearty Chicken Noodle as prep	1 serv (6 oz)	60	1	0	15	3	10	0	0	590	—	0	16	0
Ring Noodle as prep	1 serv (6 oz)	50	1	0	10	2	9	0	0	560	—	0	16	0

FOOD	PORTION	CALORIES	FAT	SAT FAT	CHOL	PROTEIN	CARBO	FIBER	CALCIUM	SOD	POTAS	VIT C	FOLIC	VIT A
CUP-A-SOUP (CONT.)														
Spring Vegetable as prep	1 serv (6 oz)	45	1	0	10	2	21	tr	0	500	—	0	16	0
Tomato as prep	1 serv (6 oz)	100	1	0	5	2	20	tr	100	510	—	4	—	200
EMES														
Beef Base	1 tsp	18	tr	0	0	3	2	—	7	10	19	—	—	50
Chicken Base	1 tsp	18	tr	0	0	3	2	—	7	10	19	—	—	50
FANTASTIC														
Cha-Cha Chili Low Fat	1 pkg	220	1	0	0	18	37	13	100	470	—	15	—	2000
GOLDEN DIPT														
Lobster Bisque	¼ pkg	30	1	—	2	1	5	—	—	560	—	—	—	—
Manhattan Clam Chowder	¼ pkg	80	2	—	3	2	13	—	—	700	—	5	—	—
New England Clam Chowder	¼ pkg	24	2	—	2	2	12	—	—	680	—	5	—	—
Seafood Chowder	¼ pkg	70	2	—	2	2	12	—	—	730	—	5	—	—
Shrimp Bisque	¼ pkg	30	1	—	2	1	5	—	—	570	—	—	—	—
GOODMAN'S														
Cup Of Soup Beef	1 pkg (1½ cups)	180	3	1	45	7	32	2	0	1640	—	0	—	400
Cup Of Soup Chicken Noodle	1 pkg (1½ cups)	180	3	1	45	7	31	2	0	1360	—	0	—	1000
Cup Of Soup Vegetable	1 pkg (1½ cups)	180	3	1	40	8	32	2	0	1500	—	0	—	1000
Matzo Ball & Soup	1 cup	40	1	0	0	2	9	1	20	1040	—	0	—	0
Matzo Ball & Soup 50% Less Salt	1 serv	50	1	0	0	2	10	1	20	640	—	0	—	0
Noodleman	1 cup	45	1	0	10	2	9	0	0	990	—	0	—	0
Noodleman Low Sodium	1 cup	50	1	0	10	2	9	1	20	95	—	0	—	0
Onion	1 cup	30	1	1	0	1	5	1	0	1280	—	0	—	0
Onion Low Sodium	1 cup	30	1	0	0	1	6	1	0	115	—	0	—	0
HAIN														
Cheese & Broccoli	¾ cup	310	22	—	—	7	19	—	200	980	340	—	—	300
Cheese Savory	¾ cup	250	16	—	—	6	20	—	150	890	310	—	—	—
Savory Lentil	¾ cup	130	2	—	—	4	20	—	40	810	150	2	—	—
Savory Minestrone	¾ cup	110	1	—	—	4	20	—	40	870	240	1	—	200
Savory Mushroom	¾ cup	210	15	—	—	4	11	—	80	710	230	1	—	300
Savory Mushroom No Salt Added	¾ cup	250	20	—	—	5	15	—	100	180	280	1	—	—
Savory Onion	¾ cup	50	2	—	—	2	6	—	20	900	100	2	—	—
Savory Onion No Salt Added	¾ cup	50	1	—	—	1	9	—	20	470	50	2	—	—
Savory Potato Leek	¾ cup	260	18	—	—	4	20	—	—	690	240	1	—	—
Savory Split Pea	¾ cup	310	10	—	—	4	16	—	40	940	200	—	—	200
Savory Tomato	¾ cup	220	14	—	—	3	19	—	80	770	440	6	—	—

FOOD	PORTION	CALORIES	FAT	SAT FAT	CHOL	PROTEIN	CARBO	FIBER	CALCIUM	SOD	POTAS	VIT C	FOLIC	VIT A
HAIN (CONT.)														
Savory Vegetable	¾ cup	80	1	—	—	2	13	—	20	730	180	1	—	200
Savory Vegetable No Salt Added	¾ cup	80	1	—	—	2	13	—	20	330	170	1	—	400
HERB-OX														
Beef Bouillon	1 cube (3.5 g)	5	0	0	0	0	tr	0	0	900	—	0	—	0
Beef Instant Bouillon Powder	1 tsp (4 g)	5	0	0	0	0	tr	0	0	1020	—	0	—	0
Beef Instant Broth & Seasoning Pack	1 pkg (4.5 g)	5	0	0	0	0	tr	0	0	1020	—	0	—	0
Beef Instant Broth & Seasoning Pack Low Sodium	1 pkg (4 g)	10	0	0	0	0	2	0	0	5	—	0	—	0
Chicken Bouillon	1 cube (4 g)	5	0	0	0	0	tr	0	0	1100	—	0	—	0
Chicken Instant Bouillon Powder	1 tsp (4 g)	5	0	0	0	0	tr	0	0	1100	—	0	—	0
Chicken Instant Broth & Seasoning Pack	1 pkg (4 g)	5	0	0	0	0	tr	0	0	1100	—	0	—	0
Chicken Instant Broth & Seasoning Pack Low Sodium	1 pkg (4 g)	10	0	0	0	0	2	0	0	5	—	0	—	0
Vegetable Bouillon	1 cube (4 g)	5	0	0	0	0	tr	0	0	980	—	0	—	0
HODGSON MILL														
13 Bean not prep	1.5 oz	100	1	0	0	9	14	12	40	0	—	0	—	0
HURST														
15 Bean Soup Beef	1 serv (6 oz)	120	1	0	0	8	20	9	40	310	—	0	—	100
15 Bean Soup Cajun	1 serv	120	1	0	0	8	20	9	40	100	—	0	—	100
15 Bean Soup Chicken	1 serv (6 oz)	120	1	0	0	8	20	9	40	250	—	0	—	100
15 Bean Soup Chili	1 serv (6 oz)	120	1	0	0	8	20	9	40	170	—	0	—	100
15 Bean Soup Ham	1 serv	120	1	0	0	8	20	9	40	70	—	0	—	100
HamBeens Great Northern Bean	1 serv	120	1	0	0	7	22	11	60	470	—	1	—	0
HamBeens Navy Bean	1 serv	120	1	0	0	8	21	11	40	470	—	0	—	0
Pasta Fagioli	1 serv	120	1	0	0	8	23	9	40	540	—	0	—	0
Spanish American Pinto Bean	1 serv	120	1	0	0	7	22	6	40	350	—	2	—	0
Spanish-American Black Bean	1 serv	120	1	0	0	7	22	8	40	280	—	0	—	0
KA-ME														
Won Ton Chicken not prep	1 pkg (1.25 oz)	180	11	3	0	4	18	1	0	770	—	—	—	—
Won Ton Pork not prep	1 pkg (1.25 oz)	180	11	3	0	4	18	1	—	770	—	—	—	—

FOOD	PORTION	CALORIES	FAT	SAT FAT	CHOL	PROTEIN	CARBO	FIBER	CALCIUM	SOD	POTAS	VIT C	FOLIC	VIT A
KNORR														
Black Bean Cup-A-Soup as prep	1 pkg	200	1	0	0	11	37	9	0	690	—	9	—	500
Broccoli as prep	8 fl oz	160	8	—	—	6	16	—	200	1050	—	18	—	500
Cauliflower as prep	8 fl oz	100	3	—	—	5	13	—	100	750	—	21	—	—
Chef's Series Wild Mushroom as prep	8 fl oz	100	3	—	—	3	14	—	20	800	—	1	—	—
Chick 'N Pasta as prep	8 fl oz	90	2	—	—	4	16	—	20	850	—	6	—	1250
Chicken Bouillon as prep	8 fl oz	16	1	—	—	tr	tr	—	—	1200	—	—	—	—
Chicken Flavored Noodle as prep	8 fl oz	100	2	—	—	4	18	—	—	710	—	—	—	—
Chicken Noodle Instant as prep	6 fl oz	25	tr	—	5	1	4	—	—	870	—	—	—	—
Fine Herb as prep	8 fl oz	130	6	—	—	4	15	—	80	990	—	1	—	100
Fish Bouillon as prep	8 fl oz	10	tr	—	—	1	tr	—	—	1130	—	—	—	—
French Onion as prep	8 fl oz	50	1	—	—	1	9	—	—	970	—	1	—	—
Hearty Minestrone Cup-A-Soup as prep	1 pkg	150	1	1	2	5	29	1	80	720	—	21	—	1000
Lentil Cup-A-Soup as prep	1 pkg	220	0	0	0	13	40	6	40	900	—	4	—	750
Mushroom as prep	8 fl oz	100	4	—	—	4	12	—	80	870	—	2	—	—
Navy Bean Cup-A-Soup as prep	1 pkg	140	0	0	0	7	27	5	20	870	—	4	—	750
Oriental Hot And Sour as prep	8 fl oz	50	1	—	—	1	9	—	5	670	—	1	—	35
Oxtail Hearty Beef as prep	8 fl oz	70	2	—	—	2	10	—	—	1120	—	12	—	200
Potato Leek Cup-A-Soup as prep	1 pkg	120	0	0	0	4	24	1	150	970	—	2	—	750
Spinach as prep	8 fl oz	100	5	—	—	3	11	—	100	890	—	1	—	400
Spring Vegetable With Herbs as prep	8 fl oz	30	tr	—	—	1	6	—	—	710	—	—	—	—
Tomato Basil as prep	8 fl oz	90	3	—	—	2	14	—	40	940	—	54	—	1250
Tortellini In Brodo as prep	8 fl oz	60	1	—	—	2	11	—	—	820	—	—	—	—
Vegetable Cup-A-Soup as prep	1 pkg	100	0	0	0	3	21	0	40	840	—	12	—	500
Vegetable as prep	8 fl oz	35	1	—	—	1	7	—	40	840	—	12	—	1250
Vegetarian Vegetable Bouillon as prep	8 fl oz	16	1	—	—	tr	1	—	—	990	—	—	—	—

FOOD	PORTION	CALORIES	FAT	SAT FAT	CHOL	PROTEIN	CARBO	FIBER	CALCIUM	SOD	POTAS	VIT C	FOLIC	VIT A
KOJEL														
Hearty Potato With Vegetables Instant	1 serv (6 fl oz)	60	0	0	0	1	15	2	20	650	—	12	—	150
Noodle Soup Chicken Flavor Instant	1 serv (6 fl oz)	70	1	0	0	4	11	2	80	590	—	0	—	500
Split Pea Instant	1 serv (6 fl oz)	60	tr	0	0	3	14	3	20	380	110	0	—	375
Tomato Instant	1 serv (6 fl oz)	50	0	0	0	1	15	1	20	540	—	9	—	500
Vegetable Chicken Couscous Instant	1 serv (6 fl oz)	80	1	tr	0	4	18	2	40	530	140	2	—	150
LIPTON														
Chicken Noodle w/ White Chicken Meat as prep	1 cup	80	2	1	15	3	11	0	0	690	—	0	24	0
Extra Noodle w/ Chicken Broth as prep	1 cup	90	2	1	25	3	15	tr	0	680	—	0	32	0
Giggle Noodle w/ Chicken Broth as prep	1 cup	70	2	1	20	2	11	0	0	750	—	0	16	0
Recipe Secrets Beefy Mushroom	1½ tbsp (0.4 oz)	35	0	0	0	1	7	0	0	640	—	0	—	0
Recipe Secrets Beefy Onion	1 tbsp (0.3 oz)	25	1	0	0	1	5	0	0	610	—	0	—	0
Recipe Secrets Fiesta Herb w/ Red Pepper as prep	1 cup	30	0	0	0	1	6	0	0	560	—	0	—	0
Recipe Secrets Golden Herb w/ Lemon as prep	1 cup	35	1	0	0	tr	7	0	0	510	—	0	—	0
Recipe Secrets Golden Onion	1⅔ tbsp (0.5 oz)	50	1	0	0	1	9	0	0	700	—	0	—	0
Recipe Secrets Italian Herb w/ Tomato as prep	1 cup	40	1	0	0	tr	9	0	0	510	—	2	—	100
Recipe Secrets Onion as prep	1 cup	20	0	0	0	0	4	tr	0	610	—	0	—	0
Recipe Secrets Onion Mushroom as prep	1 cup	30	1	0	0	1	5	0	0	640	—	0	—	0
Recipe Secrets Savory Herb With Garlic as prep	1 cup	30	0	0	0	1	6	0	0	480	—	0	—	0
Recipe Secrets Vegetable as prep	1 cup	30	0	0	0	tr	7	1	0	600	—	2	—	200
Ring-O-Noodle w/ Chicken Broth as prep	1 cup	70	2	1	15	2	10	0	0	720	—	0	24	0

FOOD	PORTION	CALORIES	FAT	SAT FAT	CHOL	PROTEIN	CARBO	FIBER	CALCIUM	SOD	POTAS	VIT C	FOLIC	VIT A
LIPTON (CONT.)														
Soup Secrets Chicken 'N Onion as prep	1 cup	120	2	0	5	4	24	1	40	740	—	1	24	0
Soup Secrets Chicken w/ Pasta & Beans as prep	1 cup	110	2	0	5	5	19	3	40	700	—	1	32	500
Soup Secrets Country Chicken w/ Pasta & Herbs as prep	1 cup	100	2	0	5	4	18	1	20	740	—	0	32	0
Soup Secrets Honestyle Lentil w/ Bow Tie Pasta as prep	1 cup	130	1	0	0	7	22	5	0	750	—	0	32	500
Soup Secrets Minestrone as prep	1 cup	110	1	0	0	4	21	4	40	750	—	4	49	500
Spiral Pasta w/ Chicken Broth as prep	1 cup	60	1	0	0	2	11	0	0	660	—	0	24	0
LITE LINE														
Beef Bouillon Instant Low Sodium	1 tsp	12	tr	—	—	tr	2	—	—	5	590	—	—	—
Chicken Bouillon Instant Low Sodium	1 tsp	12	tr	—	—	tr	2	—	—	5	560	—	—	—
MARUCHAN														
Instant Lunch Oriental Noodles Beef	1 pkg (2.25 oz)	290	13	—	1	6	37	—	20	1260	—	—	—	200
Instant Lunch Oriental Noodles Chicken	1 pkg (2.25 oz)	290	13	7	4	6	36	2	40	1270	—	—	—	200
Instant Lunch Oriental Noodles Chicken Mushroom	1 pkg (2.25 oz)	280	13	—	0	6	34	—	—	1380	—	—	—	100
Instant Lunch Oriental Noodles Mushroom	1 pkg (2.25 oz)	290	13	—	0	6	35	—	—	1310	—	—	—	100
Instant Lunch Oriental Noodles Pork	1 pkg (2.25 oz)	290	13	—	0	6	35	—	—	1390	—	—	—	200
Instant Lunch Oriental Noodles Shrimp	1 pkg (2.25 oz)	290	13	—	8	7	37	—	—	1260	—	—	—	200
Instant Lunch Oriental Noodles Toast Onion	1 pkg (2.25 oz)	270	12	—	0	6	34	—	20	1290	—	—	—	0

FOOD	PORTION	CALORIES	FAT	SAT FAT	CHOL	PROTEIN	CARBO	FIBER	CALCIUM	SOD	POTAS	VIT C	FOLIC	VIT A
MARUCHAN (CONT.)														
Instant Lunch Oriental Noodles Vegetable Beef	1 pkg (2.25 oz)	290	12	—	0	6	34	—	20	1340	—	—	—	—
Instant Wonton Chicken	1 pkg (1.49 oz)	200	12	—	5	5	19	—	20	1440	—	—	—	—
Instant Wonton Hot & Sour	1 pkg (1.49 oz)	200	11	—	0	4	21	—	—	1070	—	—	—	100
Instant Wonton Oriental	1 pkg (1.49 oz)	190	12	—	0	5	19	—	20	1340	—	—	—	—
Instant Wonton Pork	1 pkg (1.49 oz)	200	12	—	0	5	19	—	—	1450	—	—	—	—
Instant Wonton Shrimp	1 pkg (1.49 oz)	200	12	—	10	6	19	—	—	1120	—	—	—	—
Oriental Noodle Picante Style Beef	1 pkg (2.25 oz)	290	15	—	0	7	37	—	—	950	—	4	—	750
Oriental Noodle Picante Style Chicken	1 pkg (2.25 oz)	290	15	—	5	7	38	—	—	920	—	2	—	1250
Oriental Noodle Picante Style Shrimp	1 pkg (2.25 oz)	300	16	—	5	7	36	—	20	1120	—	5	—	1500
Ramen Beef	½ pkg (1.5 oz)	190	9	—	0	5	26	—	20	770	—	—	—	—
Ramen Chicken	½ pkg (1.5 oz)	190	8	—	0	5	20	—	—	780	—	—	—	—
Ramen Chicken Mushroom	½ pkg (1.5 oz)	190	8	—	0	4	25	—	—	780	—	—	—	—
Ramen Chili	½ pkg (1.5 oz)	190	9	—	0	5	26	—	—	710	—	—	—	—
Ramen Mushroom	½ pkg (1.5 oz)	190	9	—	0	5	25	—	—	910	—	—	—	—
Ramen Oriental	½ pkg (1.5 oz)	190	9	—	0	5	26	—	—	990	—	—	—	—
Ramen Pork	½ pkg (1.5 oz)	190	9	—	0	5	25	—	—	890	—	—	—	—
Ramen Shrimp	½ pkg (1.5 oz)	190	9	—	tr	5	26	—	—	820	—	2	—	—
Wonton Beef	⅓ pkg (0.68 oz)	90	5	—	0	2	8	—	—	890	—	2	—	750
Wonton Chicken	⅓ pkg (0.67 oz)	90	5	—	0	2	8	—	—	810	—	—	—	750
Wonton Pork	⅓ pkg (0.68 oz)	90	5	—	0	2	9	—	—	930	—	1	—	750
Wonton Vegetable	⅓ pkg (0.7 oz)	90	6	—	0	2	9	—	—	980	—	1	—	1000
MORGA														
Vegetable Bouillon No Salt Added	½ cube (5 g)	25	2	1	0	tr	1	0	0	115	—	0	—	0
Vegetable Broth Fat Free	1 tsp (4 g)	10	0	0	0	tr	2	0	0	710	—	0	—	0
NILE SPICE														
Couscous Almondine	1 pkg	200	3	0	0	7	37	2	60	490	—	1	—	0
Couscous Garbanzo	1 pkg	220	3	0	0	9	39	2	60	500	—	4	—	0

FOOD	PORTION	CALORIES	FAT	SAT FAT	CHOL	PROTEIN	CARBO	FIBER	CALCIUM	SOD	POTAS	VIT C	FOLIC	VIT A
NILE SPICE (CONT.)														
Couscous Lentil Curry	1 pkg	200	2	0	0	10	36	4	40	730	—	2	—	0
Couscous Minestrone	1 pkg	180	2	0	0	8	34	2	60	590	—	15	—	100
Couscous Parmesan	1 pkg	200	3	2	10	8	34	2	80	570	—	15	—	400
Homestyle Black Bean	1 pkg	190	2	0	0	11	34	2	80	570	—	12	—	400
Homestyle Chicken Flavored Vegetable	1 pkg	120	2	1	5	4	20	4	40	600	—	1	—	0
Homestyle Lentil	1 pkg	180	2	0	0	12	31	3	60	500	—	48	—	750
Homestyle Minestrone	1 pkg	160	2	0	0	8	29	4	80	550	—	4	—	200
Homestyle Red Beans & Rice	1 pkg	190	2	0	0	9	36	3	40	560	—	1	—	0
Homestyle Split Pea	1 pkg	200	2	0	0	13	35	6	60	710	—	0	—	0
Homestyle Sweet Corn Chowder	1 pkg	120	3	1	0	3	20	0	40	420	—	12	—	750
Italian Tomato	1 pkg	140	4	3	10	4	21	2	60	670	—	4	—	300
Potato Leek	1 pkg	150	6	4	20	4	21	2	80	490	—	9	—	0
Potato Romano	1 pkg	140	5	4	15	5	19	3	100	550	—	6	—	300
RAMEN NOODLE														
Beef Low Fat as prep	8 oz	160	1	—	—	5	32	—	—	890	—	—	—	—
Beef as prep	8 oz	190	8	—	—	5	26	—	20	1010	—	—	—	—
Chicken Low Fat as prep	8 oz	160	1	—	—	5	32	—	—	940	—	—	—	—
Chicken as prep	8 oz	190	8	—	—	5	26	—	20	970	—	—	—	—
Oriental Low Fat as prep	8 oz	150	1	—	—	5	31	—	—	940	—	—	—	—
Oriental as prep	8 oz	190	8	—	—	5	26	—	20	930	—	—	—	—
Pork Low Fat as prep	8 oz	150	1	—	—	4	31	—	—	1140	—	—	—	—
Pork as prep	8 oz	200	8	—	—	5	26	—	—	860	—	—	—	—
ULTRA SLIM-FAST														
Beef Noodle	6 oz	45	tr	—	5	4	7	2	100	700	130	6	40	500
Chicken Leek	6 oz	50	tr	—	<2	5	7	2	100	1070	100	6	40	500
Chicken Noodle	6 oz	45	tr	—	5	5	6	2	100	970	110	6	40	500
Creamy Broccoli	6 oz	75	tr	—	0	5	14	2	100	800	100	6	40	500
Creamy Tomato	6 oz	60	tr	—	0	5	10	2	100	800	250	6	40	500
Hearty Vegetable	6 oz	50	tr	—	0	5	7	2	100	750	150	6	40	500
Onion	6 oz	45	tr	—	0	4	7	2	100	930	150	6	40	500
Potato Leek	6 oz	80	tr	—	0	5	15	2	100	780	100	6	40	500

FOOD	PORTION	CALORIES	FAT	SAT FAT	CHOL	PROTEIN	CARBO	FIBER	CALCIUM	SOD	POTAS	VIT C	FOLIC	VIT A
WEIGHT WATCHERS														
Instant Beef Broth	1 pkg (0.16 oz) mix	10	0	0	0	0	2	0	0	800	—	0	—	0
Instant Chicken Broth	1 pkg (0.16 oz)	10	0	0	0	0	2	0	0	830	—	0	—	0
WYLER'S														
Beef Bouillon Instant	1 tsp	6	tr	—	—	tr	1	—	—	930	10	—	—	—
Beef Bouillon Instant Cube	1	6	tr	—	—	tr	1	—	—	930	10	—	—	—
Chicken Bouillon Instant	1 tsp	8	tr	—	—	tr	1	—	—	900	<5	—	—	—
Chicken Bouillon Instant Cube	1	8	tr	—	—	tr	1	—	—	900	<5	—	—	—
Onion Bouillon Instant	1 tsp	10	tr	—	—	tr	1	—	—	910	10	—	—	—
Vegetable Bouillon Instant	1 tsp	6	tr	—	—	tr	1	—	—	910	10	—	—	—
SHELF-STABLE														
HORMEL														
Micro Cup Bean & Ham	1 cup (7.5 oz)	190	4	1	15	9	29	7	20	680	—	1	—	400
Micro Cup Beef Vegetable	1 cup (7.5 oz)	90	1	0	10	6	15	1	20	790	—	0	—	2500
Micro Cup Broccoli Cheese w/ Ham	1 cup (7.5 oz)	170	13	5	40	4	10	1	60	710	—	6	—	300
Micro Cup Chicken & Rice	1 cup (7.5 oz)	110	3	1	15	5	17	1	20	950	—	1	—	1750
Micro Cup Chicken Noodle	1 cup (7.5 oz)	110	3	2	35	8	13	0	20	790	—	0	—	100
Micro Cup New England Clam Chowder	1 cup (7.5 oz)	130	5	3	25	5	17	1	20	820	—	0	—	0
Micro Cup Potato Cheese w/ Ham	1 cup (7.5 oz)	190	13	5	50	4	15	1	60	750	—	0	—	100
LUNCH BUCKET														
Chicken Noodle	1 pkg (7.25 oz)	90	2	—	25	4	13	—	—	810	—	—	—	—
Country Vegetable	1 pkg (7.25 oz)	70	1	—	0	1	15	—	—	740	—	—	—	—
TAKE-OUT														
beef stew soup	1 cup (8.8 oz)	221	5	2	60	23	20	—	32	461	527	14	25	6626
black bean turtle soup	1 cup	241	1	tr	0	15	45	—	103	6	801	0	158	11
brunswick stew soup	1 cup (8.5 oz)	232	6	2	71	27	17	—	39	438	509	14	21	433
gazpacho	1 cup	46	tr	—	0	1	5	—	28	63	—	—	—	—
hot & sour	1 serv (14 oz)	173	8	2	87	15	8	1	50	475	197	1	9	124

FOOD	PORTION	CALORIES	FAT	SAT FAT	CHOL	PROTEIN	CARBO	FIBER	CALCIUM	SOD	POTAS	VIT C	FOLIC	VIT A
pasta e fagiole	1 cup (8.8 oz)	194	5	1	3	9	30	—	62	790	522	12	49	1878
ratatouille	1 cup (7.5 oz)	266	25	3	0	2	12	—	56	329	485	41	34	815

SOUR CREAM

(see also SOUR CREAM SUBSTITUTES)

FOOD	PORTION	CALORIES	FAT	SAT FAT	CHOL	PROTEIN	CARBO	FIBER	CALCIUM	SOD	POTAS	VIT C	FOLIC	VIT A
sour cream	1 tbsp (0.4 oz)	26	3	2	5	tr	1	—	14	6	17	tr	1	95
sour cream	1 cup (8 oz)	493	48	30	102	7	10	—	268	123	331	2	25	1817
BREAKSTONE'S														
Free	2 tbsp (1.1 oz)	35	0	0	<5	2	6	0	40	25	70	0	—	200
Reduced Fat	2 tbsp (1.1 oz)	45	4	3	15	1	2	0	40	20	65	0	—	100
Sour Cream	2 tbsp (1 oz)	60	5	4	20	tr	1	0	20	15	45	0	—	200
CABOT														
Light	1 oz	33	2	—	7	1	2	—	41	72	—	—	—	—
Sour Cream	1 oz	60	6	4	13	1	1	—	34	15	—	—	—	200
FRIENDSHIP														
Light	2 tbsp (1 oz)	35	3	2	10	1	2	0	40	30	—	0	—	100
Sour Cream	2 tbsp (1 oz)	60	5	4	20	1	2	0	40	15	—	0	—	200
HELUVA GOOD CHEESE														
Fat-Free	2 tbsp (1.1 oz)	20	0	0	0	1	3	0	40	45	—	0	—	200
Light	2 tbsp (1.1 oz)	40	3	2	10	1	3	0	40	20	—	0	—	200
Sour Cream	2 tbsp (1.1 oz)	60	5	4	20	1	2	0	40	15	—	0	—	200
HOOD														
Fat Free	2 tbsp (1 oz)	20	0	0	0	1	3	0	60	25	—	0	—	200
Light	2 tbsp (1 oz)	40	3	2	10	1	2	0	40	20	—	0	—	200
Sour Cream	2 tbsp (1 oz)	60	5	4	20	1	2	0	40	20	—	0	—	200
KNUDSEN														
Free	2 tbsp (1.1 oz)	35	0	0	<5	2	6	0	40	25	70	0	—	200
Hampshire	2 tbsp (1 oz)	60	6	4	25	tr	1	0	20	15	45	0	—	200
Light	2 tbsp (1.1 oz)	50	3	2	10	2	2	0	60	10	70	0	—	200
NATURALLY YOURS														
No Fat	2 tbsp (1 fl oz)	15	0	0	0	3	1	—	20	15	—	0	—	200

SOUR CREAM SUBSTITUTES

FOOD	PORTION	CALORIES	FAT	SAT FAT	CHOL	PROTEIN	CARBO	FIBER	CALCIUM	SOD	POTAS	VIT C	FOLIC	VIT A
nondairy	1 oz	59	6	5	0	1	2	—	1	29	46	0	0	0
nondairy	1 cup	479	45	41	0	6	15	—	6	235	369	0	0	0
PET														
Imitation	1 tbsp	25	2	—	tr	tr	tr	—	—	25	—	—	—	—
TOFUTTI														
Better Than Sour Cream Sour Supreme	1 oz	50	5	2	0	1	1	—	—	120	—	—	—	—

SOURSOP

FOOD	PORTION	CALORIES	FAT	SAT FAT	CHOL	PROTEIN	CARBO	FIBER	CALCIUM	SOD	POTAS	VIT C	FOLIC	VIT A
fresh	1	416	2	—	0	6	105	—	88	87	1739	129	—	15
fresh cut up	1 cup	150	1	—	0	2	38	—	32	31	626	46	—	5

SOY

(see also CHEESE SUBSTITUTES, ICE CREAM AND FROZEN DESSERTS, MILK SUBSTITUTES, MISO, SOY SAUCE, SOYBEANS, TEMPH, TOFU, AND YOGURT FROZEN)

FOOD	PORTION	CALORIES	FAT	SAT FAT	CHOL	PROTEIN	CARBO	FIBER	CALCIUM	SOD	POTAS	VIT C	FOLIC	VIT A
soy milk	1 cup	79	5	1	0	7	4	—	10	30	338	0	4	77

FOOD	PORTION	CALORIES	FAT	SAT FAT	CHOL	PROTEIN	CARBO	FIBER	CALCIUM	SOD	POTAS	VIT C	FOLIC	VIT A
LOMA LINDA														
Soyagen All Purpose	¼ cup (1 oz)	130	6	1	0	6	12	3	100	150	270	5	—	1250
Soyagen Carob	¼ cup (1 oz)	130	6	1	0	6	13	2	100	170	270	5	—	1000
Soyagen No Sucrose	¼ cup (1 oz)	130	6	1	0	6	12	3	100	160	270	2	—	1250

SOY SAUCE

FOOD	PORTION	CALORIES	FAT	SAT FAT	CHOL	PROTEIN	CARBO	FIBER	CALCIUM	SOD	POTAS	VIT C	FOLIC	VIT A
shoyu	1 tbsp	9	tr	tr	0	1	2	—	3	1029	32	0	3	0
soy sauce	1 tbsp	7	tr	tr	0	tr	1	—	1	1024	27	0	2	0
tamari	1 tbsp	11	tr	tr	0	2	1	—	4	1005	38	0	3	0
EDEN														
Shoyu Organic	1 tbsp (0.5 oz)	15	0	0	0	2	2	0	0	1040	75	0	—	0
Shoyu Traditional	1 tbsp (0.5 oz)	15	0	0	0	2	2	0	0	1010	85	0	—	0
Tamari Organic Domestic	1 tbsp (0.5 oz)	15	0	0	0	2	2	0	0	970	—	0	—	0
Tamari Organic Imported	1 tbsp (0.5 oz)	15	0	0	0	2	2	0	0	1130	—	0	—	0
HOUSE OF TSANG														
Dark	1 tbsp (0.6 oz)	10	0	0	0	1	1	0	0	860	—	0	—	0
Ginger Flavored	1 tbsp (0.6 oz)	20	0	0	0	1	4	0	0	730	—	0	—	0
Light	1 tbsp (0.6 oz)	5	0	0	0	1	0	0	0	900	—	0	—	0
Low Sodium	1 tbsp (0.6 oz)	5	0	0	0	0	0	0	0	280	—	0	—	0
Low Sodium Ginger	1 tbsp (0.6 oz)	10	0	0	0	0	2	0	0	280	—	0	—	0
Low Sodium Mushroom	1 tbsp (0.6 oz)	10	0	0	0	0	2	0	0	280	—	0	—	0
KA-ME														
Chinese Dark	1 tbsp (0.5 fl oz)	10	0	0	0	0	3	0	—	1020	—	—	—	—
Chinese Light	1 tbsp (0.5 fl oz)	5	0	0	0	0	1	0	—	1170	—	—	—	—
Dark	1 tbsp (0.5 fl oz)	10	0	0	0	0	3	0	—	1020	—	—	—	—
Japanese	1 tbsp (0.5 fl oz)	5	0	0	0	0	1	0	—	520	—	—	—	—
Light	1 tbsp (0.5 oz)	5	0	0	0	0	1	0	—	1170	—	—	—	—
Mild	1 tbsp (0.5 fl oz)	5	0	0	0	1	0	0	—	490	—	—	—	—
LA CHOY														
Lite	½ tsp	1	tr	—	0	tr	tr	tr	—	110	65	—	—	—
Soy Sauce	½ tsp	2	tr	—	0	tr	tr	tr	—	230	10	—	—	—
TRAPPEY														
Chef Magic	1 tbsp (0.5 oz)	23	tr	tr	0	1	4	tr	3	952	—	3	—	1
TREE OF LIFE														
Shoyu	1 tbsp (0.5 oz)	15	0	0	0	2	1	—	—	960	—	—	—	—
Tamari Reduced Sodium	1 tbsp (0.5 oz)	20	0	0	0	2	1	—	—	700	—	—	—	—

FOOD	PORTION	CALORIES	FAT	SAT FAT	CHOL	PROTEIN	CARBO	FIBER	CALCIUM	SOD	POTAS	VIT C	FOLIC	VIT A
TREE OF LIFE (CONT.)														
Tamari Wheat Free	1 tbsp (0.5 oz)	15	0	0	0	2	1	—	—	940	—	—	—	—

SOYBEANS

(*see also* MILK SUBSTITUTES, MISO, SOY, SOY SAUCE, TEMPH, TOFU)

FOOD	PORTION	CALORIES	FAT	SAT FAT	CHOL	PROTEIN	CARBO	FIBER	CALCIUM	SOD	POTAS	VIT C	FOLIC	VIT A
dried cooked	1 cup	298	15	2	0	29	17	—	175	1	886	3	93	15
dry-roasted	½ cup	387	19	3	0	34	28	—	232	2	1173	4	176	20
green cooked	½ cup	127	6	1	0	11	10	4	—	13	485	—	100	—
honey toasted	¼ cup (1 oz)	130	4	1	0	6	19	0	0	45	—	0	—	0
roasted	½ cup	405	22	3	0	30	29	—	119	140	1264	2	182	172
roasted & toasted	1 oz	129	7	1	0	11	9	—	39	1	417	1	64	57
roasted & toasted	1 cup	490	26	3	0	40	33	—	149	4	1588	2	244	216
roasted & toasted salted	1 cup	490	26	3	0	40	33	—	149	176	1588	2	244	216
roasted & toasted salted	1 oz	129	7	1	0	11	9	—	39	54	417	1	64	57

SPAGHETTI

(*see* PASTA, PASTA DINNERS, PASTA SALAD, SPAGHETTI SAUCE)

SPAGHETTI SAUCE

(*see also* PIZZA, TOMATO)

JARRED

FOOD	PORTION	CALORIES	FAT	SAT FAT	CHOL	PROTEIN	CARBO	FIBER	CALCIUM	SOD	POTAS	VIT C	FOLIC	VIT A
marinara sauce	1 cup	171	8	tr	0	4	25	—	44	1572	1061	32	—	2403
spaghetti sauce	1 cup	272	12	2	0	12	40	—	70	1236	957	28	—	3055
CLASSICO														
Beef & Pork	4 fl oz	80	4	—	10	3	7	—	40	540	460	6	—	400
Four Cheese	4 fl oz	70	4	—	<5	2	7	—	20	440	320	6	—	750
Ripe Olives & Mushrooms	4 fl oz	50	2	—	0	2	7	—	40	470	380	5	—	400
Spicy Red Pepper	4 fl oz	50	2	—	0	2	6	—	60	250	380	6	—	300
Sweet Peppers & Onions	4 fl oz	50	4	—	0	1	7	—	20	360	320	6	—	500
Tomato & Basil	4 fl oz	60	3	—	0	2	6	—	20	340	430	6	—	300
CONTADINA														
Italian	¼ cup	15	0	0	0	tr	4	1	—	320	—	6	—	300
Sauce	¼ cup	20	0	0	0	tr	4	tr	—	280	—	—	—	300
Thick & Zesty	¼ cup	15	0	0	0	tr	4	1	—	330	—	6	—	500
DEL MONTE														
Traditional	½ cup (4.4 oz)	80	1	0	0	2	15	tr	40	470	—	21	—	500
Traditional No Sugar Added	½ cup (4.4 oz)	60	1	0	0	2	11	tr	40	470	—	21	—	500
With Garlic & Onion	½ cup (4.4 oz)	70	1	0	0	2	15	tr	40	440	—	24	—	750
With Green Peppers & Mushrooms	½ cup (4.4 oz)	70	1	0	0	2	13	tr	40	320	—	24	—	750
With Meat	½ cup (4.4 oz)	40	2	0	0	3	13	tr	40	390	—	21	—	750
With Mushrooms	½ cup (4.4 oz)	80	2	0	0	2	15	tr	40	520	—	18	—	500

FOOD	PORTION	CALORIES	FAT	SAT FAT	CHOL	PROTEIN	CARBO	FIBER	CALCIUM	SOD	POTAS	VIT C	FOLIC	VIT A
EDEN														
Organic No Salt Added	½ cup (4.4 oz)	80	3	0	0	3	12	3	31	10	530	11	—	2350
ENRICO'S														
Fat Free Organic Basil	½ cup (4 oz)	50	0	0	0	5	8	4	90	220	—	tr	—	100
Fat Free Organic Garlic	½ cup (4 oz)	50	0	0	0	3	9	5	40	340	—	tr	—	150
Fat Free Organic Hot Pepper	½ cup (4 oz)	50	0	0	0	4	8	5	40	350	—	tr	—	100
Fat Free Organic Mushroom	½ cup (4 oz)	60	0	0	0	3	10	7	50	400	—	tr	—	100
Fat Free Organic Traditional	½ cup (4 oz)	45	0	0	0	7	4	6	40	280	—	tr	—	100
HEALTHY CHOICE														
Extra Chunky Garlic & Onion	½ cup (4.4 oz)	43	tr	0	0	2	8	1	56	368	—	1	—	153
Extra Chunky Italian Vegetable	½ cup (4.4 oz)	39	tr	0	0	2	8	1	45	380	—	1	—	250
Extra Chunky Mushroom	½ cup (4.4 oz)	41	tr	0	0	2	8	1	50	352	—	1	—	160
Garlic & Herbs	½ cup (4.4 oz)	47	1	—	—	2	10	2	40	391	—	14	—	140
Super Chunky Mushroom & Sweet Peppers	½ cup (4.4 oz)	44	tr	0	0	2	9	1	37	366	—	1	—	125
Super Chunky Tomato, Mushroom & Garlic	½ cup (4.4 oz)	46	tr	0	0	3	9	2	37	411	—	10	—	161
Super Chunky Vegetable Primavera	½ cup (4.4 oz)	46	tr	0	0	2	9	1	38	358	—	1	—	200
Traditional	½ cup (4.4 oz)	47	1	0	0	2	10	2	40	391	—	14	—	140
With Meat	½ cup (4.4 oz)	47	1	tr	2	2	8	2	42	384	—	11	—	182
With Mushrooms	½ cup (4.4 oz)	47	1	—	—	2	10	3	40	391	—	14	—	140
HUNT'S														
Chunky Marinara	½ cup (4.4 oz)	60	2	tr	0	1	12	2	31	526	—	18	—	112
Chunky Tomato Garlic & Onion	½ cup (4.4 oz)	61	1	tr	0	1	13	2	31	526	—	18	—	117
Chunky Vegetable	½ cup (4.4 oz)	63	1	tr	0	2	13	2	32	528	—	29	—	203
Classic Garlic & Onion	½ cup (4.4 oz)	58	2	tr	0	2	10	2	3	598	—	9	—	89
Classic Tomato & Basil	½ cup (4.4 oz)	48	2	tr	0	2	8	4	31	613	—	9	—	82
Classic Italian With Parmesan	½ cup (4.4 oz)	50	2	tr	0	2	8	2	4	634	—	5	—	29
Home Style With Meat	½ cup (4.4 oz)	56	2	1	2	2	7	2	3	596	—	12	—	67

FOOD	PORTION	CALORIES	FAT	SAT FAT	CHOL	PROTEIN	CARBO	FIBER	CALCIUM	SOD	POTAS	VIT C	FOLIC	VIT A
HUNT'S (CONT.)														
Home Style With Mushrooms	½ cup (4.4 oz)	56	2	tr	0	2	7	2	3	586	—	12	—	162
Homestyle Traditional	½ cup (4.4 oz)	56	3	tr	0	2	7	2	3	596	—	12	—	67
Italian Cheese & Garlic	½ cup (4.5 oz)	65	2	1	1	3	9	2	52	690	—	11	—	162
Italian Sausage	½ cup (4.5 oz)	77	3	1	2	2	12	2	31	596	—	11	—	164
Old Country Garlic & Herbs	½ cup (4.4 oz)	63	3	tr	0	2	9	3	3	522	—	12	—	44
Old Country Italian Style Vegetables	½ cup (4.4 oz)	64	3	tr	0	2	9	3	3	616	—	12	—	52
Old Country Traditional	½ cup (4.4 oz)	53	3	tr	0	2	7	3	3	542	—	17	—	50
Old Country With Meat	½ cup (4.4 oz)	56	3	1	tr	2	7	3	3	474	—	18	—	40
Old Country With Mushrooms	½ cup (4.4 oz)	53	3	tr	0	2	7	3	3	542	—	17	—	50
Original Traditional	½ cup (4.4 oz)	65	2	tr	0	2	11	4	3	621	—	22	—	26
Original With Meat	½ cup (4.4 oz)	65	2	1	3	2	11	2	9	604	—	22	—	26
Original With Mushrooms	½ cup (4.4 oz)	65	2	tr	0	2	11	2	3	604	—	22	—	26
MAMA RIZZO'S														
Mushroom Onion	½ cup (4.3 oz)	60	2	0	0	2	9	1	40	290	—	1	—	1000
Pepper Mushroom Onion	½ cup (4.3 oz)	60	2	0	0	2	9	1	40	290	—	1	—	1000
Pepper Primavera Vegetable	½ cup (4.2 oz)	50	2	0	0	2	8	2	60	220	—	7	—	2000
Pepper Tomato Basil Garlic	½ cup (4.7 oz)	60	2	0	0	2	10	1	40	490	—	2	—	750
Primavera Vegetable	½ cup (4.2 oz)	50	2	0	0	2	8	2	60	220	—	7	—	2000
Tomato Basil Garlic	½ cup (4.6 oz)	60	2	0	0	2	8	2	80	500	—	4	—	750
MUIR GLEN														
Organic Cabernet Marinara	½ cup (4.4 oz)	45	0	—	0	2	10	2	40	350	—	18	—	750
Organic Chunky Style	½ cup (4.5 oz)	80	2	—	0	2	13	3	20	300	—	6	—	500
Organic Fat Free Tomato Basil	½ cup (4.3 oz)	50	0	0	0	2	10	2	100	300	—	5	—	500
Organic Garlic Onion	½ cup (4.3 oz)	50	0	—	0	2	11	3	60	300	—	2	—	500
Organic Garlic Roasted Garlic	½ cup (4.4 oz)	45	0	—	0	2	10	2	40	350	—	18	—	750
Organic Green Pepper & Mushroom	½ cup (4.5 oz)	70	2	—	0	2	10	4	20	360	—	9	—	500
Organic Italian Herb	½ cup (4.5 oz)	60	0	—	0	2	13	2	20	300	—	18	—	750

FOOD	PORTION	CALORIES	FAT	SAT FAT	CHOL	PROTEIN	CARBO	FIBER	CALCIUM	SOD	POTAS	VIT C	FOLIC	VIT A
MUIR GLEN (CONT.)														
Organic Romano Cheese	½ cup (4.5 oz)	90	3	—	0	2	14	4	20	300	—	6	—	1000
Organic Sun Dried Tomato	½ cup (4.4 oz)	40	0	—	0	2	9	2	40	360	—	18	—	750
Organic Sweet Pepper Onion	½ cup (4.4 oz)	40	0	—	0	2	8	1	80	300	—	18	—	500
Organic Tomato Basil	½ cup (4.3 oz)	50	0	—	0	2	10	2	100	300	—	5	—	500
NEWMAN'S OWN														
Marinara Ventian	½ cup (4.4 oz)	60	2	0	0	2	9	3	60	590	—	0	—	750
Marinara Ventian w/ Mushrooms	½ cup (4.4 oz)	60	2	0	0	2	9	3	60	590	—	0	—	750
Pasta Sauce Bambolina	½ cup (4.5 oz)	100	5	1	0	1	15	5	40	590	—	0	—	750
Pasta Sauce Roasted Garlic & Red & Green Peppers	½ cup (4.7 oz)	70	3	0	0	2	11	4	0	460	—	0	—	1000
Pasta Sauce Say Cheese	½ cup (4.4 oz)	90	3	2	<5	3	14	3	60	510	—	0	—	750
Sockarooni	½ cup (4.4 oz)	60	2	0	0	2	9	3	60	590	—	0	—	750
PREGO														
Chunky Sausage & Green Peppers	4 oz	160	8	—	—	3	19	—	40	500	—	18	—	1000
Extra Chunky Garden Combination	4 oz	80	2	—	—	2	14	—	20	420	—	24	—	1000
Extra Chunky Mushroom & Tomato	4 oz	110	5	—	—	1	14	—	20	500	—	12	—	500
Extra Chunky Mushroom & Green Pepper	4 oz	100	4	—	—	2	14	—	20	410	—	12	—	750
Extra Chunky Mushroom & Onion	4 oz	100	4	—	—	2	13	—	20	490	—	12	—	500
Extra Chunky Mushroom With Extra Spice	4 oz	100	3	—	—	2	17	—	40	450	—	21	—	750
Extra Chunky Tomato & Onion	4 oz	110	5	—	—	2	14	—	20	490	—	12	—	500
Marinara	4 oz	100	6	—	—	2	10	—	20	620	—	18	—	750
Meat Flavored	4 oz	140	6	—	—	2	20	—	40	660	—	15	—	1000
Mushroom	4 oz	130	5	—	—	2	20	—	40	630	—	15	—	1000
Onion & Garlic	4 oz	110	4	—	—	1	16	—	20	510	—	5	—	1000
Regular	4 oz	130	5	—	—	2	20	—	40	630	—	18	—	1000
Three Cheese	4 oz	100	2	—	—	3	17	—	40	410	—	21	—	750
Tomato & Basil	4 oz	100	2	—	—	2	18	—	40	370	—	21	—	1000

FOOD	PORTION	CALORIES	FAT	SAT FAT	CHOL	PROTEIN	CARBO	FIBER	CALCIUM	SOD	POTAS	VIT C	FOLIC	VIT A
PRITIKIN														
Chunky Garden	½ cup (4 oz)	50	1	0	0	—	12	—	—	30	470	—	—	—
Marinara	½ cup (4 oz)	60	0	0	0	—	13	—	—	260	430	—	—	—
Original	½ cup (4 oz)	60	1	0	0	—	13	—	—	30	490	—	—	—
PROGRESSO														
Marinara	½ cup (4.3 oz)	90	5	1	<5	2	8	2	20	480	—	0	—	500
Meat Flavored	½ cup (4.4 oz)	100	5	1	5	4	12	3	40	610	—	0	—	300
Mushroom	½ cup (4.4 oz)	100	5	1	<5	3	12	4	40	580	—	0	—	200
Sauce	½ cup (4.4 oz)	100	5	1	<5	3	12	2	20	620	—	2	—	750
RAGU														
Fino Italian Garden Medley	½ cup (4.5 oz)	90	3	0	0	2	14	2	40	580	—	2	—	500
Fino Italian Garlic & Basil	½ cup (4.5 oz)	90	3	0	0	2	15	2	40	580	—	2	—	750
Fino Italian Parmesan	½ cup (4.5 oz)	100	3	1	<5	3	15	2	100	580	—	2	—	750
Fino Italian Sliced Mushroom	½ cup (4.5 oz)	90	3	0	0	2	14	2	40	580	—	2	—	750
Fino Italian Tomato & Herb	½ cup (4.5 oz)	90	3	0	0	2	15	2	40	580	—	2	—	750
Fino Italian Zesty Tomato	½ cup (4.5 oz)	90	3	0	0	2	14	2	40	580	—	2	—	750
Gardenstyle Chunky Garden Combination	½ cup (4.5 oz)	120	4	1	0	2	18	3	60	540	—	4	—	1000
Gardenstyle Chunky Green & Red Pepper	½ cup (4.5 oz)	120	4	1	0	2	19	2	40	570	—	6	—	1250
Gardenstyle Chunky Mushroom & Green Pepper	½ cup (4.5 oz)	120	4	1	0	2	18	3	40	570	—	2	—	1000
Gardenstyle Chunky Mushroom & Onion	½ cup (4.5 oz)	120	4	1	0	2	19	3	40	560	—	2	—	1000
Gardenstyle Chunky Tomato Garlic & Onion	½ cup (4.5 oz)	120	4	1	0	2	19	3	60	550	—	4	—	1000
Gardenstyle Super Mushroom	½ cup (4.5 oz)	120	4	1	0	3	19	3	40	540	—	2	—	1000
Gardenstyle Super Vegetable Primavera	½ cup (4.5 oz)	110	4	1	0	2	17	4	40	480	—	6	—	1750
Homestyle Mushroom	½ cup (4.5 oz)	120	4	1	0	3	18	3	40	650	—	2	—	1000
Homestyle Tomato & Herb	½ cup (4.5 oz)	120	4	1	0	3	18	3	40	650	—	2	—	1000

FOOD	PORTION	CALORIES	FAT	SAT FAT	CHOL	PROTEIN	CARBO	FIBER	CALCIUM	SOD	POTAS	VIT C	FOLIC	VIT A
RAGU (CONT.)														
Homestyle With Meat	½ cup (4.5 oz)	130	4	1	<5	3	18	3	40	650	—	2	—	1000
Light Chunky Mushroom	½ cup (4.4 oz)	50	0	0	0	2	10	2	20	410	—	2	—	750
Light Garden Harvest	½ cup (4.4 oz)	50	0	0	0	2	11	2	20	410	—	2	—	1000
Light No Sugar Added	½ cup (4.4 oz)	60	0	0	0	3	9	3	20	410	—	2	—	1000
Light Tomato & Herb	½ cup (4.4 oz)	50	0	0	0	2	10	2	20	410	—	2	—	1000
Old World Style Marinara	½ cup (4.4 oz)	90	5	1	0	2	9	3	40	820	—	1	—	1000
Old World Style Mushrooms	½ cup (4.4 oz)	80	3	1	0	2	10	3	40	820	—	1	—	1000
Old World Style Traditional	½ cup (4.4 oz)	80	3	1	0	2	10	3	40	820	—	1	—	1000
Old World Style With Meat	½ cup (4.4 oz)	90	5	1	<5	3	9	3	40	820	—	1	—	1000
Sauce	4 fl oz	80	4	—	0	2	9	—	20	740	—	6	—	750
Thick & Hearty Mushroom	½ cup (4.5 oz)	120	3	1	0	3	19	3	40	580	—	2	—	1000
Thick & Hearty Spaghetti Sauce	4 oz	100	3	—	0	2	15	—	40	460	—	9	—	750
Thick & Hearty Tomato & Herb	½ cup (4.5 oz)	120	3	1	0	3	19	3	40	580	—	2	—	1000
Thick & Hearty With Meat	1.2 cup (4.5 oz)	130	5	1	<5	4	19	3	40	580	—	2	—	1000
TREE OF LIFE														
Pasta Sauce	½ cup (4 oz)	50	2	—	0	2	9	—	20	290	—	15	—	500
Pasta Sauce Calabrese	½ cup (3.9 oz)	60	3	—	—	2	9	—	80	310	—	42	—	1250
Pasta Sauce Fat Free Classic	½ cup (3.9 oz)	40	0	0	0	2	8	0	20	250	—	18	—	1250
Pasta Sauce Fat Free Mushroom & Basil	½ cup (3.9 oz)	30	0	0	0	1	7	0	0	300	—	12	—	750
Pasta Sauce Fat Free Onion & Garlic	½ cup (3.9 oz)	30	0	0	0	1	7	0	0	240	—	12	—	1000
Pasta Sauce Fat Free Sweet Pepper	½ cup (3.9 oz)	30	0	0	0	1	7	0	0	280	—	18	—	1000
Pasta Sauce No Salt	½ cup (3.9 oz)	50	2	—	0	2	9	—	20	0	—	15	—	500
MIX														
DURKEE														
American Style as prep	½ cup	15	0	0	0	0	6	0	0	170	—	4	—	300
Family Style as prep	½ cup	20	0	0	0	1	4	0	0	560	—	0	—	200

FOOD	PORTION	CALORIES	FAT	SAT FAT	CHOL	PROTEIN	CARBO	FIBER	CALCIUM	SOD	POTAS	VIT C	FOLIC	VIT A
DURKEE (CONT.)														
Spaghetti Sauce as prep	½ cup	15	0	0	0	0	5	0	0	390	—	1	—	100
With Mushrooms as prep	½ cup	15	0	0	0	1	4	0	0	520	—	0	—	200
Zesty as prep	½ cup	20	0	0	0	1	5	0	10	350	—	15	—	500
FRENCH'S														
All American as prep	½ cup	20	0	0	0	0	7	0	0	200	—	4	—	300
Italian as prep	½ cup	16	0	0	0	0	5	0	0	390	—	1	—	100
Mushroom as prep	½ cup	20	1	0	2	1	4	0	40	760	—	2	—	0
Thick as prep	½ cup	10	0	0	0	0	4	0	0	630	—	0	—	0
Zesty Pasta as prep	½ cup	20	0	0	0	1	5	0	20	350	—	15	—	500
REFRIGERATED														
CONTADINA														
Alfredo	½ cup (4.2 fl oz)	400	38	21	80	7	8	0	200	510	—	0	—	0
Four Cheese Sauce With White Wine & Shallots	½ cup (4.2 fl oz)	320	25	14	70	8	8	0	250	480	—	0	—	0
Light Alfredo	½ cup (4.2 fl oz)	190	13	7	40	8	10	0	250	560	—	0	—	0
Light Chunky Tomato	½ cup (4.4 fl oz)	45	0	0	0	2	8	3	60	470	—	0	—	1750
Light Garden Vegetable	½ cup (4.4 fl oz)	45	1	0	0	2	8	3	60	540	—	1	—	1250
Marinara	½ cup (4.4 fl oz)	80	4	1	0	2	8	2	40	470	—	0	—	750
Pesto With Basil	¼ cup (2 oz)	310	30	5	10	6	5	0	150	440	—	0	—	400
Pesto With Sun Dried Tomatoes	¼ cup (2 oz)	250	24	4	0	3	6	3	40	520	—	0	—	400
Plum Tomato With Basil	½ cup (4.4 fl oz)	70	3	1	0	2	8	3	40	450	—	0	—	750
Spicy Italian Sausage & Bell Pepper	½ cup (4.4 fl oz)	100	5	1	40	4	9	3	40	540	—	0	—	500
DI GIORNO														
Alfredo	¼ cup (2.2 oz)	180	18	7	25	3	3	0	80	600	65	0	0	400
Basil Pesto	¼ cup (2.2 oz)	320	31	6	15	7	2	tr	250	530	100	0	8	500
Four Cheese	¼ cup (2.2 oz)	160	15	7	30	5	3	0	150	410	75	0	0	500
Garlic Pesto	¼ cup (2.1 oz)	340	33	7	15	7	3	tr	250	540	65	0	0	200
Light Alfredo Sauce	¼ cup (2.4 oz)	140	9	6	30	5	9	0	100	600	90	0	0	750
Marinara	½ cup (4.5 oz)	70	0	0	0	2	15	2	40	220	400	0	0	500
Plum Tomato Cream Sauce	½ cup (4.4 oz)	160	13	7	40	3	8	2	100	370	360	1	0	750
Plum Tomato & Mushroom	½ cup (4.4 oz)	60	0	0	0	2	13	2	40	260	400	0	0	500

FOOD	PORTION	CALORIES	FAT	SAT FAT	CHOL	PROTEIN	CARBO	FIBER	CALCIUM	SOD	POTAS	VIT C	FOLIC	VIT A
DI GIORNO (CONT.)														
Roasted Red Bell Pepper Cream Sauce	¼ cup (2.3 oz)	140	10	6	35	4	8	0	80	510	70	0	0	1000

SPANISH FOOD

(see also BEANS, CHILI, CHIPS, DINNER, PEPPERS, SALSA, SAUCE, SNACKS, TORTILLA)

CANNED

FOOD	PORTION	CALORIES	FAT	SAT FAT	CHOL	PROTEIN	CARBO	FIBER	CALCIUM	SOD	POTAS	VIT C	FOLIC	VIT A
CHI-CHI'S														
Pico De Gallo	2 tbsp (1.2 oz)	10	0	0	0	0	2	0	0	170	—	2	—	100
DERBY														
Tamales	2	160	7	3	24	8	15	1	12	570	150	1	—	65
EL MOLINO														
Enchilada Sauce Hot	2 tbsp	16	1	—	—	0	2	—		100	45	—	—	1000
Green Chili Sauce Mild	2 tbsp	10	0	0	0	0	2	—		210	60	—	—	400
GEBHARDT														
Enchiladas	2	310	24	9	58	5	20	2	21	460	210	3	—	25
Tamales	2	290	22	8	54	5	19	2	34	730	190	2	—	100
Tamales Jumbo	2	400	30	11	75	7	26	3	47	1025	270	3	—	139
GUILTLESS GOURMET														
Picante Mild	1 oz	6	0	0	0	0	1	tr	—	133	—	—	—	—
Queso Mild Cheddar	1 oz	22	tr	—	tr	tr	5	tr	—	150	—	—	—	—
HORMEL														
Tamales Beef	3 (7.5 oz)	280	21	8	35	6	20	3	20	1010	—	0	—	750
Tamales Chicken	3 (7.5 oz)	210	11	4	50	6	22	2	40	1020	—	1	—	0
Tamales Hot Spicy Beef	3 (7.5 oz)	280	21	8	35	6	20	3	20	1010	—	0	—	750
Tamales Jumbo Beef	2 (6.9 oz)	270	20	8	35	5	18	3	20	940	—	0	—	500
OLD EL PASO														
Tamales	3 (7.2 oz)	330	19	7	30	7	31	5	40	590	—	0	—	0
ROSARITA														
Enchilada Sauce Mild	2.5 oz	25	1	tr	0	tr	3	tr	7	230	110	6	—	150
Picante Chunky Hot	3 tbsp (2 fl oz)	18	tr	—	0	tr	4	tr	14	515	90	45	—	45
Picante Chunky Medium	3 tbsp (2 fl oz)	16	tr	—	0	tr	4	tr	12	650	130	10	—	45
Picante Chunky Mild	3 tbsp (2 oz)	25	tr	—	0	1	5	tr	15	630	140	33	—	56
VAN CAMP'S														
Tamales	2 (5.1 oz)	210	13	5	20	6	20	3	20	610	180	—	8	750
FROZEN														
AMY'S ORGANIC														
Black Bean Vegetable Enchilada	1 (4.75 oz)	130	4	0	0	4	20	2	—	390	—	—	—	—

FOOD	PORTION	CALORIES	FAT	SAT FAT	CHOL	PROTEIN	CARBO	FIBER	CALCIUM	SOD	POTAS	VIT C	FOLIC	VIT A
AMY'S ORGANIC (CONT.)														
Burritos Bean & Cheese	1 (6 oz)	280	8	3	10	10	43	6	—	460	—	—	—	—
Burritos Bean & Rice Non-Dairy	1 (6 oz)	250	5	tr	0	9	44	6	—	450	—	—	—	—
Burritos Black Bean Vegetable	1 (6 oz)	320	8	1	0	9	54	4	—	480	—	—	—	—
Burritos Breakfast	1 (6 oz)	230	5	tr	0	9	38	5	—	480	—	—	—	—
Cheese Enchilada	1 (4.7 oz)	210	9	3	20	11	16	2	150	390	—	9	—	300
Mexican Tamale Pie	1 (8 oz)	220	3	0	0	10	41	11	—	480	—	—	—	—
Pocket Sandwich Tamale	1 (4.5 oz)	250	7	3	10	8	39	3	—	580	—	—	—	—
Whole Meals Cheese Enchilada	1 pkg (9 oz)	330	14	7	30	15	38	6	—	680	—	—	—	—
Whole Meals Enchilada	1 pkg (10 oz)	250	8	1	0	7	41	5	—	680	—	—	—	—
BANQUET														
Beef Enchilada	1 pkg (11 oz)	320	12	5	15	15	54	10	150	1330	—	0	—	750
Chimichanga Meal	1 pkg (9.5 oz)	470	23	7	15	13	56	9	60	1180	—	6	—	400
Enchilada Cheese	1 pkg (11 oz)	350	6	3	15	15	56	9	200	1500	—	4	—	750
Enchilada Chicken	1 pkg (11 oz)	360	10	3	20	15	54	9	150	1580	—	0	—	750
Family Entree Beef Enchilada w/ Cheese	1 serv (4.67 oz)	130	4	2	5	45	19	3	100	690	—	1	—	500
CHI-CHI'S														
Burro Beef	1 pkg (15.9 oz)	590	19	8	55	27	76	11	250	2060	—	3	—	1250
Burro Chicken	1 pkg (15.9 oz)	540	14	5	55	26	77	10	200	2110	—	9	—	500
Chimichanga Beef	1 pkg (15.9 oz)	630	24	9	55	28	75	10	200	2050	—	9	—	1250
Chimichanga Chicken	1 pkg (15.9 oz)	580	19	6	50	25	78	10	200	2100	—	12	—	1000
Enchilada Chicken Suprema	1 pkg (15.9 oz)	600	20	9	70	26	80	11	200	2310	—	4	—	750
Enchilida Baja	1 pkg (15.9 oz)	590	20	9	50	27	75	15	200	1920	—	5	—	1250
HEALTHY CHOICE														
Beef Burrito Ranchero Medium	1 (5.4 oz)	290	7	3	15	13	44	6	20	500	—	4	—	200
Beef Burrito Ranchero Mild	1 (5.4 oz)	300	7	3	15	13	45	7	20	480	—	5	—	200
Beef Enchilada Rio Grande	1 meal (13.4 oz)	410	8	3	15	14	70	9	200	480	—	156	—	1000
Burrito Chicken Con Queso	1 (5.4 oz)	280	6	2	10	12	43	5	40	600	—	15	—	200

FOOD	PORTION	CALORIES	FAT	SAT FAT	CHOL	PROTEIN	CARBO	FIBER	CALCIUM	SOD	POTAS	VIT C	FOLIC	VIT A
HEALTHY CHOICE (CONT.)														
Chicken Enchilada Supreme	1 meal (13.4 oz)	390	9	5	30	17	60	8	250	390	—	66	—	400
Enchiladas Suiza Chicken	1 meal (10 oz)	270	4	2	25	14	43	5	150	440	—	2	—	300
Fiesta Chicken Fajitas	1 meal (7 oz)	260	4	1	30	21	36	5	20	410	—	36	—	750
JIMMY DEAN														
Burrito Breakfast Bacon	1 (4 oz)	260	8	3	70	11	37	1	—	680	—	—	—	—
Burrito Breakfast Sausage	1 (4 oz)	250	8	3	45	10	36	2	—	580	—	—	—	—
LE MENU														
Entree LightStyle Enchiladas Chicken	8 oz	280	8	—	35	21	32	—	200	530	—	9	—	100
LEAN CUISINE														
Chicken Enchilada Suiza w/ Mexican Style Rice	1 pkg (9 oz)	280	5	2	25	11	48	3	150	520	340	2	—	200
LIFE CHOICE														
Burrito Black Bean	1 meal (13.2 oz)	410	2	0	0	12	86	13	150	570	—	9	—	500
Vegetable Enchilada Sonora	1 meal (14 oz)	420	2	0	0	12	89	11	100	600	—	9	—	1750
LIGHTLIFE														
Vegetarian Taco	2 oz	51	1	tr	0	5	4	—	—	280	—	—	—	—
OLD EL PASO														
Burrito Bean & Cheese	1 (4.9 oz)	290	9	5	15	12	44	3	150	840	—	5	—	200
Burrito Beef & Bean Hot	1 (5 oz)	320	10	4	15	12	45	3	60	850	—	2	—	0
Burrito Beef & Bean Medium	1 (5 oz)	320	10	4	15	12	46	3	60	800	—	0	—	0
Burrito Beef & Bean Mild	1 (5 oz)	330	9	3	15	12	48	4	60	690	—	0	—	0
Chimichanga Beef	1 (4.5 oz)	370	20	5	10	9	37	3	40	470	—	0	—	0
Chimichanga Chicken	1 (4.5 oz)	350	16	4	20	11	39	2	60	540	—	0	—	0
PATIO														
Burrito Bean & Cheese	1 (5 oz)	270	5	2	5	9	46	7	60	530	—	5	—	200
Burrito Chicken	1 (5 oz)	260	4	2	15	12	44	3	60	740	—	1	—	0
Burrito Red Chili	1 (5 oz)	270	6	2	10	11	42	6	20	850	—	4	—	400
Burritos Beef & Bean	1 (5 oz)	280	7	3	15	10	45	7	0	660	—	1	—	300
Burritos Beef & Bean Green Chili	1 (5 oz)	260	5	2	10	11	44	7	20	890	—	1	—	0

FOOD	PORTION	CALORIES	FAT	SAT FAT	CHOL	PROTEIN	CARBO	FIBER	CALCIUM	SOD	POTAS	VIT C	FOLIC	VIT A
PATIO (CONT.)														
Burritos Beef & Bean Red Chili	1 (5 oz)	260	5	2	10	11	42	7	20	640	—	5	—	200
Enchilada Beef Dinner	1 meal (12 oz)	320	8	3	15	12	52	9	150	1810	—	4	—	500
Enchilada Cheese Dinner	1 meal (12 oz)	330	8	3	15	13	52	10	200	1570	—	5	—	500
Enchilada Chicken	1 pkg (12 oz)	380	9	3	25	14	58	9	200	1470	—	5	—	300
Family Entree Beef Enchilada	2 (5.7 oz)	170	4	2	10	6	27	5	100	940	—	1	—	400
Family Entree Enchilada Beef	2 (5.3 oz)	250	7	3	15	12	35	8	100	1350	—	0	—	1000
Family Entree Enchilada Beef & Cheese	2 (5.3 oz)	250	6	3	20	12	35	9	150	1130	—	4	—	750
Family Entree Enchilada Cheese	2 (5.7 oz)	170	4	2	10	6	26	4	100	880	—	1	—	400
Fiesta Dinner	1 meal (12 oz)	340	9	4	15	13	51	11	150	1760	—	4	—	500
Mexican Dinner	1 meal (13.25 oz)	440	15	6	20	15	59	13	100	1840	—	6	—	500
Salis Con Queso	1 pkg (11 oz)	390	20	11	40	18	33	10	100	1570	—	5	—	300
PATIO BRITOS														
Beef & Bean	10 (6 oz)	420	19	7	20	11	51	7	40	800	—	2	—	500
Nacho Beef	10 (6 oz)	410	18	5	20	13	48	5	60	1050	—	1	—	100
Nacho Cheese	10 (6 oz)	360	13	4	15	10	52	3	150	500	—	2	—	0
Spicy Chicken	10 (6 oz)	400	16	4	25	13	52	3	100	640	—	0	—	0
RUDY'S FARM														
Burrito Beef/Bean	1 (5 oz)	326	12	4	15	12	43	5	—	765	—	—	—	—
Burrito Hot Beef/ Bean	1 (5 oz)	305	9	3	11	12	44	5	—	844	—	—	—	—
SENOR FELIX'S														
Burrito Black Bean	1 (10 oz)	540	18	9	40	26	70	7	450	510	—	6	—	750
Burrito Black Bean Soy	1 (5 oz)	240	7	1	0	12	36	3	150	360	—	21	—	200
Burrito Chicken	1 (10 oz)	520	20	4	65	32	51	3	400	1240	—	30	—	1500
Burrito Hot Potato	1 (10 oz)	560	24	9	40	19	67	5	400	470	—	81	—	750
Burrito Soy Hot	1 (10 oz)	520	20	3	0	18	70	5	250	470	—	81	—	400
Burritos Charbroiled Chicken	1 + 4 tsp sauce (6.7 oz)	320	11	3	20	15	40	7	60	910	—	15	—	3250
Burritos Sonora Style	1 + 4 tsp sauce (6.7 oz)	280	8	2	10	10	45	3	250	240	—	46	—	400
Burritos Yucatan Style	1 + 4 tsp sauce (6.7 oz)	310	9	2	10	14	46	5	300	500	—	36	—	500
Empanadas Chicken	1 (4.7 oz)	340	15	30	30	11	41	13	20	650	—	6	—	5000

FOOD	PORTION	CALORIES	FAT	SAT FAT	CHOL	PROTEIN	CARBO	FIBER	CALCIUM	SOD	POTAS	VIT C	FOLIC	VIT A
SENOR FELIX'S (CONT.)														
Empanadas Corn & Rice	1 (4.7 oz)	280	13	4	25	9	37	6	100	530	—	4	—	400
Empanadas Pumpkin & Mushroom	1 (4.7 oz)	260	11	4	25	10	32	6	150	520	—	1	—	1250
Empanadas Spinach & Ricotta	1 (4.7 oz)	260	12	4	30	10	32	6	200	520	—	5	—	3000
Enchilada Red Pepper	1 (10 oz)	420	19	5	25	18	51	8	450	640	—	42	—	1750
Enchilada Soy Verda	1 (10 oz)	430	24	3	0	14	41	6	250	1230	—	30	—	400
Enchilada Supreme Soy Cheese	1 (10 oz)	460	23	4	0	20	48	6	350	490	—	30	—	1250
Enchilada Verde	1 (5 oz)	423	23	5	25	16	41	6	400	1140	—	27	—	750
Tamales Blue Corn & Soy Cheese	2 + 4 tsp sauce (5.7 oz)	240	10	3	15	8	28	3	200	830	—	30	—	500
Tamales Chicken	2 + 4 tsp sauce (5.7 oz)	240	9	2	20	10	30	8	40	480	—	6	—	1000
Tamales Gourmet Vegetarian	2 + 4 tsp sauce	240	9	2	20	10	30	8	40	480	—	6	—	1000
Taquitos Blue Corn Soy	3 + 4 tsp sauce (5.2 oz)	230	11	2	0	7	27	3	100	560	—	20	—	200
Taquitos Chicken	2 + 4 tsp sauce (5.7 oz)	240	10	3	15	8	28	3	200	830	—	30	—	500
STOUFFER'S														
Chicken Enchilada	1 serv (4.8 oz)	230	11	5	30	7	25	3	150	530	220	0	—	100
SWANSON														
Enchiladas Beef	13¾ oz	480	21	—	—	17	55	—	200	1350	—	4	—	1250
Mexican Style Combination	14¼ oz	490	18	—	—	19	62	—	200	1760	—	—	—	1500
Mexican Style Hungry Man	20¼ oz	820	41	—	—	25	88	—	300	2080	—	6	—	2000
TODAY'S TAMALES														
Cheese & Chili	1 pkg (7 oz)	390	21	10	30	12	38	6	300	630	—	9	—	200
Del Sol	1 pkg (6.5 oz)	310	15	2	0	5	40	15	150	650	—	2	—	1500
Original Bean	1 pkg (7 oz)	330	11	1	0	9	49	10	90	520	—	tr	—	<100
Spicy Taco	1 pkg (7 oz)	310	15	1	0	12	41	10	150	570	—	tr	—	<100
TYSON														
Fajita Kit Beef	3.84 oz	160	4	—	—	9	21	—	—	240	—	—	—	—
Fajita Kit Chicken	4 oz	80	2	—	—	7	2	—	—	240	—	—	—	—
WEIGHT WATCHERS														
Smart Ones Chicken Enchiladas Suiza	1 pkg (9 oz)	270	9	5	40	14	33	4	250	540	—	2	—	200

FOOD	PORTION	CALORIES	FAT	SAT FAT	CHOL	PROTEIN	CARBO	FIBER	CALCIUM	SOD	POTAS	VIT C	FOLIC	VIT A
WEIGHT WATCHERS (CONT.)														
Smart Ones Santa Fe Style Rice & Beans	1 pkg (10 oz)	290	8	4	5	12	41	10	200	670	—	1	—	100
MIX														
GEBHARDT														
Menudo Mix	1 tsp	5	tr	—	0	tr	1	tr	5	310	2	—	—	—
HAIN														
Taco Seasoning Mix	¹⁄₁₀ pkg	10	0	0	0	1	2	—	—	200	50	—	—	200
OLD EL PASO														
Burrito Seasoning Mix	2 tsp (6 g)	20	0	0	0	tr	3	1	20	290	—	0	—	100
Dinner Kit Burrito as prep	1	280	7	3	66	—	35	3	60	840	—	0	—	100
Dinner Kit Soft Taco as prep	2	380	10	4	63	—	45	3	100	1340	—	0	—	100
Dinner Kit Taco as prep	2	270	13	5	60	—	21	4	100	910	—	0	—	100
Enchilada Sauce Mix	2 tsp (4 g)	10	0	0	0	0	2	tr	0	540	—	0	—	300
Taco Mix 40% Less Sodium	2 tsp (6 g)	20	0	0	0	0	4	0	0	330	—	0	—	200
Taco Seasoning Mix	2 tsp (6 g)	20	0	0	0	0	5	0	0	550	—	0	—	200
ORTEGA														
Taco Meat Seasoning Mix Mild	1 filled taco	90	1	0	0	2	18	—	40	999	120	1	—	750
TACO BELL														
Home Originals Chicken Fajita Dinner as prep	2 (6.9 oz)	340	9	2	40	21	45	3	60	1120	—	27	—	400
Home Originals Chicken Fajita Seasoning Mix	1 tbsp (8 g)	25	0	0	0	tr	5	2	0	540	—	1	—	200
Home Originals Soft Taco Dinner as prep	2 (6.3 oz)	410	18	4	60	21	41	2	40	1090	—	0	—	500
Home Originals Taco Dinner as prep	2 (4.4 oz)	280	15	5	50	16	19	2	40	580	—	0	—	500
Home Originals Taco Seasoning Mix	2 tsp (6 g)	20	0	0	0	tr	3	tr	0	450	—	0	—	300
Home Originals Ultimate Bean Burrito Dinner as prep	1 (4.4 oz)	200	5	2	0	6	34	3	40	710	—	0	—	100
Home Originals Ultimate Nachos as prep	12 pieces (4.6 oz)	240	11	3	0	6	31	4	100	680	—	0	—	100

FOOD	PORTION	CALORIES	FAT	SAT FAT	CHOL	PROTEIN	CARBO	FIBER	CALCIUM	SOD	POTAS	VIT C	FOLIC	VIT A
READY-TO-EAT														
taco shell baked	1 med (0.5 oz)	61	3	tr	0	1	8	tr	21	48	23	0	1	—
taco shell baked w/o salt	1 med (½ oz)	61	3	tr	0	1	8	tr	21	2	23	0	1	—
CASA FIESTA														
Taco Shells	3.5 oz	480	23	—	—	9	60	—	67	10	—	tr	—	106
CHI-CHI'S														
Taco Shells White Corn	2 (1.2 oz)	170	8	2	0	3	22	2	0	0	—	0	—	0
Taco Shells Yellow Corn	2 shells (1.2 oz)	170	8	0	0	2	22	2	0	0	—	0	—	0
GEBHARDT														
Taco Shells	1	50	2	2	0	1	7	tr	12	tr	25	—	—	—
OLD EL PASO														
Taco Shells Mini	7 (1.1 oz)	160	10	2	0	2	18	2	40	130	—	0	—	0
Taco Shells Regular	3 (1.1 oz)	170	10	2	0	2	18	2	40	130	—	0	—	0
Taco Shells Super	2 (1.3 oz)	190	12	2	0	3	21	2	40	150	—	0	—	0
Taco Shells White Corn	3 (1.1 oz)	170	10	2	0	2	18	2	40	30	—	0	—	0
Tostaco Shells	1 (0.8 oz)	130	7	1	0	2	14	1	40	10	—	0	—	0
Tostada Shells	3 (1.1 oz)	160	10	2	0	2	19	2	40	220	—	0	—	0
ROSARITA														
Taco Shells	1 shell (11 g)	50	2	2	0	1	7	tr	12	tr	25	—	—	—
Tostada Shells	1 shell (14 g)	60	3	2	0	1	8	tr	15	tr	35	—	—	—
TACO BELL														
Home Originals Taco Shells	3 (1.1 oz)	150	6	1	0	2	21	2	0	5	—	0	—	100
TAKE-OUT														
burrito w/ apple	1 sm (2.6 oz)	231	10	5	3	3	35	—	15	211	104	tr	4	405
burrito w/ apple	1 lg (5.4 oz)	484	20	7	7	5	73	—	32	443	218	2	4	849
burrito w/ beans	2 (7.6 oz)	448	14	7	5	14	71	—	113	986	653	2	118	332
burrito w/ beans & cheese	2 (6.5 oz)	377	12	7	27	15	55	—	214	1166	496	2	81	1250
burrito w/ beans & chili peppers	2 (7.2 oz)	413	15	8	33	16	58	—	100	1043	580	1	118	205
burrito w/ beans & meat	2 (8.1 oz)	508	18	8	48	22	66	—	105	1335	656	2	73	636
burrito w/ beans cheese & beef	2 (7.1 oz)	331	13	7	125	15	40	—	131	990	410	5	61	799
burrito w/ beans cheese & chili peppers	2 (11.8 oz)	663	23	11	158	33	85	—	288	2060	810	7	146	1596
burrito w/ beef	2 (7.7 oz)	523	21	10	65	27	59	—	84	1492	739	1	39	277
burrito w/ beef & chili peppers	2 (7.1 oz)	426	17	8	54	22	49	—	87	1116	499	2	37	463
burrito w/ beef cheese & chili peppers	2 (10.7 oz)	634	25	10	170	41	64	—	223	2091	667	4	58	972

FOOD	PORTION	CALORIES	FAT	SAT FAT	CHOL	PROTEIN	CARBO	FIBER	CALCIUM	SOD	POTAS	VIT C	FOLIC	VIT A
burrito w/ cherry	1 sm (2.6 oz)	231	10	5	3	3	35	—	15	211	104	tr	4	405
burrito w/ cherry	1 lg (5.4 oz)	484	20	7	7	5	73	—	32	443	218	2	4	849
chimichanga w/ beef	1 (6.1 oz)	425	20	9	9	20	43	—	63	910	587	5	31	147
chimichanga w/ beef & cheese	1 (6.4 oz)	443	23	11	51	20	39	—	238	956	203	3	34	540
chimichanga w/ beef & red chili peppers	1 (6.7 oz)	424	19	8	9	18	46	—	71	1169	613	tr	34	262
chimichanga w/ beef cheese & red chili peppers	1 (6.3 oz)	364	18	8	50	15	38	—	218	895	330	2	33	702
enchilada eggplant	1	142	5	—	7	—	—	—	124	—	—	—	—	—
enchilada w/ cheese	1 (5.7 oz)	320	19	11	44	10	29	—	324	784	240	tr	34	1160
enchilada w/ cheese & beef	1 (6.7 oz)	324	18	9	40	12	30	—	228	1320	574	1	192	1135
enchirito w/ cheese beef & beans	1 (6.8 oz)	344	16	8	49	18	34	—	217	1251	560	5	254	1015
frijoles w/ cheese	1 cup (5.9 oz)	226	8	4	36	11	29	—	188	882	605	2	111	457
nachos w/ cheese	6 to 8 (4 oz)	345	19	8	18	9	36	—	272	816	172	1	10	559
nachos w/ cheese & jalapeno peppers	6 to 8 (7.2 oz)	607	34	14	83	17	60	—	620	1736	292	tr	19	4061
nachos w/ cheese beans ground beef & peppers	6 to 8 (8.9 oz)	568	31	12	21	20	56	—	384	1800	451	5	39	3401
nachos w/ cinnamon & sugar	6 to 8 (3.8 oz)	592	36	18	39	7	63	—	85	439	75	8	7	108
taco	1 sm (6 oz)	370	21	11	57	21	27	—	221	802	473	2	23	855
taco salad	1½ cups	279	15	7	44	13	24	—	192	763	416	4	40	589
taco salad w/ chili con carne	1½ cups	288	13	6	4	17	27	—	246	886	393	3	64	1573
tostada w/ beans & cheese	1 (5.1 oz)	223	10	5	30	10	27	—	211	543	403	1	75	622
tostada w/ beans beef & cheese	1 (7.9 oz)	334	17	11	75	16	30	—	190	870	490	4	97	1275
tostada w/ beef & cheese	1 (5.7 oz)	315	16	10	41	19	23	—	217	896	572	3	15	713
tostada w/ guacamole	2 (9.2 oz)	360	23	10	39	12	32	—	424	789	649	4	110	1752

SPARE RIBS

(see PORK)

SPELT

ARROWHEAD

Spelt	1 oz	83	1	tr	—	4	20	4	2	1	119	—	—	—

SPICES

(see individual names, HERBS/SPICES)

SPINACH

CANNED

spinach	½ cup	25	1	tr	0	3	4	—	135	29	370	15	105	9390

FOOD	PORTION	CALORIES	FAT	SAT FAT	CHOL	PROTEIN	CARBO	FIBER	CALCIUM	SOD	POTAS	VIT C	FOLIC	VIT A
DEL MONTE														
50% Less Salt	½ cup (4 oz)	30	0	0	0	2	4	2	100	180	—	24	—	3000
Chopped	½ cup (4 oz)	30	0	0	0	2	4	2	100	360	—	24	—	2500
No Salt Added	½ cup (4 oz)	30	0	0	0	2	4	2	100	85	—	24	—	3000
Whole Leaf	½ cup (4 oz)	30	0	0	0	2	4	2	100	360	—	24	—	2500
POPEYE														
Chopped	½ cup (4.1 oz)	40	1	0	0	2	6	4	100	310	—	12	—	8000
Leaf	½ cup (4.2 oz)	45	1	0	0	2	7	4	150	310	—	15	—	8000
Low Sodium	½ cup (4.2 oz)	35	1	0	0	2	4	3	150	35	—	15	—	8000
SUNSHINE														
Chopped	½ cup (4.1 oz)	40	1	0	0	2	6	4	100	310	—	12	—	8000
FRESH														
malabar cooked	1 cup (1.5 oz)	10	tr	—	0	1	1	1	55	24	113	1	50	510
mustard chopped cooked	½ cup	14	tr	—	0	2	3	—	142	—	—	59	—	7380
mustard raw chopped	½ cup	17	tr	—	0	2	3	—	158	—	—	98	—	7425
new zealand chopped cooked	½ cup	11	tr	tr	0	1	2	—	43	97	92	14	—	3260
new zealand raw	½ cup	4	tr	tr	0	tr	1	—	16	36	36	8	—	1232
raw chopped	1 pkg (10 oz)	46	1	tr	0	6	7	—	202	160	1139	57	397	13699
DOLE														
Spinach	3 oz	9	tr	—	0	3	tr	8	—	107	379	21	—	4751
FRESH EXPRESS														
Spinach	1½ cups (3 oz)	40	0	0	0	2	10	5	60	160	—	15	—	3500
FROZEN														
cooked	½ cup	27	tr	tr	0	3	5	—	139	82	283	12	102	7395
AMY'S ORGANIC														
Pocket Sandwich Spinach Feta	1 (4.5 oz)	200	7	3	15	9	27	2	—	420	—	—	—	—
BIRDS EYE														
Creamed	½ cup (4.3 oz)	100	7	3	35	3	7	1	80	630	—	5	—	4500
Whole Leaf	1 cup (2.8 oz)	20	0	0	0	2	2	2	60	110	—	6	—	5500
BUDGET GOURMET														
Au Gratin	1 pkg (5.5 oz)	160	11	—	25	5	9	—	150	600	240	21	—	750
FRESH LIKE														
Cut Leaf	3.5 oz	21	tr	—	—	3	4	1	108	81	344	26	—	8194
GREEN GIANT														
Butter Sauce	½ cup (3.4 oz)	40	2	1	<5	2	5	2	100	280	—	18	—	2250
Creamed	½ cup (3.8 oz)	80	3	2	0	4	10	2	100	520	—	15	—	1500
Cut Leaf	¾ cup (2.6 oz)	25	0	0	0	3	3	3	100	65	—	12	—	3000
Harvest Fresh	½ cup (3.5 oz)	25	0	0	0	3	3	2	100	240	—	21	—	3500
STOUFFER'S														
Creamed	1 serv (4.5 oz)	160	12	4	15	4	8	2	100	380	410	5	—	2500
Souffle	1 serv (4 oz)	150	10	2	120	6	9	0	100	480	430	1	—	1750

FOOD	PORTION	CALORIES	FAT	SAT FAT	CHOL	PROTEIN	CARBO	FIBER	CALCIUM	SOD	POTAS	VIT C	FOLIC	VIT A
TABATCHNICK														
Creamed	7.5 oz	60	2	1	5	2	8	2	60	270	—	9	—	750
TAKE-OUT														
indian saag	1 serv	28	2	tr	0	2	2	1	—	44	—	—	—	—
spanakopita spinach pie	1 cup (6 oz)	196	3	2	30	14	35	4	250	590	—	9	—	1750

SPORTS DRINKS

(*see also* NUTRITIONAL SUPPLEMENTS)

FOOD	PORTION	CALORIES	FAT	SAT FAT	CHOL	PROTEIN	CARBO	FIBER	CALCIUM	SOD	POTAS	VIT C	FOLIC	VIT A
GATORADE														
Citrus Cooler	1 cup (8 oz)	50	0	0	0	0	14	—	—	110	25	—	—	—
Fruit Punch	1 cup (8 oz)	50	0	0	0	0	14	—	—	110	25	—	—	—
Grape	1 cup (8 oz)	50	0	0	0	0	14	—	—	110	25	—	—	—
Iced Tea Cooler	1 cup (8 oz)	50	0	0	0	0	14	—	—	110	25	—	—	—
Lemon-Lime	1 cup (8 oz)	50	0	0	0	0	14	—	—	110	25	—	—	—
Lemonade	1 cup (8 oz)	50	0	0	0	0	14	—	—	110	25	—	—	—
Orange	1 cup (8 oz)	50	0	0	0	0	14	—	—	110	25	—	—	—
Tropical Fruit	1 cup (8 oz)	50	0	0	0	0	14	—	—	110	25	—	—	—
POWERADE														
Fruit Punch	8 fl oz	72	0	0	0	0	19	—	—	28	32	—	—	—
Grape	8 fl oz	73	0	0	0	0	19	—	—	28	32	—	—	—
Lemon-Lime	8 fl oz	70	0	0	0	0	19	—	—	55	30	—	—	—
Orange	8 fl oz	72	0	0	0	0	19	—	—	28	32	—	—	—
SLICE														
All Sport Diet Lemon Lime	8 fl oz	1	0	0	0	tr	0	—	—	40	48	tr	—	—
All Sport Lemon Lime	8 fl oz	72	0	0	0	tr	19	—	—	55	57	tr	—	—
All Sport Orange	8 fl oz	74	0	0	0	tr	19	—	—	55	57	tr	—	—
All Sport Punch	8 fl oz	81	0	0	0	tr	22	—	—	55	57	tr	—	—
SNAPPLE														
Sport Fruit	1 bottle	80	0	0	0	0	20	—	0	60	50	24	—	0
Sport Lemon	1 bottle	80	0	0	0	0	20	—	0	60	50	24	—	0
Sport Lemon Lime	1 bottle	80	0	0	0	0	20	—	0	60	50	24	—	0
Sport Orange	1 bottle	80	0	0	0	0	20	—	0	60	50	24	—	0
ULTRA FUEL														
Lemon Lime	16 fl oz	400	0	0	0	0	100	—	—	55	99	60	—	—

SQUAB

FOOD	PORTION	CALORIES	FAT	SAT FAT	CHOL	PROTEIN	CARBO	FIBER	CALCIUM	SOD	POTAS	VIT C	FOLIC	VIT A
breast w/o skin raw	1 (3.5 oz)	135	5	1	91	22	0	—	—	—	—	—	—	—
w/ skin raw	1 squab (6.9 oz)	584	47	17	—	37	0	—	—	—	—	—	—	—
w/o skin raw	1 squab (5.9 oz)	239	13	3	—	29	0	—	—	—	—	—	—	—

FOOD	PORTION	CALORIES	FAT	SAT FAT	CHOL	PROTEIN	CARBO	FIBER	CALCIUM	SOD	POTAS	VIT C	FOLIC	VIT A
SQUASH														
(*see also* ZUCCHINI)														
CANNED														
crookneck sliced	½ cup	14	tr	tr	0	1	3	—	13	5	104	3	11	130
ALLEN														
Yellow	½ cup (4.2 oz)	25	0	0	0	0	5	2	40	160	—	1	—	0
SUNSHINE														
Yellow	½ cup (4.2 oz)	25	0	0	0	0	5	2	40	160	—	1	—	0
FRESH														
NATURE'S PASTA														
Spaghetti Squash	1 cup (5.5 oz)	20	0	0	0	1	4	2	40	30	180	48	—	200
FROZEN														
crookneck sliced cooked	½ cup	24	tr	tr	0	1	5	—	19	6	243	7	12	187
SEEDS														
dried	1 oz	154	13	2	0	7	5	—	12	5	229	—	—	108
dried	1 cup	747	63	12	0	34	25	—	59	24	1114	—	—	525
roasted	1 oz	148	12	2	0	9	4	—	12	5	229	—	—	—
roasted	1 cup	1184	96	18	0	75	31	—	97	40	1829	—	—	—
salted & roasted	1 cup	1184	96	18	0	75	31	—	97	1294	1829	—	—	—
salted & roasted	1 oz	148	12	2	0	9	4	—	12	5	229	—	—	—
whole roasted	1 oz	127	6	1	0	5	15	—	16	5	261	—	—	—
whole roasted	1 cup	285	12	2	0	12	34	—	35	12	588	—	—	—
whole salted roasted	1 cup	285	12	2	0	12	34	—	35	368	588	—	—	—
whole salted roasted	1 oz	127	6	1	0	6	15	—	16	191	261	—	—	—
SQUID														
fried	3 oz	149	6	2	221	15	7	—	33	260	237	4	—	—
raw	3 oz	78	1	tr	198	13	3	—	27	37	209	4	—	—
STAR FRUIT														
fresh	1	42	tr	—	0	1	10	—	6	2	207	27	—	626
SONOMA														
Dried	7-9 pieces (1.4 oz)	140	0	0	0	1	34	0	0	0	—	0	—	0
STRAWBERRIES														
CANNED														
in heavy syrup	½ cup	117	tr	tr	0	1	30	—	16	5	109	40	36	33
FRESH														
strawberries	1 pint	97	1	tr	0	2	22	—	45	4	530	182	57	87
DOLE														
Strawberries	8	50	0	—	0	1	13	3	—	0	230	95	—	—
FROZEN														
sweetened sliced	1 cup	245	tr	tr	0	1	66	—	29	8	249	106	38	61
sweetened sliced	1 pkg (10 oz)	273	tr	tr	0	2	74	—	31	9	277	118	42	68

FOOD	PORTION	CALORIES	FAT	SAT FAT	CHOL	PROTEIN	CARBO	FIBER	CALCIUM	SOD	POTAS	VIT C	FOLIC	VIT A
unsweetened	1 cup	52	tr	tr	0	1	14	—	23	3	220	61	25	66
whole sweetened	1 pkg (10 oz)	223	tr	tr	0	1	60	—	32	3	277	112	11	78
whole sweetened	1 cup	200	tr	tr	0	1	54	—	29	3	249	101	10	70
BIG VALLEY														
Strawberries	⅔ cup (4.9 oz)	50	0	0	0	tr	12	2	0		0	36	—	0
BIRDS EYE														
Halves	½ cup (4.7 oz)	120	0	0	0	tr	31	1	—	0	—	36	—	—
Halves In Lite Syrup	½ cup (4.6 oz)	70	0	0	0	tr	17	1	—	0	—	36	—	—
Whole	½ cup (4.5 oz)	100	0	0	0	tr	25	1	—	0	—	36	—	—

STRAWBERRY JUICE

FOOD	PORTION	CALORIES	FAT	SAT FAT	CHOL	PROTEIN	CARBO	FIBER	CALCIUM	SOD	POTAS	VIT C	FOLIC	VIT A
CAPRI SUN														
Strawberry Cooler Drink	1 pkg (7 oz)	90	0	0	0	0	25	0	0	20	20	0	—	0
KERN'S														
Nectar	6 fl oz	110	0	0	0	0	28	—	20	0	60	24	—	—
KOOL-AID														
Drink as prep w/ sugar	1 serv (8 oz)	100	0	0	0	0	25	0	0	30	0	6	—	0
Drink Mix as prep	1 serv (8 oz)	60	0	0	0	0	16	0	0	0	0	6	—	0
LIBBY														
Nectar	1 can (11.5 fl oz)	210	0	0	0	0	52	—	40	10	140	60	—	—
VERYFINE														
Juice-Ups	8 fl oz	140	0	0	0	0	36	0	0	15	—	60	—	0

STUFFING/DRESSING

FOOD	PORTION	CALORIES	FAT	SAT FAT	CHOL	PROTEIN	CARBO	FIBER	CALCIUM	SOD	POTAS	VIT C	FOLIC	VIT A
MIX														
bread dry as prep	½ cup	178	9	2	—	3	22	3	32	543	74	—	17	—
cornbread as prep	½ cup	179	9	2	0	3	22	—	26	455	62	1	8	353
ARNOLD														
All Purpose Seasoned	½ oz	50	0	0	0	2	9	1	—	200	—	—	—	—
Corn	½ oz	50	1	0	0	2	9	1	—	140	—	—	—	—
Herb Seasoned	½ oz	50	tr	—	0	10	2	1	—	150	—	—	—	—
Sage & Onion	½ oz	50	tr	0	0	2	9	1	—	230	—	—	—	—
BROWNBERRY														
Corn	1 oz	103	2	—	0	4	19	2	21	350	—	—	—	—
Herb	1 oz	100	1	—	0	3	19	2	17	297	—	—	—	—
Sage & Onion	1 oz	97	1	—	0	4	18	2	30	450	—	—	—	—
KELLOGG'S														
Croutettes	1 cup (1.2 oz)	120	0	0	0	5	25	0	40	460	50	0	—	0
PEPPERIDGE FARM														
Corn Bread	1 oz	110	1	—	—	3	22	—	20	320	—	—	—	—
Country Style	1 oz	100	1	—	—	4	21	—	40	400	—	—	—	—
Cube	1 oz	110	1	—	—	3	22	—	40	400	—	—	—	—

FOOD	PORTION	CALORIES	FAT	SAT FAT	CHOL	PROTEIN	CARBO	FIBER	CALCIUM	SOD	POTAS	VIT C	FOLIC	VIT A
PEPPERIDGE FARM (CONT.)														
Distinctive Apple Raisin	1 oz	110	1	—	—	3	21	—	20	410	—	1	—	—
Distinctive Classic Chicken	1 oz	110	1	—	—	4	20	—	40	410	—	5	—	300
Distinctive Country Garden Herb	1 oz	120	4	—	—	4	18	—	40	300	—	2	—	—
Distinctive Vegetable & Almond	1 oz	110	3	—	—	4	19	—	40	250	—	6	—	—
Distinctive Wild Rice & Mushroom	1 oz	130	5	—	—	4	17	—	20	310	—	5	—	—
Herb Seasoned	1 oz	110	1	—	—	3	22	—	40	380	—	—	—	—
STOVE TOP														
Chicken as prep w/ margarine	½ cup (3.6 oz)	170	9	2	0	4	20	tr	20	510	90	0	16	300
Cornbread as prep w/ margarine	½ cup (3.6 oz)	170	8	2	0	3	21	1	20	580	85	0	16	300
Flexible Serve Chicken as prep w/ margarine	½ cup (3.3 oz)	170	8	2	0	3	19	tr	20	520	70	0	16	300
Flexible Serve Cornbread as prep w/ margarine	½ cup (3.3 oz)	160	8	2	0	3	19	1	0	560	70	0	16	300
Flexible Serve Homestyle Herb as prep w/ margarine	½ cup (3.3 oz)	170	8	2	0	3	19	1	20	500	75	0	16	300
For Beef as prep w/ margarine	½ cup (3.7 oz)	180	9	2	0	4	22	1	20	540	100	0	16	500
For Pork as prep w/ margarine	½ cup (3.6 oz)	170	9	2	0	4	20	1	20	530	95	0	24	400
For Turkey as prep w/ margarine	½ cup (3.6 oz)	170	9	2	0	4	20	tr	20	530	90	0	16	300
Long Grain & Wild Rice as prep w/ margarine	½ cup (3.7 oz)	180	9	2	0	4	22	tr	20	500	75	0	16	300
Lower Sodium Chicken as prep w/ margarine	½ cup (3.6 oz)	180	9	2	0	4	21	tr	20	340	90	0	16	300
Microwave Chicken as prep w/ margarine	½ cup (3.5 oz)	160	7	2	0	4	20	tr	20	480	70	0	16	200
Microwave Homestyle Cornbread as prep w/ margarine	½ cup (3 oz)	160	7	2	0	3	20	tr	0	480	70	0	16	200
Mushroom & Onion as prep w/ margarine	½ cup (3.6 oz)	180	9	2	0	4	20	tr	20	480	85	0	16	300

FOOD	PORTION	CALORIES	FAT	SAT FAT	CHOL	PROTEIN	CARBO	FIBER	CALCIUM	SOD	POTAS	VIT C	FOLIC	VIT A
STOVE TOP (CONT.)														
San Francisco Style as prep w/ margarine	½ cup (3.6 oz)	170	9	2	0	4	20	1	20	530	100	0	24	500
Savory Herb as prep w/ margarine	½ cup (3.6 oz)	170	9	2	0	4	20	1	40	530	95	0	16	300
Traditional Sage as prep w/ margarine	½ cup (3.6 oz)	180	9	2	0	4	21	1	20	530	110	0	16	500
WONDER														
Seasoned Stuffing	1 cup (0.9 oz)	60	1	0	0	2	12	tr	40	135	30	—	—	—
TAKE-OUT														
bread	½ cup (3½ oz)	195	8	2	0	4	26	3	74	534	152	2	19	349
STURGEON														
cooked	3 oz	115	4	1	—	18	0	—	—	—	309	—	—	687
raw	3 oz	90	3	1	—	14	0	—	—	—	241	—	—	595
roe raw	3.5 oz	207	10	—	—	25	1	—	—	—	—	18	—	—
smoked	3 oz	147	4	1	—	27	0	—	—	—	—	—	—	—
smoked	1 oz	48	1	tr	—	9	0	—	—	—	—	—	—	—
SUGAR														
(*see also* FRUCTOSE, SUGAR SUBSTITUTES, SYRUP)														
brown packed	1 cup (7.7 oz)	828	0	0	0	0	214	—	167	86	762	0	1	0
brown unpacked	1 cup (5.1 oz)	546	0	0	0	0	141	—	123	57	502	0	1	0
maple	1 piece (1 oz)	100	tr	—	0	0	26	—	26	3	78	0	0	0
powdered	1 tbsp (0.3 oz)	31	0	0	0	0	8	—	0	0	0	0	0	0
powdered unsifted	1 cup (4.2 oz)	467	tr	—	0	tr	119	—	1	2	3	0	0	0
white	1 cup (7 oz)	773	0	0	0	0	200	—	2	3	4	0	0	0
white	1 packet (6 g)	25	0	0	0	0	6	—	tr	tr	tr	0	—	0
white	1 tbsp	45	0	0	0	0	12	—	tr	tr	tr	0	—	0
white	1 tsp (4 g)	15	0	0	0	0	4	—	0	0	0	0	0	0
C&H														
White	1 tsp	16	0	0	0	0	4	—	—	—	—	—	—	—
DOMINO														
White	1 tsp	16	0	0	0	0	4	—	—	0	—	—	—	—
HAIN														
Turbinado	1 tbsp	50	0	0	0	0	12	—	—	0	—	—	—	—
HOLLYWOOD														
Turbinado	1 tbsp	50	0	0	0	0	12	—	—	0	—	—	—	—
SUGAR SUBSTITUTES														
(*see also* FRUCTOSE)														
MRS. BATEMAN'S														
Sugarlike	1 tsp (4 g)	4	0	0	0	0	4	0	0	0	—	0	—	0
NATRATASTE														
Packet	1 pkg (1 g)	0	0	0	0	0	1	—	—	0	—	—	—	—
SWEET ONE														
Packet	1 pkg (1 g)	4	0	0	0	0	1	—	—	0	—	—	—	—

FOOD	PORTION	CALORIES	FAT	SAT FAT	CHOL	PROTEIN	CARBO	FIBER	CALCIUM	SOD	POTAS	VIT C	FOLIC	VIT A
SWEET'N LOW														
Granulated	1 pkg (1g)	4	0	0	0	—	—	—	1	1	1	—	—	—
WEIGHT WATCHERS														
Sweetner	1 serv (1 g)	5	0	0	0	0	1	0	0	30	—	0	—	0
SUGAR-APPLE														
fresh	1	146	tr	—	0	3	37	—	37	15	384	66	—	9
fresh cut up	1 cup	236	1	—	0	5	59	—	59	24	619	91	—	15
SUNCHOKE														
fresh raw sliced	½ cup	57	tr	0	0	2	13	—	10	—	—	3	—	15
SUNDAE TOPPINGS														
(*see* ICE CREAM TOPPINGS)														
SUNFLOWER														
seeds dried	1 oz	162	14	7	0	33	5	—	33	1	196	—	—	72
seeds dried	1 cup	821	71	7	0	33	27	—	168	4	992	—	—	72
seeds dry roasted	1 oz	165	14	1	0	5	7	—	20	1	241	—	—	—
seeds dry roasted	1 cup	745	64	7	0	25	31	—	90	4	1088	—	—	—
seeds dry roasted salted	1 oz	165	14	1	0	5	7	—	20	195	241	—	—	—
seeds dry roasted salted	1 cup	745	64	7	0	25	31	—	90	975	1088	—	—	—
seeds oil roasted	1 cup	830	78	8	0	29	20	—	76	4	652	2	316	—
seeds oil roasted salted	1 cup	830	78	8	0	29	20	—	76	804	6528	2	316	—
seeds oil roasted salted	1 oz	175	16	2	0	6	4	—	16	201	137	tr	67	—
seeds toasted	1 oz	176	16	2	0	5	6	—	16	1	139	—	—	—
seeds toasted	1 cup	826	76	8	0	23	28	—	76	4	658	—	—	—
seeds toasted salted	1 oz	176	16	2	0	5	6	—	16	204	139	—	—	—
seeds toasted salted	1 cup	826	76	8	0	23	28	—	76	817	658	—	—	—
sunflower butter	1 tbsp	93	8	1	0	3	4	—	19	82	12	tr	—	—
sunflower butter w/o salt	1 tbsp	93	8	1	0	3	4	—	19	1	12	tr	—	—
FISHER														
Seeds Oil Roasted	1 oz	170	15	2	0	8	6	—	20	170	—	—	—	—
Seeds Salted In Shell shelled	1 oz	160	14	1	0	6	6	—	20	100	—	—	—	—
Seeds Salted In Shell unshelled	1 oz	170	15	2	0	8	6	—	20	110	—	—	—	—
FRITO LAY														
Seeds	1 oz	160	14	—	0	7	6	—	20	265	—	—	—/	—
PLANTERS														
Kernels	1 pkg (1.7 oz)	290	25	3	0	11	9	7	60	260	340	—	—	—
Kernels	1 pkg (2 oz)	340	29	3	0	13	11	8	60	310	400	—	—	100
Kernels Barbecue	1 pkg (1.7 oz)	290	25	3	0	11	10	6	60	180	350	—	—	—
Kernels Honey Roasted	1 pkg (1.7 oz)	280	22	3	0	10	15	6	60	105	300	—	—	—

FOOD	PORTION	CALORIES	FAT	SAT FAT	CHOL	PROTEIN	CARBO	FIBER	CALCIUM	SOD	POTAS	VIT C	FOLIC	VIT A
PLANTERS (CONT.)														
Kernels Salted	1 oz	170	14	2	0	7	4	4	40	140	200	—	—	—
Munch'N Go Singles Dry Roasted	1 pkg	120	11	1	0	4	4	1	—	70	150	—	—	—
Nuts Dry Roasted	¼ cup (1.1 oz)	190	17	2	0	7	6	4	20	230	210	—	—	—
Original With Shell Dry Roasted	¾ cup	160	15	2	0	6	5	2	20	35	190	—	—	—
STONE-BUHR														
Seeds Raw	4 tsp (1 oz)	170	14	2	0	7	6	6	40	10	—	0	—	0

SUSHI

TAKE-OUT

FOOD	PORTION	CALORIES	FAT	SAT FAT	CHOL	PROTEIN	CARBO	FIBER	CALCIUM	SOD	POTAS	VIT C	FOLIC	VIT A
california roll	1 piece (0.8 oz)	28	1	tr	1	1	4	—	13	37	37	1	5	39
kim chi	⅓ cup (5.8 oz)	18	tr	tr	0	1	4	—	75	2143	188	21	60	510
sashimi	1 serv (6 oz)	198	7	1	63	24	4	—	25	718	668	4	8	1035
tuna roll	1 piece (0.7 oz)	23	tr	tr	3	2	3	—	2	33	24	tr	1	255
vegetable roll	1 piece (1.2 oz)	27	1	tr	0	1	5	—	20	47	60	3	16	371
vinegared ginger	⅓ cup (1.6 oz)	48	tr	tr	0	1	12	—	8	6	189	2	5	0
wasabi	2 tsp (0.3 oz)	5	tr	0	0	tr	1	—	6	124	28	0	0	0
yellowtail roll	1 piece (0.6 oz)	25	1	tr	0	1	3	—	12	32	14	1	3	57

SWAMP CABBAGE

FOOD	PORTION	CALORIES	FAT	SAT FAT	CHOL	PROTEIN	CARBO	FIBER	CALCIUM	SOD	POTAS	VIT C	FOLIC	VIT A
chopped cooked	½ cup	10	tr	—	0	1	2	—	26	60	139	8	—	2548
raw chopped	1 cup	11	tr	—	0	1	2	—	43	63	174	31	—	3528

SWEET POTATO

(*see also* YAM)

CANNED

FOOD	PORTION	CALORIES	FAT	SAT FAT	CHOL	PROTEIN	CARBO	FIBER	CALCIUM	SOD	POTAS	VIT C	FOLIC	VIT A
in syrup	½ cup	106	tr	tr	0	1	25	—	16	38	189	11	—	7014
pieces	1 cup	183	tr	tr	0	3	42	—	44	107	625	53	33	15965
PRINCELLA														
Mashed	⅔ cup (5.1 oz)	120	1	0	0	1	28	3	20	30	—	0	—	26500
ROYAL PRINCE														
Candied	½ cup (4.9 oz)	210	1	0	0	1	50	2	20	50	—	4	—	7500
Halves	3 pieces (5.7 oz)	190	1	0	0	1	46	4	40	40	—	4	—	27000
Orange Pineapple	½ cup (4.8 oz)	210	1	0	0	1	43	3	0	30	—	1	—	8500
SUGARY SAM														
Mashed	⅔ cup (5.1 oz)	120	1	0	0	1	28	3	20	30	—	0	—	26500
FRESH														
leaves cooked	½ cup	11	tr	tr	0	1	2	—	8	4	153	1	—	293
FROZEN														
cooked	½ cup	88	tr	tr	0	2	21	—	31	7	332	8	20	14441

FOOD	PORTION	CALORIES	FAT	SAT FAT	CHOL	PROTEIN	CARBO	FIBER	CALCIUM	SOD	POTAS	VIT C	FOLIC	VIT A
MRS. PAUL'S														
Candied Sweet Potatoes	4 oz	170	0	—	—	1	42	—	80	40	—	12	—	1750
Candied Sweets 'N Apples	4 oz	160	0	—	—	1	38	—	80	60	—	30	—	1250
TAKE-OUT														
candied	3½ oz	144	3	1	0	1	29	—	27	73	198	7	12	4399
SWEETBREADS														
beef braised	3 oz	230	15	—	—	23	0	—	14	51	209	17	—	0
lamb braised	3 oz	199	13	6	340	19	0	—	10	44	247	17	11	—
veal braised	3 oz	218	12	—	—	25	0	—	—	—	—	5	—	—
SWISS CHARD														
cooked	½ cup	18	tr	—	0	2	4	—	51	158	483	16	—	2762
raw chopped	½ cup	3	tr	—	0	tr	1	—	9	38	68	5	—	594
SWORDFISH														
cooked	3 oz	132	4	1	43	22	0	—	5	98	314	1	—	117
raw	3 oz	103	3	1	33	17	0	—	4	76	245	1	—	101
SYRUP														
(see also ICE CREAM TOPPINGS, PANCAKE/WAFFLE SYRUP)														
corn	2 tbsp	122	0	0	0	0	32	—	1	19	7	0	—	0
corn dark	1 tbsp (0.7 oz)	56	0	—	0	0	15	—	4	31	9	0	0	0
corn dark	1 cup (11.5 oz)	925	tr	—	0	0	251	—	58	608	144	0	0	0
corn light	1 cup (11.5 oz)	925	tr	—	0	0	251	—	10	395	13	0	0	0
corn light	1 tbsp (0.7 oz)	56	0	—	0	0	15	—	1	24	1	0	0	0
malt	1 tbsp (0.8 oz)	76	0	—	0	2	17	—	15	8	77	0	3	0
malt	1 cup (13 oz)	1222	tr	—	0	24	274	—	234	134	1229	0	46	0
maple	1 tbsp (0.8 oz)	52	0	—	0	0	13	—	13	2	41	0	0	—
maple	1 cup (11.1 oz)	824	1	—	0	tr	212	—	211	27	643	0	1	—
rose hip	3.5 oz	33	0	0	—	0	8	0	—	—	—	—	—	—
sorghum	1 cup (11.6 oz)	957	0	0	0	0	247	—	495	28	3300	—	—	—
sorghum	1 tbsp (0.7 oz)	61	0	0	0	0	16	—	31	2	210	—	—	—
ESTEE														
Blueberry Lite	¼ cup (2.4 oz)	80	0	0	0	0	20	—	—	70	—	—	—	—
MCILHENNY														
Cane	2 tbsp (1.4 oz)	130	0	0	0	tr	32	tr	22	20	—	tr	—	4
QUIK														
Strawberry	2 tbsp (1.5 oz)	110	0	0	0	0	27	0	0	0	5	0	—	0
RED WING														
Strawberry	2 tbsp (1.4 oz)	110	0	0	0	0	28	0	0	5	—	0	—	0
TREE OF LIFE														
Maple	¼ cup (2.1 oz)	200	0	0	0	0	53	—	60	7	—	—	—	—

FOOD	PORTION	CALORIES	FAT	SAT FAT	CHOL	PROTEIN	CARBO	FIBER	CALCIUM	SOD	POTAS	VIT C	FOLIC	VIT A
TREE OF LIFE (CONT.)														
Rice Syrup	2 tbsp (1 oz)	120	1	—	—	0	29	—	—	5	—	—	—	100
WHISTLING WINGS														
Blueberry	1 oz	45	tr	—	—	tr	10	tr	5	1	19	tr	—	—
Raspberry	1 oz	60	tr	—	—	tr	14	0	3	2	25	tr	—	—
TACO														
(*see* SPANISH FOOD)														
TAHINI														
(*see* SESAME)														
TAMARIND														
fresh	1	5	tr	tr	0	tr	1	—	1	1	13	tr	—	1
fresh cut up	1 cup	287	1	tr	0	3	75	—	89	33	753	4	—	36
TANGERINE														
CANNED														
in light syrup	½ cup	76	tr	tr	0	1	20	—	9	8	99	25	—	1058
juice pack	½ cup	46	tr	tr	0	1	12	—	14	7	165	43	—	1056
FRESH														
sections	1 cup	86	tr	tr	0	1	22	—	27	3	305	60	40	1794
tangerine	1	37	tr	tr	0	1	9	—	12	1	132	26	17	773
DOLE														
Tangerine	2	70	1	—	0	1	19	2	—	2	—	—	—	—
TANGERINE JUICE														
canned sweetened	1 cup	125	1	tr	0	1	30	—	45	2	443	55	—	1046
fresh	1 cup	106	tr	tr	0	1	25	—	44	2	440	77	—	1037
frzn sweetened as prep	1 cup	110	tr	tr	0	1	27	—	18	2	273	58	11	1382
frzn sweetened not prep	6 oz	344	1	tr	0	3	83	—	57	7	850	182	35	4310
AFTER THE FALL														
Juice	1 can (12 oz)	170	0	0	0	2	40	0	20	35	35	1	—	0
DOLE														
Mandarin frzn as prep	8 fl oz	140	0	0	0	1	35	0	20	30	380	60	0	200
FRESH SAMANTHA														
Fresh Juice	1 cup (8 oz)	106	1	0	0	2	24	1	40	0	—	66	8	1000
MINUTE MAID														
Frozen	8 fl oz	120	0	0	0	0	29	—	0	0	—	60	—	—
TAPIOCA														
pearl dry	⅓ cup	174	0	0	0	tr	45	1	10	0	6	0	2	—
MINUTE														
Minute Tapioca	1½ tsp (6 g)	20	0	0	0	0	5	0	0	0	0	0	—	0
TARO														
chips	1 oz	141	7	2	0	1	19	—	17	97	214	1	—	0
chips	10 (0.8 oz)	115	6	1	0	1	16	—	14	79	174	1	—	0

FOOD	PORTION	CALORIES	FAT	SAT FAT	CHOL	PROTEIN	CARBO	FIBER	CALCIUM	SOD	POTAS	VIT C	FOLIC	VIT A
leaves cooked	½ cup	18	tr	tr	0	2	3	—	63	2	341	26	—	3136
raw sliced	½ cup	56	tr	tr	0	1	14	—	22	6	307	2	—	0
shoots sliced cooked	½ cup	10	tr	tr	0	1	2	—	9	1	240	—	—	—
sliced cooked	½ cup (2.3 oz)	94	tr	tr	0	tr	23	—	12	10	319	3	—	0
tahitian sliced cooked	½ cup	30	tr	tr	0	3	5	—	101	37	423	26	—	1200

TARRAGON

ground	1 tsp	5	tr	—	0	tr	1	—	18	1	48	—	—	67

TEA/HERBAL TEA

(*see also* ICED TEA)

HERBAL

BIGELOW

Almond Orange	5 fl oz	tr	tr	—	0	tr	tr	—	1	tr	10	—	—	—
Apple Orchard	5 fl oz	5	tr	—	0	tr	1	—	5	tr	32	—	—	—
Apple Spice	5 fl oz	tr	tr	—	0	tr	tr	—	2	1	22	—	—	—
Chamomile	5 fl oz	tr	tr	—	0	tr	—	—	2	2	23	—	—	—
Chamomile Mint	5 fl oz	tr	tr	—	0	tr	tr	—	2	1	20	—	—	—
Cinnamon Orange	5 fl oz	tr	tr	—	0	tr	tr	—	5	tr	23	—	—	—
Early Riser	5 fl oz	3	tr	—	0	tr	1	—	1	tr	32	—	—	—
Feeling Free	5 fl oz	1	tr	—	0	tr	tr	—	13	1	44	—	—	—
Fruit & Almond	5 fl oz	1	tr	—	0	tr	tr	—	1	tr	10	—	—	—
Hibiscus & Rose Hips	5 fl oz	1	tr	—	0	tr	tr	—	13	1	44	—	—	—
I Love Lemon	5 fl oz	1	tr	—	0	tr	tr	—	3	tr	20	—	—	—
Lemon & C	5 fl oz	tr	tr	—	0	tr	tr	—	3	tr	14	—	—	—
Looking Good	5 fl oz	1	tr	—	0	tr	1	—	10	1	48	—	—	—
Mint Blend	5 fl oz	tr	tr	—	0	tr	tr	—	8	3	36	—	—	—
Mint Medley	5 fl oz	1	tr	—	0	tr	tr	—	8	3	36	—	—	—
Orange & C	5 fl oz	tr	tr	—	0	tr	tr	—	3	tr	16	—	—	—
Orange & Spice	5 fl oz	1	tr	—	0	tr	tr	—	4	1	20	—	—	—
Peppermint	5 fl oz	tr	tr	—	0	tr	tr	—	6	2	38	—	—	—
Roasted Grains & Carob	5 fl oz	3	tr	—	0	tr	1	—	2	1	27	—	—	—
Spearmint	5 fl oz	tr	tr	—	0	tr	tr	—	8	tr	19	—	—	—
Sweet Dreams	5 fl oz	1	tr	—	0	tr	tr	—	4	1	31	—	—	—
Take-A-Break	5 fl oz	3	tr	—	0	tr	1	—	2	1	27	—	—	—

CELESTIAL SEASONINGS

Almond Sunset	8 fl oz	3	tr	—	0	tr	1	—	—	2	20	—	—	—
Bengal Spice	8 fl oz	5	tr	—	0	1	tr	—	—	3	14	—	—	—
Caffeine Free	8 fl oz	2	tr	—	0	tr	1	—	—	5	26	—	—	—
Chamomile	8 fl oz	2	tr	—	0	tr	1	—	0	1	26	—	—	—
Cinnamon Apple Spice	8 fl oz	<3	tr	—	0	tr	tr	—	0	1	26	—	—	—
Cinnamon Rose	8 fl oz	<4	tr	—	0	tr	1	—	—	1	24	—	—	—

FOOD	PORTION	CALORIES	FAT	SAT FAT	CHOL	PROTEIN	CARBO	FIBER	CALCIUM	SOD	POTAS	VIT C	FOLIC	VIT A
CELESTIAL SEASONINGS (CONT.)														
Country Peach Spice	8 fl oz	3	tr	—	0	—	1	—	—	1	22	—	—	—
Cranberry Cove	8 fl oz	2	tr	—	0	tr	1	—	—	1	34	—	—	—
Emperor's Choice	8 fl oz	4	tr	—	0	tr	1	—	—	2	16	—	—	—
Ginseng Plus	8 fl oz	3	tr	—	0	tr	1	—	—	4	22	—	—	—
Grandma's Tummy Mint	8 fl oz	2	tr	—	0	tr	tr	—	—	7	31	—	—	—
Lemon Mist	8 fl oz	3	tr	—	0	tr	tr	—	—	3	35	—	—	—
Lemon Zinger	8 fl oz	4	tr	—	0	tr	1	—	—	1	38	—	—	—
Mama Bear's Cold Care	8 fl oz	6	tr	—	0	1	tr	—	—	2	21	—	—	—
Mandarin Orange Spice	8 fl oz	5	tr	—	0	tr	1	—	—	2	39	—	—	—
Mellow Mint	8 fl oz	2	tr	—	0	tr	tr	—	—	5	33	—	—	—
Mint Magic	8 fl oz	1	tr	—	0	tr	tr	—	—	13	13	—	—	—
Orange Zinger	8 fl oz	6	tr	—	0	tr	1	—	—	1	26	—	—	—
Peppermint	8 fl oz	2	tr	—	0	tr	1	—	—	9	38	—	—	—
Raspberry Patch	8 fl oz	4	tr	—	0	tr	1	—	—	1	29	—	—	—
Red Zinger	8 fl oz	4	tr	—	0	tr	1	—	—	2	49	—	—	—
Roastaroma	8 fl oz	10	tr	—	0	tr	2	—	—	3	22	—	—	—
Sleepytime	8 fl oz	4	tr	—	0	tr	1	—	—	2	31	—	—	—
Spearmint	8 fl oz	5	1	—	0	tr	tr	—	—	6	40	—	—	—
Strawberry Fields	8 fl oz	4	tr	—	0	tr	1	—	—	1	28	—	—	—
Sunburst C	8 fl oz	3	tr	—	0	tr	1	—	—	6	34	—	—	—
Tropical Escape	8 fl oz	1	tr	—	0	tr	tr	—	—	7	22	—	—	—
Wild Forest Blackberry	8 fl oz	2	tr	—	0	tr	1	—	—	1	21	—	—	—
LIPTON														
Bedtime Story	1 tea bag	0	0	0	0	0	0	—	—	0	—	0	—	—
Cinnamon Apple	1 tea bag	0	0	0	0	0	0	—	—	0	—	0	—	—
Country Cranberry	1 tea bag	0	0	0	0	0	0	—	—	0	—	0	—	—
Gentle Orange	1 tea bag	0	0	0	0	0	0	—	—	0	—	0	—	—
Ginger Twist	1 tea bag	0	0	0	0	0	0	—	—	0	—	0	—	—
Golden Lemon Honey	1 tea bag	0	0	0	0	0	tr	—	—	0	—	0	—	—
Lemon Soother	1 tea bag	0	0	0	0	0	tr	—	—	0	—	0	—	—
Peppermint Breeze	1 tea bag	0	0	0	0	0	0	—	—	0	—	0	—	—
REGULAR														
brewed tea	6 oz	2	0	0	0	0	tr	—	0	5	66	0	9	0
instant unsweetened as prep w/ water	8 oz	2	0	0	0	tr	tr	—	5	8	47	0	1	0
BIGELOW														
Chinese Fortune	5 fl oz	1	tr	—	0	tr	tr	—	1	tr	26	—	—	—
Cinnamon Stick	5 fl oz	1	tr	—	0	tr	tr	—	tr	tr	22	—	—	—

FOOD	PORTION	CALORIES	FAT	SAT FAT	CHOL	PROTEIN	CARBO	FIBER	CALCIUM	SOD	POTAS	VIT C	FOLIC	VIT A
BIGELOW (CONT.)														
Constant Comment	5 fl oz	1	tr	—	0	tr	tr	—	tr	tr	15	—	—	—
Darjeeling Blend	5 fl oz	1	tr	—	0	tr	tr	—	tr	tr	28	—	—	—
Earl Gray	5 fl oz	1	tr	—	0	tr	tr	—	tr	tr	23	—	—	—
English Teatime	5 fl oz	1	tr	—	0	tr	tr	—	tr	tr	31	—	—	—
Lemon Lift	5 fl oz	1	tr	—	0	tr	tr	—	tr	tr	18	—	—	—
Orange Pekoe	5 fl oz	1	tr	—	0	tr	tr	—	tr	tr	30	—	—	—
Peppermint Stick	5 fl oz	1	tr	—	0	tr	tr	—	1	1	14	—	—	—
Plantation Mint	5 fl oz	1	tr	—	0	tr	tr	—	tr	1	17	—	—	—
Raspberry Royale	5 fl oz	1	tr	—	0	tr	tr	—	tr	tr	26	—	—	—
CELESTIAL SEASONINGS														
Cinnamon Vienna	8 fl oz	2	tr	—	0	tr	1	—	—	1	21	—	—	—
Earl Grey Extraordinary	8 fl oz	3	tr	—	0	tr	1	—	—	tr	23	—	—	—
English Breakfast Classic	8 fl oz	3	tr	—	0	tr	tr	—	—	tr	30	—	—	—
Lemon	8 fl oz	7	tr	—	0	1	1	—	—	1	23	—	—	—
Mint	8 fl oz	4	tr	—	0	tr	tr	—	—	1	28	—	—	—
Morning Thunder	8 fl oz	3	tr	—	0	tr	tr	—	—	1	40	—	—	—
Naturally Decaffeinated	8 fl oz	10	1	—	0	1	tr	—	—	1	36	—	—	—
Orange Spice	8 fl oz	7	tr	—	0	1	1	—	—	1	26	—	—	—
Orange Spice Decaff	8 fl oz	7	tr	—	0	tr	1	—	—	1	31	—	—	—
Organically Grown	8 fl oz	12	tr	—	0	1	1	—	—	1	38	—	—	—
Raspberry	8 fl oz	7	tr	—	0	1	1	—	—	1	26	—	—	—
GENERAL FOODS														
International Instant Tea Decaffeinated English Breakfast Creme	1 serv (8 oz)	70	2	1	0	0	13	0	0	105	220	0	—	0
International Instant Tea Decaffeinated Viennese Cinnamon Creme	1 serv (8 oz)	70	2	1	0	0	13	0	0	105	220	0	—	0
International Instant Tea English Breakfast Creme as prep	1 serv (8 oz)	70	2	1	0	0	13	0	0	65	70	0	—	0
International Instant Tea English Raspberry Creme as prep	1 serv (8 oz)	70	2	1	0	0	13	0	0	65	80	0	—	0
International Instant Tea Island Orange Creme as prep	1 serv (8 oz)	70	2	1	0	0	13	0	0	65	80	0	—	0

FOOD	PORTION	CALORIES	FAT	SAT FAT	CHOL	PROTEIN	CARBO	FIBER	CALCIUM	SOD	POTAS	VIT C	FOLIC	VIT A
GENERAL FOODS (CONT.)														
International Instant Tea Viennese Cinnamon Creme as prep	1 serv (8 oz)	70	2	1	0	0	13	0	0	65	80	0	—	0
LIPTON														
Brisk Tea as prep	1 serv	0	0	0	0	0	0	0	0	0	—	0	—	0
Decaffeinated Brisk Tea as prep	1 serv	0	0	0	0	0	0	0	0	0	—	0	—	0
English Blend as prep	1 cup	0	0	0	0	0	0	0	0	0	—	0	—	0
Flavored Blackberry	1 tea bag	0	0	0	0	0	0	—	—	0	—	0	—	—
Flavored Decaffeinated Orange & Spice	1 tea bag	0	0	0	0	0	0	—	—	0	—	0	—	—
Flavored Honey & Lemon	1 tea bag	0	0	0	0	0	0	—	—	0	—	0	—	—
Flavored Mint	1 tea bag	0	0	0	0	0	0	—	—	0	—	0	—	—
Flavored Orange & Spice	1 tea bag	0	0	0	0	0	0	—	—	0	—	0	—	—
Flavored Raspberry	1 tea bag	0	0	0	0	0	0	—	—	0	—	0	—	—
Green Tea	1 tea bag	0	0	0	0	0	0	—	—	0	—	0	—	—
Loose Tea	1 tsp (2 g)	0	0	0	0	0	0	0	—	0	—	0	—	—
TETLEY														
Tea Bag as prep	1	0	0	0	0	0	0	0	—	0	28	—	—	—
TEFF														
ARROWHEAD														
Whole Grain	¼ cup (1.6 oz)	160	1	0	0	5	32	6	80	5	220	0	—	0
TEMPEH														
tempeh	½ cup	165	6	1	0	16	14	—	77	5	305	0	43	569
LIGHTLIFE														
Garden Vege	4 oz	142	4	1	0	18	9	2	140	125	—	5	—	250
Tempeh	4 oz	182	6	1	0	24	9	—	—	10	—	—	—	—
WHITE WAVE														
Burger	1 patty (3 oz)	110	3	0	0	12	10	6	20	270	—	2	—	0
Lemon Broil	1 patty (2 oz)	130	6	1	0	8	11	4	20	340	—	1	—	0
Organic Wild Rice	⅓ block (2.7 oz)	140	4	1	0	13	12	6	20	10	—	0	—	0
Teriyaki Burger	1 patty (3 oz)	110	2	0	0	10	11	6	20	340	—	1	—	0
THYME														
ground	1 tsp	4	tr	tr	0	tr	1	—	26	1	11	—	—	53
WATKINS														
Thyme	¼ tsp (0.5 oz)	0	0	0	0	0	0	0	0	0	—	0	—	0
TILEFISH														
cooked	½ fillet (5.3 oz)	220	7	1	—	37	0	—	39	88	768	—	—	—

FOOD	PORTION	CALORIES	FAT	SAT FAT	CHOL	PROTEIN	CARBO	FIBER	CALCIUM	SOD	POTAS	VIT C	FOLIC	VIT A
cooked	3 oz	125	4	1	—	21	0	—	22	50	435	—	—	—
raw	3 oz	81	2	tr	—	15	0	—	22	45	368	—	—	—

TOFU

AZUMAYA

Blue Label	3.5 oz	46	1	—	—	5	4	—	25	2	—	2	—	—
Green Label	3.5 oz	68	2	—	—	9	4	—	168	2	—	1	—	30
Name Age Fried	3.5 oz	144	4	—	—	17	9	—	162	2	—	1	—	130
Red Label	3.5 oz	68	1	—	—	9	5	—	164	3	—	1	—	—

CASBAH

Gyro as prep w/ tofu	1 patty (2 oz)	105	3	0	0	2	15	tr	90	480	—	0	—	50

LONG LIFE

Tofu	3 oz	60	3	0	0	6	2	1	100	10	—	0	—	0

MORI-NU

Extra Firm	1 in slice (3 oz)	55	2	0	0	7	2	—	20	60	—	0	—	0
Firm	1 in slice (3 oz)	50	3	0	0	6	2	—	20	30	—	0	—	0
Lite Extra Firm	1 in slice (3 oz)	35	1	0	0	6	1	—	20	80	—	0	—	0
Lite Firm	1 in slice (3 oz)	35	1	0	0	5	1	—	20	70	—	0	—	0
Soft	1 in slice (3 oz)	45	3	0	0	4	2	—	20	5	—	0	—	0

NASOYA

Chinise 5 Spice	¼ block (3 oz)	68	4	1	0	7	1	1	32	121	119	0	—	13
Extra Firm	⅕ block (3.2 oz)	92	5	1	0	11	1	tr	47	9	151	tr	—	9
Firm	⅕ block (3.2 oz)	76	4	1	0	9	2	tr	131	8	164	tr	—	8
French Country	⅕ block (3 oz)	68	4	1	tr	8	1	1	32	130	119	—	—	14
Silken	⅕ block (3.2 oz)	48	2	tr	0	5	2	tr	66	12	198	1	—	9
Soft	⅕ block (3.2 oz)	63	3	tr	0	7	2	tr	126	6	175	tr	—	6

TREE OF LIFE

Baked	⅕ block (3.2 oz)	150	8	1	0	16	5	0	250	310	—	—	—	—
Firm	⅕ block (3.2 oz)	100	5	—	0	9	2	0	150	5	—	—	—	—
Raw Firm	⅕ block (3.2 oz)	100	5	—	0	9	2	0	150	5	—	—	—	—
Ready Ground Hot & Spicy	⅓ pkg (3 oz)	60	4	1	0	7	2	0	100	10	—	0	—	0
Ready Ground Original	⅓ pkg (3 oz)	60	4	1	0	7	2	0	100	10	—	0	—	0
Ready Ground Savory Garlic	⅓ pkg (3 oz)	60	4	1	0	7	2	0	100	10	—	0	—	0

FOOD	PORTION	CALORIES	FAT	SAT FAT	CHOL	PROTEIN	CARBO	FIBER	CALCIUM	SOD	POTAS	VIT C	FOLIC	VIT A
TREE OF LIFE (CONT.)														
Reduced Fat	1/5 block (3.2 oz)	90	4	—	0	10	4	2	40	5	—	—	—	—
Savory Baked	1/5 block (3.2 oz)	140	8	1	0	15	4	0	250	310	—	—	—	—
Smoked Hot'N Spicy	1/2 block (3 oz)	120	5	1	0	18	3	0	20	120	—	0	—	0
Smoked Original	1/2 block (3 oz)	120	5	1	0	18	3	0	20	120	—	0	—	0
WHITE WAVE														
Baked Tofus Teriyaki Oriental Style	1/4 block (2 oz)	120	6	1	0	13	3	1	40	240	—	1	—	1250
Hard	4 oz	120	7	—	0	12	1	—	150	15	—	—	—	—
International Baked Italian Garlic Herb	1/4 pkg (2 oz)	120	6	1	0	13	3	1	40	240	—	1	—	1250
International Baked Mexican Jalapeno	1/4 pkg (2 oz)	120	6	1	0	13	3	1	40	240	—	1	—	1250
International Baked Oriental Teriyaki	1/4 pkg (2 oz)	120	6	1	0	13	3	1	40	240	—	1	—	1250
International Baked Thai Sesame Peanut	1/4 pkg (2 oz)	120	6	1	0	13	3	1	40	240	—	1	—	1250
Soft	4 oz	120	7	—	0	12	1	—	150	15	—	—	—	—
YOGURT														
STIR FRUITY														
Black Cherry	6 oz	141	2	—	—	6	25	—	117	51	—	2	—	196
Blueberry	6 oz	140	1	—	—	6	26	—	72	43	—	5	—	43
Lemon Chiffon	6 oz	152	3	—	—	6	26	—	111	43	—	3	—	—
Mixed Berry	6 oz	149	2	—	—	6	26	—	100	34	—	6	—	—
Orange	6 oz	143	2	—	—	6	26	—	115	51	—	5	—	34
Peach	6 oz	160	3	—	—	6	27	—	104	34	—	1	—	—
Pina Colada	6 oz	162	3	—	—	6	28	—	199	43	—	5	—	—
Raspberry	6 oz	155	2	—	—	6	29	—	144	34	—	3	—	—
Spiced Apple	6 oz	167	2	—	—	6	31	—	119	43	—	2	—	—
Strawberry	6 oz	140	2	—	—	6	25	—	113	51	—	3	—	34
Tropical Fruit	6 oz	170	2	—	—	6	32	—	150	43	—	4	—	—

TOMATO

(*see also* PIZZA, SPAGHETTI SAUCE)

FOOD	PORTION	CALORIES	FAT	SAT FAT	CHOL	PROTEIN	CARBO	FIBER	CALCIUM	SOD	POTAS	VIT C	FOLIC	VIT A
CANNED														
red whole	1/2 cup	24	tr	tr	0	1	5	—	32	195	265	18	—	725
sauce w/ mushrooms	1/2 cup	42	tr	tr	0	2	10	—	16	552	464	15	—	1165
sauce w/ onion	1/2 cup	52	tr	tr	0	1	12	—	20	672	504	16	—	1038
stewed	1/2 cup	34	tr	tr	0	1	8	—	47	325	307	17	—	710
w/ green chiles	1/2 cup	18	tr	tr	0	1	4	—	24	481	129	8	—	468
wedges in tomato juice	1/2 cup	34	tr	tr	0	1	8	—	34	285	329	19	—	757

FOOD	PORTION	CALORIES	FAT	SAT FAT	CHOL	PROTEIN	CARBO	FIBER	CALCIUM	SOD	POTAS	VIT C	FOLIC	VIT A
AMORE														
Sun-Dried Tomato Paste	1 tsp (6 g)	15	1	0	0	0	tr	0	0	115	—	0	—	200
CONTADINA														
Crushed	¼ cup	20	0	0	0	tr	4	1	20	150	—	6	—	400
Italian Paste	2 tbsp	40	1	—	—	1	7	1	—	320	—	6	—	300
Italian Style Pear	½ cup	25	0	0	0	1	4	1	20	220	—	12	—	500
Italian Style Stewed	½ cup	40	0	0	0	1	8	1	40	260	—	2	—	300
Mexican Style Stewed	½ cup	40	0	0	0	1	9	1	40	220	—	2	—	300
Pasta Ready Primavera	½ cup	50	2	1	—	1	8	1	60	600	—	9	—	750
Pasta Ready Tomatoes	½ cup	50	2	0	—	1	7	1	20	550	—	15	—	500
Pasta Ready With Crushed Red Pepper	½ cup	60	3	1	—	1	8	1	80	690	—	9	—	500
Pasta Ready With Mushrooms	½ cup	50	2	1	—	1	9	1	60	640	—	9	—	500
Pasta Ready With Olives	½ cup	60	3	1	—	1	8	1	80	640	—	9	—	500
Pasta Ready With Three Cheeses	½ cup	70	4	0	<5	1	8	tr	100	650	—	9	—	500
Paste	2 tbsp	30	0	0	0	2	6	1	—	20	—	6	—	500
Peeled Whole	½ cup	25	0	0	0	1	4	1	20	220	—	12	—	500
Puree	¼ cup	20	0	0	0	tr	4	tr	—	15	—	9	—	500
Recipe Ready	½ cup	25	0	0	0	1	5	3	40	200	—	9	—	750
Stewed	½ cup	40	0	0	0	1	9	1	40	250	—	9	—	400
DEL MONTE														
Paste	2 tbsp (1.2 oz)	30	0	0	0	1	7	2	0	25	—	9	—	750
Peeled Diced	½ cup (4.4 oz)	25	0	0	0	1	6	2	20	160	—	15	—	500
Puree	¼ cup (2.2 oz)	30	0	0	0	1	7	1	0	25	—	9	—	750
Sauce	¼ cup (2.1 oz)	20	0	0	0	tr	4	tr	0	340	—	5	—	200
Sauce No Salt Added	¼ cup (2.1 oz)	20	0	0	0	tr	4	tr	0	20	—	5	—	200
Stewed Cajun Style	½ cup (4.4 oz)	35	0	0	0	1	9	2	20	460	—	15	—	500
Stewed Chunky Chili	½ cup (4.5 oz)	30	0	0	0	1	8	2	20	600	—	15	—	500
Stewed Chunky Pasta	½ cup (4.5 oz)	45	0	0	0	1	11	2	20	560	—	15	—	500
Stewed Chunky Pizza	½ cup (4.5 oz)	35	0	0	0	1	9	2	20	670	—	15	—	500
Stewed Chunky Salsa	½ cup (4.5 oz)	35	0	0	0	1	8	2	20	560	—	15	—	500
Stewed Italian Style	½ cup (4.4 oz)	30	0	0	0	1	8	2	20	420	—	15	—	500
Stewed Mexican Style	½ cup (4.4 oz)	35	0	0	0	1	9	2	20	400	—	15	—	500
Stewed Original	½ cup (4.4 oz)	35	0	0	0	1	9	2	20	360	—	15	—	500

FOOD	PORTION	CALORIES	FAT	SAT FAT	CHOL	PROTEIN	CARBO	FIBER	CALCIUM	SOD	POTAS	VIT C	FOLIC	VIT A
DEL MONTE (CONT.)														
Stewed Original No Salt Added	½ cup (4.4 oz)	35	0	0	0	1	9	2	20	50	—	15	—	500
Wedges	½ cup (4.4 oz)	35	0	0	0	1	9	2	20	380	—	15	—	500
Whole Peeled	½ cup (4.4 oz)	25	0	0	0	1	6	2	20	160	—	15	—	500
EDEN														
Crushed Organic	¼ cup (2.1 oz)	20	0	0	0	1	3	1	6	0	170	10	—	641
Sauce Lightly Seasoned	¼ cup (2.1 oz)	25	0	0	0	1	5	1	9	45	260	10	—	738
HEALTH VALLEY														
Sauce	1 cup	70	1	—	0	2	13	tr	25	460	594	tr	2	4916
Sauce Low Sodium	1 cup	70	1	—	0	2	13	1	25	35	594	tr	2	4916
HEBREW NATIONAL														
Pickled	⅓ tomato (1 oz)	4	0	0	0	0	1	—	—	280		—		—
HUNT'S														
Choice Cut	½ cup (4.2 oz)	22	tr	0	0	1	5	1	30	325	—	14	—	145
Choice Cut Diced Tomatoes & Green Chiles	2 tbsp (0.4 oz)	1	0	0	0	tr	tr	tr	4	24	—	tr	—	15
Choice Cut Diced Tomatoes & Italian Herb	½ cup (4.2 oz)	24	—	—	—	1	5	1	27	600	—	18	—	145
Choice Cut Diced Tomatoes & Roasted Garlic	½ cup (4.2 oz)	24	0	0	0	1	5	1	27	505	—	18	—	145
Crushed	½ cup (4.2 oz)	29	tr	0	0	1	7	2	19	286	—	11	—	264
Crushed Angela Mia	½ cup (4.2 oz)	27	tr	0	0	2	6	2	25	380	—	3	—	101
Paste	2 tbsp (1.2 oz)	30	tr	0	0	1	6	2	13	88	—	7	—	121
Paste Italian	2 tbsp (1.2 oz)	27	tr	0	0	1	6	2	17	264	—	8	—	114
Paste No Salt Added	2 tbsp (1.2 oz)	30	tr	0	0	1	6	2	10	7	—	7	—	121
Paste With Garlic	2 tbsp (1.2 oz)	28	tr	0	0	1	6	2	17	281	—	7	—	77
Pear Shaped	½ cup (4.6 oz)	20	tr	0	0	1	4	1	3	360	—	28	—	46
Puree	¼ cup (2.2 oz)	24	tr	0	0	1	5	2	24	98	—	14	—	157
Ready Sauce Chunky Chili	¼ cup (2.2 oz)	22	tr	0	0	1	4	1	4	320	—	5	—	49
Ready Sauce Chunky Italian	¼ cup (2.2 oz)	26	tr	0	0	1	5	1	1	251	—	8	—	47
Ready Sauce Chunky Mexican	¼ cup (2.2 oz)	21	tr	0	0	1	4	1	12	390	—	7	—	116
Ready Sauce Chunky Special	¼ cup (2.2 oz)	21	tr	0	0	1	4	1	1	144	—	9	—	27
Ready Sauce Chunky Tomato	¼ cup (2.2 oz)	15	0	0	0	1	3	1	9	403	—	7	—	63
Ready Sauce Country Herb	¼ cup (2.2 oz)	33	1	tr	0	1	5	1	2	255	—	4	—	27

FOOD	PORTION	CALORIES	FAT	SAT FAT	CHOL	PROTEIN	CARBO	FIBER	CALCIUM	SOD	POTAS	VIT C	FOLIC	VIT A
HUNT'S (CONT.)														
Ready Sauce Garlic	¼ cup (2.2 oz)	29	1	tr	0	1	5	2	2	269	—	12	—	35
Ready Sauce Garlic & Herb	¼ cup (2.2 oz)	26	tr	0	0	1	5	1	47	202	—	5	—	105
Ready Sauce Meatloaf Fixins	¼ cup (2.2 oz)	23	tr	0	0	1	4	1	1	600	—	4	—	30
Ready Sauce Original	¼ cup (2.2 oz)	30	1	0	0	1	4	1	17	179	—	5	—	115
Ready Sauce Salsa	¼ cup (2.2 oz)	18	tr	0	0	1	3	1	27	357	—	4	—	63
Sauce	¼ cup (2.2 oz)	16	tr	0	0	1	3	1	8	366	—	7	—	160
Sauce Italian	¼ cup (2.2 oz)	32	1	0	0	1	5	1	18	210	—	3	—	160
Sauce No Salt Added	¼ cup (2.2 oz)	16	tr	0	0	1	3	1	18	12	—	7	—	160
Sauce With Herb	¼ cup (2.2 oz)	32	1	0	0	1	5	1	1	271	—	4	—	81
Stewed	½ cup (4.2 oz)	33	tr	0	0	1	7	2	28	357	—	7	—	123
Stewed Italian	4 oz	40	tr	—	0	2	9	tr	37	370	260	20	—	133
Tomatoes	½ cup (4.2 oz)	33	tr	0	0	1	7	2	36	31	—	7	—	124
Whole	2 (5.2 oz)	22	tr	0	0	2	4	1	34	403	—	19	—	50
MUIR GLEN														
Organic Chunky Sauce	¼ cup (2.3 oz)	20	0	0	0	tr	4	1	0	160	—	2	—	500
Organic Crushed With Basil	¼ cup (2.3 oz)	25	0	0	0	1	4	1	0	85	—	9	—	300
Organic Diced	½ cup (4.5 oz)	25	0	—	0	1	4	1	0	290	—	15	—	500
Organic Diced No Salt Added	½ cup (4.5 oz)	25	0	0	0	1	4	1	0	45	—	15	—	500
Organic Ground Peeled	¼ cup (2.3 oz)	10	0	0	0	tr	2	1	0	100	—	1	—	400
Organic Italian Style Diced	½ cup (4.4 oz)	25	0	0	0	1	4	1	0	290	—	15	—	500
Organic Paste	2 tbsp (1.2 oz)	30	0	0	0	2	6	1	0	20	—	6	—	500
Organic Puree	¼ cup (2.2 oz)	20	0	0	0	1	5	1	0	20	—	4	—	1000
Organic Sauce	¼ cup (2.2 oz)	20	0	0	0	tr	5	1	0	190	—	2	—	300
Organic Sauce No Salt Added	¼ cup (2.2 oz)	20	0	0	0	tr	5	1	0	30	—	2	—	300
Organic Stewed	½ cup (4.5 oz)	30	0	0	0	1	7	tr	40	290	—	15	—	200
Organic Stewed Italian Style	½ cup (4.4 oz)	30	0	0	0	1	7	tr	40	290	—	15	—	200
Organic Stewed Mexican Style	½ cup (4.4 oz)	30	0	0	0	1	7	tr	40	290	—	15	—	200
Organic Whole Peeled	½ cup (4.6 oz)	30	0	0	0	1	5	1	0	260	—	15	—	750
OLD EL PASO														
Tomatoes & Jalapenos	¼ cup (2 oz)	15	0	0	0	1	3	1	0	290	—	0	—	0
Tomatoes & Green Chilies	¼ cup (2 oz)	10	0	—	0	0	2	0	0	310	—	2	—	100

FOOD	PORTION	CALORIES	FAT	SAT FAT	CHOL	PROTEIN	CARBO	FIBER	CALCIUM	SOD	POTAS	VIT C	FOLIC	VIT A
PROGRESSO														
Crushed	¼ cup (2.1 oz)	20	0	0	0	1	4	1	20	95	—	6	—	300
Paste	2 tbsp (1.2 oz)	30	0	0	0	2	6	1	0	20	—	6	—	500
Peeled Whole	½ cup (4.2 oz)	25	0	0	0	1	4	1	20	220	—	12	—	500
Peeled w/ Basil	½ cup (4.2 oz)	25	0	0	0	1	4	1	20	220	—	12	—	500
Puree	¼ cup (2.2 oz)	25	0	0	0	1	5	1	0	15	—	9	—	750
Puree Thick Style	¼ cup (2.2 oz)	30	0	0	0	1	5	1	0	15	—	9	—	750
Sauce	¼ cup (2.1 oz)	20	0	0	0	1	4	1	0	260	—	2	—	300
RO-TEL														
Diced Tomatoes & Green Chilies	½ cup (4.4 oz)	20	0	0	0	tr	4	1	80	370	—	4	—	300
ROSOFF'S														
Pickled	⅓ tomato (1 oz)	5	0	0	0	0	1	—	—	290	—	—	—	—
SCHORR'S														
Pickled	⅓ tomato (1 oz)	4	0	0	0	0	1	—	—	280	—	—	—	—
SONOMA														
Dried Spice Medley oil drained	1 tbsp (0.5 oz)	50	4	0	0	1	3	1	0	200	—	0	—	0
Pesto	¼ cup (2 oz)	110	9	2	2	3	6	1	0	125	—	0	—	200
Tapenade	1 tbsp (0.7 oz)	70	6	1	0	1	4	1	0	5	—	0	—	100
TREE OF LIFE														
Sauce	¼ cup (2 oz)	20	0	0	0	1	4	—	0	9	—	9	—	300
DRIED														
SONOMA														
Bits	2-3 tsp (5 g)	15	0	0	0	1	3	1	0	5	—	0	—	0
Dried	2-3 halves (5 g)	15	0	0	0	1	3	1	—	5	—	—	—	—
Halves	2-3 halves (5 g)	15	0	0	0	1	3	1	0	5	—	0	—	0
Julienne	7-9 pieces (5 g)	15	0	0	0	1	3	1	0	5	—	0	—	0
Pasta Toss	½ cup (0.7 oz)	70	0	0	0	4	13	3	20	75	—	0	—	300
Season It	2-3 tsp (5 g)	20	0	0	0	1	3	1	0	25	—	0	—	0
FRESH														
green	1	30	tr	tr	0	1	6	—	16	16	251	29	—	789
TOMATO JUICE														
beef broth & tomato	5½ oz	61	tr	tr	—	1	14	—	19	220	162	2	—	215
clam & tomato	1 can (5½ oz)	77	tr	tr	—	1	18	—	21	664	149	7	—	357
tomato juice	6 oz	32	tr	tr	0	1	8	—	16	658	400	33	36	1012
tomato juice	½ cup	21	tr	tr	0	1	5	—	10	441	268	22	24	678
CAMPBELL														
Juice	6 oz	40	0	—	0	1	8	—	—	540	—	16	—	750

FOOD	PORTION	CALORIES	FAT	SAT FAT	CHOL	PROTEIN	CARBO	FIBER	CALCIUM	SOD	POTAS	VIT C	FOLIC	VIT A
DEL MONTE														
Snap-E-Tom	6 fl oz	40	0	0	0	2	8	1	0	500	—	12	—	2500
Snap-E-Tom	8 fl oz	50	0	0	0	2	11	2	20	670	—	18	—	3500
Snap-E-Tom	10 fl oz	60	0	0	0	3	13	2	20	840	—	20	—	4000
HUNT'S														
Juice	8 fl oz	22	tr	0	0	1	5	1	13	452	—	15	—	62
No Salt Added	8 fl oz	34	tr	0	0	2	8	2	10	12	—	22	—	94
MOTT'S														
Beefamato	8 fl oz	80	0	0	0	1	20	1	0	780	120	0	—	200
Clamato	8 fl oz	100	0	0	0	1	24	2	0	720	70	1	—	100
Clamato Caesar	8 fl oz	100	0	0	0	0	24	0	20	780	190	1	—	500
MUIR GLEN														
Organic	8 oz	40	0	—	0	3	7	tr	0	550	—	21	—	750
TONGUE														
beef simmered	3 oz	241	18	8	91	19	tr	—	6	51	153	tr	4	—
lamb braised	3 oz	234	17	7	161	18	0	—	8	57	134	6	2	—
pork braised	3 oz	230	16	5	124	20	0	0	16	93	—	1	3	0
TOPPINGS														
(*see* ICE CREAM TOPPINGS)														
TORTILLA														
(*see also* CHIPS TORTILLA, SPANISH FOOD)														
corn	1 (6 in diam)	56	1	tr	0	1	12	1	44	40	39	0	4	—
corn w/o salt	1-6 in diam (.9 oz)	56	1	tr	0	1	12	1	44	3	39	0	4	—
flour w/o salt	1-8 in diam (1.2 oz)	114	3	tr	0	3	20	1	44	167	46	0	4	0
ALVARADO ST. BAKERY														
Burrito Size	1 (2.2 oz)	170	4	0	0	5	30	1	—	480	—	—	—	—
Fajita Size	1 (1.6 oz)	130	3	0	0	4	23	1	—	370	—	—	—	—
OLD EL PASO														
Flour	1 (1.4 oz)	150	3	1	0	4	27	0	0	340	—	0	—	0
Soft Taco Tortilla	2 (1.8 oz)	180	4	1	0	5	33	0	0	410	—	0	—	0
TYSON														
Burrito Style Flour	1	170	4	—	0	5	29	—	—	40	—	—	—	—
Burrito Style Hand Stretched Small Flour	1	106	2	—	0	3	19	—	—	50	—	—	—	—
Burrito Style Heat Pressed Large Flour	1	182	4	—	0	5	33	—	—	90	—	—	—	—
Enchilada Style Corn	1	54	tr	—	0	1	11	—	—	4	—	—	—	—
Fajito Style Flour	1	89	2	—	0	3	15	—	—	21	—	—	—	—
Soft Taco Flour	1	121	3	—	0	4	20	—	—	28	—	—	—	—
Whole Wheat	1	120	3	—	0	4	20	—	—	32	—	—	—	—

FOOD	PORTION	CALORIES	FAT	SAT FAT	CHOL	PROTEIN	CARBO	FIBER	CALCIUM	SOD	POTAS	VIT C	FOLIC	VIT A
WONDER														
Low Fat Wheat	1 (1.4 oz)	120	2	1	0	3	24	1	60	280	—	—	—	—
Low Fat White	1 (1.4 oz)	110	2	1	0	3	22	1	60	280	—	—	—	—
ZAPATA														
Tortilla	1 (1.2 oz)	100	2	0	0	33	18	tr	0	250	—	0	—	0

TORTILLA CHIPS

(*see* CHIPS)

TREE FERN

FOOD	PORTION	CALORIES	FAT	SAT FAT	CHOL	PROTEIN	CARBO	FIBER	CALCIUM	SOD	POTAS	VIT C	FOLIC	VIT A
chopped cooked	½ cup	28	tr	—	0	tr	8	—	6	3	3	21	—	142

TRITICALE

FOOD	PORTION	CALORIES	FAT	SAT FAT	CHOL	PROTEIN	CARBO	FIBER	CALCIUM	SOD	POTAS	VIT C	FOLIC	VIT A
dry	½ cup	323	2	tr	0	13	69	17	36	5	318	0	70	—
triticale not prep	3.5 oz	329	2	—	—	13	64	7	38	26	444	—	17	—

TROUT

FOOD	PORTION	CALORIES	FAT	SAT FAT	CHOL	PROTEIN	CARBO	FIBER	CALCIUM	SOD	POTAS	VIT C	FOLIC	VIT A
rainbow cooked	3 oz	129	4	1	62	22	0	—	73	29	539	3	—	63
CLEAR SPRINGS														
Rainbow	3.5 oz	140	7	—	75	20	tr	—	90	35	410	—	—	—

TUMERIC

FOOD	PORTION	CALORIES	FAT	SAT FAT	CHOL	PROTEIN	CARBO	FIBER	CALCIUM	SOD	POTAS	VIT C	FOLIC	VIT A
ground	1 tsp	8	tr	—	0	tr	1	—	4	1	56	1	—	—

TUNA

(*see also* TUNA DISHES)

FOOD	PORTION	CALORIES	FAT	SAT FAT	CHOL	PROTEIN	CARBO	FIBER	CALCIUM	SOD	POTAS	VIT C	FOLIC	VIT A
CANNED														
light in oil	1 can (6 oz)	399	14	3	30	50	0	—	23	606	354	—	9	134
light in oil	3 oz	169	7	1	15	25	0	—	11	301	176	—	5	66
white in oil	3 oz	158	7	—	26	23	0	—	4	336	283	—	4	—
white in oil	1 can (6.2 oz)	331	14	—	55	47	0	—	8	704	593	—	8	—
BUMBLE BEE														
Chunk Light In Oil	2 oz	160	12	3	30	12	0	—	—	250	120	—	—	—
Chunk Light In Water	2 oz	60	1	1	30	12	0	—	—	250	120	—	—	—
Chunk White In Oil	2 oz	160	12	3	30	12	0	—	—	250	120	—	—	—
Chunk White In Water	2 oz	70	2	1	30	12	0	—	—	250	130	—	—	—
Chunk White In Water Diet	2 oz	60	1	—	—	13	0	—	—	30	—	—	—	—
Solid White In Oil	2 oz	130	8	2	30	14	0	—	—	250	130	—	—	—
Solid White In Water	2 oz	70	2	1	30	14	0	—	—	250	130	—	—	—
PROGRESSO														
In Olive Oil	¼ cup (2 oz)	160	12	2	30	13	0	0	0	250	—	0	—	0
TREE OF LIFE														
Tongol In Spring Water	2 oz	60	0	0	30	13	0	0	0	310	—	0	—	0
Tongol In Spring Water No Salt Water	2 oz	70	0	0	0	13	0	0	0	95	—	0	—	0

FOOD	PORTION	CALORIES	FAT	SAT FAT	CHOL	PROTEIN	CARBO	FIBER	CALCIUM	SOD	POTAS	VIT C	FOLIC	VIT A
FRESH														
bluefin cooked	3 oz	157	5	1	42	25	0	—	—	43	275	—	—	2142
bluefin raw	3 oz	122	4	1	32	20	0	—	—	33	214	—	—	1856

TUNA DISHES

MIX

BUMBLE BEE

FOOD	PORTION	CALORIES	FAT	SAT FAT	CHOL	PROTEIN	CARBO	FIBER	CALCIUM	SOD	POTAS	VIT C	FOLIC	VIT A
Tuna Mix-ins Classic Italian	⅓ pkg (0.17 oz)	25	0	0	0	0	5	—	—	5	—	—	—	—
Tuna Mix-ins Garden & Herb	⅓ pkg (0.17 oz)	25	0	—	0	0	5	—	—	5	—	—	—	—
Tuna Mix-ins Lemon Herb	⅓ pkg (0.17 oz)	25	0	0	0	0	6	—	—	5	—	—	—	—
Tuna Mix-ins Zesty Tomato	⅓ pkg (0.17 oz)	25	0	0	0	0	5	—	—	5	—	—	—	—

TUNA HELPER

FOOD	PORTION	CALORIES	FAT	SAT FAT	CHOL	PROTEIN	CARBO	FIBER	CALCIUM	SOD	POTAS	VIT C	FOLIC	VIT A
AuGratin 50% Less Fat Recipe as prep	1 cup	250	6	2	<15	30	36	1	100	870	270	0	60	400
AuGratin as prep	1 cup	310	12	3	20	30	36	1	100	930	270	0	60	400
Cheesy Pasta 50% Less Fat Recipe as prep	1 cup	230	5	2	15	26	32	tr	100	850	270	0	60	400
Cheesy Pasta as prep	1 cup	280	11	3	20	26	32	tr	100	890	270	0	60	400
Creamy Broccoli 50% Less Fat Recipe as prep	1 cup	240	5	2	15	28	35	1	80	820	290	0	60	400
Creamy Broccoli as prep	1 cup	280	11	3	20	28	35	1	80	880	290	0	60	400
Creamy Pasta 50% Less Fat Recipe as prep	1 cup	230	6	2	15	26	31	1	80	840	290	0	40	500
Creamy Pasta as prep	1 cup	300	13	4	20	26	31	1	80	910	290	0	40	500
Fettuccine Alfredo 50% Less Fat Recipe as prep	1 cup	240	6	2	15	14	32	1	80	870	260	0	60	400
Fettuccine Alfredo as prep	1 cup	310	14	4	15	14	32	1	80	950	260	0	60	400
Garden Cheddar 50% Less Fat Recipe as prep	1 cup	250	6	2	20	16	35	1	100	980	290	0	60	500
Garden Cheddar as prep	1 cup	310	12	3	20	16	35	1	100	1040	290	0	60	500
Pasta Salad Low Fat Recipe as prep	⅔ cup	230	2	0	10	10	26	1	20	790	160	0	40	100
Pasta Salad as prep	⅔ cup	380	27	3	10	10	26	1	20	730	160	0	40	100
Tetrazzini 50% Less Fat Recipe as prep	1 cup	240	5	2	20	17	33	1	60	930	250	0	60	400
Tetrazzini as prep	1 cup	310	12	3	20	17	33	1	60	1010	250	0	60	400

FOOD	PORTION	CALORIES	FAT	SAT FAT	CHOL	PROTEIN	CARBO	FIBER	CALCIUM	SOD	POTAS	VIT C	FOLIC	VIT A
TUNA HELPER (CONT.)														
Tuna Melt Reduced Fat Recipe as prep	1 cup	240	6	2	15	14	34	0	100	870	310	0	60	400
Tuna Melt as prep	1 cup	300	12	4	20	14	34	0	100	930	310	0	60	400
Tuna Pot Pie as prep	1 cup	440	24	7	110	18	40	1	150	1080	390	0	60	1250
Tuna Romanoff 50% Less Fat Recipe as prep	1 cup	240	3	1	20	15	38	1	40	740	270	0	60	200
Tuna Romanoff as prep	1 cup	280	8	2	20	15	38	1	40	800	270	0	60	200
READY-TO-EAT														
WAMPLER LONGACRE														
Salad	1 oz	60	4	—		5	2	3	—	—	130	—	—	—
TAKE-OUT														
tuna salad	3 oz	159	8	1	11	14	8	—	15	342	151	1	6	82
tuna salad	1 cup	383	19	3	27	33	19	—	35	824	365	5	15	199
tuna salad submarine sandwich w/ lettuce & oil	1	584	28	5	47	30	55	—	74	1294	335	4	58	188

TURKEY

(*see also* DINNER, HOT DOG, TURKEY DISHES, TURKEY SUBSTITUTES)

FOOD	PORTION	CALORIES	FAT	SAT FAT	CHOL	PROTEIN	CARBO	FIBER	CALCIUM	SOD	POTAS	VIT C	FOLIC	VIT A
CANNED														
w/ broth	½ can (2.5 oz)	116	5	1	—	17	0	—	9	332	—	1	—	0
w/ broth	1 can (5 oz)	231	10	3	—	34	0	—	17	663	—	3	—	0
ARMOUR														
Turkey Loaf	2 oz	110	8	—	40	8	1	—	—	390	—	—	—	—
HORMEL														
Chunk Turkey Ham	2 oz	70	4	2	40	9	0	0	0	600	—	1	—	0
SWANSON														
White	2½ oz	80	1	—	—	17	1	—	—	260	—	—	—	—
UNDERWOOD														
Chunky Light	2.08 oz	75	2	tr	25	11	2	—	—	330	160	—	—	—
FRESH														
back w/ skin roasted	½ back (9 oz)	637	38	11	238	70	0	—	87	191	682	0	21	0
breast w/ skin roasted	4 oz	212	8	2	83	32	0	—	24	70	323	0	7	0
dark meat w/ skin roasted	3.6 oz	230	12	4	93	29	0	—	34	79	285	0	9	0
dark meat w/o skin roasted	1 cup (5 oz)	262	10	3	119	40	0	—	45	110	406	0	13	0
dark meat w/o skin roasted	3 oz	170	7	2	78	26	0	—	19	72	264	0	9	0
leg w/ skin roasted	2.5 oz	147	7	2	61	20	0	—	23	55	199	0	6	0
leg w/ skin roasted	1 (1.2 lbs)	1133	54	17	466	152	0	—	176	420	1530	0	49	0

FOOD	PORTION	CALORIES	FAT	SAT FAT	CHOL	PROTEIN	CARBO	FIBER	CALCIUM	SOD	POTAS	VIT C	FOLIC	VIT A
light meat w/ skin roasted	from ½ turkey (2.3 lbs)	2069	87	25	794	87	0	—	225	658	2996	0	61	0
light meat w/ skin roasted	4.7 oz	268	11	3	103	39	0	—	29	85	388	0	8	0
light meat w/o skin roasted	4 oz	183	4	1	81	35	0	—	23	75	356	0	7	0
neck simmered	1 (5.3 oz)	274	11	4	186	41	0	—	56	84	226	0	12	0
skin roasted	from ½ turkey (9 oz)	1096	98	26	281	49	0	—	87	132	396	0	10	0
skin roasted	1 oz	141	13	3	36	13	0	—	11	17	51	0	1	0
w/ skin roasted	½ turkey (4 lbs)	3857	181	53	1514	522	0	—	488	1269	5207	0	130	0
w/ skin roasted	8.4 oz	498	23	7	196	67	0	—	63	164	673	0	17	0
w/ skin neck & giblets roasted	½ turkey (8.8 lbs)	4123	190	56	1920	190	1	—	525	1358	5473	1	409	4631
w/o skin roasted	7.3 oz	354	10	3	159	61	0	—	52	147	621	0	16	0
w/o skin roasted	1 cup (5 oz)	238	7	2	107	41	0	—	35	99	418	0	10	0
wing w/ skin roasted	1 (6.5 oz)	426	23	6	150	51	0	—	44	114	494	0	10	0
BUTTERBALL														
Ground All White Meat	3 oz	100	3	—	45	19	tr	—	—	55	—	—	—	—
LOUIS RICH														
Ground	4 oz	190	12	4	90	20	0	0	20	140	—	0	—	0
Patties White	1 (4 oz)	170	10	3	65	19	0	0	0	440	—	0	—	0
MR. TURKEY														
Ground 85% Fat Free	3.5 oz	210	16	—	110	18	0	—	—	90	—	—	—	—
Ground 91% Fat Free	3.5 oz	170	10	—	95	18	1	—	—	90	—	—	—	—
PERDUE														
Breast Tenderloins Cooked	3 oz	110	1	1	55	26	0	—	—	35	—	—	—	—
Breast Boneless Cooked	3 oz	110	1	0	55	26	0	—	—	35	—	—	—	—
Breast Cutlets Thin Sliced Cooked	1 (2.5 oz)	90	1	1	50	21	0	—	—	25	—	—	—	—
Breast Fillets Cooked	3 oz	110	1	1	55	26	0	—	—	50	—	—	—	—
Burger Cooked	1 (3 oz)	170	9	3	110	21	0	—	—	65	—	—	—	—
Cubed Steak Cooked	3 oz	120	3	1	85	24	0	—	—	60	—	—	—	—
Dark Cooked	3 oz	200	14	5	95	19	0	—	—	55	—	—	—	—
Drumsticks Roasted	3 oz	150	7	2	100	22	0	—	—	70	—	—	—	—
Drumsticks Cooked	3 oz	150	7	2	100	22	0	—	—	70	—	—	—	—
Ground Cooked	3 oz	170	9	3	110	21	0	—	—	65	—	—	—	—
Ground Breast Cooked	3 oz	110	2	1	55	24	0	—	—	40	—	—	—	—

FOOD	PORTION	CALORIES	FAT	SAT FAT	CHOL	PROTEIN	CARBO	FIBER	CALCIUM	SOD	POTAS	VIT C	FOLIC	VIT A
PERDUE (CONT.)														
Half Breast Cooked	3 oz	170	8	3	65	24	0	—	—	35	—	—	—	—
Thighs Cooked	3 oz	180	11	4	100	20	0	—	—	55	—	—	—	—
Tom Wings Cooked	3 oz	160	8	3	90	23	0	—	—	90	—	—	—	—
White Cooked	3 oz	170	9	3	70	22	0	—	—	35	—	—	—	—
Whole Breast Cooked	3 oz	170	8	3	65	23	0	—	—	30	—	—	—	—
Wings Roasted	1 (3 oz)	180	10	3	95	22	0	—	—	60	—	—	—	—
Wings Drummettes Roasted	1 (3.5 oz)	180	9	3	100	24	0	—	—	65	—	—	—	—
SHADY BROOK														
Cutlets	4 oz	130	1	0	70	28	—	—	—	55	—	—	—	—
Drumstick	4 oz	170	9	3	70	22	—	—	—	80	—	—	—	—
Ground Breast	4 oz	120	1	0	70	28	—	—	—	55	—	—	—	—
Ground Lean	4 oz	170	9	3	90	20	—	—	—	105	—	—	—	—
Ground Turkey 85%	4 oz	220	15	5	75	21	—	—	—	75	—	—	—	—
Mesquite Seasoned Tenderloin	4 oz	110	1	0	50	23	—	—	—	360	—	—	—	—
OnlyOne Boneless Breast Roast	4 oz	130	1	0	70	28	—	—	—	55	—	—	—	—
Split Breast	4 oz	190	9	3	70	24	—	—	—	60	—	—	—	—
Tenderloin	4 oz	130	1	0	70	28	—	—	—	55	—	—	—	—
Teriyaki Seasoned Tenderloin	4 oz	120	1	0	50	24	—	—	—	460	—	—	—	—
Thigh	4 oz	220	15	5	75	21	—	—	—	75	—	—	—	—
Turkey Burgers	4 oz	170	9	3	90	20	—	—	—	105	—	—	—	—
Turkey Meatloaf Lean	4 oz	150	7	2	95	18	—	—	—	400	—	—	—	—
Whole Breast	4 oz	190	9	3	70	24	—	—	—	60	—	—	—	—
Whole Turkey	4 oz	180	9	3	75	23	—	—	—	75	—	—	—	—
Wing	4 oz	220	14	4	80	23	—	—	—	60	—	—	—	—
Zesty Lemon Seasoned Tenderlion	4 oz	120	1	0	50	24	—	—	—	200	—	—	—	—
SWIFT-ECKRICH														
Ground All White	3 oz	100	3	—	45	19	tr	—	—	55	—	—	—	—
THE TURKEY STORE														
Seasoned Cuts Turkey Breast Roast	4 oz	110	1	0	45	22	4	—	—	530	—	—	—	—
WAMPLER LONGACRE														
Ground raw	1 oz	60	4	—	30	5	0	—	—	20	—	—	—	—
FROZEN														
roast boneless seasoned light & dark meat roasted	1 pkg (1.7 lbs)	1213	45	—	413	167	24	—	40	5320	2332	—	—	—

FOOD	PORTION	CALORIES	FAT	SAT FAT	CHOL	PROTEIN	CARBO	FIBER	CALCIUM	SOD	POTAS	VIT C	FOLIC	VIT A
EMPIRE														
Patties	1 (3.1 oz)	200	10	2	5	13	14	1	0	280	—	0	—	0
READY-TO-EAT														
bologna	1 oz	57	4	—	28	4	tr	—	24	249	56	—	—	—
breast	1 slice (0.75 oz)	23	tr	tr	9	5	0	—	1	301	58	0	—	0
diced light & dark seasoned	1 oz	39	2	1	—	5	tr	—	0	241	88	—	—	—
diced light & dark seasoned	½ lb	313	14	4	—	42	2	—	2	1928	703	—	—	—
ham thigh meat	2 oz	73	3	1	—	11	tr	—	5	565	184	—	—	—
ham thigh meat	1 pkg (8 oz)	291	12	4	—	43	1	—	22	2260	738	—	—	—
pastrami	2 oz	80	4	1	—	10	1	—	5	698	147	—	—	—
pastrami	1 pkg (8 oz)	320	14	4	—	42	4	—	20	2372	589	—	—	—
patties battered & fried	1 (2.3 oz)	181	12	—	—	9	10	—	9	512	176	—	—	—
patties battered & fried	1 (3.3 oz)	266	17	—	—	13	15	—	13	752	259	—	—	—
patties breaded & fried	1 (3.3 oz)	266	17	—	—	13	15	—	13	752	259	—	—	—
patties breaded & fried	1 (2.3 oz)	181	12	—	—	9	10	—	9	512	176	—	—	—
poultry salad sandwich spread	1 tbsp	109	2	tr	4	2	1	—	1	49	24	0	1	18
poultry salad sandwich spread	1 oz	238	4	1	9	4	2	—	3	107	52	0	1	39
prebasted breast w/ skin roasted	1 breast (3.8 lbs)	2175	60	17	718	383	0	—	149	6868	4281	0	—	0
prebasted breast w/ skin roasted	½ breast (1.9 lbs)	1087	30	8	359	191	0	—	75	3434	2141	0	—	0
prebasted thigh w/ skin roasted	1 thigh (11 oz)	494	27	8	194	59	0	—	25	1371	758	—	—	0
roll light & dark meat	1 oz	42	2	1	16	5	1	—	9	166	77	—	—	—
roll light meat	1 oz	42	2	1	12	5	2	—	11	139	71	—	—	—
salami cooked	2 oz	111	8	—	46	9	tr	—	11	569	138	—	—	—
salami cooked	1 pkg (8 oz)	446	31	—	186	37	1	—	44	2278	553	—	—	—
turkey loaf breast meat	1 pkg (6 oz)	187	3	1	69	38	0	—	12	2433	473	0	—	0
turkey loaf breast meat	2 slices (1.5 oz)	47	1	tr	17	10	0	—	3	608	118	0	—	0
turkey sticks battered & fried	1 stick (2.3 oz)	178	11	—	—	9	11	—	9	536	166	—	—	—
turkey sticks breaded & fried	1 stick (2.3 oz)	178	11	—	—	9	11	—	9	536	166	—	—	—
ALPINE LACE														
Breast Fat Free	2 oz	50	0	25	0	12	0	—	—	290	—	—	—	—

FOOD	PORTION	CALORIES	FAT	SAT FAT	CHOL	PROTEIN	CARBO	FIBER	CALCIUM	SOD	POTAS	VIT C	FOLIC	VIT A
CARL BUDDIG														
Honey Turkey	1 oz	40	2	1	15	5	1	—	0	360	55	0	—	0
Turkey	1 oz	50	3	1	15	5	1	0	20	340	55	0	—	0
Turkey Ham	1 oz	40	2	1	15	5	1	0	0	430	85	0	—	0
EMPIRE														
Barbecue Whole	5 oz	250	12	4	100	35	0	0	0	320	—	2	—	500
Bologna	3 slices (1.8 oz)	90	6	2	30	8	3	0	40	430	—	0	—	0
Oven Prepared Breast Slices	3 slices (1.8 oz)	50	1	0	15	10	1	0	0	200	—	0	—	0
Pastrami	3 slices (1.8 oz)	60	2	5	30	9	0	1	0	270	—	0	—	0
Salami	3 slices (1.8 oz)	70	4	1	35	9	1	0	0	350	—	0	—	0
Smoked Breast Slices	3 slices (1.8 oz)	40	0	0	15	8	0	0	0	350	—	0	—	0
FALLS														
BBQ	3 oz	140	8	—	55	17	—	—	—	300	—	—	—	—
Gourmet Breast	3 oz	80	1	—	35	18	—	—	—	320	—	—	—	—
Premium Cooked Breast	3 oz	100	2	—	40	20	—	—	—	240	—	—	—	—
HEALTHY CHOICE														
Deli-Thin Honey Roast & Smoked	6 slices (2 oz)	70	2	1	25	10	2	0	0	410	—	0	—	0
Deli-Thin Roasted Breast	6 slices (2 oz)	60	2	1	25	11	1	0	0	550	—	0	—	0
Deli-Thin Smoked Breast	6 slices (2 oz)	60	2	1	25	11	1	0	0	420	—	0	—	0
Deli-Thin Turkey Ham	6 slices (2 oz)	60	2	1	40	11	1	0	0	550	—	0	—	0
Fresh-Trak Honey Roast & Smoked Breast	1 slice (1 oz)	35	1	0	10	5	1	0	0	200	—	0	—	0
Fresh-Trak Oven Roasted Breast	1 slice (1 oz)	35	1	0	15	6	1	0	0	270	—	0	—	0
Honey Roasted & Smoked	1 slice (1 oz)	35	1	0	15	5	1	0	0	220	—	0	—	0
Oven Roasted Breast	1 slice (1 oz)	35	1	0	15	6	1	0	0	270	—	0	—	0
Smoked Breast	1 slice (1 oz)	30	1	0	10	6	0	0	0	230	—	0	—	0
Variety Pack Regular	3 slices (2.2 oz)	70	2	1	30	13	2	0	0	530	—	0	—	0
HEBREW NATIONAL														
Deli Thin Hickory Smoked	1.8 oz	55	1	—	25	11	—	—	—	310	—	—	—	—
Deli Thin Lemon Garlic	1.8 oz	50	1	—	20	11	—	—	—	400	—	—	—	—

FOOD	PORTION	CALORIES	FAT	SAT FAT	CHOL	PROTEIN	CARBO	FIBER	CALCIUM	SOD	POTAS	VIT C	FOLIC	VIT A
HEBREW NATIONAL (CONT.)														
Deli Thin Oven Roasted	1.8 oz	80	1	—	20	11	—	—	—	420	—	—	—	—
HILLSHIRE														
Deli Select Honey Roasted Breast	1 slice	10	tr	—	—	2	tr	—	—	90	—	—	—	—
Deli Select Oven Roasted Breast	1 slice	10	tr	—	—	2	tr	—	—	105	—	—	—	—
Deli Select Smoked Breast	1 slice	10	tr	—	—	2	tr	—	—	100	—	—	—	—
Deli Select Turkey Ham	1 slice	10	tr	—	—	2	tr	—	—	95	—	—	—	—
Flavor Pack 90-99% Fat Free Honey Roasted Breast	1 slice (0.75 oz)	20	tr	—	—	4	1	—	—	200	—	—	—	—
Flavor Pack 90-99% Fat Free Oven Roasted Breast	1 slice (0.75 oz)	20	tr	—	—	4	1	—	—	230	—	—	—	—
Flavor Pack 90-99% Fat Free Smoked Breast	1 slice (0.75 oz)	20	tr	—	—	4	tr	—	—	220	—	—	—	—
Honey Cured Breast	1 oz	35	1	—	—	5	2	—	—	340	—	—	—	—
Lunch 'N Munch Smoked Turkey/ Cheddar	1 pkg (4.5 oz)	350	21	—	—	21	20	—	—	1130	—	—	—	—
Lunch 'N Munch Smoked Turkey/ Cheddar/ Brownie	1 pkg (4.5 oz)	400	22	—	—	17	34	—	—	1240	—	—	—	—
Lunch 'N Munch Turkey/Cheddar/ Brownie/Hi-C	1 pkg (4.5 oz + 6 fl oz)	500	22	—	—	17	58	—	—	1260	—	—	—	—
Smoked Breast	1 oz	35	1	—	—	6	1	—	—	340	—	—	—	—
HORMEL														
Light & Lean 97 Breast Sliced	1 slice (1 oz)	30	1	0	15	5	0	0	0	380	—	0	—	0
Light & Lean 97 Mesquite Smoked Breast	1 slice (1 oz)	30	1	0	15	5	0	0	0	370	—	0	—	0
turkey pepperoni	17 slices (1 oz)	80	4	2	40	9	0	0	0	550	—	0	—	100
JORDAN'S														
Healthy Trim Fat Free Oven Roasted Breast	1 slice (1 oz)	20	0	0	15	4	0	0	0	180	—	0	—	0
Healthy Trim Fat Free Oven Roasted Smoked Breast	1 slice (1 oz)	20	0	0	15	4	0	0	0	180	—	0	—	0

FOOD	PORTION	CALORIES	FAT	SAT FAT	CHOL	PROTEIN	CARBO	FIBER	CALCIUM	SOD	POTAS	VIT C	FOLIC	VIT A
LOUIS RICH														
Bologna	1 slice (28 g)	50	4	1	20	3	1	0	40	270	—	0	—	0
Breaded Nuggets	4 (3.2 oz)	260	16	3	35	13	15	0	0	640	—	0	—	0
Breaded Patties	1 (3 oz)	220	13	3	35	12	13	0	0	530	—	0	—	0
Breaded Sticks	3 (3 oz)	230	15	3	35	12	12	0	0	580	—	0	—	0
Breast Skinless Hickory Smoked	2 oz	50	0	0	25	11	1	0	0	720	—	0	—	0
Breast Skinless Honey Roasted	2 oz	60	0	0	20	11	3	0	0	660	—	0	—	0
Breast Skinless Oven Roasted	2 oz	50	0	0	20	11	1	0	0	660	—	0	—	0
Breast Skinless Rotisserie	2 oz	50	0	0	20	11	1	0	0	670	—	0	—	0
Breast Slices Hickory Smoked	1 slice (2 oz)	50	0	0	25	11	1	0	0	720	—	0	—	0
Breast Slices Honey Roasted	1 slice (2 oz)	60	0	0	20	11	3	0	0	660	—	0	—	0
Breast Slices Oven Roasted	1 slice (2 oz)	50	0	0	20	11	1	0	0	660	—	0	—	0
Breast Slices Rotisserie	1 slice (2 oz)	50	0	0	20	11	1	0	0	670	—	0	—	0
Carving Board Hickory Smoked	2 slices (1.6 oz)	40	1	0	20	9	0	0	0	540	—	0	—	0
Carving Board Oven Roasted Thin	6 slices (2.1 oz)	60	1	0	25	12	1	0	0	710	—	0	—	0
Carving Board Oven Roasted Traditional	2 slices (1.6 oz)	40	1	0	20	9	0	0	0	540	—	0	—	0
Carving Board Rotisserie	2 slices (1.6 oz)	40	1	0	20	9	0	0	0	460	—	0	—	0
Cotto Salami	1 slice (28 g)	40	3	1	25	4	0	0	0	280	—	0	—	0
Deli-Thin Oven Roasted	4 slices (1.8 oz)	50	1	0	20	9	2	0	0	580	—	0	—	0
Deli-Thin Smoked	4 slices (1.8 oz)	50	2	1	20	9	1	0	0	480	—	0	—	0
Fat Free Hickory Smoked Breast	1 slice (1 oz)	25	0	0	10	4	1	0	0	300	—	0	—	0
Fat Free Oven Roasted Breast	1 slice (1 oz)	25	0	0	10	4	1	0	0	330	—	0	—	0
Fat Free Oven Roasted Deli-Thin Breast	4 slices (1.8 oz)	45	0	0	15	8	2	0	0	620	—	0	—	0
Fat Free Turkey Ham Honey	2 slices (1.7 oz)	35	0	0	15	7	2	0	0	600	—	0	—	0
Fat Free Turkey Ham Smoked	2 slices (1.7 oz)	35	0	0	15	7	1	0	0	580	—	0	—	0
Hickory Smoked	1 slice (1 oz)	30	1	0	10	5	1	0	0	260	—	0	—	0
Oven Roasted	1 slice (1 oz)	30	1	0	10	5	1	0	0	310	—	0	—	0

FOOD	PORTION	CALORIES	FAT	SAT FAT	CHOL	PROTEIN	CARBO	FIBER	CALCIUM	SOD	POTAS	VIT C	FOLIC	VIT A
LOUIS RICH (CONT.)														
Pastrami	1 slice (1 oz)	30	1	0	20	5	1	0	0	380	—	0	—	0
Salami	1 slice (28 g)	40	3	1	20	4	0	0	0	280	—	0	—	0
Smoked	1 slice (1 oz)	30	1	0	15	5	0	0	0	280	—	0	—	0
Turkey Ham	1 slice (1 oz)	30	1	0	20	5	1	0	0	380	—	0	—	0
Turkey Ham Chopped	1 slice (1 oz)	45	3	1	20	5	1	0	0	350	—	0	—	0
Turkey Ham Honey Cured	1 slice (1 oz)	30	1	0	20	5	1	0	0	350	—	0	—	0
MR. TURKEY														
Deli Cuts Hardwood Smoked Breast	3 slices	30	1	—	13	5	1	—	—	340	—	—	—	—
Deli Cuts Honey Roasted Breast	3 slices	30	1	—	15	5	2	—	—	310	—	—	—	—
Deli Cuts Oven Roasted Breast	3 slices	30	1	—	13	5	2	—	—	270	—	—	—	—
Deli Cuts Turkey Ham	3 slices	35	2	—	20	5	1	—	—	310	—	—	—	—
Deli Cuts Turkey Pastrami	3 slices	35	1	—	20	5	1	—	—	255	—	—	—	—
Hardwood Smoked Breast	1 slice	30	1	—	15	5	2	—	—	280	—	—	—	—
Hardwood Smoked Turkey Ham	1 slice	35	2	—	20	5	0	—	—	320	—	—	—	—
Honey Cured Turkey Ham	1 slice	30	1	—	20	5	1	—	—	320	—	—	—	—
Oven Roasted Breast	1 slice	30	1	—	15	5	2	—	—	270	—	—	—	—
Smoked Breakfast Turkey Ham	1 oz	30	1	—	18	5	1	—	—	325	—	—	—	—
Turkey Bologna	1 slice	70	5	—	25	3	1	—	—	370	—	—	—	—
Turkey Cotto Salami	1 slice	50	4	—	20	4	1	—	—	240	—	—	—	—
Turkey Ham	1 slice	35	2	—	20	5	0	—	—	320	—	—	—	—
Turkey Pastrami	1 slice	30	1	—	15	4	1	—	—	290	—	—	—	—
OSCAR MAYER														
Free Oven Roasted Breast	4 slices (1.8 oz)	40	0	0	15	8	2	0	0	670	—	0	—	0
Free Smoked Breast	4 slices (1.8 oz)	40	0	0	15	8	2	0	0	570	—	0	—	0
Lunchables Fun Pack Turkey/ Pacific Cooler	1 pkg (11.2 oz)	460	21	10	50	16	53	tr	200	1310	—	0	—	300
Lunchables Fun Pack Turkey/ Surger Cooler	1 pkg (11.2 oz)	440	16	8	45	14	60	0	200	1220	—	9	—	400
Lunchables Turkey/ Cheddar	1 pkg (4.5 oz)	360	22	11	70	20	20	1	300	1650	—	0	—	300

FOOD	PORTION	CALORIES	FAT	SAT FAT	CHOL	PROTEIN	CARBO	FIBER	CALCIUM	SOD	POTAS	VIT C	FOLIC	VIT A
OSCAR MAYER (CONT.)														
Oven Roasted White	1 slice (1 oz)	30	1	0	10	4	1	0	0	300	—	0	—	0
Smoked White	1 slice (1 oz)	30	1	0	10	4	1	0	0	310	—	0	—	0
PERDUE														
Nuggets Dinosaur	3 (3 oz)	200	12	3	35	9	15	2	—	390	—	—	—	—
SARA LEE														
Hardwood Smoked Breast Of Turkey	2 oz	60	1	0	20	13	0	—	—	550	—			
Hardwood Smoked Turkey Ham	2 oz	60	2	1	40	10	1	—	—	620	—	15	—	
Honey Roasted Breast Of Turkey	2 oz	60	0	0	20	12	2	—	—	550	—	9	—	
Honey Roasted Turkey Ham	2 oz	70	3	1	40	9	2	—	—	660	—	15	—	
Mesquite Smoked Breast Of Turkey	2 oz	60	2	1	30	12	0	—	—	510	—	—	—	
Oven Roasted Breast Of Turkey	2 oz	60	2	1	25	12	0	—	—	370	—	—	—	
Peppered Breast Of Turkey	2 oz	50	0	0	20	10	2	—	—	420	—	—	—	
Seasoned Breast Of Turkey Pastrami	2 oz	60	1	0	30	12	2	—	—	510	—	5	—	—
SHADY BROOK														
Black Forest Turkey Ham	2 oz	70	3	1	30	10	—	—	—	470	—	—	—	—
Browned Homestyle Oven Roasted Breast	2 oz	60	1	0	20	11	—	—	—	400	—	—	—	—
Browned Slow Roasted Breast	2 oz	60	0	0	20	11	—	—	—	400	—	—	—	—
Carved Breast Italian Seasoned	2 oz	60	0	0	20	12	—	—	—	490	—	—	—	—
Carved Breast Natural Roast	2 oz	60	0	0	20	12	—	—	—	470	—	—	—	—
Carved Breast Peppered	2 oz	60	0	0	20	12	—	—	—	450	—	—	—	—
Hickory Smoked Breast	2 oz	50	0	0	25	11	—	—	—	470	—	—	—	—
Honey Roasted Breast	2 oz	60	1	0	30	11	—	—	—	400	—	—	—	—
Honey Roasted Breast Covered w/ Cracked Pepper	2 oz	60	0	0	25	11	—	—	—	470	—	—	—	—
Meatballs Italian Style	3 oz	130	7	3	45	12	350	—	—	350	—	—	—	—
Smoked Drumstick	3 oz	180	8	3	70	22	—	—	—	620	—	—	—	—
Smoked Neck	3 oz	150	6	2	65	22	—	—	—	700	—	—	—	—

FOOD	PORTION	CALORIES	FAT	SAT FAT	CHOL	PROTEIN	CARBO	FIBER	CALCIUM	SOD	POTAS	VIT C	FOLIC	VIT A
SHADY BROOK (CONT.)														
Smoked Whole Turkey	3 oz	150	4	2	60	24	—	—	—	660	—	—	—	—
Smoked Wing	3 oz	200	10	3	65	22	—	—	—	680	—	—	—	—
TYSON														
Breast	1 slice	20	tr	—	—	4	tr	—	—	136	—	—	—	—
Ham	1 slice	23	tr	—	—	3	1	—	—	182	—	—	—	—
WAMPLER LONGACRE														
Bologna	1 oz	60	5	—	20	4	tr	—	—	260	—	—	—	—
Breast Chops	1 serv (4 oz)	120	1	—	50	22	0	—	—	90	—	—	—	—
Breast Sliced	1 slice (1 oz)	35	tr	—	30	3	1	—	—	310	—	—	—	—
Breast Sliced Smoked	1 slice (0.75 oz)	20	tr	—	10	4	1	—	—	210	—	—	—	—
Burger	1 (3 oz)	170	13	—	90	15	0	—	—	70	—	—	—	—
Burger	1 (4 oz)	230	17	—	120	20	0	—	—	90	—	—	—	—
Burger Barbecue	1 (4 oz)	240	17	—	120	19	4	—	—	280	—	—	—	—
Chef Select Breast Skinless	1 oz	35	tr	—	15	6	tr	—	—	220	—	—	—	—
Chef Select Breast Smoked	1 oz	35	1	—	15	6	1	—	—	240	—	—	—	—
Chunk Dark Smoked Cured	1 oz	45	3	—	25	4	1	—	—	300	—	—	—	—
Chunk Ham 12% Water Smoked	1 oz	45	3	—	15	4	tr	—	—	200	—	—	—	—
Chunk Ham 20% Water	1 oz	40	2	—	20	4	2	—	—	370	—	—	—	—
Chunk Pastrami	1 oz	35	2	—	20	6	tr	—	—	280	—	—	—	—
Cook-In-The-Bag Breast	1 oz	30	1	—	15	6	1	—	—	125	—	—	—	—
Cook-In-The-Bag Breast Mini	1 oz	30	1	—	10	6	tr	—	—	105	—	—	—	—
Cook-In-The-Bag Combo Roast	1 oz	35	1	—	15	7	tr	—	—	125	—	—	—	—
Cook-In-The-Bag Thigh Roast	1 oz	40	2	—	15	6	1	—	—	130	—	—	—	—
Dark Smoked Cured	1 oz	45	3	—	25	4	1	—	—	3000	—	—	—	—
Deli Chef Breast And White Meat No Skin	1 oz	40	2	—	15	4	1	—	—	240	—	—	—	—
Gourmet Breast	1 oz	35	1	—	15	5	1	—	—	300	—	—	—	—
Gourmet Breast Mini	1 oz	35	1	—	15	5	1	—	—	300	—	—	—	—
Gourmet Breast Mini Smoked	1 oz	35	1	—	15	6	1	—	—	240	—	—	—	—
Gourmet Breast Smoked	1 oz	30	tr	—	15	6	1	—	—	230	—	—	—	—

FOOD	PORTION	CALORIES	FAT	SAT FAT	CHOL	PROTEIN	CARBO	FIBER	CALCIUM	SOD	POTAS	VIT C	FOLIC	VIT A
WAMPLER LONGACRE (CONT.)														
Gourmet Brown & Glazed Breast	1 oz	35	1	—	15	5	1	—	—	240	—	—	—	—
Gourmet Brown & Roasted Breast	1 oz	35	1	—	15	5	1	—	—	260	—	—	—	—
Gourmet Honey Cured Breast	1 oz	30	1	—	15	5	1	—	—	210	—	—	—	—
Lean-Lite Breast Skinless	1 oz	35	tr	—	15	6	0	—	—	160	—	—	—	—
Lean-Lite Deli Breast	1 oz	35	1	—	15	6	0	—	—	160	—	—	—	—
Lean-Lite Deli Breast Smoked	1 oz	35	1	—	15	6	1	—	—	170	—	—	—	—
Old Fashioned Brown & Roasted Breast	1 oz	35	tr	—	15	6	tr	—	—	160	—	—	—	—
Pastrami	1 oz	35	2	—	20	6	tr	—	—	280	—	—	—	—
Premium Breast Skinless	1 oz	30	tr	—	15	4	1	—	—	250	—	—	—	—
Premium Brown & Roasted Breast Skinless	1 oz	16	1	—	15	5	1	—	—	300	—	—	—	—
Roll Combo	1 oz	44	3	—	17	4	tr	—	—	187	—	—	—	—
Roll Sliced Breast	1 slice (0.75 oz)	30	tr	—	30	4	1	—	—	250	—	—	—	—
Roll White	1 oz	45	3	—	15	4	tr	—	—	200	—	—	—	—
Salami	1 oz	50	3	—	20	5	1	—	—	280	—	—	—	—
Salt Watchers Breast Skinless	1 oz	35	1	—	15	7	0	—	—	20	—	—	—	—
Seasoned Roast	1 oz	40	2	—	15	6	0	—	—	90	—	—	—	—
Sliced Salami	1 slice (0.8 oz)	45	3	—	20	3	1	—	—	240	—	—	—	—
Tenderlings BBQ	1 serv (4 oz)	110	tr	—	40	24	0	—	—	520	—	—	—	—
Tenderlings Cajun	1 serv (4 oz)	110	tr	—	40	24	0	—	—	560	—	—	—	—
Tenderlings Garlic & Pepper	1 serv (4 oz)	110	tr	—	40	24	0	—	—	600	—	—	—	—
Tenderlings Original	1 serv (4 oz)	110	tr	—	40	24	0	—	—	480	—	—	—	—
Turkey Ham 12% Water Baked	1 oz	45	3	—	15	4	tr	—	—	200	—	—	—	—
Turkey Ham 20% Water Baked	1 oz	40	2	—	20	4	1	—	—	370	—	—	—	—
Unseasoned Roast	1 oz	40	2	—	15	6	0	—	—	15	—	—	—	—
Whole Browned & Roasted	1 oz	60	3	—	20	7	tr	—	—	100	—	—	—	—
WEIGHT WATCHERS														
Deli Thin Smoked Breast	5 slices (1/3 oz)	10	tr	—	5	2	tr	—	—	80	—	—	—	—

FOOD	PORTION	CALORIES	FAT	SAT FAT	CHOL	PROTEIN	CARBO	FIBER	CALCIUM	SOD	POTAS	VIT C	FOLIC	VIT A
WEIGHT WATCHERS (CONT.)														
Oven Roasted Breast	2 slices (¾ oz)	25	1	—	10	4	tr	—	—	200	—	—	—	—
Oven Roasted Turkey Ham	2 slices (¾ oz)	25	1	—	10	4	tr	—	—	210	—	—	—	—
Roasted & Smoked Breast	2 slices (¾ oz)	25	1	—	10	4	tr	—	—	170	—	—	—	—

TURKEY DISHES

(*see also* DINNER, TURKEY SUBSTITUTES)

CANNED

FOOD	PORTION	CALORIES	FAT	SAT FAT	CHOL	PROTEIN	CARBO	FIBER	CALCIUM	SOD	POTAS	VIT C	FOLIC	VIT A
DINTY MOORE														
Stew	1 cup (8.5 oz)	140	3	1	20	10	19	2	20	910	—	2	—	750
FROZEN														
gravy & turkey	1 cup (8.4 oz)	160	6	2	—	14	11	—	33	1328	—	—	—	100
gravy & turkey	1 pkg (5 oz)	95	4	1	—	8	7	—	20	786	—	—	—	59
HOT POCKET														
Stuffed Sandwich Turkey & Ham With Cheese	1 (4.5 oz)	320	13	6	35	14	38	1	300	680	—	0	—	200
LEAN POCKETS														
Stuffed Sandwich Turkey & Ham With Cheddar	1 (4.5 oz)	260	7	3	35	15	35	4	150	810	—	12	—	300
Stuffed Sandwich Turkey Broccoli & Cheese	1 (4.5 oz)	260	8	3	35	12	35	4	200	710	—	0	—	500
LUIGINO'S														
Gravy Dressing & Turkey	1 pkg (8 oz)	340	15	4	40	16	36	2	80	910	—	0	—	100
READY-TO-EAT														
SHADY BROOK														
Meatloaf	1 serv (16 oz)	470	17	10	175	38	—	—	—	900	—	—	—	—
WAMPLER LONGACRE														
Meatloaf Italian	1 serv (4 oz)	114	5	—	56	17	5	—	—	640	—	—	—	—
Meatloaf Mexican	1 serv (4 oz)	114	5	—	56	17	4	—	—	680	—	—	—	—
Meatloaf Original	1 serv (4 oz)	126	5	—	80	18	10	—	—	620	—	—	—	—
Salad	1 oz	60	4	—	10	4	3	—	—	140	—	—	—	—
Salad Turkey Ham	1 oz	50	4	—	10	2	3	—	—	190	—	—	—	—
Teriyaki	1 serv (4 oz)	112	tr	—	25	11	14	—	—	640	—	—	—	—
SHELF-STABLE														
DINTY MOORE														
Microwave Cup Stew	1 pkg (7.5 oz)	130	3	1	10	9	16	2	20	760	—	4	—	500

TURKEY SUBSTITUTES

FOOD	PORTION	CALORIES	FAT	SAT FAT	CHOL	PROTEIN	CARBO	FIBER	CALCIUM	SOD	POTAS	VIT C	FOLIC	VIT A
HARVEST DIRECT														
TVP Poultry Chunks	3.5 oz	280	1	tr	0	52	32	18	—	15	2200	—	—	—

FOOD	PORTION	CALORIES	FAT	SAT FAT	CHOL	PROTEIN	CARBO	FIBER	CALCIUM	SOD	POTAS	VIT C	FOLIC	VIT A
HARVEST DIRECT (CONT.)														
TVP Poultry Ground	3.5 oz	280	1	tr	0	52	32	18	—	15	2200	—	—	—
SOY IS US														
Turkey Not!	½ cup (1.75 oz)	140	2	1	0	25	15	9	160	5	—	0	—	0
WHITE WAVE														
Meatless Sandwich Slices	2 slices (1.6 oz)	80	0	0	0	13	7	1	0	400	—	0	—	0
WORTHINGTON														
Smoked Turkey Meatless	3 slices (2 oz)	140	10	2	0	10	3	2	0	620	70	0	—	0
Turkee Slices	3 slices (3.3 oz)	130	14	3	0	13	3	2	0	580	45	0	—	0
TURNIPS														
CANNED														
greens	½ cup	17	tr	tr	0	2	3	—	138	325	165	18	48	4196
ALLEN														
Chopped Greens And Diced Turnip	½ cup (4.2 oz)	30	1	0	0	1	5	tr	100	20	—	9	—	5500
Greens	½ cup (4.2 oz)	25	1	0	0	2	3	2	100	15	—	9	—	5500
SUNSHINE														
Chopped Greens And Diced Turnip	½ cup (4.2 oz)	30	1	0	0	1	5	tr	100	20	—	9	—	5500
Greens	½ cup (4.2 oz)	25	1	0	0	2	3	2	100	15	—	9	—	5500
FRESH														
cooked mashed	½ cup (4.2 oz)	47	tr	tr	0	2	10	—	58	25	391	23	19	674
cubed cooked	½ cup (3 oz)	33	tr	tr	0	1	7	—	41	17	277	17	13	477
raw cubed	½ cup (2.4 oz)	25	tr	tr	0	1	6	—	39	14	236	18	14	406
FROZEN														
BIRDS EYE														
Chopped Greens	1 cup (3.1 oz)	30	0	0	0	1	1	1	80	20	—	15	—	2250
VANILLA														
VIRGINIA DARE														
Vanilla Extract	1 tsp	10	0	—	0	—	—	—	0	—	—	—	—	—
VEAL														
(see also DINNER, VEAL DISHES)														
FRESH														
cutlet lean only braised	3 oz	172	4	2	115	31	0	—	7	57	329	—	15	—
cutlet lean only fried	3 oz	156	4	1	91	28	0	—	6	65	375	—	14	—
ground broiled	3 oz	146	6	3	87	21	0	—	14	70	287	—	10	—
loin chop w/ bone lean & fat braised	1 chop (2.8 oz)	227	14	5	94	24	0	—	22	64	224	—	11	—
loin chop w/ bone lean only braised	1 chop (2.4 oz)	155	6	2	86	23	0	—	22	58	205	—	10	—

FOOD	PORTION	CALORIES	FAT	SAT FAT	CHOL	PROTEIN	CARBO	FIBER	CALCIUM	SOD	POTAS	VIT C	FOLIC	VIT A
shoulder w/ bone lean only braised	3 oz	169	5	1	110	29	0	—	31	83	271	—	14	—
sirloin w/ bone lean & fat roasted	3 oz	171	9	4	87	21	0	—	11	71	299	—	13	—
sirloin w/ bone lean only roasted	3 oz	143	5	2	89	22	0	—	12	72	310	—	13	—

VEGETABLE JUICE

FOOD	PORTION	CALORIES	FAT	SAT FAT	CHOL	PROTEIN	CARBO	FIBER	CALCIUM	SOD	POTAS	VIT C	FOLIC	VIT A
vegetable juice cocktail	6 fl oz	34	tr	tr	0	1	8	—	20	664	351	50	—	2130
vegetable juice cocktail	½ cup	22	tr	tr	0	1	6	—	13	442	234	34	—	1416
MOTT'S														
Vegetable Juice as prep	8 fl oz	60	0	0	0	2	13	2	20	800	710	2	—	7000
MUIR GLEN														
Organic	8 oz	70	0	—	0	2	15	3	80	620	—	60	—	7000
Organic Reduced Sodium	8 oz	70	0	—	0	2	15	3	80	465	—	60	—	7000
ODWALLA														
Vegetable Cocktail	8 fl oz	70	0	0	0	4	18	2	60	290	—	9	—	29500
V8														
No Salt Added	6 fl oz	35	0	—	0	1	8	—	20	45	—	20	—	2500
Original	6 fl oz	35	0	—	0	1	8	—	20	560	—	20	—	2250
Spicy Hot	6 fl oz	35	0	—	0	1	8	—	20	650	—	24	—	2500
Splash Tropical Blend	8 fl oz	120	0	0	0	0	30	—	—	20	—	60	—	5000

VEGETABLES MIXED

(*see also* VEGETABLE JUICE)

CANNED

FOOD	PORTION	CALORIES	FAT	SAT FAT	CHOL	PROTEIN	CARBO	FIBER	CALCIUM	SOD	POTAS	VIT C	FOLIC	VIT A
mixed vegetables	½ cup	39	tr	tr	0	2	8	—	22	122	239	4	19	9551
peas & carrots	½ cup	48	tr	tr	0	3	11	—	29	332	128	8	24	7386
peas & onions	½ cup	30	tr	tr	0	2	5	—	10	265	57	2	—	96
succotash	½ cup	102	1	tr	0	4	23	—	15	325	243	9	59	187
ALLEN														
Green Beans And Potatoes	½ cup (4.2 oz)	35	0	0	0	1	7	2	40	220	—	4	—	200
Okra & Tomatoes	½ cup (4 oz)	25	0	0	0	1	5	3	60	380	—	6	—	400
Okra Tomatoes & Corn	½ cup (4.1 oz)	30	0	0	0	tr	6	4	60	280	—	6	—	750
CHI-CHI'S														
Diced Tomatoes & Green Chilies	¼ cup (2.5 oz)	20	0	0	0	0	4	0	20	340	—	1	—	200
DEL MONTE														
Mixed	½ cup (4.4 oz)	40	0	0	0	2	8	2	20	360	—	6	—	2250
Peas And Carrots	½ cup (4.5 oz)	60	0	0	0	2	11	2	20	360	—	12	—	5000
GREEN GIANT														
Garden Medley	½ cup (4.2 oz)	40	0	0	0	1	9	2	0	360	—	0	—	2000

FOOD	PORTION	CALORIES	FAT	SAT FAT	CHOL	PROTEIN	CARBO	FIBER	CALCIUM	SOD	POTAS	VIT C	FOLIC	VIT A
GREEN GIANT (CONT.)														
Mixed	½ cup (4.3 oz)	60	0	0	0	2	12	2	0	460	—	5	—	1000
Sweet Peas & Carrots	½ cup (4.3 oz)	50	0	0	0	2	11	3	0	410	—	5	—	2000
Sweet Peas & Tiny Pearl Onion	½ cup (4.4 oz)	60	0	0	0	4	11	4	20	520	—	6	—	300
HOUSE OF TSANG														
Vegetables & Sauce Cantonese Classic	½ cup (4.2 oz)	70	1	0	0	1	14	1	0	960	—	0	—	400
Vegetables & Sauce Hong Kong Sweet & Sour	½ cup (4.5 oz)	160	0	0	0	0	40	0	0	580	—	1	—	300
Vegetables & Sauce Szechuan Hot & Spicy	½ cup (4.2 oz)	70	1	0	0	1	14	1	20	1130	—	1	—	400
Vegetables & Sauce Tokyo Teriyaki	½ cup (4.4 oz)	100	0	0	0	1	23	1	20	1240	—	1	—	500
KA-ME														
Stir Fry	½ cup (4.5 oz)	20	0	0	0	1	4	2	—	10	—	—	—	—
LA CHOY														
Chop Suey Vegetables	½ cup	10	tr	tr	0	1	2	tr	13	320	60	6	—	80
LESUEUR														
Early Peas w/ Mushrooms & Pearl Onions	½ cup (4.3 oz)	60	0	0	0	3	11	2	20	380	—	9	—	300
SENECA														
Peas & Carrots	½ cup	60	0	0	0	4	9	4	20	408	140	9	—	6500
Succotash	½ cup	90	0	0	0	2	18	2	0	240	210	6	—	0
SUNSHINE														
Green Beans And Potatoes	½ cup (4.2 oz)	35	0	0	0	1	7	2	40	220	—	4	—	200
TRAPPEY														
Okra & Tomatoes	½ cup (4 oz)	25	0	0	0	1	5	3	60	380	—	6	—	400
Okra Tomatoes & Corn	½ cup (4.1 oz)	30	0	0	0	tr	6	4	60	280	—	6	—	750
FROZEN														
peas & carrots cooked	½ cup	38	tr	tr	0	3	8	—	18	55	127	7	21	6209
peas & onions cooked	½ cup	40	tr	tr	0	2	8	—	13	—	—	6	—	313
succotash cooked	½ cup	79	1	tr	0	4	17	—	13	38	225	5	28	196
AMY'S ORGANIC														
Pocket Sandwich Mediterranean Vegetables	1 (4.5 oz)	220	7	4	15	9	33	3	—	540	—	—	—	—

FOOD	PORTION	CALORIES	FAT	SAT FAT	CHOL	PROTEIN	CARBO	FIBER	CALCIUM	SOD	POTAS	VIT C	FOLIC	VIT A
AMY'S ORGANIC (CONT.)														
Pocket Sandwich Roasted Vegetables	1 (4.5 oz)	220	8	2	0	6	35	4	—	480	—	—	—	—
Pocket Sandwich Vegetable Pie	1 (5 oz)	230	6	1	0	7	37	2	—	420	—	—	—	—
BIG VALLEY														
California Blend	¾ cup (3 oz)	25	0	0	0	2	6	3	20	20	—	36	—	3750
Italian Blend	¾ cup (3 oz)	30	0	0	0	2	5	2	20	20	—	27	—	2000
Oriental Blend	¾ cup (3 oz)	25	0	0	0	2	5	3	20	10	—	24	—	750
Stew Vegetables	⅔ cup (3 oz)	40	0	0	0	1	10	2	0	30	—	9	—	300
Winter Blend	¾ cup (3 oz)	25	0	0	0	2	4	2	20	15	—	42	—	60
BIRDS EYE														
Baby Bean & Carrot Blend	1 cup (2.9 oz)	30	0	0	0	1	5	2	20	25	—	0	—	2000
Broccoli Cauliflower Carrots w/ Cheese	½ cup (3.9 oz)	70	4	1	5	3	7	2	60	460	—	18	—	1250
Brussels Sprouts Cauliflower Carrots	½ cup (3.1 oz)	30	0	0	0	2	7	3	20	20	—	42	—	4000
Chicken Viola Garlic	2 cups (6.2 oz)	260	11	3	25	14	27	1	40	540	—	12	—	1250
Chicken Viola Pesto	2¼ cups (6.6 oz)	250	9	3	25	16	25	1	100	720	—	12	—	1500
Chicken Viola Three Cheese	1¾ cups (6.2 oz)	240	9	3	25	16	26	9	100	630	—	18	—	1000
Chicken Voila Teriyaki	2 ⅓ cups (6.1 oz)	230	6	2	15	15	26	2	60	610	—	12	—	1500
Farm Fresh Broccoli Carrots Water Chestnuts	½ cup (3.3 oz)	30	0	0	0	2	7	3	20	30	—	30	—	7000
Farm Fresh Broccoli Cauliflower	½ cup (3.2 oz)	20	0	0	0	2	4	2	20	20	—	54	—	400
Farm Fresh Broccoli Cauliflower Carrots	½ cup (3.2 oz)	25	0	0	0	2	5	2	20	30	—	42	—	4500
Farm Fresh Broccoli Cauliflower Red Peppers	½ cup (3.3 oz)	20	0	0	0	2	5	2	20	20	—	54	—	1000
Farm Fresh Broccoli Corn Red Peppers	½ cup (3.6 oz)	50	0	0	0	3	12	3	20	15	—	36	—	750
Farm Fresh Broccoli Red Peppers Onions Mushrooms	½ cup (3.5 oz)	25	0	0	0	2	5	2	20	20	—	48	—	1000
Farm Fresh Brussels Sprouts Cauliflower Carrots	½ cup (3.1 oz)	30	0	0	0	2	7	3	20	20	—	42	—	4000

FOOD	PORTION	CALORIES	FAT	SAT FAT	CHOL	PROTEIN	CARBO	FIBER	CALCIUM	SOD	POTAS	VIT C	FOLIC	VIT A
BIRDS EYE (CONT.)														
Farm Fresh Cauliflower Carrots Snow Peas Pods	½ cup (3.2 oz)	30	0	0	0	2	6	2	20	25	—	24	—	7500
For Soup	⅔ cup (3 oz)	45	0	0	0	1	9	2	0	45	—	2	—	1250
For Stew	¾ cup (2.9 oz)	40	0	0	0	1	9	1	0	40	—	1	—	2000
Gumbo Blend	¾ cup (3 oz)	40	0	0	0	2	10	2	40	30	—	2	—	100
Internationals Bavarian Style	1 cup (5.5 oz)	150	8	4	30	5	15	3	60	460	—	1	—	300
Internationals California Style	½ cup (3 oz)	100	5	2	10	3	9	3	20	240	—	6	—	1000
Internationals French Country Style	⅔ cup (4.4 oz)	110	6	3	10	2	10	2	20	290	—	15	—	2000
Internationals Italian Style	1 cup (5.8 oz)	150	10	3	15	3	12	3	40	380	—	18	—	500
Internationals New England Style	1 pkg (9 oz)	260	14	5	15	6	29	3	40	480	—	24	—	500
Internationals Oriental Style	½ cup (3 oz)	60	4	2	10	2	4	2	0	260	—	18	—	400
Internationals Stir Fry Style	½ cup 3.6 oz)	60	4	2	10	2	5	1	0	270	—	9	—	1000
Peas & Carrots	⅔ cup (3 oz)	50	0	0	0	3	9	3	0	65	—	6	—	2500
Peas & Pearl Onions	⅔ cup (4.2 oz)	90	1	0	0	5	18	5	0	520	—	12	—	400
Peas & Potatoes In Cream Sauce	½ cup (4.4 oz)	90	3	1	10	4	13	2	60	350	—	6	—	200
Seasoning Blend	¾ cup (2.9 oz)	20	0	0	0	1	5	1	0	25	—	6	—	200
Stir Fry Asparagus	2 cups (5.8 oz)	90	1	0	0	5	16	3	40	35	—	21	—	2250
Stir Fry Broccoli	1 cup (3.3 oz)	30	0	0	0	2	5	2	0	30	—	21	—	1250
Stir Fry Pepper	1 cup (2.9 oz)	25	0	0	0	1	5	2	0	15	—	15	—	400
Stir Fry Sugar Snap	¾ cup (2.6 oz)	35	0	0	0	1	5	1	0	20	—	1	—	1500
Stir Fry Whole Green Bean	1¾ cup (5.3 oz)	100	1	0	0	4	19	2	20	30	—	18	—	1500
BUDGET GOURMET														
Mandarin Vegetables	1 pkg (5.25 oz)	160	11	—	10	3	13	—	40	440	190	15	—	4500
New England Recipe Vegetables	1 pkg (5.5 oz)	230	13	—	25	5	21	—	40	380	210	15	—	750
Spring Vegetables In Cheese Sauce	1 pkg (5 oz)	130	8	—	20	5	9	—	150	370	220	30	—	3000
FRESH LIKE														
California Blend	3.5 oz	31	tr	—	—	2	7	1	38	21	206	40	—	6797
Chuckwagon Blend	3.5 oz	71	1	—	—	3	17	1	7	5	174	17	—	209
Italian Blend	3.5 oz	33	tr	—	—	2	7	1	27	21	182	17	—	5222
Midwestern Blend	3.5 oz	42	tr	—	—	2	9	1	33	32	224	32	—	5388

FOOD	PORTION	CALORIES	FAT	SAT FAT	CHOL	PROTEIN	CARBO	FIBER	CALCIUM	SOD	POTAS	VIT C	FOLIC	VIT A
FRESH LIKE (CONT.)														
Mixed	3.5 oz	69	tr	—	—	30	14	1	24	48	212	10	—	5199
Oriental Blend	3.5 oz	26	tr	—	—	3	5	1	43	11	214	55	—	1362
Peas & Carrots	3.5 oz	63	tr	—	—	3	12	1	26	63	193	12	—	9561
Winter Blend	3.5 oz	26	tr	—	—	3	5	1	43	26	214	55	—	1362
GREEN GIANT														
American Mixtures Broccoli Carrots Cauliflower	¾ cup (2.6 oz)	25	0	0	0	1	5	2	20	30	—	15		3000
American Mixtures Broccoli Carrots Waterchestnuts	¾ cup (3 oz)	30	0	0	0	1	6	3	20	30	—	15		2500
American Mixtures Carrots Green Bean Cauliflower	¾ cup (2.7 oz)	25	0	0	0	1	5	2	20	20	—	9		1500
American Mixtures Cauliflower Broccoli Sugar Snap & Sweet Pea	¾ cup (2.8 oz)	35	0	0	0	2	7	3	20	45	—	12		1500
American Mixtures Corn Broccoli Red Pepper	¾ cup (3.1 oz)	60	0	0	0	2	13	2	0	10	—	12		200
American Mixtures Green Beans Potatoes Onions Red Peppers	¾ cup (2.8 oz)	45	1	0	0	1	8	2	20	15	—	6		200
American Mixtures Sweet Peas Potatoes Carrots	⅔ cup (3 oz)	70	2	0	0	2	12	3	0	70	—	6		2500
Butter Sauce Broccoli Cauliflower Carrots Corn Sweet Peas	¾ cup (3.6 oz)	60	2	2	<5	2	8	2	20	300	—	18		1250
Butter Sauce Broccoli Pasta Sweet Peas Corn Red Peppers	¾ cup (3.5 oz)	70	2	2	<5	3	11	2	20	280	—	21		300
Butter Sauce Mixed	¾ cup (3.6 oz)	70	2	1	<5	2	11	3	20	240	—	2		2000
Cheese Sauce Broccoli Cauliflower Carrots	⅔ cup (4.3 oz)	80	3	2	<5	3	11	2	60	560	—	15		3000
Harvest Fresh Broccoli Cauliflower Carrots	1 cup (3.4 oz)	30	0	0	0	2	5	3	20	125	—	24		2000
Harvest Fresh Mixed Vegetables	⅔ cup (3.1 oz)	50	0	0	0	2	10	3	0	125	—	5		1500

FOOD	PORTION	CALORIES	FAT	SAT FAT	CHOL	PROTEIN	CARBO	FIBER	CALCIUM	SOD	POTAS	VIT C	FOLIC	VIT A
GREEN GIANT (CONT.)														
Harvest Fresh Sweet Peas & Pearl Onions	½ cup (2.7 oz)	55	0	0	0	3	10	3	0	170	—	9	—	300
Mixed	¾ cup (2.9 oz)	50	0	0	0	2	11	3	20	35	—	6	—	1500
LA CHOY														
Mixed Fancy	½ cup	12	tr	tr	0	1	2	1	5	30	45	9	—	20
ORE IDA														
Stew Vegetables	⅔ cup (3 oz)	50	0	0	0	1	11	tr	0	50	200	4	—	750
SOGLOWEK														
Golden Vegetarian Nuggets	4 pieces (2.5 oz)	190	11	2	0	14	9	1	200	220	—	12	—	1250
TREE OF LIFE														
Mixed	½ cup (3 oz)	65	0	0	0	3	13	3	20	60	—	6	—	200
VEG-ALL														
Country Wisconsin Blend	3.5 oz	52	tr	—	—	2	13	1	26	16	180	7	—	6877
Scandinavian Blend	3.5 oz	48	tr	—	—	2	9	1	27	32	173	11	—	4996
Vegetables For Soup (Eight)	3.5 oz	34	tr	—	—	2	12	1	24	44	200	8	—	7508
Vegetables For Soup (Potatoes)	3.5 oz	53	tr	—	—	2	12	1	25	44	200	8	—	8103
Vegetables For Stew 4-Way	3.5 oz	51	tr	—	—	1	12	1	20	42	203	6	—	8962
Vegetables For Stew 5-Way	3.5 oz	54	tr	—	—	2	12	1	20	42	199	7	—	8988
TAKE-OUT														
caponata	¼ cup	28	1	—	0	—	—	—	16	—	—	—	—	—
gyoza potstickers vegetable	8 (4.9 oz)	210	4	1	0	8	34	5	40	500	—	0	—	500
succotash	½ cup	111	1	tr	0	5	23	—	16	16	393	8	—	282
VENISON														
roasted	3 oz	134	3	1	95	26	0	—	6	46	285	—	—	—
BROKEN ARROW RANCH														
Antelope Chili Meat	3.5 oz	115	2	1	70	23	1	—	—	76	—	—	—	—
Antelope Ground Venison	3.5 oz	110	2	1	73	23	tr	—	—	69	—	—	—	—
Antelope Stew Meat	3.5 oz	110	2	1	72	22	2	—	—	54	—	—	—	—
Nilgai Chili Meat	3.5 oz	115	2	1	70	23	1	—	—	76	—	—	—	—
Nilgai Leg	3.5 oz	100	1	tr	65	23	1	—	—	55	—	—	—	—
Nilgai Stew Meat	3.5 oz	110	2	1	72	22	2	—	—	54	—	—	—	—
Venison & Beef Smoked Sausage	6 oz	432	30	—	—	36	4	—	—	—	—	—	—	—
Venison Meat Chunks	6 oz	175	2	—	—	40	0	—	—	—	—	—	—	—

FOOD	PORTION	CALORIES	FAT	SAT FAT	CHOL	PROTEIN	CARBO	FIBER	CALCIUM	SOD	POTAS	VIT C	FOLIC	VIT A
BROKEN ARROW RANCH (CONT.)														
Venison Salami	6 oz	252	8	—	—	44	0	—	—	—	—	—	—	—
VINEGAR														
balsamic	1 tbsp (0.5 oz)	5	0	0	0	0	2	—	0	0	—	0	—	0
cider	1 tbsp	tr	0	0	0	tr	1	—	1	tr	15	0	—	0
HAIN														
Cider	1 tbsp	2	0	0	0	0	4	—	—	1	15	—	—	—
KA-ME														
Chinese Seasoned	1 tbsp (0.5 fl oz)	5	0	0	0	0	1	0	0	60	—	—	—	—
Rice Wine Chinese	1 tbsp (0.5 fl oz)	5	0	0	0	0	1	0	0	0	—	—	—	—
Rice Wine Japanese	1 tbsp (0.5 oz)	0	0	0	0	0	1	0	0	0	—	—	—	—
Seasoned Rice Japanese	1 tbsp (0.5 fl oz)	10	0	0	0	0	3	0	0	180	—	—	—	—
NAKANO														
Rice	1 tbsp	0	0	0	0	tr	0	—	—	1	—	—	—	—
REGINA														
Red Wine	1 oz	4	0	0	0	0	0	—	—	0	20	—	—	—
TREE OF LIFE														
Apple Cider Organic	1 tbsp (0.5 oz)	0	0	0	0	0	tr	—	—	0	—	—	—	—
Brown Rice	1 tbsp (0.5 oz)	2	0	0	0	0	0	—	—	45	—	—	—	—
VICTORIA														
Balsamic	1 tbsp (0.5 oz)	5	0	0	0	0	2	—	0	0	—	0	—	0
WAFFLES														
FROZEN														
buttermilk	1 4 in sq (1.2 oz)	88	3	tr	—	2	14	1	77	262	43	0	17	448
plain	1 4 in sq (1.2 oz)	88	3	tr	—	2	14	1	77	262	43	0	17	448
AUNT JEMIMA														
Blueberry	2 (2.5 oz)	190	7	2	10	4	28	1	200	530	95	0	—	0
Buttermilk	2 (2.5 oz)	170	6	2	10	4	27	1	200	410	90	0	—	0
Cinnamon	2 (2.5 oz)	180	6	2	10	4	28	1	200	470	100	0	—	0
Oatmeal	2 (2.5 oz)	170	7	1	0	4	27	3	200	660	105	0	—	0
Whole Grain	2 (2.5 oz)	170	7	1	0	5	24	2	150	450	120	0	—	0
BELGIAN CHEF														
Belgian	2 (2.5 oz)	140	3	1	0	3	24	1	60	340	—	0	—	0
DOWNYFLAKE														
Blueberry	2	180	4	—	0	4	32	—	200	570	65	—	—	—
Buttermilk	2	190	5	—	0	5	32	—	—	750	85	—	—	—
Multi-Grain	2	250	14	—	0	6	28	4	600	500	190	—	—	—
Oat Bran	2	260	13	—	0	6	30	3	1000	650	190	—	—	—
Regular	2	120	3	—	0	3	20	—	—	420	50	—	—	—
Regular Jumbo	2	170	4	—	0	4	30	—	—	570	75	—	—	—

FOOD	PORTION	CALORIES	FAT	SAT FAT	CHOL	PROTEIN	CARBO	FIBER	CALCIUM	SOD	POTAS	VIT C	FOLIC	VIT A
DOWNYFLAKE (CONT.)														
Rice Bran	2	210	11	—	0	5	25	4	60	230	125	—	—	—
Roman Meal	2	280	14	—	4	5	33	3	40	680	130	—	—	—
Waffles	2	180	6	—	—	4	27	—	200	620	75	—	—	—
EGGO														
Apple Cinnamon	2 (2.7 oz)	220	8	2	20	5	33	0	40	450	40	0	80	1000
Blueberry	2 (2.7 oz)	220	8	2	20	5	33	0	40	450	40	0	80	1000
Buttermilk	2 (2.7 oz)	220	8	2	25	5	30	0	40	480	65	0	80	1000
Common Sense Oat Bran	2 (2.7 oz)	200	7	2	0	6	27	3	40	350	35	0	80	1000
Common Sense Oat Bran With Fruit & Nut	2 (2.9 oz)	220	8	2	0	6	32	4	40	340	70	0	80	1000
Homestyle	2 (2.7 oz)	220	8	2	25	5	30	0	40	470	40	0	80	1000
Minis Blueberry	12 (3 oz)	240	8	2	25	6	37	0	40	510	45	0	120	1500
Minis Cinnamon Toast	12 (3.2 oz)	280	9	2	25	5	40	0	40	470	40	0	120	1500
Minis Homestyle	12 (1.8 oz)	240	8	2	25	6	34	0	40	520	45	0	120	1500
Nut & Honey	2 (2.7 oz)	240	10	2	25	6	32	0	40	480	40	0	80	1000
Nutri-Grain	2 (2.7 oz)	190	6	1	0	5	30	4	40	430	50	0	80	1000
Nutri-Grain Multi-Bran	2 (2.7 oz)	180	6	1	0	5	32	6	40	400	45	0	80	1000
Nutri-Grain Raisin & Bran	2 (3 oz)	210	6	1	0	5	36	5	40	390	110	0	80	1000
Special K	2 (2 oz)	140	0	0	0	6	29	0	40	250	30	0	80	1000
Strawberry	2 (2.7 oz)	220	8	2	20	5	32	0	40	460	40	0	80	1000
GREAT STARTS														
Belgian Waffles And Sausage	2.85 oz	280	19	—	—	7	21	—	40	420	—	1	—	—
Belgian Waffles Strawberries And Sausage	3.5 oz	210	8	—	—	3	31	—	40	240	—	2	—	—
Waffle With Bacon	2.2 oz	230	14	—	—	7	19	—	40	710	—	—	—	—
VAN'S														
7 Grain Belgain	2	152	4	0	0	7	9	8	—	160	—	—	—	—
Belgian Original	2	145	4	0	0	5	30	2	—	108	—	—	—	—
Belgian Original Toaster	2	145	4	0	0	5	24	2	—	92	—	—	—	—
Blueberry Toaster	2	157	4	0	0	5	24	2	—	92	—	—	—	—
Blueberry Wheat Free Toaster	2	225	5	1	0	4	32	5	—	390	—	—	—	—
Fat Free	2	155	2	0	0	5	30	7	—	230	—	—	—	—
Mini	4	107	4	0	0	3	18	6	—	275	—	—	—	—
Multigrain Toaster	2	160	4	0	0	6	25	6	—	135	—	—	—	—
Organic Whole Wheat	2	190	5	0	0	6	30	6	—	230	—	—	—	—

FOOD	PORTION	CALORIES	FAT	SAT FAT	CHOL	PROTEIN	CARBO	FIBER	CALCIUM	SOD	POTAS	VIT C	FOLIC	VIT A
VAN'S (CONT.)														
Organic Whole Wheat Blueberry	2	190	5	0	0	6	30	6	—	230	—	—	—	—
Wheat Free Cinnamon Apple Toaster	2	220	5	1	0	4	32	5	—	390	—	—	—	—
Wheat Free Toaster	2	220	5	1	0	4	32	5	—	390	—	—	—	—
HOME RECIPE														
plain	1 (7 in diam)	218	11	2	52	6	25	—	191	383	119	tr	—	140
MIX														
plain as prep	1 7 in diam (2.6 oz)	218	10	2	39	5	26	1	93	458	134	tr	9	68

WALNUTS

FOOD	PORTION	CALORIES	FAT	SAT FAT	CHOL	PROTEIN	CARBO	FIBER	CALCIUM	SOD	POTAS	VIT C	FOLIC	VIT A
black dried chopped	1 cup	759	71	5	0	30	15	—	72	2	655	—	—	370
PLANTERS														
Black	1 pkg (2 oz)	340	31	2	0	14	8	3	40	0	350	2	—	200
Gold Measure Halves	1 pkg (2 oz)	380	38	4	0	8	8	2	40	0	220	2	—	—
Halves	⅓ cup (1.2 oz)	220	22	3	0	5	5	1	20	0	130	1	—	—
Pieces	¼ cup (1 oz)	190	20	2	0	4	4	1	20	0	115	2	—	—

WASABI

FOOD	PORTION	CALORIES	FAT	SAT FAT	CHOL	PROTEIN	CARBO	FIBER	CALCIUM	SOD	POTAS	VIT C	FOLIC	VIT A
root raw	1 (5.9 oz)	184	1	—	0	8	40	12	216	29	960	71	30	78
root raw sliced	1 cup (4.6 oz)	142	1	—	0	6	31	10	166	22	738	71	23	60

WATER

(*see* MINERAL/BOTTLED WATER)

WATER CHESTNUTS

FOOD	PORTION	CALORIES	FAT	SAT FAT	CHOL	PROTEIN	CARBO	FIBER	CALCIUM	SOD	POTAS	VIT C	FOLIC	VIT A
CANNED														
chinese sliced	½ cup	35	tr	—	0	1	9	—	3	6	82	1	—	3
KA-ME														
Whole In Water	½ cup (4.5 oz)	45	0	0	0	2	11	4	—	10	—	—	—	—
LA CHOY														
Sliced	¼ cup	18	tr	tr	0	tr	4	tr	2	3	41	—	—	tr
Whole	4	14	tr	tr	0	tr	4	tr	1	2	35	—	—	tr
FRESH														
sliced	½ cup	66	tr	—	0	1	15	—	7	9	362	3	—	0

WATERCRESS

(*see also* CRESS)

WATERMELON

FOOD	PORTION	CALORIES	FAT	SAT FAT	CHOL	PROTEIN	CARBO	FIBER	CALCIUM	SOD	POTAS	VIT C	FOLIC	VIT A
SEEDS														
dried	1 oz	158	13	3	0	8	4	—	15	28	184	—	16	0
dried	1 cup	602	51	3	0	8	17	—	15	28	184	0	16	0

FOOD	PORTION	CALORIES	FAT	SAT FAT	CHOL	PROTEIN	CARBO	FIBER	CALCIUM	SOD	POTAS	VIT C	FOLIC	VIT A
WATERMELON JUICE														
KOOL-AID														
Splash Drink	1 serv (8 oz)	110	0	0	0	0	30	0	0	35	15	0	—	0
WAX BEANS														
CANNED														
DEL MONTE														
Cut Golden	½ cup (4.3 oz)	20	0	0	0	1	4	2	20	360	—	6	—	0
SENECA														
Cuts Natural Pack	½ cup	25	0	0	0	1	6	2	20	0	105	9	—	0
Wax Beans	½ cup	25	0	0	0	1	6	2	40	360	140	6	—	0
WHALE														
raw	3.5 oz	134	3	—	—	23	0	—	12	100	300	—	—	120
WHEAT														
(*see also* BULGUR, BRAN, CEREAL, COUSCOUS, FLOUR, WHEAT GERM)														
sprouted	1 cup (3.8 oz)	214	1	tr	0	8	46	1	30	17	183	3	41	0
ARROWHEAD														
Kamut Grain	¼ cup (1.7 oz)	140	1	0	0	6	32	5	0	0	190	0	—	0
Seitan Quick Mix	⅓ cup (1.4 oz)	150	1	0	0	21	14	2	0	20	65	0	—	0
HODGSON MILL														
Vital Wheat Gluten Plus Ascorbic Acid	1 tbsp (0.3 oz)	30	0	0	0	6	2	1	0	0	—	24	—	0
NEAR EAST														
Taboule Salad Mix as prep	⅔ cup	120	3	1	0	3	23	3	—	340	190	—	8	400
Wheat Pilaf as prep	1 cup	220	5	1	0	6	42	5	—	690	210	—	8	200
SONOMA														
Wheat Nuts Salted	2 tbsp (0.5 oz)	60	3	0	0	0	8	1	0	140	—	0	—	0
WHITE WAVE														
Seitan	½ pkg (4 oz)	140	0	0	0	31	4	1	0	240	—	0	—	0
Seitan Fajita Strips	⅓ cup (1.8 oz)	60	0	0	0	14	2	1	0	105	—	0	—	0
Seitan Marinated Slices	3 slices (1.8 oz)	60	0	0	0	14	2	1	0	105	—	0	—	0
WHEAT GERM														
plain toasted	¼ cup	108	3	tr	0	8	14	4	13	1	269	2	100	—
plain untoasted	¼ cup	104	3	tr	0	7	15	4	11	4	259	0	82	—
ARROWHEAD														
Wheat Germ	3 tbsp (0.5 oz)	50	1	0	0	3	10	2	20	0	125	0	—	0
HODGSON MILL														
Wheat Germ	2 tbsp (0.5 oz)	55	1	0	0	4	7	4	0	0	—	0	—	0
STONE-BUHR														
Untoasted	2 tbsp (0.5 oz)	58	2	0	0	4	7	2	0	0	—	0	—	0
WHEY														
acid dry	1 tbsp (3 g)	10	tr	tr	—	tr	2	—	59	28	66	tr	1	2
acid fluid	1 cup (8 fl oz)	59	tr	tr	—	25	13	—	253	118	352	tr	5	17

FOOD	PORTION	CALORIES	FAT	SAT FAT	CHOL	PROTEIN	CARBO	FIBER	CALCIUM	SOD	POTAS	VIT C	FOLIC	VIT A
sweet dry	1 tbsp (8 g)	26	tr	tr	—	1	6	—	59	80	155	tr	1	3
sweet fluid	1 cup (8 fl oz)	66	1	1	—	2	13	—	115	132	396	tr	2	39
whey cheese	3.5 oz	440	27	18	—	15	33	0	340	511	—	1	—	1245

WHIPPED TOPPINGS

(see also CREAM*)*

FOOD	PORTION	CALORIES	FAT	SAT FAT	CHOL	PROTEIN	CARBO	FIBER	CALCIUM	SOD	POTAS	VIT C	FOLIC	VIT A
cream pressurized	1 tbsp (3 g)	8	tr	tr	2	tr	tr	—	3	4	4	0	—	27
cream pressurized	1 cup (2.1 oz)	154	13	8	46	2	7	—	61	78	88	0	—	548
nondairy frzn	1 tbsp	13	1	1	0	tr	1	—	tr	1	1	0	0	34
nondairy powdered as prep w/ whole milk	1 cup	151	10	9	8	3	13	—	72	53	121	1	3	289
nondairy powdered as prep w/ whole milk	1 tbsp (4 g)	8	tr	tr	tr	tr	1	—	4	3	6	tr	tr	14
nondairy pressurized	1 tbsp (4 g)	11	1	1	0	tr	1	—	tr	2	1	0	0	19
nondairy pressurized	1 cup	184	16	13	0	1	11	—	4	43	13	0	0	331
COOL WHIP														
Extra Creamy	2 tbsp (0.3 oz)	25	2	2	0	0	2	0	0	5	0	0	—	0
Free	2 tbsp (0.3 oz)	15	0	0	0	0	3	0	0	5	0	0	—	0
Lite	2 tbsp (0.3 oz)	20	1	1	0	0	2	0	0	0	0	0	—	0
Original	2 tbsp (0.3 oz)	25	2	2	0	0	2	0	0	0	0	—	0	0
DREAM WHIP														
Mix as prep	2 tbsp (0.3 oz)	20	1	1	0	0	2	0	0	5	15	0	—	0
ESTEE														
Whipped Topping Sugar Free as prep	2 tbsp	10	1	—	—	0	1	—	—	5	10	—	—	—
HOOD														
Instant	2 tbsp	20	2	1	<5	0	1	0	0	0	—	0	—	0
Light Instant	2 tbsp	15	1	0	<5	0	1	0	0	0	—	0	—	0
KRAFT														
Dairy Whip Light Cream	2 tbsp (0.2 oz)	10	1	1	<5	0	tr	0	0	0	5	0	—	0
Fat Free	1 tbsp (0.3 oz)	15	0	0	0	0	2	0	0	5	10	0	—	0
LA CREME														
Topping	1 tbsp	16	1	—	tr	0	1	—	—	5	0	—	—	—
PET														
Whip	1 tbsp	14	1	—	0	0	1	—	—	0	0	—	—	—
REDDIWIP														
Lite	2 tbsp (8 g)	15	1	0	0	0	2	—	—	5	—	—	—	—
Non-Dairy	2 tbsp (8 g)	20	2	1	0	0	2	—	—	5	—	—	—	—
Real Whipped Heavy Cream	2 tbsp (8 g)	30	3	2	10	0	tr	—	—	0	—	—	—	100

FOOD	PORTION	CALORIES	FAT	SAT FAT	CHOL	PROTEIN	CARBO	FIBER	CALCIUM	SOD	POTAS	VIT C	FOLIC	VIT A
REDDIWIP (CONT.)														
Real Whipped Light Cream	2 tbsp (8 g)	20	2	1	<5	0	tr	—	—	0	—	—	—	—
WHITE BEANS														
CANNED														
white beans	1 cup	306	1	tr	0	19	58	—	191	13	1189	0	171	0
GOYA														
Spanish Style	7.5 oz	130	1	—	0	13	29	12	195	990	760	2	—	844
PROGRESSO														
Cannellini	½ cup (4.6 oz)	100	1	0	0	5	18	5	40	270	—	0	—	0
DRIED														
regular cooked	1 cup	249	1	tr	0	17	45	—	161	11	1003	0	145	0
small cooked	1 cup	253	1	tr	0	16	46	—	131	4	828	0	245	0
WHITEFISH														
smoked	3 oz	92	1	tr	28	20	0	—	15	866	360	—	6	162
smoked	1 oz	39	tr	tr	9	7	0	—	5	285	118	—	2	53
WHITING														
cooked	3 oz	98	1	tr	71	20	0	—	53	113	369	—	13	97
raw	3 oz	77	1	tr	57	16	0	—	41	61	212	—	11	84
WILD RICE														
cooked	1 cup (5.7 oz)	166	1	tr	0	7	35	3	5	5	166	0	43	0
HADDON HOUSE														
Extra Fancy	¼ cup (1.6 oz)	170	1	0	0	6	35	2	0	0	120	0	—	0
WINE														
(*see also* CHAMPAGNE, WINE COOLERS)														
madeira	3.5 oz	169	0	—	—	0	10	0	8	—	—	—	—	0
port	3.5 oz	156	0	—	—	tr	11	0	4	4	—	0	—	0
red	3½ oz	74	0	0	0	tr	2	—	8	6	115	0	2	0
rose	3½ oz	73	0	0	0	tr	2	—	9	5	102	0	1	—
sweet dessert	2 oz	90	0	0	0	tr	7	—	5	5	54	0	tr	—
white	3½ oz	70	0	0	0	tr	1	—	9	5	82	0	tr	0
BOONE'S														
Country Kwencher	1 fl oz	24	0	0	0	0	3	—	—	1	—	—	—	—
Delicious Apple	1 fl oz	21	0	0	0	0	3	—	—	1	—	—	—	—
Sangria	1 fl oz	22	0	0	0	0	3	—	—	1	—	—	—	—
Snow Creek Berry	1 fl oz	18	0	0	0	0	3	—	—	tr	—	—	—	—
Strawberry Hill	1 fl oz	22	0	0	0	0	3	—	—	1	—	—	—	—
Sun Peak Peach	1 fl oz	18	0	0	0	0	3	—	—	1	—	—	—	—
Wild Island	1 fl oz	18	0	0	0	0	3	—	—	tr	—	—	—	—
CARLO ROSSI														
Blush	1 fl oz	21	0	0	0	0	1	—	—	1	—	—	—	—
Burgundy	1 fl oz	22	0	0	0	0	tr	—	—	1	—	—	—	—
Chablis	1 fl oz	21	0	0	0	0	tr	—	—	1	—	—	—	—
Paisano	1 fl oz	23	0	0	0	0	tr	—	—	3	—	—	—	—

FOOD	PORTION	CALORIES	FAT	SAT FAT	CHOL	PROTEIN	CARBO	FIBER	CALCIUM	SOD	POTAS	VIT C	FOLIC	VIT A
CARLO ROSSI (CONT.)														
Red Sangria	1 fl oz	24	0	0	0	0	2	—	—	1	—	—	—	—
Rhine	1 fl oz	21	0	0	0	0	1	—	—	1	—	—	—	—
Vin Rosé	1 fl oz	21	0	0	0	0	1	—	—	1	—	—	—	—
White Grenache	1 fl oz	20	0	0	0	0	1	—	—	tr	—	—	—	—
FAIRBANKS														
Cream Sherry	1 fl oz	42	0	0	0	0	4	—	—	1	—	—	—	—
Port	1 fl oz	44	0	0	0	0	4	—	—	1	—	—	—	—
Sherry	1 fl oz	34	0	0	0	0	2	—	—	2	—	—	—	—
White Port	1 fl oz	44	0	0	0	0	4	—	—	1	—	—	—	—
GALLO														
Blush Chablis	1 fl oz	22	0	0	0	0	1	—	—	2	—	—	—	—
Burgundy	1 fl oz	22	0	0	0	0	tr	—	—	1	—	—	—	—
Cabernet Sauvignon	1 fl oz	22	0	0	0	0	0	—	—	tr	—	—	—	—
Chablis Blanc	1 fl oz	20	0	0	0	0	tr	—	—	1	—	—	—	—
Chardonnay	1 fl oz	23	0	0	0	0	tr	—	—	1	—	—	—	—
Classic Burgundy	1 fl oz	21	0	0	0	0	0	—	—	tr	—	—	—	—
French Colombard	1 fl oz	21	0	0	0	0	1	—	—	1	—	—	—	—
Hearty Burgundy	1 fl oz	22	0	0	0	0	tr	—	—	1	—	—	—	—
Johannisbery Riesling '88	1 fl oz	20	0	0	0	0	1	—	—	1	—	—	—	—
Pink Chablis	1 fl oz	20	0	0	0	0	1	—	—	1	—	—	—	—
Red Rosé	1 fl oz	23	0	0	0	0	1	—	—	2	—	—	—	—
Rhine	1 fl oz	22	0	0	0	0	1	—	—	1	—	—	—	—
Sauvignon Blanc '90	1 fl oz	20	0	0	0	0	tr	—	—	1	—	—	—	—
White Grenache '92	1 fl oz	20	0	0	0	0	1	—	—	1	—	—	—	—
White Grenache New Vintage	1 fl oz	20	0	0	0	0	1	—	—	tr	—	—	—	—
White Zinfandel '91	1 fl oz	18	0	0	0	0	tr	—	—	1	—	—	—	—
White Zinfandel New Vintage	1 fl oz	18	0	0	0	0	tr	—	—	1	—	—	—	—
Zinfandel '87	1 fl oz	23	0	0	0	0	0	—	—	tr	—	—	—	—
KA-ME														
Chinese Cooking	2 tbsp (1 fl oz)	20	0	0	0	0	5	0	0	170	—	—	—	—
SHEFFIELD CELLARS														
Sherry	1 fl oz	44	0	0	0	0	4	—	—	1	—	—	—	—
Tawny Port	1 fl oz	45	0	0	0	0	4	—	—	2	—	—	—	—
Vermouth Extra Dry	1 fl oz	28	0	0	0	0	1	—	—	1	—	—	—	—
Vermouth Sweet	1 fl oz	43	0	0	0	0	4	—	—	2	—	—	—	—

FOOD	PORTION	CALORIES	FAT	SAT FAT	CHOL	PROTEIN	CARBO	FIBER	CALCIUM	SOD	POTAS	VIT C	FOLIC	VIT A
SHEFFIELD CELLARS (CONT.)														
Very Dry Sherry	1 fl oz	32	0	0	0	0	1	—	—	2	—	—	—	—
WINE COOLERS														
BARTLES & JAYMES														
Berry	12 fl oz	210	0	0	0	0	32	—	—	0	62	—	—	—
Margarita	12 fl oz	260	0	0	0	0	46	—	—	40	174	—	—	—
Original	12 fl oz	190	0	0	0	0	28	—	—	10	48	—	—	—
Peach	12 fl oz	210	0	0	0	0	33	—	—	5	58	—	—	—
Pina Colada	12 fl oz	280	0	0	0	0	49	—	—	0	66	—	—	—
Planter's Punch	12 fl oz	230	0	0	0	0	36	—	—	0	66	—	—	—
Strawberry	12 fl oz	210	0	0	0	0	32	—	—	0	73	—	—	—
Strawberry Daquiri	12 fl oz	230	0	0	0	0	37	—	—	5	68	—	—	—
Tropical	12 fl oz	230	0	0	0	0	38	—	—	0	56	—	—	—
WINGED BEANS														
dried cooked	1 cup	252	10	1	0	18	26	—	244	22	481	0	18	0
YAM														
(*see also* SWEET POTATO)														
CANNED														
ALLEN														
Cut	⅔ cup (5.8 oz)	160	1	0	0	0	40	3	20	35	—	5	—	20000
BRUCE														
Cut	½ cup	139	1	—	—	1	20	—	—	27	—	9	—	6500
Mashed	½ cup	130	1	—	—	1	29	—	—	50	—	9	—	10000
Vacuum Pack	½ cup	122	1	—	—	1	28	—	—	30	—	18	—	7500
Whole	½ cup	139	1	—	—	tr	31	—	—	27	—	9	—	6500
PRINCELLA														
Cut	⅔ cup (5.8 oz)	160	1	0	0	0	40	3	20	40	—	5	—	20000
ROYAL PRINCE														
Whole	4 pieces (5.9 oz)	200	1	0	0	1	48	4	40	40	—	6	—	28000
SUGARY SAM														
Cut	⅔ cup (5.8 oz)	160	1	0	0	0	40	3	20	35	—	5	—	20000
TRAPPEY														
Whole	4 pieces (5.9 oz)	200	1	0	0	1	48	4	40	40	—	6	—	28000
FRESH														
mountain yam hawaii cooked	½ cup	59	tr	tr	0	1	14	—	6	9	356	0	—	0
yam cubed cooked	½ cup	79	tr	tr	0	1	19	—	9	6	455	8	11	0
YARDLONG BEANS														
dried cooked	1 cup	202	1	tr	0	14	36	—	72	9	539	1	249	27
YAUTIA (TANNIER)														
raw sliced	1 cup (4.7 oz)	132	1	—	0	2	32	2	12	28	807	16	23	15
root raw	1 (10.7 oz)	299	1	—	0	4	72	5	27	64	1824	16	52	34

FOOD	PORTION	CALORIES	FAT	SAT FAT	CHOL	PROTEIN	CARBO	FIBER	CALCIUM	SOD	POTAS	VIT C	FOLIC	VIT A
YEAST														
baker's compressed	1 cake (0.6 oz)	18	tr	tr	0	1	3	2	3	5	102	—	133	—
baker's dry	1 pkg (¼ oz)	21	tr	tr	0	3	3	—	5	—	140	—	—	—
baker's dry	1 tbsp	35	1	tr	0	5	5	3	8	—	240	—	—	—
brewer's dry	1 tbsp	25	tr	tr	0	3	3	—	17	10	152	tr	—	tr
FLEISCHMANN'S														
Active Dry	1 pkg (¼ oz)	20	0	0	0	3	3	—	—	10	150	—	—	—
Fresh Active	1 pkg (0.6 oz)	15	0	0	0	2	2	—	—	5	100	—	—	—
Household Yeast	½ oz	15	0	0	0	2	2	—	—	5	85	—	—	—
RapidRise	1 pkg (¼ oz)	20	0	0	0	3	3	—	—	10	150	—	—	—
RED STAR														
Yeast	4 tbsp (0.5 oz)	47	tr	0	0	8	5	4	10	5	—	0	—	0
Yeast Flakes	3 tbsp (0.5 oz)	47	tr	0	0	8	5	4	10	5	—	0	—	0
YELLOW BEANS														
dried cooked	1 cup	254	2	tr	0	16	45	—	110	8	576	3	143	4
fresh cooked	½ cup	22	tr	tr	0	1	5	—	29	2	185	6	21	50
fresh raw	½ cup	17	tr	tr	0	1	4	—	21	3	115	9	20	59
YELLOWEYE BEANS														
CANNED														
B&M														
Baked	½ cup (4.6 oz)	170	2	1	<5	8	28	7	60	460	—	0	—	0
DRIED														
BEAN CUISINE														
Dried	½ cup	115	1	—	0	8	—	5	—	5	310	—	62	—
YOGURT														
(*see also* YOGURT FROZEN)														
coffee lowfat	8 oz	194	3	2	11	11	31	—	389	149	498	2	24	123
fruit lowfat	4 oz	113	1	1	5	5	21	—	157	60	201	1	10	56
fruit lowfat	8 oz	225	3	2	10	9	42	—	314	121	402	1	19	111
plain	8 oz	139	7	5	29	8	11	—	274	105	351	1	17	279
plain lowfat	8 oz	144	4	2	14	12	16	—	415	159	531	2	25	150
plain no fat	8 oz	127	tr	tr	4	13	17	—	452	174	579	2	28	16
vanilla lowfat	8 oz	194	3	2	11	11	31	—	389	149	498	2	24	123
BREYERS														
Blended Blueberry	4.4 oz	130	1	1	10	4	25	0	100	60	180	0	—	0
Blended Peach	4.4 oz	130	1	1	10	4	26	0	100	65	180	0	—	0
Blended Strawberry	4.4 oz	130	1	1	10	4	26	0	100	60	180	0	—	0
Light Nonfat Apple Pie A La Mode	8 oz	120	0	0	10	7	22	0	200	105	300	0	—	0
Light Nonfat Berry Banana Split	8 oz	120	0	0	10	8	21	0	200	105	320	0	—	0
Light Nonfat Black Cherry Jubilee	8 oz	120	0	0	10	8	23	0	200	100	330	0	—	0

FOOD	PORTION	CALORIES	FAT	SAT FAT	CHOL	PROTEIN	CARBO	FIBER	CALCIUM	SOD	POTAS	VIT C	FOLIC	VIT A
BREYERS (CONT.)														
Light Nonfat Blueberries N' Cream	8 oz	120	0	0	10	8	23	0	200	100	310	0	—	0
Light Nonfat Cherry Bon-Bon	8 oz	120	0	0	10	8	22	0	200	105	300	0	—	0
Light Nonfat Cherry Vanilla Cream	8 oz	120	0	0	10	8	22	0	200	105	320	0	—	0
Light Nonfat Classic Strawberry	8 oz	120	0	0	10	8	22	0	200	100	320	0	—	0
Light Nonfat Key Lime Pie	8 oz	120	0	0	10	8	22	0	200	100	300	0	—	0
Light Nonfat Lemon Chiffon	8 oz	120	0	0	10	7	22	0	200	100	310	0	—	0
Light Nonfat Peaches 'N Cream	8 oz	120	0	0	10	8	22	0	200	115	340	0	—	0
Light Nonfat Raspberries 'N Cream	8 oz	120	0	0	10	8	22	0	200	105	330	0	—	0
Light Nonfat Strawberry Cheesecake	8 oz	120	0	0	10	8	22	tr	200	100	320	0	—	0
Lowfat Black Cherry	8 oz	240	3	2	15	9	44	0	300	125	450	0	—	0
Lowfat Blueberry	8 oz	230	3	2	15	9	43	0	300	125	430	0	—	0
Lowfat Mixed Berry	8 oz	320	3	2	15	9	43	0	300	125	440	0	—	0
Lowfat Peach	8 oz	240	3	2	15	9	43	0	300	125	440	0	—	0
Lowfat Pineapple	8 oz	240	3	2	15	9	45	0	300	125	430	0	—	0
Lowfat Red Raspberry	8 oz	230	3	2	15	9	43	2	300	125	450	0	—	0
Lowfat Strawberry	8 oz	230	3	2	15	9	43	0	300	125	440	0	—	0
Lowfat Strawberry Banana	8 oz	240	3	2	15	9	44	tr	300	125	470	0	—	0
Lowfat Vanilla	8 oz	220	3	2	20	10	38	0	350	135	480	0	—	100
Smooth & Creamy Apple Cobbler	8 oz	230	2	1	20	8	46	0	250	140	390	0	—	0
Smooth & Creamy Black Cherry Parfait	4.4 oz	130	1	1	10	5	26	0	150	70	210	0	—	0
Smooth & Creamy Black Cherry Parfait	8 oz	240	2	1	20	9	46	0	250	130	390	0	—	0
Smooth & Creamy Blueberries 'N Cream	4.4 oz	130	1	1	10	5	26	0	150	70	210	0	—	0
Smooth & Creamy Blueberries 'N Cream	8 oz	240	2	1	20	9	46	0	250	125	380	0	—	0

FOOD	PORTION	CALORIES	FAT	SAT FAT	CHOL	PROTEIN	CARBO	FIBER	CALCIUM	SOD	POTAS	VIT C	FOLIC	VIT A
BREYERS (CONT.)														
Smooth & Creamy Classic Strawberry	4.4 oz	130	1	1	10	5	25	0	150	70	220	0	—	0
Smooth & Creamy Classic Strawberry	8 oz	230	2	1	20	9	45	0	250	125	400	0	—	0
Smooth & Creamy Orange Vanilla Cream	8 oz	230	2	1	20	9	45	0	250	125	380	0	—	0
Smooth & Creamy Peaches 'N Cream	4.4 oz	130	1	1	10	5	25	0	150	70	220	0	—	0
Smooth & Creamy Peaches 'N Cream	8 oz	230	2	1	20	9	46	0	250	125	390	0	—	0
Smooth & Creamy Raspberries 'N Cream	8 oz	230	2	1	20	9	45	0	250	135	400	0	—	0
Smooth & Creamy Strawberry Banana Split	8 oz	240	2	1	10	8	48	tr	250	125	390	0	—	0
Smooth & Creamy Strawberry Cheesecake	8 oz	240	2	1	20	9	46	0	250	125	400	0	—	0
CABOT														
All Flavors	8 oz	220	3	2	10	9	42	—	314	120	—	1	—	100
Plain	8 oz	140	4	2	14	12	16	—	415	160	—	2	—	200
COLOMBO														
Banana Strawberry	8 oz	210	4	2	15	6	39	0	200	110	—	0	—	0
Black Cherry	8 oz	200	4	2	15	6	36	0	200	115	—	0	—	0
Blueberry	8 oz	200	4	2	15	6	36	0	200	110	—	0	—	0
Fat Free Apples 'n Spice	8 oz	190	0	0	5	8	39	0	300	130	—	0	—	0
Fat Free Apricot	8 oz	190	0	0	5	8	39	0	300	130	—	4	—	—
Fat Free Banana Strawberry	8 oz	200	0	0	5	8	42	0	300	130	—	0	—	0
Fat Free Blueberry	8 oz	190	0	0	5	8	39	0	300	130	—	0	—	0
Fat Free Cappuccino	8 oz	180	0	0	<5	9	35	0	300	140	—	0	—	0
Fat Free Cherry	8 oz	190	0	0	5	8	39	0	300	135	—	0	—	0
Fat Free Cranberry Strawberry	8 oz	200	0	0	5	8	43	0	250	120	—	0	—	0
Fat Free French Roast	8 oz	180	0	0	<5	9	35	0	300	140	—	0	—	0
Fat Free Fruit Cocktail	8 oz	190	0	0	5	8	39	0	300	130	—	0	—	0
Fat Free Lemon	8 oz	170	0	0	<5	10	33	0	350	150	—	0	—	0
Fat Free Peach	8 oz	190	0	0	5	8	33	0	300	130	—	0	—	0
Fat Free Plain	8 oz	110	0	0	5	11	16	0	400	170	—	0	—	0
Fat Free Raspberry	8 oz	190	0	0	5	8	39	0	300	130	—	0	—	0
Fat Free Strawberry	8 oz	190	0	0	5	8	39	0	300	130	—	6	—	0

FOOD	PORTION	CALORIES	FAT	SAT FAT	CHOL	PROTEIN	CARBO	FIBER	CALCIUM	SOD	POTAS	VIT C	FOLIC	VIT A
COLOMBO (CONT.)														
Fat Free Strawberry Pineapple Orange	8 oz	190	0	0	5	8	38	0	300	125	—	0	—	0
Fat Free Vanilla	8 oz	170	0	0	5	10	32	0	350	150	—	0	—	0
French Vanilla	8 oz	180	4	3	20	7	29	0	250	130	—	0	—	0
Light 100 Blueberry	8 oz	100	0	0	<5	8	16	0	250	140	—	0	—	0
Light 100 Cherry Vanilla	8 oz	100	0	0	<5	8	16	0	250	120	—	0	—	0
Light 100 Coffee & Cream	8 oz	100	0	0	<5	8	16	0	250	120	—	0	—	0
Light 100 Creamy Vanilla	8 oz	100	0	0	<5	8	16	0	250	130	—	0	—	0
Light 100 Fruit Medley	8 oz	100	0	0	<5	8	16	0	250	120	—	0	—	0
Light 100 Juicy Peach	8 oz	100	0	0	<5	8	16	0	250	140	—	0	—	0
Light 100 Lemon Creme	8 oz	100	0	0	<5	8	16	0	250	160	—	0	—	0
Light 100 Mandarin Orange	8 oz	100	0	0	<5	8	16	0	250	120	—	0	—	0
Light 100 Mixed Berries	8 oz	100	0	0	<5	8	16	0	250	110	—	0	—	0
Light 100 Raspberry	8 oz	100	0	0	<5	8	16	0	250	140	—	0	—	0
Light 100 Strawberry	8 oz	100	0	0	<5	8	16	0	250	140	—	0	—	0
Peach Melba	8 oz	200	4	2	15	6	36	0	200	115	—	0	—	0
Plain	8 oz	120	5	3	20	8	12	0	300	150	—	0	—	0
Raspberry	8 oz	200	4	2	15	6	36	0	200	115	—	0	—	0
Strawberry	8 oz	200	4	2	15	6	36	0	200	110	—	6	—	0
DANNON														
Chunky Fruit Nonfat Apple Cinnamon	6 oz	160	0	0	5	7	33	0	200	100	320	2	—	0
Chunky Fruit Nonfat Blueberry	6 oz	160	0	0	5	7	32	0	200	110	310	2	—	0
Chunky Fruit Nonfat Cherry Vanilla	6 oz	160	0	0	5	7	31	0	200	100	360	5	—	0
Chunky Fruit Nonfat Peach	6 oz	160	0	0	5	7	33	0	200	100	330	2	—	0
Chunky Fruit Nonfat Strawberry	6 oz	160	0	0	5	7	32	0	200	105	350	12	—	0
Chunky Fruit Nonfat Strawberry Banana	6 oz	160	0	0	5	7	32	0	200	105	350	12	—	0
Daniamls Lowfat Tropical Punch	4.4 oz	130	1	1	5	6	25	0	200	95	250	1	—	0

FOOD	PORTION	CALORIES	FAT	SAT FAT	CHOL	PROTEIN	CARBO	FIBER	CALCIUM	SOD	POTAS	VIT C	FOLIC	VIT A
DANNON (CONT.)														
Danimals Lowfat Blueberry	4.4 oz	130	1	1	5	6	24	0	200	100	250	1	—	0
Danimals Lowfat Grape Lemonade	4.4 oz	120	1	1	5	6	22	0	200	90	270	1	—	0
Danimals Lowfat Lemon Ice	4.4 oz	120	1	1	5	6	22	0	200	100	270	4	—	0
Danimals Lowfat Orange Banana	4.4 oz	130	1	1	5	6	24	0	200	90	260	2	—	0
Danimals Lowfat Strawberry	4.4 oz	130	1	1	5	6	24	0	200	90	250	4	—	0
Danimals Lowfat Vanilla	4.4 oz	120	1	1	5	6	23	0	200	90	270	1	—	0
Danimals Lowfat Wild Raspberry	4.4 oz	120	1	1	5	6	22	0	200	90	270	2	—	0
Double Delights Banana Creme Strawberry	6 oz	160	1	1	10	7	32	0	200	100	330	15	—	0
Double Delights Bavarian Creme Raspberry	6 oz	170	1	1	10	7	34	0	200	125	330	6	—	200
Double Delights Cheesecake Cherry	6 oz	170	1	1	10	7	34	0	200	100	340	4	—	0
Double Delights Cheesecake Strawberry	6 oz	170	1	1	10	7	33	0	200	100	340	15	—	0
Double Delights Chocolate Cheesecake	6 oz	220	1	1	10	8	45	0	250	150	350	6	—	0
Double Delights Chocolate Dipped Strawberry	6 oz	210	1	1	10	8	45	0	250	150	350	15	—	0
Double Delights Chocolate Eclair	6 oz	220	1	1	10	8	45	0	250	150	350	6	—	0
Double Delights Vanilla Strawberry	6 oz	170	1	1	10	7	33	0	200	100	340	15	—	0
Double Delights Vanilla Peach & Apricot	6 oz	170	1	1	10	7	33	0	200	100	330	2	—	400
Fruit On The Bottom Lowfat Apple Cinnamon	8 oz	240	3	2	15	9	46	1	350	140	460	2	—	100
Fruit On The Bottom Lowfat Blueberry	8 oz	240	3	2	15	9	46	1	350	140	460	5	—	100
Fruit On The Bottom Lowfat Boysenberry	8 oz	240	3	2	15	9	45	1	350	150	450	4	—	100

FOOD	PORTION	CALORIES	FAT	SAT FAT	CHOL	PROTEIN	CARBO	FIBER	CALCIUM	SOD	POTAS	VIT C	FOLIC	VIT A
DANNON (CONT.)														
Fruit On The Bottom Lowfat Cherry	8 oz	240	3	2	15	9	46	1	350	135	500	6	—	200
Fruit On The Bottom Lowfat Minipack Mixed Berry	4.4 oz	130	2	1	10	5	25	tr	200	80	250	4	—	100
Fruit On The Bottom Lowfat Minipack Strawberry	4.4 oz	130	2	1	10	5	25	tr	200	75	260	6	—	100
Fruit On The Bottom Lowfat Mixed Berries	8 oz	240	3	2	15	9	45	1	350	150	450	6	—	100
Fruit On The Bottom Lowfat Orange	8 oz	240	3	2	15	9	45	0	350	135	470	15	—	100
Fruit On The Bottom Lowfat Peach	8 oz	240	3	2	15	9	45	1	350	140	450	2	—	100
Fruit On The Bottom Lowfat Raspberry	8 oz	240	3	2	15	9	45	1	350	150	460	6	—	100
Fruit On The Bottom Lowfat Strawberry	8 oz	240	3	2	15	9	46	1	350	135	470	12	—	100
Fruit On The Bottom Lowfat Strawberry Banana	8 oz	240	3	2	15	9	43	1	350	140	480	15	—	100
Light 'N Crunchy Mint Chocolate Chip	8 oz	140	0	0	5	8	27	0	250	150	330	0	—	0
Light 'N Crunchy Nonfat Caramel Apple Crunch	8 oz	140	0	0	<5	8	26	0	250	340	160	0	—	0
Light 'N Crunchy Nonfat Lemon Blueberry Cobbler	8 oz	140	0	0	<5	8	25	0	250	135	350	0	—	0
Light 'N Crunchy Nonfat Mocha Cappuccino	8 oz	140	0	0	<5	8	26	0	250	150	330	0	—	0
Light 'N Crunchy Nonfat Raspberry w/ Granola	8 oz	140	0	0	<5	9	26	2	250	120	340	2	—	0
Light 'N Crunchy Nonfat Vanilla Chocolate Crunch	8 oz	130	0	0	<5	8	23	0	250	140	340	0	—	0
Light Duets Cherry Cheesecake	6 oz	90	0	0	0	5	18	0	260	70	260	4	—	0

FOOD	PORTION	CALORIES	FAT	SAT FAT	CHOL	PROTEIN	CARBO	FIBER	CALCIUM	SOD	POTAS	VIT C	FOLIC	VIT A
DANNON (CONT.)														
Light Duets Peaches N' Cream	6 oz	90	0	0	0	5	18	0	150	70	260	4	—	0
Light Duets Raspberry Royale	6 oz	90	0	0	0	5	17	0	150	75	240	5	—	0
Light Duets Strawberry Cheesecake	6 oz	90	0	0	0	5	18	0	150	70	240	15	—	0
Light Nonfat Banana Cream Pie	8 oz	100	0	0	<5	8	15	0	250	120	350	0	—	0
Light Nonfat Blueberry	8 oz	100	0	0	<5	8	18	0	250	115	360	0	—	0
Light Nonfat Cappuccino	8 oz	100	0	0	5	8	16	0	250	120	340	0	—	0
Light Nonfat Cherry Vanilla	8 oz	100	0	0	<5	8	18	0	250	120	390	0	—	0
Light Nonfat Coconut Cream Pie	8 oz	100	0	0	5	8	16	0	250	120	350	0	—	0
Light Nonfat Creme Caramel	8 oz	100	0	0	<5	8	15	0	250	120	350	0	—	0
Light Nonfat Lemon Chiffon	8 oz	100	0	0	5	8	15	0	250	120	340	0	—	0
Light Nonfat Mint Chocolate Cream Pie	8 oz	100	0	0	<5	8	17	0	250	120	350	0	—	0
Light Nonfat Peach	8 oz	100	0	0	<5	8	16	0	250	115	370	0	—	0
Light Nonfat Raspberry	8 oz	100	0	0	<5	8	17	0	250	120	350	2	—	0
Light Nonfat Strawberry	8 oz	100	0	0	<5	8	16	0	250	115	370	12	—	0
Light Nonfat Strawberry Banana	8 oz	100	0	0	<5	8	17	0	250	120	380	4	—	0
Light Nonfat Strawberry Kiwi	8 oz	100	0	0	5	8	16	0	250	120	360	9	—	0
Light Nonfat Tangerine Chiffon	8 oz	100	0	0	5	8	15	0	250	120	350	0	—	0
Light Nonfat Vanilla	8 oz	100	0	0	<5	8	15	0	250	120	340	0	—	0
Lowfat Coffee	8 oz	210	3	2	15	10	36	0	400	160	510	2	—	200
Lowfat Cranberry Raspberry	8 oz	210	3	2	15	10	36	0	400	160	510	2	—	200
Lowfat Lemon	8 oz	210	3	2	15	10	36	0	400	160	510	2	—	200
Lowfat Vanilla	8 oz	210	3	2	15	10	36	0	400	160	510	2	—	200
Minipack Blended Nonfat Blueberry	4.4 oz	120	0	0	5	5	25	0	150	80	260	2	—	0
Minipack Blended Nonfat Cherry	4.4 oz	110	0	0	5	5	24	0	150	80	270	2	—	0

FOOD	PORTION	CALORIES	FAT	SAT FAT	CHOL	PROTEIN	CARBO	FIBER	CALCIUM	SOD	POTAS	VIT C	FOLIC	VIT A
DANNON (CONT.)														
Minipack Blended Nonfat Peach	4.4 oz	120	0	0	5	5	23	0	150	80	260	4	—	0
Minipack Blended Nonfat Raspberry	4.4 oz	120	0	0	5	5	24	0	150	80	260	4	—	0
Minipack Blended Nonfat Strawberry	4.4 oz	120	0	0	5	5	23	0	150	85	240	1	—	0
Minipack Blended Nonfat Strawberry Banana	4.4 oz	120	0	0	5	5	23	0	150	85	250	4	—	0
Sprinkl'ins Cherry Vanilla	1 (4.1 oz)	130	2	1	5	5	24	0	150	85	250	2	—	0
Sprinkl'ins Strawberry	1 (4.1 oz)	130	2	1	5	5	24	0	150	85	250	2	—	0
Sprinkl'ins Strawberry Banana	1 (4.1 oz)	130	2	1	5	5	24	0	150	80	250	2	—	0
Sprinkl'ins Vanilla w/ Cherry Crystals	1 (4.1 oz)	110	1	1	5	5	21	0	150	85	240	9	—	0
Sprinkl'ins Vanilla w/ Orange Crystals	1 (4.1 oz)	110	1	1	5	5	21	0	150	85	240	9	—	0
FRIENDSHIP														
Coffee	8 oz	210	3	2	20	11	30	0	350	170	—	0	—	100
Fruit Crunch Peach	6 oz	190	5	2	10	8	31	0	250	125	—	2	—	300
Fruit Crunch Strawberry	6 oz	190	5	2	10	8	31	0	250	125	—	4	—	300
Fruit Crunch Strawberry Banana	6 oz	190	4	2	10	6	32	0	250	125	—	4	—	300
Plain	8 oz	150	3	2	20	12	13	0	300	190	—	0	—	100
HOOD														
Fat Free Blueberry	1 (8 oz)	190	0	0	5	8	40	1	300	120	—	6	—	0
Fat Free Cherry	1 (8 oz)	190	0	0	5	8	40	1	300	120	—	5	—	0
Fat Free Peach	1 (8 oz)	190	0	0	5	8	40	1	300	120	—	4	—	100
Fat Free Plain	1 (8 oz)	130	0	0	5	12	18	0	450	190	—	4	—	0
Fat Free Raspberry	1 (8 oz)	190	0	0	5	8	40	1	300	120	—	6	—	0
Fat Free Strawberry	1 (8 oz)	190	0	0	5	8	39	1	300	120	—	6	—	0
Fat Free Strawberry Banana	1 (8 oz)	190	0	0	5	8	40	1	300	120	—	12	—	0
Fat Free Vanilla	1 (8 oz)	190	0	0	5	11	34	1	400	170	—	2	—	0
Fat Free Swiss Blueberry	1 (8 oz)	210	0	0	5	7	45	0	250	110	—	2	—	0
Fat Free Swiss Lemon	1 (8 oz)	210	0	0	5	7	45	0	250	110	—	2	—	0
Fat Free Swiss Raspberry	1 (8 oz)	210	0	0	5	7	45	0	250	110	—	4	—	0
Fat Free Swiss Strawberry	1 (8 oz)	210	0	0	5	7	45	0	250	105	—	6	—	0
Fat Free Swiss Strawberry Banana	1 (8 oz)	210	0	0	5	7	45	0	250	110	—	5	—	0

FOOD	PORTION	CALORIES	FAT	SAT FAT	CHOL	PROTEIN	CARBO	FIBER	CALCIUM	SOD	POTAS	VIT C	FOLIC	VIT A
HOOD (CONT.)														
Fat Free Swiss Vanilla	1 (8 oz)	210	0	0	5	7	45	0	250	105	—	2	—	0
JELL-O														
Lowfat Cherry	4.4 oz	130	1	1	10	4	25	0	100	65	200	0	—	0
Lowfat Grape	4.4 oz	130	1	1	10	4	25	0	100	65	200	0	—	0
Lowfat Raspberry	4.4 oz	130	1	1	10	4	25	0	100	65	200	0	—	0
Lowfat Tropical Berry Twist	4.4 oz	130	1	1	10	4	25	0	100	65	200	0	—	0
Lowfat Tropical Punch	4.4 oz	130	1	1	10	4	25	0	100	65	200	0	—	0
Lowfat Watermelon	4.4 oz	130	1	1	10	4	25	0	100	65	200	0	—	0
Lowfat Wild Berry	4.4 oz	130	1	1	10	4	25	0	100	65	200	0	—	0
Lowfat Wild Strawberry	4.4 oz	130	1	1	10	4	25	0	100	65	200	0	—	0
LA YOGURT														
French Style Banana	6 oz	180	3	2	10	6	32	0	200	100	—	2	—	200
French Style Blueberry	6 oz	180	3	2	10	6	32	1	200	100	—	4	—	200
French Style Cherry	6 oz	180	3	2	10	6	32	0	200	100	—	2	—	100
French Style Cherry Vanilla	6 oz	190	3	2	10	6	35	0	200	95	—	2	—	100
French Style Guava	6 oz	180	3	2	10	6	32	1	200	100	—	24	—	200
French Style Key Lime	6 oz	180	3	2	10	6	32	0	200	100	—	1	—	100
French Style Mango	6 oz	180	3	2	10	6	32	0	200	100	—	4	—	400
French Style Mixed Berry	6 oz	180	3	2	10	7	32	0	250	100	—	4	—	200
French Style Nonfat Blueberry	6 oz	70	0	0	5	6	12	0	200	90	—	4	—	0
French Style Nonfat Cherry	6 oz	75	0	0	5	6	13	0	200	90	—	2	—	0
French Style Nonfat Raspberry	6 oz	70	0	0	5	6	12	0	200	90	—	4	—	0
French Style Nonfat Strawberry	6 oz	70	0	0	5	6	12	0	200	90	—	9	—	0
French Style Nonfat Strawberry Banana	6 oz	70	0	0	5	6	12	0	200	90	—	6	—	0
French Style Peach	6 oz	180	3	2	10	6	32	0	200	100	—	2	—	200
French Style Pina Colada	6 oz	180	3	2	10	6	32	0	200	100	—	2	—	100
French Style Raspberry	6 oz	180	3	2	10	6	32	1	250	100	—	4	—	200
French Style Strawberry	6 oz	180	3	2	10	6	32	0	250	100	—	9	—	100

FOOD	PORTION	CALORIES	FAT	SAT FAT	CHOL	PROTEIN	CARBO	FIBER	CALCIUM	SOD	POTAS	VIT C	FOLIC	VIT A
LA YOGURT (CONT.)														
French Style Strawberry Banana	6 oz	180	3	2	10	6	32	0	250	100	—	4	—	100
French Style Strawberry Fruit Cup	6 oz	180	3	2	10	6	32	0	250	100	—	6	—	200
French Style Tropical Orange	6 oz	180	4	2	10	6	32	0	200	100	—	2	—	200
French Style Vanilla	6 oz	170	3	2	15	7	28	0	250	110	—	2	—	200
Latin Style Banana	6 oz	190	3	2	10	6	34	0	250	105	—	4	—	100
Latin Style Guava	6 oz	190	3	2	10	6	34	0	250	105	—	2	—	100
Latin Style Mango	6 oz	190	3	2	10	6	34	0	250	105	—	2	—	100
Latin Style Papaya	6 oz	190	3	2	10	6	34	0	250	105	—	2	—	100
Latin Style Passion Fruit	6 oz	190	3	2	10	6	34	0	250	105	—	1	—	100
Latin Style Strawberry Kiwi	6 oz	180	3	2	10	6	32	0	200	100	—	5	—	100
LIGHT N'LIVELY														
Free Blueberry	4.4 oz	70	0	0	5	4	13	0	100	55	170	0	—	0
Free Peach	4.4 oz	70	0	0	5	4	12	0	100	65	190	0	—	0
Free Strawberry	4.4 oz	70	0	0	5	4	12	0	100	55	180	0	—	0
Free Strawberry Banana Cream	4.4 oz	70	0	0	5	4	13	0	100	55	190	0	—	0
Free Strawberry Fruit Cup	4.4 oz	70	0	0	5	4	13	0	100	55	180	0	—	0
Lowfat Blueberry	4.4 oz	130	1	1	10	4	25	0	100	60	180	0	—	0
Lowfat Peach	4.4 oz	130	1	1	10	4	26	0	100	65	180	0	—	0
Lowfat Pineapple	4.4 oz	130	1	1	10	4	26	0	100	60	230	0	—	0
Lowfat Red Raspberry	4.4 oz	120	1	1	10	5	23	0	100	65	200	0	—	0
Lowfat Strawberry	4.4 oz	130	1	1	10	4	26	0	100	60	180	0	—	0
Lowfat Strawberry Banana Cream	4.4 oz	130	1	1	10	4	25	0	100	60	190	0	—	0
Lowfat Strawberry Fruit Cup	4.4 oz	130	1	1	10	4	25	0	100	60	200	0	—	0
LITE LINE														
Swiss Style Cherry Vanilla	1 cup	240	2	—	—	10	45	—	300	150	350	—	—	—
Swiss Style Peach	1 cup	230	2	—	—	10	42	—	300	150	450	—	—	—
Swiss Style Plain	1 cup	140	2	—	—	12	16	—	400	150	450	—	—	—
Swiss Style Strawberry	1 cup	240	2	—	—	10	46	—	300	150	450	—	—	—
MEADOW GOLD														
Plain	1 cup	160	5	—	—	12	16	—	400	160	—	—	—	100
Sundae Style Raspberry	1 cup	250	4	—	—	10	42	—	350	160	—	—	—	100
MOUNTAIN HIGH														
Blueberry	1 cup	220	6	—	—	10	31	—	350	140	—	—	—	200

FOOD	PORTION	CALORIES	FAT	SAT FAT	CHOL	PROTEIN	CARBO	FIBER	CALCIUM	SOD	POTAS	VIT C	FOLIC	VIT A
MOUNTAIN HIGH (CONT.)														
Plain	1 cup	200	9	—	—	12	16	—	400	140	—	—	—	300
WEIGHT WATCHERS														
Ultimate 90 Blueberries 'n Creme	1 cup	90	0	0	5	8	14	3	250	140	240	0	—	0
Ultimate 90 Cappuccino	1 cup	90	0	0	5	8	14	0	250	140	—	0	—	0
Ultimate 90 Cherries Jubilee	1 cup	90	0	0	5	8	14	3	250	140	280	0	—	0
Ultimate 90 Cranberry Raspberry	1 cup	90	0	0	5	8	14	0	250	140	8	0	—	0
Ultimate 90 Lemon Chiffon	1 cup	90	0	0	5	8	14	1	250	140	305	0	—	0
Ultimate 90 Plain	1 cup	90	0	0	5	8	14	0	300	150	320	0	—	0
Ultimate 90 Raspberries 'n Creme	1 cup	90	0	0	5	8	14	0	250	140	210	0	—	0
Ultimate 90 Strawberry	1 cup	90	0	0	5	8	14	2	250	140	290	0	—	0
Ultimate 90 Strawberry Banana	1 cup	90	0	0	5	8	14	2	250	140	305	0	—	0
Ultimate 90 Vanilla	1 cup	90	0	0	5	8	14	0	250	140	260	0	—	0
Utlimate 90 Peach	1 cup	90	0	0	5	8	14	0	250	140	—	0	—	0
YOPLAIT														
Custard Style Banana	6 oz	190	4	—	20	7	32	—	200	95	290	—	—	100
Custard Style Blueberry	6 oz	190	4	—	20	7	32	—	200	95	290	—	—	100
Custard Style Cherry	6 oz	180	4	—	20	7	30	—	200	95	330	—	—	—
Custard Style Lemon	6 oz	190	4	—	20	7	32	—	200	95	290	—	—	100
Custard Style Mixed Berry	6 oz	180	4	—	20	7	30	—	200	95	330	—	—	—
Custard Style Raspberry	6 oz	190	4	—	20	7	32	—	200	95	290	—	—	100
Custard Style Strawberry	6 oz	190	4	—	20	7	32	—	200	95	290	—	—	100
Custard Style Strawberry	4 oz	130	3	—	15	5	21	—	150	60	190	—	—	—
Custard Style Strawberry Banana	6 oz	190	4	—	20	7	32	—	200	95	290	—	—	100
Custard Style Strawberry Banana	4 oz	130	3	—	15	5	21	—	150	60	190	—	—	—
Custard Style Vanilla	6 oz	180	4	—	20	7	30	—	250	110	300	—	—	100

FOOD	PORTION	CALORIES	FAT	SAT FAT	CHOL	PROTEIN	CARBO	FIBER	CALCIUM	SOD	POTAS	VIT C	FOLIC	VIT A
YOPLAIT (CONT.)														
Custard Style Vanilla	4 oz	130	3	—	15	5	20	—	150	70	200	—	—	—
Fat Free Blueberry	6 oz	150	0	—	5	7	31	—	250	95	390	—	—	—
Fat Free Cherry	6 oz	150	0	—	5	7	31	—	250	95	390	—	—	—
Fat Free Mixed Berry	6 oz	150	0	—	5	7	31	—	250	95	390	—	—	—
Fat Free Peach	6 oz	150	0	—	5	7	31	—	250	95	390	—	—	—
Fat Free Raspberry	6 oz	150	0	—	5	7	31	—	250	95	390	—	—	—
Fat Free Strawberry	6 oz	150	0	—	5	7	31	—	250	95	390	—	—	—
Fat Free Strawberry Banana	6 oz	150	0	—	5	7	31	—	250	95	390	—	—	—
Light Blueberry	6 oz	80	0	—	<5	7	13	—	150	80	270	—	—	—
Light Blueberry	4 oz	60	0	—	<5	5	9	—	100	75	230	—	—	—
Light Cherry	6 oz	80	0	—	<5	7	13	—	150	80	270	—	—	—
Light Cherry	4 oz	60	0	—	<5	5	9	—	100	75	230	—	—	—
Light Peach	4 oz	60	0	—	<5	5	9	—	100	75	230	—	—	—
Light Peach	6 oz	80	0	—	<5	7	13	—	150	80	270	—	—	—
Light Raspberry	4 oz	60	0	—	<5	5	9	—	100	75	230	—	—	—
Light Raspberry	6 oz	80	0	—	<5	7	13	—	150	80	270	—	—	—
Light Strawberry	4 oz	60	0	—	<5	5	9	—	100	75	230	—	—	—
Light Strawberry	6 oz	80	0	—	<5	7	13	—	150	110	350	—	—	—
Light Strawberry Banana	4 oz	60	0	—	<5	5	9	—	100	75	230	—	—	—
Light Strawberry Banana	6 oz	80	0	—	<5	7	13	—	150	80	270	—	—	—
Nonfat Plain	8 oz	120	0	—	5	13	18	—	450	160	590	—	—	—
Nonfat Vanilla	8 oz	180	0	—	5	11	35	—	400	140	500	—	—	—
Original Apple	6 oz	190	3	—	10	8	32	—	250	110	350	—	—	—
Original Blueberry	4 oz	120	2	—	5	5	21	—	150	75	230	—	—	—
Original Blueberry	6 oz	190	3	—	10	8	32	—	250	110	350	—	—	—
Original Boysenberry	6 oz	190	3	—	10	8	32	—	250	110	350	—	—	—
Original Cherry	6 oz	190	3	—	10	8	32	—	250	110	350	—	—	—
Original Lemon	6 oz	190	3	—	10	8	32	—	250	110	350	—	—	—
Original Mixed Berry	6 oz	190	3	—	10	8	32	—	250	110	350	—	—	—
Original Orange	6 oz	190	3	—	10	8	32	—	250	110	350	—	—	—
Original Peach	6 oz	190	3	—	10	8	32	—	250	110	350	—	—	—
Original Peach	4 oz	120	2	—	5	5	21	—	150	75	230	—	—	—
Original Pina Colada	6 oz	190	3	—	10	8	32	—	250	110	350	—	—	—
Original Pineapple	6 oz	190	3	—	10	8	32	—	250	110	350	—	—	—
Original Plain	6 oz	130	3	—	15	10	15	—	300	140	370	—	—	100
Original Raspberry	6 oz	190	3	—	10	8	32	—	250	110	350	—	—	—
Original Raspberry	4 oz	120	2	—	5	5	21	—	150	75	230	—	—	—

FOOD	PORTION	CALORIES	FAT	SAT FAT	CHOL	PROTEIN	CARBO	FIBER	CALCIUM	SOD	POTAS	VIT C	FOLIC	VIT A
YOPLAIT (CONT.)														
Original Strawberry	4 oz	120	2	—	5	5	21	—	150	75	230	—	—	—
Original Strawberry	6 oz	190	3	—	10	8	32	—	250	110	350	—	—	—
Original Strawberry Banana	6 oz	190	3	—	10	8	32	—	250	110	350	—	—	—
Original Strawberry Rhubarb	6 oz	190	3	—	10	8	32	—	250	110	350	—	—	—
Original Vanilla	6 oz	180	3	—	10	9	29	—	250	120	390	—	—	—
YOGURT FROZEN														
(*see also* TOFU YOGURT)														
chocolate soft serve	½ cup (4 fl oz)	115	4	3	3	3	18	—	106	71	188	tr	8	—
vanilla soft serve	½ cup (4 fl oz)	114	4	2	2	3	17	—	103	63	152	1	4	152
BEN & JERRY'S														
Cherry Garcia	½ cup (3.7 oz)	170	3	2	10	4	31	0	150	70	—	1	—	200
Chocolate Fudge Brownie	½ cup (3.7 oz)	190	4	2	10	6	35	2	150	130	—	1	—	200
Coffee Almond Fudge	½ cup (3.7 oz)	200	7	2	15	6	30	1	150	85	—	1	—	300
English Toffee Crunch	½ cup (3.7 oz)	190	6	3	10	4	32	0	150	110	—	0	—	300
No Fat Cappuccino	½ cup (3.3 oz)	140	0	0	0	3	32	0	100	85	—	0	—	100
Pop Cherry Garcia	1 (3.8 oz)	290	16	10	20	6	34	2	60	60	—	6	—	200
BREYERS														
Chocolate	½ cup (2.6 oz)	130	3	2	10	3	23	tr	100	45	—	0	—	100
Fat Free Chocolate	½ cup (2.6 oz)	100	0	0	<5	3	23	0	100	40	—	0	—	0
Fat Free Cookies N Cream	½ cup (2.6 oz)	110	0	0	0	3	25	tr	100	75	—	0	—	0
Fat Free Peach	½ cup (2.6 oz)	90	0	0	0	3	20	0	100	40	—	0	—	0
Fat Free Strawberry	½ cup (2.6 oz)	100	0	0	0	2	22	0	80	40	—	9	—	0
Fat Free Take Two Vanilla Chocolate	½ cup (2.6 oz)	100	0	0	0	2	23	tr	80	45	—	0	—	0
Fat Free Vanilla	½ cup (2.6 oz)	100	0	0	0	3	23	tr	100	50	—	0	—	0
Fat Free Vanilla Fudge Twirl	½ cup (2.6 oz)	110	0	0	0	3	25	0	80	45	—	0	—	0
Vanilla	½ cup (2.6 oz)	120	3	2	10	3	22	0	100	40	—	0	—	0
Vanilla Chocolate Strawberry	½ cup (2.6 oz)	120	3	2	10	3	22	0	100	40	—	1	—	0
DANNON														
Light Cappuccino	½ cup (2.8 oz)	80	0	0	0	4	20	0	100	60	180	0	—	0
Light Cherry Vanilla Swirl	½ cup (2.8 oz)	90	0	0	0	4	21	0	100	55	170	0	—	0
Light Chocolate	½ cup (2.7 oz)	80	0	0	0	4	21	tr	100	55	160	0	—	0
Light Mint Chocolate Fudge	½ cup (2.8 oz)	90	0	0	0	4	23	0	100	60	190	0	—	0
Light Peach Raspberry Melba	½ cup (2.8 oz)	90	0	0	0	4	20	0	100	60	180	0	—	0

FOOD	PORTION	CALORIES	FAT	SAT FAT	CHOL	PROTEIN	CARBO	FIBER	CALCIUM	SOD	POTAS	VIT C	FOLIC	VIT A
DANNON (CONT.)														
Light Strawberry Cheesecake	½ cup (2.8 oz)	90	0	0	0	3	21	0	100	70	150	0	—	0
Light Vanilla	½ cup (2.8 oz)	80	0	0	0	4	20	0	100	60	180	0	—	0
Light Duets Strawberry Sundae	6 oz	90	0	0	0	5	18	0	150	70	230	15	—	0
Light Nonfat Cappuccino	8 oz	100	0	0	<5	9	17	0	350	140	430	2	—	0
Light'N Crunchy Banana Cream Pie	½ cup (2.8 oz)	110	1	0	0	3	23	0	100	65	170	0	—	0
Light'N Crunchy Carmel Toffee Crunch	½ cup (2.8 oz)	110	1	1	0	3	26	0	100	75	160	0	—	0
Light'N Crunchy Mocha Chocolate Chunk	½ cup (2.8 oz)	110	1	1	0	4	23	0	100	60	170	0	—	0
Light'N Crunchy Peanut Chocolate Crunch	½ cup (2.8 oz)	110	1	1	0	4	24	0	100	65	180	0	—	0
Light'N Crunchy Rocky Road	½ cup (2.8 oz)	110	1	0	0	3	27	tr	100	60	140	0	—	0
Light'N Crunchy Triple Chocolate	½ cup (2.8 oz)	110	1	1	0	4	25	tr	100	60	160	0	—	0
Light'N Crunchy Vanilla Streusel	½ cup (2.8 oz)	110	1	1	0	3	25	0	100	80	150	0	—	0
EDY'S														
Banana Strawberry	3 oz	80	1	—	5	2	15	—	6	40	—	—	—	—
Blueberry	3 oz	80	1	—	5	2	15	—	6	40	—	—	—	—
Cherry	3 oz	80	1	—	5	2	15	—	6	40	—	—	—	—
Chocolate	3 oz	80	1	—	5	2	15	—	6	40	—	—	—	—
Chocolate Chip	3 oz	100	1	—	5	3	20	—	6	55	—	—	—	—
Citrus Heights	3 oz	80	1	—	5	2	15	—	6	40	—	—	—	—
Cookies'N'Cream	3 oz	100	1	—	5	3	20	—	6	55	—	—	—	—
Marble Fudge	3 oz	100	1	—	5	3	20	—	6	55	—	—	—	—
Perfectly Peach	3 oz	80	1	—	5	2	15	—	6	40	—	—	—	—
Raspberry	3 oz	80	1	—	5	2	15	—	6	40	—	—	—	—
Raspberry Vanilla Swirl	3 oz	80	1	—	5	2	15	—	6	45	—	—	—	—
Strawberry	3 oz	80	1	—	5	2	15	—	6	40	—	—	—	—
Vanilla	3 oz	80	1	—	5	2	15	—	6	50	—	—	—	—
ELAN														
Blueberry	4 oz	130	3	—	11	3	23	—	130	50	—	—	—	100
Caramel Almond Praline	4 oz	150	4	—	10	4	26	—	120	90	—	—	—	100
Chocolate	4 oz	130	3	—	10	4	24	—	150	50	—	—	—	100
Chocolate Almond	4 oz	160	6	—	10	5	22	—	120	50	—	—	—	100
Coffee	4 oz	130	3	—	11	4	22	—	130	60	—	—	—	100

FOOD	PORTION	CALORIES	FAT	SAT FAT	CHOL	PROTEIN	CARBO	FIBER	CALCIUM	SOD	POTAS	VIT C	FOLIC	VIT A
ELAN (CONT.)														
Coffee Decaffeinated	4 oz	130	3	—	11	4	22	—	130	60	—	—	—	100
Peach	4 oz	130	3	—	10	4	23	—	130	50	—	—	—	—
Rum Raisin	4 oz	135	3	—	12	3	25	—	130	55	—	—	—	100
Strawberry	4 oz	125	3	—	10	3	22	—	130	50	—	—	—	100
Vanilla	4 oz	130	3	—	11	4	22	—	130	60	—	—	—	100
FI-BAR														
Chocolate	1	190	7	—	0	4	26	4	—	160	—	—	—	—
Strawberry	1	190	7	—	0	4	26	4	—	150	—	—	—	—
Vanilla	1	190	7	—	0	4	26	4	—	150	—	—	—	—
FRIENDLY'S														
Apple Bettie	½ cup (2.6 oz)	140	3	2	10	3	25	0	—	75	—	—	—	—
Fabulous Fudge Swirl	½ cup (2.6 oz)	140	3	3	10	4	23	0	—	80	—	—	—	—
Fudge Berry Swirl	½ cup (2.6 oz)	150	4	3	10	4	25	0	—	75	—	—	—	—
Lowfat Perfectly Peach	½ cup (2.6 oz)	110	2	1	10	3	21	0	—	55	—	—	—	—
Lowfat Purely Chocolate	½ cup (2.6 oz)	120	3	2	10	4	20	0	—	65	—	—	—	—
Lowfat Raspberry Delight	½ cup (2.6 oz)	120	3	2	10	4	21	0	—	60	—	—	—	—
Lowfat Simply Vanilla	½ cup (2.6 oz)	120	3	2	10	4	19	0	—	70	—	—	—	—
Lowfat Strawberry Patch	½ cup (2.6 oz)	110	2	1	10	3	20	0	—	55	—	—	—	—
Mint Chocolate Chip	½ cup (2.6 oz)	130	4	2	10	4	21	0	—	65	—	—	—	—
Strawberry Cheesecake Blast	½ cup (2.6 oz)	140	4	2	15	4	22	0	—	75	—	—	—	—
Toffee Almond Crunch	½ cup (2.6 oz)	160	5	2	15	4	24	tr	—	85	—	—	—	—
GOOD HUMOR														
Creamsicle Raspberry	1 (2.8 oz)	100	1	1	<5	1	23	0	20	20	—	0	—	0
Frista Cup	1 (6.2 oz)	220	5	4	15	7	38	1	200	125	—	0	—	200
HAAGEN-DAZS														
Banana Nut Blast	½ cup (3.5 oz)	220	8	4	40	8	29	1	200	65	—	0	—	100
Bars Cherry Chocolate Fudge	1 (2.6 oz)	240	13	8	35	5	26	1	100	45	—	0	—	200
Bars Peach	1 (2.5 oz)	90	1	1	15	2	19	0	60	20	—	2	—	0
Bars Pina Colada	1 (2.5 oz)	100	1	1	15	3	19	0	40	45	—	2	—	0
Bars Raspberry & Vanilla	1 (2.5 oz)	90	1	0	15	3	19	0	80	25	—	2	—	0
Bars Strawberry Daiquiri	1 (2.5 oz)	90	1	1	15	3	18	0	20	20	—	4	—	0
Chocolate	½ cup (3.4 oz)	160	3	2	30	8	26	tr	200	60	—	0	—	100

FOOD	PORTION	CALORIES	FAT	SAT FAT	CHOL	PROTEIN	CARBO	FIBER	CALCIUM	SOD	POTAS	VIT C	FOLIC	VIT A
HAAGEN-DAZS (CONT.)														
Coffee	½ cup (3.4 oz)	160	3	2	45	8	26	0	250	55	—	0	—	0
Fat Free Bar Raspberry & Vanilla	1 (2.5 oz)	90	0	—	0	2	20	0	60	15	—	0	—	0
Fat Free Cherry Vanilla	½ cup (3.3 oz)	140	0	—	<5	6	30	0	0	40	—	1	—	100
Fat Free Chocolate	½ cup (3.3 oz)	140	0	—	<5	6	28	tr	200	45	—	0	—	0
Fat Free Coffee	½ cup (3.3 oz)	140	0	—	<5	6	29	0	200	45	—	0	—	0
Fat Free Vanilla	½ cup (3.3 oz)	140	0	—	<5	6	29	0	200	45	—	0	—	0
Fat Free Vanilla Fudge	½ cup (3.3 oz)	160	0	—	<5	6	34	0	150	100	—	0	—	0
Orange Tango	½ cup (3.5 oz)	130	1	1	20	4	26	0	100	25	—	6	—	100
Pina Colada	½ cup (3.4 oz)	130	2	1	25	3	26	0	100	25	—	6	—	100
Raspberry Randevous	½ cup (3.5 oz)	130	2	1	20	4	26	1	100	25	—	2	—	0
Strawberry Cheesecake Craze	½ cup (3.6 oz)	220	8	4	65	7	31	0	150	140	—	2	—	100
Strawberry Duet	½ cup (3.4 oz)	130	2	1	25	3	26	tr	80	25	—	9	—	100
Vanilla	½ cup (3.4 oz)	160	3	2	45	8	26	0	250	55	—	0	—	0
HOOD														
Bavarian Truffle & Twist	½ cup (2.6 oz)	150	4	3	10	2	26	0	100	60	—	0	—	0
Coffee Toffee Chunk Sundae	½ cup (2.6 oz)	150	4	3	10	2	27	0	100	75	—	0	—	100
Combo Bars	1 (2.2 oz)	90	2	1	5	2	17	0	80	40	—	0	—	0
Cookies & Cream	½ cup (2.6 oz)	140	4	2	10	3	25	0	100	75	—	0	—	0
Grandma's Raisin Oatmeal Cookie Dough	½ cup (2.6 oz)	140	3	2	10	3	25	0	100	75	—	0	—	0
Mixed Berry Swirl	½ cup (2.6 oz)	120	2	2	10	2	24	0	100	45	—	0	—	0
Natural Strawberry	½ cup (2.6 oz)	110	3	2	10	2	21	0	100	50	—	2	—	0
Natural Strawberry Banana	½ cup (2.6 oz)	110	3	2	10	2	21	0	100	50	—	2	—	0
Natural Vanilla	½ cup (2.6 oz)	120	3	2	10	3	22	0	100	55	—	0	—	0
Nonfat Caramel & Brownie Sundae	½ cup (2.6 oz)	120	0	0	0	3	28	0	100	60	—	0	—	0
Nonfat Chocolate Marshmallow	½ cup (2.6 oz)	110	0	0	0	2	26	0	100	60	—	0	—	0
Nonfat Double Raspberry	½ cup (2.6 oz)	120	0	0	0	2	26	0	100	55	—	0	—	0
Nonfat Mocha Fudge	½ cup (2.6 oz)	120	0	0	0	3	27	0	100	55	—	0	—	0
Nonfat Olde Fashioned Vanilla	½ cup (2.6 oz)	110	0	0	0	3	24	0	100	55	—	0	—	0
Nonfat Peach Cobbler A La Mode	½ cup (2.6 oz)	110	0	0	0	3	25	0	100	50	—	0	—	0

FOOD	PORTION	CALORIES	FAT	SAT FAT	CHOL	PROTEIN	CARBO	FIBER	CALCIUM	SOD	POTAS	VIT C	FOLIC	VIT A
HOOD (CONT.)														
Nonfat Strawberry	½ cup (2.6 oz)	100	0	0	0	2	23	0	100	50	—	0	—	0
Nonfat Vanilla Fudge	½ cup (2.6 oz)	120	0	0	0	3	27	0	100	55	—	0	—	0
Raspberry Swirl	½ cup (2.6 oz)	130	2	2	10	2	25	0	100	55	—	0	—	0
Sundae Cups Chocolate & Strawberry	1 (2.2 oz)	110	2	1	5	1	24	1	60	55	—	0	—	0
Vanilla Chocolate Strawberry	½ cup (2.6 oz)	120	3	2	10	3	22	0	100	50	—	0	—	0
Vanilla Swiss Almond Sundae	½ cup (2.6 oz)	150	4	2	10	3	25	0	100	60	—	0	—	0
SEALTEST														
Chocolate	½ cup (2.7 oz)	120	2	1	5	3	24	tr	100	45	—	0	—	0
Mocha Fudge	½ cup (2.6 oz)	130	2	2	10	3	25	tr	100	45	—	0	—	0
Vanilla	½ cup (2.6 oz)	120	2	1	10	3	24	0	100	45	—	0	—	0
TOFUTTI														
Better Than Yogurt Chocolate Fudge	4 fl oz	120	2	1	0	2	25	0	—	98	38	—	—	—
Better Than Yogurt Coffee Mashmallow Swirl	4 fl oz	100	1	0	0	1	24	0	—	77	7	—	—	—
Better Than Yogurt Passion Island Fruit	4 fl oz	100	1	0	0	1	21	0	—	100	13	—	—	—
Better Than Yogurt Peach Mango	4 fl oz	100	1	0	0	1	23	0	—	102	10	—	—	—
Better Than Yogurt Strawberry Banana	4 fl oz	100	1	0	0	1	23	0	—	92	13	—	—	—
Better Than Yogurt Vanilla Fudge	4 fl oz	120	2	0	0	2	24	0	—	90	8	—	—	—
TURKEY HILL														
Chocolate Cherry Cordial	½ cup (2.6 oz)	130	3	2	10	3	22	0	100	60	—	0	—	100
Chocolate Chip Cookie Dough	½ cup (2.6 oz)	140	5	3	10	3	23	0	100	120	—	0	—	100
Death By Chocolate	½ cup (2.6 oz)	150	4	3	10	3	25	0	100	90	—	0	—	100
Nonfat Chocolate Cherry Cordial	½ cup (2.4 oz)	100	0	0	0	4	24	0	100	70	—	0	—	0
Nonfat Chocolate Marshmallow	½ cup (2.4 oz)	130	0	0	0	3	30	0	80	40	—	0	—	0
Nonfat Coffee Cappuccino	½ cup (2.4 oz)	110	0	0	0	3	23	0	100	60	—	0	—	0
Nonfat Mint Cookie 'N Cream	½ cup (2.4 oz)	110	0	0	0	4	24	0	100	80	—	0	—	0
Nonfat Neapolitan	½ cup (2.4 oz)	100	0	0	0	3	22	0	100	50	—	0	—	0
Nonfat Raspberry Chocolate Bliss	½ cup (2.4 oz)	110	0	0	0	3	25	0	100	100	—	0	—	0

FOOD	PORTION	CALORIES	FAT	SAT FAT	CHOL	PROTEIN	CARBO	FIBER	CALCIUM	SOD	POTAS	VIT C	FOLIC	VIT A
TURKEY HILL (CONT.)														
Nonfat Southern Lemon Pie	½ cup (2.4 oz)	110	0	0	0	3	25	0	100	90	—	0	—	0
Nonfat Vanilla Fudge	½ cup (2.4 oz)	110	0	0	0	3	24	0	100	80	—	0	—	0
Peach Raspberry	½ cup (2.6 oz)	110	2	2	10	3	20	0	100	60	—	0	—	100
Strawberry	½ cup (2.6 oz)	110	2	2	10	3	20	0	100	60	—	0	—	100
Tin Roof Sundae	½ cup (2.6 oz)	140	5	3	10	4	21	0	100	100	—	0	—	100
Vanilla & Chocolate	½ cup (2.6 oz)	110	3	2	10	3	19	0	100	70	—	0	—	100
Vanilla Bean	½ cup (2.6 oz)	110	3	2	10	4	17	0	100	70	—	0	—	100
ZUCCHINI														
CANNED														
italian style	½ cup	33	tr	tr	0	1	8	—	19	427	312	3	—	615
DEL MONTE														
With Italian Tomato Sauce	½ cup (4.2 oz)	30	0	0	0	1	7	1	0	490	—	9	—	300
PROGRESSO														
Italian Style	½ cup (4.2 oz)	40	2	0	0	2	7	2	20	400	—	6	—	1000
FROZEN														
cooked	½ cup	19	tr	tr	0	1	4	—	19	2	218	4	9	483
BIG VALLEY														
Zucchini	¾ cup (3 oz)	10	0	0	0	1	2	1	20	0	—	9	—	200
EMPIRE														
Breaded	1 (2.9 oz)	100	0	0	0	5	18	1	0	280	—	0	—	200
TAKE-OUT														
indian paalkora	1 serv	46	2	tr	1	2	7	2	—	141	—	—	—	—

PART TWO

RESTAURANT CHAINS

ARBY'S

FOOD	PORTION	CALORIES	FAT	SAT FAT	CHOL	PROTEIN	CARBO	FIBER	CALCIUM	SOD	POTAS	VIT C	FOLIC	VIT A
BREAKFAST SELECTIONS														
Bacon	2 strips (0.53 oz)	90	7	3	15	5	0	0	—	220	—	—	—	—
Biscuit Plain	1 (2.9 oz)	280	15	3	0	6	34	1	—	730	—	—	—	—
Blueberry Muffin	1 (2.3 oz)	230	9	2	25	2	35	0	—	290	—	—	—	—
Cinnamon Nut Danish	1 (3.5 oz)	360	11	1	0	6	60	1	—	105	—	—	—	—
Croissant Plain	1 (2 oz)	220	12	7	25	4	25	0	—	230	—	—	—	—
Egg Portion	1 serv (1.6 oz)	95	8	2	180	1	1	0	—	54	—	—	—	—
Ham	1 serv (1.5 oz)	45	1	1	20	7	0	0	—	405	—	—	—	—
Sausage	1 (1.3 oz)	163	15	6	25	7	0	0	—	321	—	—	—	—
Swiss	1 serv (0.5 oz)	45	3	2	12	4	1	0	—	175	—	—	—	—
Table Syrup	1 serv (1 oz)	100	0	0	0	0	25	0	—	30	—	—	—	—
Toastix	6 pieces (4.4 oz)	430	21	5	0	10	52	3	—	550	—	—	—	—
DESSERTS														
Apple Turnover	1 (3.2 oz)	330	14	7	0	4	48	0	—	180	—	—	—	—
Cheesecake Plain	1 serv (3 oz)	320	23	14	95	5	23	0	—	240	—	—	—	—
Cherry Turnover	1 (3.2 oz)	320	13	5	0	4	46	0	—	190	—	—	—	—
Chocolate Chip Cookie	1 (1 oz)	125	6	2	10	2	16	0	—	85	—	—	—	—
Polar Swirl Butterfinger	1 (11.6 oz)	457	18	8	28	15	62	0	—	318	—	—	—	—
Polar Swirl Heath	1 (11.6 oz)	543	22	5	39	15	76	0	—	346	—	—	—	—
Polar Swirl Oreo	1 (11.6 oz)	329	22	10	35	15	66	0	—	521	—	—	—	—
Polar Swirl Peanut Butter Cup	1 (11.6 oz)	517	24	8	34	20	61	1	—	385	—	—	—	—
Polar Swirl Snickers	1 (11.6 oz)	511	19	7	33	15	73	1	—	351	—	—	—	—
MAIN MENU SELECTIONS														
Arby's Sauce	1 serv (0.5 oz)	15	tr	0	0	tr	4	0	—	113	—	—	—	—
Baked Potato Broccoli 'n Cheddar	1 (15.7 oz)	571	20	5	12	14	89	9	—	565	—	—	—	—
Baked Potato Deluxe	1 (15.3 oz)	736	36	16	59	19	86	7	—	499	—	—	—	—
Baked Potato Plain	1 (11.5 oz)	355	tr	0	0	7	82	7	—	26	—	—	—	—
Baked Potato w/ Margarine & Sour Cream	1 (14 oz)	578	24	9	25	9	85	7	—	209	—	—	—	—
Barbeque Sauce	1 serv (0.5 oz)	30	0	0	0	0	7	0	—	185	—	—	—	—
Beef Stock Au Jus	1 serv (2 oz)	10	0	0	0	0	1	0	—	440	—	—	—	—
Breaded Chicken Fillet	1 (7.2 oz)	536	28	5	45	28	46	5	—	1016	—	—	—	—
Cheddar Cheese Sauce	1 serv (0.75 oz)	35	3	1	4	1	1	0	—	139	—	—	—	—

FOOD	PORTION	CALORIES	FAT	SAT FAT	CHOL	PROTEIN	CARBO	FIBER	CALCIUM	SOD	POTAS	VIT C	FOLIC	VIT A
Cheddar Curly Fried	1 serv (4.25 oz)	333	18	4	3	5	40	0	—	1016	—	—	—	—
Chicken Cordon Bleu	1 (8.5 oz)	623	33	8	77	38	46	5	—	1504	—	—	—	—
Chicken Finger	2 (3.6 oz)	290	16	2	32	16	20	1	—	677	—	—	—	—
Curly Fries	1 serv (3.5 oz)	300	15	3	0	4	38	0	—	853	—	—	—	—
Fish Fillet Sandwich	1 (7.7 oz)	529	27	7	43	23	50	2	—	864	—	—	—	—
French Fries	1 serv (2.5 oz)	246	13	3	0	2	30	0	—	114	—	—	—	—
Garden Salad	1 (11.9 oz)	61	1	0	0	3	12	5	—	40	—	—	—	—
Grilled Chicken BBQ	1 (7.1 oz)	388	13	3	43	23	47	2	—	1002	—	—	—	—
Grilled Chicken Deluxe	1 (8.1 oz)	430	20	4	61	23	41	3	—	848	—	—	—	—
Ham 'n Cheese Sandwich	1 (5.9 oz)	359	14	5	53	24	34	2	—	1283	—	—	—	—
Ham 'n Cheese Melt	1 (4.9 oz)	329	13	4	40	20	34	2	—	1013	—	—	—	—
Honey Mayonnaise Reduced Calorie	1 serv (0.5 oz)	70	7	1	20	0	1	0	—	135	—	—	—	—
Horsey Sauce	1 serv (0.5 oz)	60	5	1	5	0	2	0	—	150	—	—	—	—
Italian Sub	1 (10.1 oz)	675	36	13	836	30	46	2	—	2089	—	—	—	—
Italian Sub Sauce	1 serv (0.5 oz)	70	7	1	0	0	1	0	—	240	—	—	—	—
Ketchup	1 serv (0.5 oz)	16	0	0	0	tr	4	0	—	143	—	—	—	—
Light Roast Beef Deluxe	1 (6.4 oz)	296	10	3	42	18	33	6	—	826	—	—	—	—
Light Roast Chicken Deluxe	1 (6.8 oz)	276	6	2	33	20	33	4	—	777	—	—	—	—
Light Roast Chicken Salad	1 serv (14.4 oz)	149	2	1	29	20	12	5	—	418	—	—	—	—
Light Roast Turkey Deluxe	1 (6.8 oz)	260	7	2	33	20	33	4	—	1262	—	—	—	—
Mayonnaise	1 serv (0.5 oz)	110	12	7	5	0	0	0	—	80	—	—	—	—
Mayonnaise Light Cholesterol Free	1 serv (0.25 oz)	12	1	0	0	0	1	1	—	64	—	—	—	—
Mustard German Style	1 serv (0.16 oz)	5	0	0	0	0	1	0	—	70	—	—	—	—
Parmesan Cheese Sauce	1 serv (0.5 oz)	70	7	1	5	1	2	0	—	130	—	—	—	—
Potato Cakes	2 (3 oz)	204	12	2	0	2	20	0	—	397	—	—	—	—
Roast Beef Arby's Melt w/ Cheddar	1 (5.2 oz)	368	18	6	31	18	36	2	—	936	—	—	—	—
Roast Beef Arby-Q	1 (6.4 oz)	431	18	6	37	22	48	3	—	1321	—	—	—	—
Roast Beef Bac'n Cheddar Deluxe	1 (8.1 oz)	539	34	10	44	22	38	3	—	1140	—	—	—	—
Roast Beef Beef 'n Cheddar	1 (6.7 oz)	487	28	9	50	25	40	2	—	1216	—	—	—	—
Roast Beef Gaint	1 (8.1 oz)	555	28	11	71	35	43	5	—	1561	—	—	—	—

FOOD	PORTION	CALORIES	FAT	SAT FAT	CHOL	PROTEIN	CARBO	FIBER	CALCIUM	SOD	POTAS	VIT C	FOLIC	VIT A
Roast Beef Junior	1 (4.4 oz)	324	14	5	30	17	35	2	—	779	—	—	—	—
Roast Beef Regular	1 (5.4 oz)	388	19	7	43	23	33	3	—	1009	—	—	—	—
Roast Beef Sub	1 (10.8 oz)	700	42	14	846	38	44	4	—	2034	—	—	—	—
Roast Beef Super	1 (8.7 oz)	523	27	9	43	25	50	5	—	1189	—	—	—	—
Roast Chicken Club	1 (8.5 oz)	546	31	9	58	31	37	2	—	1103	—	—	—	—
Roast Chicken Deluxe	1 (7.6 oz)	433	22	5	34	24	36	2	—	763	—	—	—	—
Roast Chicken Santa Fe	1 (6.4 oz)	436	22	6	54	29	35	1	—	816	—	—	—	—
Side Salad	1 (5 oz)	23	tr	0	0	1	4	2	—	15	—	—	—	—
Sub Roll French Dip	1 (6.8 oz)	475	22	8	55	30	40	3	—	1411	—	—	—	—
Sub Roll Hot Ham 'n Swiss	1 (9.3 oz)	500	23	7	68	30	43	2	—	1664	—	—	—	—
Sub Roll Pilly Beef 'n Swiss	1 (10.4 oz)	755	47	15	91	39	48	3	—	2025	—	—	—	—
Sub Roll Triple Cheese Melt	1 (8.4 oz)	720	45	16	91	37	46	2	—	1797	—	—	—	—
Tartar Sauce	1 serv (1 oz)	140	15	2	30	0	0	0	—	220	—	—	—	—
Turkey Sub	1 (9.8 oz)	550	27	7	65	31	47	2	—	2084	—	—	—	—
SALAD DRESSINGS														
Blue Cheese	1 serv (2 oz)	290	31	6	50	2	2	0	—	580	—	—	—	—
Buttermilk Ranch Reduced Calorie	1 serv (2 oz)	50	0	0	0	0	12	0	—	710	—	—	—	—
Honey French	1 serv (2 oz)	280	23	3	0	0	18	0	—	400	—	—	—	—
Italian Reduced Calorie	1 serv (2 oz)	20	1	0	0	0	3	0	—	1000	—	—	—	—
Red Ranch	1 serv (0.5 oz)	75	6	1	0	0	5	0	—	115	—	—	—	—
Thousand Island	1 serv (2 oz)	260	26	4	30	0	7	0	—	420	—	—	—	—
SOUPS														
Boston Clam Chowder	1 serv (8 oz)	190	9	3	25	9	18	1	—	965	—	—	—	—
Cream of Broccoli	1 serv (8 oz)	160	8	4	25	7	15	2	—	1000	—	—	—	—
Lumberjack Mixed Vegetable	1 serv (8 oz)	90	4	2	5	2	10	1	—	1150	—	—	—	—
Old Fashioned Chicken Noodle	1 serv (8 oz)	80	2	0	20	6	11	1	—	850	—	—	—	—
Potato w/ Bacon	1 serv (8 oz)	170	7	3	20	6	23	—	—	905	—	—	—	—
Timberline Chili	1 serv (8 oz)	220	10	4	30	18	17	7	—	1130	—	—	—	—
Wisconsin Cheese	1 serv (8 oz)	280	18	7	35	10	20	2	—	1065	—	—	—	—

AU BON PAIN

FOOD	PORTION	CALORIES	FAT	SAT FAT	CHOL	PROTEIN	CARBO	FIBER	CALCIUM	SOD	POTAS	VIT C	FOLIC	VIT A
BAKED SELECTIONS														
Apple Coffee Cake	1 piece (4.6 oz)	480	24	12	96	6	60	2	90	285	—	2	—	1350
Bagel Chocolate Chip	1 (5 oz)	380	7	4	5	12	69	3	60	480	—	0	—	0

FOOD	PORTION	CALORIES	FAT	SAT FAT	CHOL	PROTEIN	CARBO	FIBER	CALCIUM	SOD	POTAS	VIT C	FOLIC	VIT A
Bagel Dutch Apple w/ Walnut Streussel	1 (5 oz)	360	5	0	0	11	77	4	40	480	—	1	—	0
Baguette Loaf	1 slice (1.8 oz)	140	5	0	0	5	29	1	80	350	—	5	—	0
Biscotti	1 (1.5 oz)	200	10	4	35	4	24	1	40	45	—	0	—	200
Biscotti Chocolate	1 (1.7 oz)	240	13	6	35	5	28	2	40	50	—	0	—	200
Braided Roll	1 (1.8 oz)	170	5	—	0	5	26	1	40	320	—	6	—	0
Cinnamon Roll	1 (7 oz)	710	26	10	100	12	110	3	100	740	—	1	—	1000
Cookie Chocolate Chip	1 (2.1 oz)	280	13	8	40	3	40	2	20	85	—	0	—	400
Cookie Oatmeal Raisin	1 (2.1 oz)	250	10	4	30	3	40	2	20	240	—	0	—	400
Cookie Peanut Butter	1 (2.1 oz)	280	15	5	30	7	32	1	20	260	—	0	—	300
Cookie Shortbread	1 (2.4 oz)	390	25	15	65	3	39	1	20	190	—	0	—	1000
Croissant Almond	1 (4.3 oz)	560	37	15	105	12	50	4	150	260	—	0	—	1000
Croissant Apple	1 (3.4 oz)	280	10	6	25	4	46	1	60	180	—	6	—	400
Croissant Chocolate	1 (3.4 oz)	440	23	15	30	7	53	4	60	230	—	1	—	500
Croissant Cinnamon Raisin	1 (3.7 oz)	380	13	8	35	7	61	2	80	290	—	1	—	500
Croissant Plain	1 (2.1 oz)	270	15	9	40	6	30	1	60	240	—	0	—	500
Croissant Raspberry Cheese	1 (3.5 oz)	380	19	11	60	6	47	1	80	300	—	0	—	500
Croissant Sweet Cheese	1 (3.6 oz)	390	22	12	75	7	42	1	80	330	—	0	—	500
Danish Cheese Swirl	1 (3.8 oz)	450	28	14	95	7	46	1	150	410	—	6	—	750
Danish Lemon Swirl	1 (4 oz)	450	24	12	80	7	53	1	150	410	—	6	—	1250
Danish Raspberry	1 (3.6 oz)	370	21	10	65	7	42	2	100	350	—	12	—	750
Danish Sweet Cheese	1 (3.6 oz)	420	26	13	90	7	42	1	150	380	—	6	—	750
Four Grain Loaf	1 slice (1.8 oz)	130	1	0	0	5	25	1	80	280	—	9	—	0
French Sandwich Roll	1 (1.8 oz)	120	5	0	0	4	25	1	60	320	—	4	—	0
Hazelnut Fudge Brownie	1 (4 oz)	380	18	11	100	5	56	4	20	150	—	0	—	750
Holiday Cookie Cranberry Almond Macaroon	1 (1.5 oz)	160	8	5	0	2	22	2	20	115	—	0	—	0
Holiday Cookie Cranberry Almond Macaroon w/ Chocolate	1 (1.9 oz)	210	11	9	0	3	27	2	20	120	—	0	—	0
Holiday Cookie English Toffee	1 (1.8 oz)	220	12	7	45	2	28	0	20	110	—	0	—	400
Holiday Cookie Ginger Pecan	1 (2 oz)	260	15	6	40	5	30	1	20	115	—	1	—	400

FOOD	PORTION	CALORIES	FAT	SAT FAT	CHOL	PROTEIN	CARBO	FIBER	CALCIUM	SOD	POTAS	VIT C	FOLIC	VIT A
Mochaccino Bar	1 (4 oz)	404	24	10	37	5	44	1	20	294	—	0	—	700
Muffin Blueberry	1 (4.5 oz)	410	15	3	85	8	64	1	80	380	—	1	—	100
Muffin Carrot	1 (5 oz)	480	23	5	55	8	61	3	80	650	—	4	—	6500
Muffin Chocolate Chip	1 (4.5 oz)	490	20	7	35	8	70	2	60	560	—	0	—	200
Muffin Corn	1 (4.6 oz)	470	18	3	65	8	70	2	150	570	—	0	—	200
Muffin Pumpkin w/ Streusel Topping	1 (5.5 oz)	470	18	3	60	8	74	2	150	550	—	1	—	300
Muffin Low Fat Chocolate Cake	1 (4 oz)	290	3	1	20	4	68	3	40	630	—	0	—	0
Muffin Low Fat Triple Berry	1 (4.2 oz)	270	3	1	25	5	60	2	60	560	—	5	—	0
Multigrain Loaf	1 slice (1.8 oz)	130	1	0	0	5	26	1	100	340	—	6	—	0
Parisienne Loaf	1 slice (1.8 oz)	120	5	0	0	4	25	1	80	300	—	5	—	0
Pear Ginger Tea Cake	1 piece (4 oz)	380	20	3	0	3	47	1	0	202	—	0	—	0
Pecan Roll	1 (6.8 oz)	900	48	16	50	11	111	4	150	480	—	1	—	1000
Roll 3 Seed Pecan Raisin	1 (2.7 oz)	250	6	1	0	9	43	3	80	240	—	15	—	0
Roll Hearth Sandwich	1 (2.8 oz)	220	2	0	0	9	43	2	150	410	—	12	—	0
Rolls Petit Pan	1 (2.5 oz)	200	1	0	0	7	41	1	100	570	—	6	—	0
Rye Loaf	1 slice (1.8 oz)	110	2	0	0	5	21	2	100	310	—	6	—	0
Scone Cinnamon	1 (4.1 oz)	520	28	14	145	10	60	1	80	230	—	0	—	1000
Scone Current	1 (3.7 oz)	430	23	13	155	10	47	2	60	230	—	21	—	1000
Scone Orange	1 (4.1 oz)	440	23	13	155	10	53	2	60	240	—	9	—	1000
Sourdough Bagel Asiago Cheese	1 (4.2 oz)	380	6	4	15	17	66	3	200	690	—	0	—	0
Sourdough Bagel Cinnamon Raisin	1 (4.5 oz)	390	1	0	0	14	83	4	40	550	—	1	—	0
Sourdough Bagel Cranberry Walnut	1 (5 oz)	460	4	1	0	15	93	7	40	590	—	6	—	0
Sourdough Bagel Everything	1 (4.2 oz)	360	3	0	0	14	72	3	40	710	—	0	—	0
Sourdough Bagel Honey 8 Grain	1 (4.2 oz)	360	2	0	0	14	72	6	40	580	—	0	—	0
Sourdough Bagel Mocha Chip Swirl	1 (5 oz)	370	4	2	0	12	72	3	40	480	—	0	—	0
Sourdough Bagel Plain	1 (4 oz)	350	1	0	0	13	71	3	0	540	—	0	—	0
Sourdough Bagel Sesame	1 (4.2 oz)	380	4	1	0	15	71	3	40	540	—	0	—	0
Sourdough Bagel Wild Blueberry	1 (4.5 oz)	380	2	0	0	14	80	4	20	570	—	0	—	0
Valentine Cookie Chocolate Dipped Shortbread	1 (2.8 oz)	410	27	19	55	4	41	2	20	160	—	0	—	750

FOOD	PORTION	CALORIES	FAT	SAT FAT	CHOL	PROTEIN	CARBO	FIBER	CALCIUM	SOD	POTAS	VIT C	FOLIC	VIT A
Valentine Cookie Red Sugar Shortbread Heart	1 (2.4 oz)	350	22	14	60	3	37	1	20	170	—	0	—	750
Valentine Cookie Shortbread	1 (2.4 oz)	340	22	14	60	3	35	1	20	170	—	0	—	750
SALAD DRESSINGS														
Bleu Cheese	1 serv (3 oz)	370	41	8	40	4	8	0	80	910	—	0	—	100
Buttermilk Ranch	1 serv (3 oz)	310	32	4	35	3	4	0	80	270	—	0	—	0
Ceasar	1 serv (3 oz)	380	39	5	25	5	3	0	150	410	—	0	—	0
Fat Free Tomato Basil	1 serv (3 oz)	70	0	0	0	1	17	1	0	650	—	5	—	400
Greek	1 serv (3 oz)	440	50	7	0	0	2	0	0	820	—	0	—	0
Lemon Basil Vinaigrette	1 serv (3 oz)	330	32	2	0	0	15	0	0	460	—	0	—	0
Lite Honey Mustard	1 serv (3 oz)	280	17	3	40	2	30	1	20	560	—	2	—	0
Lite Italian	1 serv (3 oz)	230	20	2	0	0	15	0	0	570	—	0	—	0
Sesame French	1 serv (3 oz)	370	30	5	0	1	26	1	20	1010	—	4	—	500
SALADS AND SALAD BARS														
Caesar	1 serv (8.9 oz)	270	10	6	20	19	27	5	500	800	—	54	—	5500
Chicken Caesar	1 serv (11.4 oz)	360	11	6	65	36	28	5	500	910	—	54	—	5500
Garden	1 lg (10.6 oz)	160	2	0	0	7	34	6	150	290	—	60	—	14000
Garden	1 sm (7.5 oz)	100	1	0	0	5	20	4	100	150	—	42	—	11500
Mozzarella & Roasted Pepper Salad	1 serv (13.7 oz)	340	18	10	60	22	25	10	900	135	—	534	—	22000
Pesto Chicken Salad	1 serv (10.7 oz)	230	11	2	45	20	11	4	100	250	—	48	—	10000
Tuna	1 serv (15 oz)	490	27	5	45	26	40	7	200	750	—	78	—	16000
SANDWICHES AND FILLINGS														
Bagel Spreads Lite Strawberry	1 serv (2 oz)	150	11	7	35	5	6	1	100	210	—	6	—	500
Bagel Spreads Lite Vanilla Hazelnut	1 serv (2 oz)	150	11	7	35	5	6	1	40	210	—	0	—	500
Cheddar	½ serv (1.5 oz)	170	14	9	45	11	1	0	400	260	—	0	—	500
Chicken Tarragon	1 serv (4 oz)	240	17	3	65	20	1	0	20	170	—	0	—	0
Club Sandwich Hot Roasted Turkey	1 (14.9 oz)	950	50	16	135	50	80	4	150	2240	—	27	—	1250
Country Ham	1 serv (3.7 oz)	150	7	3	55	21	1	0	0	1370	—	1	—	0
Cracked Pepper Chicken	1 serv (3.9 oz)	140	2	0	72	27	2	0	0	184	—	19	—	160
Cream Cheese Lite	1 serv (2 oz)	130	12	8	35	5	2	1	40	230	—	0	—	500
Cream Cheese Lite Honey Walnut	1 serv (2 oz)	260	12	5	20	4	8	—	80	260	—	0	—	1000
Cream Cheese Lite Raspberry	1 serv (2 oz)	200	8	5	20	6	10	—	80	280	—	0	—	1000

FOOD	PORTION	CALORIES	FAT	SAT FAT	CHOL	PROTEIN	CARBO	FIBER	CALCIUM	SOD	POTAS	VIT C	FOLIC	VIT A
Cream Cheese Lite Sun-Dried Tomato	1 serv (2 oz)	130	11	8	35	5	2	1	40	230	—	1	—	750
Cream Cheese Plain	1 serv (2 oz)	190	18	12	55	3	2	—	40	210	—	0	—	600
Cream Cheese Veggie Lite	1 serv (2 oz)	100	10	5	20	6	6	—	80	300	—	2	—	6000
Grilled Chicken	1 serv (3.9 oz)	140	2	0	72	27	2	0	0	184	—	19	—	160
Hot Croissant Ham & Cheese	1 (4.2 oz)	380	20	12	70	16	36	1	200	690	—	1	—	750
Hot Croissants Spinach & Cheese	1 (3.6 oz)	270	16	9	40	9	27	2	200	330	—	9	—	3000
Provolone	½ serv (1.5 oz)	150	11	7	30	11	1	0	300	370	—	0	—	300
Roast Beef	1 serv (3.7 oz)	140	5	0	50	22	1	0	20	550	—	0	—	0
Sandwich Arizona Chicken	1 (12.7 oz)	720	33	12	125	49	57	4	350	1190	—	18	—	2250
Sandwich Buffalo Chicken	1 (13.7 oz)	640	19	4	85	41	76	3	150	1650	—	21	—	1250
Sandwich California Chicken	1 (13.2 oz)	820	44	12	135	51	55	4	600	1200	—	15	—	1750
Sandwich Fresh Mozzarella Tomato & Pesto	1 (10.5 oz)	650	30	12	55	30	69	4	900	1090	—	21	—	4000
Sandwich Honey Dijon Chicken	1 (15.3 oz)	730	18	6	135	57	85	4	350	1990	—	21	—	1250
Sandwich Parmesan Chicken	1 (11.1 oz)	740	24	9	70	42	91	5	400	1620	—	5	—	1000
Sandwich Steak & Cheese Melt	1 (11.7 oz)	750	32	8	90	40	79	2	200	1600	—	1	—	1000
Sandwich Thai Chicken	1 (8.3 oz)	420	6	1	20	20	72	3	200	1320	—	15	—	500
Swiss	½ serv (1.5 oz)	160	12	8	40	12	1	0	80	110	—	0	—	400
Tuna Salad	1 serv (4.5 oz)	360	29	5	50	21	3	1	20	520	—	1	—	4000
Turkey Breast	1 serv (3.7 oz)	120	1	0	20	24	1	0	0	1110	—	0	—	0
Wraps Chicken Caesar	1 (9.9 oz)	630	31	8	80	36	46	2	500	1140	—	21	—	2500
Wraps Southwestern Tuna	1 (14.4 oz)	950	64	17	110	41	53	4	350	1230	—	36	—	11000
Wraps Summer Turkey	1 (11.7 oz)	340	9	1	35	29	36	9	60	1380	—	510	—	20000
SOUPS														
Beef Barley	1 serv (16 oz)	150	4	2	25	12	22	5	40	1310	—	6	—	6500
Beef Barley	1 serv (12 oz)	112	3	1	18	9	16	3	40	980	—	5	—	4500
Beef Barley	1 serv (8 oz)	75	2	1	15	6	11	2	20	660	—	4	—	3000
Beef Stew	1 serv (8 oz)	140	7	3	25	9	14	2	20	840	—	12	—	2250

FOOD	PORTION	CALORIES	FAT	SAT FAT	CHOL	PROTEIN	CARBO	FIBER	CALCIUM	SOD	POTAS	VIT C	FOLIC	VIT A
Bohemian Cabbage	1 serv (8 oz)	70	3	1	0	3	11	2	50	650	—	1	—	550
Bohemian Cabbage	1 serv (12 oz)	110	5	2	0	4	17	4	70	960	—	2	—	850
Bohemian Cabbage	1 serv (16 oz)	140	6	2	0	5	22	5	90	1280	—	2	—	1100
Bread Bowl	1 (9 oz)	640	4	1	0	27	131	5	20	1950	—	21	—	0
Broccoli & Cheddar	1 serv (8 oz)	260	22	11	50	9	13	1	100	690	—	21	—	1500
Broccoli & Cheddar	1 serv (16 oz)	520	44	22	100	17	25	2	250	1380	—	42	—	3000
Broccoli & Cheddar	1 serv (12 oz)	390	33	17	75	13	19	2	150	1030	—	30	—	2250
Caribbean Black Bean	1 serv (16 oz)	250	2	0	10	13	43	16	100	1540	—	2	—	2500
Caribbean Black Bean	1 serv (12 oz)	180	2	0	10	10	32	12	80	1150	—	1	—	2000
Caribbean Black Bean	1 serv (8 oz)	120	1	0	5	7	22	8	60	770	—	1	—	1250
Chicken Chili	1 serv (12 oz)	350	18	10	65	21	31	5	100	2030	—	12	—	1500
Chicken Chili	1 serv (8 oz)	240	12	7	45	14	21	4	60	1350	—	9	—	1000
Chicken Chili	1 serv (16 oz)	470	24	13	90	28	41	8	150	2700	—	15	—	1750
Chicken Noodle	1 serv (16 oz)	170	3	1	35	16	19	2	40	1340	—	5	—	7000
Chicken Noodle	1 serv (8 oz)	80	2	0	15	8	10	1	20	670	—	2	—	3500
Chicken Noodle	1 serv (12 oz)	120	2	1	25	12	14	2	40	1000	—	4	—	5000
Chili	1 serv (12 oz)	340	14	6	50	22	32	7	40	910	—	48	—	1750
Chili	1 serv (8 oz)	230	10	4	35	15	22	5	40	610	—	36	—	1250
Chili	1 serv (16 oz)	460	19	7	70	30	43	9	60	1220	—	66	—	2500
Clam Chowder	1 serv (16 oz)	540	39	18	125	22	32	1	300	1460	—	6	—	1500
Clam Chowder	1 serv (8 oz)	270	19	9	65	11	16	0	150	730	—	4	—	750
Clam Chowder	1 serv (12 oz)	400	29	14	95	16	24	1	250	1090	—	5	—	1000
Corn Chowder	1 serv (8 oz)	260	16	10	50	5	29	1	100	760	—	6	—	1250
Corn Chowder	1 serv (12 oz)	390	24	14	70	8	43	2	150	1150	—	9	—	1750
Corn Chowder	1 serv (16 oz)	530	33	19	95	11	58	3	200	1530	—	12	—	2250
Cream Of Broccoli	1 serv (16 oz)	440	37	17	80	10	28	3	250	1550	—	60	—	2000
Cream Of Broccoli	1 serv (8 oz)	220	18	9	40	5	14	1	150	770	—	30	—	1000
Cream Of Broccoli	1 serv (12 oz)	330	28	13	60	8	21	2	200	1160	—	48	—	1500
Cream Of Chicken With Wild Rice	1 serv (16 oz)	330	19	11	90	19	33	1	200	1310	—	6	—	4000
French Onion	1 serv (12 oz)	120	5	1	0	4	17	3	40	1910	—	9	—	100
French Onion	1 serv (16 oz)	170	7	1	0	5	23	4	60	2550	—	15	—	200
French Onion	1 serv (8 oz)	80	4	1	0	2	12	2	20	1280	—	6	—	100
In A Bread Bowl Beef Barley	1 serv (21 oz)	760	7	2	20	36	147	8	60	2940	—	27	—	4500
In A Bread Bowl Carribean Black Bean	1 serv (21 oz)	830	5	1	10	36	163	17	100	3100	—	24	—	2000
In A Bread Bowl Chicken Chili	1 serv (21 oz)	990	22	11	65	48	162	12	100	3970	—	12	—	1500
In A Bread Bowl Chicken Noodle	1 serv (21 oz)	760	6	1	20	39	146	7	60	2950	—	27	—	5000
In A Bread Bowl Clam Chowder	1 serv (21 oz)	1050	32	15	100	43	155	5	250	3040	—	27	—	1000

FOOD	PORTION	CALORIES	FAT	SAT FAT	CHOL	PROTEIN	CARBO	FIBER	CALCIUM	SOD	POTAS	VIT C	FOLIC	VIT A
In A Bread Bowl Cream of Broccoli	1 serv (21 oz)	970	31	15	60	34	152	7	250	3100	—	66	—	1500
In A Bread Bowl French Onion	1 serv (21 oz)	760	8	2	0	30	148	8	60	3860	—	9	—	100
In A Bread Bowl New England Potato & Cheese w/ Ham	1 serv (21 oz)	860	15	9	40	34	152	9	80	3170	—	66	—	750
In A Bread Bowl Tomato Florentine	1 serv (21 oz)	760	5	2	10	33	150	8	100	3490	—	42	—	1500
In A Bread Bowl Vegetarian Chili	1 serv (21 oz)	870	7	1	0	36	171	8	80	3550	—	66	—	750
Louisiana Beans & Rice	1 serv (16 oz)	360	9	2	20	18	50	3	130	1320	—	2	—	500
Louisiana Beans & Rice	1 serv (8 oz)	180	5	1	10	9	25	1	70	660	—	1	—	550
Louisiana Beans & Rice	1 serv (12 oz)	280	7	2	15	13	37	2	100	960	—	2	—	400
New England Potato & Cheese w/ Ham	1 serv (8 oz)	150	8	5	25	5	14	3	0	820	—	1	—	300
New England Potato & Cheese w/ Ham	1 serv (12 oz)	220	12	8	40	7	21	4	0	1220	—	1	—	500
New England Potato & Cheese w/ Ham	1 serv (16 oz)	290	15	11	55	10	28	5	0	1630	—	2	—	750
Potato Leek	1 serv (12 oz)	320	20	12	70	6	28	2	—	1700	—	18	—	1500
Potato Leek	1 serv (8 oz)	200	13	8	45	4	18	2	—	1060	—	12	—	750
Potato Leek	1 serv (16 oz)	400	25	15	85	7	36	3	—	2120	—	21	—	1250
Sante Fe Chicken Tortilla	1 serv (16 oz)	300	13	4	30	12	42	4	150	1900	—	2	—	900
Sante Fe Chicken Tortilla	1 serv (8 oz)	150	7	2	15	6	21	2	70	950	—	1	—	450
Sante Fe Chicken Tortilla	1 serv (12 oz)	230	10	3	25	9	32	3	110	1430	—	1	—	700
Seafood Gumbo	1 serv (16 oz)	260	12	2	35	14	28	3	60	1160	—	48	—	750
Seafood Gumbo	1 serv (12 oz)	190	9	1	25	10	21	2	40	870	—	36	—	500
Seafood Gumbo	1 serv (8 oz)	130	6	1	20	7	14	1	40	580	—	24	—	400
Tomato Florentine	1 serv (8 oz)	61	1	1	5	4	13	2	60	1030	—	12	—	1000
Tomato Florentine	1 serv (16 oz)	122	2	1	5	8	27	3	100	2070	—	27	—	1750
Tomato Florentine	1 serv (12 oz)	90	2	1	5	6	20	2	80	1550	—	18	—	1250
Tomato Tortellini	1 serv (16 oz)	110	2	1	10	6	20	3	80	1770	—	21	—	500
Tomato Tortellini	1 serv (8 oz)	60	1	0	5	3	11	2	40	950	—	12	—	300
Tomato Tortellini	1 serv (12 oz)	90	2	1	5	4	15	2	60	1320	—	15	—	400
Vegetable Stew	1 serv (16 oz)	130	2	1	5	6	22	5	150	1950	—	54	—	4500
Vegetable Stew	1 serv (12 oz)	100	2	1	5	5	16	4	100	1460	—	42	—	3000
Vegetable Stew	1 serv (8 oz)	60	1	0	5	3	11	2	60	980	—	27	—	2250

FOOD	PORTION	CALORIES	FAT	SAT FAT	CHOL	PROTEIN	CARBO	FIBER	CALCIUM	SOD	POTAS	VIT C	FOLIC	VIT A
Vegetarian Lentil	1 serv (8 oz)	130	0	0	0	10	24	2	40	790	—	5	—	3000
Vegetarian Lentil	1 serv (16 oz)	270	1	0	0	21	47	5	60	1580	—	9	—	6000
Vegetarian Lentil	1 serv (12 oz)	200	1	0	0	16	35	4	40	1180	—	6	—	4500
Vegetarian Chili	1 serv (8 oz)	139	3	0	0	6	27	2	40	1070	—	30	—	500
Vegetarian Chili	1 serv (12 oz)	210	4	0	0	9	40	3	60	1610	—	42	—	750
Vegetarian Chili	1 serv (16 oz)	278	·5	1	0	13	53	4	80	2150	—	60	—	1000
Vegetarian Corn & Green Chili Bisque	1 serv (8 oz)	190	10	6	30	4	21	3	—	1140	—	54	—	2000
Vegetarian Corn & Green Chili Bisque	1 serv (16 oz)	380	20	12	60	8	41	5	—	2290	—	114	—	4000
Vegetarian Corn & Green Chili Bisque	1 serv (12 oz)	300	16	9	45	7	30	4	—	1830	—	90	—	3000

BASKIN-ROBBINS

FROZEN YOGURT

FOOD	PORTION	CALORIES	FAT	SAT FAT	CHOL	PROTEIN	CARBO	FIBER	CALCIUM	SOD	POTAS	VIT C	FOLIC	VIT A
Maui Brownie Madness	½ cup	140	3	1	5	4	26	1	100	80	—	0	—	0
Perils Of Pauline	½ cup	140	3	2	5	4	25	0	100	105	—	0	—	0

ICE CREAM

FOOD	PORTION	CALORIES	FAT	SAT FAT	CHOL	PROTEIN	CARBO	FIBER	CALCIUM	SOD	POTAS	VIT C	FOLIC	VIT A
Banana Strawberry	½ cup	130	7	5	25	2	17	0	60	40	—	1	—	300
Baseball Nut	½ cup	160	9	5	30	2	18	0	60	55	—	2	—	300
Black Walnut	½ cup	160	11	5	30	3	13	1	60	45	—	0	—	300
Cherries Jubilee	½ cup	140	7	5	30	2	16	0	60	40	—	0	—	300
Chocolate	½ cup	150	9	6	30	2	18	0	60	60	—	0	—	300
Chocolate Almond	½ cup	180	11	5	30	3	17	1	60	55	—	0	—	300
Chocolate Chip	½ cup	150	10	6	35	2	15	0	60	45	—	0	—	300
Chocolate Chip Cookie Dough	½ cup	170	9	6	35	2	20	0	60	70	—	0	—	300
Chocolate Fudge	½ cup	160	9	6	30	2	21	0	60	80	—	0	—	300
Chocolate Mousse Royale	½ cup	170	10	5	25	2	20	1	60	60	—	0	—	300
Chocolate Raspberry Truffle	½ cup	180	9	6	30	3	23	0	80	60	—	0	—	300
Chunky Heath Bar	½ cup	170	10	6	30	2	19	0	60	70	—	0	—	300
Cookies N Cream	½ cup	170	11	7	30	2	16	0	60	80	—	0	—	300
Dirt 'N Worms	½ cup	160	8	5	25	2	22	0	60	80	—	0	—	200
Egg Nog	½ cup	150	8	5	40	2	16	0	60	45	—	0	—	300
Everybody's Favorite Candy Bar	½ cup	170	9	5	30	2	20	2	80	30	—	0	—	300
French Vanilla	½ cup	160	10	6	70	2	14	0	80	45	—	0	—	400
French Vanilla	½ cup	170	11	7	55	2	15	—	90	50	—	0	—	450
Fudge Brownie	½ cup	170	11	6	25	3	19	1	60	75	—	0	—	300
Fudge Brownie	½ cup	180	10	7	20	3	20	—	60	—	—	0	—	300

FOOD	PORTION	CALORIES	FAT	SAT FAT	CHOL	PROTEIN	CARBO	FIBER	CALCIUM	SOD	POTAS	VIT C	FOLIC	VIT A
German Chocolate Cake	½ cup	180	10	6	25	3	20	0	80	75	—	0	—	300
Gold Medal Ribbon	½ cup	150	8	5	30	2	20	0	60	95	—	0	—	300
Gold Medal Ribbon	½ cup	150	7	5	20	2	20	—	110	—	—	0	—	300
Jamoca	½ cup	140	9	5	35	2	14	0	60	45	—	0	—	300
Jamoca Almond Fudge	½ cup	150	8	5	20	3	17	—	60	65	—	0	—	250
Jomoca Almond Fudge	½ cup	140	9	5	25	3	17	0	60	40	—	0	—	300
Lemon Custard	½ cup	150	8	5	45	2	16	0	80	55	—	0	—	300
Lowfat Carmel Apple AlaMod	½ cup	100	2	1	5	3	20	0	100	75	—	2	—	0
Lowfat Espresso 'N Cream	½ cup	100	3	1	5	3	18	1	100	60	—	0	—	0
Mint Chocolate Chip	½ cup	150	10	6	35	3	15	0	60	35	—	0	—	300
No Sugar Added Call Me Nuts	½ cup	110	2	1	5	3	21	1	100	55	—	0	—	0
No Sugar Added Cherry Cordial	½ cup	100	2	2	5	3	18	0	100	55	—	0	—	0
No Sugar Added Mad About Chocolate	½ cup	100	2	1	5	3	19	0	80	40	—	0	—	0
No Sugar Added Pineapple Coconut	½ cup	90	2	1	5	3	16	0	100	60	—	1	—	0
No Sugar Added Thin Mint	½ cup	100	3	2	5	3	16	0	150	65	—	0	—	0
Nonfat Berry Innocent Cheese	½ cup	110	0	0	0	3	24	0	100	100	—	0	—	0
Nonfat Check-It-Out Cherry	½ cup	100	0	0	0	3	22	0	100	90	—	0	—	0
Nonfat Jamoca Swirl	½ cup	110	0	0	5	3	23	0	100	105	—	0	—	0
Ocean Commotion	½ cup	150	7	5	25	1	20	0	60	40	—	0	—	300
Old Fashion Butter Pecan	½ cup	160	11	6	35	2	13	0	60	35	—	0	—	300
Oregon Blueberry	½ cup	140	8	5	30	2	16	0	60	50	—	0	—	300
Peanut Butter 'N Chocolate	½ cup	180	12	6	30	3	16	1	60	95	—	0	—	300
Pink Bubblegum	½ cup	150	8	5	30	2	19	0	60	40	—	0	—	300
Pistachio Almond	½ cup	170	12	5	30	3	13	1	60	45	—	0	—	300
Pralines 'N Cream	½ cup	160	9	5	30	2	19	0	60	85	—	0	—	300
Pumpkin Pie	½ cup	130	7	5	30	2	16	0	60	50	—	0	—	300
Quarterback Crunch	½ cup	160	10	7	30	2	18	0	80	75	—	0	—	300
Reeses Peanut Butter	½ cup	180	11	6	30	3	17	0	60	70	—	0	—	300

FOOD	PORTION	CALORIES	FAT	SAT FAT	CHOL	PROTEIN	CARBO	FIBER	CALCIUM	SOD	POTAS	VIT C	FOLIC	VIT A
Rocky Road	½ cup	170	10	5	30	3	19	0	60	60	—	0	—	300
Rum Raisin	½ cup	140	7	5	30	2	18	0	60	40	—	0	—	300
Strawberry Cheesecake	½ cup	150	9	5	35	2	17	0	60	65	—	1	—	300
Triple Chocolate Passion	½ cup	180	11	7	35	3	21	0	80	70	—	0	—	300
Vanilla	½ cup	140	8	5	40	3	14	0	100	40	—	0	—	300
Very Berry Strawberry	½ cup	130	7	4	25	1	16	0	60	40	—	6	—	300
Winter White Chocolate	½ cup	150	9	6	25	2	18	0	60	50	—	2	—	200
World Class Chocolate	½ cup	160	9	5	30	2	18	0	60	55	—	0	—	300
ICES AND ICE POPS														
Daiquiri Ice	½ cup	110	0	0	0	0	28	0	0	10	—	0	—	0
Sherbet Blue Raspberry	½ cup	120	2	1	5	1	25	0	40	30	—	0	—	0
Sherbet Orange	½ cup	120	2	1	5	1	26	0	40	25	—	2	—	0
Sherbet Rainbow	½ cup	120	2	1	5	1	26	0	40	25	—	1	—	0
Sorbet Pink Raspberry Lemon	½ cup	120	0	0	0	0	29	0	0	10	—	0	—	0
The Mask Ice	½ cup	120	0	0	0	0	29	0	0	10	—	2	—	0
Watermelon Ice	½ cup	110	0	0	0	0	28	0	0	10	—	0	—	0
Watermelon Ice	½ cup	110	0	0	0	0	28	0	0	10	—	0	—	0

BEN & JERRY'S

FOOD	PORTION	CALORIES	FAT	SAT FAT	CHOL	PROTEIN	CARBO	FIBER	CALCIUM	SOD	POTAS	VIT C	FOLIC	VIT A
Sugar Cone	1	48	tr	tr	0	1	10	tr	1	42	—	0	—	0
FROZEN YOGURT														
Cherry Garcia	½ cup (3.3 oz)	150	3	2	15	4	29	tr	150	60	—	0	—	100
Chocolate Chip Cookie Dough	½ cup (3.3 oz)	190	4	3	25	4	34	0	150	110	—	0	—	100
Chocolate Fudge Brownie	½ cup (3.3 oz)	180	3	2	15	8	32	1	150	100	—	0	—	100
No Fat Black Raspberry	½ cup (3.4 oz)	140	0	0	5	4	30	0	150	60	—	2	—	0
No Fat Vanilla	½ cup (3.4 oz)	140	0	0	5	4	28	0	200	75	—	0	—	0
No Fat Vanilla Swirl	½ cup (3.4 oz)	130	0	0	0	3	29	0	100	70	—	0	—	100
Peach Raspberry Trifle	½ cup (3.3 oz)	150	2	1	20	8	30	tr	100	65	—	2	—	100
Vanilla w/ Heath Toffee Crunch	½ cup (3.3 oz)	190	6	3	20	4	30	0	150	115	—	0	—	100
ICE CREAM														
Butter Pecan	½ cup (3.1 oz)	270	21	9	60	4	17	tr	100	105	—	0	—	500
Cherry Garcia	½ cup (3.1 oz)	210	12	9	55	3	20	tr	100	45	—	0	—	400
Chocolate Chip Cookie Dough	½ cup (3.1 oz)	180	11	8	55	3	17	0	100	45	—	0	—	400
Chocolate Fudge Brownie	½ cup (3.1 oz)	230	11	7	35	4	28	2	100	80	—	0	—	400

FOOD	PORTION	CALORIES	FAT	SAT FAT	CHOL	PROTEIN	CARBO	FIBER	CALCIUM	SOD	POTAS	VIT C	FOLIC	VIT A
Chubby Hubby	½ cup (3.1 oz)	280	17	10	50	5	26	1	100	135	—	0	—	400
Chunky Monkey	½ cup (3.1 oz)	220	13	9	50	3	25	0	100	45	—	1	—	400
Coffee Coffee Buzz Buzz	½ cup (3.1 oz)	240	16	11	55	3	23	tr	100	60	—	0	—	400
Coffee Ole	½ cup (3.1 oz)	200	13	9	65	3	18	0	100	50	—	0	—	500
Coffee w/ Heath Toffee Crunch	½ cup (3.1 oz)	250	16	9	55	3	25	0	100	105	—	0	—	400
Cool Britannia	½ cup (3.1 oz)	210	12	8	55	3	23	0	100	55	—	4	—	400
Deep Deep Chocolate	½ cup (3.1 oz)	210	12	8	40	4	22	2	100	40	—	0	—	400
Holy Cannoli	½ cup (3.1 oz)	240	16	9	55	4	20	tr	100	55	—	0	—	500
Low Fat Blond Brownie Sundae	½ cup (3.1 oz)	160	3	2	25	4	32	tr	150	80	—	0	—	300
Low Fat Coffee & Biscotti	½ cup (3.1 oz)	160	3	2	30	5	30	tr	150	85	—	0	—	300
Low Fat Sweet Cream & Cookies	½ cup (3.1 oz)	160	3	2	25	4	30	0	150	100	—	0	—	300
Low Fat Vanilla & Chocolate Mint Patty	½ cup (3.1 oz)	170	3	2	20	4	32	tr	150	65	—	0	—	300
Maple Walnut	½ cup (3.1 oz)	240	13	8	55	3	19	0	100	40	—	0	—	400
Mint Chocolate Chunk	½ cup (3.1 oz)	240	16	11	60	3	24	0	100	55	—	0	—	500
Mint Chocolate Cookie	½ cup (3.1 oz)	230	14	8	60	4	24	tr	100	110	—	0	—	500
New York Super Fudge Chunk	½ cup (3.1 oz)	250	16	9	35	4	25	0	100	45	—	0	—	400
Peanut Butter Cup	½ cup (3.1 oz)	270	18	10	55	5	21	1	100	95	—	0	—	400
Peanut Butter & Jelly	½ cup (3.1 oz)	230	14	7	50	4	23	tr	100	85	—	0	—	400
Phish Food	½ cup (3.1 oz)	230	12	8	30	3	30	1	100	70	—	0	—	300
Pistachio Pistachio	½ cup (3.1 oz)	230	16	9	60	5	18	tr	100	45	—	0	—	500
Rainforest Crunch	½ cup (3.1 oz)	250	16	9	60	4	21	0	100	105	—	0	—	500
Southern Peach	½ cup (3.1 oz)	180	10	7	50	3	20	0	100	40	—	2	—	500
Strawberry	½ cup (3.1 oz)	180	10	7	50	3	20	tr	100	40	—	9	—	400
Sweet Cream Cookie	½ cup (3.1 oz)	230	14	8	60	4	23	tr	100	110	—	0	—	500
Vanilla Caramel Fudge	½ cup (3.1 oz)	230	13	8	60	3	25	0	100	85	—	0	—	500
Vanilla Chocolate Chunk	½ cup (3.1 oz)	240	16	11	60	3	23	0	100	55	—	0	—	500
Vanilla Fudge Brownie	½ cup (3.1 oz)	210	12	7	60	4	23	0	80	80	—	0	—	500
Vanilla World's Best	½ cup (3.1 oz)	200	13	9	65	3	17	0	150	50	—	0	—	500
Vanilla w/ Heath Toffee Crunch	½ cup (3.1 oz)	250	16	9	60	3	25	0	100	110	—	0	—	400
Wavy Gravy	½ cup (3.1 oz)	260	17	8	50	5	24	1	150	75	—	0	—	400
White Russian	½ cup (3.1 oz)	200	13	9	65	3	18	0	100	45	—	0	—	500

FOOD	PORTION	CALORIES	FAT	SAT FAT	CHOL	PROTEIN	CARBO	FIBER	CALCIUM	SOD	POTAS	VIT C	FOLIC	VIT A
SORBETS														
Cranberry Orange	½ cup (3.2 oz)	110	0	0	0	0	26	0	20	10	—	9	—	0
Doonesberry	½ cup (3.2 oz)	100	0	0	0	0	27	0	20	10	—	5	—	0
Mango Lime	½ cup (3.2 oz)	110	0	0	0	0	27	0	20	10	—	6	—	750
Pina Colada	½ cup (3.2 oz)	110	0	0	0	0	26	0	20	10	—	2	—	0
Purple Passion Fruit	½ cup (3.2 oz)	100	0	0	0	0	27	0	20	10	—	4	—	0
Strawberry Kiwi	½ cup (3.2 oz)	110	0	0	0	0	27	tr	20	10	—	12	—	0

BIG BOY

FOOD	PORTION	CALORIES	FAT	SAT FAT	CHOL	PROTEIN	CARBO	FIBER	CALCIUM	SOD	POTAS	VIT C	FOLIC	VIT A
DESSERTS														
Frozen Yogurt Fat Free	1 serv	118	0	—	0	3	27	—	—	60	—	—	—	—
Frozen Yogurt Shake	1	156	1	—	2	7	33	—	—	120	—	—	—	—
MAIN MENU SELECTIONS														
Baked Cod w/ Salad Baked Potato Roll & Margarine	1 meal	744	21	—	76	57	82	—	—	655	—	—	—	—
Baked Potato	1	163	2	—	0	6	37	—	—	7	—	—	—	—
Breast of Chicken Pita w/ Mozzarella & Ranch Dressing	1	361	11	—	84	41	23	—	—	369	—	—	—	—
Breast of Chicken w/ Mozzarella Salad Baked Potato Roll & Margarine	1 meal	697	20	—	76	50	80	—	—	613	—	—	—	—
Cabbage Soup	1 bowl	40	5	—	0	1	7	—	—	347	—	—	—	—
Cabbage Soup	1 cup	34	4	—	0	1	6	—	—	295	—	—	—	—
Cajun Cod w/ Salad Baked Potato Roll & Margarine	1 meal	736	21	—	76	56	80	—	—	745	—	—	—	—
Chicken & Pasta Primavera w/ Salad Roll & Margarine	1 meal	676	14	—	65	53	83	—	—	875	—	—	—	—
Chicken 'n Vegetable Stir Fry w/ Salad Baked Potato Roll & Margarine	1 meal	795	18	—	65	51	109	—	—	845	—	—	—	—
Dinner Roll	1	210	5	—	0	0	36	—	—	340	—	—	—	—
Plain Egg Beaters Omelette w/ Whole Wheat Bread & Margarine	1 meal	305	10	—	0	19	36	—	—	603	—	—	—	—
Promise Margarine	1 pat	25	3	—	0	0	0	—	—	35	—	—	—	—

FOOD	PORTION	CALORIES	FAT	SAT FAT	CHOL	PROTEIN	CARBO	FIBER	CALCIUM	SOD	POTAS	VIT C	FOLIC	VIT A
Rice Pilaf	1 serv	153	4	—	10	3	25	—	—	688	—	—	—	—
Scrambled Egg Beaters w/ Whole Wheat Bread & Margarine	1 meal	305	10	—	0	19	36	—	—	603	—	—	—	—
Southwest Chicken w/ Salad Baked Potato Roll & Margarine	1 meal	702	18	—	76	50	85	—	—	948	—	—	—	—
Spaghetti Marinara w/ Salad Roll & Margarine	1 meal	754	11	—	8	17	105	—	—	754	—	—	—	—
Turkey Pita w/ Ranch Dressing	1	245	6	—	83	25	23	—	—	938	—	—	—	—
Vegetable Stir Fry w/ Salad Baked Potato Roll & Margarine	1 meal	616	14	—	0	17	109	—	—	774	—	—	—	—
Vegetarian Egg Beaters Omelette w/ Whole Wheat Bread & Margarine	1 meal	330	10	—	0	21	40	—	—	618	—	—	—	—
SALAD DRESSINGS														
Italian Fat Free	1 oz	11	0	—	0	0	3	—	—	191	—	—	—	—
Lo Cal Oriental	1 oz	20	2	—	0	1	4	—	—	189	—	—	—	—
Lo Cal Ranch	1 oz	41	3	—	8	1	3	—	—	151	—	—	—	—
SALADS AND SALAD BARS														
Chicken Breast Salad w/ Roll & Margarine	1 serv	523	16	—	73	44	50	—	—	654	—	—	—	—
Oriental Chicken Breast Salad w/ Dinner Roll & Margarine	1 serv	660	20	—	65	48	73	—	—	855	—	—	—	—
Tossed Salad	1	35	2	—	0	2	7	—	—	71	—	—	—	—

BLIMPIE

6 INCH SUB

FOOD	PORTION	CALORIES	FAT	SAT FAT	CHOL	PROTEIN	CARBO	FIBER	CALCIUM	SOD	POTAS	VIT C	FOLIC	VIT A
5 Meatball	1 (7.8 oz)	500	22	8	25	23	52	2	100	970	—	2	—	750
Blimpie Best	1 (8.5 oz)	410	13	5	50	26	47	4	150	1480	—	5	—	750
Cheese Trio	1 (8.2 oz)	510	23	13	60	26	51	2	250	1060	—	0	—	500
Club	1 (9.8 oz)	450	13	6	40	30	53	3	500	1350	—	6	—	1250
Grilled Chicken	1 (9.1 oz)	400	9	2	30	28	52	2	80	950	—	2	—	500
Ham & Swiss	1 (8.2 oz)	400	13	7	35	25	47	5	400	970	—	5	—	1000
Ham Salami Provolone	1 (9.8 oz)	590	28	11	70	32	52	3	300	1880	—	6	—	500
Roast Beef	1 (8.5 oz)	340	5	1	20	27	47	2	80	870	—	0	—	200
Steak & Cheese	1 (7.1 oz)	550	26	4	70	27	51	2	0	1080	—	0	—	0

FOOD	PORTION	CALORIES	FAT	SAT FAT	CHOL	PROTEIN	CARBO	FIBER	CALCIUM	SOD	POTAS	VIT C	FOLIC	VIT A
Tuna	1 (10.2 oz)	570	32	5	50	21	50	2	0	790	—	21	—	500
Turkey	1 (8.2 oz)	320	5	1	10	19	51	3	80	890	—	5	—	300
SALADS AND SALAD BARS														
Grilled Chicken Salad	1 serv (16.2 oz)	350	12	0	150	47	13	0	0	1190	—	36	—	750

BOJANGLES

FOOD	PORTION	CALORIES	FAT	SAT FAT	CHOL	PROTEIN	CARBO	FIBER	CALCIUM	SOD	POTAS	VIT C	FOLIC	VIT A
BAKED SELECTIONS														
Biscuit	1	243	12	3	2	4	29	2	—	663	—	—	—	—
Multi-Grain Roll	1	150	3	0	0	6	26	3	—	210	—	—	—	—
Sweet Biscuit Apple Cinnamon	1	330	13	3	tr	4	48	1	—	540	—	—	—	—
Sweet Biscuit Bo*Berry	1	220	10	3	tr	3	29	1	—	410	—	—	—	—
Sweet Biscuit Cinnamon	1	320	18	4	tr	4	37	1	—	560	—	—	—	—
MAIN MENU SELECTIONS														
Biscuit Sandwich Bacon	1	290	17	5	10	8	26	1	—	810	—	—	—	—
Biscuit Sandwich Bacon Egg & Cheese	1	550	42	14	160	17	27	1	—	1250	—	—	—	—
Biscuit Sandwich Cajun Filet	1	454	21	6	41	20	46	1	—	949	—	—	—	—
Biscuit Sandwich Country Ham	1	270	15	4	20	9	26	1	—	1010	—	—	—	—
Biscuit Sandwich Egg	1	400	30	6	120	8	26	1	—	630	—	—	—	—
Biscuit Sandwich Sausage	1	350	23	7	20	9	26	1	—	810	—	—	—	—
Biscuit Sandwich Smoked Sausage	1	380	26	9	20	10	27	1	—	940	—	—	—	—
Biscuit Sandwich Steak	1	649	49	13	34	14	13	1	—	1126	—	—	—	—
Bo Rounds	1 serv	235	11	4	13	3	31	3	—	328	—	—	—	—
Buffalo Bites	1 serv	180	5	2	105	27	5	0	—	720	—	—	—	—
Cajun Pintos	1 serv	110	0	0	0	6	18	6	—	480	—	—	—	—
Cajun Roast Skinfree Breast	1 serv	143	5	—	84	24	tr	tr	—	562	—	—	—	—
Cajun Roast Skinfree Leg	1 serv	161	8	—	125	23	tr	tr	—	566	—	—	—	—
Cajun Roast Skinfree Thigh	1 serv	215	15	—	95	20	tr	tr	—	428	—	—	—	—
Cajun Roast Wing	1 serv	231	15	—	117	22	3	tr	—	617	—	—	—	—
Cajun Spiced Breast	1 serv	278	17	—	75	18	12	tr	—	565	—	—	—	—
Cajun Spiced Leg	1 serv	310	23	—	67	15	11	tr	—	465	—	—	—	—
Cajun Spiced Thigh	1 serv	264	16	—	96	19	11	tr	—	530	—	—	—	—

FOOD	PORTION	CALORIES	FAT	SAT FAT	CHOL	PROTEIN	CARBO	FIBER	CALCIUM	SOD	POTAS	VIT C	FOLIC	VIT A
Cajun Spiced Wing	1 serv	355	25	—	94	21	11	tr	—	630	—	—	—	—
Chicken Supremes	1 serv	337	16	6	58	21	26	1	—	629	—	—	—	—
Corn On The Cob	1 serv	140	2	0	0	5	34	2	—	20	—	—	—	—
Dirty Rice	1 serv	166	6	2	10	5	24	1	—	762	—	—	—	—
Green Beans	1 serv	25	0	0	0	5	25	2	—	710	—	—	—	—
Macaroni & Cheese	1 serv	198	14	5	26	7	12	tr	—	418	—	—	—	—
Marinated Cole Slaw	1 serv	136	3	0	0	1	26	3	—	454	—	—	—	—
Potatoes w/o Gravy	1 serv	80	1	0	0	2	16	1	—	380	—	—	—	—
Sandwich Cajun Filet w/ Mayonnaise	1	437	22	7	55	22	41	3	—	506	—	—	—	—
Sandwich Cajun Filet w/o Mayonnaise	1	337	11	5	45	22	41	3	—	401	—	—	—	—
Sandwich Cajun Steak w/ Horseradish Sauce & Pickles	1	434	26	8	55	18	39	2	—	985	—	—	—	—
Sandwich Grilled Filet w/ Mayonnaise	1	335	16	5	61	23	25	2	—	645	—	—	—	—
Sandwich Grilled Filet w/o Mayonnaise	1 serv (5.2 oz)	329	7	—	59	27	37	—	—	418	—	—	—	—
Seasoned Fries	1 serv.	344	19	5	13	5	39	4	—	480	—	—	—	—
Southern Style Breast	1 serv	261	16	—	76	16	12	tr	—	702	—	—	—	—
Southern Style Leg	1 serv	254	15	—	94	19	11	tr	—	446	—	—	—	—
Southern Style Thigh	1 serv	308	21	—	78	16	14	tr	—	630	—	—	—	—
Southern Style Wing	1 serv	337	21	—	86	17	19	tr	—	684	—	—	—	—

BOSTON MARKET

BAKED SELECTIONS

FOOD	PORTION	CALORIES	FAT	SAT FAT	CHOL	PROTEIN	CARBO	FIBER	CALCIUM	SOD	POTAS	VIT C	FOLIC	VIT A
Brownie	1 (3.3 oz)	450	27	7	80	6	47	3	20	190	—	0	—	100
Cookie Chocolate Chip	1 (2.8 oz)	340	17	6	25	4	48	1	40	240	—	0	—	300
Cookie Oatmeal Raisin	1 (2.8 oz)	320	13	3	25	4	48	1	40	260	—	0	—	100
Honey Wheat Roll	½ roll (2 oz)	150	2	0	0	5	29	2	40	280	—	0	—	0

MAIN MENU SELECTIONS

FOOD	PORTION	CALORIES	FAT	SAT FAT	CHOL	PROTEIN	CARBO	FIBER	CALCIUM	SOD	POTAS	VIT C	FOLIC	VIT A
½ Chicken w/ Skin	1 serv (10 oz)	630	37	19	370	74	2	0	100	960	—	1	—	0
¼ Dark Meat Chicken No Skin	1 serv (3.6 oz)	210	10	3	150	28	1	0	20	320	—	1	—	100
¼ Dark Meat Chicken w/ Skin	1 serv (4.6 oz)	330	22	6	180	31	2	0	20	460	—	2	—	0

FOOD	PORTION	CALORIES	FAT	SAT FAT	CHOL	PROTEIN	CARBO	FIBER	CALCIUM	SOD	POTAS	VIT C	FOLIC	VIT A
¼ White Meat Chicken No Skin Or Wing	1 serv (3.6 oz)	160	4	1	95	31	0	0	0	350	—	1	—	0
¼ White Meat Chicken w/ Skin	1 serv (5.4 oz)	330	18	5	175	43	2	0	20	530	—	2	—	0
BBQ Baked Beans	¾ cup (7.1 oz)	330	9	3	10	11	53	9	100	630	—	6	—	300
Butternut Squash Low Fat	¾ cup (6.8 oz)	160	6	4	15	2	25	3	80	580	—	24	—	6000
Caesar Salad Entree	1 serv (10 oz)	520	43	12	40	20	16	3	500	1420	—	30	—	2500
Caesar Salad w/o Dressing	1 serv (8 oz)	240	13	7	25	19	14	3	500	780	—	30	—	2500
Caesar Side Salad	1 (4 oz)	210	17	5	20	8	6	1	200	560	—	12	—	1000
Chicken Caesar Salad	1 serv (13 oz)	670	47	13	120	45	16	3	500	1860	—	30	—	2500
Chicken Gravy	1 serv (1 oz)	15	1	0	0	0	2	0	0	170	—	0	—	0
Chicken Salad Sandwich	1 (10.7 oz)	680	30	5	120	39	63	4	100	1360	—	12	—	200
Chicken Sandwich w/ Cheese & Sauce	1 (12.4 oz)	750	33	12	135	41	72	5	400	1860	—	9	—	750
Chicken Sandwich w/o Cheese & Sauce Low Fat	1 (10 oz)	430	4	1	65	34	62	5	100	910	—	9	—	200
Chunky Chicken Salad	¾ cup (5.5 oz)	370	27	5	120	28	3	1	20	800	—	4	—	100
Cole Slaw	¾ cup (6.5 oz)	280	16	3	25	2	32	3	60	520	—	36	—	750
Corn Bread	1 (2.4 oz)	200	6	2	25	3	33	1	0	390	—	0	—	0
Cranberry Relish Low Fat	¾ cup (7.9 oz)	370	5	1	0	2	84	5	20	5	—	0	—	0
Creamed Spinach	¾ cup (6.4 oz)	280	21	13	65	9	12	2	250	820	—	12	—	4500
Fruit Salad Low Fat	¾ cup (5.5 oz)	70	1	0	0	1	17	2	20	10	—	60	—	1750
Green Bean Casserole	¾ cup (6 oz)	170	5	2	5	2	10	2	20	580	—	5	—	200
Ham & Turkey Club w/ Cheese & Sauce	1 (13.3 oz)	890	44	20	150	48	76	4	800	2350	—	9	—	1250
Ham & Turkey Club w/o Cheese & Sauce	1 (9.3 oz)	430	6	2	55	29	64	4	80	1330	—	9	—	200
Ham Sandwich w/ Cheese & Sauce	1 (11.8 oz)	760	35	13	100	38	71	5	500	1880	—	9	—	750
Ham Sandwich w/o Cheese & Sauce	1 (9.3 oz)	450	9	3	45	25	66	4	80	1600	—	9	—	200
Ham w/ Cinnamon Apples	1 serv (8 oz)	350	13	5	75	25	35	2	0	1750	—	0	—	100

FOOD	PORTION	CALORIES	FAT	SAT FAT	CHOL	PROTEIN	CARBO	FIBER	CALCIUM	SOD	POTAS	VIT C	FOLIC	VIT A
Homestyle Mashed Potatoes & Gravy	¾ cup (6.6 oz)	200	9	5	25	3	27	2	40	560	—	6	—	300
Hot Cinnamon Apples	¾ cup (6.4 oz)	250	5	1	0	0	56	3	20	45	—	0	—	0
Macaroni & Cheese	¾ cup (6.7 oz)	280	10	6	20	36	12	1	200	760	—	0	—	300
Mashed Potatoes	⅔ cup (5.6 oz)	180	8	5	25	3	25	2	40	390	—	9	—	300
Meat Loaf & Brown Gravy	1 serv (7 oz)	390	22	8	120	30	19	1	20	1040	—	5	—	300
Meat Loaf & Chunky Tomato Sauce	1 serv (8 oz)	370	18	8	120	30	22	2	40	1170	—	18	—	750
Meat Loaf Sandwich w/ Cheese	1 (13.8 oz)	860	33	16	165	46	95	6	400	2270	—	15	—	1000
Meat Loaf Sandwich w/o Cheese	1 (12.3 oz)	690	21	7	120	40	86	6	100	1610	—	15	—	500
Mediterranean Pasta Salad	¾ cup (4.5 oz)	170	10	3	10	4	16	2	60	490	—	9	—	1750
New Potatoes Low Fat	¾ cup (4.6 oz)	130	3	0	0	3	25	2	0	150	—	12	—	0
Original Chicken Pot Pie	1 serv (14.9 oz)	750	34	9	115	34	78	9	100	2380	—	12	—	6000
Rice Pilaf	⅔ cup (5.1 oz)	180	5	1	0	5	32	2	40	600	—	4	—	200
Rotisserie Turkey Breast Skinless Low Fat	1 serv (5 oz)	170	1	1	100	36	1	0	20	850	—	0	—	0
Steamed Vegetables Low Fat	⅔ cup (3.7 oz)	35	1	0	0	2	7	3	20	35	—	20	—	4000
Stuffing	¾ cup (6.1 oz)	310	12	2	0	6	44	3	80	1140	—	1	—	1500
Tortellini Salad	¾ cup (5.6 oz)	380	24	5	90	14	29	2	250	530	—	9	—	200
Turkey Sandwich w/ Cheese & Sauce	1 (11.8 oz)	710	28	10	110	45	68	4	500	1390	—	9	—	750
Turkey Sandwich w/o Cheese & Sauce	1 (9.3 oz)	400	4	1	60	32	61	4	100	1070	—	9	—	200
Whole Kernel Corn Low Fat	¾ cup (5.8 oz)	180	4	1	0	6	30	2	0	170	—	5	—	200
Zucchini Marinara	¾ cup (6.6 oz)	80	4	1	0	2	10	2	40	470	—	12	—	300
SOUPS														
Chicken Low Fat	¾ cup (6.8 oz)	80	3	1	25	9	4	1	20	470	—	2	—	1500
Chicken Tortilla	1 cup (8.4 oz)	220	11	4	35	10	19	2	80	1410	—	12	—	500

BROWN'S CHICKEN

FOOD	PORTION	CALORIES	FAT	SAT FAT	CHOL	PROTEIN	CARBO	FIBER	CALCIUM	SOD	POTAS	VIT C	FOLIC	VIT A
Breadsticks w/ Garlic Butter	1	199	4	—	tr	6	36	—	—	2213	—	—	—	—
Breast	3.5 oz	284	15	—	67	26	12	—	—	529	—	tr	—	141
Coleslaw	3.5 oz	131	10	—	6	2	9	—	—	211	—	32	—	221

FOOD	PORTION	CALORIES	FAT	SAT FAT	CHOL	PROTEIN	CARBO	FIBER	CALCIUM	SOD	POTAS	VIT C	FOLIC	VIT A
Corn Fritters	3.5 oz	415	25	—	4	5	42	—	—	552	—	tr	—	318
Corn On Cob	1 ear (3 inch)	126	3	—	1	3	22	—	—	23	—	8	—	332
Fettucini Alfredo	1 serv (12 oz)	1507	64	—	51	56	173	—	—	3018	—	—	—	—
French Fries	3.5 oz	503	22	—	1	5	44	—	—	235	—	8	—	88
Gizzard	3.5 oz	387	20	—	88	24	26	—	—	795	—	tr	—	154
Leg	3.5 oz	287	16	—	52	26	9	—	—	542	—	tr	—	254
Liver	3.5 oz	341	19	—	147	23	19	—	—	704	—	11	—	8652
Mostaccioli w/ Meat	1 serv (12 oz)	835	14	—	17	27	44	—	—	898	—	—	—	—
Mostaccioli w/o Meat	1 serv (12 oz)	792	10	—	0	24	146	—	—	842	—	—	—	—
Mushrooms	3.5 oz	289	16	—	1	6	30	—	—	671	—	4	—	79
Potato Salad	3.5 oz	94	4	—	11	2	13	—	—	639	—	6	—	111
Ravioli w/ Meat	1 serv (12 oz)	865	20	—	17	30	138	—	—	934	—	—	—	—
Ravioli w/o Meat	1 serv (12 oz)	822	16	—	0	27	140	—	—	878	—	—	—	—
Shrimp	3.5 oz	277	10	—	31	13	34	—	—	778	—	tr	—	69
Thigh	3.5 oz	355	24	—	63	21	13	—	—	574	—	tr	—	318
Wing	3.5 oz	385	25	—	81	23	17	—	—	654	—	tr	—	274

BRUEGGER'S BAGELS

FOOD	PORTION	CALORIES	FAT	SAT FAT	CHOL	PROTEIN	CARBO	FIBER	CALCIUM	SOD	POTAS	VIT C	FOLIC	VIT A
Blueberry	1 (3.5 oz)	300	2	0	0	10	60	2	20	480	—	0	—	0
Cinnamon Raisin	1 (3.5 oz)	290	2	0	0	10	60	3	40	400	—	0	—	0
Egg	1 (3.5 oz)	280	1	1	25	10	67	3	20	510	—	0	—	0
Everything	1 (3.6 oz)	290	2	0	0	11	55	2	40	700	—	0	—	0
Garlic	1 (3.6 oz)	280	2	0	0	10	57	2	20	440	—	0	—	0
Honey Grain	1 (3.6 oz)	300	3	1	0	11	58	3	40	390	—	0	—	0
Onion	1 (3.6 oz)	280	2	0	0	10	57	2	20	430	—	0	—	0
Orange Cranberry	1 (3.5 oz)	290	1	0	0	10	61	2	40	470	—	8	—	0
Pesto	1 (3.5 oz)	280	2	0	0	10	55	2	40	480	—	0	—	100
Plain	1 (3.5 oz)	280	2	0	0	10	56	2	0	430	—	0	—	0
Poppy Seed	1 (3.6 oz)	280	2	0	0	11	57	2	20	440	—	0	—	0
Pumpernickel	1 (3.5 oz)	280	2	0	0	11	56	4	20	390	—	0	—	0
Salt	1 (3.6 oz)	270	2	0	0	10	55	2	0	1670	—	0	—	0
Sesame	1 (3.6 oz)	290	3	1	0	11	57	2	20	440	—	0	—	0
Spinach	1 (3.5 oz)	280	1	0	0	11	56	3	60	490	—	6	—	1750
Sun Dried Tomato	1 (3.5 oz)	280	2	0	0	10	58	3	20	490	—	0	—	300
Wheat Bran	1 (3.5 oz)	280	2	0	0	10	55	5	20	410	—	0	—	0

BURGER KING

BREAKFAST SELECTIONS

FOOD	PORTION	CALORIES	FAT	SAT FAT	CHOL	PROTEIN	CARBO	FIBER	CALCIUM	SOD	POTAS	VIT C	FOLIC	VIT A
AM Express Grape Jam	1 serv (0.4 oz)	30	0	0	0	0	7	0	0	0	—	0	—	0
AM Express Strawberry Jam	1 serv (0.4 oz)	30	0	0	0	0	8	0	0	5	—	0	—	0
AM Express Dip	1 serv (1 oz)	80	0	0	0	0	21	0	—	20	—	—	—	—
Biscuit	1 (3.3 oz)	330	18	4	2	6	37	1	60	950	—	0	—	0
Biscuit w/ Bacon Egg & Cheese	1 (6 oz)	510	31	10	225	19	39	1	150	1530	—	0	—	400

FOOD	PORTION	CALORIES	FAT	SAT FAT	CHOL	PROTEIN	CARBO	FIBER	CALCIUM	SOD	POTAS	VIT C	FOLIC	VIT A
Biscuit w/ Egg	1 (5.3 oz)	420	24	6	205	13	38	1	100	1110	—	0	—	300
Biscuit w/ Sausage	1 (4.8 oz)	530	36	11	35	13	38	1	60	1350	—	0	—	0
Croissan'wich Sausage Egg & Cheese	1 (5.7 oz)	550	42	14	250	20	22	1	150	1110	—	0	—	300
Croissan'wich w/ Sausage & Cheese	1 (3.7 oz)	450	35	12	54	13	21	1	100	940	—	0	—	200
French Toast Sticks	1 serv (4.9 oz)	500	27	7	0	4	60	1	60	490	—	0	—	0
Hash Browns	1 sm (2.6 oz)	240	15	6	0	2	25	2	0	440	—	0	—	0
Land O'Lakes Whipped Classic Blend	1 serv (0.4 oz)	65	7	1	0	0	0	0	—	75	—	—	—	400
MAIN MENU SELECTIONS														
American Cheese	2 slices (0.9 oz)	90	8	5	25	6	0	0	—	420	—	—	—	—
BK Big Fish Sandwich	1 (8.8 oz)	720	43	9	80	23	59	3	80	1180	—	0	—	100
BK Broiler Chicken Sandwich	1 (8.7 oz)	530	16	5	105	29	45	2	60	1060	—	6	—	300
Bacon Bits	1 serv (3 g)	15	1	0	3	1	0	0	—	70	—	—	—	—
Big King Sandwich	1 (7.9 oz)	660	43	18	135	40	29	1	250	920	—	0	—	400
Broiled Chicken Salad w/o Dressing	1 serv (10.6 oz)	190	8	4	75	20	9	3	150	500	—	15	—	5000
Bull's Eye Barbecue Sauce	1 serv (0.5 oz)	20	0	0	0	0	5	0	—	140	—	—	—	—
Cheeseburger	1 (5 oz)	380	19	9	65	23	28	1	150	770	—	0	—	300
Chicken Sandwich	1 (8 oz)	710	43	9	60	26	54	2	100	1400	—	0	—	0
Chicken Tenders	8 pieces (4.3 oz)	350	22	7	65	22	17	1	20	940	—	0	—	0
Coated French Fries Salted	1 med (4.1 oz)	400	21	8	0	3	50	4	0	820	—	0	—	0
Croutons	1 serv (0.2 oz)	30	1	0	0	tr	5	0	—	90	—	—	—	—
Dipping Sauce Barbecue	1 serv (1 oz)	35	0	0	0	0	9	0	—	400	—	—	—	—
Dipping Sauce Honey	1 serv (1 oz)	90	0	0	0	0	23	0	—	10	—	—	—	—
Dipping Sauce Ranch	1 serv (1 oz)	170	17	3	0	0	2	0	—	200	—	—	—	—
Dipping Sauce Sweet & Sour	1 serv (1 oz)	45	0	0	0	0	11	0	—	50	—	—	—	—
Double Cheeseburger	1 (7.5 oz)	600	36	17	135	41	28	1	200	1060	—	0	—	400
Double Cheeseburger w/ Bacon	1 (7.6 oz)	640	39	18	145	44	28	1	200	1240	—	0	—	400
Double Whopper	1 (12.3 oz)	870	56	19	170	46	45	3	80	940	—	9	—	500
Double Whopper w/ Cheese	1 (13.2 oz)	960	63	24	195	52	46	3	250	1420	—	9	—	750

FOOD	PORTION	CALORIES	FAT	SAT FAT	CHOL	PROTEIN	CARBO	FIBER	CALCIUM	SOD	POTAS	VIT C	FOLIC	VIT A
Dutch Apple Pie	1 serv (4 oz)	300	15	3	0	3	39	2	0	230	—	6	—	0
French Fries Salted	1 med (4.1 oz)	370	20	5	0	5	43	3	0	240	—	4	—	0
Garden Salad w/o Dressing	1 (7.5 oz)	100	5	3	15	6	7	3	150	110	—	30	—	5500
Hamburger	1 (4.5 oz)	330	15	6	55	20	28	1	40	530	—	0	—	100
Ketchup	1 serv (0.5 oz)	15	0	0	0	0	4	0	—	180	—	—	—	—
King Sauce	1 serv (0.5 oz)	70	7	1	4	0	2	0	—	70	—	—	—	—
Lettuce	1 leaf (0.7 oz)	0	0	0	0	0	0	0	—	0	—	—	—	—
Mayonnaise	1 serv (1 oz)	210	23	3	20	0	tr	0	—	160	—	—	—	—
Mustard	1 serv (3 g)	0	0	0	0	0	0	0	—	40	—	—	—	—
Onion	1 serv (0.5 oz)	5	0	0	0	0	1	0	—	0	—	—	—	—
Onion Rings	1 serv (4.4 oz)	310	14	2	0	4	41	6	100	810	—	0	—	0
Pickles	4 slices (0.5 oz)	0	0	0	0	0	0	0	—	140	—	—	—	—
Side Salad w/o Dressing	1 (4.7 oz)	60	3	2	5	3	4	2	80	55	—	12	—	2500
Tartar Sauce	1 serv (1 oz)	180	19	3	15	0	0	0	—	220	—	—	—	—
Tomato	2 slices (1 oz)	5	0	0	0	0	1	0	—	0	—	—	—	—
Whopper	1 (9.5 oz)	640	39	11	90	27	45	3	80	870	—	9	—	500
Whopper Jr.	1 (5.9 oz)	420	24	8	60	21	29	2	60	530	—	5	—	200
Whopper Jr. w/ Cheese	1 (6.3 oz)	460	28	10	75	23	29	2	150	770	—	5	—	400
Whopper w/ Cheese	1 (10.3 oz)	730	46	16	115	33	46	3	250	1350	—	9	—	750
SALAD DRESSINGS														
Bleu Cheese	1 serv (1 oz)	160	16	4	30	2	1	tr	—	260	—	—	—	—
French	1 serv (1 oz)	140	10	2	0	0	11	0	—	190	—	—	—	—
Ranch	1 serv (1 oz)	180	19	4	10	tr	2	tr	—	170	—	—	—	—
Reduced Calorie Light Italian	1 serv (1 oz)	15	1	0	0	0	3	0	—	360	—	—	—	—
Thousand Island	1 serv (1 oz)	140	12	3	15	0	7	tr	—	190	—	—	—	—

CAPTAIN D'S

FOOD	PORTION	CALORIES	FAT	SAT FAT	CHOL	PROTEIN	CARBO	FIBER	CALCIUM	SOD	POTAS	VIT C	FOLIC	VIT A
DESSERTS														
Carrot Cake	1 piece (4 oz)	434	23	—	32	8	49	0	—	414	—	—	—	—
Cheesecake	1 piece (4 oz)	420	31	—	141	7	30	0	—	480	—	—	—	—
Chocolate Cake	1 piece (4 oz)	303	10	—	20	4	49	0	—	259	—	—	—	—
Lemon Pie	1 piece (4 oz)	351	10	—	45	7	59	0	—	135	—	—	—	—
Pecan Pie	1 piece (4 oz)	458	20	—	4	5	64	4	—	373	—	—	—	—
MAIN MENU SELECTIONS														
Baked Potato	1	278	0	0	0	6	—	—	—	—	—	—	—	—
Breadstick	1	113	4	0	0	3	—	—	—	—	—	—	—	—
Broiled Chicken Lunch	1 serv	503	9	2	82	39	—	—	—	—	—	—	—	—
Broiled Chicken Platter	1 serv	802	10	2	82	46	—	—	—	—	—	—	—	—
Broiled Chicken Sandwich	1 (8.2 oz)	451	19	—	105	40	29	—	—	858	—	—	—	—

FOOD	PORTION	CALORIES	FAT	SAT FAT	CHOL	PROTEIN	CARBO	FIBER	CALCIUM	SOD	POTAS	VIT C	FOLIC	VIT A
Broiled Fish & Chicken Platter	1 serv	777	10	1	66	41	—	—	—	—	—	—	—	—
Broiled Fish & Chicken Lunch	1 serv	478	8	1	66	34	—	—	—	—	—	—	—	—
Broiled Fish Lunch	1 serv	435	7	1	49	28	—	—	—	—	—	—	—	—
Broiled Fish Platter	1 serv	734	7	1	49	36	—	—	—	—	—	—	—	—
Broiled Shrimp Lunch	1 serv	421	7	1	155	25	—	—	—	—	—	—	—	—
Broiled Shrimp Platter	1 serv	720	8	1	155	32	—	—	—	—	—	—	—	—
Cheese	1 slice (1 oz)	54	5	—	14	3	tr	0	—	206	—	—	—	—
Cob Corn	1 serv (9.5 oz)	251	2	—	0	9	60	—	—	13	—	—	—	—
Cocktail Sauce	1 serv (1 fl oz)	137	tr	—	0	2	34	0	—	1007	—	—	—	—
Cocktail Sauce	1 lg serv (1 fl oz)	34	tr	—	0	tr	8	0	—	252	—	—	—	—
Cole Slaw	1 serv (4 oz)	158	12	—	16	3	12	2	—	246	—	—	—	—
Cole Slaw	1 pt (16 oz)	633	47	—	66	10	47	8	—	454	—	—	—	—
Crackers	4 (0.5 oz)	50	1	—	3	1	8	tr	—	147	—	—	—	—
Cracklins	1 serv (1 oz)	218	17	—	0	1	16	0	—	741	—	—	—	—
Dinner Salad w/o Dressing	1 (2.5 oz)	27	1	—	1	1	3	1	—	67	—	—	—	—
French Fried Potatoes	1 serv (3.5 oz)	302	10	—	0	3	50	0	—	152	—	—	—	—
Fried Okra	1 serv (4 oz)	300	16	—	0	7	34	0	—	445	—	—	—	—
Green Beans Seasoned	1 serv (4 oz)	46	2	—	4	2	5	1	—	752	—	—	—	—
Hushpuppies	6 (6.7 oz)	756	25	—	0	13	119	1	—	2790	—	—	—	—
Hushpuppy	1 (1.1 oz)	126	4	—	0	2	20	tr	—	465	—	—	—	—
Imitation Sour Cream	1 serv	29	3	3	0	0	—	—	—	—	—	—	—	—
Margarine	1 serv	102	12	7	0	0	—	—	—	—	—	—	—	—
Non-Dairy Creamer	1 serv	14	1	—	0	tr	1	0	—	8	—	—	—	—
Rice	1 serv (4 oz)	124	0	0	0	3	28	1	—	9	—	—	—	—
Stuffed Crab	1 serv	91	7	—	—	8	16	—	—	250	—	—	—	—
Sugar	1 pkg	18	0	0	0	0	3	0	—	0	—	—	—	—
Sweet & Sour Sauce	1 serv (1.8 fl oz)	52	0	0	0	0	13	0	—	5	—	—	—	—
Sweet & Sour Sauce	1 lg serv (4 fl oz)	206	0	0	0	tr	52	0	—	18	—	—	—	—
Tartar Sauce	1 lg serv (4 fl oz)	298	27	—	41	1	13	0	—	633	—	—	—	—
Tartar Sauce	1 serv (1 fl oz)	75	7	—	10	tr	3	0	—	158	—	—	—	—
Vegetable Medley	1 serv	36	1	0	0	1	—	—	—	—	—	—	—	—
White Beans	1 serv (4 oz)	126	1	—	2	8	22	3	—	99	—	—	—	—
SALAD DRESSINGS														
Blue Cheese	1 pkg (1 fl oz)	105	12	—	14	tr	tr	0	—	101	—	—	—	—
French	1 pkg (1 fl oz)	111	11	—	7	tr	4	0	—	187	—	—	—	—

FOOD	PORTION	CALORIES	FAT	SAT FAT	CHOL	PROTEIN	CARBO	FIBER	CALCIUM	SOD	POTAS	VIT C	FOLIC	VIT A
Light Italian	1 serv	16	1	0	0	0	—	—	—	—	—	—	—	—
Ranch	1 pkg (1 fl oz)	92	10	—	15	tr	tr	0	—	230	—	—	—	—

CARL'S JR.

BAKED SELECTIONS

FOOD	PORTION	CALORIES	FAT	SAT FAT	CHOL	PROTEIN	CARBO	FIBER	CALCIUM	SOD	POTAS	VIT C	FOLIC	VIT A
Cheese Danish	1 (4.1 oz)	400	22	5	15	5	49	1	60	390	—	0	—	750
Cheesecake Strawberry Swirl	1 serv (3.5 oz)	300	17	9	55	6	31	0	100	220	—	2	—	500
Chocolate Cake	1 serv (3 oz)	300	10	3	13	3	49	4	80	260	—	0	—	400
Chocolate Chip Cookie	1 (2.5 oz)	370	19	8	25	3	49	1	0	350	—	0	—	100
Cinnamon Roll	1 (4.2 oz)	420	13	4	15	9	68	4	60	570	—	0	—	500
Muffin Blueberry	1 (4.2 oz)	340	14	2	40	5	49	1	150	340	—	2	—	100
Muffin Bran	1 (4.7 oz)	370	13	2	45	7	61	6	100	410	—	1	—	100

BREAKFAST SELECTIONS

FOOD	PORTION	CALORIES	FAT	SAT FAT	CHOL	PROTEIN	CARBO	FIBER	CALCIUM	SOD	POTAS	VIT C	FOLIC	VIT A
Bacon	2 strips (0.3 oz)	40	4	2	10	3	0	0	0	125	—	0	—	0
Breakfast Burrito	1 (5.3 oz)	430	26	12	460	22	29	tr	300	810	—	0	—	1000
Breakfast Quesadilla Cheese	1 (5.2 oz)	300	14	6	225	14	27	1	150	750	—	0	—	500
English Muffin w/ Margarine	1 (2.6 oz)	230	10	2	0	5	30	2	150	330	—	0	—	400
French Toast Dips w/o Syrup	1 serv (3.7 oz)	410	25	6	0	6	40	3	60	380	—	0	—	0
Grape Jelly	1 serv (0.5 oz)	35	0	0	0	0	9	0	0	0	—	0	—	0
Hash Brown Nuggets	1 serv (3.3 oz)	270	17	4	0	3	27	2	0	410	—	0	—	0
Sausage	1 patty (1.8 oz)	200	18	7	35	7	0	0	40	530	—	0	—	0
Scrambed Eggs	1 serv (3.5 oz)	160	11	4	425	13	1	0	40	125	—	0	—	500
Strawberry Jam	1 serv (0.5 oz)	35	0	0	0	0	9	0	0	0	—	2	—	0
Sunrise Sandwich	1 (4.6 oz)	370	21	6	225	14	31	2	250	710	—	0	—	1000
Table Syrup	1 serv (1 oz)	90	0	0	0	0	22	0	0	22	—	0	—	0

MAIN MENU SELECTIONS

FOOD	PORTION	CALORIES	FAT	SAT FAT	CHOL	PROTEIN	CARBO	FIBER	CALCIUM	SOD	POTAS	VIT C	FOLIC	VIT A
American Cheese	1 slice (0.5 oz)	60	5	3	15	3	0	0	100	270	—	0	—	200
BBQ Chicken Sandwich	1 (6.7 oz)	310	6	2	55	31	34	3	80	830	—	1	—	200
BBQ Sauce	1 serv (1.1 oz)	50	0	0	0	tr	11	0	0	270	—	0	—	0
Big Burger	1 (6.8 oz)	470	20	8	55	25	46	2	80	810	—	2	—	200
Breadstick	1 (0.3 oz)	35	1	0	0	1	7	1	0	60	—	0	—	0
Carl's Catch Fish Sandwich	1 (7.5 oz)	560	30	7	60	17	54	5	150	1220	—	0	—	0
Chicken Club Sandwich	1 (8.8 oz)	550	29	8	85	35	37	3	200	1160	—	1	—	400
Chicken Stars	6 pieces (3 oz)	230	14	3	85	13	11	0	<20	450	—	0	—	0
CrissCut Fries	1 lg (5.7 oz)	550	34	9	0	7	55	3	0	1280	—	1	—	0
Croutons	1 serv (7 g)	35	1	0	0	tr	5	0	0	65	—	0	—	0

FOOD	PORTION	CALORIES	FAT	SAT FAT	CHOL	PROTEIN	CARBO	FIBER	CALCIUM	SOD	POTAS	VIT C	FOLIC	VIT A
Double Western Bacon Cheeseburger	1 (11.5 oz)	970	57	27	145	56	58	2	300	1810	—	1	—	400
Famous Big Star Hamburger	1 (8.6 oz)	610	38	11	70	26	42	2	100	890	—	4	—	200
French Fries	1 reg (4.4 oz)	370	20	7	0	4	44	3	0	240	—	9	—	0
Great Stuff Potato Bacon & Cheese	1 (14.2 oz)	630	29	7	40	20	76	6	150	1720	—	30	—	750
Great Stuff Potato Broccoli & Cheese	1 (14.2 oz)	530	22	5	15	11	76	8	150	930	—	66	—	1250
Great Stuff Potato Plain	1 (9.4 oz)	290	0	0	0	6	68	6	20	40	—	26	—	0
Great Stuff Potato Sour Cream & Chive	1 (10.9 oz)	430	14	3	10	8	70	6	80	160	—	36	—	750
Hamburger	1 (3.1 oz)	200	8	4	25	11	23	1	60	500	—	tr	—	100
Honey Sauce	1 serv (1 oz)	90	0	0	0	0	23	0	0	5	—	0	—	0
Hot & Crispy Sandwich	1 (5 oz)	400	22	5	45	14	35	2	100	980	—	0	—	0
Mustard Sauce	1 serv (1 oz)	45	1	0	0	0	10	0	0	150	—	0	—	0
Onion Rings	1 serv (5.3 oz)	520	26	6	0	8	63	3	20	840	—	0	—	0
Salsa	1 serv (0.9 oz)	10	0	0	0	0	2	0	0	160	—	1	—	100
Sante Fe Chicken Sandwich	1 (7.9 oz)	530	30	7	85	30	36	3	150	1230	—	5	—	200
Super Star Hamburger	1 (11.2 oz)	820	53	20	120	43	41	2	100	1030	—	6	—	300
Sweet N' Sour Sauce	1 serv (1 oz)	50	0	0	0	0	11	0	0	60	—	2	—	100
Swiss Cheese	1 slice (0.5 oz)	45	4	3	10	3	0	0	100	220	—	0	—	100
Western Bacon Cheeseburger	1 (8.1 oz)	870	35	16	90	34	59	2	200	1490	—	1	—	200
Zucchini	1 serv (5.9 oz)	380	23	6	0	7	38	3	60	1040	—	0	—	400
SALAD DRESSINGS														
1000 Island	2 fl oz	250	24	4	20	tr	7	0	0	540	—	0	—	0
Blue Cheese	2 fl oz	310	34	6	25	2	1	0	60	360	—	0	—	100
French Fat Free	2 fl oz	70	0	0	0	0	18	1	0	760	—	1	—	0
House	2 fl oz	220	22	4	20	1	3	0	40	440	—	0	—	0
Italian Fat Free	2 fl oz	15	0	0	0	0	4	0	0	800	—	1	—	0
SALADS AND SALAD BARS														
Salad-To-Go Charbroiled Chicken	1 serv (12 oz)	260	9	5	70	28	11	4	150	530	—	5	—	6000
Salad-To-Go Garden	1 (4.8 oz)	50	3	2	5	3	4	2	80	75	—	1	—	3000

CARVEL

FROZEN YOGURT

FOOD	PORTION	CALORIES	FAT	SAT FAT	CHOL	PROTEIN	CARBO	FIBER	CALCIUM	SOD	POTAS	VIT C	FOLIC	VIT A
Vanilla Low Fat No Sugar Added	4 fl oz	110	2	—	—	4	22	—	150	90	—	—	—	—

FOOD	PORTION	CALORIES	FAT	SAT FAT	CHOL	PROTEIN	CARBO	FIBER	CALCIUM	SOD	POTAS	VIT C	FOLIC	VIT A
ICE CREAM														
Brown Bonnet Cone	1 (4.7 oz)	380	21	15	40	6	43	1	150	150	—	1	—	300
Brown Bonnet Cone No Fat Vanilla	1 (4.7 oz)	300	11	9	—	5	47	—	150	95	—	1	—	100
Cake	1 pkg (7 oz)	450	23	15	45	8	54	1	200	230	—	1	—	400
Cake	1 pkg (4 oz)	270	14	9	30	5	33	tr	150	160	—	1	—	300
Cake Cheesecake	1 serv (4 oz)	280	14	9	30	5	34	—	150	190	—	1	—	200
Cake Chocolate Vanilla Chocolate Crunchies	1/15 cake (3.4 oz)	230	12	8	35	4	27	1	100	95	—	1	—	0
Cake Cookies & Cream	1 serv (4 oz)	270	14	8	35	5	32	1	150	160	—	1	—	300
Cake Fudge Drizzle	1/8 cake (4 oz)	310	17	10	30	6	35	1	100	170	—	0	—	0
Cake Fudgie The Whale	1/14 cake (3.6 oz)	290	16	7	30	5	33	1	100	180	—	0	—	0
Cake Holiday	1/15 cake (3.4 oz)	240	12	8	30	4	30	1	100	100	—	0	—	—
Cake S'mores	1 serv (4 oz)	270	14	9	25	5	33	1	150	150	—	1	—	200
Cake Sinfully Chocolate	1 serv (4 oz)	280	14	9	25	5	34	1	150	150	—	1	—	200
Cake Strawberries & Cream	1/8 cake (3.8 oz)	240	12	8	35	4	31	1	100	100	—	5	—	0
Chocolate	4 fl oz	190	10	6	25	4	22	0	150	100	—	1	—	300
Chocolate No Fat	4 fl oz	120	0	0	0	2	28	0	80	40	—	0	—	100
Flying Saucer Chocolate	1 (4 oz)	230	9	5	30	5	33	2	100	140	—	1	—	0
Flying Saucer Chocolate w/ Sprinkles	1 (4 oz)	330	14	7	30	5	49	2	100	150	—	0	—	0
Flying Saucer Low Fat Chocolate	1 (4 oz)	190	3	1	0	3	38	1	60	130	—	0	—	100
Flying Saucer Low Fat Vanilla	1 (4 oz)	180	3	1	0	4	36	1	100	140	—	0	—	100
Flying Saucer Vanilla	1 (4 oz)	240	10	5	40	5	33	1	100	150	—	1	—	0
Flying Saucer Vanilla w/ Sprinkles	1 (4 oz)	340	14	7	40	5	49	1	100	160	—	1	—	0
Nature's Crunch	1 (4.2 g)	450	25	14	20	5	55	2	100	240	—	1	—	200
Olde Fashion Sundae Butterscotch	1 (8 oz)	500	17	10	60	7	80	1	300	340	—	2	—	500
Olde Fashion Sundae Chocolate	1 (8 oz)	470	19	12	55	8	71	1	300	280	—	2	—	400

FOOD	PORTION	CALORIES	FAT	SAT FAT	CHOL	PROTEIN	CARBO	FIBER	CALCIUM	SOD	POTAS	VIT C	FOLIC	VIT A
Olde Fashion Sundae Strawberry	1 (8 oz)	420	15	9	55	7	64	2	300	230	—	2	—	400
Sheet Cake Chocolate Vanilla Chocolate Crunchies	¹/₂₆ cake (3.3 oz)	230	12	8	35	4	27	1	100	100	—	1	—	0
Sinful Love Bar	1 (4.2 oz)	460	29	14	20	8	48	3	150	240	200	1	8	200
Thick Shake Chocolate	1 (16 oz)	719	31	18	116	18	96	tr	631	418	689	5	9	947
Thick Shake Low Fat Chocolate	1 (16 oz)	490	1	1	15	16	108	1	500	330	—	2	—	1000
Thick Shake Low Fat Strawberry	1 (16 oz)	460	1	1	15	15	96	1	500	290	—	2	—	1000
Thick Shake Low Fat Vanilla	1 (16 oz)	460	1	1	15	15	98	1	500	280	—	2	—	1000
Thick Shake No Fat Chocolate	1 (16 oz)	524	8	4	36	17	100	1	570	346	735	4	9	948
Thick Shake No Fat Strawberry	1 (16 oz)	453	7	4	36	16	82	1	542	285	628	4	9	947
Thick Shake No Fat Vanilla	1 (16 oz)	462	7	4	36	16	84	1	542	278	628	4	9	947
Thick Shake Strawberry	1 (16 oz)	648	30	18	116	17	77	tr	603	358	581	5	9	947
Thick Shake Vanilla	1 (16 oz)	657	30	18	116	17	79	tr	603	350	581	5	9	947
Vanilla	4 fl oz	200	10	6	40	5	21	0	150	110	—	1	—	300
Vanilla No Fat	4 fl oz	120	0	0	0	4	25	0	150	55	—	1	—	100
SHERBET														
Black Raspberry	½ cup (3.4 oz)	150	1	1	5	1	33	0	60	35	—	0	—	0
Blueberry	½ cup (3.4 oz)	150	1	1	5	1	33	0	40	30	—	0	—	0
Lemon	½ cup (3.5 oz)	150	1	1	5	1	31	0	60	30	—	0	—	0
Lime	½ cup (3.5 oz)	150	1	1	5	1	31	0	60	30	—	0	—	0
Mango	½ cup (3.5 oz)	140	1	1	5	1	30	0	40	25	—	2	—	400
Orange	½ cup (3.5 oz)	150	1	1	5	1	31	0	60	30	—	0	—	0
Peach	½ cup (3.4 oz)	150	1	1	5	1	32	0	60	35	—	0	—	0
Pineapple	½ cup (3.5 oz)	150	1	1	5	1	33	0	40	40	—	0	—	0
Strawberry	½ cup (3.5 oz)	150	1	1	5	1	32	0	60	35	—	0	—	0

CHICK-FIL-A

FOOD	PORTION	CALORIES	FAT	SAT FAT	CHOL	PROTEIN	CARBO	FIBER	CALCIUM	SOD	POTAS	VIT C	FOLIC	VIT A
DESSERTS														
Cheesecake	1 slice (3.1 oz)	270	21	9	10	13	7	0	20	510	—	0	—	300
Cheesecake w/ Blueberry Topping	1 slice (4.1 oz)	290	23	10	10	14	9	0	40	550	—	2	—	400
Cheesecake w/ Strawberry Topping	1 slice (4.1 oz)	290	23	10	10	14	8	0	40	580	—	6	—	400
Fudge Nut Brownie	1 (2.6 oz)	350	16	3	30	10	41	0	0	650	—	0	—	400
Icedream Cone	1 sm (4.5 oz)	140	4	1	40	11	16	0	40	240	—	0	—	400

FOOD	PORTION	CALORIES	FAT	SAT FAT	CHOL	PROTEIN	CARBO	FIBER	CALCIUM	SOD	POTAS	VIT C	FOLIC	VIT A
Icedream Cup	1 sm (7.5 oz)	350	10	3	70	16	50	0	80	390	—	0	—	500
Lemon Pie	1 slice (4 oz)	320	16	5	135	7	40	1	150	280	—	5	—	750
MAIN MENU SELECTIONS														
Carrot & Raisin Salad	1 sm (2.7 oz)	150	2	0	6	5	28	2	40	650	—	6	—	1000
Chargrilled Chicken Club Sandwich w/o Dressing	1 (8.2 oz)	390	12	5	70	33	38	2	80	980	—	8	—	700
Chargrilled Chicken Deluxe Sandwich	1 (7.4 oz)	290	3	1	40	28	38	2	0	640	—	5	—	500
Chargrilled Chicken Garden Salad	1 serv (14 oz)	170	3	1	25	26	10	5	60	650	—	13	—	1200
Chargrilled Chicken Sandwich	1 (5.3 oz)	280	3	1	40	27	36	1	0	640	—	1	—	400
Chargrilled Chicken w/o Bun Or Pickles	1 piece (2.8 oz)	130	3	1	30	27	0	0	0	630	—	0	—	300
Chick-n-Strips	4 (4.2 oz)	230	8	2	20	29	10	0	0	380	—	0	—	300
Chick-n-Strips Salad	1 serv (15.9 oz)	290	9	2	20	32	21	5	0	430	—	13	—	1000
Chicken Sandwich	1 (5.9 oz)	290	9	2	50	24	29	1	0	870	—	0	—	400
Chicken Deluxe Sandich	1 (8 oz)	300	9	2	50	25	31	2	0	870	—	5	—	750
Chicken Salad Plate	1 serv (16.5 oz)	290	21	0	35	21	40	6	60	570	—	10	—	800
Chicken Salad Sandwich On Whole Wheat	1 (5.9 oz)	320	5	2	10	25	42	1	0	810	—	0	—	500
Chicken w/o Bun Or Pickles	1 piece (3.7 oz)	160	8	2	45	21	1	0	0	690	—	0	—	300
Cole Slaw	1 sm (2.8 oz)	130	6	1	15	6	11	1	20	430	—	6	—	700
Hearty Breast of Chicken Soup	1 cup (7.6 oz)	110	1	0	45	16	10	1	0	760	—	2	—	700
Nuggets	8 (3.9 oz)	290	14	3	60	28	12	0	0	770	—	0	—	400
Tossed Salad	1 serv (4.6 oz)	70	5	0	0	5	13	1	0	0	—	8	—	500
Waffle Potato Fries	1 sm (3 oz)	290	10	4	5	1	49	0	0	960	—	0	—	0
Waffle Potato Fries w/o Salt	1 sm (3 oz)	290	10	4	5	1	49	0	0	80	—	0	—	0

CHILI'S

FOOD	PORTION	CALORIES	FAT	SAT FAT	CHOL	PROTEIN	CARBO	FIBER	CALCIUM	SOD	POTAS	VIT C	FOLIC	VIT A
DESSERTS														
Diet By Chocolate Cake	1 serv	370	2	1	0	10	79	8	19	670	—	0	—	0
Diet By Chocolate Cake w/ Yogurt	1 serv	465	2	1	3	13	99	8	133	622	—	1	—	15

FOOD	PORTION	CALORIES	FAT	SAT FAT	CHOL	PROTEIN	CARBO	FIBER	CALCIUM	SOD	POTAS	VIT C	FOLIC	VIT A
Diet By Chocolate Cake w/ Yogurt & Fudge Topping	1 serv	534	3	1	3	14	116	8	163	703	—	1	—	32
MAIN MENU SELECTIONS														
Guiltless Grill Chicken Fijitas	1 serv	726	13	4	44	45	108	24	487	4759	—	73	—	5010
Guiltless Grill Chicken Platter	1 serv	563	7	3	58	38	83	12	172	3284	—	33	—	3678
Guiltless Grill Chicken Salad w/ Dressing	1 serv	254	3	1	47	29	27	6	36	1475	—	16	—	2082
Guiltless Grill Chicken Sandwich	1	527	7	2	43	44	70	18	306	2923	—	26	—	3102
Guiltless Grill Veggie Pasta	1 serv	590	11	3	55	25	98	16	245	964	—	7	—	3096
Guiltless Grill Veggie Pasta w/ Chicken	1 serv	696	13	4	97	44	102	17	249	1399	—	7	—	3163
CHURCH'S CHICKEN														
Apple Pie	1 serv (3.1 oz)	280	12	—	<5	2	41	1	0	340	—	0	—	0
Biscuit	1 (2.1 oz)	250	16	—	<5	2	26	1	40	640	—	0	—	0
Breast	1 serv (2.8 oz)	200	12	—	65	19	4	0	0	510	—	0	—	300
Cajun Rice	1 serv (3.1 oz)	130	7	—	5	1	16	tr	0	260	—	0	—	1250
Cole Slaw	1 serv (3 oz)	92	6	—	0	4	8	2	0	230	—	5	—	0
Corn On The Cob	1 serv (5.7 oz)	139	3	—	0	4	24	9	0	15	—	1	—	0
French Fries	1 serv (2.7 oz)	210	11	—	0	3	29	2	0	60	—	0	—	0
Leg	1 serv (2 oz)	140	9	—	45	13	2	0	0	160	—	0	—	200
Okra	1 serv (2.8 oz)	210	16	—	0	3	19	4	80	520	—	1	—	0
Potatoes & Gravy	1 serv (3.7 oz)	90	3	—	0	1	14	1	0	520	—	0	—	0
Tender Strip	1 (1.1 oz)	80	4	—	15	6	5	1	0	140	—	0	—	0
Thigh	1 serv (2.8 oz)	230	16	—	80	16	5	0	0	520	—	0	—	200
Wing	1 serv (3.1 oz)	250	16	—	60	19	8	0	40	540	—	0	—	500
COLOMBO FROZEN YOGURT														
Alpine Strawberry Nonfat	4 fl oz	100	0	0	0	4	22	0	100	60	—	—	—	—
Banana Strawberry Nonfat	4 fl oz	50	0	0	0	3	12	—	80	10	—	—	—	0
Brazlian Banana Nonfat	4 fl oz	100	0	0	0	4	22	0	100	60	—	—	—	—
Butter Pecan Nonfat	4 fl oz	100	0	0	0	4	22	0	100	60	—	—	—	—
Cappuccino Nonfat	4 fl oz	100	0	0	0	4	22	0	100	60	—	—	—	—
Cherry Amaretto Nonfat	4 fl oz	50	0	0	0	3	12	—	80	10	—	—	—	0
Cherry Vanilla Nonfat	4 fl oz	100	0	0	0	4	22	0	100	60	—	—	—	—
Chocolate Nonfat	4 fl oz	50	0	0	0	3	12	—	80	10	—	—	—	0

FOOD	PORTION	CALORIES	FAT	SAT FAT	CHOL	PROTEIN	CARBO	FIBER	CALCIUM	SOD	POTAS	VIT C	FOLIC	VIT A
Coconut Cooler Nonfat	4 fl oz	100	0	0	0	4	22	0	100	60	—	—	—	—
Cool Berry Blue Nonfat	4 fl oz	100	0	0	0	4	22	0	100	60	—	—	—	—
Country Pumpkin Nonfat	4 fl oz	100	0	0	0	4	22	0	100	60	—	—	—	—
Double Dutch Chocolate Nonfat	4 fl oz	100	0	0	0	4	22	0	100	60	—	—	—	—
Egg Nog Nonfat	4 fl oz	100	0	0	0	4	22	0	100	60	—	—	—	—
French Vanilla Lowfat	4 fl oz	110	2	1	5	3	22	0	100	60	—	—	—	—
French Vanilla Nonfat	4 fl oz	100	0	0	0	4	22	0	100	60	—	—	—	—
Georgia Peach Nonfat	4 fl oz	100	0	0	0	4	22	0	100	60	—	—	—	—
German Fudge Chocolate Nonfat	4 fl oz	100	0	0	0	4	22	0	100	60	—	—	—	—
Hawaiian Pineapple Nonfat	4 fl oz	100	0	0	0	4	22	0	100	60	—	—	—	—
Hazelnut Amaretto Nonfat	4 fl oz	100	0	0	0	4	22	0	100	60	—	—	—	—
Honey Almond Nonfat	4 fl oz	100	0	0	0	4	22	0	100	60	—	—	—	—
Irish Cream Nonfat	4 fl oz	100	0	0	0	4	22	0	100	60	—	—	—	—
New York Cheesecake Nonfat	4 fl oz	100	0	0	0	4	22	0	100	60	—	—	—	—
Old World Chocolate Lowfat	4 fl oz	110	2	1	5	3	22	0	100	60	—	—	—	—
Orange Bavarian Creme Nonfat	4 fl oz	100	0	0	0	4	22	0	100	60	—	—	—	—
Peanut Butter Lowfat	4 fl oz	110	2	1	5	3	22	0	100	60	—	—	—	—
Pecan Praline Nonfat	4 fl oz	100	0	0	0	4	22	0	100	60	—	—	—	—
Pina Colada Nonfat	4 fl oz	100	0	0	0	4	22	0	100	60	—	—	—	—
Raspberry Nonfat	4 fl oz	50	0	0	0	3	12	—	80	10	—	—	—	0
Rockin' Raspberry Nonfat	4 fl oz	100	0	0	0	4	22	0	100	60	—	—	—	—
Simply Vanilla Lowfat	4 fl oz	110	2	1	5	3	22	0	100	60	—	—	—	—
Simply Vanilla Nonfat	4 fl oz	100	0	0	0	4	22	0	100	60	—	—	—	—
Strawberry Nonfat	4 fl oz	50	0	0	0	3	12	—	80	10	—	—	—	0
Tropical Tango Nonfat	4 fl oz	100	0	0	0	4	22	0	100	60	—	—	—	—
Vanilla Nonfat	4 fl oz	50	0	0	0	3	12	—	80	10	—	—	—	0
White Chocolate Almond Nonfat	4 fl oz	100	0	0	0	4	22	0	100	60	—	—	—	—

FOOD	PORTION	CALORIES	FAT	SAT FAT	CHOL	PROTEIN	CARBO	FIBER	CALCIUM	SOD	POTAS	VIT C	FOLIC	VIT A
Wild Strawberry Lowfat	4 fl oz	110	2	1	5	3	22	0	100	60	—	—	—	—

D'ANGELO'S SANDWICH SHOPS

SALADS AND SALAD BARS

FOOD	PORTION	CALORIES	FAT	SAT FAT	CHOL	PROTEIN	CARBO	FIBER	CALCIUM	SOD	POTAS	VIT C	FOLIC	VIT A
Antipasto Salad w/o Dressing	1	420	14	—	40	—	56	—	—	1400	—	—	—	—
Caesar Salad w/ Dressing	1	740	45	—	70	—	61	—	—	2270	—	—	—	—
Caesar Salad w/o Dressing	1	490	20	—	15	—	60	—	—	1310	—	—	—	—
Chicken Caesar Salad w/ Dressing	1	860	48	—	130	—	62	—	—	2820	—	—	—	—
Chicken Caesar Salad w/o Dressing	1	600	23	—	70	—	60	—	—	1870	—	—	—	—
Chicken Salad w/o Dressing	1	390	5	—	60	—	56	—	—	1200	—	—	—	—
Greek Salad w/ Dressing	1	940	71	—	50	—	63	—	—	1320	—	—	—	—
Greek Salad w/ Tuna & Dressing	1	1010	72	—	65	—	63	—	—	1510	—	—	—	—
Greek Salad w/ Tuna w/o Dressing	1	490	15	—	65	—	58	—	—	1510	—	—	—	—
Greek Salad w/o Dressing	1	420	15	—	50	—	58	—	—	1310	—	—	—	—
Roast Beef Salad w/o Dressing	1	400	6	—	50	—	55	—	—	920	—	—	—	—
Tossed Garden Salad w/o Dressing	1	270	2	—	0	—	55	—	—	650	—	—	—	—
Tuna Salad w/o Dressing	1	330	3	—	15	—	55	—	—	840	—	—	—	—
Turkey Salad w/o Dressing	1	400	3	—	80	—	55	—	—	700	—	—	—	—

SANDWICHES

FOOD	PORTION	CALORIES	FAT	SAT FAT	CHOL	PROTEIN	CARBO	FIBER	CALCIUM	SOD	POTAS	VIT C	FOLIC	VIT A
BLT w/ Cheese	1	1170	62	—	165	—	88	—	—	3310	—	—	—	—
BLT w/ Cheese Medium Sub	1	870	47	—	125	—	64	—	—	2490	—	—	—	—
BLT w/ Cheese Pokket	1	570	31	—	90	—	41	—	—	1690	—	—	—	—
BLT w/ Cheese Small Sub	1	600	33	—	90	—	—	—	—	1730	—	—	—	—
Barbecue Curls	1	480	19	—	70	—	45	—	—	650	—	—	—	—
Buffalo Chicken Wrap w/ Blue Cheese Dressing	1	621	28	—	93	—	51	—	—	1831	—	—	—	—
Buffalo Chicken Wrap w/o Dressing	1	417	13	—	78	—	48	—	—	1551	—	—	—	—

FOOD	PORTION	CALORIES	FAT	SAT FAT	CHOL	PROTEIN	CARBO	FIBER	CALCIUM	SOD	POTAS	VIT C	FOLIC	VIT A
Caesar Salad w/ Dressing Pokket	1	590	26	—	40	—	68	—	—	1690	—	—	—	—
Caesar Salad w/o Dressing Pokket	1	460	13	—	10	—	68	—	—	1210	—	—	—	—
Caesar Salad w/ Chicken w/ Dressing Pokket	1	570	16	—	70	—	68	—	—	1760	—	—	—	—
Caesar Salad w/ Chicken w/ Dressing Pokket	1	700	28	—	100	—	69	—	—	2240	—	—	—	—
Caesar Wrap w/ Dressing	1	484	15	—	10	—	66	—	—	2135	—	—	—	—
Caesar Wrap w/ Fat Free Dressing	1	484	15	—	10	—	66	—	—	2135	—	—	—	—
Capicola Ham & Cheese Large Sub	1	740	23	—	85	—	89	—	—	2540	—	—	—	—
Capicola Ham & Cheese Medium Sub	1	550	17	—	65	—	64	—	—	1900	—	—	—	—
Capicola Ham & Cheese Pokket	1	350	11	—	45	—	41	—	—	1260	—	—	—	—
Capicola Ham & Cheese Small Sub	1	390	13	—	45	—	45	—	—	1310	—	—	—	—
Cheeseburger Large Sub	1	1060	49	—	165	—	87	—	—	2090	—	—	—	—
Cheeseburger Medium Sub	1	780	37	—	125	—	63	—	—	1560	—	—	—	—
Cheeseburger Pokket	1	490	23	—	80	—	40	—	—	1000	—	—	—	—
Cheeseburger Small Sub	1	530	25	—	80	—	44	—	—	1040	—	—	—	—
Chicken Salad Large Sub	1	1370	78	—	155	—	89	—	—	1570	—	—	—	—
Chicken Salad Medium Sub	1	970	55	—	110	—	64	—	—	1120	—	—	—	—
Chicken Salad Pokket	1	650	38	—	80	—	41	—	—	740	—	—	—	—
Chicken Salad Small Sub	1	690	39	—	80	—	44	—	—	790	—	—	—	—
Chicken Stir Fry D'Lite Pokket	1	360	5	—	70	—	46	—	—	1240	—	—	—	—
Chicken Stir Fry D'Lite Sub	1	280	6	—	70	—	47	—	—	1280	—	—	—	—
Chicken Stir Fry Large Sub	1	800	12	—	160	—	93	—	—	2730	—	—	—	—

FOOD	PORTION	CALORIES	FAT	SAT FAT	CHOL	PROTEIN	CARBO	FIBER	CALCIUM	SOD	POTAS	VIT C	FOLIC	VIT A
Chicken Stir Fry Medium Sub	1	560	9	—	110	—	68	—	—	1890	—	—	—	—
Classic Vegetable Large Sub	1	860	33	—	80	—	104	—	—	2450	—	—	—	—
Classic Vegetable Medium Sub	1	610	23	—	55	—	74	—	—	1700	—	—	—	—
Classic Vegetable Pokket	1	400	15	—	40	—	48	—	—	1180	—	—	—	—
Classic Vegetable Small Sub	1	430	15	—	40	—	52	—	—	1220	—	—	—	—
Crunchy Vegetable Large Sub	1	880	33	—	80	—	106	—	—	2520	—	—	—	—
Crunchy Vegetable Pokket	1	410	15	—	40	—	50	—	—	1220	—	—	—	—
Crunchy Vegetables Medium Sub	1	620	23	—	55	—	76	—	—	1750	—	—	—	—
Crunchy Vegetables Small Sub	1	440	16	—	40	—	53	—	—	1260	—	—	—	—
Greek Pokket	1	910	71	—	50	—	57	—	—	1120	—	—	—	—
Grilled Steak Cheese Large Sub	1	1160	54	—	195	—	87	—	—	1970	—	—	—	—
Grilled Steak Cheese Medium Sub	1	820	38	—	135	—	63	—	—	1460	—	—	—	—
Grilled Steak Cheese Pokket	1	550	26	—	100	—	40	—	—	1010	—	—	—	—
Grilled Steak Cheese Small Sub	1	580	28	—	100	—	44	—	—	1050	—	—	—	—
Grilled Steak Combo Large Sub	1	1170	54	—	195	—	92	—	—	2200	—	—	—	—
Grilled Steak Combo Medium Sub	1	830	38	—	135	—	67	—	—	1630	—	—	—	—
Grilled Steak Combo Pokket	1	550	26	—	100	—	43	—	—	1120	—	—	—	—
Grilled Steak Combo Small Sub	1	590	28	—	100	—	46	—	—	1170	—	—	—	—
Grilled Steak Large Sub	1	990	40	—	155	—	87	—	—	1320	—	—	—	—
Grilled Steak Medium Sub	1	680	27	—	105	—	63	—	—	940	—	—	—	—
Grilled Steak Mushrooms Large Sub	1	1000	40	—	155	—	—	—	—	1570	—	—	—	—
Grilled Steak Mushrooms Medium Sub	1	690	27	—	105	—	65	—	—	1120	—	—	—	—
Grilled Steak Mushrooms Pokket	1	450	18	—	70	—	41	—	—	720	—	—	—	—

FOOD	PORTION	CALORIES	FAT	SAT FAT	CHOL	PROTEIN	CARBO	FIBER	CALCIUM	SOD	POTAS	VIT C	FOLIC	VIT A
Grilled Steak Mushrooms Small Sub	1	480	19	—	70	—	45	—	—	770	—	—	—	—
Grilled Steak Onion Large Sub	1	1000	40	—	155	—	91	—	—	1330	—	—	—	—
Grilled Steak Onion Medium Sub	1	700	27	—	105	—	66	—	—	940	—	—	—	—
Grilled Steak Onion Small Sub	1	480	19	—	70	—	45	—	—	650	—	—	—	—
Grilled Steak Onions Pokket	1	450	17	—	70	—	42	—	—	600	—	—	—	—
Grilled Steak Peppers	1	690	27	—	105	—	65	—	—	940	—	—	—	—
Grilled Steak Peppers Large Sub	1	1000	40	—	155	—	90	—	—	1330	—	—	—	—
Grilled Steak Peppers Pokket	1	540	17	—	70	—	42	—	—	600	—	—	—	—
Grilled Steak Pokket	1	440	17	—	70	—	40	—	—	600	—	—	—	—
Grilled Steak Small Sub	1	470	19	—	70	—	43	—	—	650	—	—	—	—
Ham & Cheese Large Sub	1	760	25	—	105	—	88	—	—	3030	—	—	—	—
Ham & Cheese Medium Sub	1	550	19	—	75	—	63	—	—	2170	—	—	—	—
Ham & Cheese Pokket	1	370	13	—	55	—	40	—	—	1550	—	—	—	—
Ham & Cheese Small Sub	1	400	14	—	55	—	44	—	—	1600	—	—	—	—
Ham Salami & Cheese Large Sub	1	870	36	—	110	—	88	—	—	3000	—	—	—	—
Ham Salami & Cheese Medium Sub	1	630	27	—	80	—	64	—	—	2190	—	—	—	—
Ham Salami & Cheese Pokket	1	420	18	—	60	—	41	—	—	1500	—	—	—	—
Ham Salami & Cheese Smalle Sub	1	450	20	—	60	—	44	—	—	1550	—	—	—	—
Hamburger Large Sub	1	920	38	—	130	—	87	—	—	1570	—	—	—	—
Hamburger Medium Sub	1	680	28	—	95	—	63	—	—	1150	—	—	—	—
Hamburger Pokket	1	430	18	—	65	—	40	—	—	740	—	—	—	—
Hamburger Small Sub	1	460	19	—	65	—	43	—	—	780	—	—	—	—
Italian Cold Cut Large Sub	1	1130	61	—	155	—	92	—	—	3580	—	—	—	—

FOOD	PORTION	CALORIES	FAT	SAT FAT	CHOL	PROTEIN	CARBO	FIBER	CALCIUM	SOD	POTAS	VIT C	FOLIC	VIT A
Italian Cold Cut Medium Sub	1	820	44	—	110	—	68	—	—	2600	—	—	—	—
Meatball Large Sub	1	1010	42	—	135	—	102	—	—	2600	—	—	—	—
Meatball Medium Sub	1	750	32	—	100	—	76	—	—	1980	—	—	—	—
Meatball Pokket	1	480	20	—	65	—	50	—	—	1360	—	—	—	—
Meatball Small Sub	1	520	21	—	65	—	54	—	—	1400	—	—	—	—
Meatball w/ Cheese Large Sub	1	1170	54	—	165	—	103	—	—	3000	—	—	—	—
Meatball w/ Cheese Medium Sub	1	880	41	—	125	—	77	—	—	2300	—	—	—	—
Meatball w/ Cheese Pokket	1	580	28	—	85	—	51	—	—	1600	—	—	—	—
Meatball w/ Cheese Small Sub	1	620	29	—	85	—	54	—	—	1650	—	—	—	—
Pastrami Large Sub	1	1250	69	—	175	—	87	—	—	2920	—	—	—	—
Pastrami Medium Sub	1	860	46	—	115	—	63	—	—	2010	—	—	—	—
Pastrami Pokket	1	550	30	—	75	—	40	—	—	1310	—	—	—	—
Pastrami Small Sub	1	580	31	—	75	—	44	—	—	1350	—	—	—	—
Pastrami w/ Cheese Large Sub	1	1640	102	—	270	—	89	—	—	4420	—	—	—	—
Pastrami w/ Cheese Medium Sub	1	1170	73	—	195	—	64	—	—	3210	—	—	—	—
Pastrami w/ Cheese Pokket	1	780	49	—	135	—	41	—	—	2210	—	—	—	—
Pastrami w/ Cheese Small Sub	1	820	51	—	135	—	45	—	—	2250	—	—	—	—
Seafood Salad Large Sub	1	1210	68	—	50	—	118	—	—	2890	—	—	—	—
Seafood Salad Medium Sub	1	860	48	—	35	—	85	—	—	2050	—	—	—	—
Seafood Salad Pokket	1	570	33	—	25	—	56	—	—	1400	—	—	—	—
Seafood Salad Small Sub	1	610	34	—	25	—	59	—	—	1440	—	—	—	—
Stuffed Turkey Large Sub	1	1070	19	—	165	—	146	—	—	1850	—	—	—	—
Stuffed Turkey Medium Sub	1	790	14	—	120	—	107	—	—	1360	—	—	—	—
Tuna Salad Large Sub	1	1510	102	—	120	—	90	—	—	2200	—	—	—	—
Tuna Salad Medium Sub	1	1070	72	—	85	—	65	—	—	1570	—	—	—	—
Tuna Salad Pokket	1	720	50	—	60	—	41	—	—	1060	—	—	—	—
Tuna Salad Small Sub	1	760	51	—	60	—	45	—	—	1100	—	—	—	—
Turkey Large Sub	1	710	7	—	160	—	87	—	—	1070	—	—	—	—

FOOD	PORTION	CALORIES	FAT	SAT FAT	CHOL	PROTEIN	CARBO	FIBER	CALCIUM	SOD	POTAS	VIT C	FOLIC	VIT A
Turkey Medium Sub	1	520	5	—	115	—	63	—	—	780	—	—	—	—
Turkey Club Large Sub	1	860	20	—	180	—	87	—	—	1470	—	—	—	—
Turkey Club Medium Sub	1	630	15	—	130	—	63	—	—	1080	—	—	—	—
Turkey Club Pokket	1	400	9	—	90	—	40	—	—	690	—	—	—	—
Turkey Club Small Sub	1	430	10	—	90	—	43	—	—	740	—	—	—	—

DAIRY QUEEN

FOOD SELECTIONS

FOOD	PORTION	CALORIES	FAT	SAT FAT	CHOL	PROTEIN	CARBO	FIBER	CALCIUM	SOD	POTAS	VIT C	FOLIC	VIT A
Chicken Breast Fillet Sandwich	1 (6.7 oz)	430	20	4	55	24	37	2	40	760	—	0	—	0
Chicken Strip Basket	1 serv (14.5 oz)	1000	50	13	55	35	102	5	60	2260	—	9	—	200
Chili 'n' Cheese Dog	1 (5 oz)	330	21	9	45	14	22	2	150	1090	—	4	—	750
DQ Homestyle Bacon Double Cheeseburger	1 (8.9 oz)	610	36	18	130	41	31	2	250	1380	—	6	—	750
DQ Homestyle Cheeseburger	1 (5.3 oz)	340	17	8	55	20	29	2	150	850	—	4	—	500
DQ Homestyle Double Cheeseburger	1 (7.7 oz)	540	31	16	115	35	30	2	250	1130	—	4	—	750
DQ Homestyle Hamburger	1 (4.8 oz)	290	12	5	45	17	29	2	60	630	—	4	—	200
DQ Ultimate Burger	1 (9.4 oz)	670	43	19	135	40	29	2	250	1210	—	9	—	750
French Fries	1 med (3.9 oz)	350	18	4	0	4	42	3	20	630	—	4	—	0
French Fries	1 lg (4.9 oz)	440	23	5	0	5	53	4	40	790	—	5	—	0
Grilled Chicken Sandwich	1 (6.5 oz)	310	10	3	50	24	30	3	200	1040	—	0	—	0
Hot Dog	1 (3.5 oz)	240	14	5	25	9	19	1	60	730	—	4	—	100
Onion Rings	1 serv (4 oz)	320	16	4	0	5	39	3	20	180	—	0	—	0

ICE CREAM

FOOD	PORTION	CALORIES	FAT	SAT FAT	CHOL	PROTEIN	CARBO	FIBER	CALCIUM	SOD	POTAS	VIT C	FOLIC	VIT A
Banana Split	1 (12.9 oz)	510	12	8	30	8	96	3	250	180	—	15	—	1000
Blizzard Chocolate Sandwich Cookie	1 med (11.4 oz)	640	23	11	45	12	97	1	400	500	—	1	—	1250
Blizzard Chocolate Sandwich Cookie	1 sm (12 oz)	520	18	9	40	10	79	1	350	380	—	1	—	1000
Blizzard Chocolate Chip Cookie Dough	1 med (15.4 oz)	950	36	19	75	17	143	2	450	660	—	1	—	1750
Blizzard Chocolate Chip Cookie Dough	1 sm (12 oz)	660	24	13	55	12	99	1	350	440	—	1	—	1250
Breeze Heath	1 med (14.2 oz)	710	18	11	20	15	123	1	450	580	—	2	—	100

FOOD	PORTION	CALORIES	FAT	SAT FAT	CHOL	PROTEIN	CARBO	FIBER	CALCIUM	SOD	POTAS	VIT C	FOLIC	VIT A
Breeze Heath	1 sm (10.2 oz)	470	10	6	10	11	85	1	350	380	—	2	—	0
Breeze Strawberry	1 sm (12 oz)	320	1	1	5	10	68	1	350	190	—	6	—	0
Breeze Strawberry	1 med (13.4 oz)	460	1	1	10	13	99	1	450	270	—	9	—	0
Buster Bar	1 (5.2 oz)	450	28	12	15	10	41	2	150	280	—	0	—	400
Chocolate Malt	1 med (19.9 oz)	880	22	14	70	19	153	0	600	500	—	2	—	2000
Chocolate Malt	1 sm (14.7 oz)	650	16	10	55	15	111	0	450	370	—	2	—	1500
Cone Chocolate	1 med (6.9 oz)	340	11	7	30	8	53	0	250	160	—	1	—	750
Cone Chocolate	1 sm (5 oz)	240	8	5	20	6	37	0	150	115	—	0	—	750
Cone Vanilla	1 sm (5 oz)	230	7	5	20	6	38	0	200	115	—	1	—	500
Cone Vanilla	1 med (6.9 oz)	330	9	6	30	8	53	0	250	160	—	2	—	750
Cone Vanilla	1 lg (8.9 oz)	410	12	8	40	10	65	0	350	200	—	2	—	1000
Cone Yogurt	1 med (6.9 oz)	260	1	1	5	9	56	0	250	160	—	2	—	0
Cone Dipped	1 med (7.7 oz)	490	24	13	30	9	59	1	250	190	—	2	—	750
Cone Dipped	1 sm (5.5 oz)	340	17	9	20	6	42	1	200	130	—	1	—	500
Cup Of Yogurt	1 med (6.7 oz)	230	1	0	5	8	48	0	250	150	—	1	—	0
DQ 8 Inch Round Cake Undecorated	1/8 of cake (6.2 oz)	340	12	7	25	7	53	1	200	250	—	0	—	750
DQ Fudge Bar No Sugar Added	1 (2.3 oz)	50	0	0	0	4	13	0	100	70	—	0	—	300
DQ Lemon Freez'r	1/2 cup (3.2 oz)	80	0	0	0	0	20	0	0	10	—	0	—	0
DQ Nonfat Frozen Yogurt	1/2 cup (3 oz)	100	0	0	<5	3	21	0	100	70	—	0	—	0
DQ Sandwich	1 (2.1 oz)	150	5	2	5	3	24	1	60	115	—	0	—	200
DQ Soft Serve Chocolate	1/2 cup (3.3 oz)	150	5	4	15	4	22	0	100	75	—	0	—	500
DQ Soft Serve Vanilla	1/2 cup (3.3 oz)	140	5	3	15	3	22	0	150	70	—	0	—	500
DQ Treatzza Pizza Heath	1/8 of pie (2.3 oz)	180	7	4	5	3	28	1	60	160	—	0	—	200
DQ Treatzza Pizza M&M	1/8 of pie (2.4 oz)	190	7	4	5	3	29	1	60	160	—	0	—	200
DQ Vanilla Orange Bar No Sugar Added	1 (2.3 oz)	60	0	0	0	2	17	0	60	40	—	0	—	100
Dilly Bar Chocolate	1 (3 oz)	210	13	7	10	3	21	0	100	75	—	0	—	300
Fudge Cake Supreme	1 serv (11.2 oz)	890	38	22	65	11	124	3	200	960	—	0	—	1000
Misty Slush	1 med (20.9 oz)	290	0	0	0	0	74	0	0	30	—	0	—	0
Misty Slush	1 sm (15.9 oz)	220	0	0	0	0	56	0	0	20	—	0	—	0
Peanut Buster Parfait	1 (10.7 oz)	730	31	17	35	16	99	2	300	400	—	1	—	750
Shake Chocolate	1 med (18.9 oz)	770	20	13	70	17	130	0	600	420	—	2	—	2000
Shake Chocolate	1 sm (13.9 oz)	560	15	10	50	13	94	0	450	310	—	2	—	1500

FOOD	PORTION	CALORIES	FAT	SAT FAT	CHOL	PROTEIN	CARBO	FIBER	CALCIUM	SOD	POTAS	VIT C	FOLIC	VIT A
Starkiss	1 (3 oz)	80	0	—	0	0	21	0	0	10	—	0	—	0
Strawberry Shortcake	1 (8.5 oz)	430	14	9	60	7	70	1	250	360	—	6	—	500
Sundae Chocolate	1 med (8.2 oz)	400	10	6	30	8	71	0	250	210	—	0	—	750
Sundae Chocolate	1 sm (5.7 oz)	280	7	5	20	5	49	0	200	140	—	0	—	500
Yogurt Sundae Strawberry	1 med (8.2 oz)	280	1	0	5	8	61	1	300	160	—	6	—	0

DELTACO

BREAKFAST SELECTIONS

FOOD	PORTION	CALORIES	FAT	SAT FAT	CHOL	PROTEIN	CARBO	FIBER	CALCIUM	SOD	POTAS	VIT C	FOLIC	VIT A
Burrito Beef And Egg	1	529	27	10	328	29	43	—	—	929	—	—	—	—
Burrito Breakfast	1	256	11	4	90	9	30	—	—	409	—	—	—	—
Burrito Egg And Cheese	1	443	22	8	305	22	40	—	—	792	—	—	—	—
Burrito Egg and Bean	1	470	22	8	305	24	45	—	—	1035	—	—	—	—
Burrito Steak And Egg	1	500	25	9	337	30	41	—	—	1068	—	—	—	—

CHILDREN'S MENU SELECTIONS

FOOD	PORTION	CALORIES	FAT	SAT FAT	CHOL	PROTEIN	CARBO	FIBER	CALCIUM	SOD	POTAS	VIT C	FOLIC	VIT A
Kid's Meal Hamburger	1 meal	617	20	7	29	14	96	—	—	799	—	—	—	—
Kid's Meal Taco	1 meal	532	17	6	16	8	87	—	—	373	—	—	—	—

MAIN MENU SELECTIONS

FOOD	PORTION	CALORIES	FAT	SAT FAT	CHOL	PROTEIN	CARBO	FIBER	CALCIUM	SOD	POTAS	VIT C	FOLIC	VIT A
American Cheese	1 slice	53	4	3	14	3	tr	—	—	203	—	—	—	—
Beans And Cheese	1	122	3	2	9	7	17	—	—	892	—	—	—	—
Burrito Chicken	1	264	10	4	36	13	32	—	—	771	—	—	—	—
Burrito Combination	1	413	17	7	49	21	46	—	—	1035	—	—	—	—
Burrito Del Beef	1	440	20	9	63	23	43	—	—	878	—	—	—	—
Burrito Deluxe Chicken	1	549	34	10	83	21	40	—	—	978	—	—	—	—
Burrito Deluxe Combo	1	453	20	9	59	22	49	—	—	1047	—	—	—	—
Burrito Deluxe Del Beef	1	479	23	10	73	25	45	—	—	890	—	—	—	—
Burrito Green	1	229	8	3	15	9	32	—	—	714	—	—	—	—
Burrito Green Regular	1	330	11	5	22	14	46	—	—	1149	—	—	—	—
Burrito Macho Beef	1	893	41	18	139	49	84	—	—	1969	—	—	—	—
Burrito Macho Combo	1	774	31	15	100	38	87	—	—	2180	—	—	—	—
Burrito Red	1	235	8	4	17	10	32	—	—	656	—	—	—	—
Burrito Red Regular	1	342	12	5	26	15	46	—	—	1033	—	—	—	—
Burrito Spicy Chicken	1	392	11	3	35	16	59	—	—	1243	—	—	—	—
Burrito The Works	1	448	18	6	27	15	60	—	—	1248	—	—	—	—
Cheeseburger	1	284	13	6	42	14	26	—	—	852	—	—	—	—

FOOD	PORTION	CALORIES	FAT	SAT FAT	CHOL	PROTEIN	CARBO	FIBER	CALCIUM	SOD	POTAS	VIT C	FOLIC	VIT A
Chicken Salad	1	254	19	6	58	12	8	—	—	476	—	—	—	—
Chicken Salad Deluxe	1	716	47	15	98	26	55	—	—	1419	—	—	—	—
Del Burger	1	385	20	6	42	14	35	—	—	1065	—	—	—	—
Del Cheeseburger	1	439	25	9	55	18	35	—	—	1268	—	—	—	—
Double Del Cheeseburger	1	618	39	16	108	29	36	—	—	1638	—	—	—	—
French Fries	1 lg	566	26	9	0	8	76	—	—	318	—	—	—	—
French Fries	1 reg	404	19	6	0	5	54	—	—	227	—	—	—	—
French Fries	1 sm	242	11	4	0	3	32	—	—	136	—	—	—	—
Fries Chili Cheese	1 serv	562	30	13	38	15	58	—	—	846	—	—	—	—
Fries Deluxe Chili Cheese	1 serv	600	33	15	48	16	61	—	—	855	—	—	—	—
Fries Nacho	1 serv	669	34	11	2	10	80	—	—	926	—	—	—	—
Guacamole	1 oz	60	6	0	0	1	2	—	—	130	—	—	—	—
Hamburger	1	231	8	3	29	11	26	—	—	649	—	—	—	—
Hot Sauce	1 pkg	2	tr	0	0	tr	tr	—	—	38	—	—	—	—
Nacho Cheese Sauce	1 side order	100	8	2	2	2	4	—	—	401	—	—	—	—
Nachos	1 serv	390	32	4	2	6	39	—	—	504	—	—	—	—
Nachos Macho	1	1089	61	13	46	26	110	—	—	1740	—	—	—	—
Quesadilla	1	257	12	6	30	11	26	—	—	455	—	—	—	—
Quesadilla Chicken	1	544	31	16	113	30	38	—	—	1147	—	—	—	—
Quesadilla Regular	1	483	27	16	75	23	37	—	—	871	—	—	—	—
Quesadilla Spicy Jack	1	254	12	6	30	11	26	—	—	402	—	—	—	—
Quesadilla Spicy Jack Chicken	1	537	30	17	114	31	38	—	—	1214	—	—	—	—
Quesadilla Spicy Jack Regular	1	476	27	16	76	23	37	—	—	938	—	—	—	—
Salsa	2 oz	14	tr	0	tr	tr	3	—	—	308	—	—	—	—
Salsa Dressing	1 oz	33	3	2	10	tr	1	—	—	85	—	—	—	—
Soft Taco	1	146	6	3	16	5	17	—	—	223	—	—	—	—
Soft Taco Chicken	1	197	11	3	35	7	16	—	—	401	—	—	—	—
Soft Taco Deluxe Double Beef	1	211	11	5	35	8	20	—	—	283	—	—	—	—
Soft Taco Double Beef	1	178	8	3	25	7	18	—	—	274	—	—	—	—
Sour Cream	1 oz	60	6	4	20	tr	tr	—	—	15	—	—	—	—
Taco	1	140	8	3	16	6	10	—	—	99	—	—	—	—
Taco Chicken	1	186	13	3	35	8	10	—	—	276	—	—	—	—
Taco Deluxe Double Beef	1	205	13	5	35	9	13	—	—	159	—	—	—	—
Taco Double Beef	1	172	10	3	25	8	12	—	—	150	—	—	—	—
Taco Salad	1	235	19	6	31	9	9	—	—	268	—	—	—	—
Taco Salad Deluxe	1	741	49	16	83	26	57	—	—	1280	—	—	—	—
Tostada	1	140	8	3	15	6	12	—	—	333	—	—	—	—

DENNY'S

BREAKFAST SELECTIONS

FOOD	PORTION	CALORIES	FAT	SAT FAT	CHOL	PROTEIN	CARBO	FIBER	CALCIUM	SOD	POTAS	VIT C	FOLIC	VIT A
All American Slam	1 serv (15 oz)	1028	87	21	724	48	24	2	500	1942	—	5	—	3600
Applesauce	1 serv (3 oz)	60	0	0	0	0	15	1	0	13	—	0	—	0
Bacon	4 strips (1 oz)	162	18	5	36	12	1	0	0	640	—	1	—	0
Bagel Dry	1 (3 oz)	235	1	0	0	9	46	0	0	495	—	0	—	0
Banana	1 (4 oz)	110	0	0	0	1	29	4	0	0	—	9	—	50
Banana Strawberry Medley	1 serv (4 oz)	108	1	0	0	1	27	2	0	6	—	5	—	0
Biscuit Plain	1 (3 oz)	375	22	5	0	5	40	0	0	750	—	0	—	0
Biscuit w/ Sausage Gravy	1 serv (7 oz)	570	38	10	24	11	45	0	0	1475	—	0	—	50
Blueberry Topping	1 serv (3 oz)	106	0	0	0	0	26	0	0	15	—	0	—	0
Canadian Bacon	1 serv (3 oz)	110	5	2	43	17	1	0	0	1039	—	10	—	0
Cantaloup	1 serv (3 oz)	32	0	0	0	1	8	1	10	16	—	30	—	315
Cheddar Cheese Omelette	1 serv (13 oz)	770	62	20	675	34	24	2	480	1133	—	7	—	3500
Cherry Topping	1 serv (3 oz)	86	0	0	0	0	21	0	0	5	—	0	—	2450
Chicken Fried Steak & Eggs	1 serv (14 oz)	723	56	18	452	28	31	8	70	1505	—	7	—	1800
Country Scramble	1 serv (16 oz)	795	50	11	409	20	67	2	60	1819	—	7	—	1700
Cream Cheese	1 oz	100	10	6	31	2	1	0	20	6	—	0	—	600
Egg	1 (2 oz)	134	12	3	205	6	1	0	20	61	—	0	—	500
Egg Beaters	1 serv (2.3 oz)	71	5	1	1	5	1	0	20	138	—	0	—	1850
Eggs Benedict	1 serv (19 oz)	860	56	23	525	35	55	3	150	1943	—	7	—	5000
English Muffin Dry	1 (4 oz)	125	1	0	0	5	24	1	80	198	—	0	—	0
Farmer's Omelette	1 serv (18 oz)	912	69	19	633	34	38	3	160	1816	—	22	—	2750
French Slam	1 serv (14 oz)	1029	71	20	777	44	58	2	120	1428	—	0	—	2650
French Toast	2 pieces (8 oz)	510	25	6	317	19	51	2	70	413	—	0	—	1000
Fresh Fruit Mix	1 serv (3 oz)	36	0	0	0	1	9	1	0	16	—	18	—	75
Grapefruit	½ (5 oz)	60	0	0	0	1	16	6	20	0	—	66	—	750
Grapes	1 serv (3 oz)	55	1	0	0	1	15	1	10	0	—	9	—	50
Grits	1 serv (4 oz)	80	0	0	0	2	18	0	0	520	—	0	—	0
Ham	1 serv (3 oz)	94	3	1	23	15	2	0	0	761	—	0	—	0
Ham'n'Cheddar Omelette	1 serv (14 oz)	743	55	10	657	36	24	2	290	1518	—	7	—	2900
Hashed Browns	1 serv (4 oz)	218	14	2	0	2	20	2	10	424	—	7	—	150
Hashed Browns Covered	1 serv (6 oz)	318	23	7	30	9	21	2	220	604	—	7	—	650
Hashed Browns Covered & Smothered	1 serv (8 oz)	359	26	7	30	9	26	2	220	790	—	8	—	650
Honeydew	1 serv (3 oz)	31	0	0	0	1	8	1	0	22	—	16	—	50
Junior Meals Basic Breakfast	1 serv (9 oz)	558	39	9	230	18	38	3	70	1103	—	8	—	950
Junior Meals Junior French Slam	1 serv (7 oz)	461	35	10	386	21	18	1	50	663	—	0	—	1300

FOOD	PORTION	CALORIES	FAT	SAT FAT	CHOL	PROTEIN	CARBO	FIBER	CALCIUM	SOD	POTAS	VIT C	FOLIC	VIT A
Junior Meals Junior Grand Slam	1 serv (5 oz)	397	25	7	230	17	33	1	80	1118	—	0	—	800
Junior Meals Junior Waffle Supreme	1 serv (4 oz)	190	11	2	73	3	20	0	60	102	—	13	—	600
Meat Lover's Sampler	1 serv (14 oz)	806	62	17	481	42	24	2	70	2211	—	7	—	1800
Moon Over My Hammy	1 serv (12 oz)	807	48	8	430	44	46	2	60	2247	—	0	—	2100
Muffin Blueberry	1 (3 oz)	309	14	0	0	4	42	0	70	190	—	1	—	100
Oatmeal	1 serv (4 oz)	100	2	0	0	5	18	3	10	175	—	0	—	0
Original Grand Slam	1 serv (10 oz)	795	50	14	460	34	65	2	160	2237	—	0	—	1650
Pancakes	3 (5 oz)	491	7	1	0	12	95	3	150	1818	—	0	—	0
Pork Chop & Eggs	1 serv (12 oz)	555	36	9	469	33	21	2	80	968	—	8	—	1050
Porterhouse Steak & Eggs	1 serv (18 oz)	1223	95	32	570	70	21	2	160	1369	—	7	—	1750
Ready To Eat Cereal	1 serv (1 oz)	100	0	0	0	2	23	1	0	276	—	10	—	175
Sausage	4 links (3 oz)	354	32	2	64	16	0	0	10	944	—	0	—	200
Sausage Cheddar Omelette	1 serv (16 oz)	1036	86	29	721	46	24	2	500	1841	—	7	—	3650
Scram Slam	1 serv (18 oz)	974	80	23	694	42	30	4	300	1750	—	37	—	3250
Senior Belgian Waffle Slam	1 serv (6 oz)	399	33	8	302	16	12	0	90	612	—	1	—	1400
Senior Omelette	1 serv (12 oz)	623	47	10	439	23	27	3	130	1194	—	16	—	2100
Senior Starter	1 serv (7 oz)	336	24	5	205	11	36	2	30	541	—	7	—	900
Senior Triple Play	1 serv (8 oz)	537	25	6	409	20	64	2	150	1445	—	0	—	1500
Sirloin Steak & Eggs	1 serv (13 oz)	808	64	18	474	37	21	2	100	952	—	7	—	1750
Slim Slam	1 serv (14 oz)	638	12	3	34	34	98	1	110	1772	—	0	—	500
Southern Slam	1 serv (13 oz)	1065	84	23	484	37	47	0	60	2449	—	4	—	1600
Strawberries w/ Sugar	1 serv (3 oz)	115	1	0	0	1	26	1	0	12	—	1	—	0
Strawberry Topping	1 serv (3 oz)	115	1	0	0	1	26	1	10	12	—	1	—	0
Sunshine Slam	1 serv (8 oz)	537	25	6	409	20	64	2	150	1445	—	0	—	1500
Super Play It Again Slam	1 serv (15 oz)	1192	75	21	690	51	98	3	240	3555	—	1	—	2400
Syrup	3 tbsp (1.5 oz)	143	0	0	0	0	36	0	0	26	—	0	—	0
Syrup Reduced Calorie	1 serv (1.5 oz)	25	0	0	0	0	6	0	0	96	—	0	—	0
T-Bone Steak & Eggs	1 serv (16 oz)	1045	82	26	530	56	21	2	130	1191	—	7	—	1750
Toast Dry	1 slice (1 oz)	92	1	0	0	3	17	1	30	166	—	0	—	0
Ultimate Omelette	1 serv (17 oz)	780	62	14	639	31	29	4	90	1360	—	38	—	2700
Vegggie Cheese Omelette	1 serv (16 oz)	714	53	10	644	28	29	4	290	955	—	35	—	3050
Waffle	1 (6 oz)	304	21	3	146	7	23	0	120	200	—	2	—	1200

FOOD	PORTION	CALORIES	FAT	SAT FAT	CHOL	PROTEIN	CARBO	FIBER	CALCIUM	SOD	POTAS	VIT C	FOLIC	VIT A
Whipped Margarine	1 serv (0.5 oz)	87	10	2	0	0	0	0	0	117	—	0	—	0
Whipped Cream	1 serv (2 oz)	23	2	0	7	0	2	0	0	3	—	0	—	100
DESSERTS														
Apple Pie	1 serv (7 oz)	430	20	5	<5	3	59	1	0	390	—	0	—	0
Apple Pie w/ Equal	1 serv (7 oz)	370	20	5	<5	3	43	2	0	360	—	0	—	0
Banana Split	1 serv (19 oz)	894	43	19	78	15	121	6	240	177	—	23	—	1250
Blueberry Topping	1 serv (3 oz)	106	0	0	0	0	26	0	0	15	—	0	—	0
Cheesecake Pie	1 serv (4 oz)	470	27	13	90	8	48	0	80	280	—	0	—	750
Cherry Topping	1 serv (3 oz)	86	0	0	0	0	21	0	0	5	—	0	—	2450
Cherry Pie	1 serv (7 oz)	540	21	5	<5	5	83	2	0	430	—	0	—	1000
Chocolate Topping	1 serv (2 oz)	317	25	0	0	2	27	0	0	83	—	0	—	0
Chocolate Cake	1 serv (4 oz)	370	17	4	29	4	53	2	20	374	—	0	—	200
Chocolate Pecan Pie	1 serv (6 oz)	790	37	9	70	6	107	3	20	460	—	0	—	400
Chocolate Shake	1 serv (10 oz)	579	27	17	108	12	77	0	380	278	—	6	—	1400
Coconut Cream Pie	1 serv (7 oz)	480	26	16	15	5	58	1	80	440	—	0	—	0
Double Scoop Sundae	1 serv (6 oz)	375	27	12	74	6	29	0	130	86	—	0	—	900
Dutch Apple Pie	1 serv (7 oz)	440	19	5	0	3	65	1	0	290	—	0	—	0
French Silk Pie	1 serv (6 oz)	650	43	26	165	6	60	2	20	220	—	0	—	750
Fudge Topping	1 serv (2 oz)	201	10	7	3	1	30	1	30	96	—	0	—	0
German Chocolate Pie	1 serv (7 oz)	580	33	18	15	7	66	2	100	460	—	0	—	0
Hot Fudge Cake Sundae	1 serv (8 oz)	687	38	11	62	9	83	3	110	486	—	0	—	750
Ice Cream Float	1 serv (12 oz)	280	10	6	39	3	47	0	120	109	—	0	—	400
Key Lime Pie	1 serv (6 oz)	600	27	15	35	10	79	0	300	300	—	0	—	750
Lemon Meringue Pie	1 serv (7 oz)	460	17	4	95	5	71	1	20	310	—	0	—	200
Pecan Pie	1 serv (6 oz)	600	28	4	50	5	81	2	0	430	—	0	—	0
Single Scoop Sundae	1 serv (3 oz)	188	14	6	37	3	14	0	60	43	—	0	—	450
Strawberry Topping	1 serv (3 oz)	115	1	0	0	1	26	1	10	12	—	1	—	0
Vanilla Shake	1 serv (11 oz)	581	27	17	108	11	77	0	380	236	—	6	—	1400
MAIN MENU SELECTIONS														
BBQ Sauce	1 serv (1.5 oz)	47	1	0	0	0	11	0	10	595	—	2	—	350
Bacon Cheddar Burger	1 (14 oz)	935	63	25	164	53	43	3	430	1732	—	11	—	1600
Bacon Lettuce & Tomato Sandwich	1 (6 oz)	634	46	8	54	18	37	3	70	1116	—	17	—	300
Baked Potato Plain	1 (6 oz)	186	0	0	0	4	43	4	10	14	—	22	—	0
Battered Cod Dinner w/ Tartar Sauce	1 serv (9 oz)	732	47	7	105	30	48	3	0	1335	—	0	—	0
Broccoli In Butter Sauce	2 serv (4 oz)	50	2	2	5	3	7	3	60	280	—	48	—	2250

FOOD	PORTION	CALORIES	FAT	SAT FAT	CHOL	PROTEIN	CARBO	FIBER	CALCIUM	SOD	POTAS	VIT C	FOLIC	VIT A
Brown Gravy	1 serv (1 oz)	13	0	0	0	0	2	0	0	184	—	0	—	0
Buffalo Chicken Strips	1 serv (10 oz)	734	42	4	96	48	43	0	20	1673	—	22	—	1100
Buffalo Wings	12 pieces (15 oz)	856	54	17	500	92	1	1	190	5552	—	29	—	900
Carrots In Honey Glaze	2 serv (4 oz)	80	3	1	0	1	12	3	40	220	—	3	—	19000
Charleston Chicken Sandwich	1 (11 oz)	632	32	7	81	35	53	4	140	1967	—	10	—	850
Chicken Quesadilla	1 serv (16 oz)	827	55	23	181	50	43	2	640	1982	—	54	—	3150
Chicken Fried Chicken	1 serv (6 oz)	327	18	4	65	25	16	1	30	993	—	1	—	50
Chicken Fried Steak w/ Gravy	1 serv (4 oz)	265	17	8	27	15	14	1	10	668	—	0	—	0
Chicken Gravy	1 serv (1 oz)	14	1	0	2	0	2	0	0	139	—	0	—	0
Chicken Melt Sandwich	1 (7 oz)	520	29	5	39	26	43	2	10	1096	—	12	—	750
Chicken Strip w/ Dressing	1 serv (10 oz)	635	25	1	95	47	55	0	20	1510	—	0	—	0
Chicken Strips	5 pieces (10 oz)	720	33	4	95	47	56	0	20	1666	—	0	—	0
Classic Burger	1 (11 oz)	673	40	15	106	37	42	3	130	1142	—	11	—	1000
Classic Burger w/ Cheese	1 (13 oz)	836	53	19	137	47	43	3	340	1595	—	11	—	1050
Club Sandwich	1	485	35	6	90	29	40	—	—	1385	—	—	—	—
Corn In Butter Sauce	2 serv (4 oz)	120	4	2	5	3	19	5	0	260	—	1	—	400
Cornbread Stuffing Plain	1 serv (2 oz)	182	9	0	0	4	20	0	0	405	—	0	—	0
Cottage Cheese	1 serv (3 oz)	72	3	2	10	9	2	0	40	281	—	0	—	150
Country Gravy	1 serv (1 oz)	17	1	0	0	0	2	0	0	93	—	0	—	0
Delidinger Sandwich	1 (14 oz)	852	45	6	80	56	62	3	30	3142	—	12	—	1050
Deluxe Grilled Cheese Sandwich	1 (7 oz)	482	26	2	1	18	44	2	10	1135	—	7	—	900
Dinner Roll	1 (1.5 oz)	132	2	0	0	4	26	1	20	265	—	0	—	0
French Fries Unsalted	1 serv (4 oz)	323	14	3	0	5	44	0	0	130	—	0	—	0
Fried Fish Sandwich	1 (11 oz)	905	56	8	69	29	74	4	40	1704	—	1	—	650
Gardenburger Patty	1 patty (3.4 oz)	160	3	0	10	11	22	3	—	390	—	—	—	—
Gardenburger Patty w/ Bun & Fat Free Honey Mustard Dressing	1 serv (11.1 oz)	653	32	6	26	21	72	6	110	1017	—	10	—	1150
Green Beans w/ Bacon	2 serv (4 oz)	60	4	2	5	1	6	3	40	390	—	6	—	500

FOOD	PORTION	CALORIES	FAT	SAT FAT	CHOL	PROTEIN	CARBO	FIBER	CALCIUM	SOD	POTAS	VIT C	FOLIC	VIT A
Green Peas In Butter Sauce	2 serv (4 oz)	100	2	2	5	5	14	4	20	360	—	15	—	1000
Grilled Mushrooms	1 serv (2 oz)	14	0	0	0	2	2	1	0	0	—	1	—	0
Grilled Alaskan Salmon	1 serv (7 oz)	296	14	2	102	43	1	0	20	257	—	0	—	0
Grilled Chicken Breast	1 serv (4 oz)	130	4	1	67	24	0	0	10	566	—	1	—	50
Grilled Chicken Dinner	1 serv (4 oz)	130	4	1	67	24	0	0	10	560	—	1	—	50
Grilled Chicken Sandwich	1 (11 oz)	509	19	5	83	34	52	3	120	1809	—	10	—	850
Grilled Chopped Steak w/ Gravy	1 serv (10 oz)	400	26	11	91	30	12	2	20	447	—	0	—	0
Ham & Swiss On Rye	1 (9 oz)	533	31	4	36	23	40	5	70	1638	—	8	—	300
Hashed Browns	1 serv (4 oz)	218	14	2	0	2	20	2	10	424	—	7	—	150
Herb Toast	1 serv (2 oz)	200	11	2	0	4	21	1	50	372	—	0	—	0
Horseradish Sauce	1 serv (1.5 oz)	170	20	3	43	1	3	0	0	227	—	0	—	0
Junior Meals Junior Burger	1 serv (3 oz)	261	15	4	41	14	16	0	10	115	—	0	—	300
Junior Meals Junior Chicken Strips	1 serv (5 oz)	318	12	1	48	25	28	0	10	755	—	0	—	0
Junior Meals Junior Fried Fish	1 serv (5 oz)	465	34	5	68	15	25	1	0	743	—	0	—	0
Junior Meals Junior Grilled Cheese	1 serv (4 oz)	375	22	3	1	12	35	1	60	811	—	0	—	600
Junior Meals Junior Shrimp Basket	1 serv (4 oz)	291	16	3	60	10	27	2	30	774	—	0	—	150
Lunch Basket Charleston Chicken Ranch Melt	1 serv (14 oz)	975	59	10	96	47	68	4	80	2479	—	11	—	1050
Lunch Basket Chicken Strips	1 serv (8 oz)	568	26	4	70	34	45	0	20	1239	—	0	—	0
Lunch Basket Classic Burger	1 serv (12 oz)	674	39	13	121	38	42	3	120	1161	—	11	—	1000
Lunch Basket Delidinger	1 serv (14 oz)	852	45	6	80	56	62	3	30	3142	—	12	—	1100
Lunch Basket Five Star Philly	1 serv (10 oz)	657	29	8	97	41	55	4	60	652	—	40	—	100
Lunch Basket Patty Melt	1 serv (8 oz)	696	42	12	129	39	39	2	200	1026	—	1	—	1200
Mashed Potatoes Plain	1 serv (6 oz)	105	1	0	0	3	21	2	20	378	—	5	—	0
Mayonnaise	2 tbsp (1 oz)	200	22	3	16	0	1	0	0	159	—	0	—	100
Mozzarella Sticks w/ Sauce	8 pieces (10 oz)	756	43	24	48	37	56	7	790	5423	—	8	—	600
Onion Ring Basket	1 serv (5 oz)	439	27	7	7	6	44	1	20	1158	—	2	—	50
Onion Rings	1 serv (3 oz)	264	16	4	4	3	27	0	10	695	—	1	—	0

FOOD	PORTION	CALORIES	FAT	SAT FAT	CHOL	PROTEIN	CARBO	FIBER	CALCIUM	SOD	POTAS	VIT C	FOLIC	VIT A
Patty Melt Sandwich	1 (8 oz)	695	44	13	114	38	39	2	200	1007	—	1	—	1200
Pork Chop Dinner w/ Gravy	1 serv (8 oz)	386	24	8	121	39	0	0	40	844	—	2	—	0
Porterhouse Steak	1 (14 oz)	708	54	24	161	56	0	0	130	713	—	0	—	900
Pot Roast Dinner w/ Gravy	1 serv (7 oz)	260	11	4	140	39	5	0	10	1085	—	0	—	0
Rice Pilaf	1 serv (3 oz)	112	2	0	0	2	21	0	0	328	—	0	—	100
Roast Turkey & Stuffing	1 serv (12 oz)	701	27	1	100	47	63	0	20	2346	—	2	—	0
Sampler	1 serv (15 oz)	1120	59	19	69	44	104	5	450	3430	—	11	—	1050
Seasoned Fries	1 serv (4 oz)	261	12	3	0	5	35	0	10	556	—	0	—	0
Senior Battered Cod	1 serv (5 oz)	465	34	5	68	15	25	1	0	743	—	0	—	0
Senior Chicken Fried Steak	1 serv (8 oz)	341	18	8	27	16	29	2	30	943	—	3	—	0
Senior Grilled Cheese Sandwich	1 serv	360	25	10	50	16	21	—	—		1190	—	—	—	—
Senior Grilled Chicken Breast	1 serv (6 oz)	219	6	1	67	26	16	0	10	880	—	1	—	200
Senior Liver w/ Bacon & Onions	1 serv (8 oz)	322	19	5	270	22	20	2	40	643	—	10	—	>2000
Senior Pork Chop	1 serv (4 oz)	193	12	4	60	19	0	0	20	422	—	1	—	0
Senior Pot Roast	1 serv (5 oz)	149	6	2	71	20	6	0	0	818	—	0	—	0
Senior Roast Turkey & Stuffing	1 serv (8 oz)	596	25	1	51	29	61	0	10	1750	—	1	—	0
Senior Turkey Sandwich	1	340	27	3	75	24	26	—	—		1000	—	—	—	—
Senior Sandwich Ham & Swiss	1 serv (9 oz)	497	30	4	36	22	34	4	60	1537	—	8	—	450
Shrimp Dinner	1 serv (8 oz)	558	32	6	135	19	49	3	60	1114	—	0	—	350
Sirloin Steak Dinner	1 serv (5.5 oz)	271	21	9	62	22	0	0	30	273	—	0	—	0
Sliced Tomatoes	3 slices (2 oz)	13	0	0	0	1	3	1	0	6	—	11	—	150
Sour Cream	1 serv (1.5 oz)	91	9	6	19	1	2	0	40	23	—	0	—	500
Steak & Shrimp Dinner w/ Gravy	1 serv (9 oz)	645	42	14	150	36	31	2	80	1143	—	0	—	200
Super Bird Sandwich	1 (9 oz)	620	32	5	60	35	48	2	80	1880	—	12	—	750
T-Bone Steak Dinner	1 serv (10 oz)	530	40	18	121	42	0	0	70	534	—	0	—	0
Turkey Breast On Multigrain	1 (9 oz)	476	26	3	57	23	39	5	90	1107	—	8	—	300
SALAD DRESSINGS														
Bleu Cheese	1 oz	124	12	4	18	4	4	0	0	405	—	0	—	0
Caesar	1 oz	142	15	2	2	1	1	0	20	340	—	0	—	0
Creamy Italian	1 oz	106	10	2	0	0	4	0	0	306	—	0	—	0

FOOD	PORTION	CALORIES	FAT	SAT FAT	CHOL	PROTEIN	CARBO	FIBER	CALCIUM	SOD	POTAS	VIT C	FOLIC	VIT A
Fat Free Honey Mustard	1 oz	38	0	0	0	0	9	0	0	121	—	0	—	0
French	1 oz	106	10	2	7	0	3	0	0	274	—	0	—	0
Oriental Peanut Dressing	1 serv (1 oz)	106	8	1	0	1	6	0	0	399	—	4	—	100
Ranch	1 oz	101	11	2	8	1	1	0	20	215	—	0	—	150
Reduced Calorie French	1 oz	76	5	1	0	0	8	0	0	265	—	0	—	0
Reduced Calorie Italian	1 oz	32	1	0	0	0	3	0	0	515	—	0	—	0
Thousand Island	1 oz	104	10	2	21	0	2	0	0	208	—	0	—	0
SALADS AND SALAD BARS														
Buffalo Chicken Salad	1 serv (17 oz)	615	37	8	88	39	36	3	280	1258	—	53	—	4300
Fried Chicken Salad	1 serv (13 oz)	506	31	8	94	38	30	3	260	1174	—	33	—	3300
Garden Chicken Delight Salad	1 serv (16 oz)	277	5	1	67	30	30	6	80	785	—	44	—	6900
Grilled Chicken Caesar Salad w/ Dressing	1 serv (13 oz)	655	47	9	86	37	23	4	320	1728	—	43	—	2500
Oriental Chicken Salad w/ Dressing	1 serv (20 oz)	568	26	5	67	33	49	7	100	1656	—	76	—	3400
Side Caesar w/ Dressing	1 serv (6 oz)	338	25	5	7	8	20	3	160	725	—	27	—	1550
Side Garden Salad w/ Dressing	1 serv (7 oz)	113	4	1	0	3	16	3	40	147	—	16	—	1800
SOUPS														
Cheese	1 serv (8 oz)	293	23	13	19	6	13	4	120	895	—	0	—	350
Chicken Noodle	1 serv (8 oz)	60	2	0	10	2	8	0	10	640	—	0	—	50
Clam Chowder	1 serv (8 oz)	214	11	9	5	5	22	1	10	903	—	0	—	0
Cream Of Broccoli	1 serv (8 oz)	193	12	9	0	4	15	2	60	818	—	8	—	0
Cream of Potato	1 serv (8 oz)	222	12	9	0	4	23	2	30	761	—	1	—	0
Split Pea	1 serv (8 oz)	146	6	2	5	8	18	2	20	819	—	0	—	0
Vegetable Beef	1 serv (8 oz)	79	1	1	5	6	11	2	20	820	—	1	—	0

DOMINO'S PIZZA

FOOD	PORTION	CALORIES	FAT	SAT FAT	CHOL	PROTEIN	CARBO	FIBER	CALCIUM	SOD	POTAS	VIT C	FOLIC	VIT A
12 INCH MEDIUM PIZZAS														
Add A Topping Anchovies	1 topping serv	23	1	tr	9	3	0	0	25	395	—	0	—	8
Add A Topping Bacon	1 topping serv	81	7	2	12	4	tr	0	2	226	—	5	—	0
Add A Topping Banana Peppers	1 topping serv	3	tr	—	—	tr	1	—	3	92	—	3	—	21
Add A Topping Canned Mushrooms	1 topping serv	4	tr	tr	0	tr	1	tr	2	75	—	0	—	0
Add A Topping Cheddar Cheese	1 topping serv	57	5	3	15	4	tr	0	102	88	—	0	—	150

FOOD	PORTION	CALORIES	FAT	SAT FAT	CHOL	PROTEIN	CARBO	FIBER	CALCIUM	SOD	POTAS	VIT C	FOLIC	VIT A
Add A Topping Cooked Beef	1 topping serv	56	5	2	11	3	tr	tr	2	154	—	0	—	tr
Add A Topping Extra Cheese	1 topping serv	48	4	2	7	3	1	tr	80	150	—	tr	—	147
Add A Topping Fresh Mushrooms	1 topping serv	4	tr	tr	0	tr	1	tr	1	1	—	1	—	0
Add A Topping Green Olives	1 topping serv	12	1	tr	0	tr	tr	tr	6	255	—	0	—	32
Add A Topping Green Peppers	1 topping serv	3	tr	—	0	tr	1	tr	1	tr	—	14	—	56
Add A Topping Ham	1 topping serv	18	1	tr	7	2	tr	0	2	162	—	tr	—	tr
Add A Topping Italian Sausage	1 topping serv	55	4	2	11	2	2	tr	8	171	—	tr	—	21
Add A Topping Onion	1 topping serv	4	tr	—	0	tr	1	tr	3	tr	—	1	—	0
Add A Topping Pepperoni	1 topping serv	62	6	2	13	3	tr	tr	5	199	—	tr	—	11
Add A Topping Pineapple Tidbits	1 topping serv	10	0	0	0	tr	2	tr	2	1	—	2	—	0
Add A Topping Ripe Olives	1 topping serv	14	1	tr	0	tr	1	tr	8	71	—	0	—	0
Deep Dish Cheese	2 slices (6.3 oz)	477	22	8	19	18	50	3	232	1085	—	3	—	589
Hand Tossed Cheese	2 slices (5.2 oz)	347	11	5	15	14	49	3	179	723	—	6	—	526
Thin Crust Cheese	¼ pie (3.7 oz)	271	12	5	15	12	31	2	218	809	—	3	—	496
14 INCH LARGE PIZZAS														
Add A Topping Anchovies	1 topping serv	23	1	tr	tr	3	0	0	25	395	—	0	—	8
Add A Topping Anchovies	1 topping serv	23	1	tr	9	3	0	0	25	395	—	0	—	8
Add A Topping Bacon	1 topping serv	75	6	2	11	4	tr	0	2	207	—	4	—	0
Add A Topping Banana Peppers	1 topping serv	3	tr	—	—	tr	1	—	3	81	—	3	—	19
Add A Topping Canned Mushrooms	1 topping serv	3	tr	tr	0	tr	1	tr	1	50	—	0	—	0
Add A Topping Cheddar Cheese	1 topping serv	48	4	2	12	3	tr	0	85	73	—	0	—	125
Add A Topping Cheddar Cheese	1 topping serv	48	4	2	12	3	tr	0	85	73	—	0	—	125
Add A Topping Cooked Beef	1 topping serv	44	4	2	8	2	tr	tr	1	123	—	0	—	tr
Add A Topping Extra Cheese	1 topping serv	45	4	2	7	3	1	tr	75	140	—	0	—	137
Add A Topping Extra Cheese	1 topping serv	45	4	2	7	3	1	tr	75	140	—	tr	—	137

FOOD	PORTION	CALORIES	FAT	SAT FAT	CHOL	PROTEIN	CARBO	FIBER	CALCIUM	SOD	POTAS	VIT C	FOLIC	VIT A
Add A Topping Fresh Mushrooms	1 topping serv	3	tr	tr	0	tr	1	tr	1	tr	—	tr	—	0
Add A Topping Green Olives	1 topping serv	11	1	tr	0	tr	tr	tr	7	63	—	0	—	0
Add A Topping Green Peppers	1 topping serv	2	tr	—	0	tr	1	tr	1	tr	—	1	—	12
Add A Topping Ham	1 topping serv	17	1	tr	7	2	tr	0	1	156	—	tr	—	tr
Add A Topping Italian Sausage	1 topping serv	44	3	1	9	2	1	tr	6	137	—	tr	—	22
Add A Topping Onion	1 topping serv	3	tr	—	0	tr	1	tr	2	tr	—	1	—	0
Add A Topping Pepperoni	1 topping serv	55	5	2	12	2	tr	tr	4	177	—	tr	—	10
Add A Topping Pineapple Tidbits	1 topping serv	8	0	0	0	2	tr	tr	2	1	—	1	—	0
Add A Topping Ripe Olives	1 topping serv	12	1	tr	0	tr	1	tr	7	63	—	0	—	0
Deep Dish Cheese	2 slices (6.1 oz)	455	20	8	18	18	54	3	215	1029	—	3	—	547
Hand-Tossed Cheese	2 slices (4.8 oz)	317	10	5	14	13	45	3	167	669	—	5	—	491
Thin Crust Cheese	1/6 pie (3.5 oz)	253	11	5	14	11	29	2	204	757	—	2	—	465
6 INCH DEEP DISH PIZZAS														
Add A Topping Anchovies	1 topping serv	45	2	tr	18	6	0	0	50	790	—	0	—	15
Add A Topping Bacon	1 topping serv	82	7	2	12	4	tr	0	2	226	—	5	—	0
Add A Topping Banana Peppers	1 topping serv	3	tr	—	—	tr	tr	—	2	73	—	3	—	17
Add A Topping Canned Mushrooms	1 topping serv	2	tr	0	0	tr	tr	tr	1	36	—	0	—	0
Add A Topping Cheddar Cheese	1 topping serv	86	7	4	22	5	tr	0	153	132	—	0	—	225
Add A Topping Cooked Beef	1 topping serv	44	4	2	8	2	tr	tr	1	122	—	0	—	tr
Add A Topping Extra Cheese	1 topping serv	57	5	3	9	4	1	tr	96	180	—	tr	—	176
Add A Topping Fresh Mushrooms	1 topping serv	2	tr	0	0	tr	tr	tr	tr	tr	—	tr	—	0
Add A Topping Green Olives	1 topping serv	10	1	tr	0	tr	tr	tr	5	204	—	0	—	26
Add A Topping Green Peppers	1 topping serv	2	tr	—	0	tr	tr	tr	1	tr	—	11	—	45
Add A Topping Ham	1 topping serv	17	1	tr	7	2	tr	0	1	156	—	tr	—	tr
Add A Topping Italian Sausage	1 topping serv	44	3	1	9	1	1	tr	6	137	—	tr	—	21

FOOD	PORTION	CALORIES	FAT	SAT FAT	CHOL	PROTEIN	CARBO	FIBER	CALCIUM	SOD	POTAS	VIT C	FOLIC	VIT A
Add A Topping Onion	1 topping serv	3	tr	—	0	tr	1	tr	2	tr	—	1	—	0
Add A Topping Pepperoni	1 topping serv	50	5	2	10	2	tr	tr	4	159	—	tr	—	9
Add A Topping Pineapple Tidbits	1 topping serv	5	0	0	0	tr	1	tr	1	tr	—	1	—	0
Add A Topping Ripe Olives	1 topping serv	11	1	tr	0	tr	tr	tr	7	57	—	0	—	0
Cheese	1 pie (7.6 oz)	595	27	11	23	23	68	4	284	1300	—	3	—	666
MAIN MENU SELECTIONS														
Breadstick	1 (0.8 oz)	78	3	1	0	2	11	tr	7	158	—	tr	—	9
Buffalo Wings Barbeque	1 piece (0.9 oz)	50	2	1	26	6	2	tr	6	175	—	tr	—	42
Buffalo Wings Hot	1 piece (0.9 oz)	45	2	1	26	5	1	tr	5	354	—	1	—	136
Cheesy Bread	1 piece (1 oz)	103	5	2	5	3	11	tr	47	187	—	tr	—	68
Garden Salad	1 sm (4.3 oz)	22	tr	tr	0	1	4	2	24	14	—	11	—	3793
Garden Salad	1 lg (7.7 oz)	39	tr	tr	0	2	8	3	41	26	—	20	—	7102
SALAD DRESSINGS														
Marzetti Blue Cheese	1 serv (1.5 oz)	220	24	4	40	2	2	0	20	440	—	0	—	0
Marzetti Creamy Caesar	1 serv (1.5 oz)	200	22	3	10	1	2	0	20	470	—	0	—	0
Marzetti Fat Free Ranch	1 serv (1.5 oz)	40	0	0	0	0	10	1	0	560	—	0	—	0
Marzetti Honey French	1 serv (1.5 oz)	210	18	3	0	0	14	0	0	300	—	0	—	0
Marzetti House Italian	1 serv (1.5 oz)	220	24	3	0	0	1	0	0	440	—	0	—	0
Marzetti Light Italian	1 serv (1.5 oz)	20	1	0	0	—	2	0	0	780	—	0	—	0
Marzetti Ranch	1 serv (1.5 oz)	260	29	4	5	0	1	0	0	380	—	0	—	0
Marzetti Thousand Island	1 serv (1.5 oz)	200	20	3	25	0	5	0	0	320	—	0	—	0

DUNKIN' DONUTS

FOOD	PORTION	CALORIES	FAT	SAT FAT	CHOL	PROTEIN	CARBO	FIBER	CALCIUM	SOD	POTAS	VIT C	FOLIC	VIT A
BAGELS AND CREAM CHEESE														
Bagel Blueberry	1 (4.4 oz)	330	1	0	0	11	70	3	40	640	—	4	—	0
Bagel Cinnamon Raisin	1 (4.4 oz)	340	1	0	0	11	72	4	40	470	—	4	—	0
Bagel Egg	1 (4.4 oz)	340	2	0	40	12	69	3	20	670	—	4	—	0
Bagel Everything	1 (4.4 oz)	340	2	0	0	12	68	3	40	680	—	4	—	0
Bagel Garlic	1 (4.4 oz)	330	1	0	0	12	69	3	20	670	—	4	—	0
Bagel Onion	1 (4.4 oz)	320	1	0	0	12	66	3	40	650	—	4	—	0
Bagel Plain	1 (4.4 oz)	330	1	0	0	12	68	3	20	690	—	4	—	0
Bagel Plain	1 (3 oz)	200	1	0	0	6	43	0	0	420	—	0	—	0
Bagel Poppy	1 (4.4 oz)	340	3	0	0	12	68	3	80	680	—	4	—	0
Bagel Pumpernickel	1 (4.4 oz)	340	2	0	0	11	70	3	40	660	—	4	—	0

FOOD	PORTION	CALORIES	FAT	SAT FAT	CHOL	PROTEIN	CARBO	FIBER	CALCIUM	SOD	POTAS	VIT C	FOLIC	VIT A
Bagel Salt	1 (4.4 oz)	320	1	0	0	11	65	3	40	3170	—	4	—	0
Bagel Sesame	1 (4.4 oz)	350	4	0	0	13	66	3	20	660	—	4	—	0
Bagel Whole Wheat	1 (4.4 oz)	320	2	0	0	12	13	5	40	630	—	6	—	0
Bagel Sticks Cinnamon Sugar	1 (2.9 oz)	210	1	0	0	6	45	0	20	410	—	0	—	0
Bagel Sticks Jalapeno Cheddar	1 (2.9 oz)	210	1	0	0	6	43	0	40	490	—	0	—	0
Bagel Sticks Santa Fe Ranch	1 (2.9 oz)	210	1	0	0	6	43	0	20	690	—	0	—	0
Bagel Sticks Spinach Romano	1 (2.9 oz)	210	1	0	0	6	43	0	20	520	—	1	—	300
Cream Cheese Classic Lite	2 tbsp (1 oz)	60	5	3	15	3	3	tr	60	115	—	1	—	400
Cream Cheese Classic Plain	2 tbsp (1 oz)	100	10	6	30	2	1	0	20	110	—	0	—	300
Cream Cheese Garden Veggie	2 tbsp (1 oz)	90	9	5	25	2	2	0	20	200	—	2	—	600
Cream Cheese Honey Walnut	2 tbsp (1 oz)	100	9	5	10	2	4	0	20	110	—	0	—	300
Cream Cheese Savory Chive	2 tbsp (1 oz)	100	10	6	30	2	2	0	20	125	—	4	—	600
Cream Cheese Smoked Salmon	2 tbsp (1 oz)	100	9	5	30	2	1	0	20	95	—	0	—	300
Cream Cheese Strawberry	2 tbsp (1 oz)	100	9	5	25	1	5	0	20	100	—	0	—	300
Super Bagel Glazed Apple Cinnamon	1 (4.6 oz)	350	1	0	0	9	74	1	40	550	—	1	—	0
BAKED SELECTIONS														
Bismark	1 (2.8 oz)	310	14	4	0	4	42	1	0	260	—	2	—	0
Bow Tie	1 (2.5 oz)	250	10	3	0	5	35	1	0	300	—	2	—	0
Brownie Blondie w/ Chocolate Chips	1 (2.4 oz)	300	13	3	25	4	41	1	0	150	—	0	—	0
Brownie Fudge	1 (2.4 oz)	290	13	3	35	5	37	tr	20	85	—	0	—	0
Brownie Peanut Butter Blondie	1 (2.4 oz)	330	18	4	25	6	36	1	20	300	—	0	—	0
Cake Donut Blueberry	1 (2.4 oz)	230	10	3	0	4	30	1	0	240	—	1	—	0
Cake Donut Blueberry Crumb	1 (2.6 oz)	260	11	3	0	4	36	1	0	260	—	1	—	0
Cake Donut Butternut	1 (2.6 oz)	340	20	5	0	4	35	2	0	360	—	1	—	0
Cake Donut Chocolate	1 (2.1 oz)	210	14	3	0	3	19	1	0	270	—	4	—	0
Cake Donut Chocolate Coconut	1 (2.4 oz)	250	15	5	0	3	25	2	0	270	—	4	—	0

FOOD	PORTION	CALORIES	FAT	SAT FAT	CHOL	PROTEIN	CARBO	FIBER	CALCIUM	SOD	POTAS	VIT C	FOLIC	VIT A
Cake Donut Chocolate Glazed	1 (2.5 oz)	250	14	3	0	3	29	1	0	280	—	4	—	0
Cake Donut Cinnamon	1 (2.3 oz)	300	19	4	0	3	29	1	0	350	—	1	—	0
Cake Donut Coconut	1 (2.5 oz)	320	20	5	0	3	32	1	0	360	—	1	—	0
Cake Donut Double Chocolate	1 (2.6 oz)	260	14	3	0	3	30	1	0	280	—	4	—	0
Cake Donut Old Fashioned	1 (2.1 oz)	280	19	4	0	3	24	1	0	350	—	1	—	0
Cake Donut Peanut	1 (2.6 oz)	340	22	4	0	5	32	2	0	360	—	1	—	0
Cake Donut Powdered	1 (2.4 oz)	310	19	4	0	3	30	1	0	350	—	1	—	0
Cake Donut Sugared	1 (2.4 oz)	310	20	4	0	4	28	1	0	380	—	2	—	0
Cake Donut Toasted Coconut	1 (2.5 oz)	320	19	5	0	3	33	1	0	360	—	1	—	0
Cake Donut Whole Wheat Glazed	1 (2.7 oz)	230	11	3	0	3	31	2	0	340	—	2	—	0
Coffee Roll	1 (2.6 oz)	280	13	3	0	5	35	2	0	300	—	0	—	0
Coffee Roll Chocolate Frosted	1 (2.7 oz)	290	14	3	0	5	38	2	0	300	—	0	—	0
Coffee Roll Cinnamon Raisin	1 (3.1 oz)	330	13	3	0	5	48	3	0	300	—	0	—	0
Coffee Roll Maple Frosted	1 (2.7 oz)	300	13	3	0	5	40	2	0	300	—	0	—	0
Coffee Roll Vanilla Frosted	1 (2.7 oz)	300	13	3	0	5	40	2	0	300	—	0	—	0
Cookie Chocolate Chocolate Chunk	1 (1.5 oz)	200	11	6	30	2	26	1	0	160	—	0	—	300
Cookie Chocolate Chunk	1 (1.5 oz)	200	10	6	30	2	26	1	0	150	—	0	—	300
Cookie Chocolate Chunk w/ Nut	1 (1.5 oz)	200	11	6	30	2	25	1	0	150	—	0	—	300
Cookie Chocolate White Chocolate Chunk	1 (1.5 oz)	200	11	6	30	2	25	1	0	160	—	0	—	300
Cookie Oatmeal Raisin Pecan	1 (1.5 oz)	190	9	5	25	2	27	0	0	150	—	0	—	300
Cookie Peanut Butter Chocolate Chunk w/ Nuts	1 (1.5 oz)	210	13	6	25	4	23	1	0	110	—	0	—	400
Cookie Peanut Butter Chocolate Chunk w/ Peanuts	1 (1.5 oz)	210	12	5	30	4	22	3	0	140	—	0	—	400
Croissant Almond	1 (2.7 oz)	360	21	5	10	6	38	2	60	300	—	0	—	0
Croissant Cheese	1 (2.5 oz)	240	15	3	5	6	28	0	20	260	—	0	—	0
Croissant Chocolate	1 (2.5 oz)	370	23	8	10	5	40	1	40	260	—	0	—	0

FOOD	PORTION	CALORIES	FAT	SAT FAT	CHOL	PROTEIN	CARBO	FIBER	CALCIUM	SOD	POTAS	VIT C	FOLIC	VIT A
Croissant Plain	1 (2.1 oz)	270	17	4	5	4	27	0	20	260	—	0	—	0
Crullers/Sticks Dunkin' Donut	1 (2.1 oz)	240	14	3	0	4	26	2	0	370	—	2	—	0
Crullers/Sticks Glazed	1 (3 oz)	340	14	3	0	3	49	2	20	320	—	0	—	0
Crullers/Sticks Glazed Chocolate	1 (3.2 oz)	410	24	6	0	4	46	3	20	350	—	0	—	0
Crullers/Sticks Jelly	1 (3.2 oz)	330	14	3	0	3	48	3	20	350	—	0	—	0
Crullers/Sticks Plain	1 (2.1 oz)	260	14	3	0	3	29	2	20	300	—	0	—	0
Crullers/Sticks Powdered	1 (2.3 oz)	290	14	4	0	3	35	2	20	300	—	0	—	0
Crullers/Sticks Sugar	1 (2.2 oz)	270	14	3	0	3	31	2	20	300	—	0	—	0
Eclair	1 (3.2 oz)	290	12	3	0	4	42	1	0	280	—	1	—	0
English Muffin	1 (2 oz)	130	1	1	0	4	26	1	60	520	—	0	—	0
French Roll	1 (2.1 oz)	140	1	0	0	5	27	1	0	220	—	18	—	0
Fritter Apple	1 (3.3 oz)	300	13	3	0	5	41	2	0	320	—	0	—	0
Fritter Glazed	1 (2.7 oz)	290	13	3	0	5	39	2	0	300	—	0	—	0
Muffin Banana Nut	1 (3.3 oz)	340	12	3	35	6	53	2	0	210	—	1	—	0
Muffin Blueberry	1 (3.3 oz)	310	10	2	35	5	51	2	40	190	—	0	—	0
Muffin Cherry	1 (3.3 oz)	330	11	3	35	5	53	1	40	210	—	1	—	0
Muffin Chocolate Chip	1 (3.3 oz)	400	16	6	35	5	63	2	40	190	—	0	—	0
Muffin Corn	1 (3.3 oz)	350	14	1	50	6	51	2	40	310	—	0	—	100
Muffin Cranberry Orange Nut	1 (3.5 oz)	310	11	3	30	5	51	2	40	180	—	4	—	0
Muffin Honey Raisin Bran	1 (3.3 oz)	330	10	0	15	5	57	4	40	360	—	0	—	0
Muffin Lemon Poppy Seed	1 (3.3 oz)	360	13	3	40	6	57	1	150	440	—	0	—	0
Muffin Oat Bran	1 (3.2 oz)	290	11	1	0	4	44	1	0	330	—	0	—	0
Muffin Lowfat Apple n' Spice	1 (3.3 oz)	220	2	0	0	3	50	1	0	480	—	0	—	0
Muffin Lowfat Banana	1 (3.3 oz)	240	2	0	0	3	54	1	0	380	—	1	—	0
Muffin Lowfat Blueberry	1 (3.3 oz)	230	2	0	0	3	51	1	0	370	—	0	—	0
Muffin Lowfat Bran	1 (3.3 oz)	260	2	0	0	4	59	4	60	440	—	0	—	0
Muffin Lowfat Cherry	1 (3.3 oz)	230	2	0	0	3	53	0	0	380	—	1	—	0
Muffin Lowfat Corn	1 (3.3 oz)	250	2	0	0	4	55	1	0	460	—	0	—	0
Muffin Lowfat Cranberry Orange	1 (3.3 oz)	230	2	0	0	3	53	1	0	380	—	2	—	0
Munchkins Butternut	3 (2 oz)	230	11	4	0	2	30	2	0	210	—	0	—	0

FOOD	PORTION	CALORIES	FAT	SAT FAT	CHOL	PROTEIN	CARBO	FIBER	CALCIUM	SOD	POTAS	VIT C	FOLIC	VIT A
Munchkins Chocolate Glazed	3 (2 oz)	180	10	2	0	2	22	1	0	240	—	0	—	0
Munchkins Cinnamon	4 (2 oz)	240	13	3	0	3	29	1	20	290	—	1	—	0
Munchkins Coconut	3 (1.7 oz)	200	11	4	0	2	22	1	0	220	—	0	—	0
Munchkins Glazed Cake	3 (2.1 oz)	220	9	2	0	2	32	1	0	220	—	0	—	0
Munchkins Glazed Raised	4 (2.1 oz)	210	7	2	0	3	36	1	0	170	—	0	—	0
Munchkins Jelly	3 (1.9 oz)	170	5	1	0	2	28	1	0	170	—	0	—	0
Munchkins Lemon	3 (2 oz)	160	6	1	0	2	23	1	0	160	—	0	—	0
Munchkins Plain	4 (1.8 oz)	200	12	3	0	3	21	1	0	290	—	1	—	0
Munchkins Powdered Sugar	4 (2 oz)	240	13	3	0	3	28	1	0	290	—	1	—	0
Munchkins Sugar Raised	6 (1.9 oz)	210	10	3	0	4	26	2	0	250	—	0	—	0
Munchkins Toasted Coconut	3 (1.8 oz)	210	11	3	0	2	26	1	0	220	—	0	—	0
Tart Apple	1 (3.4 oz)	310	10	3	0	5	45	1	0	330	—	2	—	0
Tart Blueberry	1 (3.4 oz)	300	10	3	0	5	48	2	0	320	—	2	—	0
Tart Lemon	1 (3.4 oz)	280	11	3	0	5	43	1	0	340	—	2	—	0
Tart Raspberry	1 (3.4 oz)	310	10	3	0	5	51	2	0	350	—	2	—	0
Tart Strawberry	1 (3.4 oz)	310	10	3	0	5	51	1	0	340	—	5	—	0
Turnover Apple	1 (3.8 oz)	350	15	4	0	5	49	2	0	340	—	2	—	0
Turnover Blueberry	1 (3.8 oz)	370	15	4	0	5	54	2	0	330	—	2	—	0
Turnover Lemon	1 (3.8 oz)	350	15	4	0	5	48	2	0	360	—	2	—	0
Turnover Raspberry	1 (3.8 oz)	380	15	4	0	5	57	2	0	370	—	4	—	0
Turnover Strawberry	1 (3.8 oz)	380	15	4	0	5	57	2	0	360	—	5	—	0
Yeast Donut Apple Crumb	1 (2.6 oz)	250	11	3	0	4	34	1	0	270	—	1	—	0
Yeast Donut Apple n' Spice	1 (2.5 oz)	230	10	3	0	4	31	1	0	250	—	1	—	0
Yeast Donut Bavarian Kreme	1 (2.5 oz)	250	11	3	0	4	33	1	0	250	—	1	—	0
Yeast Donut Black Raspberry	1 (2.4 oz)	240	10	3	0	4	32	1	0	260	—	2	—	0
Yeast Donut Boston Kreme	1 (2.8 oz)	270	11	3	0	4	38	1	0	260	—	1	—	0
Yeast Donut Chocolate Frosted	1 (2.1 oz)	210	8	2	0	4	31	1	0	230	—	1	—	0
Yeast Donut Chocolate Kreme Filled	1 (2.6 oz)	320	16	4	0	4	39	1	0	250	—	1	—	0
Yeast Donut Glazed	1 (1.6 oz)	160	7	2	0	3	23	1	0	200	—	1	—	0
Yeast Donut Jelly Filled	1 (2.4 oz)	240	10	3	0	4	32	1	0	260	—	2	—	0

FOOD	PORTION	CALORIES	FAT	SAT FAT	CHOL	PROTEIN	CARBO	FIBER	CALCIUM	SOD	POTAS	VIT C	FOLIC	VIT A
Yeast Donut Lemon	1 (2.5 oz)	240	11	3	0	4	31	1	0	250	—	1	—	0
Yeast Donut Maple Frosted	1 (2.1 oz)	210	8	2	0	4	32	1	0	230	—	1	—	0
Yeast Donut Marble Frosted	1 (2.1 oz)	210	8	2	0	4	32	1	0	230	—	1	—	0
Yeast Donut Strawberry	1 (2.4 oz)	240	10	3	0	4	32	1	0	250	—	4	—	0
Yeast Donut Strawberry Frosted	1 (2.1 oz)	220	8	2	0	4	32	1	0	230	—	1	—	0
Yeast Donut Sugar Raised	1 (1.6 oz)	170	7	2	0	4	23	1	0	220	—	1	—	0
Yeast Donut Vanilla Frosted	1 (2.1 oz)	220	8	2	0	4	32	1	0	230	—	1	—	0
BEVERAGES														
Coffee Coolatta w/ 2% Milk	1 (15.7 oz)	210	2	2	10	4	45	0	150	85	—	0	—	200
Coffee Coolatta w/ Cream	1 (15.7 oz)	370	22	14	75	3	44	0	100	70	—	0	—	750
Coffee Coolatta w/ Skim Milk	1 (15.7 oz)	190	0	0	2	4	45	0	150	85	—	0	—	200
Coffee Coolatta w/ Whole Milk	1 (15.7 oz)	230	4	3	15	4	45	0	150	80	—	1	—	200
Cream	1 serv (1 oz)	60	5	3	20	1	1	0	20	10	—	0	—	200
Dark Roast	1 serv (10 oz)	5	0	0	0	0	1	0	0	5	—	0	—	0
Decaf	1 serv (10 oz)	0	0	0	0	0	0	0	0	0	—	0	—	0
French Vanilla	1 serv (10 oz)	5	0	0	0	0	1	0	0	5	—	0	—	0
Hazelnut	1 serv (10 oz)	5	0	0	0	0	1	0	0	10	—	0	—	0
Hazelnut Coolatta w/ 2% Milk	1 (15.7 oz)	210	2	2	10	4	43	0	150	85	—	0	—	200
Hazelnut Coolatta w/ Cream	1 (15.7 oz)	370	22	13	75	3	42	0	100	70	—	0	—	750
Hazelnut Coolatta w/ Skim Milk	1 (15.7 oz)	200	0	0	2	4	43	0	150	85	—	0	—	200
Hazelnut Coolatta w/ Whole Milk	1 (15.7 oz)	230	4	3	15	4	43	0	150	80	—	1	—	200
Mocha Coolatta w/ 2% Milk	1 (15.7 oz)	220	2	2	10	4	43	0	150	80	—	0	—	200
Mocha Coolatta w/ Cream	1 (15.7 oz)	380	22	13	75	3	42	0	100	70	—	0	—	750
Mocha Coolatta w/ Skim Milk	1 (15.7 oz)	200	0	0	2	4	43	0	150	85	—	0	—	200
Mocha Coolatta w/ Whole Milk	1 (15.7 oz)	230	4	3	15	4	43	0	150	80	—	1	—	200
Regular	1 serv (10 oz)	5	0	0	0	0	1	0	0	5	—	0	—	0
Vanilla Coolatta w/ 2% Milk	1 (15.7 oz)	220	2	2	10	4	43	0	150	85	—	0	—	200

FOOD	PORTION	CALORIES	FAT	SAT FAT	CHOL	PROTEIN	CARBO	FIBER	CALCIUM	SOD	POTAS	VIT C	FOLIC	VIT A
Vanilla Coolatta w/ Cream	1 (15.7 oz)	380	22	13	75	5	42	0	100	70	—	0	—	750
Vanilla Coolatta w/ Skim Milk	1 (15.7 oz)	200	0	0	2	4	43	0	150	85	—	0	—	200
Vanilla Coolatta w/ Whole Milk	1 (15.7 oz)	230	4	3	15	4	43	0	150	80	—	1	—	200
SANDWICHES														
Croissant Sandwich Broccoli & Cheese	1 (6.1 oz)	370	21	6	20	10	36	2	150	680	—	24	—	1000
Croissant Sandwich Chicken Salad	1 (7.6 oz)	540	31	7	75	27	37	1	60	710	—	5	—	200
Croissant Sandwich Egg & Cheese	1 (5 oz)	430	27	9	280	16	30	0	150	640	—	0	—	500
Croissant Sandwich Egg, Bacon & Cheese	1 (5.4 oz)	500	34	12	290	20	30	0	150	930	—	0	—	500
Croissant Sandwich Egg, Ham & Cheese	1 (6 oz)	530	29	9	295	23	30	0	150	1080	—	9	—	500
Croissant Sandwich Egg, Sausage & Cheese	1 (6.9 oz)	630	49	15	320	24	30	0	150	1180	—	0	—	500
Croissant Sandwich Ham & Cheese	1 (6.7 oz)	710	32	13	85	33	29	0	250	1840	—	24	—	500
Croissant Sandwich Roast Beef & Cheese	1 (6 oz)	490	27	8	30	31	28	0	200	680	—	0	—	200
Croissant Sandwich Seafood Salad	1 (7.6 oz)	480	26	6	50	16	45	1	80	1020	—	0	—	0
Croissant Sandwich Tuna Salad	1 (7.5 oz)	540	30	6	50	30	39	1	60	1140	—	4	—	400
SOUPS														
Beef Barley	1 serv (8 oz)	90	1	0	10	7	15	0	0	970	—	0	—	0
Beef Noodle	1 serv (8 oz)	90	1	0	20	8	12	0	0	980	—	2	—	1250
Chicken Noodle	1 serv (8 oz)	80	2	1	15	6	12	0	0	890	—	1	—	2250
Chili	1 serv (8 oz)	170	6	3	20	8	20	0	60	860	—	9	—	400
Chili Con Carne w/ Beans	1 serv (8 oz)	300	15	0	45	17	25	0	80	690	—	12	—	1000
Cream Of Broccoli	1 serv (8 oz)	200	11	6	25	8	17	0	150	1050	—	18	—	1000
Cream Of Potato	1 serv (8 oz)	190	10	5	25	6	19	1	150	770	—	6	—	2250
Harvest Vegetable	1 serv (8 oz)	80	2	0	0	4	12	0	40	1120	—	15	—	3500
Manhattan Clam Chowder	1 serv (8 oz)	70	1	0	5	5	11	1	40	890	—	15	—	3000
Minestrone	1 serv (8 oz)	100	1	0	0	5	16	2	60	900	—	9	—	1750
New England Clam Chowder	1 serv (8 oz)	200	10	3	30	10	16	0	150	1050	—	4	—	500
Split Pea w/ Ham	1 serv (8 oz)	190	9	3	15	8	20	0	0	830	—	5	—	2500

EINSTEIN BROS. BAGELS

BAGELS

FOOD	PORTION	CALORIES	FAT	SAT FAT	CHOL	PROTEIN	CARBO	FIBER	CALCIUM	SOD	POTAS	VIT C	FOLIC	VIT A
Bagel Chips Cinnamon Raisin Swirl	1 serv (1 oz)	90	1	0	0	3	19	1	0	120	—	0	—	0
Bagel Chips Plain	1 serv (1 oz)	90	0	0	0	3	18	1	0	14	—	0	—	0
Bagel Chips Sourdough Dill	1 serv (1 oz)	90	1	0	0	3	18	1	0	120	—	0	—	0
Bagel Chips Sun Dried Tomato	1 serv (1 oz)	90	1	0	0	3	17	1	40	130	—	0	—	0
Bagel Chips Sunflower	1 serv (1 oz)	100	2	0	0	3	8	1	0	190	—	0	—	0
Bagel Chips Wild Blueberry	1 serv (1 oz)	90	1	0	0	3	19	1	0	105	—	0	—	0
Chocolate Chip	1 (4 oz)	380	3	2	0	11	78	2	20	480	—	0	—	0
Chopped Garlic	1 (4.2 oz)	377	4	1	0	14	81	5	50	593	—	0	—	0
Chopped Onion	1 (4 oz)	340	3	1	0	11	72	2	40	500	—	0	—	0
Cinnamon Raisin Swirl	1 (4 oz)	360	1	0	0	11	78	2	40	480	—	0	—	0
Cinnamon Sugar	1	330	0	0	0	10	72	2	20	510	—	0	—	0
Dark Pumpernickel	1 (3.8 oz)	330	1	0	0	11	72	5	40	710	—	0	—	0
Everything	1 (4 oz)	342	2	0	0	13	74	2	30	653	—	1	—	0
Honey 8 Grain	1 (4 oz)	320	1	0	0	11	71	4	40	500	—	0	—	0
Nutty Banana	1 (4 oz)	370	3	1	0	11	77	2	20	500	—	0	—	0
Plain	1 (3.7 oz)	330	1	0	0	11	72	2	20	520	—	0	—	0
Poppy Dip'd	1 (3.9 oz)	346	2	0	0	12	73	2	60	520	—	0	—	0
Salt	1 (3.9 oz)	330	1	0	0	11	72	2	20	1626	—	0	—	0
Sesame Dip'd	1 (4.1 oz)	381	5	1	0	11	74	3	30	523	—	0	—	0
Spinach Herb	1 (3.8 oz)	320	1	0	0	11	71	3	40	510	—	0	—	0
Sun Dried Tomato	1 (3.8 oz)	320	1	0	0	11	70	3	40	520	—	0	—	0
Veggie Confetti	1 (3.8 oz)	330	1	0	0	10	71	3	40	480	—	0	—	0
Wild Blueberry	1 (4 oz)	360	1	0	0	11	79	3	20	510	—	0	—	0

SANDWICHES AND FILLINGS

FOOD	PORTION	CALORIES	FAT	SAT FAT	CHOL	PROTEIN	CARBO	FIBER	CALCIUM	SOD	POTAS	VIT C	FOLIC	VIT A
Butter & Margarine Blend	1 serv (0.4 oz)	60	7	2	0	0	0	0	20	75	—	0	—	0
Capers	1 tbsp	0	0	0	0	0	0	0	0	320	—	0	—	0
Cheddar Cheese	1 serv (0.75 oz)	110	9	5	30	7	1	0	0	180	—	0	—	0
Classic New York Lox & Bagel	1 (11.4 oz)	560	24	13	75	24	31	3	60	1120	—	15	—	1500
Cream Cheese Cheddarpeno	1 serv (1 oz)	90	8	5	30	2	2	0	60	150	—	1	—	400
Cream Cheese Chive	1 serv (1 oz)	90	9	6	35	1	2	0	40	125	—	1	—	500
Cream Cheese Maple Walnut Raisin	1 serv (1 oz)	100	8	5	25	1	7	0	40	95	—	0	—	300

FOOD	PORTION	CALORIES	FAT	SAT FAT	CHOL	PROTEIN	CARBO	FIBER	CALCIUM	SOD	POTAS	VIT C	FOLIC	VIT A
Cream Cheese Plain	1 serv (1 oz)	100	9	6	35	1	2	0	40	130	—	0	—	400
Cream Cheese Smoked Salmon	1 serv (1 oz)	90	8	5	35	2	2	0	40	130	—	0	—	300
Cream Cheese Strawberry	1 serv (1 oz)	90	8	5	30	1	4	0	40	105	—	1	—	300
Cream Cheese Sun Dried Tomato	1 serv (1 oz)	90	8	5	35	1	3	0	40	160	—	1	—	300
Cucumbers	1 serv (1 oz)	0	0	0	0	0	1	0	0	0	—	0	—	0
Fruit Spreads	1 tbsp	40	0	0	0	0	10	0	0	10	—	0	—	0
Ham	1 serv (2.5 oz)	75	2	1	20	10	1	0	0	560	—	0	—	0
Ham & Cheese Sandwich	1 (9.9 oz)	520	15	6	70	31	63	3	200	1280	—	9	—	400
Honey	1 tbsp	64	0	0	0	0	18	0	0	1	—	0	—	0
Hummus	2 tbsp	60	3	0	0	2	4	1	0	105	—	1	—	100
Hummus Sandwich	1 (6 oz)	440	7	0	0	13	62	4	0	590	—	1	—	100
Lettuce	1 leaf	0	0	0	0	0	0	0	0	0	—	4	—	200
Lite Cream Cheese Plain	1 serv (1 oz)	60	5	3	20	2	2	0	80	150	—	0	—	200
Lite Cream Cheese Spinach Dill	1 serv (1 oz)	60	5	3	20	2	2	0	80	150	—	0	—	200
Lite Cream Cheese Veggie	1 serv (1 oz)	60	5	3	20	2	3	0	80	170	—	1	—	1250
Lite Cream Cheese Wildberry	1 serv (1 oz)	70	4	3	15	2	7	0	80	85	—	1	—	200
Lowfat Chicken Salad Sandwich	1 (11.6 oz)	440	9	2	45	26	63	3	80	940	—	18	—	300
Lowfat Tuna Salad Sandwich	1 (11.6 oz)	440	8	2	30	29	62	3	60	970	—	15	—	300
Marshall's Loz	1 serv (2 oz)	90	4	2	10	12	2	0	0	400	—	0	—	0
Mayonnaise Lite Reduced Calorie	1 serv (0.5 oz)	50	5	1	5	0	1	0	0	115	—	0	—	0
Peanut Butter	1 serv (1.1 oz)	190	16	2	0	7	8	2	20	140	—	0	—	0
Peanut Butter & Jelly Sandwich	1 (6 oz)	595	17	2	0	18	99	4	40	663	—	0	—	0
Scrambled Egg Sandwich	1 (7.7 oz)	480	17	7	385	25	56	2	200	630	—	0	—	1000
Scrambled Egg Sandwich w/ Meat & Cheese	1 (8.9 oz)	520	31	18	8	32	57	2	200	1000	—	0	—	1000
Smoked Turkey	1 serv (2.5 oz)	75	1	0	20	13	0	0	0	550	—	0	—	0
Smoked Turkey Sandwich	1 (9.9 oz)	480	14	5	45	28	59	3	150	1180	—	9	—	500
Spouts Alfalfa	1 serv (0.5 oz)	0	0	0	0	0	3	1	0	10	—	1	—	3500
Sweet Onions	1 serv (1 oz)	0	0	0	0	0	2	0	0	0	—	1	—	0
Swiss Cheese	1 serv (0.75 oz)	100	8	5	25	8	0	0	0	60	—	0	—	0

FOOD	PORTION	CALORIES	FAT	SAT FAT	CHOL	PROTEIN	CARBO	FIBER	CALCIUM	SOD	POTAS	VIT C	FOLIC	VIT A
Tasty Turkey Sandwich	1 (10 oz)	530	22	12	90	25	61	2	100	1210	—	5	—	1000
Tomato	1 serv (1.5 oz)	0	0	0	0	0	2	1	0	0	—	6	—	200
Turkey Pastrami 99% Fat Free	1 serv (2.5 oz)	75	6	1	0	12	2	0	0	510	—	5	—	0
Turkey Pastrami Sandwich	1 (9.7 oz)	460	12	5	20	29	60	3	200	—	—	9	—	500
Veg Out Sandwich	1 (8.9 oz)	350	17	6	3	12	62	3	100	570	—	12	—	1500
Whitefish Salad Sandwich	1 (9.2 oz)	630	23	4	45	22	59	3	60	1020	—	9	—	400

EL POLLO LOCO

MAIN MENU SELECTIONS

FOOD	PORTION	CALORIES	FAT	SAT FAT	CHOL	PROTEIN	CARBO	FIBER	CALCIUM	SOD	POTAS	VIT C	FOLIC	VIT A
Broccoli Slaw	1 serv (5 oz)	203	17	0	0	3	14	3	40	365	—	107	—	3650
Burrito BRC	1 (9.3 oz)	482	15	5	15	16	72	9	350	1250	—	16	—	1650
Burrito Classic Chicken	1 (9.3 oz)	556	22	7	117	30	61	8	390	1499	—	25	—	1650
Burrito Grilled Steak	1 (11.3 oz)	705	32	13	77	39	68	10	360	1689	—	17	—	1650
Burrito Loco Grande	1 (13.1 oz)	632	26	7	129	33	67	8	410	1649	—	32	—	1950
Burrito Smokey Black Bean	1 (9.3 oz)	566	22	8	22	16	78	9	310	1337	—	11	—	1100
Burrito Spicy Hot Chicken	1 (9.8 oz)	559	22	7	117	30	61	8	390	1503	—	29	—	2150
Burrito Whole Wheat Chicken	1 (10.8 oz)	592	26	9	146	31	60	8	500	1199	—	16	—	1350
Chicken Breast	1 piece (3 oz)	160	6	2	110	26	0	0	10	390	—	1	—	300
Chicken Leg	1 piece (1.75 oz)	90	5	2	75	11	0	0	0	150	—	0	—	150
Chicken Soft Taco	1 (4 oz)	224	12	4	66	16	15	0	170	585	—	8	—	550
Chicken Thigh	1 piece (2 oz)	180	12	4	130	16	0	0	30	230	—	0	—	200
Chicken Wing	1 (1.5 oz)	110	6	2	80	12	0	0	20	220	—	1	—	150
Chicken Tamale	1 (3.5 oz)	190	8	2	10	6	23	2	40	480	—	2	—	300
Cole Slaw	1 serv (5 oz)	206	16	3	11	2	12	2	30	358	—	34	—	1250
Corn-On-Cob	1 ear (5.5 oz)	146	2	0	0	5	33	2	0	18	—	0	—	500
Cornbread Stuffing	1 serv (6 oz)	281	12	2	0	6	40	6	30	832	—	8	—	750
Crispy Green Beans	1 serv (5 oz)	41	2	1	0	1	6	3	40	667	—	9	—	750
Cucumber Salad	1 serv (4.2 oz)	34	0	0	0	2	7	1	20	11	—	13	—	50
Fiesta Corn	1 serv (5 oz)	152	6	1	0	4	25	6	0	397	—	12	—	500
Flame Broiled Chicken Salad	1 serv (14.9 oz)	167	5	0	56	27	11	4	70	765	—	39	—	3000
French Fries	1 serv (4.4 oz)	323	14	3	0	5	44	0	0	330	—	0	—	0
Garden Salad	1 serv (6.4 oz)	29	0	0	0	3	6	2	30	20	—	21	—	2800
Gravy	1 serv (1 oz)	14	0	0	2	0	2	0	0	139	—	1	—	0
Honey Glazed Carrots	1 serv (5 oz)	104	6	1	0	1	14	3	40	403	—	2	—	2395
Lime Parfait	1 serv (5 oz)	125	3	3	0	1	25	0	0	107	—	0	—	0

FOOD	PORTION	CALORIES	FAT	SAT FAT	CHOL	PROTEIN	CARBO	FIBER	CALCIUM	SOD	POTAS	VIT C	FOLIC	VIT A
Macaroni & Cheese	1 serv (6 oz)	238	12	5	31	10	22	1	170	919	—	0	—	200
Mashed Potatoes	1 serv (5 oz)	97	1	0	0	3	21	2	20	369	—	4	—	0
Pinto Beans	1 serv (6 oz)	185	4	0	0	11	29	8	120	744	—	11	—	100
Polo Bowl	1 serv (19 oz)	504	13	2	56	37	69	9	160	2068	—	40	—	1900
Potato Salad	1 serv (6 oz)	256	14	2	15	3	30	3	30	527	—	18	—	150
Rainbow Pasta Salad	1 serv (5 oz)	157	1	0	0	6	30	2	10	533	—	17	—	650
Salad Shell	1 (5.6 oz)	440	27	4	0	7	42	0	—	610	—	—	—	—
Smokey Black Beans	1 serv (5 oz)	255	13	5	11	6	29	4	—	609	—	—	—	—
Southwest Cole Slaw	1 serv (5 oz)	178	13	2	8	2	15	3	30	267	—	51	—	500
Spanish Rice	1 serv (4 oz)	130	3	1	0	2	24	1	10	397	—	16	—	750
Spiced Apples	1 serv (5 oz)	146	0	0	0	0	39	0	0	139	—	1	—	0
Steak Bowl	1 serv (15.2 oz)	616	26	10	68	37	62	8	120	1743	—	35	—	1900
Taco Al Carbon Chicken	1 serv (4.4 oz)	265	12	2	28	10	30	3	30	223	—	1	—	500
Taco Al Carbon Steak	1 (4.4 oz)	394	22	7	46	20	30	3	30	473	—	1	—	450
Taquito	1 serv (5 oz)	370	17	4	25	15	43	3	20	690	—	2	—	200
Tortilla Corn	1 (1.1 oz)	70	1	0	0	1	14	1	10	35	—	0	—	150
Tortilla Flour	1 (1 oz)	90	3	0	0	3	13	0	30	224	—	0	—	0
Tortilla Wrap Chicken Caesar	1 (10.47 oz)	518	19	3	48	28	59	3	180	1709	—	24	—	1850
Tortilla Wrap Southwest	1 (11.97 oz)	632	27	4	61	30	69	5	210	1792	—	22	—	1050
Tostada Salad Chicken	1 serv (14.7 oz)	332	14	5	80	35	26	4	230	1280	—	22	—	1000
Tostado Salad Steak	1 serv (13.2 oz)	525	31	14	100	40	26	4	220	1206	—	21	—	1050
SALAD DRESSINGS														
Blue Cheese	1 serv (2 oz)	300	32	6	50	2	2	0	20	590	—	0	—	0
Light Italian	1 serv (2 oz)	25	1	1	0	0	3	0	0	990	—	0	—	0
Ranch	1 serv (2 oz)	350	39	6	5	1	2	0	0	500	—	0	—	0
Thousand Island	1 serv (2 oz)	270	27	4	30	1	9	0	0	460	—	0	—	0

FRIENDLY'S

FROZEN YOGURT

FOOD	PORTION	CALORIES	FAT	SAT FAT	CHOL	PROTEIN	CARBO	FIBER	CALCIUM	SOD	POTAS	VIT C	FOLIC	VIT A
Apple Bettie	½ cup (2.6 oz)	140	3	2	10	3	25	0	—	75	—	—	—	—
Chocolate Fudge Brownie	½ cup (2.6 oz)	160	5	3	10	4	25	0	—	80	—	—	—	—
Fabulous Fudge Swirl	½ cup (2.6 oz)	140	3	3	10	4	23	0	—	80	—	—	—	—
Fudge Berry Swirl	½ cup (2.6 oz)	150	4	3	10	4	25	0	—	75	—	—	—	—
Lowfat Perfectly Peach	½ cup (2.6 oz)	110	2	1	10	3	21	0	—	55	—	—	—	—

FOOD	PORTION	CALORIES	FAT	SAT FAT	CHOL	PROTEIN	CARBO	FIBER	CALCIUM	SOD	POTAS	VIT C	FOLIC	VIT A
Lowfat Purely Chocolate	½ cup (2.6 oz)	120	3	2	10	4	20	0	—	65	—	—	—	—
Lowfat Raspberry Delight	½ cup (2.6 oz)	120	3	2	10	4	21	0	—	60	—	—	—	—
Lowfat Simply Vanilla	½ cup (2.6 oz)	120	3	2	10	4	19	0	—	70	—	—	—	—
Lowfat Strawberry Patch	½ cup (2.6 oz)	110	2	1	10	3	20	0	—	55	—	—	—	—
Mint Chocolate Chip	½ cup (2.6 oz)	130	4	2	10	4	21	0	—	65	—	—	—	—
Strawberry Cheesecake Blast	½ cup (2.6 oz)	140	4	2	15	4	22	0	—	75	—	—	—	—
Toffee Almond Crunch	½ cup (2.6 oz)	160	5	2	15	4	24	tr	—	85	—	—	—	—
ICE CREAM														
Black Raspberry	½ cup	150	7	5	30	2	17	0	—	35	—	—	—	—
Chocolate Almond Chip	½ cup	170	10	6	35	3	18	0	—	45	—	—	—	—
Forbidden Chocolate	½ cup	150	9	5	30	3	14	0	—	40	—	—	—	—
Fudge Nut Brownie	½ cup	200	11	7	25	3	23	0	—	60	—	—	—	—
Heath English Toffee	½ cup (2.7 oz)	190	10	6	30	3	24	0	60	240	—	0	—	300
Purely Pictachio	½ cup	160	10	6	35	3	16	0	—	50	—	—	—	—
Vanilla	½ cup	150	8	5	35	26	16	0	—	40	—	—	—	—
Vienna Mocha Chunk	½ cup	180	11	7	30	3	19	0	—	50	—	—	—	—

FRULLATI CAFE

BAKED SELECTIONS

FOOD	PORTION	CALORIES	FAT	SAT FAT	CHOL	PROTEIN	CARBO	FIBER	CALCIUM	SOD	POTAS	VIT C	FOLIC	VIT A
Muffin Banana Nut	1 (4 oz)	394	15	3	31	—	—	1	—	381	—	—	—	—
Muffin Cranberry Orange	1 (4 oz)	357	12	3	31	—	—	1	—	369	—	—	—	—
Muffin Fat Free Apple Streusel	1 (4 oz)	260	0	0	0	—	—	2	—	460	—	—	—	—
Muffin Fat Free Chocolate	1 (4 oz)	260	0	0	0	—	—	2	—	580	—	—	—	—
Muffin Fat Free Very Berry	1 (4 oz)	260	0	0	0	—	—	2	—	500	—	—	—	—
Muffin Sugar Free Blueberry	1 (4 oz)	308	9	1	12	—	—	1	—	443	—	—	—	—
Muffin Wild Blueberry	1 (4 oz)	344	11	3	31	—	—	1	—	369	—	—	—	—
BEVERAGES														
Apple Juice	1 serv (12 oz)	131	tr	0	0	—	—	0	—	8	—	—	—	—
Carrot Juice	1 serv (12 oz)	111	tr	tr	0	—	—	2	—	80	—	—	—	—
Celery Juice	1 serv (12 oz)	22	tr	tr	0	—	—	2	—	393	—	—	—	—
Lemondae	1 serv	209	tr	0	0	—	—	2	—	18	—	—	—	—
Lemondae Apple	1 serv	245	tr	tr	0	—	—	3	—	18	—	—	—	—

FOOD	PORTION	CALORIES	FAT	SAT FAT	CHOL	PROTEIN	CARBO	FIBER	CALCIUM	SOD	POTAS	VIT C	FOLIC	VIT A
Lemondae Cherry	1 serv	237	tr	0	0	—	—	2	—	21	—	—	—	—
Lemondae Orange	1 serv	270	tr	tr	0	—	—	5	—	18	—	—	—	—
Lemondae Strawberry	1 serv	234	tr	0	0	—	—	2	—	19	—	—	—	—
Orange Banana Juice	1 serv (12 oz)	150	tr	tr	0	—	—	2	—	3	—	—	—	—
Orange Juice	1 serv (12 oz)	126	tr	0	0	—	—	1	—	3	—	—	—	—
Smoothie A La Frullati	1 sm	275	9	6	10	—	—	3	—	42	—	—	—	—
Smoothie A La Frullati	1 lg	426	16	12	20	—	—	3	—	82	—	—	—	—
Smoothie Affinity	1 lg	378	16	12	20	—	—	2	—	82	—	—	—	—
Smoothie Affinity	1 sm	226	8	6	10	—	—	2	—	42	—	—	—	—
Smoothie Fiesta	1 lg	257	1	tr	0	—	—	6	—	9	—	—	—	—
Smoothie Fiesta	1 sm	234	1	tr	0	—	—	6	—	8	—	—	—	—
Smoothie Peach Banana	1 sm	266	1	tr	0	—	—	5	—	13	—	—	—	—
Smoothie Peach Banana	1 lg	289	1	tr	0	—	—	5	—	13	—	—	—	—
Smoothie Pina Colada	1 sm	236	8	6	10	—	—	2	—	42	—	—	—	—
Smoothie Pina Colada	1 lg	387	16	12	82	—	—	2	—	82	—	—	—	—
Smoothie Strawberry Banana	1 sm	165	1	tr	0	—	—	4	—	3	—	—	—	—
Smoothie Strawberry Banana	1 lg	188	1	tr	0	—	—	4	—	3	—	—	—	—
Smoothie Strawberry Blueberry	1 sm	90	1	0	0	—	—	3	—	5	—	—	—	—
Smoothie Strawberry Blueberry	1 lg	113	1	0	0	—	—	3	—	5	—	—	—	—
Smoothie Strawberry Fruit	1 lg	101	1	0	0	—	—	3	—	2	—	—	—	—
Smoothie Strawberry Fruit	1 sm	79	1	0	0	—	—	3	—	2	—	—	—	—
Smoothie Strawberry Watermelon	1 lg	123	1	0	0	—	—	2	—	4	—	—	—	—
Smoothie Strawberry Watermelon	1 sm	100	1	0	0	—	—	2	—	4	—	—	—	—
DESSERTS														
Frozen Yogurt	1 reg	205	tr	tr	3	—	—	0	—	103	—	—	—	—
Frozen Yogurt	1 lg	263	tr	tr	3	—	—	0	—	132	—	—	—	—
Frozen Yogurt	1 sm	146	tr	tr	2	—	—	0	—	73	—	—	—	—
Yogurt Smoothie Cappuccino	1 serv	472	3	2	17	—	—	0	—	250	—	—	—	—

FOOD	PORTION	CALORIES	FAT	SAT FAT	CHOL	PROTEIN	CARBO	FIBER	CALCIUM	SOD	POTAS	VIT C	FOLIC	VIT A
Yogurt Smoothie Chocolate Fudge	1 serv	555	4	2	17	—	—	1	—	289	—	—	—	—
Yogurt Smoothie Fiesta	1 serv	432	4	2	17	—	—	3	—	249	—	—	—	—
Yogurt Smoothie Oreo Cookie	1 serv	566	8	4	19	—	—	2	—	398	—	—	—	—
Yogurt Smoothie Peach	1 serv	486	4	2	17	—	—	1	—	248	—	—	—	—
Yogurt Smoothie Peach Banana	1 serv	519	4	2	17	—	—	2	—	248	—	—	—	—
Yogurt Smoothie Peanut Butter	1 serv	630	18	5	17	—	—	2	—	380	—	—	—	—
Yogurt Smoothie Pina Colada	1 serv	519	1	tr	5	—	—	1	—	225	—	—	—	—
Yogurt Smoothie Strawberry Banana	1 serv	514	4	2	17	—	—	2	—	249	—	—	—	—
Yogurt Smoothie Strawberry Fruit	1 serv	487	4	2	17	—	—	2	—	249	—	—	—	—
Yogurt Smoothie Strawberry Vanilla	1 serv	462	4	2	17	—	—	0	—	248	—	—	—	—
Yogurt Smoothie Strawberry Watermelon	1 serv	503	4	2	17	—	—	2	—	250	—	—	—	—
SALADS AND SALAD BARS														
Fruit Salad	1 lg	148	1	tr	0	—	—	3	—	25	—	—	—	—
Fruit Salad	1 sm	99	1	0	0	—	—	2	—	16	—	—	—	—
Garden Salad	1 sm	56	1	tr	0	—	—	2	—	86	—	—	—	—
Garden Salad w/ Italian Fat Free Dressing	1 lg	72	2	tr	8	—	—	3	—	815	—	—	—	—
Pasta Salad	1 lg	256	2	tr	0	—	—	0	—	1078	—	—	—	—
Pasta Salad	1 sm	179	2	tr	0	—	—	0	—	741	—	—	—	—
SANDWICHES														
Chicken On Croissant	1	481	24	12	109	—	—	4	—	649	—	—	—	—
Chicken On Honey Wheat	1	297	8	2	34	—	—	6	—	854	—	—	—	—
Chicken On Jewish Rye	1	261	7	1	34	—	—	5	—	820	—	—	—	—
Chicken On Pita	1	281	6	1	34	—	—	4	—	797	—	—	—	—
Chicken On White	1	291	7	2	35	—	—	4	—	825	—	—	—	—
Ham & Cheese On Croissant	1	797	50	22	192	—	—	3	—	1051	—	—	—	—
Ham & Cheese On Honey Wheat	1	613	34	11	117	—	—	5	—	1262	—	—	—	—
Ham & Cheese On Jewish Rye	1	577	32	11	117	—	—	4	—	1227	—	—	—	—
Ham & Cheese On Pita	1	597	32	11	117	—	—	3	—	1205	—	—	—	—

FOOD	PORTION	CALORIES	FAT	SAT FAT	CHOL	PROTEIN	CARBO	FIBER	CALCIUM	SOD	POTAS	VIT C	FOLIC	VIT A
Ham & Cheese On White	1	607	33	11	118	—	—	3	—	1232	—	—	—	—
Roast Beef On Croissant	1	631	36	15	155	—	—	3	—	814	—	—	—	—
Roast Beef On Honey Wheat	1	348	8	2	72	—	—	5	—	947	—	—	—	—
Roast Beef On Jewish Rye	1	312	7	2	72	—	—	4	—	912	—	—	—	—
Roast Beef On Pita	1	332	7	2	72	—	—	3	—	889	—	—	—	—
Roast Beef On White	1	342	8	2	72	—	—	3	—	917	—	—	—	—
Tuna On Croissant	1	480	23	12	90	—	—	4	—	881	—	—	—	—
Tuna On Honey Wheat	1	295	6	1	16	—	—	7	—	1086	—	—	—	—
Tuna On Jewish Rye	1	259	6	1	16	—	—	5	—	1051	—	—	—	—
Tuna On Pita	1	280	5	1	16	—	—	4	—	1028	—	—	—	—
Tuna On White	1	289	6	1	16	—	—	4	—	1056	—	—	—	—
Turkey On Croissant	1	566	33	14	122	—	—	3	—	1578	—	—	—	—
Turkey On Honey Wheat	1	342	9	3	56	—	—	5	—	962	—	—	—	—
Turkey On Jewish Rye	1	306	8	3	56	—	—	4	—	927	—	—	—	—
Turkey On Pita	1	326	7	3	56	—	—	3	—	904	—	—	—	—
Turkey On White	1	338	9	3	57	—	—	3	—	932	—	—	—	—
Veggie On Croissant	1	510	35	14	83	—	—	4	—	764	—	—	—	—
Veggie On Honey Wheat	1	227	7	1	0	—	—	6	—	897	—	—	—	—
Veggie On Jewish Rye	1	191	6	1	0	—	—	5	—	862	—	—	—	—
Veggie On Pita	1	211	5	1	0	—	—	4	—	839	—	—	—	—
Veggie On White	1	221	7	1	0	—	—	4	—	867	—	—	—	—
GODFATHER'S PIZZA														
Golden Crust Cheese	1/8 med (3.1 oz)	212	8	—	12	10	26	—	170	311	51	2	—	150
Golden Crust Cheese	1/10 lg (3.5 oz)	242	9	—	14	12	28	—	200	363	57	3	—	200
Golden Crust Combo	1/8 med (4.4 oz)	271	12	—	22	13	28	—	180	562	154	3	—	150
Golden Crust Combo	1/10 lg (4.9 oz)	305	14	—	25	16	31	—	220	674	176	4	—	200
Original Crust Cheese	1/10 jumbo (5.8 oz)	382	9	—	27	22	53	—	360	580	106	4	—	350
Original Crust Cheese	1/4 mini (1.9 oz)	131	3	—	8	7	19	—	110	183	36	1	—	100
Original Crust Cheese	1/8 med (3.5 oz)	231	5	—	14	13	24	—	190	338	64	2	—	200

FOOD	PORTION	CALORIES	FAT	SAT FAT	CHOL	PROTEIN	CARBO	FIBER	CALCIUM	SOD	POTAS	VIT C	FOLIC	VIT A
Original Crust Cheese	¹/₁₀ lg (4 oz)	258	6	—	18	15	36	—	240	396	72	3	—	200
Original Crust Combo	¹/₁₀ lg (5.6 oz)	338	12	—	31	19	38	—	270	740	217	4	—	250
Original Crust Combo	⅛ med (5.1 oz)	306	11	—	27	17	36	—	220	660	200	3	—	200
Original Crust Combo	¹/₁₀ jumbo (8.3 oz)	503	18	—	47	29	56	—	400	1096	325	5	—	350
Original Crust Combo	¼ mini (2.9 oz)	176	7	—	16	10	21	—	130	382	127	1	—	100

GODIVA

FOOD	PORTION	CALORIES	FAT	SAT FAT	CHOL	PROTEIN	CARBO	FIBER	CALCIUM	SOD	POTAS	VIT C	FOLIC	VIT A
Almond Butter Dome	3 pieces (1.5 oz)	240	17	6	5	4	19	0	80	20	—	0	—	0
Bouchee Au Chocolat	1 piece (1.5 oz)	210	11	6	5	3	25	0	20	40	—	0	—	0
Bouchee Ivory Raspberry	1 pieces (1 oz)	160	9	3	5	2	17	0	20	25	—	0	—	0
Gold Ballotin	3 pieces (1.5 oz)	210	10	4	5	2	27	0	40	15	—	0	—	0
Truffle Amaretto Di Saronno	2 pieces (1.5 oz)	210	12	6	5	2	24	0	40	25	—	0	—	0
Truffle Deluxe Liqueur	2 pieces (1.5 oz)	210	13	6	5	2	23	0	20	25	—	0	—	0

HAAGEN-DAZS

FROZEN YOGURT

FOOD	PORTION	CALORIES	FAT	SAT FAT	CHOL	PROTEIN	CARBO	FIBER	CALCIUM	SOD	POTAS	VIT C	FOLIC	VIT A
Brownie Nut Blast	½ cup (3.5 oz)	215	8	3	41	8	29	1	195	66	—	1	—	140
Chocolate	½ cup (3.4 oz)	160	3	1	33	8	26	1	222	59	—	1	—	119
Coffee	½ cup (3.4 oz)	161	3	1	45	8	26	tr	233	56	—	1	—	0
Orange Tango	½ cup (3.5 oz)	132	1	1	20	4	27	tr	106	26	—	7	—	102
Pina Colada	½ cup (3.4 oz)	139	2	1	25	4	27	tr	99	27	—	8	—	103
Raspberry Randezvous	½ cup (3.5 oz)	132	1	1	20	4	26	1	109	27	—	3	—	92
Soft Serve Coffee	½ cup (3.3 oz)	145	4	3	38	5	22	tr	165	79	—	1	—	314
Soft Serve Nonfat Chocolate	½ cup (3.3 oz)	116	tr	tr	2	5	24	1	147	68	—	1	—	178
Soft Serve Nonfat Chocolate Mousse	½ cup (3.3 oz)	86	tr	tr	2	5	26	1	148	70	—	1	—	178
Soft Serve Nonfat Vanilla	½ cup (3.3 oz)	114	tr	tr	2	5	23	tr	170	76	—	1	—	213
Soft Serve Nonfat Vanilla Mousse	½ cup (3.3 oz)	78	tr	tr	2	4	24	tr	143	66	—	1	—	178
Strawberry Cheesecake Craze	½ cup (3.6 oz)	213	7	4	64	7	30	tr	168	64	—	2	—	120
Strawberry Duet	½ cup (3.4 oz)	135	2	1	25	3	27	1	78	24	—	11	—	119
Vanilla	½ cup (3.4 oz)	162	3	1	44	8	26	0	238	58	—	1	—	0
Vanilla Almond Crunch	½ cup (3.4 oz)	198	5	2	41	9	30	1	227	88	—	1	—	100

FOOD	PORTION	CALORIES	FAT	SAT FAT	CHOL	PROTEIN	CARBO	FIBER	CALCIUM	SOD	POTAS	VIT C	FOLIC	VIT A
ICE CREAM														
Bar Chocolate	1 (2.7 oz)	247	17	10	108	5	21	1	120	73	—	1	—	533
Bar Coffee	1 (2.7 oz)	249	17	10	111	5	20	tr	134	81	—	1	—	577
Bar Vanilla	1 (2.7 oz)	251	17	10	111	4	20	0	134	81	—	1	—	578
Belgian Chocolate Chocolate	½ cup (3.6 oz)	315	21	12	84	5	28	3	103	59	—	1	—	429
Brownies A La Mode	½ cup (3.5 oz)	284	18	11	103	5	25	1	117	134	—	1	—	417
Butter Pecan	½ cup (3.7 oz)	304	23	10	100	5	19	1	123	136	—	1	—	530
Cappuccino Commotion	½ cup (3.6 oz)	305	21	12	98	5	24	1	123	102	—	1	—	521
Caramel Cone Explosion	½ cup (3.6 oz)	298	20	12	93	5	26	1	120	127	—	1	—	500
Chocolate	½ cup (3.7 oz)	249	17	10	110	5	21	1	121	71	—	1	—	554
Chocolate Chocolate Chip	½ cup (3.7 oz)	282	19	11	97	5	25	2	111	65	—	1	—	476
Chocolate Chocolate Mint	½ cup (3.6 oz)	285	20	11	94	5	25	1	108	64	—	1	—	465
Coffee	½ cup (3.7 oz)	251	17	10	113	5	20	tr	135	80	—	1	—	580
Coffee Chip	½ cup (3.6 oz)	285	19	11	98	5	24	1	123	72	—	1	—	513
Cookie Dough Dynamo	½ cup (3.6 oz)	298	19	11	92	4	28	tr	109	134	—	1	—	487
Cookies & Cream	½ cup (3.6 oz)	264	17	10	107	5	23	tr	129	112	—	1	—	566
Deep Chocolate Peanut Butter	½ cup (3.7 oz)	339	23	11	81	8	25	4	107	95	—	1	—	420
Macadamia Brittle	½ cup (3.7 oz)	282	19	11	103	4	23	tr	122	112	—	1	—	555
Macadamia Nut	½ cup (3.6 oz)	309	24	11	109	5	19	tr	126	114	—	1	—	521
Midnight Cookies & Cream	½ cup (3.6 oz)	285	18	11	89	5	28	1	111	131	—	1	—	453
Peanut Butter Burst	½ cup (2.6 oz)	314	21	11	91	6	25	1	113	144	—	1	—	491
Pralines & Cream	½ cup (3.6 oz)	278	17	9	94	4	26	tr	121	174	—	1	—	519
Rum Raisin	½ cup (3.7 oz)	256	16	10	102	4	21	tr	113	70	—	1	—	533
Strawberry	½ cup (3.7 oz)	242	16	9	91	4	22	1	124	74	—	1	—	540
Strawberry Cheesecake Craze	½ cup (3.7 oz)	273	17	10	97	4	27	1	103	151	—	2	—	520
Swiss Chocolate Almond	½ cup (3.6 oz)	288	20	11	97	6	23	2	122	65	—	1	—	491
Triple Brownie Overload	½ cup (3.5 oz)	298	20	11	91	5	26	1	103	101	—	1	—	484
Vanilla	½ cup (3.7 oz)	252	17	10	113	5	20	0	132	80	—	1	—	582
Vanilla Chip	½ cup (3.6 oz)	286	19	12	99	5	24	1	122	73	—	1	—	514
Vanilla Fudge	½ cup (3.7 oz)	268	17	11	98	4	24	tr	129	101	—	1	—	519
Vanilla Swiss Almond	½ cup (3.7 oz)	288	20	11	101	6	21	1	134	73	—	1	—	533
SORBET														
Mango	½ cup (4 oz)	107	tr	0	0	tr	26	1	4	1	—	10	—	1437
Raspberry	½ cup (4 oz)	110	tr	0	0	tr	27	2	8	3	—	6	—	15

FOOD	PORTION	CALORIES	FAT	SAT FAT	CHOL	PROTEIN	CARBO	FIBER	CALCIUM	SOD	POTAS	VIT C	FOLIC	VIT A
Soft Serve Lemonade	½ cup (3.3 oz)	113	0	0	0	tr	28	1	2	5	—	3	—	0
Soft Serve Mango	½ cup (3.3 oz)	107	tr	0	0	tr	26	1	4	1	—	10	—	956
Soft Serve Raspberry	½ cup (3.3 oz)	108	tr	0	0	tr	26	2	9	3	—	6	—	14
Strawberry	½ cup (4 oz)	118	tr	0	0	tr	29	1	6	1	—	13	—	16
Zesty Lemon	½ cup (4 oz)	111	0	0	0	tr	28	1	2	5	—	3	—	0

HARDEE'S

BREAKFAST SELECTIONS

FOOD	PORTION	CALORIES	FAT	SAT FAT	CHOL	PROTEIN	CARBO	FIBER	CALCIUM	SOD	POTAS	VIT C	FOLIC	VIT A
Apple Cinnamon 'N' Raisin Biscuit	1 (2.18 oz)	200	8	2	0	2	30	—	—	350				
Bacon & Egg Biscuit	1 (5.5 oz)	570	33	11	275	22	45	—	—	1400				
Bacon Egg & Cheese Biscuit	1 (5.9 oz)	610	37	13	280	24	45	—	—	1630				
Big Country Breakfast Bacon	1 serv (9.4 oz)	820	49	15	535	33	62	—	—	1870				
Big Country Breakfast Sausage	1 serv (11.4 oz)	1000	66	38	570	41	62	—	—	3210				
Biscuit 'N' Gravy	1 (7.8 oz)	510	28	9	15	10	55	—	—	1500				
Country Ham Biscuit	1 (3.8 oz)	430	22	5	25	15	45	—	—	1930				
Frisco Breakfast Sandwich Ham	1 (7.4 oz)	500	25	9	290	24	46	—	—	1370				
Ham Biscuit	1 (4 oz)	400	20	6	15	9	47	—	—	1340				
Ham Egg & Cheese Biscuit	1 (6.5 oz)	540	30	11	285	20	48	—	—	1660				
Hash Rounds	1 serv (2.8 oz)	230	14	3	0	3	24	—	—	560	—	—	—	—
Jelly Biscuit	1 (3.5 oz)	440	21	6	0	6	57	—	—	1000				
Rise 'N' Shine Biscuit	1 (2.9 oz)	390	21	6	0	6	44	—	—	1000				
Sausage Biscuit	1 (4.1 oz)	510	31	10	25	14	44	—	—	1360				
Sausage & Egg Biscuit	1 (6.3 oz)	630	40	22	285	23	45	—	—	1480				
Three Pancakes	1 serv (4.8 oz)	280	2	1	15	8	56	—	—	890				
Ultimate Omelet Biscuit	1 (5.8 oz)	570	33	12	120	22	45	—	—	1370	—	—	—	—

DESSERTS

FOOD	PORTION	CALORIES	FAT	SAT FAT	CHOL	PROTEIN	CARBO	FIBER	CALCIUM	SOD	POTAS	VIT C	FOLIC	VIT A
Big Cookie	1 (2.0 oz)	280	12	4	15	4	41	—	—	150	—	—	—	—
Cone Chocolate	1 (4.1 oz)	180	2	1	15	5	34	—	—	110	—	—	—	—
Cone Vanilla	1 (4.1 oz)	170	2	1	10	4	34	—	—	130	—	—	—	—
Cool Twist Cone Vanilla/ Chocolate	1 (4.1 oz)	180	2	1	10	4	34	—	—	120	—	—	—	—
Peach Cobbler	1 serv (6 oz)	310	7	1	0	2	60	—	—	360	—	—	—	—
Sundae Hot Fudge	1 (5.5 oz)	290	6	3	20	7	51	—	—	310	—	—	—	—
Sundae Strawberry	1 (5.8 oz)	210	2	1	10	5	43	—	—	140	—	—	—	—

FOOD	PORTION	CALORIES	FAT	SAT FAT	CHOL	PROTEIN	CARBO	FIBER	CALCIUM	SOD	POTAS	VIT C	FOLIC	VIT A
MAIN MENU SELECTIONS														
Baked Beans	1 serv (5 oz)	170	1	0	0	8	32	—	—	600	—	—	—	—
Big Roast Beef Sandwich	1 (6.5 oz)	460	24	9	70	26	35	—	—	1230	—	—	—	—
Cheeseburger	1 (4.3 oz)	310	14	6	40	16	30	—	—	890	—	—	—	—
Chicken Fillet Sandwich	1 (7.5 oz)	480	18	3	55	26	54	—	—	1280	—	—	—	—
Cole Slaw	1 serv (4 oz)	240	20	3	10	2	13	—	—	340	—	—	—	—
Cravin' Bacon Cheeseburger	1 (8.1 oz)	690	46	15	95	30	38	—	—	1150	—	—	—	—
Fisherman's Fillet	1 (8.3 oz)	560	27	7	65	26	54	—	—	1330	—	—	—	—
French Fries	1 lg (6 oz)	430	18	5	0	6	59	—	—	190	—	—	—	—
French Fries	1 sm (3.4 oz)	240	10	3	0	4	33	—	—	100	—	—	—	—
French Fries	1 med (5 oz)	350	15	4	0	5	49	—	—	150	—	—	—	—
Fried Chicken Breast	1 piece (5.2 oz)	370	15	4	75	29	29	—	—	1190	—	—	—	—
Fried Chicken Leg	1 piece (2.4 oz)	170	7	2	45	13	15	—	—	570	—	—	—	—
Fried Chicken Thigh	1 piece (4.2 oz)	330	15	4	60	19	30	—	—	1000	—	—	—	—
Fried Chicken Wing	1 piece (2.3 oz)	200	8	2	30	10	23	—	—	740	—	—	—	—
Frisco Burger	1 (8.1 oz)	720	46	16	95	33	43	—	—	1340	—	—	—	—
Gravy	1 serv (1.5 oz)	20	tr	tr	0	tr	3	—	—	260	—	—	—	—
Grilled Chicken Sandwich	1 (7.1 oz)	350	11	2	65	25	38	—	—	950	—	—	—	—
Hamburger	1 (3.9 oz)	270	11	3	35	14	29	—	—	670	—	—	—	—
Hot Ham 'N' Cheese	1 (5.1 oz)	310	12	6	50	16	34	—	—	1410	—	—	—	—
Mashed Potatoes	1 serv (4 oz)	70	tr	tr	0	2	14	—	—	330	—	—	—	—
Mesquite Bacon Cheeseburger	1 (4.5 oz)	370	18	7	45	19	32	—	—	970	—	—	—	—
Mushroom 'N' Swiss Burger	1 (6.8 oz)	490	25	12	80	28	39	—	—	1100	—	—	—	—
Quarter Pound Double Cheeseburger	1 (6 oz)	470	27	11	80	27	31	—	—	1290	—	—	—	—
Regular Roast Beef	1 (4.3 oz)	320	16	6	43	17	26	—	—	820	—	—	—	—
The Boss	1 (7 oz)	570	33	12	85	37	42	—	—	910	—	—	—	—
The Works Burger	1 (8.1 oz)	530	30	12	80	25	41	—	—	1030	—	—	—	—
SALAD DRESSINGS														
Fat Free French	1 serv (2 oz)	70	0	0	0	0	17	4	—	580	—	—	—	—
Ranch	1 serv (2 oz)	290	29	4	25	1	6	—	—	510	—	—	—	—
Thousand Island	1 serv (2 oz)	250	23	3	35	1	9	—	—	540	—	—	—	—
SALADS AND SALAD BARS														
Garden Salad	1 (10.2 oz)	220	13	9	40	12	11	—	—	350	—	—	—	—
Grilled Chicken Salad	1 (11.5 oz)	150	3	1	60	20	11	—	—	610	—	—	—	—
Side Salad	1 (4.6 oz)	25	tr	tr	0	1	4	—	—	45	—	—	—	—

FOOD	PORTION	CALORIES	FAT	SAT FAT	CHOL	PROTEIN	CARBO	FIBER	CALCIUM	SOD	POTAS	VIT C	FOLIC	VIT A
H.SALT SEAFOOD														
Chicken	3 oz	108	6	—	69	20	—	—	—	2	—	—	—	—
Cod	3 oz	62	2	—	18	14	—	—	—	57	—	—	—	—
Hamburger	3 oz	228	18	—	65	15	—	—	—	40	—	—	—	—
Pork Loin	3 oz	254	21	—	55	15	—	—	—	55	—	—	—	—
Sirloin Steak	3 oz	239	20	—	58	15	—	—	—	36	—	—	—	—
IHOP														
Pancake Buckwheat	1 (2.5 oz)	134	5	1	61	4	19	1	55	372	94	tr	—	140
Pancake Buttermilk	1 (2 oz)	108	3	1	31	3	17	tr	109	459	44	24	—	52
Pancake Country Griddle	1 (2.25 oz)	134	4	1	38	4	22	1	162	497	79	0	—	311
Pancake Egg	1 (2 oz)	102	5	1	66	2	12	tr	12	213	13	tr	—	108
Pancake Harvest Grain 'N Nut	1 (2.25 oz)	160	8	1	38	4	18	1	120	391	113	59	—	69
Waffle	1 (4 oz)	305	15	3	70	6	37	1	57	468	87	47	—	115
Waffle Belgian	1 (6 oz)	408	20	11	146	9	49	1	73	882	122	64	—	795
Waffle Belgian Harvest Grain 'N Nut	1 (6 oz)	445	28	12	147	10	40	3	88	876	201	129	—	805
JACK IN THE BOX														
BREAKFAST SELECTIONS														
Breakfast Jack	1 (4.2 oz)	300	12	5	185	18	30	0	0	890	220	9	—	400
Country Crock Spread	1 pat (5 g)	25	3	1	0	0	0	0	0	40	0	0	—	200
Grape Jelly	1 serv (0.5 oz)	40	0	0	0	0	9	0	0	5	0	0	—	0
Hash Browns	1 serv (2 oz)	160	11	11	—	1	14	1	0	310	190	6	—	0
Pancake Syrup	1 serv (1.5 oz)	120	0	0	0	0	30	0	0	5	10	0	—	0
Pancakes w/ Bacon	1 serv (5.6 oz)	400	12	3	30	13	59	3	80	980	280	0	—	0
Sausage Croissant	1 (6.4 oz)	670	48	19	250	21	39	2	150	940	180	1	—	1000
Sourdough Breakfast Sandwich	1 (5.2 oz)	380	21	8	355	21	31	0	250	1120	260	9	—	750
Supreme Croissant	1 (6 oz)	570	20	7	235	21	39	2	100	1240	300	12	—	750
Ultimate Breakfast Sandwich	1 (8.5 oz)	620	36	15	245	36	39	tr	250	1800	450	9	—	750
DESSERTS														
Carrot Cake	1 serv (3.5 oz)	370	16	3	35	3	54	2	20	340	150	0	—	5500
Cheesecake	1 serv (3.5 oz)	310	18	9	65	8	29	2	100	210	15	0	—	0
Double Fudge Cake	1 serv (3 oz)	300	10	3	50	3	50	1	40	320	250	0	—	300
Hot Apple Turnover	1 (3.8 oz)	340	18	4	0	4	41	2	0	510	85	12	—	100
MAIN MENU SELECTIONS														
¼ lb Burger	1 (6 oz)	510	27	10	65	26	39	0	150	1080	300	0	—	300
American Cheese	1 slice (0.4 oz)	45	4	3	10	2	0	0	60	200	15	0	—	200
Bacon & Cheddar Potato Wedges	1 serv (9.3 oz)	800	58	16	55	20	49	4	350	1470	960	12	—	500

FOOD	PORTION	CALORIES	FAT	SAT FAT	CHOL	PROTEIN	CARBO	FIBER	CALCIUM	SOD	POTAS	VIT C	FOLIC	VIT A
Bacon Ultimate Cheeseburger	1 (10.4 oz)	1150	89	30	230	57	31	0	300	1770	610	1	—	500
Barbeque Dipping Sauce	1 serv (1 fl oz)	45	0	0	0	1	11	0	0	300	75	0	—	0
Cheeseburger	1 (4 oz)	330	15	6	60	15	32	2	150	760	210	—	—	400
Chicken & Fries	1 serv (9.3 oz)	730	34	7	65	26	79	5	40	1690	1100	9	—	200
Chicken Caesar Sandwich	1 (8.3 oz)	520	26	6	55	27	44	4	250	1050	490	2	—	400
Chicken Fajita Pita	1 (6.6 oz)	280	9	4	75	24	25	3	150	840	410	0	—	500
Chicken Sandwich	1 (5.9 oz)	450	26	5	45	16	38	2	80	1030	265	1	—	200
Chicken Strips Breaded	5 pieces (5.3 oz)	360	17	3	80	27	24	1	20	970	430	1	—	200
Chicken Supreme Sandwich	1 (8.2 oz)	680	45	11	85	23	46	4	250	1500	400	9	—	750
Chili Cheese Curly Fries	1 serv (8.1 oz)	650	41	12	25	12	60	13	100	1640	810	—	—	1250
Double Cheeseburger	1 (5.3 oz)	450	24	12	75	24	35	0	250	970	320	0	—	500
Egg Rolls	3 pieces (6 oz)	440	24	6	35	15	40	4	80	1020	500	12	—	750
Egg Rolls	5 pieces (10 oz)	730	41	10	60	25	67	7	150	1700	830	18	—	1250
Fish & Chips	1 serv (9 oz)	720	35	8	35	19	81	6	20	1580	1060	12	—	100
French Fries	1 reg (4.1 oz)	360	17	4	0	4	48	3	0	740	610	24	—	0
Grilled Chicken Fillet Sandwich	1 (8.1 oz)	520	26	6	140	27	42	4	200	1240	510	0	—	500
Hamburger	1 (3.6 oz)	280	12	4	45	13	32	2	80	560	200	0	—	200
Jumbo Fries	1 serv (5 oz)	430	20	5	0	4	58	4	0	890	740	27	—	0
Jumbo Jack	1 (7.8 oz)	560	36	12	80	28	31	4	100	680	350	9	—	—
Jumbo Jack w/ Cheese	1 (8.6 oz)	650	43	16	105	32	32	4	250	1090	380	9	—	500
Ketchup	1 pkg (0.3 oz)	10	0	0	0	0	3	0	0	100	30	1	—	200
Monster Taco	1 (4 oz)	290	18	6	40	11	21	3	200	550	290	5	—	400
Onion Rings	1 serv (4.2 oz)	460	25	5	0	7	50	3	40	780	150	18	—	200
Pilly Cheesesteak Sandwich	1 (7.6 oz)	520	25	9	155	33	41	4	300	1980	420	0	—	750
Salsa	1 serv (1 oz)	10	0	0	0	0	2	0	tr	200	70	tr	—	100
Seasoned Curly Fries	1 serv (4.5 oz)	420	24	5	0	6	46	4	40	1030	630	0	—	400
Sour Cream	1 serv (1 oz)	60	6	4	20	1	1	0	20	30	40	0	—	200
Sourdough Jack	1 (7.8 oz)	670	43	16	110	32	39	0	200	1180	510	6	—	750
Soy Sauce	1 serv (0.3 oz)	5	0	0	0	tr	tr	0	0	480	35	0	—	0
Spicy Crispy Chicken Sandwich	1 (7.9 oz)	560	27	5	50	24	55	0	100	1020	470	5	—	200
Stuffed Jalapenos	10 pieces (7.6 oz)	680	40	15	75	20	59	5	500	2220	270	30	—	1500
Stuffed Jalapenos	7 pieces (5.3 oz)	470	28	11	50	14	41	3	300	1560	190	18	—	1000

FOOD	PORTION	CALORIES	FAT	SAT FAT	CHOL	PROTEIN	CARBO	FIBER	CALCIUM	SOD	POTAS	VIT C	FOLIC	VIT A
Super Scoop French Fries	1 serv (7 oz)	610	28	6	0	6	82	5	20	1250	1040	42	—	0
Sweet & Sour Dipping Sauce	1 serv (1 oz)	40	0	0	0	tr	11	0	0	160	10	0	—	0
Swiss-Style Cheese	1 slice (0.4 oz)	40	3	2	10	3	0	0	100	190	10	0	—	100
Taco	1 (2.7 oz)	190	11	4	20	7	15	2	100	410	240	0	—	0
Tartar Dipping Sauce	1 pkg (1.5 oz)	220	23	4	20	1	2	0	20	240	25	0	—	0
Teriyaki Bowl Chicken	1 serv (17.6 oz)	670	4	1	15	29	128	5	150	1620	620	0	—	3000
Ultimate Cheeseburger	1 (9.8 oz)	1030	79	26	205	50	30	0	300	1200	520	1	—	500
SALAD DRESSINGS														
Blue Cheese	1 serv (2 fl oz)	210	18	4	15	1	11	0	0	750	35	0	—	0
Buttermilk House	1 serv (2 fl oz)	290	30	11	20	1	6	0	20	560	70	4	—	100
Buttermilk House Dipping Sauce	1 serv (0.9 oz)	130	13	5	10	tr	3	tr	0	240	30	1	—	0
Low Calorie Italian	1 serv (2 fl oz)	25	2	0	0	0	2	0	0	670	40	0	—	0
Thousand Island	1 serv (2 fl oz)	250	24	4	20	1	10	0	0	570	65	0	—	0
SALADS AND SALAD BARS														
Croutons	1 serv (0.4 oz)	50	2	1	0	1	8	0	0	105	20	0	—	0
Garden Chicken Salad	1 serv (8.9 oz)	200	9	4	65	23	8	3	200	420	560	12	—	3500
Side Salad	1 (3 oz)	50	3	2	10	2	3	1	80	75	160	0	—	750

KENNY ROGERS ROASTERS

MAIN MENU SELECTIONS

FOOD	PORTION	CALORIES	FAT	SAT FAT	CHOL	PROTEIN	CARBO	FIBER	CALCIUM	SOD	POTAS	VIT C	FOLIC	VIT A
½ Chicken w/ Skin	1 serv (9.06 oz)	515	28	7	301	65	2	—	59	1129	—	—	—	—
½ Chicken w/o Skin & Wing	1 serv (7.03 oz)	313	10	3	221	56	1	—	38	876	—	—	—	—
¼ Chicken Dark Meat w/ Skin	1 serv (4.35 oz)	271	17	4	165	29	1	—	26	524	—	—	—	—
¼ Chicken Dark Meat w/o Skin & Wing	1 serv (3.29 oz)	169	7	2	130	25	1	—	15	454	—	—	—	—
¼ Chicken White Meat w/ Skin	1 serv (4.71 oz)	244	11	3	136	35	1	—	33	604	—	—	—	—
¼ Chicken White Meat w/o Skin & Wing	1 serv (3.74 oz)	144	2	1	92	31	tr	—	23	422	—	—	—	—
Baked Sweet Potato	1 (9 oz)	263	tr	0	0	4	62	1	—	26	—	—	—	—
Chicken Caesar Salad	1 serv (9.4 oz)	285	9	3	122	34	18	1	—	704	—	—	—	—
Cinnamon Apples	1 serv (5.27 oz)	199	5	3	13	0	41	3	—	3	—	—	—	—

FOOD	PORTION	CALORIES	FAT	SAT FAT	CHOL	PROTEIN	CARBO	FIBER	CALCIUM	SOD	POTAS	VIT C	FOLIC	VIT A
Cole Slaw	1 serv (5.05 oz)	225	16	3	13	1	18	2	—	288	—	—	—	—
Corn Muffin	1 (2 oz)	175	8	2	0	2	24	1	—	210	—	—	—	—
Corn On The Cob	1 (2.25 oz)	68	1	tr	0	2	14	2	—	11	—	—	—	—
Corn Stuffing	1 serv (7.1 oz)	326	19	3	5	7	34	tr	—	765	—	—	—	—
Creamy Parmesan Spinach	1 serv (5.3 oz)	119	69	3	12	10	10	tr	—	547	—	—	—	—
Garlic Parsley Potatoes	1 serv (6.5 oz)	259	12	5	16	3	37	3	—	867	—	—	—	—
Honey Baked Beans	1 serv (5 oz)	148	1	tr	0	6	32	tr	—	787	—	—	—	—
Italian Green Beans	1 serv (6.1 oz)	116	8	1	0	2	10	tr	—	374	—	—	—	—
Macaroni & Cheese	1 serv (5.51 oz)	197	6	3	26	6	24	1	—	661	—	—	—	—
Pasta Salad	1 serv (5 oz)	236	12	2	40	6	28	1	—	296	—	—	—	—
Pita BBQ Chicken	1 (7.33 oz)	401	7	1	112	33	51	—	—	1307	—	—	—	—
Pita Chicken Caesar	1 (9.2 oz)	606	35	3	122	36	34	1	—	829	—	—	—	—
Pita Roasted Chicken	1 (10.8 oz)	685	35	3	159	47	42	tr	—	1620	—	—	—	—
Pot Pie Chicken	1 (12 oz)	708	33	11	69	26	78	tr	—	1500	—	—	—	—
Potato Salad	1 serv (7.01 oz)	390	27	3	0	3	34	2	—	628	—	—	—	—
Real Mashed Potatoes	1 serv (8 oz)	295	14	3	2	4	39	1	—	478	—	—	—	—
Rice Pilaf	1 serv (5 oz)	173	5	1	0	3	43	0	—	146	—	—	—	—
Roasted Chicken Salad	1 serv (16.9 oz)	292	10	2	218	35	19	6	—	573	—	—	—	—
Sandwich Turkey	1 (9.2 oz)	385	12	2	88	39	30	1	—	923	—	—	—	—
Side Salad	1 serv (4.73 oz)	23	1	0	0	1	5	2	—	16	—	—	—	—
Sour Cream & Dill Pasta Salad	1 serv (5 oz)	233	16	3	16	4	20	1	—	432	—	—	—	—
Steamed Vegetables	1 serv (4.25 oz)	48	tr	0	0	3	8	4	—	59	—	—	—	—
Sweet Corn Niblets	1 serv (5 oz)	112	1	tr	0	3	28	1	—	385	—	—	—	—
Tomato Cucumber Salad	1 serv (6 oz)	123	2	1	0	1	10	1	—	794	—	—	—	—
Turkey Sliced Breast	1 serv (4.5 oz)	158	2	1	78	34	—	—	—	586	—	—	—	—
Zucchini & Squash Santa Fe	1 serv (5 oz)	70	5	1	0	1	8	1	—	209	—	—	—	—
SALAD DRESSINGS														
Blue Cheese	1 serv (2.47 oz)	370	39	7	65	3	3	0	—	720	—	—	—	—
Buttermilk Ranch	1 serv (2.47 oz)	430	48	7	10	1	2	0	—	620	—	—	—	—
Caesar	1 serv (2.47 oz)	340	36	5	15	1	3	0	—	780	—	—	—	—

FOOD	PORTION	CALORIES	FAT	SAT FAT	CHOL	PROTEIN	CARBO	FIBER	CALCIUM	SOD	POTAS	VIT C	FOLIC	VIT A
Honey French	1 serv (2.47 oz)	350	29	4	0	0	22	0	—	490	—	—	—	—
Honey Mustard	1 serv (2.47 oz)	320	28	4	40	1	18	1	—	410	—	—	—	—
Italian Fat Free	1 serv (2.47 oz)	35	0	0	0	0	8	0	—	1040	—	—	—	—
Thousand Island	1 serv (2.47 oz)	330	33	5	40	1	8	0	—	550	—	—	—	—
SOUPS														
Chicken Noodle	1 bowl (10 oz)	91	2	tr	22	7	12	tr	—	931	—	—	—	—
Chicken Noodle	1 cup (6 oz)	55	1	tr	13	4	7	1	—	559	—	—	—	—
KFC														
BBQ Baked Beans	1 serv (5.5 oz)	190	3	1	5	6	33	6	80	760	—	—	—	400
Biscuit	1 (2 oz)	180	10	3	0	4	20	tr	20	560	—	—	—	—
Chicken Pot Pie	1 (13 oz)	770	42	13	70	29	69	5	100	2160	—	1	—	4000
Chicken Twister	1 (8.7 oz)	550	32	7	85	26	40	1	—	980	—	5	—	400
Cole Slaw	1 serv (5 oz)	180	9	2	5	2	21	3	40	280	—	36	—	—
Corn On The Cob	1 ear (5.7 oz)	150	2	0	0	5	35	2	—	20	—	4	—	100
Cornbread	1 (2 oz)	228	13	2	42	3	25	1	60	194	—	—	—	—
Crispy Strips Colonel's	3 (3.25 oz)	261	16	4	40	20	10	3	—	658	—	—	—	—
Crispy Strips Spicy Buffalo	3 (4.2 oz)	350	19	4	35	22	22	2	20	1110	—	—	—	—
Extra Tasty Crispy Breast	1 (5.9 oz)	470	28	7	80	31	25	1	40	930	—	—	—	—
Extra Tasty Crispy Drumstick	1 (2.4 oz)	190	11	3	60	13	8	tr	—	260	—	—	—	—
Extra Tasty Crispy Thigh	1 (4.2 oz)	370	25	6	70	19	18	2	20	540	—	—	—	—
Extra Tasty Crispy Whole Wing	1 (1.9 oz)	200	13	4	45	10	10	tr	—	290	—	—	—	—
Green Beans	1 serv (4.7 oz)	45	2	1	5	1	7	3	40	730	—	2	—	200
Hot & Spicy Breast	1 (6.5 oz)	530	35	8	110	32	23	2	40	1110	—	—	—	—
Hot & Spicy Drumstick	1 (2.3 oz)	190	11	3	50	13	10	tr	—	300	—	—	—	—
Hot & Spicy Thigh	1 (3.8 oz)	370	27	7	90	18	13	1	—	570	—	—	—	—
Hot & Spicy Whole Wing	1 (1.9 oz)	210	15	4	50	10	9	tr	40	340	—	—	—	—
Hot Wings	6 (4.8 oz)	471	33	8	150	27	18	2	40	1230	—	—	—	—
Macaroni & Cheese	1 serv (5.4 oz)	180	8	3	10	7	21	2	150	860	—	—	—	1000
Mashed Potatoes With Gravy	1 serv (4.8 oz)	120	6	1	tr	1	17	2	—	440	—	—	—	—
Mean Greens	1 serv (5.4 oz)	70	3	1	10	4	11	5	200	650	—	6	—	3000
Original Recipe Breast	1 (5.4 oz)	400	24	6	135	29	16	1	40	1116	—	—	—	—
Original Recipe Chicken Sandwich	1 (7.3 oz)	497	22	5	52	29	46	3	100	1213	—	—	—	—

FOOD	PORTION	CALORIES	FAT	SAT FAT	CHOL	PROTEIN	CARBO	FIBER	CALCIUM	SOD	POTAS	VIT C	FOLIC	VIT A
Original Recipe Drumstick	1 (2.2 oz)	140	9	2	75	13	4	0	—	422	—	—	—	—
Original Recipe Thigh	1 (3.2 oz)	250	18	5	95	16	6	1	20	747	—	—	—	—
Original Recipe Whole Wing	1 (1.6 oz)	140	10	3	55	9	5	0	—	414	—	—	—	—
Potato Salad	1 serv (5.6 oz)	230	14	2	15	4	23	3	20	540	—	—	—	500
Potato Wedges	1 serv (4.8 oz)	280	13	4	5	5	28	5	20	750	—	1	—	—
Tender Roast Breast w/ Skin	1 (4.9 oz)	251	11	3	151	37	1	0	—	830	—	—	—	—
Tender Roast Breast w/o Skin	1 (4.2 oz)	169	4	1	112	31	1	0	—	797	—	—	—	—
Tender Roast Drumstick w/ Skin	1 (1.9 oz)	97	4	1	85	15	tr	0	—	271	—	—	—	—
Tender Roast Drumstick w/o Skin	1 (1.2 oz)	67	2	1	63	11	tr	0	—	259	—	—	—	—
Tender Roast Thigh w/ Skin	1 (3.2 oz)	207	12	4	120	19	<2	0	—	504	—	—	—	—
Tender Roast Thigh w/o Skin	1 (2.1 oz)	106	6	2	84	13	tr	0	—	312	—	—	—	—
Tender Roast Wing w/ Skin	1 (1.8 oz)	121	8	2	74	12	1	0	—	331	—	—	—	—
Value BBQ Chicken Sandwich	1 (5.3 oz)	256	8	1	57	17	28	2	60	782	—	4	—	—

KRYSTAL

BREAKFAST SELECTIONS

FOOD	PORTION	CALORIES	FAT	SAT FAT	CHOL	PROTEIN	CARBO	FIBER	CALCIUM	SOD	POTAS	VIT C	FOLIC	VIT A
Biscuit	1 (2.5 oz)	244	12	2	2	3	31	—	—	437	98	—	—	—
Biscuit Bacon	1 (2.9 oz)	306	17	5	14	8	32	—	—	726	147	—	—	—
Biscuit Bacon, Egg & Cheese	1 (4.7 oz)	421	26	8	153	14	33	—	—	899	204	—	—	400
Biscuit Country Ham	1 (3.7 oz)	334	17	4	23	14	31	—	—	1147	214	—	—	—
Biscuit Egg	1 (4 oz)	327	19	4	134	8	32	—	—	481	149	—	—	400
Biscuit Gravy	1 (7.5 oz)	419	26	7	23	7	40	—	—	980	99	—	—	—
Biscuit Sausage	1 (4.1 oz)	437	30	8	49	10	31	—	—	668	230	—	—	—
Sunriser	1 (3.8 oz)	259	17	5	162	14	17	—	—	544	163	—	—	1250

DESSERTS

FOOD	PORTION	CALORIES	FAT	SAT FAT	CHOL	PROTEIN	CARBO	FIBER	CALCIUM	SOD	POTAS	VIT C	FOLIC	VIT A
Apple Pie	1 serv (4.5 oz)	300	10	4	0	3	49	—	—	420	81	—	—	—
Donut Plain	1 (1.3 oz)	150	9	2	5	2	17	—	—	135	43	—	—	—
Donut w/ Chocolate Icing	1 (1.8 oz)	212	11	3	5	2	27	—	—	165	43	—	—	—
Donut w/ Vanilla Icing	1 (1.8 oz)	198	9	2	5	2	29	—	—	135	43	—	—	—
Lemon Meringue Pie	1 serv (4 oz)	340	9	3	50	7	57	—	—	190	57	—	—	—
Pecan Pie	1 serv (4 oz)	450	23	6	55	5	56	—	—	290	107	—	—	100

FOOD	PORTION	CALORIES	FAT	SAT FAT	CHOL	PROTEIN	CARBO	FIBER	CALCIUM	SOD	POTAS	VIT C	FOLIC	VIT A
MAIN MENU SELECTIONS														
Bacon Cheeseburger	1 (7.4 oz)	521	34	14	89	26	29	—	—	1083	441	—	—	150
Big K	1 (8 oz)	540	35	14	93	29	29	—	—	1283	487	—	—	150
Burger Plus	1 (6.5 oz)	415	26	10	63	20	28	—	—	614	397	—	—	150
Burger Plus w/ Cheese	1 (7.1 oz)	473	31	13	77	23	28	—	—	867	410	—	—	150
Cheese Krystal	1 (2.5 oz)	187	10	4	29	11	16	—	—	453	105	—	—	—
Chili	1 lg (12 oz)	327	12	5	28	16	41	—	—	1283	582	—	—	800
Chili	1 reg (8 oz)	218	8	3	19	11	27	—	—	855	388	—	—	550
Chili Cheese Pup	1 (2.7 oz)	211	13	7	31	9	14	—	—	642	59	—	—	250
Chili Pup	1 (2.5 oz)	182	10	6	24	7	13	—	—	597	52	—	—	—
Corn Pup	1 (2.3 oz)	214	14	6	24	6	17	—	—	710	92	—	—	—
Crispy Crunchy Chicken Sandwich	1 (5.75 oz)	467	24	7	56	16	48	—	—	949	235	—	—	—
Double Cheese Krystal	1 (4.5 oz)	337	19	8	57	21	25	—	—	815	190	—	—	—
Double Krystal	1 (4 oz)	277	14	4	43	18	24	—	—	547	177	—	—	—
Fries	1 reg (4.1 oz)	358	18	6	12	4	45	—	—	157	478	—	—	—
Fries	1 sm (3 oz)	262	13	5	9	3	33	—	—	115	350	—	—	—
Fries	1 lg (5.3 oz)	463	23	8	16	5	59	—	—	203	618	—	—	—
Krys Kross Fries	1 serv (4.3 oz)	486	29	11	31	5	52	—	—	604	345	—	—	—
Krys Kross Fries Chili Cheese	1 serv (6.8 oz)	625	39	16	61	12	57	—	—	1111	408	—	—	—
Krys Kross Fries w/ Cheese	1 serv (5.3 oz)	515	31	12	31	5	54	—	—	803	349	—	—	—
Krystal	1 (2.2 oz)	158	7	2	22	10	16	—	—	324	99	—	—	—
Plain Pup	1 (1.9 oz)	160	9	5	20	6	12	—	—	470	38	—	—	—

LITTLE CAESARS

FOOD	PORTION	CALORIES	FAT	SAT FAT	CHOL	PROTEIN	CARBO	FIBER	CALCIUM	SOD	POTAS	VIT C	FOLIC	VIT A
MAIN MENU SELECTIONS														
Crazy Bread	1 piece (1.4 oz)	106	3	1	0	3	16	1	10	114	—	—	—	135
Crazy Sauce	1 serv (6 oz)	170	tr	0	0	5	14	5	30	381	—	—	—	645
Deli-Style Sandwich Ham & Cheese	1 (11.6 oz)	728	35	13	54	30	71	3	496	1602	—	22	—	1205
Deli-Style Sandwich Italian	1 (11.9 oz)	740	37	12	62	29	71	3	267	1831	—	32	—	830
Deli-Style Sandwich Veggie	1 (11.9 oz)	647	29	9	29	22	74	4	347	1195	—	34	—	1020
Hot Oven-Baked Sandwich Cheeser	1 (12.1 oz)	822	39	20	580	40	75	5	655	2244	—	—	—	1175
Hot Oven-Baked Sandwich Meatsa	1 (15 oz)	1036	56	24	130	55	75	5	538	3302	—	28	—	1030
Hot Oven-Baked Sandwich Pepperoni	1 (11.2 oz)	899	47	23	58	43	74	4	654	2428	—	—	—	1175

FOOD	PORTION	CALORIES	FAT	SAT FAT	CHOL	PROTEIN	CARBO	FIBER	CALCIUM	SOD	POTAS	VIT C	FOLIC	VIT A
Hot Oven-Baked Sandwich Supreme	1 (13.1 oz)	894	46	21	700	41	77	5	528	2367	—	15	—	1035
Hot Oven-Baked Sandwich Veggie	1 (13.7 oz)	669	23	14	58	33	79	6	661	1534	—	32	—	1490
PIZZA														
Baby Pan!Pan!	1 serv (8.4 oz)	616	24	12	47	33	67	4	561	1466	—	—	—	855
Pan!Pan! Cheese	1 med slice (2.9 oz)	181	6	3	15	9	22	1	185	379	—	—	—	265
Pan!Pan! Pepperoni	1 med slice (3 oz)	199	8	4	15	11	22	1	187	452	—	—	—	285
Pizza!Pizza! Cheese	1 med slice (3.2 oz)	201	7	4	17	11	24	1	189	281	—	—	—	295
Pizza!Pizza! Pepperoni	1 med slice (3.3 oz)	220	9	4	17	12	24	1	190	358	—	—	—	295
SALAD DRESSINGS														
1000 Island	1 serv (1.5 oz)	183	17	3	30	—	6	—	—	542	—	—	—	—
Blue Cheese	1 serv (1.5 oz)	160	14	2	17	—	8	—	—	600	—	—	—	—
Caesar	1 serv (1.5 oz)	255	27	4	13	—	3	—	—	404	—	—	—	—
French	1 serv (1.5 oz)	166	16	2	0	—	5	—	—	553	—	—	—	—
Greek	1 serv (1.5 oz)	268	30	8	9	—	tr	—	—	202	—	—	—	—
Italian	1 serv (1.5 oz)	200	21	3	12	—	3	—	—	468	—	—	—	—
Italian Fat Free	1 serv (1.5 oz)	15	0	0	0	—	3	—	—	420	—	—	—	—
Ranch	1 serv (1.5 oz)	221	22	3	18	—	5	—	—	340	—	—	—	—
SALADS AND SALAD BARS														
Antipasto Salad	1 serv (8.4 oz)	176	12	2	19	12	7	2	212	542	—	35	—	1390
Caesar Salad	1 serv (5 oz)	140	5	3	11	9	14	2	247	372	—	27	—	1630
Greek Salad	1 serv (10.3 oz)	168	10	tr	37	9	12	3	261	653	—	36	—	1210
Tossed Salad	1 serv (8.5 oz)	116	3	tr	0	5	19	3	71	170	—	41	—	3215

LONG JOHN SILVER'S

FOOD	PORTION	CALORIES	FAT	SAT FAT	CHOL	PROTEIN	CARBO	FIBER	CALCIUM	SOD	POTAS	VIT C	FOLIC	VIT A
MAIN MENU SELECTIONS														
Batter-Dipped Chicken	1 piece (2 oz)	120	6	2	15	8	11	3	—	400	—	—	—	—
Batter-Dipped Fish	1 piece (3 oz)	170	11	3	30	11	12	5	—	470	—	—	—	—
Batter-Dipped Shrimp	1 piece (0.4 oz)	35	3	1	10	1	2	0	—	95	—	—	—	—
Breaded Chicken Strips	1 piece (1.15 oz)	100	5	1	10	6	6	0	—	360	—	—	—	—
Breaded Clams	1 serv (3 oz)	300	17	4	40	11	31	5	—	670	—	—	—	—
Breaded Fish	1 piece (1.6 oz)	110	5	1	20	5	11	0	—	340	—	—	—	—
Cheese Sticks	1 serv (1.6 oz)	160	9	4	10	6	12	tr	—	360	—	—	—	—
Chicken Salsa	1 reg (11 oz)	690	32	7	20	18	81	5	—	1690	—	—	—	—
Corn Cobbette w/ Butter	1 piece (3.3 oz)	140	8	2	0	3	19	0	—	0	—	—	—	—

FOOD	PORTION	CALORIES	FAT	SAT FAT	CHOL	PROTEIN	CARBO	FIBER	CALCIUM	SOD	POTAS	VIT C	FOLIC	VIT A
Corn Cobbette w/o Butter	1 (3.1 oz)	80	1	0	0	3	19	0	—	0	—	—	—	—
Fish Cajun	1 lg (23 oz)	1450	70	15	60	18	85	10	—	3630	—	—	—	—
Flavorbaked Chicken	1 piece (2.6 oz)	110	3	1	55	19	tr	tr	—	600	—	—	—	—
Flavorbaked Fish	1 piece (2.3 oz)	90	3	1	35	14	1	0	—	320	—	—	—	—
Fries	1 reg (3 oz)	250	15	3	0	3	28	3	—	500	—	—	—	—
Fries	1 lg (5 oz)	420	24	4	0	5	46	4	—	830	—	—	—	—
Honey Mustard Sauce	1 serv (0.4 oz)	20	0	0	0	0	5	0	—	60	—	—	—	—
Hushpuppy	1 (0.8 oz)	60	3	0	0	1	9	0	—	25	—	—	—	—
Ketchup	1 serv (.32 oz)	10	0	0	0	0	2	0	—	110	—	—	—	—
Popcorn Chicken Munchers	1 serv (4 oz)	380	23	4	35	23	20	2	—	1030	—	—	—	—
Popcorn Fish Munchers	1 serv (4 oz)	300	14	3	50	14	29	tr	—	1220	—	—	—	—
Popcorn Shrimp Munchers	1 serv (4 oz)	320	15	3	85	15	33	1	—	1440	—	—	—	—
Rice	1 serv (3 oz)	140	3	1	0	3	26	tr	—	210	—	—	—	—
Sandwich Batter Dipped Fish No Sauce	1 (5.4 oz)	320	13	4	30	17	40	6	—	800	—	—	—	—
Sandwich Flavorbaked Chicken	1 (5.8 oz)	290	10	2	60	24	27	2	—	970	—	—	—	—
Sandwich Flavorbaked Fish	1 (6 oz)	320	14	7	55	23	28	2	—	930	—	—	—	—
Sandwich Ultimate Fish	1 (6.4 oz)	430	21	7	35	18	44	3	—	1340	—	—	—	—
Shrimp Sauce	1 serv (0.4 oz)	15	0	0	0	0	3	0	—	180	—	—	—	—
Side Salad	1 (4.3 oz)	25	0	0	0	1	4	tr	—	15	—	—	—	—
Slaw	1 serv (3.4 oz)	140	6	—	0	1	20	3	—	260	—	—	—	—
Sweet'N'Sour Sauce	1 serv (0.4 oz)	20	0	0	0	0	5	0	—	45	—	—	—	—
Tartar Sauce	1 serv (0.4 oz)	35	2	—	0	0	5	0	—	35	—	—	—	—
Wraps Chicken Cajun	1 reg (11 oz)	720	35	7	25	18	83	5	—	1860	—	—	—	—
Wraps Chicken Cajun	1 lg (22 oz)	1440	71	14	50	37	165	11	—	3730	—	—	—	—
Wraps Chicken Ranch	1 reg (11 oz)	730	36	7	25	18	82	5	—	1810	—	—	—	—
Wraps Chicken Ranch	1 lg (22 oz)	1450	72	14	50	36	165	10	—	3620	—	—	—	—
Wraps Chicken Salsa	1 lg (22 oz)	1370	64	13	35	36	162	10	—	3370	—	—	—	—
Wraps Chicken Tartar	1 lg (22 oz)	1450	72	14	45	36	165	11	—	3560	—	—	—	—

FOOD	PORTION	CALORIES	FAT	SAT FAT	CHOL	PROTEIN	CARBO	FIBER	CALCIUM	SOD	POTAS	VIT C	FOLIC	VIT A
Wraps Chicken Tartar	1 reg (11 oz)	730	36	7	25	18	83	6	—	1780	—	—	—	—
Wraps Fish Cajun	1 reg (11.5 oz)	730	35	8	30	18	85	5	—	1820	—	—	—	—
Wraps Fish Ranch	1 reg (11.5 oz)	730	36	8	30	18	85	5	—	1760	—	—	—	—
Wraps Fish Ranch	1 lg (23 oz)	1460	72	15	60	35	170	10	—	3520	—	—	—	—
Wraps Fish Salsa	1 lg (23 oz)	1380	64	14	45	35	167	10	—	3280	—	—	—	—
Wraps Fish Salsa	1 reg (11.5 oz)	690	32	7	25	18	84	5	—	1640	—	—	—	—
Wraps Fish Tartar	1 lg (23 oz)	1470	72	15	55	35	170	10	—	3460	—	—	—	—
Wraps Fish Tartar	1 reg (11.5 oz)	730	36	8	25	18	85	5	—	1730	—	—	—	—
Wraps Popcorn Shrimp Cajun	1 lg (22 oz)	1450	71	18	95	32	172	10	—	3660	—	—	—	—
Wraps Popcorn Shrimp Cajun	1 reg (11 oz)	720	35	9	50	16	86	5	—	1830	—	—	—	—
Wraps Popcorn Shrimp Ranch	1 lg (22 oz)	1460	72	18	100	32	171	10	—	3560	—	—	—	—
Wraps Popcorn Shrimp Ranch	1 reg (11 oz)	720	35	9	50	16	86	5	—	1830	—	—	—	—
Wraps Popcorn Shrimp Salsa	1 lg (22 oz)	1380	64	17	85	32	169	9	—	3310	—	—	—	—
Wraps Popcorn Shrimp Salsa	1 reg (11 oz)	690	32	9	40	16	84	5	—	1660	—	—	—	—
Wraps Popcorn Shrimp Tartar	1 reg (11 oz)	730	36	9	45	16	86	5	—	1750	—	—	—	—
Wraps Popcorn Shrimp Tartar	1 lg (22 oz)	1460	72	18	95	32	172	10	—	3500	—	—	—	—
SALAD DRESSINGS														
Fat-Free French	1 serv (1.5 oz)	50	0	0	0	0	14	—	—	360	—	—	—	—
Fat-Free Ranch	1 serv (1.5 oz)	50	0	0	0	2	13	—	—	380	—	—	—	—
Italian	1 serv (1 oz)	130	14	2	0	0	2	—	—	280	—	—	—	—
Malt Vinegar	1 serv (0.3 oz)	0	0	0	0	0	0	0	—	15	—	—	—	—
Ranch Dressing	1 serv (1 oz)	170	18	3	5	0	1	—	—	260	—	—	—	—
Thousand Island	1 serv (1 oz)	110	10	2	15	0	5	—	—	280	—	—	—	—

LYONS RESTAURANTS

MAIN MENU SELECTIONS

FOOD	PORTION	CALORIES	FAT	SAT FAT	CHOL	PROTEIN	CARBO	FIBER	CALCIUM	SOD	POTAS	VIT C	FOLIC	VIT A
Light & Healthy Halibut Brochette	1 serv	502	7	—	47	—	—	—	—	—	—	—	—	—
Light & Healthy Lime & Cilantro Chicken	1 serv	511	9	—	101	—	—	—	—	—	—	—	—	—

MACHEEZMO MOUSE

CHILDREN'S MENU SELECTIONS

FOOD	PORTION	CALORIES	FAT	SAT FAT	CHOL	PROTEIN	CARBO	FIBER	CALCIUM	SOD	POTAS	VIT C	FOLIC	VIT A
El Bento Kid	1 serv (7 oz)	235	1	—	63	23	35	—	—	330	—	—	—	—
Quesadilla Kid Cheese	1 serv (5 oz)	360	13	—	40	21	42	—	—	535	—	—	—	—
Quesadilla Kid Chicken	1 serv (7 oz)	430	15	—	100	34	42	—	—	565	—	—	—	—

FOOD	PORTION	CALORIES	FAT	SAT FAT	CHOL	PROTEIN	CARBO	FIBER	CALCIUM	SOD	POTAS	VIT C	FOLIC	VIT A
Taco Kid Cheese	1 serv (6 oz)	285	5	—	20	15	47	—	—	344	—	—	—	—
Taco Kid Chicken	1 (8 oz)	355	7	—	80	28	47	—	—	374	—	—	—	—
MAIN MENU SELECTIONS														
Beans	1 oz	35	0	—	0	2	7	—	—	30	—	—	—	—
Bento Stick	1 oz	30	1	—	63	7	0	—	—	68	—	—	—	—
Boss Sauce	1 oz	30	0	—	0	0	8	—	—	140	—	—	—	—
Broccoli	1 oz	4	0	—	0	0	1	—	—	5	—	—	—	—
Burrito Chicken	1 (13 oz)	580	11	—	110	39	85	—	—	748	—	—	—	—
Burrito Combo	1 (14 oz)	630	12	—	124	48	87	—	—	933	—	—	—	—
Burrito Vegetarian	1 (14 oz)	655	8	—	20	26	123	—	—	890	—	—	—	—
Cheese	1 oz	81	5	—	20	8	1	—	—	180	—	—	—	—
Chicken	1 oz	35	1	—	30	7	0	—	—	15	—	—	—	—
Chili	1 oz	43	1	—	22	8	1	—	—	100	—	—	—	—
Chips	1 oz	140	6	—	0	2	19	—	—	80	—	—	—	—
Cilantro	1 oz	8	0	—	0	1	1	—	—	15	—	—	—	—
Dinner Rice, Beans, Broccoli	1 serv (10 oz)	328	tr	—	0	11	72	—	—	330	—	—	—	—
Dinner Rice, Beans, Salad	1 serv (12 oz)	344	tr	—	0	11	76	—	—	370	—	—	—	—
El Bento	1 serv (16 oz)	600	2	—	63	30	121	—	—	776	—	—	—	—
El Bento Deluxe	1 serv (20 oz)	740	7	—	65	35	136	—	—	902	—	—	—	—
Enchilada Chicken	1 (12 oz)	533	13	—	92	35	71	—	—	825	—	—	—	—
Enchilada Chili	1 (12 oz)	549	13	—	76	37	73	—	—	995	—	—	—	—
Enchilada Veggie	1 (14 oz)	623	11	—	32	27	106	—	—	955	—	—	—	—
Enchilada Sauce	1 oz	6	0	—	0	0	2	—	—	65	—	—	—	—
Fresh Greens	1 oz	2	0	—	0	0	0	—	—	5	—	—	—	—
Green Sauce	1 oz	5	0	—	0	0	1	—	—	110	—	—	—	—
Guacamole	1 oz	100	3	—	0	0	19	—	—	110	—	—	—	—
Marinated Veggies	1 oz	10	tr	—	0	0	3	—	—	20	—	—	—	—
Mexican Cheese	1 oz	100	8	—	24	7	0	—	—	280	—	—	—	—
Mustard Dressing	1 oz	25	tr	—	0	1	3	—	—	200	—	—	—	—
Power Salad Chicken	1 serv (16 oz)	275	1	—	63	23	44	—	—	444	—	—	—	—
Power Salad Veggie	1 serv (13 oz)	200	tr	—	0	6	44	—	—	275	—	—	—	—
Rice	1 oz	45	tr	—	0	1	11	—	—	50	—	—	—	—
Salad Chicken	1 serv (15 oz)	430	8	—	110	33	56	—	—	655	—	—	—	—
Salad Veggie Taco	1 serv (16 oz)	655	14	—	20	21	110	—	—	755	—	—	—	—
Salsa	1 oz	4	0	—	0	0	1	—	—	45	—	—	—	—
Snack Famouse #5	1 serv (14 oz)	585	5	—	20	23	114	—	—	747	—	—	—	—
Snack Nacho Grande	1 serv (9 oz)	841	41	—	62	35	84	—	—	960	—	—	—	—
Snack Quesadilla Cheese	1 serv (6 oz)	377	13	—	42	22	42	—	—	610	—	—	—	—
Snack Quesadilla Chicken	1 serv (10 oz)	450	15	—	102	35	42	—	—	650	—	—	—	—

FOOD	PORTION	CALORIES	FAT	SAT FAT	CHOL	PROTEIN	CARBO	FIBER	CALCIUM	SOD	POTAS	VIT C	FOLIC	VIT A
Snack Tacos Chicken	1 serv (6 oz)	290	8	—	82	25	34	—	—	295	—	—	—	—
Snack Tacos Chili	1 serv (6 oz)	314	8	—	66	28	36	—	—	465	—	—	—	—
Snack Tacos Veggie	1 serv (6 oz)	290	6	—	22	16	48	—	—	325	—	—	—	—
Sour Cream	1 oz	23	0	—	0	2	4	—	—	25	—	—	—	—
Tortilla Corn	3 (1 oz)	60	0	—	0	2	15	—	—	5	—	—	—	—
Tortilla Flour	1 oz	80	3	—	0	2	16	—	—	70	—	—	—	—
Tortilla Wheat	1 oz	80	3	—	0	3	15	—	—	65	—	—	—	—
Veggie Deluxe	1 serv (18 oz)	665	6	—	2	17	136	—	—	733	—	—	—	—
Yogurt Nonfat	1 oz	20	tr	—	0	2	2	—	—	22	—	—	—	—

MANHATTAN BAGEL

FOOD	PORTION	CALORIES	FAT	SAT FAT	CHOL	PROTEIN	CARBO	FIBER	CALCIUM	SOD	POTAS	VIT C	FOLIC	VIT A
Blueberry	1 (4 oz)	260	tr	0	0	9	54	2	20	560	—	0	—	0
Cheddar Cheese	1 (4 oz)	270	4	2	10	11	48	2	80	560	—	0	—	0
Chocolate Chip	1 (4 oz)	290	3	2	0	9	56	2	40	530	—	0	—	0
Cinnamon Raisin	1 (4 oz)	280	tr	0	0	10	57	3	40	560	—	0	—	0
Egg	1 (4 oz)	270	2	0	0	10	53	2	40	710	—	0	—	0
Everything	1 (4 oz)	290	3	0	0	11	54	3	60	2000	—	1	—	0
Garlic	1 (4 oz)	270	tr	0	0	10	55	2	40	560	—	2	—	0
Jalapeno Cheddar	1 (4 oz)	260	2	0	0	16	53	2	40	310	—	1	—	0
Marble	1 (4 oz)	260	tr	0	0	10	52	3	40	540	—	0	—	0
Oat Bran	1 (4 oz)	260	1	0	0	10	53	3	20	470	—	0	—	0
Oat Bran Raisin Walnut	1 (4 oz)	270	3	0	0	10	54	3	20	450	—	0	—	0
Onion	1 (4 oz)	270	tr	0	0	10	55	2	40	560	—	2	—	0
Plain	1 (4 oz)	260	tr	0	0	10	52	2	20	560	—	0	—	0
Poppy	1 (4 oz)	300	4	1	0	11	54	5	150	560	—	0	—	0
Pumpernickel	1 (4 oz)	250	1	0	0	10	52	3	20	530	—	0	—	0
Rye	1 (4 oz)	260	1	0	0	10	52	3	40	560	—	0	—	0
Salt	1 (4 oz)	260	tr	0	0	10	53	2	150	7100	—	0	—	0
Sesame	1 (4 oz)	310	5	1	0	11	55	3	100	560	—	0	—	0
Spinach	1 (4 oz)	270	tr	0	0	10	54	3	40	580	—	2	—	250
Sun-Dried Tomato	1 (4 oz)	260	1	0	0	10	53	3	40	340	—	1	—	0
Whole Wheat	1 (4 oz)	260	tr	0	0	10	52	3	20	470	—	0	—	0

MAX & IRMA'S

FOOD	PORTION	CALORIES	FAT	SAT FAT	CHOL	PROTEIN	CARBO	FIBER	CALCIUM	SOD	POTAS	VIT C	FOLIC	VIT A
Black Bean Roll Up	1 serv	401	8	3	13	—	—	—	—	534	—	—	—	—
Fat Free French	2 tbsp	126	tr	0	0	—	—	—	—	1034	—	—	—	—
Fat Free Honey Mustard	2 tbsp	60	0	0	0	—	—	—	—	280	—	—	—	—
Fruit Smoothie	1 serv	114	tr	tr	0	—	—	—	—	3	—	—	—	—
Garden Grill	1 serv	467	7	3	12	—	—	—	—	911	—	—	—	—
Garlic Breadstick	1	156	6	0	0	—	—	—	—	293	—	—	—	—
Gourmet Garden Grill	1 serv	484	8	3	12	—	—	—	—	912	—	—	—	—
Grilled Zucchini & Mushroom Pasta	1 serv	448	10	4	13	—	—	—	—	—	—	—	—	—

FOOD	PORTION	CALORIES	FAT	SAT FAT	CHOL	PROTEIN	CARBO	FIBER	CALCIUM	SOD	POTAS	VIT C	FOLIC	VIT A
Grilled Zucchini & Mushroom Pasta w/ Chicken	1 serv	621	18	6	78	—	—	—	—	—	—	—	—	—
Hula Bowl w/ Fat Free Honey Mustard Dressing	1 serv	526	8	1	91	—	—	—	—	1309	—	—	—	—
Lo-Cal Ranch	2 tbsp	54	6	1	7	—	—	—	—	141	—	—	—	—
Tijuana Tortilla Wrap	1	692	15	3	54	—	—	—	—	1958	—	—	—	—

MCDONALD'S

BAKED SELECTIONS

FOOD	PORTION	CALORIES	FAT	SAT FAT	CHOL	PROTEIN	CARBO	FIBER	CALCIUM	SOD	POTAS	VIT C	FOLIC	VIT A
Apple Pie Baked	1 (2.7 oz)	260	13	4	0	3	34	tr	20	200	—	24	—	—
Chocolate Chip Cookie	1 (1.2 oz)	170	10	6	20	2	22	1	20	120	—	—	—	200
Cinnamon Roll	1 (3.3 oz)	400	20	5	75	7	47	2	80	340	—	—	—	500
Danish Apple	1 (3.7 oz)	360	16	5	40	5	51	1	80	290	—	—	—	500
Danish Cheese	1 (3.7 oz)	410	22	8	70	7	47	0	80	340	—	—	—	750
Lowfat Muffin Apple Bran	1 (4 oz)	300	3	1	0	6	61	3	100	380	—	—	—	—
McDonaldland Cookies	1 pkg (1.5 oz)	180	5	1	0	3	32	1	20	190	—	—	—	—

BREAKFAST SELECTIONS

FOOD	PORTION	CALORIES	FAT	SAT FAT	CHOL	PROTEIN	CARBO	FIBER	CALCIUM	SOD	POTAS	VIT C	FOLIC	VIT A
Bacon Egg & Cheese Biscuit	1 (5.5 oz)	470	25	8	235	18	36	1	100	1250	—	—	—	500
Biscuit	1 (2.9 oz)	290	15	3	0	5	34	1	60	780	—	—	—	—
Breakfast Burrito	1 (4.1 oz)	320	19	7	195	13	23	1	80	600	—	9	—	500
Egg McMuffin	1 (4.8 oz)	290	14	5	235	17	27	1	150	710	—	1	—	500
English Muffin	1 (1.9 oz)	140	2	0	0	4	25	1	100	210	—	—	—	—
Hash Browns	1 serv (1.9 oz)	130	8	2	0	1	14	1	—	330	—	2	—	—
Hotcakes Margarine & Syrup	2 serv (7.8 oz)	570	16	3	15	9	100	2	100	750	—	—	—	400
Hotcakes Plain	1 serv (5.3 oz)	310	7	2	15	9	53	2	100	610	—	—	—	—
Sausage	1 (1.5 oz)	170	16	5	35	6	0	0	—	290	—	—	—	—
Sausage Biscuit	1 (4.5 oz)	470	31	9	35	11	35	1	80	1080	—	—	—	—
Sausage Biscuit With Egg	1 (6.2 oz)	550	37	10	245	18	35	1	100	1160	—	—	—	300
Sausage McMuffin	1 (3.9 oz)	360	23	8	45	13	26	1	150	740	—	—	—	200
Sausage McMuffin With Egg	1 (5.7 oz)	440	28	10	255	19	27	1	150	810	—	—	—	500
Scrambled Eggs	2 (3.6 oz)	160	11	4	425	13	1	0	40	170	—	—	—	500

DESSERTS

FOOD	PORTION	CALORIES	FAT	SAT FAT	CHOL	PROTEIN	CARBO	FIBER	CALCIUM	SOD	POTAS	VIT C	FOLIC	VIT A
Nuts For Sundaes	1 serv (7 g)	40	4	0	0	2	2	0	—	0	—	—	—	—
Reduced Fat Ice Cream Cone Vanilla	1 (3.2 oz)	150	5	3	20	4	23	0	100	75	—	1	—	300
Sundae Hot Caramel	1 (6.4 oz)	360	10	6	35	7	61	0	250	180	—	1	—	500

FOOD	PORTION	CALORIES	FAT	SAT FAT	CHOL	PROTEIN	CARBO	FIBER	CALCIUM	SOD	POTAS	VIT C	FOLIC	VIT A
Sundae Hot Fudge	1 (6.3 oz)	340	12	9	30	8	52	1	250	170	—	1	—	500
Sundae Strawberry	1 (6.2 oz)	290	7	5	30	7	50	tr	300	95	—	1	—	500
MAIN MENU SELECTIONS														
Arch Deluxe	1 (8.4 oz)	550	31	11	55	38	39	4	60	1010	—	6	—	500
Arch Deluxe With Bacon	1 (8.7 oz)	590	34	12	60	32	39	4	60	1150	—	6	—	500
Barbeque Sauce	1 pkg (1 oz)	45	0	0	0	0	10	0	—	250	—	4	—	—
Big Mac	1 (7.5 oz)	560	31	10	85	26	45	3	200	1070	—	4	—	300
Cheeseburger	1 (4.2 oz)	320	13	6	40	15	35	2	150	820	—	2	—	300
Chicken McNuggets	4 pieces (2.5 oz)	190	11	3	40	12	10	0	—	340	—	—	—	—
Chicken McNuggets	6 pieces (3.7 oz)	290	17	4	60	18	15	0	20	510	—	—	—	—
Chicken McNuggets	9 pieces (5.6 oz)	430	26	5	90	27	23	0	20	770	—	—	—	—
Crispy Chicken Deluxe	1 (7.8 oz)	500	25	4	55	26	43	3	60	1100	—	5	—	300
Fish Filet Deluxe	1 (8 oz)	560	28	6	30	23	54	4	80	1060	—	2	—	300
French Fries	1 sm (2.4 oz)	210	10	2	0	3	26	2	—	135	—	9	—	—
French Fries	1 lg (5.2 oz)	450	22	4	0	6	57	5	20	290	—	18	—	—
French Fries	1 super (6.2 oz)	540	26	5	0	8	68	6	20	350	—	21	—	—
Grilled Chicken Deluxe	1 (7.8 oz)	440	20	3	60	27	38	3	60	1040	—	5	—	300
Grilled Chicken Deluxe Plain w/o Mayonnaise	1 (7.2 oz)	300	5	1	50	27	38	3	60	930	—	5	—	200
Grilled Chicken Salad Deluxe	1 serv (9 oz)	120	2	0	45	21	7	2	40	240	—	24	—	6000
Hamburger	1 (3.7 oz)	260	9	4	30	13	34	2	150	580	—	2	—	—
Honey	1 pkg (0.5 oz)	45	0	0	0	0	12	0	—	0	—	—	—	—
Honey Mustard	1 pkg (0.5 oz)	40	5	1	10	0	3	0	—	85	—	—	—	—
Hot Mustard	1 pkg (1 oz)	60	4	0	5	1	7	tr	—	240	—	—	—	—
Light Mayonnaise	1 pkg (0.4 oz)	40	4	1	5	0	tr	0	0	85	—	0	—	0
Quarter Pounder	1 (6 oz)	420	21	8	70	23	37	2	150	820	—	2	—	100
Quarter Pounder With Cheese	1 (7 oz)	530	30	13	95	28	38	2	150	1290	—	2	—	500
Sweet 'N Sour Sauce	1 pkg (1 oz)	50	0	0	0	0	11	0	—	140	—	—	—	300
SALAD DRESSINGS														
Caesar	1 pkg (2.1 oz)	160	14	3	20	2	7	0	60	450	—	—	—	100
Fat Free Herb Vinaigrette	1 pkg (2.1 oz)	50	0	0	0	0	11	0	—	330	—	1	—	—
Ranch	1 pkg (2.1 oz)	230	21	3	20	1	10	0	40	550	—	1	—	—
Reduced Calorie Red French	1 pkg (2.1 oz)	160	8	1	0	0	23	0	—	490	—	4	—	200

FOOD	PORTION	CALORIES	FAT	SAT FAT	CHOL	PROTEIN	CARBO	FIBER	CALCIUM	SOD	POTAS	VIT C	FOLIC	VIT A
SALADS AND SALAD BARS														
Croutons	1 pkg (0.4 oz)	50	2	0	0	2	7	tr	—	80	—	—	—	—
Garden Salad	1 serv (6.2 oz)	35	0	0	0	2	7	2	40	20	—	24	—	6000

MORRISON'S

FOOD	PORTION	CALORIES	FAT	SAT FAT	CHOL	PROTEIN	CARBO	FIBER	CALCIUM	SOD	POTAS	VIT C	FOLIC	VIT A
DESSERTS														
Boston Cream Cake	1 slice	218	4	—	—	—	—	—	—	171	—	—	—	—
MAIN MENU SELECTIONS														
Baked Potato	1	220	tr	—	—	—	—	—	—	16	—	—	—	—
Broccoli	1 serv (4 oz)	37	2	—	—	—	—	—	—	310	—	—	—	—
Cabbage	1 serv (4 oz)	36	tr	—	—	—	—	—	—	190	—	—	—	—
Cantaloupe Compote	1 serv (4 oz)	130	1	—	—	—	—	—	—	30	—	—	—	—
Cauliflower	1 serv (4 oz)	68	5	—	—	—	—	—	—	178	—	—	—	—
Chicken Stew & Dumplings	1 serv (7 oz)	362	14	—	—	—	—	—	—	468	—	—	—	—
Chicken Teriyaki	1 serv (5.5 oz)	232	10	—	—	—	—	—	—	1187	—	—	—	—
French Bread	1 slice	207	2	—	—	—	—	—	—	413	—	—	—	—
Grilled Chicken Pecan Salad	1 serv (6 oz)	298	8	—	—	—	—	—	—	635	—	—	—	—
Lima Beans	1 serv (4 oz)	170	4	—	—	—	—	—	—	300	—	—	—	—
Okra & Tomatoes	1 serv (5 oz)	40	2	—	—	—	—	—	—	233	—	—	—	—
Pinto Beans	1 serv (4 oz)	105	4	—	—	—	—	—	—	332	—	—	—	—
Plain Jello	1 serv (3 oz)	131	tr	—	—	—	—	—	—	109	—	—	—	—
Rutabagas	1 serv (4 oz)	33	1	—	—	—	—	—	—	147	—	—	—	—
Sliced Tomato	4 slices	40	1	—	—	—	—	—	—	20	—	—	—	—
Soft Roll	1 (2 oz)	170	4	—	—	—	—	—	—	200	—	—	—	—
Strawberries & Banana Bowl	1 serv (6 oz)	203	1	—	—	—	—	—	—	4	—	—	—	—
Strawberries Peaches & Bananas	1 serv (6 oz)	203	1	—	—	—	—	—	—	4	—	—	—	—
Turnip Greens	1 serv (4 oz)	30	2	—	—	—	—	—	—	365	—	—	—	—
Watermelon	1 serv (6 oz)	102	1	—	—	—	—	—	—	6	—	—	—	—
Yellow Squash	1 serv (4 oz)	22	1	—	—	—	—	—	—	179	—	—	—	—
SALADS AND SALAD BARS														
Garden Salad	1 serv (2.5 oz)	75	2	—	—	—	—	—	—	163	—	—	—	—
Tossed Salad	1 serv (3 oz)	30	tr	—	—	—	—	—	—	18	—	—	—	—

MRS. FIELDS

FOOD	PORTION	CALORIES	FAT	SAT FAT	CHOL	PROTEIN	CARBO	FIBER	CALCIUM	SOD	POTAS	VIT C	FOLIC	VIT A
Brownie Double Fudge	1 (3.1 oz)	420	20	11	35	5	56	3	20	125	—	0	—	500
Brownie Fudge Walnut	1 (3.4 oz)	500	29	10	40	7	54	4	40	135	—	1	—	400
Brownie Pecan Fudge	1 (2.8 oz)	390	21	9	40	4	48	2	20	135	—	1	—	300
Brownie Pecan Pie	1 (3 oz)	400	21	7	55	5	48	4	60	160	—	1	—	400

FOOD	PORTION	CALORIES	FAT	SAT FAT	CHOL	PROTEIN	CARBO	FIBER	CALCIUM	SOD	POTAS	VIT C	FOLIC	VIT A
Cookie Chewy Fudge	1 (1.7 oz)	230	12	7	25	3	32	1	20	100	—	0	—	200
Cookie Coconut Macadamia	1 (1.7 oz)	250	15	7	35	3	28	1	20	230	—	0	—	300
Cookie Milk Chocolate Chip	1 (1.7 oz)	240	12	7	35	3	32	1	40	210	—	0	—	300
Cookie Milk Chocolate Macadamia	1 (1.7 oz)	250	14	7	30	3	29	1	40	190	—	0	—	300
Cookie Milk Chocolate w/ Walnuts	1 (1.7 oz)	250	13	7	30	3	30	1	40	200	—	0	—	300
Cookie Oatmeal Raisin	1 (1.7 oz)	220	10	5	30	3	31	2	20	230	—	0	—	300
Cookie Peanut Butter	1 (1.7 oz)	240	13	6	40	4	27	1	20	280	—	0	—	300
Cookie Semi-Sweet Chocolate	1 (1.7 oz)	230	12	7	30	3	32	1	40	210	—	0	—	300
Cookie Semi-Sweet Chocolate w/ Walnuts	1 (1.8 oz)	240	13	7	30	3	30	2	20	190	—	0	—	200
Cookie Triple Chocolate	1 (1.7 oz)	230	12	7	30	3	31	1	30	210	—	0	—	300
Cookie White Chunk Macadamia	1 (1.7 oz)	260	15	7	30	3	29	tr	40	190	—	0	—	300
Muffin Banana Walnut	1 (3.9 oz)	460	24	5	45	9	53	5	60	390	—	1	—	400
Muffin Blueberry	1 (4 oz)	390	15	6	45	6	58	2	60	470	—	0	—	500
Muffin Chocolate Chip	1 (4 oz)	450	19	8	40	7	65	5	60	470	—	1	—	300
Muffin Mandarin Orange	1 (4 oz)	420	17	7	45	6	59	1	40	490	—	1	—	500
Peanut Butter Dream Bar	1 (5 oz)	750	40	18	40	11	85	8	80	270	—	0	—	750
PRETZELS														
Hot Sam Bavarian	1 reg (2.5 oz)	200	0	0	0	7	42	2	20	390	—	0	—	0
Hot Sam Bavarian	1 lg (5.1 oz)	390	0	0	0	14	83	4	40	780	—	0	—	0
Hot Sam Bavarian Stix	10 (5 oz)	390	0	0	0	14	83	4	40	780	—	0	—	0
Hot Sam Sweet Dough	1 (4.5 oz)	360	3	1	0	11	73	4	40	780	—	0	—	0
Hot Sam Sweet Dough Blueberry	1 (4.5 oz)	400	4	2	0	11	81	2	40	610	—	0	—	0

MY FAVORITE MUFFIN

FOOD	PORTION	CALORIES	FAT	SAT FAT	CHOL	PROTEIN	CARBO	FIBER	CALCIUM	SOD	POTAS	VIT C	FOLIC	VIT A
Basic Muffin	⅓ muffin	220	10	2	0	3	30	0	0	190	—	0	—	0
Double Chocolate	⅓ muffin	190	8	2	0	2	30	2	0	230	—	0	—	0
Fat Free Bavarian	⅓ muffin	100	0	0	0	2	24	1	0	140	—	0	—	0

FOOD	PORTION	CALORIES	FAT	SAT FAT	CHOL	PROTEIN	CARBO	FIBER	CALCIUM	SOD	POTAS	VIT C	FOLIC	VIT A
Fat Free Bavarian Chocolate	⅓ muffin	130	0	0	0	3	31	3	0	200	—	0	—	0

NATHAN'S

MAIN MENU SELECTIONS

FOOD	PORTION	CALORIES	FAT	SAT FAT	CHOL	PROTEIN	CARBO	FIBER	CALCIUM	SOD	POTAS	VIT C	FOLIC	VIT A
Breaded Chicken Sandwich	1 (7.2 oz)	510	25	4	56	23	48	—	123	927	—	4	—	185
Charbroiled Chicken Sandwich	1 (4.5 oz)	288	5	1	53	35	24	—	64	861	—	2	—	51
Cheese Steak Sandwich	1 (6.1 oz)	485	26	10	73	26	37	—	122	579	—	2	—	104
Chicken 2 Pieces	1 serv (7.1 oz)	693	44	9	211	48	26	—	67	958	—	0	—	81
Chicken 4 Pieces	1 serv (14.2 oz)	1382	88	18	422	96	52	—	134	1912	—	0	—	162
Chicken Platter 2 Pieces	1 serv (14.8 oz)	1096	66	14	212	54	72	—	102	1413	—	13	—	93
Chicken Platter 4 Pieces	1 serv (21.9 oz)	1788	109	23	425	102	99	—	188	2369	—	13	—	169
Chicken Salad	1 serv (12.7 oz)	154	4	1	49	20	9	—	76	345	—	8	—	436
Double Burger	1 (7.3 oz)	671	41	18	154	44	32	—	67	460	—	0	—	0
Filet of Fish Platter	1 serv (22 oz)	1455	74	10	147	61	137	—	213	1837	—	32	—	878
Filet of Fish Sandwich	1 (5.2 oz)	403	15	2	32	20	46	—	60	714	—	2	—	238
Frank Nuggets	11 pieces (5.1 oz)	563	38	10	73	15	40	—	71	1173	—	0	—	0
Frank Nuggets	15 pieces (6.9 oz)	764	52	13	99	20	54	—	97	1594	—	0	—	0
Frank Nuggets	7 pieces (3.2 oz)	357	24	6	46	9	25	—	45	744	—	0	—	0
Frankfurter	1 (3.2 oz)	310	19	8	45	13	22	—	72	820	—	0	—	0
French Fries	1 serv (8.6 oz)	514	26	4	0	9	62	—	39	61	—	0	—	0
Fried Clam Platter	1 serv (13.1 oz)	1024	51	7	49	23	119	—	120	1826	—	15	—	285
Fried Clam Sandwich	1 (5.4 oz)	620	29	4	44	17	72	—	68	1417	—	2	—	186
Fried Shrimp	1 serv (4.4 oz)	348	11	2	71	15	47	—	210	869	—	0	—	0
Fried Shrimp Platter	1 serv (12.6 oz)	796	34	5	83	23	100	—	443	1436	—	14	—	11
Hamburger	1 (4.7 oz)	434	23	10	77	25	32	—	131	281	—	0	—	0
Knish	1 (5.9 oz)	318	7	2	2	10	53	—	111	822	—	3	—	67
Pastrami Sandwich	1 (4.1 oz)	325	12	4	48	21	34	—	67	1013	—	0	—	0
Sauteed Onions	1 serv (3.5 oz)	39	1	0	0	1	6	—	34	16	—	1	—	0
Super Burger	1 (7.6 oz)	533	32	9	86	27	34	—	74	525	—	5	—	239
Turkey Sandwich	1 (4.9 oz)	270	2	0	27	28	34	—	45	1458	—	2	—	28

SALADS AND SALAD BARS

FOOD	PORTION	CALORIES	FAT	SAT FAT	CHOL	PROTEIN	CARBO	FIBER	CALCIUM	SOD	POTAS	VIT C	FOLIC	VIT A
Garden Salad	1 serv (10.9 oz)	193	13	7	36	10	10	—	401	261	—	6	—	498

FOOD	PORTION	CALORIES	FAT	SAT FAT	CHOL	PROTEIN	CARBO	FIBER	CALCIUM	SOD	POTAS	VIT C	FOLIC	VIT A

NEWPORT CREAMERY

ICE CREAM

FOOD	PORTION	CALORIES	FAT	SAT FAT	CHOL	PROTEIN	CARBO	FIBER	CALCIUM	SOD	POTAS	VIT C	FOLIC	VIT A
Reduced Fat No Sugar Added Chocolate	½ cup (2.6 oz)	110	3	2	0	4	22	1	100	80	—	0	—	100
Reduced Fat No Sugar Added Coffee	½ cup (2.6 oz)	100	4	2	15	4	18	0	150	70	—	0	—	100
Soft Serve Nonfat Frozen Yogurt Cone or Dish	1 reg (5 oz)	125	0	0	0	—	—	—	—	—	—	—	—	—
SALAD DRESSINGS														
Corn Oil & Vinegar	1 tbsp	45	6	0	0	—	—	—	—	—	—	—	—	—
Fat Free Ranch	1½ oz	48	0	0	0	—	—	—	—	—	—	—	—	—
Low-Cal French	1½ oz	48	0	0	0	—	—	—	—	—	—	—	—	—
SALADS AND SALAD BARS														
Chef's Salad	1 serv	215	8	—	50	—	—	—	—	—	—	—	—	—
Chicken Fajita	1 serv	295	20	—	44	—	—	—	—	—	—	—	—	—
Grilled Chicken	1 serv	247	13	—	48	—	—	—	—	—	—	—	—	—
SANDWICHES														
Lite Chicken Salad	1	379	19	—	63	—	—	—	—	—	—	—	—	—
Lite Grilled Cheese	1	274	17	—	30	—	—	—	—	—	—	—	—	—
Lite Grilled Chicken Breast Pocket	1	327	12	—	74	—	—	—	—	—	—	—	—	—
Lite Sliced Turkey	1	288	12	—	32	—	—	—	—	—	—	—	—	—
Lite Tuna Salad	1	358	21	—	23	—	—	—	—	—	—	—	—	—
Lite Vegetarian Pocket Broccoli Mushrooms Onions Peppers Cheese	1	211	5	—	15	—	—	—	—	—	—	—	—	—
Lite Vegetarian Pocket Broccoli Cheese	1	214	5	—	15	—	—	—	—	—	—	—	—	—
Lite Vegetarian Pocket Peppers Onions Mushrooms Cheese	1	230	6	—	15	—	—	—	—	—	—	—	—	—
Low Fat Cheese	1 slice	73	4	—	15	—	—	—	—	—	—	—	—	—
Mayonnaise	2 tsp	71	8	—	5	—	—	—	—	—	—	—	—	—
Smart Sides Broccoli	1 serv	23	tr	—	0	—	—	—	—	—	—	—	—	—
Smart Sides Cottage Cheese	1 serv	90	4	—	13	—	—	—	—	—	—	—	—	—
Smart Sides Side Salad	1 serv	30	0	0	0	—	—	—	—	—	—	—	—	—

FOOD	PORTION	CALORIES	FAT	SAT FAT	CHOL	PROTEIN	CARBO	FIBER	CALCIUM	SOD	POTAS	VIT C	FOLIC	VIT A
OLIVE GARDEN														
Garden Fare Apple Carmellina	1 serv (12.2 oz)	560	2	1	5	6	131	—	—	190	—	—	—	—
Garden Fare Dinner Capellini Pomodoro	1 serv (21.1 oz)	610	16	3	5	19	98	—	—	940	—	—	—	—
Garden Fare Dinner Capellini Primavera	1 serv (20.1 oz)	400	7	4	15	18	68	—	—	950	—	—	—	—
Garden Fare Dinner Capellini Primavera w/ Chicken	1 serv (23.8 oz)	560	10	5	95	47	71	—	—	1030	—	—	—	—
Garden Fare Dinner Chicken Giardino	1 serv (20.6 oz)	550	11	4	85	42	71	—	—	1000	—	—	—	—
Garden Fare Dinner Linguine Alla Marinara	1 serv (16.3 oz)	500	9	2	0	16	89	—	—	160	—	—	—	—
Garden Fare Dinner Penne Fra Diavolo	1 serv (14.3 oz)	420	7	3	10	13	77	—	—	940	—	—	—	—
Garden Fare Dinner Shrimp Primavera	1 serv (28.4 oz)	740	15	5	290	48	104	—	—	1630	—	—	—	—
Garden Fare Lunch Capellini Pamodoro	1 serv (11.7 oz)	360	9	2	5	12	57	—	—	540	—	—	—	—
Garden Fare Lunch Capellini Primavera	1 serv (11.2 oz)	260	5	3	15	12	42	—	—	560	—	—	—	—
Garden Fare Lunch Capellini Primavera w/ Chicken	1 serv (14.9 oz)	420	8	4	90	41	45	—	—	640	—	—	—	—
Garden Fare Lunch Chicken Giardino	1 serv (12.8 oz)	360	9	4	50	23	47	—	—	900	—	—	—	—
Garden Fare Lunch Linguine Alla Marinara	1 serv (10.2 oz)	310	6	1	0	10	54	—	—	105	—	—	—	—
Garden Fare Lunch Penne Fra Diavolo	1 serv (10.2 oz)	300	5	2	10	9	57	—	—	640	—	—	—	—
Garden Fare Lunch Shrimp Primavera	1 serv (15.2 oz)	410	8	3	145	25	60	—	—	840	—	—	—	—
Minestrone Soup	1 serv (6 oz)	80	1	0	0	4	15	—	—	450	—	—	—	—
PERKINS														
Low Fat Brownie	1 (5.4 oz)	260	1	—	—	—	—	—	—	—	—	—	—	—
Low Fat Muffin Banana	1 (5.8 oz)	330	3	—	—	—	—	—	—	—	—	—	—	—

FOOD	PORTION	CALORIES	FAT	SAT FAT	CHOL	PROTEIN	CARBO	FIBER	CALCIUM	SOD	POTAS	VIT C	FOLIC	VIT A
Low Fat Muffin Blueberry	1 (5.8 oz)	270	3	—	—	—	—	—	—	—	—	—	—	—
Low Fat Muffin Honey Bran	1 (5.8 oz)	270	3	—	—	—	—	—	—	—	—	—	—	—
Low Fat Muffin Plain	1 (5.8 oz)	300	3	—	—	—	—	—	—	—	—	—	—	—

PICCADILLY CAFETERIA

BAKED SELECTIONS

FOOD	PORTION	CALORIES	FAT	SAT FAT	CHOL	PROTEIN	CARBO	FIBER	CALCIUM	SOD	POTAS	VIT C	FOLIC	VIT A
Corn Sticks	1 (2 oz)	165	10	—	26	3	17	tr	63	385	44	0	4	46
French Bread	1 slice	132	2	—	6	4	24	4	11	199	53	0	57	9
Garlic Bread	1 serv (15.8 oz)	1154	24	—	48	35	195	34	95	1718	432	0	454	530
Mexican Corn Bread	1 piece	220	14	—	31	4	21	1	80	547	76	8	7	124
Roll	1 (2 oz)	130	2	—	0	4	23	4	19	195	53	0	33	0
Roll Whole Wheat	1 (1.7 oz)	117	1	—	19	4	22	3	9	159	31	0	33	29
Texas Toast	1 serv (15.5 oz)	1088	17	—	48	35	195	34	91	1633	425	0	454	209

DESSERTS

FOOD	PORTION	CALORIES	FAT	SAT FAT	CHOL	PROTEIN	CARBO	FIBER	CALCIUM	SOD	POTAS	VIT C	FOLIC	VIT A
Apple Pie	1 slice (7.2 oz)	439	19	—	0	4	67	3	33	476	137	5	2	165
Cantaloupe	1 serv (9 oz)	89	1	—	0	2	21	3	28	23	788	108	43	8226
Cantaloupe	1 serv (5.5 oz)	55	tr	—	0	1	13	2	17	14	482	66	27	5027
Chocolate Cream Pie	1 slice (7.5 oz)	512	25	—	66	9	65	tr	141	655	243	1	12	202
Custard	1 cup (5.4 oz)	183	1	—	25	6	39	0	183	358	262	1	10	41
Custard Pie	1 slice (6.2 oz)	412	18	—	18	8	54	tr	156	630	221	1	7	29
Dole Whip Topping	1 serv (3 oz)	68	1	—	0	0	15	0	0	14	19	10	0	0
Fresh Fruit Plate	1 serv (21.1 oz)	389	5	—	11	13	81	9	101	306	1373	159	65	6437
Gelatin	1 serv (4.75 oz)	128	4	—	14	2	22	0	6	94	8	0	0	146
Honeydew Melon	1 serv (5.5 oz)	55	tr	—	0	1	14	1	9	16	423	39	—	62
Honeydew Melon	1 serv (9 oz)	89	tr	—	0	1	23	2	15	26	691	63	—	102
Lemon Chiffon Pie	1 slice (6.3 oz)	481	20	—	32	14	61	tr	43	645	185	4	13	119
Pound Cake	1 slice (3.8 oz)	371	17	—	76	5	51	0	92	744	59	1	9	352
Watermelon	1 serv (11 oz)	100	1	—	0	2	22	1	25	6	362	30	7	1141

MAIN MENU SELECTIONS

FOOD	PORTION	CALORIES	FAT	SAT FAT	CHOL	PROTEIN	CARBO	FIBER	CALCIUM	SOD	POTAS	VIT C	FOLIC	VIT A
Au Jus	1 serv (3 oz)	5	tr	—	0	tr	1	0	0	537	13	0	0	0
Baby Lima Beans	1 serv (4.5 oz)	151	6	—	0	5	19	4	30	371	345	8	33	377
Baked Potato	1	218	tr	—	0	4	50	4	20	16	836	26	22	—
Baked Potato w/ Topping	1	350	15	—	33	5	51	4	43	119	864	26	24	487
Beef Chopped Steak Fried	1 serv (4 oz)	311	23	—	59	22	4	0	12	457	305	0	6	6
Beef Leg Roast	1 serv (4 oz)	311	18	—	92	34	1	tr	14	472	490	1	11	1187
Beef Liver Fried	1 serv (4.5 oz)	430	29	—	418	25	15	2	15	404	333	20	196	31460

FOOD	PORTION	CALORIES	FAT	SAT FAT	CHOL	PROTEIN	CARBO	FIBER	CALCIUM	SOD	POTAS	VIT C	FOLIC	VIT A
Beef Tips Braised	1 serv (10 oz)	470	26	—	56	30	41	3	59	828	782	9	25	16006
Black-eyed Peas w/ Pork Jowls	1 serv (4 oz)	108	6	—	7	4	9	0	14	386	14	4	0	33
Broccoli Buttered	1 serv (4 oz)	77	6	—	0	3	5	3	41	273	230	62	86	1531
Broccoli & Rice Au Gratin	½ cup	184	9	—	18	7	20	1	153	577	131	17	24	863
Carrots Young Buttered	½ cup	90	6	—	0	1	9	1	38	512	312	8	0	10213
Cauliflower Buttered	1 serv	80	6	—	0	2	6	2	36	260	406	81	75	253
Chicken Baked w/o Skin	¼ chicken	352	11	—	168	59	tr	0	32	401	489	1	9	74
Chicken Teriyaki	1 serv (4 oz)	445	22	—	124	45	14	tr	37	1432	461	3	6	177
Chicken Teriyaki Polynesian	1 serv (4 oz)	537	27	—	104	39	34	1	50	2051	219	9	8	432
Corn	1 serv (4.5 oz)	128	7	—	0	3	17	0	5	423	3	5	0	396
Cornbread Stuffing	1 serv (4.5 oz)	164	9	—	26	9	12	tr	44	597	139	2	7	47
Crackers	4 (0.4 oz)	51	1	—	—	1	8	tr	18	172	20	—	—	—
Cranberry Sauce	1 serv (1.5 oz)	64	tr	—	0	tr	17	tr	2	12	11	1	—	9
Eggplant Escalloped	½ cup	180	10	—	15	4	19	1	130	928	308	3	17	316
Fish Baked	1 serv (7 oz)	195	10	—	54	24	3	tr	73	532	550	18	1	183
Green Beans	1 serv (4.5 oz)	77	6	—	7	2	5	1	32	552	143	7	24	424
Ham Baked	1 serv (4 oz)	224	10	—	67	26	6	0	14	1703	485	26	3	0
Macaroni & Cheese	½ cup	317	11	—	22	15	38	2	343	1752	364	1	19	509
Mashed Potatoes	1 serv (4.8 oz)	120	3	—	0	3	20	0	31	62	374	5	0	117
Meatballs Baked & Spaghetti	1 serv (11.5 oz)	108	5	—	23	9	7	tr	66	419	177	4	9	402
New Potatoes Boiled	½ cup	148	12	—	0	2	12	tr	41	852	284	14	6	495
Okra Smothered	1 serv (4 oz)	121	10	—	0	2	9	1	69	633	356	26	49	639
Onion Sauce	1 serv (4 oz)	152	7	—	0	5	30	1	20	481	119	9	13	6
Rice	½ cup	99	tr	—	0	2	22	tr	9	9	25	0	3	0
Rice Polynesian	1 serv (4 oz)	140	6	—	0	2	20	tr	17	627	92	4	6	282
Spaghetti Baked	1 serv (9.5 oz)	256	10	—	13	9	33	2	74	448	387	23	33	1548
Squash Baked Italian	1 serv (4.75 oz)	73	3	—	8	4	8	1	89	1072	182	16	11	707
Squash Mixed Yellow & Zucchini	1 serv (4 oz)	72	5	—	0	1	6	1	28	390	166	7	6	2523
Squash Yellow Baked French Style	⅓ cup	86	5	—	5	3	9	1	27	405	235	13	12	357
Turkey Breast	1 serv (3 oz)	99	2	—	—	20	tr	tr	4	612	294	—	—	—
Vegetables Unseasoned	1 serv (5 oz)	29	tr	—	0	2	6	2	31	23	303	53	46	8977
SALADS AND SALAD BARS														
Broccoli Salad	1 serv (4 oz)	202	20	—	13	2	6	2	47	252	166	27	33	1052

FOOD	PORTION	CALORIES	FAT	SAT FAT	CHOL	PROTEIN	CARBO	FIBER	CALCIUM	SOD	POTAS	VIT C	FOLIC	VIT A
Cabbage Combination Salad	1 serv (4.5 oz)	50	tr	—	0	1	15	1	32	1164	214	35	27	526
Carrot & Raisin Salad	1 serv (4.5 oz)	321	23	—	10	2	30	2	41	280	401	11	1	6826
Cole Slaw w/ Cream	1 serv (4 oz)	182	18	—	9	2	5	1	51	344	216	39	42	659
Cucumber & Celery Salad	1 serv (4 oz)	82	6	—	0	1	6	1	26	686	177	9	10	222
Fruit Salad	1 serv (6 oz)	59	1	—	0	1	14	2	18	6	315	58	15	866
Neptune Salad	1 serv	361	34	—	25	10	3	1	494	659	148	7	28	432
Spinach Tossed Salad	1 serv (4 oz)	88	6	—	44	3	6	2	103	147	333	14	72	4850
Spring Salad Bowl	1 serv (4 oz)	22	tr	—	0	1	5	1	22	21	245	14	45	3762
SOUPS														
Gumbo Chicken	1 serv (8 oz)	92	2	—	22	9	9	1	22	1033	192	6	12	1626
Gumbo Seafood	1 serv (8 oz)	98	2	—	45	10	10	1	42	1300	296	15	12	510
Vegetable	1 serv (8 oz)	49	tr	—	0	2	10	tr	28	998	303	16	21	2093

PIZZA HUT

MAIN MENU SELECTIONS

FOOD	PORTION	CALORIES	FAT	SAT FAT	CHOL	PROTEIN	CARBO	FIBER	CALCIUM	SOD	POTAS	VIT C	FOLIC	VIT A
Bread Stick	1 (1.3 oz)	130	4	1	0	3	20	1	—	170	—	—	—	—
Bread Stick Dipping Sauce	1 serv (1.2 oz)	30	1	0	0	tr	5	tr	—	170	—	—	—	200
Cavatini Pasta	1 serv (12.5 oz)	480	14	6	25	21	66	9	150	1170	—	—	—	1250
Cavatini Supreme Pasta	1 serv (13.9 oz)	560	19	8	30	24	73	10	150	1400	—	—	—	1500
Garlic Bread	1 slice (1.3 oz)	150	8	2	0	3	16	1	40	240	—	—	—	500
Ham & Cheese Sandwich	1 (9.7 oz)	550	21	7	65	23	19	4	300	2150	—	—	—	500
Hot Buffalo Wings	4 pieces (2.1 oz)	210	12	3	130	22	4	tr	20	900	—	—	—	1000
Spaghetti Marinara	1 serv (16.6 oz)	490	6	1	0	18	91	8	150	730	—	—	—	1000
Spaghetti Meat Sauce	1 serv (16.4 oz)	600	13	5	25	23	98	9	100	910	—	—	—	1750
Spaghetti Meatballs	1 serv (18.8 oz)	850	24	10	50	37	120	10	150	1120	—	—	—	2000
Supreme Sandwich	1 (10.2 oz)	640	28	10	85	34	62	4	300	2150	—	—	—	750
Wild Buffalo Wings	5 pieces (2.9 oz)	200	12	4	150	23	tr	0	20	510	—	—	—	300
PIZZA														
Beef Topping Hand Tossed	1 slice (3.9 oz)	280	10	5	20	15	32	3	150	860	—	—	—	1000
Beef Topping Pan	1 slice (3.9 oz)	310	14	5	20	14	31	2	150	720	—	—	—	1000
Beef Topping Stuffed Crust	1 slice (5.6 oz)	410	14	6	30	20	49	4	250	1270	—	—	—	1250

FOOD	PORTION	CALORIES	FAT	SAT FAT	CHOL	PROTEIN	CARBO	FIBER	CALCIUM	SOD	POTAS	VIT C	FOLIC	VIT A
Beef Topping Thin 'N Crispy	1 slice (3.1 oz)	240	11	5	20	13	22	2	100	790	—	—	—	1000
Cheese Hand Tossed	1 slice (3.9 oz)	280	10	5	25	16	32	2	250	770	—	—	—	1250
Cheese Pan	1 slice (3.9 oz)	300	14	6	25	15	30	2	250	610	—	—	—	1000
Cheese Stuffed Crust	1 slice (5.4 oz)	380	11	5	25	21	49	4	350	1160	—	—	—	1250
Cheese Thin 'N Crispy	1 slice (2.6 oz)	210	9	5	20	12	21	2	200	530	—	—	—	1000
Chicken Supreme Pan	1 slice (4.1 oz)	280	11	4	25	14	32	3	100	570	—	—	—	750
Chicken Supreme Stuffed Crust	1 slice (6.4 oz)	390	13	6	40	21	46	4	300	1130	—	—	—	1250
Chicken Supreme Thin 'N Crispy	1 slice (4.2 oz)	240	6	3	25	14	31	3	150	660	—	—	—	750
Dessert Apple	1 slice (2.8 oz)	250	5	1	0	3	48	2	—	230	—	—	—	—
Dessert Cherry	1 slice (2.8 oz)	250	5	1	0	3	47	3	—	220	—	—	—	450
Ham Hand Tossed	1 slice (3.4 oz)	230	6	3	25	13	30	2	150	710	—	—	—	1000
Ham Pan	1 slice (3.4 oz)	250	9	4	10	12	31	2	100	590	—	—	—	750
Ham Stuffed Crust	1 slice (5.4 oz)	380	14	6	45	22	43	4	250	1250	—	—	—	1500
Ham Thin 'N Crispy	1 slice (2.4 oz)	190	6	3	15	10	23	1	100	560	—	—	—	750
Italian Sausage Hand Tossed	1 slice (4 oz)	300	12	5	30	15	32	3	150	780	—	—	—	750
Italian Sausage Pan	1 slice (4.3 oz)	350	18	6	40	16	31	3	150	740	—	—	—	1000
Italian Sausage Stuffed Crust	1 slice (5.7 oz)	430	19	8	35	20	46	4	300	1200	—	—	—	1750
Italian Sausage Thin 'N Crispy	1 slice (3.4 oz)	300	16	6	35	15	34	3	150	740	—	—	—	1500
Meat Lover's Hand Tossed	1 slice (3.9 oz)	290	11	5	35	15	32	3	150	820	—	—	—	750
Meat Lover's Pan	1 slice (4.4 oz)	360	19	6	40	17	30	3	150	870	—	—	—	1000
Meat Lover's Stuffed Crust	1 slice (6.6 oz)	500	23	10	60	25	47	4	300	1510	—	—	—	1500
Meat Lover's Thin 'N Crispy	1 slice (3.7 oz)	310	16	7	35	16	25	3	150	900	—	—	—	1500
Pepperoni Hand Tossed	1 slice (3.4 oz)	260	9	4	30	12	31	3	150	750	—	—	—	1250
Pepperoni Lover's Hand Tossed	1 slice (4 oz)	320	13	6	35	17	31	4	200	910	—	—	—	1500
Pepperoni Lover's Pan	1 slice (4.1 oz)	350	17	8	20	17	32	2	200	800	—	—	—	1250
Pepperoni Lover's Stuffed Crust	1 slice (6.1 oz)	480	22	9	60	24	47	4	300	1440	—	—	—	2000
Pepperoni Lover's Thin 'N Crispy	1 slice (3.1 oz)	270	12	6	25	15	26	2	150	780	—	—	—	1000
Pepperoni Pan	1 slice (3.4 oz)	280	12	5	20	12	31	3	150	640	—	—	—	1000

FOOD	PORTION	CALORIES	FAT	SAT FAT	CHOL	PROTEIN	CARBO	FIBER	CALCIUM	SOD	POTAS	VIT C	FOLIC	VIT A
Pepperoni Stuffed Crust	1 slice (5.3 oz)	410	17	7	40	20	46	4	250	1250	—	—	—	1750
Pepperoni Thin 'N Crispy	1 slice (2.3 oz)	220	9	4	20	10	22	2	100	610	—	—	—	1000
Personal Pan Cheese	1 pie (8.1 oz)	630	24	11	45	28	76	4	350	1160	—	—	—	1500
Personal Pan Pepperoni	1 pie (8.1 oz)	670	29	12	60	29	73	4	250	1250	—	—	—	2500
Personal Pan Supreme	1 pie (9.5 oz)	710	31	13	60	32	76	5	250	1380	—	—	—	2500
Pork Topping Hand Tossed	1 slice (3.9 oz)	290	11	5	25	14	33	3	150	850	—	—	—	1000
Pork Topping Pan	1 slice (3.6 oz)	300	13	5	30	14	31	3	150	720	—	—	—	1000
Pork Topping Stuffed Crust	1 slice (5.6 oz)	420	16	7	30	22	46	4	300	1290	—	—	—	1250
Pork Topping Thin 'N Crispy	1 slice (3.2 oz)	270	13	6	25	14	22	2	150	780	—	—	—	1000
Super Supreme Hand Tossed	1 slice (4.7 oz)	290	10	5	35	15	34	4	150	830	—	—	—	750
Super Supreme Pan	1 slice (4.6 oz)	340	16	5	30	15	33	4	150	790	—	—	—	1250
Super Supreme Stuffed Crust	1 slice (7.2 oz)	470	20	8	50	24	49	5	300	1440	—	—	—	1500
Super Supreme Thin 'N Crispy	1 slice (4 oz)	280	13	5	30	15	26	4	150	810	—	—	—	1500
Supreme Hand Tossed	1 slice (3.9 oz)	270	9	5	25	13	32	3	150	760	—	—	—	1000
Supreme Pan	1 slice (4 oz)	300	13	5	25	13	32	3	150	670	—	—	—	1000
Supreme Stuffed Crust	1 slice (6.4 oz)	440	16	7	40	23	51	4	300	1380	—	—	—	1500
Supreme Thin 'N Crispy	1 slice (3.4 oz)	250	11	5	20	13	24	3	150	710	—	—	—	1000
Veggie Lover's Hand Tossed	1 slice (4 oz)	240	7	3	20	11	34	3	150	650	—	—	—	1000
Veggie Lover's Pan	1 slice (3.9 oz)	240	9	4	10	10	31	3	150	480	—	—	—	750
Veggie Lover's Stuffed Crust	1 slice (5.9 oz)	390	14	6	25	18	48	5	250	1140	—	—	—	1250
Veggie Lover's Thin 'N Crispy	1 slice (2.6 oz)	170	6	2	10	7	23	3	80	460	—	—	—	1250

PONDEROSA

ICE CREAM

FOOD	PORTION	CALORIES	FAT	SAT FAT	CHOL	PROTEIN	CARBO	FIBER	CALCIUM	SOD	POTAS	VIT C	FOLIC	VIT A
Ice Milk Chocolate	3.5 oz	152	3	—	22	4	30	—	—	70	—	—	—	—
Ice Milk Vanilla	3.5 oz	150	3	—	20	4	30	—	—	58	—	—	—	—
Topping Caramel	1 oz	100	1	—	2	tr	26	—	—	72	—	—	—	—
Topping Chocolate	1 oz	89	tr	—	0	tr	24	—	—	37	—	—	—	—
Topping Strawberry	1 oz	71	tr	—	0	tr	24	—	—	29	—	—	—	—
Topping Whipped	1 oz	80	6	—	0	0	5	—	—	16	—	—	—	—

MAIN MENU SELECTIONS

FOOD	PORTION	CALORIES	FAT	SAT FAT	CHOL	PROTEIN	CARBO	FIBER	CALCIUM	SOD	POTAS	VIT C	FOLIC	VIT A
BBQ Sauce	1 tbsp	25	0	—	0	0	5	—	—	260	—	—	—	—

FOOD	PORTION	CALORIES	FAT	SAT FAT	CHOL	PROTEIN	CARBO	FIBER	CALCIUM	SOD	POTAS	VIT C	FOLIC	VIT A
Bake 'R Broil Fish	1 serv (5.2 oz)	230	13	—	50	19	10	—	—	330	—	—	—	—
Baked Potato	1 (7.2 oz)	145	tr	—	0	4	33	—	—	6	—	—	—	—
Beans Baked	1 serv (4 oz)	170	6	—	0	6	21	—	—	330	—	—	—	—
Beans Green	1 serv (3.5 oz)	20	0	—	0	1	3	—	—	391	—	—	—	—
Breaded Cauliflower	1 serv (4 oz)	115	1	—	1	4	23	—	—	446	—	—	—	—
Breaded Okra	1 serv (4 oz)	124	1	—	1	3	23	—	—	483	—	—	—	—
Breaded Onion Rings	1 serv (4 oz)	213	9	—	2	3	30	—	—	620	—	—	—	—
Breaded Zucchini	1 serv (4 oz)	102	1	—	1	3	18	—	—	584	—	—	—	—
Carrots	1 serv (3.5 oz)	31	tr	—	0	1	7	—	—	33	—	—	—	—
Cheese Herb Garlic Spread	1 tbsp	100	10	—	0	0	0	—	—	120	—	—	—	—
Cheese Sauce	2 oz	52	2	—	4	1	6	—	—	355	—	—	—	—
Chicken Breast	1 serv (5.5 oz)	90	2	—	54	20	1	—	—	400	—	—	—	—
Chicken Wings	2	213	9	—	75	11	11	—	—	610	—	—	—	—
Chopped Steak	4 oz	225	16	—	80	19	1	—	—	150	—	—	—	—
Chopped Steak	5.3 oz	296	22	—	105	25	1	—	—	296	—	—	—	—
Corn	1 serv (3.5 oz)	90	tr	—	0	3	21	—	—	5	—	—	—	—
Fish Fried	1 serv (3.2 oz)	190	9	—	15	9	17	—	—	170	—	—	—	—
Fish Nuggets	1	31	2	—	8	2	2	—	—	52	—	—	—	—
French Fries	1 serv (3 oz)	120	4	—	3	2	17	—	—	39	—	—	—	—
Gravy Brown	2 oz	25	1	—	0	1	4	—	—	167	—	—	—	—
Gravy Turkey	2 oz	25	tr	—	0	1	5	—	—	228	—	—	—	—
Halibut Broiled	1 serv (6 oz)	170	2	—	—	36	0	—	—	68	—	—	—	—
Hot Dog	1	144	13	—	27	5	1	—	—	460	—	—	—	—
Italian Breadsticks	1	100	1	—	0	4	19	—	—	200	—	—	—	—
Kansas City Strip	5 oz	138	6	—	76	21	1	—	—	850	—	—	—	—
Macaroni And Cheese	4 oz	67	2	—	4	3	18	—	—	320	—	—	—	—
Margarine Liquid	1 tbsp	100	11	—	0	0	0	—	—	110	—	—	—	—
Mashed Potatoes	1 serv (4 oz)	62	tr	—	20	2	13	—	—	191	—	—	—	—
Meatballs	1	58	2	—	11	2	1	—	—	8	—	—	—	—
Mini Shrimp	6	47	tr	—	22	4	6	—	—	125	—	—	—	—
New York Strip Choice	10 oz	314	15	—	50	45	1	—	—	1420	—	—	—	—
New York Strip Choice	8 oz	384	11	—	62	34	2	—	—	570	—	—	—	—
Pasta Shells Plain	2 oz	78	tr	—	0	2	16	—	—	tr	—	—	—	—
Peas	1 serv (3.5 oz)	67	tr	—	0	5	12	—	—	120	—	—	—	—
Porterhouse	13 oz	441	30	—	67	43	1	—	—	1844	—	—	—	—
Porterhouse Choice	16 oz	640	31	—	82	57	3	—	—	1130	—	—	—	—
Potato Wedges	1 serv (3.5 oz)	130	6	—	—	3	16	—	—	171	—	—	—	—
Ribeye	5 oz	219	13	—	75	25	1	—	—	1130	—	—	—	—
Ribeye Choice	6 oz	281	14	—	60	29	tr	—	—	570	—	—	—	—
Rice Pilaf	1 serv (4 oz)	160	4	—	22	4	26	—	—	450	—	—	—	—

FOOD	PORTION	CALORIES	FAT	SAT FAT	CHOL	PROTEIN	CARBO	FIBER	CALCIUM	SOD	POTAS	VIT C	FOLIC	VIT A
Roll Dinner	1	184	3	—	0	5	33	—	—	311	—	—	—	—
Roll Sourdough	1	110	1	—	0	4	22	—	—	230	—	—	—	—
Roughy Broiled	1 serv (5 oz)	139	5	—	28	21	—	—	—	88	—	—	—	—
Salmon Broiled	1 serv (6 oz)	192	3	—	60	37	3	—	—	72	—	—	—	—
Sandwich Steak	4 oz	408	11	—	62	20	2	—	—	850	—	—	—	—
Scrod Baked	1 serv (7 oz)	120	1	—	65	27	0	—	—	80	—	—	—	—
Shrimp Fried	7 pieces	231	tr	—	105	22	31	—	—	612	—	—	—	—
Sirloin Choice	7 oz	241	11	—	63	35	1	—	—	570	—	—	—	—
Sirloin Tips Choice	5 oz	473	8	—	72	29	2	—	—	280	—	—	—	—
Spaghetti Plain	2 oz	78	tr	—	0	2	16	—	—	tr	—	—	—	—
Spaghetti Sauce	4 oz	110	4	—	0	2	17	—	—	520	—	—	—	—
Steak Kabobs Meat Only	3 oz	153	5	—	67	26	2	—	—	280	—	—	—	—
Stuffing	4 oz	230	11	—	22	6	27	—	—	800	—	—	—	—
Sweet/Sour Sauce	1 oz	37	1	—	0	tr	8	—	—	80	—	—	—	—
Swordfish Broiled	1 serv (6 oz)	271	9	—	85	44	0	—	—	0	—	—	—	—
T-Bone	8 oz	176	9	—	71	25	1	—	—	850	—	—	—	—
T-Bone Choice	10 oz	444	18	—	80	34	2	—	—	850	—	—	—	—
Teriyaki Steak	5 oz	174	3	—	64	32	5	—	—	1420	—	—	—	—
Tortilla Chips	1 oz	150	8	—	0	3	16	—	—	80	—	—	—	—
Trout Broiled	1 serv (5 oz)	228	4	—	110	29	1	—	—	51	—	—	—	—
Winter Mix	1 serv (3.5 oz)	25	0	—	0	2	4	—	—	33	—	—	—	—
SALAD DRESSINGS														
Blue Cheese	1 oz	130	13	—	27	1	1	—	—	266	—	—	—	—
Cole Slaw	1 oz	150	14	—	31	tr	6	—	—	284	—	—	—	—
Creamy Italian	1 oz	103	10	—	0	0	3	—	—	373	—	—	—	—
Cucumber Reduced Calorie	1 oz	69	6	—	tr	tr	3	—	—	315	—	—	—	—
Italian Reduced Calorie	1 oz	31	3	—	0	0	1	—	—	371	—	—	—	—
Parmesan Pepper	1 oz	150	15	—	9	1	2	—	—	282	—	—	—	—
Ranch	1 oz	147	15	—	3	tr	1	—	—	298	—	—	—	—
Salad Oil	1 tbsp	120	14	—	0	0	0	—	—	0	—	—	—	—
Sour Cream	1 tbsp	26	3	—	5	tr	1	—	—	6	—	—	—	—
Sweet-N-Tangy	1 oz	122	9	—	1	tr	9	—	—	347	—	—	—	—
Thousand Island	1 oz	113	10	—	1	tr	9	—	—	405	—	—	—	—
SALADS AND SALAD BARS														
Alfalfa Sprouts	1 oz	10	0	—	0	1	1	—	—	0	—	—	—	—
Apple	1	80	1	—	0	0	20	—	—	1	—	—	—	—
Apples Canned	4 oz	90	0	—	0	0	22	—	—	15	—	—	—	—
Applesauce	4 oz	80	0	—	0	0	20	—	—	20	—	—	—	—
Banana	1	87	tr	—	0	1	23	—	—	1	—	—	—	—
Banana Chips	0.2 oz	25	1	—	0	tr	3	—	—	tr	—	—	—	—
Banana Pudding	1 oz	52	2	—	0	tr	6	—	—	29	—	—	—	—
Bean Sprouts	1 oz	10	tr	—	0	1	2	—	—	1	—	—	—	—

FOOD	PORTION	CALORIES	FAT	SAT FAT	CHOL	PROTEIN	CARBO	FIBER	CALCIUM	SOD	POTAS	VIT C	FOLIC	VIT A
Beets Diced	4 oz	55	tr	—	0	tr	13	—	—	307	—	—	—	—
Breadsticks Sesame	2	35	0	—	0	0	6	—	—	60	—	—	—	—
Broccoli	1 oz	9	1	—	0	1	2	—	—	4	—	—	—	—
Cabbage Green	1 oz	9	0	—	0	1	2	—	—	7	—	—	—	—
Cabbage Red	1 oz	1	0	—	0	tr	tr	—	—	1	—	—	—	—
Cantaloupe	1 wedge	13	0	—	0	tr	3	—	—	5	—	—	—	—
Carrots	1 oz	12	tr	—	0	tr	3	—	—	13	—	—	—	—
Cauliflower	1 oz	8	tr	—	0	1	2	—	—	4	—	—	—	—
Celery	1 oz	4	0	—	0	tr	1	—	—	36	—	—	—	—
Cheese Imitation Shredded	1 oz	90	7	—	5	6	1	—	—	420	—	—	—	—
Cheese Spread	1 oz	98	7	—	26	4	4	—	—	188	—	—	—	—
Cherry Peppers	2 pieces	7	tr	—	0	tr	1	—	—	415	—	—	—	—
Chicken Salad	3.5 oz	212	15	—	42	11	8	—	—	335	—	—	—	—
Chow Mein Noodles	0.2 oz	25	1	—	0	1	3	—	—	42	—	—	—	—
Cocktail Sauce	1 oz	34	1	—	0	tr	6	—	—	453	—	—	—	—
Coconut Shredded	0.2 oz	25	2	—	0	tr	2	—	—	14	—	—	—	—
Cottage Cheese	4 oz	120	5	—	17	16	5	—	—	330	—	—	—	—
Croutons	1 oz	115	4	—	0	4	18	—	—	351	—	—	—	—
Cucumber	1 oz	4	0	—	0	tr	1	—	—	2	—	—	—	—
Eggs Diced	2 oz	94	7	—	260	7	1	—	—	75	—	—	—	—
Fruit Cocktail	4 oz	97	tr	—	0	tr	25	—	—	7	—	—	—	—
Garbanzo Beans	1 oz	102	0	—	0	6	17	—	—	7	—	—	—	—
Gelatin Plain	4 oz	71	0	—	0	1	17	—	—	73	—	—	—	—
Granola	0.2 oz	24	1	—	0	tr	3	—	—	—	—	—	—	—
Grapes	10	34	tr	—	0	tr	9	—	—	2	—	—	—	—
Green Onion	1	7	tr	—	0	tr	2	—	—	1	—	—	—	—
Green Pepper	1 oz	6	tr	—	0	tr	1	—	—	4	—	—	—	—
Ham Diced	2 oz	120	10	—	76	9	1	—	—	780	—	—	—	—
Honeydew	1 wedge	24	tr	—	0	1	6	—	—	9	—	—	—	—
Lemon	1 wedge	3	tr	—	0	tr	1	—	—	0	—	—	—	—
Lettuce	1 oz	5	0	—	0	0	2	—	—	5	—	—	—	—
Macaroni Salad	3.5 oz	335	12	—	9	8	49	—	—	431	—	—	—	—
Margarine Whipped	1 tbsp	34	1	—	0	0	0	—	—	65	—	—	—	—
Meal Mates Sesame Crackers	2	45	2	—	0	1	6	—	—	95	—	—	—	—
Melba Snacks	2	18	0	—	0	1	4	—	—	60	—	—	—	—
Mousse Chocolate	1 oz	78	4	—	0	0	7	—	—	18	—	—	—	—
Mousse Strawberry	1 oz	74	5	—	0	0	6	—	—	17	—	—	—	—
Mushrooms	1 oz	8	tr	—	0	1	1	—	—	4	—	—	—	—
Olives Black	1	4	tr	—	0	0	tr	—	—	24	—	—	—	—
Olives Green	1	3	tr	—	0	0	tr	—	—	69	—	—	—	—
Onions Red & Yellow	1 oz	11	0	—	3	tr	3	—	—	3	—	—	—	—

FOOD	PORTION	CALORIES	FAT	SAT FAT	CHOL	PROTEIN	CARBO	FIBER	CALCIUM	SOD	POTAS	VIT C	FOLIC	VIT A
Orange	1	45	tr	—	0	1	11	—	—	1	—	—	—	—
Pasta Salad	3.5 oz	269	12	—	tr	6	34	—	—	441	—	—	—	—
Peaches Canned	4 oz	70	0	—	0	0	18	—	—	10	—	—	—	—
Peanuts Chopped	0.2 oz	30	2	—	0	1	1	—	—	—	—	—	—	—
Pears Canned	4 oz	98	tr	—	0	tr	25	—	—	7	—	—	—	—
Pickles Dill Spears	0.14 oz	tr	0	—	0	0	tr	—	—	54	—	—	—	—
Pickles Sweet Chips	0.14 oz	4	0	—	0	tr	1	—	—	tr	—	—	—	—
Pineapple Tidbits	4 oz	95	tr	—	0	tr	25	—	—	2	—	—	—	—
Pineapple Fresh	1 wedge	11	tr	—	0	tr	3	—	—	tr	—	—	—	—
Potato Salad	3.5 oz	126	6	—	7	1	16	—	—	300	—	—	—	—
Radishes	1 oz	4	0	—	0	tr	1	—	—	5	—	—	—	—
Ritz	2	40	2	—	0	0	4	—	—	50	—	—	—	—
Saltine Crackers	2	25	tr	—	0	1	4	—	—	38	—	—	—	—
Spiced Apple Rings	4 oz	100	0	—	0	0	24	—	—	20	—	—	—	—
Spinach	1 oz	7	tr	—	0	1	1	—	—	20	—	—	—	—
Strawberries	2 oz	14	tr	—	—	tr	3	—	—	61	—	—	—	—
Strawberry Glaze	1 oz	37	0	—	—	0	10	—	—	4	—	—	—	—
Sunflower Seeds	0.2 oz	31	0	—	0	1	1	—	—	—	—	—	—	—
Tartar Sauce	1 oz	85	11	—	9	tr	11	—	—	477	—	—	—	—
Tomatoes	1 oz	6	tr	—	0	tr	1	—	—	1	—	—	—	—
Turkey Ham Salad	3.5 oz	186	13	—	12	8	10	—	—	655	—	—	—	—
Turkey Julienne	1 oz	29	tr	—	15	5	1	—	—	192	—	—	—	—
Vanilla Wafer	2	35	1	—	5	0	6	—	—	25	—	—	—	—
Watermelon	1 wedge	111	1	—	0	2	27	—	—	4	—	—	—	—
Yogurt Fruit	4 oz	115	1	—	5	5	23	—	—	70	—	—	—	—
Yogurt Vanilla	4 oz	110	2	—	6	5	18	—	—	75	—	—	—	—
Zucchini	1 oz	5	0	—	0	tr	1	—	—	tr	—	—	—	—

POPEYE'S

FOOD	PORTION	CALORIES	FAT	SAT FAT	CHOL	PROTEIN	CARBO	FIBER	CALCIUM	SOD	POTAS	VIT C	FOLIC	VIT A
Apple Pie	1 serv (3.1 oz)	290	16	—	10	3	37	2	40	820	—	0	—	0
Biscuit	1 serv (2.3 oz)	250	15	—	<5	4	26	1	40	430	—	0	—	400
Breast Mild	1 (3.7 oz)	270	16	—	60	23	9	2	40	660	—	0	—	300
Breast Spicy	1 (3.7 oz)	270	16	—	60	23	9	2	40	590	—	0	—	300
Cajun Rice	1 serv (3.9 oz)	150	5	—	25	10	17	3	100	1260	—	0	—	0
Cole Slaw	1 serv (4 oz)	149	11	—	3	1	14	3	20	271	—	2	—	0
Corn On The Cob	1 serv (5.2 oz)	127	3	—	0	4	21	9	0	20	—	4	—	0
French Fries	1 serv (3 oz)	240	12	—	10	4	31	3	0	610	—	0	—	0
Leg Mild	1 (1.7 oz)	120	7	—	40	10	4	0	0	240	—	0	—	200
Leg Spicy	1 (1.7 oz)	120	7	—	40	10	4	0	0	240	—	0	—	200
Nuggets	1 serv (4.2 oz)	410	32	—	55	17	18	3	20	660	—	1	—	0
Nuggets Mild Tender	1 (1.2 oz)	110	7	—	15	6	6	1	0	160	—	0	—	0
Nuggets Spicy Tender	1 (1.2 oz)	110	7	—	15	6	6	1	0	215	—	0	—	0
Onion Rings	1 serv (3.1 oz)	310	19	—	25	5	31	2	60	210	—	0	—	0
Potatoes & Gravy	1 serv (3.8 oz)	100	6	—	<5	5	11	3	40	460	—	0	—	500

FOOD	PORTION	CALORIES	FAT	SAT FAT	CHOL	PROTEIN	CARBO	FIBER	CALCIUM	SOD	POTAS	VIT C	FOLIC	VIT A
Red Beans & Rice	1 serv (5.9 oz)	270	17	—	10	8	30	7	0	680	—	0	—	0
Shrimp	1 serv (2.8 oz)	250	16	—	110	16	13	3	60	650	—	0	—	0
Thigh Mild	1 (3.1 oz)	300	23	—	70	15	9	tr	20	620	—	0	—	300
Thigh Spicy	1 (3.1 oz)	300	23	—	70	15	9	tr	20	450	—	0	—	300
Wing Mild	1 (1.6 oz)	160	11	—	40	9	7	0	0	290	—	0	—	300
Wing Spicy	1 (1.6 oz)	160	11	—	40	9	7	0	0	290	—	0	—	300

PUDGIE'S FAMOUS CHICKEN

FOOD	PORTION	CALORIES	FAT	SAT FAT	CHOL	PROTEIN	CARBO	FIBER	CALCIUM	SOD	POTAS	VIT C	FOLIC	VIT A
Fried Chicken	3.5 oz	233	13	3	81	25	4	—	35	440	—	0	—	93

QUINCY'S

BAKED SELECTIONS

FOOD	PORTION	CALORIES	FAT	SAT FAT	CHOL	PROTEIN	CARBO	FIBER	CALCIUM	SOD	POTAS	VIT C	FOLIC	VIT A
Banana Nut Bread	1 serv (2 oz)	165	7	1	5	2	22	—	—	195	—	—	—	—
Biscuit	1 (2.5 oz)	270	15	4	11	5	29	—	—	610	—	—	—	—
Cornbread	1 serv (2 oz)	140	5	1	0	3	19	—	—	340	—	—	—	—
Yeast Roll	1 (2 oz)	160	4	tr	0	1	29	—	—	285	—	—	—	—

BREAKFAST SELECTIONS

FOOD	PORTION	CALORIES	FAT	SAT FAT	CHOL	PROTEIN	CARBO	FIBER	CALCIUM	SOD	POTAS	VIT C	FOLIC	VIT A
Bacon	1 serv (0.25 oz)	35	3	1	5	2	0	—	—	100	—	—	—	—
Corned Beef Hash	1 serv (4.5 oz)	210	15	8	45	10	11	—	—	795	—	—	—	—
Country Ham	1 serv (1.5 oz)	90	6	2	35	9	1	—	—	1100	—	—	—	—
Escalloped Apples	1 serv (3.5 oz)	120	2	0	0	0	26	—	—	20	—	—	—	—
Oatmeal	1 serv (1 oz)	175	2	0	0	4	18	—	—	285	—	—	—	—
Pancakes	1 (1.5 oz)	95	3	1	30	3	12	—	—	250	—	—	—	—
Sausage Gravy	1 serv (4 oz)	70	6	2	10	2	3	—	—	150	—	—	—	—
Sausage Links	1 (2 oz)	225	22	8	20	7	0	—	—	390	—	—	—	—
Sausage Patties	1 (2 oz)	230	23	9	45	7	0	—	—	350	—	—	—	—
Scrambled Eggs	1 serv (2 oz)	95	7	2	215	7	1	—	—	270	—	—	—	—
Steak Fingers	1 serv (3.5 oz)	360	25	11	50	16	18	—	—	690	—	—	—	—
Syrup	1 oz	75	0	0	0	0	20	—	—	15	—	—	—	—

DESSERTS

FOOD	PORTION	CALORIES	FAT	SAT FAT	CHOL	PROTEIN	CARBO	FIBER	CALCIUM	SOD	POTAS	VIT C	FOLIC	VIT A
Banana Pudding	1 serv (5 oz)	240	12	9	10	3	30	—	—	240	—	—	—	—
Brownie Pudding Cake	1 serv (4 oz)	310	5	tr	0	4	66	—	—	395	—	—	—	—
Caramel Topping	1 serv (1 oz)	105	1	tr	0	0	24	—	—	120	—	—	—	—
Chocolate Chip Cookies	1 (0.5 oz)	60	8	1	5	1	8	—	—	35	—	—	—	—
Cobbler Apple	1 serv (6 oz)	255	8	2	5	1	49	—	—	285	—	—	—	—
Cobbler Cherry	1 serv (6 oz)	410	8	2	5	1	55	—	—	185	—	—	—	—
Cobbler Peach	1 serv (6 oz)	305	8	2	5	1	50	—	—	190	—	—	—	—
Frozen Yogurt	1 serv (4 oz)	135	2	1	5	5	25	—	—	85	—	—	—	—
Fudge Topping	1 serv (1 oz)	105	4	1	0	1	15	—	—	75	—	—	—	—
Sugar Cookie	1 (0.5 oz)	60	3	1	5	tr	8	—	—	30	—	—	—	—

MAIN MENU SELECTIONS

FOOD	PORTION	CALORIES	FAT	SAT FAT	CHOL	PROTEIN	CARBO	FIBER	CALCIUM	SOD	POTAS	VIT C	FOLIC	VIT A
⅓ Pound Hamburger	1 serv (8 oz)	565	33	16	66	32	32	—	—	603	—	—	—	—
BBQ Beans	1 serv (4 oz)	114	1	1	0	4	21	—	—	604	—	—	—	—

FOOD	PORTION	CALORIES	FAT	SAT FAT	CHOL	PROTEIN	CARBO	FIBER	CALCIUM	SOD	POTAS	VIT C	FOLIC	VIT A
Bacon Cheese Burger	1 (9 oz)	663	41	17	87	37	33	—	—	997	—	—	—	—
Baked Potato	1 (6 oz)	115	0	0	0	5	30	—	—	0	—	—	—	—
Broccoli	1 serv (4 oz)	34	0	0	0	3	5	—	—	50	—	—	—	—
Cheese Sauce	1 serv (1 oz)	58	5	2	11	2	1	—	—	212	—	—	—	—
Chopped Steak Steak	1 serv (8 oz)	499	42	20	89	31	0	—	—	348	—	—	—	—
Cinnamon Apples	1 serv (4 oz)	172	5	1	0	0	34	—	—	149	—	—	—	—
Corn	1 serv (4 oz)	96	1	0	0	3	24	—	—	271	—	—	—	—
Country Steak w/ Gravy	1 serv (8 oz)	530	25	7	54	32	44	—	—	1161	—	—	—	—
Cowboy Steak	1 serv (14 oz)	580	33	15	176	61	9	—	—	1308	—	—	—	—
Filet w/ Bacon	1 serv (8 oz)	340	17	7	124	48	2	—	—	311	—	—	—	—
Green Beans	1 serv (4 oz)	61	4	1	0	1	6	—	—	796	—	—	—	—
Grilled Chicken	1 reg serv (5 oz)	120	2	0	55	25	1	—	—	540	—	—	—	—
Grilled Chicken Sandwich	1 (9 oz)	324	4	1	55	33	39	—	—	1183	—	—	—	—
Grilled Salmon	1 serv (7 oz)	228	4	1	109	46	1	—	—	112	—	—	—	—
Homestyle Chicken Fillet	1 serv (3 oz)	217	9	2	25	13	21	—	—	682	—	—	—	—
Junior Sirloin Steak	1 serv (5.5 oz)	194	10	5	69	25	0	—	—	199	—	—	—	—
Large Sirloin Steak	1 serv (10 oz)	368	20	9	119	46	2	—	—	390	—	—	—	—
Mashed Potatoes	1 serv (4 oz)	54	6	1	0	1	11	—	—	195	—	—	—	—
NY Strip Steak	1 serv (10 oz)	450	26	13	148	53	1	—	—	156	—	—	—	—
Philly Cheese Steak	1 serv (11 oz)	588	30	11	87	37	38	—	—	1684	—	—	—	—
Porterhouse Steak	1 serv (17 oz)	683	46	23	154	67	0	—	—	346	—	—	—	—
Regular Sirloin Steak	1 serv (8 oz)	285	16	7	71	34	0	—	—	317	—	—	—	—
Ribeye Steak	1 serv (10 oz)	452	29	13	116	48	0	—	—	156	—	—	—	—
Rice Pilaf	1 serv (4 oz)	119	2	0	0	2	23	1	—	1283	—	—	—	—
Roasted BBQ Chicken	1 serv (14 oz)	941	65	17	340	70	21	—	—	1548	—	—	—	—
Roasted Herb Chicken	1 serv (14 oz)	875	65	17	340	70	4	—	—	1238	—	—	—	—
Sirloin Tips w/ Mushroom Gravy	1 serv (6 oz)	196	7	3	64	28	5	—	—	578	—	—	—	—
Sirloin Tips w/ Peppers & Onions	1 serv (5 oz)	203	8	3	63	27	4	—	—	793	—	—	—	—
Smothered Steak Sandwich	1 (9 oz)	429	15	6	69	34	36	—	—	846	—	—	—	—
Smothered Strip Steak	1 serv (10 oz)	622	41	16	148	55	12	—	—	239	—	—	—	—
Southern Breaded Shrimp	1 serv (7 oz)	546	31	6	135	19	47	—	—	821	—	—	—	—

FOOD	PORTION	CALORIES	FAT	SAT FAT	CHOL	PROTEIN	CARBO	FIBER	CALCIUM	SOD	POTAS	VIT C	FOLIC	VIT A
Spicy BBQ Chicken Sandwich	1 (10 oz)	368	1	1	55	34	45	—	—	1608	—	—	—	—
Steak & Shrimp	1 serv (9 oz)	677	39	12	170	48	33	—	—	816	—	—	—	—
Steak Fries	1 serv (4 oz)	358	19	6	0	5	45	—	—	245	—	—	—	—
T-Bone Steak	1 serv (13 oz)	521	35	18	118	51	0	—	—	265	—	—	—	—
SALAD DRESSINGS														
Blue Cheese	1 serv (1 oz)	155	16	3	10	2	2	—	—	165	—	—	—	—
French	1 serv (1 oz)	125	12	1	0	0	4	—	—	500	—	—	—	—
Honey Mustard	1 serv (1 oz)	100	6	tr	0	2	10	—	—	220	—	—	—	—
Italian	1 serv (1 oz)	135	14	2	0	0	3	—	—	230	—	—	—	—
Light Creamy Italian	1 serv (1 oz)	65	4	0	0	2	8	—	—	485	—	—	—	—
Light French	1 serv (1 oz)	85	4	0	0	2	13	—	—	285	—	—	—	—
Light Italian	1 serv (1 oz)	20	2	0	0	2	2	—	—	485	—	—	—	—
Light Thousand Island	1 serv (1 oz)	65	4	0	20	2	8	—	—	340	—	—	—	—
Parmesan Peppercorn	1 serv (1 oz)	150	14	0	0	1	4	—	—	280	—	—	—	—
Ranch	1 serv (1 oz)	110	11	2	10	1	1	—	—	195	—	—	—	—
SOUPS														
Chili With Beans	1 serv (6 oz)	235	11	2	15	13	21	—	—	920	—	—	—	—
Clam Chowder	1 serv (6 oz)	180	9	1	0	3	21	—	—	835	—	—	—	—
Cream Of Broccoli	1 serv (6 oz)	170	10	1	0	2	18	—	—	770	—	—	—	—
Vegetable Beef	1 serv (6 oz)	90	2	1	0	5	14	—	—	325	—	—	—	—

RALLY'S

FOOD	PORTION	CALORIES	FAT	SAT FAT	CHOL	PROTEIN	CARBO	FIBER	CALCIUM	SOD	POTAS	VIT C	FOLIC	VIT A
MAIN MENU SELECTIONS														
Big Buford	1	743	46	—	151	41	35	—	—	1860	—	—	—	—
Chicken Fillet Sandwich	1	399	15	—	42	21	43	—	—	790	—	—	—	—
Chili w/ Cheese & Onion	1 serv (13 oz)	669	41	—	137	43	37	—	—	2125	—	—	—	—
Chili w/ Cheese & Onion	1 serv (7 oz)	360	22	—	74	23	20	—	—	1144	—	—	—	—
French Fries	1 reg (4 oz)	211	11	—	7	3	26	—	—	293	—	—	—	—
French Fries	1 lg (6 oz)	317	16	—	10	5	39	—	—	439	—	—	—	—
French Fries	1 extra lg (8 oz)	423	21	—	13	7	52	—	—	585	—	—	—	—
Onion Rings	1 serv	210	2	—	0	6	45	—	—	855	—	—	—	—
Rallyburger	1	433	22	—	63	20	35	—	—	1176	—	—	—	—
Rallyburger w/ Cheese	1	488	35	—	27	23	35	—	—	1376	—	—	—	—
Spicy Chicken Sandwich	1	437	18	—	40	18	50	—	—	887	—	—	—	—
Super Barbecue Bacon	1	593	31	—	88	29	49	—	—	1709	—	—	—	—
Super Double Cheeseburger	1	762	48	—	154	41	37	—	—	1734	—	—	—	—

RAX

FOOD	PORTION	CALORIES	FAT	SAT FAT	CHOL	PROTEIN	CARBO	FIBER	CALCIUM	SOD	POTAS	VIT C	FOLIC	VIT A
DESSERTS														
Chocolate Chip Cookie	1 (2 oz)	262	12	4	6	4	36	—	—	192	96	—	—	—
MAIN MENU SELECTIONS														
Bacon	1 slice (0.1 oz)	14	1	tr	2	1	0	—	—	40	12	—	—	—
Baked Potato	1 (10 oz)	264	0	0	0	6	61	—	—	15	1111	—	—	—
Baked Potato w/ 1 Tbsp Margarine	1 (10.5 oz)	364	11	2	0	6	61	—	—	115	1116	—	—	—
Barbecue Sauce	1 pkg (0.4 oz)	11	0	0	0	0	3	—	—	158	13	—	—	—
Beef Bacon 'N Cheddar	1 (6.7 oz)	523	32	8	42	24	37	—	—	1042	340	—	—	—
Cheddar Cheese Sauce	1 fl oz	29	tr	0	0	tr	4	—	—	225	65	—	—	—
Country Fried Chicken Breast Sandwich	1 (7.4 oz)	618	29	15	45	23	49	—	—	1078	408	—	—	—
Deluxe Roast Beef	1 (7.9 oz)	498	30	7	36	21	39	—	—	864	378	—	—	—
French Fries	1 serv (3.25 oz)	282	14	4	3	3	36	—	—	75	656	—	—	—
Grilled Chicken Breast Sandwich	1 (6.9 oz)	402	23	4	69	25	26	—	—	872	330	—	—	—
Grilled Chicken Garden Salad w/ French Dressing	1 serv (12.7 oz)	477	31	6	32	19	34	—	—	1189	596	—	—	—
Grilled Chicken Garden Salad w/ Lite Italian Dressing	1 serv (12.7 oz)	264	12	3	32	19	22	—	—	1040	565	—	—	—
Mushroom Sauce	1 fl oz	16	tr	0	0	1	1	—	—	113	68	—	—	—
Philly Melt	1 (8.2 oz)	396	16	7	27	25	40	—	—	1055	463	—	—	—
Regular Rax	1 (4.7 oz)	262	10	4	15	18	25	—	—	707	270	—	—	—
Swiss Slice	1 slice (0.4 oz)	42	3	3	10	3	0	—	—	157	25	—	—	—
SALAD DRESSINGS														
French	2 fl oz	275	22	3	0	0	20	—	—	442	38	—	—	—
Lite Italian	2 fl oz	63	3	0	0	0	8	—	—	294	7	—	—	—
SALADS AND SALAD BARS														
Gourmet Garden Salad w/ French Dressing	1 serv (10.7 oz)	409	29	5	10	7	33	—	—	792	449	—	—	—
Gourmet Garden Salad w/ Lite Italian Dressing	1 serv (10.7 oz)	305	10	2	2	7	22	—	—	643	417	—	—	—
Gourmet Garden Salad w/o Dressing	1 serv (8.7 oz)	134	6	2	2	7	13	—	—	350	410	—	—	—
Grilled Chicken Garden Salad w/o Dressing	1 serv (10.7 oz)	202	9	2	32	19	14	—	—	747	558	—	—	—

FOOD	PORTION	CALORIES	FAT	SAT FAT	CHOL	PROTEIN	CARBO	FIBER	CALCIUM	SOD	POTAS	VIT C	FOLIC	VIT A
RED LOBSTER														
CHILDREN'S MENU SELECTIONS														
Cheeseburger	1 serv	1040	56	18	130	—	—	—	—	720	—	—	—	—
Fried Chicken Fingers	1 serv	680	33	6	35	—	—	—	—	630	—	—	—	—
Fried Shrimp	1 serv	650	33	6	80	—	—	—	—	510	—	—	—	—
Grilled Chicken Teneders	1 serv	580	24	4	55	—	—	—	—	400	—	—	—	—
Hamburger	1 serv	920	47	12	100	—	—	—	—	550	—	—	—	—
Popcorn Shrimp	1 serv	650	35	6	120	—	—	—	—	480	—	—	—	—
Popcorn Shrimp & Cheesesticks	1 serv	750	41	9	125	—	—	—	—	680	—	—	—	—
Spaghetti & Cheesesticks	1 serv	830	39	6	5	—	—	—	—	950	—	—	—	—
DESSERTS														
Carrot Cake	1 serv (6.5 oz)	730	31	—	—	—	—	—	—	—	—	—	—	—
Cheesecake	1 serv (5.5 oz)	530	41	—	—	—	—	—	—	—	—	—	—	—
Fudge Overboard	1 serv	620	23	12	105	—	—	—	—	110	—	—	—	—
Ice Cream	1 serv (4.5 oz)	140	7	5	30	—	—	—	—	60	—	—	—	—
Key Lime Pie	1 serv (5 oz)	450	15	—	—	—	—	—	—	—	—	—	—	—
Raspberry Cobbler	1 serv (3 oz)	530	33	—	—	—	—	—	—	—	—	—	—	—
Sensational 7	1 serv	790	41	19	140	—	—	—	—	690	—	—	—	—
MAIN MENU SELECTIONS														
Admiral's Feast	1 serv	1060	52	12	265	—	—	—	—	2400	—	—	—	—
Appetizer Calamari	1 serv	350	22	6	190	—	—	—	—	510	—	—	—	—
Appetizer Chicken Fingers	1 serv	390	18	4	65	—	—	—	—	770	—	—	—	—
Appetizer Chilled Shrimp In The Shell	1 serv (6 oz)	110	2	0	235	—	—	—	—	270	—	—	—	—
Appetizer Crab & Shrimp Cakes	1 serv	480	24	6	80	—	—	—	—	1550	—	—	—	—
Appetizer Crab Add-On	1 serv	60	1	0	55	—	—	—	—	160	—	—	—	—
Appetizer Fresh Fried Mushrooms	1 serv	790	51	13	<5	—	—	—	—	1280	—	—	—	—
Appetizer Lobster Quesadilla	1 serv	760	47	24	160	—	—	—	—	1300	—	—	—	—
Appetizer Lobster Stuffed Mushroom	1 serv	400	26	13	100	—	—	—	—	960	—	—	—	—
Appetizer Mozzarella Cheesesticks	1 serv	730	46	20	50	—	—	—	—	1570	—	—	—	—
Appetizer Parmesan Zucchini	1 serv	620	40	11	10	—	—	—	—	1200	—	—	—	—

FOOD	PORTION	CALORIES	FAT	SAT FAT	CHOL	PROTEIN	CARBO	FIBER	CALCIUM	SOD	POTAS	VIT C	FOLIC	VIT A
Appetizer Shrimp Cocktail	1 serv	50	1	0	105	—	—	—	—	120	—	—	—	—
Appetizer Stuffed Mushrooms	1 serv	420	27	13	90	—	—	—	—	940	—	—	—	—
Applesauce	1 serv (4 oz)	90	0	0	0	—	—	—	—	5	—	—	—	—
Atlantic Cod	1 serv (8 oz)	200	2	0	105	—	—	—	—	150	—	—	—	—
Atlantic Cod	1 lunch serv (5 oz)	110	1	0	60	—	—	—	—	85	—	—	—	—
Atlantic Salmon	1 lunch serv (5 oz)	200	9	2	80	—	—	—	—	60	—	—	—	—
Atlantic Salmon	1 serv (8 oz)	340	15	3	135	—	—	—	—	105	—	—	—	—
Baked Atlantic Cod	1 serv	220	6	1	100	—	—	—	—	440	—	—	—	—
Baked Atlantic Haddock	1 serv	220	6	1	100	—	—	—	—	440	—	—	—	—
Baked Flounder	1 lunch serv	190	7	1	90	—	—	—	—	440	—	—	—	—
Baked Potato	1 (8 oz)	130	0	0	0	—	—	—	—	10	—	—	—	—
Broccoli	1 serv (3 oz)	25	0	0	0	—	—	—	—	10	—	—	—	—
Broiled Fisherman's Platter	1 serv	600	23	4	250	—	—	—	—	1660	—	—	—	—
Broiled Rock Lobster Tail	1 tail	190	6	1	110	—	—	—	—	750	—	—	—	—
Broiled Seafarer's Platter	1 serv	450	19	2	190	—	—	—	—	1100	—	—	—	—
Caesar Salad w/ Dressing	1 serv	240	21	4	15	—	—	—	—	490	—	—	—	·
Catfish	1 lunch serv (5 oz)	130	2	0	75	—	—	—	—	115	—	—	—	—
Catfish	1 serv (8 oz)	220	3	1	130	—	—	—	—	200	—	—	—	—
Catfish Santa Fe	1 serv	340	9	2	165	—	—	—	—	890	—	—	—	—
Catfish Sante Fe	1 lunch serv	180	6	1	85	—	—	—	—	450	—	—	—	—
Chicken Fingers	1 lunch serv	390	18	4	64	—	—	—	—	770	—	—	—	—
Chicken Fresco	1 serv	1320	73	33	240	—	—	—	—	1990	—	—	—	—
Chicken Fresco	1 lunch serv	660	36	17	120	—	—	—	—	990	—	—	—	—
Clam Strips	1 serv	720	39	9	35	—	—	—	—	1820	—	—	—	—
Clam Strips	1 lunch serv	360	19	5	15	—	—	—	—	910	—	—	—	—
Cocktail Sauce	1 oz	30	0	0	0	—	—	—	—	380	—	—	—	—
Cole Slaw	1 serv (4 oz)	190	16	2	25	—	—	—	—	260	—	—	—	—
Crab Alfredo	1 lunch serv	590	33	17	135	—	—	—	—	980	—	—	·	—
Crab Alfredo	1 serv	1170	66	35	270	—	—	—	—	1970	—	—	—	—
Fish & Shrimp Combo	1 serv	730	35	9	230	—	—	—	—	1630	—	—	—	—
Fish Nuggets	1 lunch serv	320	14	4	95	—	—	—	—	760	—	—	—	—
Fish Seasoning Add On For Blackened Dinner	1 serv	70	5	1	0	—	—	—	—	410	—	—	—	—
Fish Seasoning Add On For Blackened Lunch	1 serv	50	4	1	0	—	—	—	—	280	—	—	—	—

FOOD	PORTION	CALORIES	FAT	SAT FAT	CHOL	PROTEIN	CARBO	FIBER	CALCIUM	SOD	POTAS	VIT C	FOLIC	VIT A
Fish Seasoning Add On For Broiled Dinner	1 serv	45	5	1	0	—	—	—	—	300	—	—	—	—
Fish Seasoning Add On For Broiled Lunch	1 serv	35	4	1	0	—	—	—	—	240	—	—	—	—
Fish Seasoning Add On For Grilled Dinner	1 serv	35	4	1	0	—	—	—	—	30	—	—	—	—
Fish Seasoning Add On For Grilled Lunch	1 serv	25	3	1	0	—	—	—	—	25	—	—	—	—
Fish Seasoning Add On For Lemon Pepper Dinner	1 serv	35	4	1	0	—	—	—	—	80	—	—	—	—
Fish Seasoning Add On For Lemon Pepper Lunch	1 serv	30	3	1	0	—	—	—	—	65	—	—	—	—
Fish Seasoning Add On For Sante Fe Style Dinner	1 serv	60	4	1	0	—	—	—	—	330	—	—	—	—
Fish Seasoning Add On For Sante Fe Style Lunch	1 serv	40	3	1	0	—	—	—	—	260	—	—	—	—
Flounder	1 serv (8 oz)	220	3	1	130	—	—	—	—	200	—	—	—	—
Flounder	1 lunch serv (5 oz)	130	2	2	75	—	—	—	—	115	—	—	—	—
French Fries	1 serv (4 oz)	350	22	3	0	—	—	—	—	180	—	—	—	—
Fried Flounder	1 lunch serv	230	10	3	60	—	—	—	—	590	—	—	—	—
Fried Shrimp	12 lg	500	27	7	290	—	—	—	—	950	—	—	—	—
Fried Shrimp	1 lunch serv	270	15	4	115	—	—	—	—	460	—	—	—	—
Garden Salad w/o Dressing	1 serv	50	1	0	0	—	—	—	—	90	—	—	—	—
Garlic Cheese Biscuit	1	140	8	3	5	—	—	—	—	320	—	—	—	—
Grilled Cheeseburger	1	580	34	15	130	—	—	—	—	540	—	—	—	—
Grilled Chicken Breasts	1 serv	230	7	2	105	—	—	—	—	280	—	—	—	—
Grilled Chicken Salad w/o Dressing	1 serv	320	10	2	70	—	—	—	—	910	—	—	—	—
Grouper	1 lunch serv (5 oz)	130	2	0	50	—	—	—	—	60	—	—	—	—
Grouper	1 serv (8 oz)	220	3	1	90	—	—	—	—	100	—	—	—	—
Haddock	1 lunch serv (5 oz)	120	1	0	80	—	—	—	—	95	—	—	—	—
Haddock	1 serv (8 oz)	210	2	0	140	—	—	—	—	160	—	—	—	—
Halibut	1 lunch serv (5 oz)	150	4	0	45	—	—	—	—	75	—	—	—	—

FOOD	PORTION	CALORIES	FAT	SAT FAT	CHOL	PROTEIN	CARBO	FIBER	CALCIUM	SOD	POTAS	VIT C	FOLIC	VIT A
Halibut	1 serv (8 oz)	260	6	1	75	—	—	—	—	130	—	—	—	—
King Salmon	1 serv (8 oz)	420	25	6	160	—	—	—	—	110	—	—	—	—
King Salmon	1 lunch serv (5 oz)	250	15	4	95	—	—	—	—	70	—	—	—	—
Lake Trout	1 serv (8 oz)	340	16	3	140	—	—	—	—	125	—	—	—	—
Lake Trout	1 lunch serv (5 oz)	200	9	2	80	—	—	—	—	75	—	—	—	—
Lemon Pepper Grilled Maki Mahi	1 serv	240	7	1	130	—	—	—	—	280	—	—	—	—
Lobster Shrimp & Scallop Scampi	1 lunch serv	430	16	3	80	—	—	—	—	450	—	—	—	—
Lobster Shrimp & Scallop Scampi	1 serv	870	33	5	135	—	—	—	—	900	—	—	—	—
Mahi Mahi	1 serv (8 oz)	220	3	1	130	—	—	—	—	200	—	—	—	—
Mahi Mahi	1 lunch serv (5 oz)	130	2	0	75	—	—	—	—	115	—	—	—	—
Maine Lobster Steamed	1 serv (1.25 lb)	160	1	0	125	—	—	—	—	670	—	—	—	—
Maine Lobster Stuffed	1 serv (2 lb)	430	10	2	210	—	—	—	—	1610	—	—	—	—
Marinara Sauce	1 serv	50	4	0	0	—	—	—	—	220	—	—	—	—
Melted Butter	1 oz	200	22	14	60	—	—	—	—	240	—	—	—	—
Neptune's Feast	1 serv	1210	62	14	290	—	—	—	—	3050	—	—	—	—
New York Strip Steak	1 serv	560	34	13	180	—	—	—	—	530	—	—	—	—
Perch	1 serv (8 oz)	220	3	1	130	—	—	—	—	200	—	—	—	—
Perch	1 lunch serv (5 oz)	130	2	0	75	—	—	—	—	120	—	—	—	—
Pollack	1 lunch serv (5 oz)	120	2	0	100	—	—	—	—	120	—	—	—	—
Pollock	1 serv (8 oz)	120	2	0	100	—	—	—	—	120	—	—	—	—
Popcorn Shrimp	1 lunch serv	380	24	6	235	—	—	—	—	580	—	—	—	—
Popcorn Shrimp	1 serv	580	37	9	360	—	—	—	—	880	—	—	—	—
Red Rockfish	1 lunch serv (5 oz)	130	2	1	50	—	—	—	—	85	—	—	—	—
Red Rockfish	1 serv (8 oz)	230	4	1	85	—	—	—	—	140	—	—	—	—
Red Snapper	1 lunch serv (5 oz)	140	2	0	50	—	—	—	—	65	—	—	—	—
Red Snapper	1 serv (8 oz)	240	3	1	90	—	—	—	—	105	—	—	—	—
Rice Pilaf	1 serv (4 oz)	180	2	0	0	—	—	—	—	790	—	—	—	—
Roasted Vegetables	1 lunch serv (4 oz)	80	3	1	0	—	—	—	—	210	—	—	—	—
Roasted Vegetables	1 serv (6 oz)	120	4	1	0	—	—	—	—	310	—	—	—	—
Sailor's Platter	1 lunch serv	250	12	2	170	—	—	—	—	440	—	—	—	—
Sandwich Blackened Catfish	1	340	9	2	85	—	—	—	—	740	—	—	—	—
Sandwich Broiled Fish	1	300	8	2	80	—	—	—	—	690	—	—	—	—

FOOD	PORTION	CALORIES	FAT	SAT FAT	CHOL	PROTEIN	CARBO	FIBER	CALCIUM	SOD	POTAS	VIT C	FOLIC	VIT A
Sandwich Cajun Grilled Chicken	1	370	14	3	55	—	—	—	—	740	—	—	—	—
Sandwich Classic Fish	1	520	23	9	90	—	—	—	—	1050	—	—	—	—
Sandwich Grilled Chicken	1	290	7	2	50	—	—	—	—	430	—	—	—	—
Sassy Sauce	1 oz	80	6	1	5	—	—	—	—	140	—	—	—	—
Seafood Broil	1 lunch serv	310	14	2	110	—	—	—	—	850	—	—	—	—
Shrimp & Chicken	1 serv	340	15	4	225	—	—	—	—	470	—	—	—	—
Shrimp Caesar Salad w/o Dressing	1 serv	240	11	4	110	—	—	—	—	580	—	—	—	—
Shrimp Carbonara	1 lunch serv	650	38	19	155	—	—	—	—	1060	—	—	—	—
Shrimp Carbonara	1 serv	1290	76	38	310	—	—	—	—	2130	—	—	—	—
Shrimp Combo	1 serv	380	23	5	210	—	—	—	—	610	—	—	—	—
Shrimp Feast	1 serv	470	24	5	390	—	—	—	—	1040	—	—	—	—
Shrimp Milano	1 serv	1190	65	35	340	—	—	—	—	1970	—	—	—	—
Shrimp Milano	1 lunch serv	590	33	17	170	—	—	—	—	990	—	—	—	—
Shrimp Scampi	1 lunch serv	110	7	1	100	—	—	—	—	150	—	—	—	—
Smothered Chicken	1 serv	530	31	15	170	—	—	—	—	740	—	—	—	—
Snow Crab Legs	1 serv	110	2	0	115	—	—	—	—	320	—	—	—	—
Sockeye Salmon	1 lunch serv (5 oz)	240	12	2	95	—	—	—	—	75	—	—	—	—
Sockeye Salmon	1 serv (8 oz)	410	21	4	165	—	—	—	—	125	—	—	—	—
Sole	1 serv (8 oz)	220	3	1	130	—	—	—	—	200	—	—	—	—
Sole	1 lunch serv (5 oz)	130	2	0	75	—	—	—	—	115	—	—	—	—
Soup Bread Salad w/o Dressing	1 lunch serv	430	18	7	40	—	—	—	—	1960	—	—	—	—
Steak & Fried Shrimp	1 serv	780	46	15	340	—	—	—	—	770	—	—	—	—
Steak & Rock Lobster Tail	1 serv	570	31	11	220	—	—	—	—	880	—	—	—	—
Swordfish	1 serv (8 oz)	290	10	3	115	—	—	—	—	150	—	—	—	—
Swordfish	1 lunch serv (5 oz)	170	6	2	70	—	—	—	—	90	—	—	—	—
Tartar Sauce	1 oz	160	17	3	15	—	—	—	—	210	—	—	—	—
Teriyaki Grilled Chicken Breast	1 serv	240	7	2	105	—	—	—	—	660	—	—	—	—
Twice Baked Potato	1	430	23	14	60	—	—	—	—	1320	—	—	—	—
Walleye	1 serv (8 oz)	210	3	1	205	—	—	—	—	120	—	—	—	—
Walleye	1 lunch serv (5 oz)	120	2	0	120	—	—	—	—	70	—	—	—	—
Yellow Lake Perch	1 serv (8 oz)	220	3	1	130	—	—	—	—	200	—	—	—	—
Yellow Lake Perch	1 lunch serv (5 oz)	130	2	0	75	—	—	—	—	120	—	—	—	—
SALAD DRESSINGS														
Blue Cheese	1 serv	170	18	3	30	—	—	—	—	200	—	—	—	—

FOOD	PORTION	CALORIES	FAT	SAT FAT	CHOL	PROTEIN	CARBO	FIBER	CALCIUM	SOD	POTAS	VIT C	FOLIC	VIT A
Buttermilk Ranch	1 serv	110	11	2	15	—	—	—	—	300	—	—	—	—
Caesar	1 serv	170	18	3	10	—	—	—	—	290	—	—	—	—
Dijon Honey Mustard	1 serv	140	13	2	20	—	—	—	—	180	—	—	—	—
Fat Free Ranch	1 serv	50	0	0	0	—	—	—	—	310	—	—	—	—
Lite Red Wine Vinaigrette	1 serv	50	3	0	0	—	—	—	—	270	—	—	—	—
SOUPS														
Bayou Style Gumbo	1 serv (6 oz)	120	4	1	65	—	—	—	—	710	—	—	—	—
Broccoli Cheese	1 serv	160	9	6	25	—	—	—	—	800	—	—	—	—
Clam Chowder	1 serv (6 oz)	130	5	3	20	—	—	—	—	820	—	—	—	—

ROY ROGERS

FOOD	PORTION	CALORIES	FAT	SAT FAT	CHOL	PROTEIN	CARBO	FIBER	CALCIUM	SOD	POTAS	VIT C	FOLIC	VIT A
BREAKFAST SELECTIONS														
3 Pancakes	1 serv (4.8 oz)	280	2	1	15	8	56	—	—	890	—	—	—	—
3 Pancakes w/ 1 Sausage	1 serv (6.2 oz)	430	16	6	40	16	56	—	—	1290	—	—	—	—
3 Pancakes w/ 2 Bacon	1 serv (5.3 oz)	350	9	3	25	13	56	—	—	1130	—	—	—	—
Bagel Cinnamon Raisin	1 (4 oz)	300	1	tr	0	10	63	—	—	490	—	—	—	—
Bagel Plain	1 (4 oz)	300	2	tr	0	10	60	—	—	520	—	—	—	—
Big Country Platters w/ Bacon	1 serv (7.6 oz)	740	43	13	305	25	61	—	—	1800	—	—	—	—
Big Country Platters w/ Ham	1 serv (9.4 oz)	710	39	11	330	24	67	—	—	2210	—	—	—	—
Big Country Platters w/ Sausage	1 serv (9.6 oz)	920	60	19	340	33	61	—	—	2230	—	—	—	—
Biscuit	1 (2.9 oz)	390	21	6	0	6	44	—	—	1000	—	—	—	—
Biscuit Bacon	1 (3.1 oz)	420	23	7	5	9	44	—	—	1140	—	—	—	—
Biscuit Bacon & Egg	1 (4.2 oz)	470	26	8	150	14	44	—	—	1190	—	—	—	—
Biscuit Cinnamon 'N' Raisin	1 (2.8 oz)	370	18	5	0	3	48	—	—	450	—	—	—	—
Biscuit Ham & Cheese	1 (4.5 oz)	450	24	8	25	11	48	—	—	1570	—	—	—	—
Biscuit Ham & Egg	1 (5.1 oz)	460	23	7	165	14	48	—	—	1395	—	—	—	—
Biscuit Ham, Egg & Cheese	1 (5.6 oz)	500	27	10	170	16	48	—	—	1620	—	—	—	—
Biscuit Sausage	1 (4.1 oz)	510	31	10	25	14	44	—	—	1360	—	—	—	—
Biscuit Sausage & Egg	1 (5.2 oz)	560	35	11	170	18	44	—	—	1400	—	—	—	—
Hashrounds	1 serv (2.8 oz)	230	14	3	0	3	24	—	—	560	—	—	—	—
Sourdough Ham, Egg & Cheese	1 (6.8 oz)	480	24	9	185	20	45	—	—	1440	—	—	—	—
DESSERTS														
Strawberry Shortcake	1 serv (6.6 oz)	480	21	5	40	8	39	—	—	330	—	—	—	—

FOOD	PORTION	CALORIES	FAT	SAT FAT	CHOL	PROTEIN	CARBO	FIBER	CALCIUM	SOD	POTAS	VIT C	FOLIC	VIT A
ICE CREAM														
Ice Cream Cone	1 (4.1 oz)	180	4	3	15	5	29	—	—	80	—	—	—	—
Sundae Hot Fudge	1 (6 oz)	320	10	5	25	8	50	—	—	260	—	—	—	—
Sundae Strawberry	1 (5.5 oz)	260	6	3	15	6	44	—	—	95	—	—	—	—
MAIN MENU SELECTIONS														
¼ Cheeseburger	1 (6 oz)	510	26	—	—	24	44	—	—	620	—	—	—	—
¼ Hamburger	1 (5.5 oz)	460	22	—	—	22	44	—	—	390	—	—	—	—
¼ Roaster Dark Meat	7.4 oz	490	34	10	225	43	2	—	—	1120	—	—	—	—
¼ Roaster Dark Meat w/ Skin Off	4 oz	190	10	3	110	24	1	—	—	400	—	—	—	—
¼ Roaster White Meat	8.6 oz	500	29	9	240	56	3	—	—	1450	—	—	—	—
¼ Roaster White Meat w/ Skin Off	4.7 oz	190	6	2	100	32	2	—	—	700	—	—	—	—
Bacon Cheeseburger	1 (5.9 oz)	520	31	—	—	27	32	—	—	740	—	—	—	—
Baked Beans	1 serv (5 oz)	160	2	1	10	6	30	—	—	560	—	—	—	—
Baked Potato	1 (3.9 oz)	130	1	0	0	3	27	—	—	65	—	—	—	—
Baked Potato w/ Margarine	1 (4.4 oz)	240	13	2	0	3	27	—	—	220	—	—	—	—
Baked Potato w/ Margarine & Sour Cream	1 (5.4 oz)	300	19	6	15	4	28	—	—	230	—	—	—	—
Cheeseburger	1 (4.2 oz)	300	13	7	25	13	34	—	—	690	—	—	—	—
Chicken Fillet Sandwich	1 (8.3 oz)	500	24	5	20	19	49	—	—	1050	—	—	—	—
Cole Slaw	1 serv (5 oz)	295	25	4	15	2	16	—	—	430	—	—	—	—
Cornbread	1 serv (2.7 oz)	310	17	3	30	4	35	—	—	260	—	—	—	—
Fisherman's Fillet	1 (6.5 oz)	490	21	5	15	21	56	—	—	1040	—	—	—	—
Fried Chicken Breast	1 (5.2 oz)	370	15	4	75	29	29	—	—	1190	—	—	—	—
Fried Chicken Leg	1 (2.4 oz)	170	7	2	45	13	15	—	—	570	—	—	—	—
Fried Chicken Thigh	1 (4.2 oz)	330	15	4	60	19	30	—	—	1000	—	—	—	—
Fried Chicken Wing	1 (2.3 oz)	200	8	2	30	10	23	—	—	740	—	—	—	—
Fry	1 lg (6.1 oz)	430	18	5	0	6	59	—	—	190	—	—	—	—
Fry	1 reg (5 oz)	350	15	4	0	5	49	—	—	150	—	—	—	—
Gravy	1 serv (1.5 fl oz)	20	tr	tr	0	tr	3	—	—	260	—	—	—	—
Grilled Chicken Sandwich	1 (8.3 oz)	340	11	2	30	25	32	—	—	910	—	—	—	—
Hamburger	1 (3.8 oz)	260	9	4	20	11	33	—	—	460	—	—	—	—
Mashed Potatoes	1 serv (5 oz)	92	tr	tr	0	2	20	—	—	320	—	—	—	—
Nuggets	9 (6.2 oz)	460	29	6	25	20	32	—	—	970	—	—	—	—
Nuggets	6 (4 oz)	290	18	4	15	12	20	—	—	610	—	—	—	—

FOOD	PORTION	CALORIES	FAT	SAT FAT	CHOL	PROTEIN	CARBO	FIBER	CALCIUM	SOD	POTAS	VIT C	FOLIC	VIT A
Pizza	1 serv (4.75 oz)	282	6	3	14	13	44	1	201	549	149	4	—	408
Roast Beef Sandwich	1 (5.7 oz)	260	4	1	60	24	30	—	—	700	—	—	—	—
Sourdough Bacon Cheeseburger	1 (9.1 oz)	770	50	—	—	33	45	—	—	1410	—	—	—	—
Sourdough Grilled Chicken	1 (10.1 oz)	500	21	6	45	30	46	—	—	1530	—	—	—	—
SALADS AND SALAD BARS														
Garden Salad	1 (9.3 oz)	190	14	9	40	12	3	—	—	280	—	—	—	—
Grilled Chicken Salad	1 serv (9.8 oz)	120	4	1	60	18	2	—	—	520	—	—	—	—
Side Salad	1 (4.9 oz)	20	tr	tr	0	1	3	—	—	20	—	—	—	—

SCHLOTZSKY'S DELI

FOOD	PORTION	CALORIES	FAT	SAT FAT	CHOL	PROTEIN	CARBO	FIBER	CALCIUM	SOD	POTAS	VIT C	FOLIC	VIT A
PIZZA														
Chicken & Pesto	1	634	18	—	—	—	—	—	—	—	—	—	—	—
Onion & Mushroom	1	577	20	—	—	—	—	—	—	—	—	—	—	—
Smoked Turkey & Jalapeno	1	589	13	—	—	—	—	—	—	—	—	—	—	—
Vegetarian	1	555	17	—	—	—	—	—	—	—	—	—	—	—
SALAD AND SALAD BARS														
Chicken Chef	1 serv	192	8	—	—	—	—	—	—	—	—	—	—	—
Turkey Club	1 serv	233	10	—	—	—	—	—	—	—	—	—	—	—
SANDWICHES														
Chicken Breast	1 sm	514	22	—	—	—	—	—	—	—	—	—	—	—
Dijon Chicken Breast	1 sm	469	16	—	—	—	—	—	—	—	—	—	—	—
Smoked Turkey	1 sm	510	22	—	—	—	—	—	—	—	—	—	—	—
The Original	1 sm	598	33	—	—	—	—	—	—	—	—	—	—	—
SOUPS														
Creole Vegetable	1 serv (8 fl oz)	120	3	—	—	—	—	—	—	—	—	—	—	—
Red Bean	1 serv (8 fl oz)	110	2	—	—	—	—	—	—	—	—	—	—	—
Shrimp & Okra	1 serv (8 fl oz)	100	3	—	—	—	—	—	—	—	—	—	—	—
Spicy Chicken	1 serv (8 fl oz)	120	3	—	—	—	—	—	—	—	—	—	—	—

SHAKEY'S

FOOD	PORTION	CALORIES	FAT	SAT FAT	CHOL	PROTEIN	CARBO	FIBER	CALCIUM	SOD	POTAS	VIT C	FOLIC	VIT A
MAIN MENU SELECTIONS														
3 Piece Fried Chicken And Potatoes	1 serv	947	56	—	—	57	51	—	—	2293	—	—	—	—
5 Piece Fried Chicken And Potatoes	1 serv	1700	90	—	—	97	130	—	—	5327	—	—	—	—
Hot Ham And Cheese	1	550	21	—	—	36	56	—	—	2135	—	—	—	—
Potatoes	15 pieces	950	36	—	—	17	120	—	—	3703	—	—	—	—

FOOD	PORTION	CALORIES	FAT	SAT FAT	CHOL	PROTEIN	CARBO	FIBER	CALCIUM	SOD	POTAS	VIT C	FOLIC	VIT A
Spaghetti With Meat Sauce And Garlic Bread	1 serv	940	33	—	—	26	134	—	—	1904	—	—	—	—
PIZZA														
Thick Crust Cheese	1 slice	170	5	—	13	9	22	—	—	421	—	—	—	—
Thick Crust Green Pepper, Black Olives, Mushrooms	1 slice	162	4	—	13	9	22	—	—	418	—	—	—	—
Thick Crust Pepperoni	1 slice	185	6	—	17	10	22	—	—	422	—	—	—	—
Thick Crust Sausage, Mushrooms	1 slice	179	6	—	15	10	22	—	—	420	—	—	—	—
Thick Crust Sausage, Pepperoni	1 slice	177	8	—	19	11	22	—	—	424	—	—	—	—
Thick Crust Shakey's Special	1 slice	208	8	—	18	13	22	—	—	423	—	—	—	—
Thin Crust Cheese	1 slice	133	5	—	14	8	13	—	—	323	—	—	—	—
Thin Crust Onion, Green Pepper, Black Olives, Mushrooms	1 slice	125	5	—	11	7	14	—	—	313	—	—	—	—
Thin Crust Pepperoni	1 slice	148	7	—	14	8	13	—	—	403	—	—	—	—
Thin Crust Sausage, Mushroom	1 slice	141	6	—	13	9	13	—	—	336	—	—	—	—
Thin Crust Sausage, Pepperoni	1 slice	166	8	—	17	9	13	—	—	397	—	—	—	—
Thin Crust Shakey's Special	1 slice	171	9	—	16	9	14	—	—	475	—	—	—	—

SHONEY'S

FOOD	PORTION	CALORIES	FAT	SAT FAT	CHOL	PROTEIN	CARBO	FIBER	CALCIUM	SOD	POTAS	VIT C	FOLIC	VIT A
BREAKFAST SELECTIONS														
100% Natural	½ cup	244	11	—	0	6	33	2	—	45	—	—	—	—
Ambrosia Salad	¼ cup	75	3	—	0	1	12	1	—	167	—	—	—	—
Apple	1	81	1	—	0	tr	21	3	—	1	—	—	—	—
Apple Butter	1 tbsp	37	tr	—	0	tr	9	0	—	0	—	—	—	—
Apple Grape Surprise	¼ cup	19	0	0	0	0	5	tr	—	2	—	—	—	—
Apple Ring	1	15	0	0	0	0	4	0	—	0	—	—	—	—
Apple sliced	1 slice	13	tr	—	0	0	3	1	—	0	—	—	—	—
Bacon	1 strip	36	3	—	5	2	0	0	—	101	—	—	—	—
Beef Stick	1	43	1	—	—	3	5	0	—	17	—	—	—	—
Biscuit	1	170	8	—	0	3	22	0	—	364	—	—	—	—
Blueberries	¼ cup	21	tr	—	0	tr	5	1	—	2	—	—	—	—

FOOD	PORTION	CALORIES	FAT	SAT FAT	CHOL	PROTEIN	CARBO	FIBER	CALCIUM	SOD	POTAS	VIT C	FOLIC	VIT A
Blueberry Muffin	1	107	4	—	17	2	18	1	—	1	—	—	—	—
Bread Pudding	1 sq	305	11	—	80	8	44	0	—	409	—	—	—	—
Breakfast Ham	1 slice	26	1	—	14	4	tr	0	—	263	—	—	—	—
Brunch Cake Apple	1 sq	160	8	—	0	2	19	0	—	150	—	—	—	—
Brunch Cake Banana	1 sq	152	7	—	0	2	21	0	—	120	—	—	—	—
Brunch Cake Carrot	1 sq	150	7	—	0	2	20	0	—	159	—	—	—	—
Brunch Cake Pineapple	1 sq	147	7	—	0	2	20	0	—	120	—	—	—	—
Brunch Cake Sour Cream	1 sq	160	8	—	0	2	21	0	—	135	—	—	—	—
Buttered Toast	2 slices	163	5	—	0	4	25	1	—	296	—	—	—	—
Cantaloupe Sliced	1 slice	8	tr	—	0	tr	2	tr	—	2	—	—	—	—
Cantaloupe Diced	½ cup	28	tr	—	0	1	7	tr	—	7	—	—	—	—
Captain Crunch Berry	½ cup	73	2	—	0	1	14	tr	—	122	—	—	—	—
Cheese Sauce	1 ladle	26	2	—	0	tr	4	0	—	166	—	—	—	—
Chicken Pieces	1 piece	40	2	—	—	4	2	0	—	28	—	—	—	—
Chocolate Pudding	¼ cup	81	2	—	7	2	16	0	—	81	—	—	—	—
Cinnamon Honey Bun	1	344	12	—	0	6	54	0	—	169	—	—	—	—
Cottage Cheese	1 tbsp	12	tr	—	1	2	1	0	—	66	—	—	—	—
Cottage Fries	¼ cup	62	2	—	0	1	10	0	—	124	—	—	—	—
Country Gravy	¼ cup	82	7	—	1	1	4	0	—	255	—	—	—	—
Croissant	1	260	16	—	2	5	22	0	—	260	—	—	—	—
Donut Mini Cinnamon	1 (14 g)	56	3	—	0	1	7	0	—	65	—	—	—	—
DoughNugget	1	157	10	—	0	2	15	0	—	194	—	—	—	—
Egg Fried	1	159	15	—	274	6	1	0	—	69	—	—	—	—
Egg Scrambled	¼ cup	95	7	—	248	6	1	0	—	155	—	—	—	—
English Muffin w/ Margarine	1	140	2	—	0	2	18	1	—	1	—	—	—	—
Fluff	¼ cup	16	0	0	0	tr	3	0	—	0	—	—	—	—
French Toast	1 slice	69	3	—	0	1	9	0	—	157	—	—	—	—
Fruit Delight	¼ cup	54	2	—	0	1	10	1	—	2	—	—	—	—
Fruit Topping All Flavors	1 tbsp	24	0	0	0	tr	6	tr	—	3	—	—	—	—
Glaced Fruit	¼ cup	51	tr	—	0	tr	13	1	—	5	—	—	—	—
Golden Pound Cake	1 slice	134	5	—	13	2	20	0	—	144	—	—	—	—
Grape Jelly	1 tbsp	60	0	0	0	0	16	0	—	0	—	—	—	—
Grapefruit Canned	¼ cup	24	tr	—	0	tr	6	tr	—	5	—	—	—	—
Grapes	25	57	1	—	0	1	14	1	—	2	—	—	—	—
Grits	¼ cup	57	3	—	0	1	6	1	—	62	—	—	—	—
Hashbrowns	¼ cup	43	2	—	0	1	7	0	—	24	—	—	—	—
Home Fries	¼ cup	53	2	—	0	1	9	0	—	24	—	—	—	—

FOOD	PORTION	CALORIES	FAT	SAT FAT	CHOL	PROTEIN	CARBO	FIBER	CALCIUM	SOD	POTAS	VIT C	FOLIC	VIT A
Honey Bun	1	265	14	—	3	4	32	0	—	33	—	—	—	—
Honeydew Sliced	1 slice	13	0	0	0	tr	3	tr	—	4	—	—	—	—
Jelly Packet	1	40	0	0	0	0	10	0	—	2	—	—	—	—
Jr. Bun Chocolate	1	141	5	—	0	2	22	0	—	70	—	—	—	—
Jr. Bun Honey	1	141	5	—	0	2	22	0	—	70	—	—	—	—
Jr. Bun Maple	1	141	5	—	0	2	22	0	—	70	—	—	—	—
Kiwi Sliced	1 slice	11	tr	—	0	tr	3	tr	—	1	—	—	—	—
Marble Cake w/ Icing	1 slice	136	5	—	0	2	22	0	—	149	—	—	—	—
Mixed Fruit	¼ cup	37	tr	—	0	tr	9	tr	—	3	—	—	—	—
Mushroom Topping	1 oz	25	2	—	0	1	1	tr	—	323	—	—	—	—
Oleo Whipped	1 tbsp	70	8	—	0	0	0	0	—	97	—	—	—	—
Omelette Topping	1 spoonful	23	2	—	3	1	1	tr	—	99	—	—	—	—
Orange	1 med	65	tr	—	0	1	16	1	—	2	—	—	—	—
Orange Sections	1 section	7	0	0	0	tr	2	tr	—	0	—	—	—	—
Oriental Salad	¼ cup	79	3	—	1	1	13	1	—	32	—	—	—	—
Pancake	1	41	tr	—	0	1	9	0	—	238	—	—	—	—
Pear	1	98	1	—	0	1	25	4	—	1	—	—	—	—
Pineapple Bits	1 tbsp	9	0	0	0	tr	2	0	—	2	—	—	—	—
Pineapple Fresh Sliced	1 slice	10	tr	—	0	tr	3	tr	—	0	—	—	—	—
Pistachio Pineapple Salad	¼ cup	98	0	—	3	1	20	0	—	39	—	—	—	—
Prunes	1 tbsp	19	0	0	0	tr	5	1	—	0	—	—	—	—
Raisin Bran	½ cup	87	1	—	0	3	22	3	—	185	—	—	—	—
Raisin English Muffin w/ Margarine	1	158	4	—	0	4	27	0	—	280	—	—	—	—
Sausage Link	1	91	9	—	13	3	tr	0	—	291	—	—	—	—
Sausage Patty	1	136	13	—	2	4	1	0	—	48	—	—	—	—
Sausage Rice	¼ cup	110	6	—	8	3	10	tr	—	211	—	—	—	—
Shortcake	1	60	2	—	0	1	13	0	—	90	—	—	—	—
Sirloin Steak Charbroiled	6 oz	357	25	—	99	32	0	0	—	160	—	—	—	—
Smoked Sausage	1	103	10	—	13	3	1	0	—	39	—	—	—	—
Snow Salad	¼ cup	72	4	—	0	1	9	tr	—	18	—	—	—	—
Strawberries	5	23	tr	—	0	1	5	1	—	1	—	—	—	—
Syrup Light	1 ladle	60	0	0	0	0	15	0	—	0	—	—	—	—
Syrup Low-Cal	2.2 oz	98	0	0	0	0	24	0	—	0	—	—	—	—
Tangerine	1	37	tr	—	0	1	9	tr	—	1	—	—	—	—
Trix	½ cup	54	tr	—	0	1	13	tr	—	89	—	—	—	—
Waldorf Salad	¼ cup	81	5	—	2	1	9	1	—	68	—	—	—	—
Watermelon Diced	½ cup	50	1	—	0	1	12	tr	—	3	—	—	—	—
Watermelon Sliced	1 slice	9	tr	—	0	tr	2	tr	—	1	—	—	—	—
Whipped Topping	1 scoop	10	1	—	0	0	1	0	—	3	—	—	—	—

FOOD	PORTION	CALORIES	FAT	SAT FAT	CHOL	PROTEIN	CARBO	FIBER	CALCIUM	SOD	POTAS	VIT C	FOLIC	VIT A
CHILDREN'S MENU SELECTIONS														
Jr. Burger All-American	1 serv	234	11	—	30	11	20	0	—	543	—	—	—	—
Kid's Chicken Dinner (fried)	1 serv	244	13	—	40	22	11	0	—	151	—	—	—	—
Kid's Fish N' Chips (includes fries)	1 serv	337	17	—	41	14	33	2	—	467	—	—	—	—
Kid's Fried Shrimp	1 serv	194	12	—	70	8	12	0	—	633	—	—	—	—
Kid's Spaghetti	1 serv	247	8	—	27	12	32	1	—	193	—	—	—	—
DESSERTS														
Apple Pie A La Mode	1 slice	492	23	—	35	6	67	—	—	574	—	—	—	—
Carrot Cake	1 slice	500	26	—	37	9	56	0	—	476	—	—	—	—
Strawberry Pie	1 slice	332	17	—	0	2	45	2	—	247	—	—	—	—
Walnut Brownie A La Mode	1	576	34	—	35	10	61	0	—	435	—	—	—	—
ICE CREAM														
Hot Fudge Cake	1 slice	522	20	—	27	7	82	0	—	485	—	—	—	—
Hot Fudge Sundae	1	451	22	—	60	7	60	0	—	226	—	—	—	—
Strawberry Sundae	1	380	19	—	69	6	48	tr	—	145	—	—	—	—
MAIN MENU SELECTIONS														
All-American Burger	1	501	33	—	86	25	27	1	—	597	—	—	—	—
BBQ Sauce	1 souffle cup	41	1	—	0	tr	8	0	—	232	—	—	—	—
Bacon Burger	1	591	40	—	86	29	29	1	—	801	—	—	—	—
Baked Fish	1 serv	170	1	—	83	35	2	0	—	1641	—	—	—	—
Baked Fish Light	1 serv	170	1	—	83	35	2	0	—	1641	—	—	—	—
Baked Ham Sandwich	1	290	10	—	42	19	28	2	—	1263	—	—	—	—
Baked Potato	10 oz	264	tr	—	0	6	61	7	—	16	—	—	—	—
Beef Patty Light	1 serv	289	23	—	82	21	0	0	—	187	—	—	—	—
Charbroiled Chicken	1 serv	239	7	—	85	39	1	0	—	592	—	—	—	—
Charbroiled Chicken Sandwich	1	451	17	—	90	43	28	1	—	1002	—	—	—	—
Chicken Fillet Sandwich	1	464	21	—	51	30	39	1	—	585	—	—	—	—
Chicken Tenders	1 serv	388	20	—	64	35	17	0	—	239	—	—	—	—
Cocktail Sauce	1 souffle cup	36	tr	—	0	tr	9	0	—	260	—	—	—	—
Country Fried Sandwich	1	588	26	—	29	25	67	1	—	1501	—	—	—	—
Country Fried Steak	1 serv	449	27	—	27	19	34	1	—	1177	—	—	—	—
Fish N' Chips (includes fries)	1 serv	639	35	—	103	32	50	3	—	873	—	—	—	—
Fish N' Shrimp	1 serv	487	26	—	127	28	37	tr	—	644	—	—	—	—
Fish Sandwich	1	323	13	—	21	12	41	tr	—	740	—	—	—	—

FOOD	PORTION	CALORIES	FAT	SAT FAT	CHOL	PROTEIN	CARBO	FIBER	CALCIUM	SOD	POTAS	VIT C	FOLIC	VIT A
French Fries	3 oz	189	8	—	0	3	29	3	—	273	—	—	—	—
French Fries	4 oz	252	10	—	0	4	39	4	—	364	—	—	—	—
Fried Fish Light	1 serv	297	14	—	65	20	22	tr	—	536	—	—	—	—
Grecian Bread	1 slice	80	2	—	0	2	13	0	—	94	—	—	—	—
Grilled Bacon & Cheese Sandwich	1	440	28	—	36	18	28	1	—	1200	—	—	—	—
Grilled Cheese Sandwich	1	302	17	—	36	12	25	1	—	880	—	—	—	—
Half O'Pound	1 serv	435	34	—	123	31	0	0	—	280	—	—	—	—
Ham Club On Whole Wheat	1	642	36	—	78	37	45	10	—	2105	—	—	—	—
Hawaiian Chicken	1 serv	262	7	—	85	39	7	tr	—	593	—	—	—	—
Italian Feast	1 serv	500	20	—	74	38	44	1	—	369	—	—	—	—
Lasagna	1 serv	297	10	—	26	8	45	3	—	870	—	—	—	—
Liver N' Onions	1 serv	411	23	—	529	15	23	1	—	321	—	—	—	48636
Mushroom Swiss Burger	1	616	42	—	106	32	29	1	—	1135	—	—	—	—
Old-Fashioned Burger	1	470	28	—	82	25	26	1	—	681	—	—	—	—
Onion Rings	1	52	3	—	2	1	5	tr	—	102	—	—	—	—
Patty Melt	1	640	42	—	171	39	30	7	—	826	—	—	—	—
Philly Steak Sandwich	1	673	44	—	103	32	37	tr	—	1242	—	—	—	—
Reuben Sandwich	1	596	35	—	138	33	32	6	—	3873	—	—	—	—
Ribeye	6 oz	605	51	—	141	35	0	0	—	141	—	—	—	—
Rice	3.5 oz	137	4	—	1	2	23	tr	—	765	—	—	—	—
Sauteed Mushrooms	3 oz	75	7	—	0	2	4	1	—	968	—	—	—	—
Sauteed Onions	2.5 oz	37	2	—	0	1	4	1	—	221	—	—	—	—
Seafood Platter	1 serv	566	28	—	127	33	46	tr	—	893	—	—	—	—
Shoney Burger	1	498	36	—	79	23	22	tr	—	782	—	—	—	—
Shrimp Bite-Size	1 serv	387	25	—	140	16	25	0	—	1266	—	—	—	—
Shrimp Broiled	1 serv	93	18	—	182	20	0	0	—	210	—	—	—	—
Shrimp Charbroiled	1 serv	138	3	—	162	25	3	0	—	170	—	—	—	—
Shrimp Sampler	1 serv	412	23	—	217	26	26	tr	—	783	—	—	—	—
Shrimper's Feast	1 serv	383	22	—	125	17	30	tr	—	216	—	—	—	—
Shrimper's Feast Large	1 serv	575	33	—	188	25	45	tr	—	324	—	—	—	—
Sirloin	6 oz	357	25	—	99	32	0	0	—	160	—	—	—	—
Slim Jim Sandwich	1	484	24	—	57	27	40	1	—	1620	—	—	—	—
Spaghetti	1 serv	496	16	—	55	24	63	2	—	387	—	—	—	—
Steak N' Shrimp (charbroiled shrimp)	1 serv	361	23	—	141	37	1	0	—	198	—	—	—	—
Steak N' Shrimp (fried shrimp)	1 serv	507	33	—	150	37	15	tr	—	249	—	—	—	—

FOOD	PORTION	CALORIES	FAT	SAT FAT	CHOL	PROTEIN	CARBO	FIBER	CALCIUM	SOD	POTAS	VIT C	FOLIC	VIT A
Sweet N' Sour Sauce	1 souffle cup	58	0	0	0	0	15	0	—	5	—	—	—	—
Tartar Sauce	1 souffle cup	84	8	—	11	tr	4	0	—	177	—	—	—	—
Turkey Club On Whole Wheat	1	635	33	—	100	44	44	10	—	1289	—	—	—	—
SALAD DRESSINGS														
Biscayne Lo-Cal	2 tbsp	62	1	—	0	6	1	0	—	334	—	—	—	—
Blue Cheese	2 tbsp	113	13	—	15	0	0	0	—	109	—	—	—	—
Creamy Italian	2 tbsp	135	15	—	0	0	1	0	—	454	—	—	—	—
French	2 tbsp	124	12	—	12	2	2	0	—	204	—	—	—	—
Golden Italian	2 tbsp	141	15	—	0	0	1	0	—	302	—	—	—	—
Honey Mustard	2 tbsp	165	17	—	18	2	2	0	—	5	—	—	—	—
Ranch	2 tbsp	95	10	—	15	0	0	0	—	10	—	—	—	—
Rue French	2 tbsp	122	10	—	0	5	2	0	—	364	—	—	—	—
Thousand Island	2 tbsp	130	13	—	12	1	2	0	—	179	—	—	—	—
W.W. Italian	2 tbsp	10	0	—	0	0	2	0	—	615	—	—	—	—
SALADS AND SALAD BARS														
Ambrosia Salad	¼ cup	75	3	—	0	1	12	1	—	167	—	—	—	—
Apple Grape Surprise	¼ cup	19	0	—	0	0	5	tr	—	2	—	—	—	—
Apple Ring	1	15	0	—	0	0	4	—	—	3	—	—	—	—
Bacon Bits	1 spoonful	15	1	—	—	1	1	—	—	—	—	—	—	—
Beet Onion Salad	¼ cup	25	1	—	0	1	3	1	—	167	—	—	—	—
Broccoli	¼ cup	4	tr	—	0	0	1	tr	—	4	—	—	—	—
Broccoli Cauliflower Carrot Salad	¼ cup	53	4	—	1	1	3	1	—	193	—	—	—	—
Broccoli Cauliflower Ranch	¼ cup	65	6	—	9	1	2	1	—	12	—	—	—	—
Broccoli & Cauliflower	¼ cup	98	9	—	0	2	4	1	—	478	—	—	—	—
Carrot	¼ cup	10	tr	—	0	tr	2	1	—	8	—	—	—	—
Carrot Apple Salad	¼ cup	99	9	—	8	1	4	1	—	10	—	—	—	—
Cauliflower	¼ cup	8	tr	—	0	1	2	1	—	5	—	—	—	—
Celery	1 tbsp	5	0	—	0	tr	tr	tr	—	7	—	—	—	—
Cheese Shredded	1 tbsp	21	2	—	2	1	tr	0	—	112	—	—	—	—
Chocolate Pudding	¼ cup	81	2	—	7	2	16	0	—	81	—	—	—	—
Chow Mein Noodles	1 spoonful	13	1	—	0	tr	tr	tr	—	0	—	—	—	—
Cole Slaw	¼ cup	69	5	—	7	1	5	1	—	106	—	—	—	—
Cottage Cheese	1 tbsp	12	tr	—	1	2	1	0	—	66	—	—	—	—
Croutons	1 spoonful	13	tr	—	0	tr	2	0	—	38	—	—	—	—
Cucumber	1 tbsp	1	0	—	0	tr	tr	tr	—	0	—	—	—	—
Cucumber Lite	¼ cup	12	tr	—	0	tr	3	tr	—	344	—	—	—	—
Don's Pasta	¼ cup	82	5	—	0	2	9	tr	—	223	—	—	—	—
Egg Diced	1 tbsp	15	1	—	54	1	tr	0	—	14	—	—	—	—

FOOD	PORTION	CALORIES	FAT	SAT FAT	CHOL	PROTEIN	CARBO	FIBER	CALCIUM	SOD	POTAS	VIT C	FOLIC	VIT A
Fruit Delight	¼ cup	54	2	—	0	1	10	1	—	2	—	—	—	—
Fruit Topping All Flavors	¼ cup	64	tr	—	0	tr	16	tr	—	8	—	—	—	—
Glaced Fruit	¼ cup	51	tr	—	0	tr	13	1	—	5	—	—	—	—
Granola	1 spoonful	25	1	—	0	1	3	—	—	—	—	—	—	—
Grapefruit	¼ cup	24	tr	—	0	1	6	tr	—	5	—	—	—	—
Green Pepper	1 tbsp	1	0	—	0	0	tr	tr	—	0	—	—	—	—
Italian Vegetable	¼ cup	11	tr	—	0	tr	3	1	—	110	—	—	—	—
Jello	¼ cup	40	0	—	0	1	9	0	—	26	—	—	—	—
Jello Fluff	¼ cup	16	tr	—	0	tr	3	0	—	0	—	—	—	—
Kidney Bean Salad	¼ cup	55	2	—	2	3	7	2	—	154	—	—	—	—
Lettuce	1.8 oz	7	tr	—	0	1	1	tr	—	5	—	—	—	—
Macaroni Salad	¼ cup	207	14	—	14	4	17	tr	—	382	—	—	—	—
Margarine Whipped	1 tsp	23	3	—	0	0	0	0	—	32	—	—	—	—
Melba Toast	2	20	0	—	0	1	4	0	—	45	—	—	—	—
Mixed Fruit Salad	¼ cup	37	tr	—	0	tr	9	tr	—	3	—	—	—	—
Mixed Squash	¼ cup	49	4	—	0	1	2	tr	—	230	—	—	—	—
Mushrooms	1 tbsp	1	0	—	0	tr	tr	tr	—	0	—	—	—	—
Oil	1 tsp	45	5	—	0	0	0	0	—	0	—	—	—	—
Olives Black	2	10	1	—	0	0	0	0	—	38	—	—	—	—
Olives Green	2	8	1	—	0	0	0	0	—	162	—	—	—	—
Onion Sliced	1 tbsp	1	0	—	0	tr	tr	tr	—	0	—	—	—	—
Oriental Salad	¼ cup	79	3	—	1	1	13	1	—	31	—	—	—	—
Pea Salad	¼ cup	73	6	—	42	3	4	2	—	89	—	—	—	—
Pepperoni	1 tbsp	30	3	—	—	3	0	0	—	81	—	—	—	—
Pickle Chips	1 slice	5	0	—	0	0	1	0	—	30	—	—	—	—
Pickle Spear	1 spear	2	0	—	0	0	tr	0	—	271	—	—	—	—
Pineapple Bits	1 tbsp	9	0	—	0	tr	2	—	—	2	—	—	—	—
Pistachio Pineapple Salad	¼ cup	98	3	—	0	1	20	0	—	39	—	—	—	—
Prunes	1 tbsp	19	0	—	0	tr	5	1	—	0	—	—	—	—
Radish	1 tbsp	1	0	—	0	0	tr	tr	—	1	—	—	—	—
Raisins	1 spoonful	26	0	—	0	tr	7	1	—	1	—	—	—	—
Rotelli Pasta	¼ cup	78	4	—	0	1	9	tr	—	82	—	—	—	—
Seign Salad	¼ cup	72	4	—	5	2	8	1	—	122	—	—	—	—
Snow Delight	¼ cup	72	4	—	0	1	9	tr	—	18	—	—	—	—
Spaghetti Salad	¼ cup	81	5	—	0	2	9	tr	—	20	—	—	—	—
Spinach	¼ cup	1	0	—	0	tr	tr	tr	—	4	—	—	—	—
Spring Pasta	¼ cup	38	3	—	0	1	2	1	—	162	—	—	—	—
Summer Salad	¼ cup	114	12	—	0	1	2	1	—	233	—	—	—	—
Sunflower Seeds	1 spoonful	40	3	—	0	2	1	0	—	2	—	—	—	—
Three Bean Salad	¼ cup	96	5	—	0	1	12	1	—	189	—	—	—	—
Trail Mix	1 spoonful	30	0	—	0	1	4	tr	—	0	—	—	—	—
Turkey Ham	1 tbsp	12	1	—	1	2	tr	0	—	121	—	—	—	—

FOOD	PORTION	CALORIES	FAT	SAT FAT	CHOL	PROTEIN	CARBO	FIBER	CALCIUM	SOD	POTAS	VIT C	FOLIC	VIT A
Waldorf	¼ cup	81	5	—	2	1	9	1	—	68	—	—	—	—
Wheat Bread	1 slice	71	1	—	0	3	14	1	—	150	—	—	—	—
SOUPS														
Bean	6 fl oz	63	1	—	4	4	10	1	—	479	—	—	—	—
Beef Cabbage	6 fl oz	86	3	—	13	6	9	2	—	503	—	—	—	—
Broccoli Cauliflower	6 fl oz	124	9	—	12	4	12	1	—	560	—	—	—	—
Cheddar Chowder	6 fl oz	91	2	—	—	3	14	—	—	948	—	—	—	—
Cheese Florentine Ham	6 fl oz	110	8	—	11	4	12	1	—	890	—	—	—	—
Chicken Gumbo	6 fl oz	60	2	—	—	4	7	—	—	1050	—	—	—	—
Chicken Noodle	6 fl oz	62	1	—	14	3	9	—	—	127	—	—	—	—
Chicken Rice	6 fl oz	72	1	—	6	3	13	1	—	117	—	—	—	—
Clam Chowder	6 fl oz	94	5	—	0	2	10	0	—	66	—	—	—	—
Corn Chowder	6 fl oz	148	5	—	—	4	22	0	—	510	—	—	—	—
Cream Of Broccoli	6 fl oz	75	5	—	1	2	11	tr	—	415	—	—	—	—
Cream Of Chicken	6 fl oz	136	9	—	11	5	14	tr	—	1164	—	—	—	—
Cream Of Chicken Vegetable	6 fl oz	79	1	—	—	4	13	—	—	714	—	—	—	—
Onion	6 fl oz	29	2	—	1	1	2	tr	—	88	—	—	—	—
Potato	6 fl oz	102	3	—	0	1	17	2	—	335	—	—	—	—
Tomato Florentine	6 fl oz	63	1	—	0	2	11	0	—	683	—	—	—	—
Tomato Vegetable	6 fl oz	46	tr	—	0	2	10	tr	—	314	—	—	—	—
Vegetable Beef	6 fl oz	82	2	—	5	4	14	tr	—	1254	—	—	—	—

SIZZLER

FOOD	PORTION	CALORIES	FAT	SAT FAT	CHOL	PROTEIN	CARBO	FIBER	CALCIUM	SOD	POTAS	VIT C	FOLIC	VIT A
DESSERTS														
Chocolate & Vanilla Soft Serve	4 oz	136	4	4	0	1	24	0	0	100	—	0	—	0
Chocolate Syrup	1 oz	90	0	0	0	0	21	0	0	15	—	0	—	0
Strawberry Topping	1 oz	70	0	0	0	0	18	0	0	5	—	0	—	0
Whipped Topping	1 tbsp	12	1	1	0	0	1	0	0	0	—	0	—	0
HOT BUFFET														
Broccoli Cheese Soup	1 serv (4 oz)	139	9	2	8	2	10	0	80	355	—	8	—	50
Chicken Noodle Soup	1 serv (4 oz)	31	1	0	7	2	4	0	0	495	—	0	—	0
Chicken Wings	1 oz	73	4	1	20	4	4	0	10	135	—	0	—	0
Clam Chowder	1 serv (4 oz)	118	6	0	6	3	11	0	30	511	—	1	—	100
Fettucine	2 oz	80	1	0	5	3	15	0	0	5	—	0	—	0
Focaccia Bread	2 pieces	108	7	1	1	2	9	0	10	134	—	0	—	0
Marinara Sauce	1 oz	13	0	0	0	0	3	0	0	90	—	5	—	100
Meatballs	4	157	11	5	30	9	5	1	20	461	—	0	—	0
Minestrone Soup	1 serv (4 oz)	36	0	0	1	1	7	2	20	443	—	5	—	700
Nacho Cheese Soup	1 serv (4 oz)	120	10	5	30	5	3	0	150	600	—	0	—	100
Potato Skins	2 oz	160	8	1	0	2	22	3	20	463	—	6	—	0

FOOD	PORTION	CALORIES	FAT	SAT FAT	CHOL	PROTEIN	CARBO	FIBER	CALCIUM	SOD	POTAS	VIT C	FOLIC	VIT A
Refried Beans	¼ cup	62	1	2	5	4	11	3	30	272	—	4	—	0
Saltine Crackers	2	25	1	0	2	1	4	0	0	74	—	0	—	0
Spaghetti	2 oz	80	0	0	0	3	16	1	0	1	—	0	—	0
Taco Filling	2 oz	103	9	4	16	2	3	1	20	232	—	4	—	200
Taco Shells	1	50	2	0	0	1	7	1	10	20	—	0	—	0
Vegetable Sirloin Soup	1 serv (4 oz)	60	2	1	10	6	6	0	0	364	—	0	—	400
MAIN MENU SELECTIONS														
Buttery Dipping Sauce	1 serv (1.5 oz)	330	37	7	0	0	0	0	0	0	—	0	—	0
Cheese Toast	1 piece	273	21	5	5	6	16	1	130	494	—	0	—	350
Cocktail Sauce	1 serv (1.5 oz)	40	0	0	0	0	8	0	0	396	—	0	—	0
Dakota Ranch Steak	1 (6 oz)	316	20	8	101	30	—	—	—	253				
Dakota Ranch Steak	1 (8 oz)	421	27	11	135	37	—	—	—	337				
Dakota Ranch Steak	1 (9.5 oz)	500	32	13	160	47	—	—	—	400				
French Fries	1 serv (4 oz)	358	12	6	0	5	45	4	10	245	—	12	—	0
Hamburger	1	626	33	12	142	45	36	1	60	335	—	6	—	150
Hibachi Chicken Breast w/ Pineapple	5 oz	193	3	1	65	28	13	1	20	666	—	5	—	0
Hibachi Sauce	1 serv (1.5 oz)	57	0	0	0	0	11	0	0	707	—	0	—	0
Lemon Herb Chicken Breast	5 oz	140	3	1	65	27	0	0	20	380	—	0	—	0
Malibu Chicken Patty	1	310	19	3	75	23	11	0	280	588	—	0	—	200
Malibu Sauce	1 serv (1.5 oz)	283	31	6	28	0	0	0	0	354	—	0	—	0
Margarine Whipped	1½ tbsp	105	12	2	0	0	0	0	0	146	—	0	—	850
Potato Baked Plain	1 (4 oz)	105	0	0	0	2	24	2	0	6	—	14	—	0
Rice Pilaf	1 serv (6 oz)	256	5	1	0	4	47	1	0	866	—	0	—	50
Salmon	8 oz	110	12	2	41	32	0	0	20	232	—	0	—	200
Sante Fe Chicken Breast	5 oz	150	3	1	65	30	0	0	20	350	—	0	—	0
Shrimp Broiled	5 oz	150	6	1	218	23	0	0	40	377	—	2	—	450
Shrimp Fried	4 pieces	223	2	0	118	18	35	2	100	706	—	0	—	0
Shrimp Mini	4 oz	152	1	0	80	13	24	1	70	480	—	0	—	0
Shrimp Scampi	5 oz	143	3	1	150	27	0	0	90	386	—	0	—	0
Sour Dressing	2 tbsp	60	6	5	0	0	0	0	0	30	—	0	—	0
Swordfish	8 oz	315	14	3	89	45	0	0	20	331	—	2	—	350
Tartar Sauce	1 serv (1.5 oz)	170	17	3	14	0	6	0	0	453	—	0	—	0
SALAD DRESSINGS														
Blue Cheese	1 oz	111	12	4	8	1	1	0	10	168	—	0	—	50
Honey Mustard	1 oz	160	16	2	10	0	4	0	0	110	—	0	—	0
Italian Lite	1 oz	14	0	0	0	0	2	0	0	350	—	0	—	0

FOOD	PORTION	CALORIES	FAT	SAT FAT	CHOL	PROTEIN	CARBO	FIBER	CALCIUM	SOD	POTAS	VIT C	FOLIC	VIT A
Japanese Rice Vinegar Fat Free	1 oz	10	0	0	0	0	2	0	0	172	—	0	—	0
Parmesan Italian	1 oz	100	10	2	0	0	2	0	0	450	—	0	—	0
Ranch	1 oz	120	12	2	10	0	2	0	0	240	—	0	—	0
Ranch Reduced Calorie	1 oz	90	8	2	10	0	4	0	0	270	—	0	—	0
Thousand Island	1 oz	143	15	2	11	0	3	0	0	125	—	1	—	100
SALADS AND SALAD BARS														
Alfafa Sprouts	¼ cup	2	0	0	0	0	0	0	0	0	—	1	—	0
Avocado	½	153	15	2	0	2	6	3	0	11	—	7	—	250
Bean Sprouts	¼ cup	8	0	0	0	1	2	0	0	2	—	3	—	0
Beets	¼ cup	13	0	0	0	0	3	1	0	117	—	1	—	0
Bell Peppers	2 oz	8	0	0	0	1	2	1	0	1	—	43	—	50
Broccoli	½ cup	12	0	0	0	1	2	1	20	12	—	41	—	300
Cabbage Red	¼ cup	5	0	0	0	0	1	0	0	2	—	10	—	0
Cantoupe	½ cup	28	0	0	0	1	7	1	0	7	—	34	—	1250
Carrot & Raisin Salad	2 oz	130	10	2	10	1	10	1	10	104	—	3	—	4500
Carrots	¼ cup	12	0	0	0	0	3	1	0	10	—	2	—	3850
Chinese Chicken Salad	2 oz	54	2	0	10	4	6	1	0	119	—	5	—	500
Chives	1 oz	62	6	1	0	1	1	1	20	181	—	0	—	0
Cottage Cheese	2 oz	51	1	1	5	8	2	0	30	230	—	0	—	50
Cucumber	2 oz	7	0	0	0	0	2	1	0	1	—	2	—	0
Eggs	1 oz	44	3	1	122	4	0	0	10	35	—	0	—	200
Garbanzo Beans	¼ cup	63	1	1	0	3	11	3	20	255	—	0	—	0
Grapes	½ cup	29	0	0	0	0	8	1	0	1	—	2	—	0
Guacamole	1 oz	42	4	1	0	0	2	0	10	425	—	7	—	0
Honeydew Melon	½ cup	30	0	0	0	0	8	1	0	9	—	21	—	0
Iceberg Lettuce	1 cup	7	0	0	0	1	1	1	10	5	—	2	—	50
Jicama	2 oz	13	0	0	0	1	3	0	0	1	—	10	—	0
Kidney Beans	¼ cup	52	0	0	0	3	10	4	10	222	—	1	—	0
Kiwifruit	2 oz	35	0	0	0	1	8	2	10	3	—	55	—	55
Mediterranean Minted Fruit Salad	2 oz	29	0	0	0	1	7	0	20	11	—	15	—	550
Mexican Fiesta Salad	2 oz	54	1	0	0	2	10	1	0	99	—	7	—	50
Mushrooms	¼ cup	4	0	0	0	0	1	0	0	1	—	1	—	0
Old Fashioned Potato Salad	2 oz	84	5	1	6	1	10	1	0	231	—	5	—	0
Onions Red	2 tbsp	8	0	0	0	0	2	0	0	1	—	1	—	0
Peaches	¼ cup	34	0	0	0	0	9	1	0	3	—	4	—	100
Peas	¼ cup	31	0	0	0	2	6	2	0	35	—	4	—	100
Pineapple	½ cup	38	0	0	0	0	10	1	0	1	—	11	—	0
Real Bacon Bits	1 tbsp	27	2	0	0	2	2	1	0	165	—	0	—	0

FOOD	PORTION	CALORIES	FAT	SAT FAT	CHOL	PROTEIN	CARBO	FIBER	CALCIUM	SOD	POTAS	VIT C	FOLIC	VIT A
Red Herb Potato Salad	2 oz	121	9	1	9	1	9	1	0	271	—	3	—	0
Romaine Lettuce	1 cup	9	0	0	0	1	1	1	20	4	—	13	—	700
Salsa	1 oz	7	0	0	0	0	2	0	0	156	—	5	—	50
Seafood Louis Pasta Salad	2 oz	64	2	0	17	3	9	1	10	139	—	3	—	50
Seafood Salad	2 oz	56	3	1	7	3	4	0	10	255	—	1	—	50
Spicy Jicama Salad	2 oz	16	0	0	0	0	4	0	0	28	—	11	—	0
Spinach	½ cup	6	0	0	0	1	1	1	20	22	—	8	—	900
Strawberries	½ cup	22	0	0	0	0	5	2	10	1	—	42	—	0
Teriyaki Beef Salad	2 oz	49	2	1	7	4	5	1	10	136	—	17	—	100
Tomatoes Cherry	¼ cup	12	0	0	0	0	3	1	0	5	—	10	—	150
Tuna Pasta Salad	2 oz	133	10	7	10	6	6	0	0	188	—	2	—	100
Turkey Ham	1 oz	62	5	2	19	4	0	0	30	376	—	0	—	0
Watermelon	½ cup	26	0	0	0	0	6	0	0	2	—	7	—	100
Zucchini	¼ cup	5	0	0	0	0	1	1	0	1	—	2	—	50

SKIPPER'S

DESSERTS

FOOD	PORTION	CALORIES	FAT	SAT FAT	CHOL	PROTEIN	CARBO	FIBER	CALCIUM	SOD	POTAS	VIT C	FOLIC	VIT A
Jell-O	1 serv (2.75 oz)	55	0	0	0	1	12	—	—	35	—	—	—	—

MAIN MENU SELECTIONS

FOOD	PORTION	CALORIES	FAT	SAT FAT	CHOL	PROTEIN	CARBO	FIBER	CALCIUM	SOD	POTAS	VIT C	FOLIC	VIT A
Baked Fish With Margarine & Seas	1 serv (4.4 oz)	147	3	—	85	30	0	—	—	475	—	—	—	—
Baked Potato	1 (6 oz)	145	0	0	0	4	32	—	—	6	—	—	—	—
Captain's Cut	1 piece (2.6 oz)	160	7	—	29	10	14	—	—	353	—	—	—	—
Cocktail Sauce	1 tbsp	20	0	0	0	0	5	—	—	216	—	—	—	—
Coleslaw	1 serv (5 oz)	289	27	—	50	2	10	—	—	329	—	—	—	—
Corn Muffin	1 (2 oz)	91	5	—	16	2	14	—	—	135	—	—	—	—
English Style Fish	1 piece (2.4 oz)	187	12	—	—	9	11	—	—	415	—	—	—	—
French Fries	1 serv (3.5 oz)	239	12	—	3	3	29	—	—	57	—	—	—	—
Green Salad (no dressing)	1 serv (4 oz)	24	0	0	0	0	4	—	—	8	—	—	—	—
Ketchup	1 tbsp	17	0	0	0	0	4	—	—	213	—	—	—	—
Margarine	1 serv (0.5 oz)	50	6	—	0	0	0	—	—	60	—	—	—	—
Shrimp Fried Cajun	1 serv (4 oz)	342	21	—	64	12	27	—	—	147	—	—	—	—
Shrimp Fried Jumbo	1 piece (.65 oz)	51	2	—	9	2	5	—	—	102	—	—	—	—
Shrimp Fried Original	1 serv (4 oz)	266	13	—	54	13	25	—	—	1089	—	—	—	—
Tartar Original	1 tbsp	65	7	—	4	0	0	—	—	102	—	—	—	—

SOUPS

FOOD	PORTION	CALORIES	FAT	SAT FAT	CHOL	PROTEIN	CARBO	FIBER	CALCIUM	SOD	POTAS	VIT C	FOLIC	VIT A
Clam Chowder	1 pint (12 fl oz)	200	7	—	24	50	19	—	—	1050	—	—	—	—
Clam Chowder	1 cup (6 fl oz)	100	4	—	12	3	14	—	—	525	—	—	—	—

SONIC DRIVE-IN

FOOD	PORTION	CALORIES	FAT	SAT FAT	CHOL	PROTEIN	CARBO	FIBER	CALCIUM	SOD	POTAS	VIT C	FOLIC	VIT A
#1 Hamburger	1 (6.6 oz)	409	27	—	58	20	23	—	77	444	—	—	—	—
#2 Hamburger	1 (6.6 oz)	323	16	—	50	20	23	—	86	549	—	—	—	—
B-L-T Sandwich	1 (6.1 oz)	327	19	—	9	8	27	—	64	600	—	—	—	—
Bacon Cheeseburger	1 (7.2 oz)	548	39	—	87	28	23	—	190	839	—	—	—	—
Chicken Sandwich Breaded	1 (7.4 oz)	455	25	—	42	23	36	—	62	755	—	—	—	—
Chili Pie	1 (3.7 oz)	327	23	—	28	12	20	—	52	313	—	—	—	—
Corn Dog	1 (3 oz)	280	15	—	35	7	30	—	49	700	—	—	—	—
Extra Long Cheese Coney	1 (8.9 oz)	635	39	—	65	24	45	—	122	632	—	—	—	—
Extra Long Cheese Coney w/ Onions	1 (9.4 oz)	640	39	—	65	25	47	—	125	632	—	—	—	—
Fish Sandwich	1 (6.1 oz)	277	7	—	6	17	38	—	58	655	—	—	—	—
French Fries	1 lg (6.7 oz)	315	11	—	11	5	50	—	5	67	—	—	—	—
French Fries	1 reg (5 oz)	233	8	—	8	3	37	—	3	50	—	—	—	—
French Fries w/ Cheese	1 lg (7.7 oz)	219	20	—	38	11	51	—	178	468	—	—	—	—
Grilled Cheese Sandwich	1 (2.8 oz)	288	17	—	36	12	25	—	64	841	—	—	—	—
Grilled Chicken Sandwich w/o Dressing	1 (6.4 oz)	215	4	—	4	21	23	—	60	716	—	—	—	—
Hickory Burger	1 (5.1 oz)	314	16	—	50	20	23	—	74	459	—	—	—	—
Jalapeno Burger Double Meat & Cheese	1 (9.1 oz)	638	41	—	136	44	22	—	328	1358	—	—	—	—
Mini Burger	1 (3.5 oz)	246	11	—	36	14	20	—	61	510	—	—	—	—
Mini Cheeseburger	1 (3.9 oz)	281	14	—	45	17	20	—	119	644	—	—	—	—
Onion Rings	1 reg (3.5 oz)	404	27	—	—	5	38	—	31	372	—	—	—	—
Onion Rings	1 lg (5 oz)	577	38	—	—	8	54	—	44	532	—	—	—	—
Regular Cheese Coney	1 (5 oz)	358	15	—	40	14	23	—	64	341	—	—	—	—
Regular Cheese Coney w/ Onions	1 (5.3 oz)	361	23	—	40	14	24	—	65	341	—	—	—	—
Regular Hot Dog	1 (3.5 oz)	258	15	—	23	8	21	—	54	241	—	—	—	—
Steak Sandwich Breaded	1 (3.9 oz)	631	42	—	50	19	46	—	103	1047	—	—	—	—
Super Sonic Burger w/ Mustard Double Meat & Cheese	1 (10.1 oz)	644	41	—	136	44	24	—	328	1128	—	—	—	—
Super Sonic Burger w/ Mayo Double Meat & Cheese	1 (10.1 oz)	730	52	—	144	44	24	—	319	1023	—	—	—	—
Tater Tots	1 serv (3 oz)	150	7	—	10	2	19	—	26	330	—	—	—	—

FOOD	PORTION	CALORIES	FAT	SAT FAT	CHOL	PROTEIN	CARBO	FIBER	CALCIUM	SOD	POTAS	VIT C	FOLIC	VIT A
Tater Tots w/ Cheese	1 serv (3.6 oz)	220	13	—	28	6	19	—	141	569	—	—	—	—

STARBUCKS

FOOD	PORTION	CALORIES	FAT	SAT FAT	CHOL	PROTEIN	CARBO	FIBER	CALCIUM	SOD	POTAS	VIT C	FOLIC	VIT A
Americano Grande	1 serv	10	0	0	0	0	3	—	20	15	—	1	—	0
Americano Short	1 serv	5	0	0	0	0	1	—	0	10	—	0	—	0
Americano Tall	1 serv	5	0	0	0	0	2	—	0	10	—	1	—	0
Cappuccino Grande Lowfat Milk	1 serv	110	4	3	15	7	12	—	250	110	—	2	—	400
Cappuccino Grande Nonfat Milk	1 serv	80	0	0	5	7	12	—	250	115	—	4	—	400
Cappuccino Grande Whole Milk	1 serv	140	7	5	30	7	12	—	250	105	—	2	—	300
Cappuccino Short Lowfat Milk	1 serv	60	2	1	10	4	6	—	150	55	—	1	—	200
Cappuccino Short Nonfat Milk	1 serv	40	0	0	0	4	6	—	150	55	—	1	—	200
Cappuccino Short Whole Milk	1 serv	70	4	2	15	4	6	—	150	55	—	1	—	100
Cappuccino Tall Lowfat Milk	1 serv	80	3	2	15	6	9	—	200	85	—	2	—	300
Cappuccino Tall Nonfat Milk	1 serv	60	0	0	5	6	9	—	200	90	—	2	—	300
Cappuccino Tall Whole Milk	1 serv	110	6	4	25	6	9	—	200	85	—	2	—	200
Cocoa w/ Whipping Cream Grande Lowfat Milk	1 serv	350	20	12	70	14	35	—	450	190	—	4	—	1000
Cocoa w/ Whipping Cream Grande Nonfat Milk	1 serv	310	15	9	50	14	35	—	450	190	—	4	—	1250
Cocoa w/ Whipping Cream Grande Whole Milk	1 serv	400	26	16	90	14	34	—	450	180	—	4	—	1000
Cocoa w/ Whipping Cream Short Lowfat Milk	1 serv	180	11	7	40	6	16	—	200	85	—	1	—	500
Cocoa w/ Whipping Cream Short Nonfat Milk	1 serv	160	8	5	30	6	17	—	200	85	—	1	—	500
Cocoa w/ Whipping Cream Short Whole Milk	1 serv	210	14	8	45	6	19	—	200	80	—	1	—	500

FOOD	PORTION	CALORIES	FAT	SAT FAT	CHOL	PROTEIN	CARBO	FIBER	CALCIUM	SOD	POTAS	VIT C	FOLIC	VIT A
Cocoa w/ Whipping Cream Tall Lowfat Milk	1 serv	270	15	9	55	10	26	—	350	140	—	2	—	750
Cocoa w/ Whipping Cream Tall Nonfat Milk	1 serv	230	11	7	35	11	26	—	350	140	—	2	—	1000
Cocoa w/ Whipping Cream Tall Whole Milk	1 serv	300	19	12	70	10	26	—	300	135	—	2	—	750
Drip Coffee Grande	1 serv	10	0	0	0	1	2	—	0	15	—	0	—	0
Drip Coffee Short	1 serv	5	0	0	0	0	1	—	0	5	—	0	—	0
Drip Coffee Tall	1 serv	10	0	0	0	1	1	—	0	10	—	0	—	0
Espresso Doppio	1 serv	5	0	0	0	0	2	—	0	0	—	1	—	0
Espresso Macchiato Doppio Lowfat Milk	1 serv	15	0	0	0	1	3	—	20	10	—	1	—	0
Espresso Macchiato Doppio Nonfat Milk	1 serv	15	0	0	0	1	3	—	20	10	—	1	—	0
Espresso Macchiato Doppio Whole Milk	1 serv	15	1	0	0	1	3	—	20	10	—	1	—	0
Espresso Macchiato Solo Lowfat Milk	1 serv	10	0	0	0	1	2	—	20	10	—	1	—	0
Espresso Macchiato Solo Nonfat Milk	1 serv	10	0	0	0	1	2	—	20	10	—	1	—	0
Espresso Macchiato Solo Whole Milk	1 serv	15	1	0	0	1	2	—	20	10	—	1	—	0
Espresso Solo	1 serv	5	0	0	0	0	1	—	0	0	—	0	—	0
Espresso Con Panna Doppio	1 serv	45	4	3	15	0	2	—	0	5	—	1	—	200
Espresso Con Panna Solo	1 serv	40	4	3	15	0	1	—	0	5	—	0	—	200
Latte Grande Lowfat Milk	1 serv	170	6	4	25	12	18	—	400	180	—	5	—	500
Latte Grande Nonfat Milk	1 serv	130	1	0	5	12	19	—	450	180	—	5	—	750
Latte Grande Whole Milk	1 serv	220	11	7	45	11	18	—	400	170	—	4	—	400
Latte Short Lowfat Milk	1 serv	80	3	2	10	5	8	—	200	80	—	2	—	300
Latte Short Nonfat Milk	1 serv	60	0	0	5	5	8	—	200	80	—	2	—	300
Latte Short Whole Milk	1 serv	100	5	3	20	5	8	—	200	75	—	2	—	200

FOOD	PORTION	CALORIES	FAT	SAT FAT	CHOL	PROTEIN	CARBO	FIBER	CALCIUM	SOD	POTAS	VIT C	FOLIC	VIT A
Latte Tall Lowfat Milk	1 serv	140	5	3	20	10	15	—	350	150	—	4	—	500
Latte Tall Nonfat Milk	1 serv	110	1	0	5	10	15	—	350	150	—	4	—	500
Latte Tall Whole Milk	1 serv	180	10	6	40	10	14	—	350	140	—	4	—	400
Latte Iced Grande Lowfat Milk	1 serv	170	6	4	25	11	18	—	400	170	—	4	—	500
Latte Iced Grande Nonfat Milk	1 serv	130	1	0	5	12	18	—	400	180	—	5	—	750
Latte Iced Grande Whole Milk	1 serv	210	11	7	45	11	18	—	400	170	—	4	—	400
Latte Iced Short Lowfat Milk	1 serv	90	3	2	15	6	10	—	200	95	—	2	—	300
Latte Iced Short Nonfat Milk	1 serv	70	0	0	5	6	10	—	250	95	—	2	—	400
Latte Iced Short Whole Milk	1 serv	120	6	4	25	6	9	—	200	90	—	2	—	200
Latte Iced Tall Lowfat Milk	1 serv	120	5	3	20	8	13	—	300	125	—	2	—	400
Latte Iced Tall Nonfat Milk	1 serv	90	0	0	5	8	13	—	300	130	—	2	—	500
Latte Iced Tall Whole Milk	1 serv	150	8	5	35	8	12	—	300	120	—	2	—	300
Mocha w/ Whipping Cream Grande Lowfat Milk	1 serv	350	20	12	70	13	35	—	400	170	—	4	—	1000
Mocha w/ Whipping Cream Grande Nonfat Milk	1 serv	310	15	9	50	13	35	—	400	180	—	4	—	1000
Mocha w/ Whipping Cream Grande Whole Milk	1 serv	390	25	15	85	13	35	—	400	170	—	4	—	750
Mocha w/ Whipping Cream Short Lowfat Milk	1 serv	170	10	6	35	5	16	—	150	70	—	1	—	500
Mocha w/ Whipping Cream Short Nonfat Milk	1 serv	150	8	5	30	5	16	—	150	70	—	1	—	500
Mocha w/ Whipping Cream Short Whole Milk	1 serv	180	12	8	45	5	16	—	150	70	—	1	—	400
Mocha w/ Whipping Cream Tall Lowfat Milk	1 serv	260	15	9	50	9	26	—	300	125	—	2	—	750

FOOD	PORTION	CALORIES	FAT	SAT FAT	CHOL	PROTEIN	CARBO	FIBER	CALCIUM	SOD	POTAS	VIT C	FOLIC	VIT A
Mocha w/ Whipping Cream Tall Nonfat Milk	1 serv	230	11	7	35	10	26	—	300	130	—	2	—	750
Mocha w/ Whipping Cream Tall Whole Milk	1 serv	290	18	11	65	9	25	—	300	125	—	2	—	750
Mocha w/o Whipping Cream Grande Lowfat Milk	1 serv	230	7	5	20	11	33	—	350	150	—	4	—	500
Mocha w/o Whipping Cream Grande Nonfat Milk	1 serv	190	3	2	5	12	33	—	350	150	—	4	—	500
Mocha w/o Whipping Cream Grande Whole Milk	1 serv	260	7	12	40	11	33	—	350	150	—	4	—	400
Mocha w/o Whipping Cream Short Lowfat Milk	1 serv	120	4	3	15	6	18	—	200	85	—	2	—	300
Mocha w/o Whipping Cream Short Nonfat Milk	1 serv	100	2	1	5	7	18	—	200	90	—	2	—	300
Mocha w/o Whipping Cream Short Whole Milk	1 serv	150	7	4	25	6	17	—	200	85	—	2	—	200
Mocha w/o Whipping Cream Tall Lowfat Milk	1 serv	170	5	4	15	8	24	—	250	110	—	2	—	400
Mocha w/o Whipping Cream Tall Nonfat Milk	1 serv	140	2	2	5	9	24	—	250	110	—	2	—	400
Mocha w/o Whipping Cream Tall Whole Milk	1 serv	190	9	5	30	8	24	—	250	105	—	2	—	300
Mocha Syrup Grande	1 serv (2 oz)	80	3	2	0	2	17	—	0	0	—	0	—	0
Mocha Syrup Short	1 serv (1 oz)	40	1	1	0	1	9	—	0	0	—	0	—	0
Mocha Syrup Tall	1 serv (1.5 oz)	60	2	1	0	1	13	—	0	0	—	0	—	0
Steamed Lowfat Milk Grande	1 serv	180	7	4	30	13	18	—	450	190	—	4	—	500

FOOD	PORTION	CALORIES	FAT	SAT FAT	CHOL	PROTEIN	CARBO	FIBER	CALCIUM	SOD	POTAS	VIT C	FOLIC	VIT A
Steamed Lowfat Milk Short	1 serv	90	3	2	15	6	9	—	200	90	—	1	—	300
Steamed Lowfat Milk Tall	1 serv	140	5	3	20	10	14	—	350	150	—	2	—	500
Steamed Nonfat Milk Grande	1 serv	130	1	0	5	13	18	—	450	190	—	4	—	750
Steamed Nonfat Milk Short	1 serv	60	0	0	5	6	9	—	250	95	—	4	—	400
Steamed Nonfat Milk Tall	1 serv	100	1	0	5	10	14	—	350	150	—	2	—	500
Steamed Whole Milk Grande	1 serv	230	13	8	50	12	17	—	450	180	—	4	—	500
Steamed Whole Milk Short	1 serv	110	6	4	25	6	9	—	200	90	—	1	—	200
Steamed Whole Milk Tall	1 serv	180	10	6	40	10	14	—	350	140	—	2	—	400
Whipping Cream Grande	1 serv (1.1 oz)	110	12	7	45	1	1	—	20	10	—	0	—	500
Whipping Cream Short	1 serv (0.7 oz)	70	7	5	25	0	1	—	20	5	—	0	—	300
Whipping Cream Tall	1 serv (0.8 oz)	80	9	5	35	0	1	—	20	10	—	0	—	400
ICE CREAM														
Biscotte Bliss	½ cup	240	12	7	55	4	30	—	199	70	—	—	—	—
Caffe Almond Fudge	½ cup	260	13	7	55	5	30	—	100	80	—	—	—	—
Caffe Almond Roast	1 bar	280	18	9	25	4	26	—	60	45	—	—	—	—
Dark Roast Expresso Swirl	½ cup	220	10	6	55	4	29	—	100	60	—	—	—	—
Frappuccino Coffee	1 bar	110	2	1	10	4	20	—	100	50	—	—	—	—
Italian Roast Coffee	½ cup	230	12	7	65	5	26	—	100	65	—	—	—	—
Javachip	½ cup	250	13	8	60	4	29	—	100	55	—	—	—	—
Low Fat Latte	½ cup	170	3	2	10	5	31	—	100	65	—	—	—	—
Low Fat Mocha Mambo	½ cup	170	3	2	10	5	32	—	100	75	—	—	—	—
Vanilla Mochachip	½ cup	270	16	10	75	5	27	—	100	60	—	—	—	—
STUFF'N TURKEY														
Chef's Salad	1 serv	288	9	3	58	31	—	3	—	976	—	—	—	—
Grilled Turkey Breast	1 serv	244	3	1	23	27	—	5	—	685	—	—	—	—
Homemade Turkey Salad	1 serv	651	29	5	110	48	—	9	—	1079	—	—	—	—
Real Fresh Roasted Turkey Breast	1 serv	384	5	1	29	32	—	8	—	628	—	—	—	—
Rotisserie Turkey Breast	1 serv	251	3	1	48	—	—	4	—	1026	—	—	—	—

FOOD	PORTION	CALORIES	FAT	SAT FAT	CHOL	PROTEIN	CARBO	FIBER	CALCIUM	SOD	POTAS	VIT C	FOLIC	VIT A
Thanksgiving Dinner On A Sandwich	1 serv	605	16	4	33	37	—	10	—	1079	—	—	—	—
Turkey Barbecue	1 serv	478	6	1	48	29	—	8	—	782	—	—	—	—
Turkey Powerhouse	1 serv	482	11	5	50	39	—	10	—	768	—	—	—	—

SUBWAY

COOKIES

FOOD	PORTION	CALORIES	FAT	SAT FAT	CHOL	PROTEIN	CARBO	FIBER	CALCIUM	SOD	POTAS	VIT C	FOLIC	VIT A
Chocolate Chip	1	210	10	—	10	2	29	—	—	140	—	—	—	—
Chocolate Chip M&M	1	210	10	—	15	2	29	—	—	140	—	—	—	—
Chocolate Chunk	1	210	10	—	10	2	29	—	—	140	—	—	—	—
Double Chocolate Brazil Nut	1	230	12	—	10	3	27	—	—	115	—	—	—	—
Oatmeal Raisin	1	200	8	—	15	3	29	—	—	160	—	—	—	—
Peanut Butter	1	220	12	—	0	3	26	—	—	180	—	—	—	—
Sugar	1	230	12	—	20	2	28	—	—	180	—	—	—	—
White Chocolate Macadamia Nut	1	230	12	—	10	2	28	—	—	140	—	—	—	—

SALAD DRESSINGS

FOOD	PORTION	CALORIES	FAT	SAT FAT	CHOL	PROTEIN	CARBO	FIBER	CALCIUM	SOD	POTAS	VIT C	FOLIC	VIT A
Creamy Italian	1 tbsp	65	6	—	4	0	2	—	—	132	—	—	—	—
Fat Free French	1 tbsp	15	0	—	0	0	4	—	—	85	—	—	—	—
Fat Free Italian	1 tbsp	5	0	—	0	0	1	—	—	152	—	—	—	—
Fat Free Ranch	1 tbsp	12	0	—	0	0	0	—	—	177	—	—	—	—
French	1 tbsp	65	5	—	0	0	5	—	—	100	—	—	—	—
Ranch	1 tbsp	87	9	—	1	0	1	—	—	117	—	—	—	—
Thousand Island	1 tbsp	65	6	—	7	0	2	—	—	107	—	—	—	—

SALADS AND SALAD BARS

FOOD	PORTION	CALORIES	FAT	SAT FAT	CHOL	PROTEIN	CARBO	FIBER	CALCIUM	SOD	POTAS	VIT C	FOLIC	VIT A
B.L.T.	1 serv	140	8	—	16	7	10	—	—	672	—	—	—	—
Bread Bowl	1 serv	330	4	—	0	12	63	—	—	760	—	—	—	—
Chicken Taco	1 serv	250	14	—	52	18	15	—	—	990	—	—	—	—
Classic Italian B.M.T.	1 serv	274	20	—	56	14	11	—	—	1379	—	—	—	—
Cold Cut Trio	1 serv	191	11	—	64	13	11	—	—	1127	—	—	—	—
Ham	1 serv	116	3	—	28	12	11	—	—	1034	—	—	—	—
Meatball	1 serv	233	14	—	33	12	16	—	—	761	—	—	—	—
Pizza	1 serv	277	20	—	50	12	13	—	—	1336	—	—	—	—
Roast Beef	1 serv	117	3	—	20	12	11	—	—	654	—	—	—	—
Roasted Chicken Breast	1 serv	162	4	—	48	20	13	—	—	693	—	—	—	—
Steak & Cheese	1 serv	212	8	—	70	22	13	—	—	832	—	—	—	—
Subway Club	1 serv	126	3	—	26	14	12	—	—	1067	—	—	—	—
Subway Melt	1 serv	195	10	—	42	16	12	—	—	1461	—	—	—	—
Subway Seafood & Crab	1 serv	244	17	—	34	13	10	—	—	575	—	—	—	—
Subway Seafood & Crab w/ Light Mayonnaise	1 serv	161	8	—	32	13	11	—	—	599	—	—	—	—

FOOD	PORTION	CALORIES	FAT	SAT FAT	CHOL	PROTEIN	CARBO	FIBER	CALCIUM	SOD	POTAS	VIT C	FOLIC	VIT A
Tuna	1 serv	356	30	—	36	12	10	—	—	601	—	—	—	—
Tuna w/ Light Mayonnaise	1 serv	205	13	—	32	12	11	—	—	654	—	—	—	—
Turkey Breast	1 serv	102	2	—	19	11	12	—	—	1117	—	—	—	—
Turkey Breast & Ham	1 serv	109	3	—	24	11	11	—	—	1076	—	—	—	—
Veggie Delight	1 serv	51	1	—	0	2	10	—	—	308	—	—	—	—
SANDWICHES														
6 Inch Cold Ham	1	302	5	—	28	19	45	—	—	1319	—	—	—	—
6 Inch Cold Tuna w/ Light Mayonnaise	1	391	15	—	32	19	46	—	—	940	—	—	—	—
6 Inch Cold Sub B.L.T.	1	327	10	—	16	14	44	—	—	957	—	—	—	—
6 Inch Cold Sub Classic Italian B.M.T.	1	460	22	—	56	21	45	—	—	1664	—	—	—	—
6 Inch Cold Sub Cold Cut Trio	1	378	13	—	64	20	46	—	—	1412	—	—	—	—
6 Inch Cold Sub Roast Beef	1	303	5	—	20	20	45	—	—	939	—	—	—	—
6 Inch Cold Sub Subway Club	1	312	5	—	26	21	46	—	—	1352	—	—	—	—
6 Inch Cold Sub Subway Seafood & Crab	1	430	19	—	34	20	44	—	—	860	—	—	—	—
6 Inch Cold Sub Subway Seafood & Crab w/ Light Mayonniase	1	347	10	—	32	20	45	—	—	884	—	—	—	—
6 Inch Cold Sub Tuna	1	542	32	—	36	19	44	—	—	886	—	—	—	—
6 Inch Cold Sub Turkey Breast	1	289	4	—	19	18	46	—	—	1403	—	—	—	—
6 Inch Cold Sub Turkey Breast & Ham	1	295	5	—	24	18	46	—	—	1361	—	—	—	—
6 Inch Cold Sub Veggie Delight	1	237	3	—	0	9	44	—	—	593	—	—	—	—
6 Inch Hot Subway Melt	1	382	12	—	42	23	46	—	—	1746	—	—	—	—
6 Inch Hot Sub Chicken Taco Sub	1	436	16	—	52	25	49	—	—	1275	—	—	—	—
6 Inch Hot Sub Meatball	1	419	16	—	33	19	51	—	—	1046	—	—	—	—
6 Inch Hot Sub Pizza Sub	1	464	22	—	50	19	48	—	—	1621	—	—	—	—
6 Inch Hot Sub Roasted Chicken Breast	1	348	6	—	48	27	47	—	—	978	—	—	—	—

FOOD	PORTION	CALORIES	FAT	SAT FAT	CHOL	PROTEIN	CARBO	FIBER	CALCIUM	SOD	POTAS	VIT C	FOLIC	VIT A
6 Inch Hot Sub Steak & Cheese	1	398	10	—	70	30	47	—	—	1117	—	—	—	—
Bacon	2 strips	45	4	—	8	2	0	—	—	182	—	—	—	—
Cheese	2 triangles	41	3	—	10	2	0	—	—	204	—	—	—	—
Deli Sandwich Bologna	1	292	12	—	20	10	38	—	—	744	—	—	—	—
Deli Sandwich Ham	1	234	4	—	14	11	37	—	—	773	—	—	—	—
Deli Sandwich Roast Beef	1	245	4	—	13	13	38	—	—	638	—	—	—	—
Deli Sandwich Tuna	1	354	18	—	18	11	37	—	—	557	—	—	—	—
Deli Sandwich Tuna w/ Light Mayonnaise	1	279	9	—	16	11	38	—	—	583	—	—	—	—
Deli Sandwich Turkey Breast	1	235	4	—	12	12	38	—	—	944	—	—	—	—
Light Mayonnaise	1 tsp	18	2	—	2	0	0	—	—	33	—	—	—	—
Mayonnaise	1 tsp	37	4	—	3	0	0	—	—	27	—	—	—	—
Mustard	2 tsp	8	0	—	0	1	1	—	—	0	—	—	—	—
Olive Oil Blend	1 tsp	45	5	—	0	0	0	—	—	0	—	—	—	—
Vinegar	1 tsp	1	0	—	0	0	0	—	—	0	—	—	—	—

TACO BELL

BREAKFAST MENU SELECTIONS

FOOD	PORTION	CALORIES	FAT	SAT FAT	CHOL	PROTEIN	CARBO	FIBER	CALCIUM	SOD	POTAS	VIT C	FOLIC	VIT A
Breakfast Quesadilla Cheese	1 (5.5 oz)	380	21	9	280	15	33	1	300	1010	—	0	—	2250
Breakfast Quesadilla w/ Bacon	1 (6 oz)	450	27	11	290	19	33	2	300	1200	—	0	—	2250
Breakfast Quesadilla w/ Sausage	1 (6 oz)	430	25	10	285	17	33	1	300	1090	—	0	—	2250
Country Breakfast Burrito	1 (4 oz)	270	14	5	195	8	26	2	100	690	—	0	—	1250
Double Bacon & Egg Burrito	1 (6.25 oz)	480	27	9	405	18	39	2	150	1240	—	0	—	2250
Fiesta Breakfast Burrito	1 (3.5 oz)	280	16	6	25	9	25	2	80	580	—	0	—	750
Grande Breakfast Burrito	1 (6.25 oz)	420	22	7	205	13	43	3	100	1050	—	0	—	2500
Hash Brown Nuggets	1 serv (3.5 oz)	280	18	5	0	2	29	1	0	570	—	0	—	0

MAIN MENU SELECTIONS

FOOD	PORTION	CALORIES	FAT	SAT FAT	CHOL	PROTEIN	CARBO	FIBER	CALCIUM	SOD	POTAS	VIT C	FOLIC	VIT A
7-Layer Burrito	1 (10 oz)	530	23	7	25	16	66	13	200	1280	—	6	—	1500
BLT Soft Taco	1 (4.5 oz)	340	23	8	40	11	22	7	100	610	—	4	—	200
Bacon Cheeseburger Burrito	1 (8.5 oz)	570	31	12	70	27	46	6	200	1460	—	5	—	1500

FOOD	PORTION	CALORIES	FAT	SAT FAT	CHOL	PROTEIN	CARBO	FIBER	CALCIUM	SOD	POTAS	VIT C	FOLIC	VIT A
Bean Burrito	1 (7 oz)	380	12	4	10	13	55	13	150	1100	—	0	—	2250
Big Beef Burrito Supreme	1 (10.5 oz)	520	23	10	55	24	54	11	150	1520	—	5	—	3000
Big Beef MexiMelt	1 (4.75 oz)	290	15	7	45	16	23	4	200	850	—	4	—	1250
Big Chicken Burrito Supreme	1 (9 oz)	510	24	7	95	23	52	4	150	1900	—	0	—	2250
Border Sauce Fire	1 serv (0.3 oz)	0	0	0	0	0	0	0	0	110	—	0	—	300
Border Sauce Hot	1 serv (0.3 oz)	0	0	0	0	0	0	0	0	85	—	0	—	300
Border Sauce Mild	1 serv (0.3 oz)	0	0	0	0	0	0	0	0	75	—	0	—	300
Burger Sauce	1 serv (0.5 oz)	60	5	1	5	0	2	0	0	110	—	0	—	200
Burrito Supreme	1 (9 oz)	440	19	8	35	17	51	10	150	1230	—	5	—	2500
Cheddar Cheese	1 serv (0.25 oz)	30	2	2	5	2	0	0	60	45	—	0	—	200
Cheese Quesadilla	1 (4.25 oz)	350	18	9	50	16	32	2	450	860	—	0	—	400
Chicken Fajita Wrap	1 (8 oz)	470	22	6	60	17	51	4	150	1290	—	4	—	1750
Chicken Fajita Wrap Supreme	1 (9 oz)	520	25	8	70	18	53	4	150	1300	—	6	—	2000
Chicken Quesadilla	1 (6 oz)	410	21	10	90	23	34	3	450	1170	—	0	—	750
Chicken Club Burrito	1 (8 oz)	540	32	10	80	20	43	4	100	1250	—	5	—	750
Chili Cheese Burrito	1 (5 oz)	330	13	6	35	14	37	5	200	870	—	0	—	3000
Choco Taco Ice Cream Dessert	1 serv (4 oz)	310	17	10	20	3	37	1	60	100	—	0	—	200
Cinnamon Twists	1 serv (1 oz)	140	6	0	0	1	19	0	0	190	—	0	—	200
Club Sauce	1 serv (0.5 oz)	80	8	1	10	0	1	0	0	105	—	0	—	0
Double Decker Taco	1 (5.75 oz)	340	15	5	25	14	38	9	100	750	—	0	—	500
Double Decker Taco Supreme	1 (7 oz)	390	19	8	35	15	40	9	150	760	—	4	—	750
Fajita Sauce	1 serv (0.5 oz)	70	7	1	5	0	1	0	0	130	—	0	—	0
Green Sauce	1 serv (1 oz)	5	0	0	0	0	1	0	0	150	—	2	—	400
Grilled Chicken Burrito	1 (7 oz)	410	15	5	55	17	50	4	150	1380	—	1	—	4000
Grilled Chicken Soft Taco	1 (4.5 oz)	240	12	4	45	12	21	3	80	1110	—	0	—	750
Grilled Steak Soft Taco	1 (4.5 oz)	230	10	3	25	15	20	2	80	1020	—	0	—	200
Grilled Steak Soft Taco Supreme	1 (5.75 oz)	290	14	5	35	16	24	3	100	1040	—	12	—	400
Guacamole	1 serv (0.75 oz)	35	3	0	0	0	1	1	0	80	—	1	—	0
Mexican Pizza	1 serv (7.75 oz)	570	35	10	45	21	42	8	250	1040	—	5	—	2000
Mexican Rice	1 serv (4.75 oz)	190	9	4	15	5	23	1	150	760	—	1	—	5000

FOOD	PORTION	CALORIES	FAT	SAT FAT	CHOL	PROTEIN	CARBO	FIBER	CALCIUM	SOD	POTAS	VIT C	FOLIC	VIT A
Nacho Cheese Sauce	2 serv (2 oz)	120	10	3	5	2	5	0	40	470	—	0	—	300
Nachos	1 serv (3.5 oz)	320	18	4	5	5	34	3	100	570	—	0	—	300
Nachos Beef Beef Supreme	1 serv (7 oz)	450	24	8	30	14	45	9	150	810	—	4	—	500
Nachos Bellgrande	1 serv (11 oz)	770	39	11	35	21	84	17	200	1310	—	4	—	750
Picante Sauce	1 serv (0.3 oz)	0	0	0	0	0	0	0	0	110	—	1	—	0
Pico De Gallo	1 serv (0.75 oz)	5	0	0	0	0	1	0	0	65	—	4	—	750
Pintos 'n Cheese	1 serv (4.5 oz)	190	9	4	15	9	18	10	150	650	—	0	—	2500
Red Sauce	1 serv (1 oz)	10	0	0	0	0	2	0	0	320	—	0	—	2000
Soft Taco	1 (3.5 oz)	220	10	5	25	11	21	3	80	580	—	0	—	500
Soft Taco Supreme	1 (5 oz)	260	14	7	35	12	23	3	100	590	—	4	—	750
Sour Cream	1 serv (0.75 oz)	40	4	3	10	1	1	0	0	10	—	0	—	0
Steak Fajita Wrap	1 (8 oz)	470	21	6	40	20	50	3	150	1190	—	4	—	1500
Steak Fajita Wrap Supreme	1 (9 oz)	510	25	8	50	21	52	3	150	1200	—	6	—	1500
Taco	1 (2.75 oz)	180	10	4	25	9	12	3	80	330	—	0	—	500
Taco Supreme	1 (4 oz)	220	14	7	35	10	14	3	100	350	—	4	—	750
Taco Salad w/ Salsa	1 (19 oz)	850	52	15	60	30	65	16	300	1780	—	24	—	8000
Taco Salad w/ Salsa w/o Shell	1 (16.5 oz)	420	22	11	60	24	32	15	250	1520	—	21	—	8000
Three Cheese Blend	1 serv (0.25 oz)	25	2	1	5	2	0	0	40	50	—	0	—	0
Tostada	1 (6.25 oz)	300	15	5	15	10	31	12	150	650	—	1	—	1200
Veggie Fajita Wrap	1 (8 oz)	420	19	5	20	10	53	3	150	980	—	4	—	1750
Veggie Fajita Wrap Supreme	1 (9 oz)	470	22	7	30	11	55	3	150	990	—	6	—	1750

TACO JOHN'S

CHILDREN'S MENU SELECTIONS

FOOD	PORTION	CALORIES	FAT	SAT FAT	CHOL	PROTEIN	CARBO	FIBER	CALCIUM	SOD	POTAS	VIT C	FOLIC	VIT A
Kid's Meal Softshell Taco	1 serv (8.5 oz)	617	33	10	35	15	64	—	132	1037	—	—	—	—
Kids's Meal Crispy Taco	1 serv (8 oz)	579	34	10	35	13	54	—	95	789	—	—	—	—

DESSERTS

FOOD	PORTION	CALORIES	FAT	SAT FAT	CHOL	PROTEIN	CARBO	FIBER	CALCIUM	SOD	POTAS	VIT C	FOLIC	VIT A
Choco Taco	1 serv (3.5 oz)	320	17	11	20	3	38	—	—	100	—	—	—	—
Churro	1 serv (1.5 oz)	147	8	2	4	2	17	—	14	160	—	—	—	—
Flauta Apple	1 serv (2 oz)	84	1	tr	0	1	19	—	13	72	—	—	—	—
Flauta Cherry	1 serv (2 oz)	143	4	1	0	2	27	—	18	110	—	—	—	—
Flauta Cream Cheese	1 serv (2 oz)	181	8	3	10	2	27	—	22	135	—	—	—	—
Italian Ice	1 serv (4 oz)	80	0	0	0	0	19	—	0	5	—	—	—	—

MAIN MENU SELECTIONS

FOOD	PORTION	CALORIES	FAT	SAT FAT	CHOL	PROTEIN	CARBO	FIBER	CALCIUM	SOD	POTAS	VIT C	FOLIC	VIT A
Bean Burrito	1 (6.5 oz)	387	11	5	18	15	57	—	226	866	—	—	—	—
Beans Refried	1 serv (9.5 oz)	357	9	2	17	18	53	—	171	1032	—	—	—	—
Beef Burrito	1 (6.5 oz)	449	20	9	52	23	44	—	212	863	—	—	—	—

FOOD	PORTION	CALORIES	FAT	SAT FAT	CHOL	PROTEIN	CARBO	FIBER	CALCIUM	SOD	POTAS	VIT C	FOLIC	VIT A
Chicken Fajita Burrito	1 (6.25)	370	12	5	49	22	45	—	191	1536	—	—	—	—
Chicken Fajita Salad w/o Dressing	1 serv (12.25 oz)	557	33	9	56	22	44	—	250	1541	—	—	—	—
Chicken Fajita Softshell	1 (4.5 oz)	200	7	3	33	13	21	—	107	903	—	—	—	—
Chili	1 serv (9.25 oz)	350	21	10	56	20	19	—	200	865	—	—	—	—
Chimichanga Platter	1 serv (18 oz)	979	38	15	59	32	127	—	429	2341	—	—	—	—
Combination Burrito	1 (6.5 oz)	418	16	7	35	19	50	—	219	865	—	—	—	—
Crispy Tacos	1 serv (3.25 oz)	182	11	4	26	9	12	—	83	272	—	—	—	—
Double Enchilada Platter	1 serv (18.25 oz)	967	42	16	89	42	106	—	405	1921	—	—	—	—
Meat & Potato Burrito	1 (7.75 oz)	503	24	7	25	17	53	—	123	1341	—	—	—	—
Mexi Rolls w/ Nacho Cheese	1 serv (9.75 oz)	863	48	11	54	30	72	—	235	1392	—	—	—	—
Mexican Rice	1 serv (8 oz)	567	18	5	0	8	40	—	118	1293	—	—	—	—
Nacho Cheese	1 serv (2 oz)	300	10	0	—	5	0	—	—	600	—	—	—	—
Nachos	1 serv (3.5 oz)	333	21	2	0	7	27	—	—	611	—	—	—	—
Potato Oles	1 serv (4.63 oz)	363	23	5	—	3	38	—	14	964	—	—	—	—
Potato Oles	1 lg serv (6.12 oz)	484	30	7	—	4	50	—	18	1285	—	—	—	—
Potato Oles Bravo	1 serv (8.88 oz)	579	38	7	7	11	47	—	52	1550	—	—	—	—
Potato Oles w/ Nacho Cheese	1 serv (6.63 oz)	483	33	5	—	8	38	—	14	1564	—	—	—	—
Ranch Burrito	1 (7 oz)	447	23	8	74	18	44	—	235	804	—	—	—	—
Sampler Platter	1 serv (25.5 oz)	1406	61	24	126	61	156	—	666	2875	—	—	—	—
Sierra Chicken Fillet Sandwich	1 (8.5 oz)	534	29	8	68	30	40	—	118	1406	—	—	—	—
Smothered Burrito Platter	1 serv (19.5 oz)	1031	40	16	70	39	132	—	432	2351	—	—	—	—
Softshell Tacos	1 serv (4.25 oz)	230	10	4	26	14	23	—	120	520	—	—	—	—
Sour Cream	1 oz	60	5	—	—	1	1	—	40	15	—	—	—	—
Super Burrito	1 (8.5 oz)	465	19	9	41	20	53	—	261	922	—	—	—	—
Super Nachos	1 serv (13 oz)	919	56	13	48	26	72	—	180	1484	—	—	—	—
Taco Bravo	1 serv (6.25 oz)	346	14	5	28	15	39	—	140	677	—	—	—	—
Taco Burger	1 (5 oz)	280	12	5	32	15	28	—	150	576	—	—	—	—
Taco Salad w/o Dressing	1 (12.4 oz)	584	38	11	46	20	43	—	264	766	—	—	—	—

TACOTIME

FOOD	PORTION	CALORIES	FAT	SAT FAT	CHOL	PROTEIN	CARBO	FIBER	CALCIUM	SOD	POTAS	VIT C	FOLIC	VIT A
Casita Burrito Meat	1 serv (12 oz)	647	31	15	89	40	54	16	—	1233	—	—	—	—
Cheddar Cheese	1 serv (0.75 oz)	86	7	4	22	5	0	0	—	132	—	—	—	—
Chicken	1 serv (2.5 oz)	109	6	2	33	11	2	0	—	402	—	—	—	—
Chips	1 serv (2 oz)	266	12	3	0	4	35	3	—	461	—	—	—	—
Crisp Burrito Bean	1 (5.25 oz)	427	18	5	12	15	53	9	—	453	—	—	—	—
Crisp Burrito Chicken	1 (4.75 oz)	422	25	8	54	17	32	2	—	795	—	—	—	—
Crisp Burrito Meat	1 (5.25 oz)	552	30	10	58	34	39	7	—	1000	—	—	—	—
Crisp Taco	1 (4 oz)	295	17	7	48	22	16	5	—	609	—	—	—	—
Crustos	1 serv (3.5 oz)	373	15	—	0	9	47	—	—	86	—	—	—	—
Double Soft Bean Burrito	1 (9.5 oz)	506	12	6	22	23	77	19	—	860	—	—	—	—
Double Soft Combination Burrito	1 (9.5 oz)	617	23	10	63	39	66	18	—	1343	—	—	—	—
Double Soft Meat Burrito	1 serv (6.5 oz)	726	33	14	99	57	55	17	—	1809	—	—	—	—
Empanada Cherry	1 (4 oz)	250	9	—	0	5	37	—	—	46	—	—	—	—
Enchilada Sauce	1 serv (1 oz)	12	0	0	0	0	3	1	—	133	—	—	—	—
Flour Tortilla 10 in	1 (2.75 oz)	213	4	1	0	6	31	6	—	393	—	—	—	—
Flour Tortilla 7 in	1 (1.75 oz)	88	1	0	0	4	16	1	—	42	—	—	—	—
Flour Tortilla 8 in	1 (1.25 oz)	107	3	1	0	5	16	2	—	33	—	—	—	—
Fried Flour Tortilla 10 in	1 (2.75 oz)	318	16	4	0	6	37	2	—	315	—	—	—	—
Fried Flour Tortilla 8 in	1 (1.35 oz)	205	11	2	0	4	24	1	—	203	—	—	—	—
Guacamole	1 serv (1 oz)	29	2	0	0	0	2	1	—	94	—	—	—	—
Hot Sauce	1 serv (1 oz)	10	0	0	0	0	2	0	—	120	—	—	—	—
Lettuce	1 serv (0.5 oz)	2	0	0	0	0	0	0	—	1	—	—	—	—
Mexi Fries	1 lg (8 oz)	532	34	—	0	6	54	—	—	1598	—	—	—	—
Mexi Fries	1 reg (4 oz)	266	17	—	0	3	27	—	—	799	—	—	—	—
Mexican Dressing No Fat	1 serv (2 oz)	20	0	—	0	0	5	—	—	130	—	—	—	—
Mexican Rice	1 serv (4 oz)	159	2	1	0	3	30	1	—	530	—	—	—	—
Nachos	1 serv (10.5 oz)	680	38	19	78	26	61	11	—	1250	—	—	—	—
Nachos Deluxe	1 serv (15.25 oz)	1048	57	23	109	46	91	17	—	2252	—	—	—	—
Natural Super Taco Meat	1 (11.25 oz)	627	27	13	82	41	60	14	—	915	—	—	—	—
Olives	1 serv (0.50 oz)	16	2	0	0	tr	1	0	—	124	—	—	—	—
Quesadilla Cheese	1 serv (3.25 oz)	205	11	6	30	11	17	1	—	255	—	—	—	—
Ranchero Salsa	1 serv (2 oz)	21	1	0	0	1	3	1	—	192	—	—	—	—

FOOD	PORTION	CALORIES	FAT	SAT FAT	CHOL	PROTEIN	CARBO	FIBER	CALCIUM	SOD	POTAS	VIT C	FOLIC	VIT A
Refritos	1 serv (2.5 oz)	97	0	0	0	6	18	6	—	101	—	—	—	—
Refritos	1 serv (7 oz)	326	10	5	22	18	44	13	—	525	—	—	—	—
Rolled Soft Flour Taco	1 (7 oz)	512	23	10	63	33	46	12	—	1111	—	—	—	—
Shredded Beef	1 serv (2.5 oz)	70	7	—	—	1	1	—	—	31	—	—	—	0
Soft Taco Chicken	1 (7 oz)	387	16	6	48	21	41	7	—	933	—	—	—	—
Sour Cream	1 serv (1 oz)	55	5	3	19	1	1	0	—	11	—	—	—	—
Sour Cream Dressing	1 serv (1.5 oz)	137	14	5	8	1	2	0	—	207	—	—	—	—
Super Shredded Beef Soft Taco	1 (8 oz)	368	11	6	22	12	38	7	—	556				
Taco Cheeseburger	1 (7.5 oz)	633	36	10	66	31	48	7	—	1291	—	—	—	—
Taco Meat	1 serv (2.5 oz)	208	11	4	38	22	7	5	—	576	—	—	—	—
Taco Salad Chicken w/o Dressing	1 serv (9 oz)	370	21	7	48	19	27	3	—	861	—	—	—	—
Taco Salad w/o Dressing	1 serv (7.75 oz)	479	28	11	63	30	30	7	—	895	—	—	—	—
Taco Shell 6 in	1 (1.25 oz)	110	6	1	0	2	14	2	—	48	—	—	—	—
Thousand Island Dressing	1 serv (1 oz)	160	16	2	10	0	4	0	—	270	—	—	—	—
Tomato	1 serv (0.5 oz)	3	0	0	0	0	1	0	—	1	—	—	—	—
Tostada Delight Salad Meat	1 (9.75 oz)	628	33	14	82	36	48	13	—	1004	—	—	—	—
Value Soft Bean Burrito	1 (6.75 oz)	380	10	4	15	16	58	13	—	715	—	—	—	—
Value Soft Meat Burrito	1 (6.75 oz)	491	21	8	56	31	48	12	—	1197	—	—	—	—
Value Soft Taco	1 (5.25 oz)	316	15	7	48	24	23	5	—	599	—	—	—	—
Veggie Burrito	1 (11 oz)	491	16	6	24	21	70	10	—	643	—	—	—	—
Wheat Tortilla 11 in	1 (3.5 oz)	175	3	1	0	8	33	2	—	84	—	—	—	—
TCBY														
Hand Dipped All Flavors 96% Fat Free	½ cup (3 oz)	140	3	2	5	3	26	0	100	26	—	0	—	0
Hand Dipped All Flavors Nonfat	½ cup (2.9 oz)	120	0	0	0	4	25	1	100	60	—	0	—	0
Lowfat Ice Cream All Flavors No Sugar Added	½ cup (2.6 oz)	110	3	2	10	3	19	0	100	60	—	0	—	400
Nonfat Ice Cream All Flavors	½ cup (2.9 oz)	120	0	0	0	3	26	1	100	55	—	1	—	400
Soft Serve All Flavors 96% Fat Free	½ cup (3.4 fl oz)	140	3	2	15	4	23	0	80	60	—	0	—	0
Soft Serve All Flavors No Sugar Added Nonfat	½ cup (2.8 oz)	80	0	0	<5	4	20	0	100	35	—	0	—	0

FOOD	PORTION	CALORIES	FAT	SAT FAT	CHOL	PROTEIN	CARBO	FIBER	CALCIUM	SOD	POTAS	VIT C	FOLIC	VIT A
Soft Serve All Flavors Nonfat	½ cup (3.4 oz)	110	0	0	<5	4	23	0	100	60	—	0	—	0
Sorbet All Flavors Nonfat & Nondairy	½ cup (3.4 oz)	100	0	0	0	0	24	0	0	30	—	0	—	0

TGI FRIDAY'S

FOOD	PORTION	CALORIES	FAT	SAT FAT	CHOL	PROTEIN	CARBO	FIBER	CALCIUM	SOD	POTAS	VIT C	FOLIC	VIT A
Chili Yogurt	1 serv	30	—	—	—	—	—	—	—	—	—	—	—	—
Corn Salsa	1 serv	175	3	—	—	—	—	—	—	—	—	—	—	—
Fresh Vegetable Medley w/ Potato	1 serv	470	8	—	25	—	—	—	—	—	—	—	—	—
Fresh Vegetable Medley w/ Rice	1 serv	407	8	—	<2	—	—	—	—	—	—	—	—	—
Friday's Gardenburger	1	445	9	—	13	—	—	—	—	—	—	—	—	—
Garden Dagwood Sandwich	1 serv	375	11	—	<2	—	—	—	—	—	—	—	—	—
Pacific Coast Chicken	1 serv	415	8	—	70	—	—	—	—	—	—	—	—	—
Pacific Coast Tuna	1 serv	410	8	—	70	—	—	—	—	—	—	—	—	—
Pea Salsa	1 serv (6.4 oz)	175	3	—	0	7	32	—	—	445	—	—	—	—
Plum Sauce	1 serv	105	0	0	—	—	—	—	—	—	—	—	—	—
Salad & Baked Potato	1 serv	250	5	—	<2	—	—	—	—	—	—	—	—	—
Turkey Burger	1 (9.8 oz)	410	19	—	95	32	27	—	—	780	—	—	—	—

TJ CINNAMONS

FOOD	PORTION	CALORIES	FAT	SAT FAT	CHOL	PROTEIN	CARBO	FIBER	CALCIUM	SOD	POTAS	VIT C	FOLIC	VIT A
Doughnuts Cake	2	454	22	—	98	5	60	tr	46	582	104	0	11	100
Doughnuts Raised	2	352	22	—	98	5	32	tr	32	198	68	0	20	60
Mini-Cinn Plain	1	75	5	—	3	1	7	tr	5	89	11	tr	7	225
Mini-Cinn With Icing	1	80	5	—	3	1	8	tr	5	89	11	tr	7	225
Original Gourmet Cinnamon Roll Plain	1	630	34	—	38	62	75	1	50	712	117	1	75	1470
Original Gourmet Cinnamon Roll With Icing	1	686	34	—	38	62	89	1	50	712	117	1	75	1470
Petite Cinnamon Roll Plain	1	185	10	—	11	2	22	tr	15	214	35	tr	22	440
Petite Cinnamon Roll With Icing	1	202	10	—	11	2	26	tr	15	214	35	tr	22	440
Sticky Bun Cinnamon Pecan	1	607	35	—	29	5	69	tr	38	589	139	tr	59	1110
Sticky Bun Petite Cinnamon Pecan	1	255	15	—	11	2	29	tr	15	241	58	tr	23	445
Triple Chocolate Classic Roll Plain	1	412	28	—	28	5	35	tr	35	543	121	tr	56	1100

FOOD	PORTION	CALORIES	FAT	SAT FAT	CHOL	PROTEIN	CARBO	FIBER	CALCIUM	SOD	POTAS	VIT C	FOLIC	VIT A
Triple Chocolate Classic Roll With Icing	1	462	31	—	28	5	42	tr	37	563	131	tr	56	1260

TROPIGRILL

(Restaurants in this chain may also be called Pollo Tropical. Menu items are the same for both.)

FOOD	PORTION	CALORIES	FAT	SAT FAT	CHOL	PROTEIN	CARBO	FIBER	CALCIUM	SOD	POTAS	VIT C	FOLIC	VIT A
Banana Tropical	1 serv (7.55 oz)	498	14	—	0	4	90	9	—	7	—	—	—	—
Black Beans (combo meal portion)	1 serv (4.78 oz)	153	2	—	0	9	24	10	—	444				
Black Beans (side)	1 serv (8.39 oz)	269	4	—	0	15	43	18	—	780	—			
Boiled Yuca	1 serv (12 oz)	334	0	—	0	1	81	5	—	456	—	—		—
Boneless Breast	1 serv (3.14 oz)	140	4	—	83	26	1	tr	—	169	—	—	—	—
Cheese Potatoes	1 serv (7.42 oz)	177	6	—	10	6	25	2	—	779	—	—	—	—
Chicken 1/4 Dark Meat	1 serv (4.52 oz)	298	18	—	187	33	1	tr	—	448	—	—	—	—
Chicken 1/4 Dark Meat w/o Skin	1 serv (3.42 oz)	170	7	—	144	26	1	tr	—	312	—	—	—	—
Chicken 1/4 White Meat	1 serv (5.09 oz)	295	14	—	170	42	1	tr	—	894	—	—	—	—
Chicken 1/4 White Meat w/o Skin	1 serv (3.82 oz)	167	3	—	117	35	tr	tr	—	401	—	—	—	—
Chicken Caesar Sandwich	1 (6.4 oz)	457	20	—	97	34	36	tr	—	931	—	—	—	—
Chicken Sandwich	1 (7.92 oz)	442	19	—	89	33	35	tr	—	702	—	—	—	—
Congri	1 serv (7.08 oz)	439	13	—	0	11	69	7	—	786	—	—	—	—
Vegetable Kabob	1 (3.07 oz)	106	1	—	0	3	22	5	—	286	—	—	—	—
White Rice	1 serv (6.82 oz)	341	6	—	0	7	65	2	—	239	—	—	—	—
Yellow Rice	1 serv (7 oz)	294	5	—	0	6	56	3	—	371	—	—	—	—
Yucatan Fries	1 serv (5.3 oz)	440	24	—	0	1	54	3	—	84	—	—	—	—

UNO RESTAURANT

FOOD	PORTION	CALORIES	FAT	SAT FAT	CHOL	PROTEIN	CARBO	FIBER	CALCIUM	SOD	POTAS	VIT C	FOLIC	VIT A
DeepDish Pizza	1 serv	770	38	13	45	39	75	6	800	1390	360	—	—	1750

VILLAGE INN

FOOD	PORTION	CALORIES	FAT	SAT FAT	CHOL	PROTEIN	CARBO	FIBER	CALCIUM	SOD	POTAS	VIT C	FOLIC	VIT A
French Toast Cinnamon Raisin	1 serv	809	16	4	9	—	—	—	—	740	—	—	—	—
Fruit & Nut Pancakes Low Cholesterol	1 serv	936	19	2	2	—	—	—	—	754	—	—	—	—
Omelette Chicken & Cheese	1 serv	721	19	4	120	—	—	—	—	705	—	—	—	—
Omelette Fresh Veggie	1 serv	704	18	4	102	—	—	—	—	883	—	—	—	—

FOOD	PORTION	CALORIES	FAT	SAT FAT	CHOL	PROTEIN	CARBO	FIBER	CALCIUM	SOD	POTAS	VIT C	FOLIC	VIT A
Omelette Mushroom & Cheese	1 serv	680	18	4	102	—	—	—	—	688	—	—	—	—
Turkey & Vegetable Scrambled Sensation	1 serv	726	19	4	124	—	—	—	—	710	—	—	—	—

WENDY'S

CHILDREN'S MENU SELECTIONS

FOOD	PORTION	CALORIES	FAT	SAT FAT	CHOL	PROTEIN	CARBO	FIBER	CALCIUM	SOD	POTAS	VIT C	FOLIC	VIT A
Kid's Meal Cheeseburger	1 (4.3 oz)	320	13	6	45	17	33	2	170	830	—	0	—	300
Kid's Meal Chicken Nuggets	4 pieces (2.1 oz)	190	13	3	25	9	9	0	20	380	—	1	—	0
Kid's Meal Hamburger	1 (3.9 oz)	270	10	4	30	15	33	2	110	610	—	0	—	100

DESSERTS

FOOD	PORTION	CALORIES	FAT	SAT FAT	CHOL	PROTEIN	CARBO	FIBER	CALCIUM	SOD	POTAS	VIT C	FOLIC	VIT A
Chocolate Chip Cookie	1 (2 oz)	270	13	6	30	3	36	1	10	120	—	0	—	0
Frosty Dairy Dessert	1 sm (12 oz)	330	8	5	35	8	56	0	310	200	—	0	—	750
Frosty Dairy Dessert	1 lg (20 fl oz)	540	14	9	60	14	91	0	500	320	—	0	—	1250
Frosty Dairy Dessert	1 med (16 fl oz)	440	11	7	50	11	73	0	410	260	—	0	—	1000

MAIN MENU SELECTIONS

FOOD	PORTION	CALORIES	FAT	SAT FAT	CHOL	PROTEIN	CARBO	FIBER	CALCIUM	SOD	POTAS	VIT C	FOLIC	VIT A
¼ lb Hamburger Patty	1 (2.6 oz)	200	14	6	65	19	0	0	20	290	—	0	—	0
2 oz Hamburger Patty	1 (1.3 oz)	100	7	3	30	9	0	0	10	150	—	0	—	0
American Cheese	1 slice (0.6 oz)	70	5	4	15	3	1	0	100	320	—	0	—	300
American Cheese Jr.	1 slice (0.4 oz)	45	4	3	10	2	0	0	70	220	—	0	—	200
Bacon	1 strip (4 g)	20	2	1	5	2	0	0	0	65	—	1	—	0
Baked Potato Bacon & Cheese	1 (13.3 oz)	530	18	4	20	17	78	7	180	1390	—	36	—	500
Baked Potato Broccoli & Cheese	1 (14.4 oz)	470	14	3	5	9	80	9	210	470	—	72	—	1750
Baked Potato Cheese	1 (13.4 oz)	570	23	8	30	14	78	7	380	640	—	36	—	1000
Baked Potato Chili & Cheese	1 (15.4 oz)	630	24	9	40	20	83	9	330	770	—	36	—	1000
Baked Potato Plain	1 (10 oz)	310	0	0	0	7	71	7	30	25	—	36	—	0
Baked Potato Sour Cream & Chives	1 (11 oz)	380	6	4	15	8	74	8	80	40	—	48	—	1500
Big Bacon Classic	1 (9.9 oz)	580	30	12	100	34	46	3	250	1460	—	15	—	750
Breaded Chicken Fillet	1 (3.5 oz)	230	12	3	55	22	10	0	10	490	—	0	—	0
Breaded Chicken Sandwich	1 (7.3 oz)	440	18	4	60	28	44	2	100	840	—	6	—	200

FOOD	PORTION	CALORIES	FAT	SAT FAT	CHOL	PROTEIN	CARBO	FIBER	CALCIUM	SOD	POTAS	VIT C	FOLIC	VIT A
Cheddar Cheese Shredded	2 tbsp (0.6 oz)	70	6	4	15	4	1	0	120	110	—	0	—	200
Chicken Club Sandwich	1 (7.6 oz)	470	20	4	70	31	44	2	110	970	—	6	—	200
Chicken Nuggets	5 pieces (2.6 oz)	230	16	3	30	11	11	0	20	470	—	1	—	0
Chili	1 lg (12 oz)	310	10	4	45	23	32	7	120	1190	—	6	—	500
Chili	1 sm (8 oz)	210	7	3	30	15	21	5	80	800	—	4	—	400
French Fries	1 Great Biggie (6.7 oz)	570	27	4	0	8	73	7	30	180	—	9	—	0
French Fries	1 sm (3.2 oz)	270	13	2	0	4	35	3	10	85	—	5	—	0
French Fries	1 Biggie (5.6 oz)	470	23	4	0	7	61	6	30	150	—	9	—	0
French Fries	1 med (4.6 oz)	390	19	3	0	5	50	5	20	120	—	6	—	0
Grilled Chicken Fillet	1 (2.9 oz)	110	3	1	60	22	0	0	10	450	—	0	—	0
Grilled Chicken Sandwich	1 (6.6 oz)	310	8	2	65	27	35	2	100	790	—	6	—	200
Honey Mustard Reduced Calorie	1 tsp (7 g)	25	2	0	0	0	2	0	0	45	—	0	—	0
Jr. Bacon Cheeseburger	1 (5.8 oz)	380	19	7	60	22	34	2	170	850	—	6	—	400
Jr. Cheeseburger	1 (4.6 oz)	320	13	6	45	17	34	2	170	830	—	1	—	300
Jr. Cheeseburger Deluxe	1 (6.3 oz)	360	17	6	50	18	36	3	180	890	—	6	—	500
Jr. Hamburger	1 (4.1 oz)	270	10	4	30	15	34	2	110	610	—	1	—	100
Kaiser Bun	1 (2.4 oz)	190	3	1	0	6	36	2	110	340	—	0	—	0
Ketchup	1 tsp (7 g)	10	0	0	0	0	2	0	0	75	—	0	—	100
Lettuce	1 leaf (0.5 oz)	0	0	0	0	0	0	0	0	0	—	0	—	0
Mayonnaise	1½ tsp (9 g)	30	3	0	5	0	1	0	0	60	—	0	—	0
Mustard	½ tsp (5 g)	5	0	0	0	0	0	0	0	50	—	0	—	0
Nuggets Sauce Barbeque	1 pkg (1 oz)	45	0	0	0	1	10	0	10	160	—	0	—	0
Nuggets Sauce Honey Mustard	1 pkg (1 oz)	130	12	2	10	0	6	0	10	220	—	0	—	0
Nuggets Sauce Sweet & Sour	1 pkg (1 oz)	50	0	0	0	0	12	0	0	120	—	1	—	0
Onion	4 rings (0.5 oz)	5	0	0	0	0	1	0	0	0	—	1	—	0
Pickles	4 slices (0.4 oz)	0	0	0	0	0	0	0	10	140	—	0	—	0
Pita Dressing Caesar Vinaigrette Reduced Fat Reduced Calorie	1 tbsp (0.6 oz)	70	7	1	0	0	1	0	10	170	—	0	—	0
Pita Dressing Garden Ranch Sauce Reduced Fat Reduced Calorie	1 tbsp (0.6 oz)	50	5	1	10	0	1	0	10	125	—	0	—	0

FOOD	PORTION	CALORIES	FAT	SAT FAT	CHOL	PROTEIN	CARBO	FIBER	CALCIUM	SOD	POTAS	VIT C	FOLIC	VIT A
Plain Single	1 (4.7 oz)	360	16	6	65	24	31	2	110	580	—	0	—	0
Saltines	2 (0.2 oz)	25	1	0	0	1	4	0	10	80	—	0	—	0
Sandwich Bun	1 (2 oz)	160	3	1	0	5	29	2	90	280	—	0	—	0
Single With Everything	1 (7.7 oz)	420	20	7	70	25	37	3	130	920	—	6	—	300
Sour Cream	1 pkt (1 oz)	60	6	4	10	1	1	0	30	15	—	0	—	200
Spicy Buffalo Wing Sauce	1 pkg (1 oz)	25	1	0	0	0	4	0	0	210	—	0	—	100
Spicy Chicken Fillet	1 (3.6 oz)	210	9	2	60	22	10	0	10	920	—	1	—	0
Spicy Chicken Sandwich	1 (7.5 oz)	410	15	3	65	28	43	2	110	1280	—	6	—	200
Stuffed Pita Chicken Caesar w/ Dressing	1 (8.3 oz)	490	18	5	65	34	48	4	330	1320	—	15	—	2500
Stuffed Pita Classic Greek w/Dressing	1 (8.2 oz)	440	20	8	35	15	50	4	320	1050	—	0	—	2500
Stuffed Pita Garden Ranch Chicken w/ Dressing	1 (9.9 oz)	480	18	4	70	30	51	5	160	1180	—	54	—	3000
Stuffed Pita Garden Veggie w/ Dressing	1 (9 oz)	400	17	4	20	11	52	5	160	760	—	54	—	3000
Tomatoes	1 slice (0.9 oz)	5	0	0	0	0	1	1	0	0	—	5	—	200
Whipped Margarine	1 pkg (0.5 oz)	60	7	2	0	0	0	0	0	115	—	0	—	500
SALAD DRESSINGS														
Blue Cheese	2 tbsp (1 oz)	180	19	4	15	1	0	0	20	180	—	0	—	100
French	2 tbsp (1 oz)	120	10	2	0	0	6	0	0	330	—	1	—	100
French Fat Free	2 tbsp (1 oz)	35	0	0	0	0	8	0	0	150	—	1	—	0
Hidden Valley Ranch	2 tbsp (1 oz)	90	10	2	10	1	1	0	10	220	—	0	—	0
Hidden Valley Ranch Reduced Fat Reduced Calorie	2 tbsp (1 oz)	60	5	1	10	1	2	0	10	240	—	0	—	0
Italian Reduced Fat Reduced Calorie	2 tbsp (1 oz)	40	3	0	0	0	2	0	0	340	—	1	—	0
Italian Caesar	2 tbsp (1 oz)	150	16	3	20	1	1	0	20	240	—	1	—	0
Salad Oil	1 tbsp (0.5 oz)	120	14	2	0	0	0	0	0	0	—	0	—	0
Thousand Island	2 tbsp (1 oz)	90	8	2	10	0	2	0	0	125	—	0	—	0
Wine Vinegar	1 tbsp (0.5 oz)	0	0	0	0	0	0	0	0	0	—	0	—	0
SALADS AND SALAD BARS														
Applesauce	2 tbsp (1.4 oz)	30	0	0	0	0	7	0	0	0	—	0	—	0
Bacon Bits	2 tbsp (0.5 oz)	45	2	1	10	6	0	0	0	550	—	0	—	0
Bananas & Strawberry Glaze	¼ cup (1.6 oz)	30	0	0	0	0	8	1	0	0	—	12	—	0

FOOD	PORTION	CALORIES	FAT	SAT FAT	CHOL	PROTEIN	CARBO	FIBER	CALCIUM	SOD	POTAS	VIT C	FOLIC	VIT A
Broccoli	¼ cup (0.5 oz)	0	0	0	0	0	1	0	0	0	—	12	—	200
Cantaloupe Sliced	1 piece (1.6 oz)	15	0	0	0	0	4	0	0	0	—	18	—	750
Carrots	¼ cup (0.6 oz)	5	0	0	0	0	2	0	0	5	—	1	—	2250
Cauliflower	¼ cup (0.6 g)	0	0	0	0	0	1	0	0	0	—	6	—	0
Ceasar Side Salad w/o Dressing	1 (3.1 oz)	100	4	2	10	8	8	1	30	620	—	15	—	1750
Cheese Shredded Imitation	2 tbsp (0.6 oz)	50	4	1	0	3	1	0	110	260	—	0	—	100
Chicken Salad	2 tbsp (1.2 oz)	70	5	1	0	4	2	0	0	135	—	1	—	0
Cottage Cheese	2 tbsp (1.1 oz)	30	2	1	5	4	1	0	20	125	—	0	—	100
Croutons	2 tbsp (0.2 oz)	25	1	0	0	1	4	0	0	65	—	0	—	0
Cucumbers	2 slices (0.5 oz)	0	0	0	0	0	0	0	0	0	—	1	—	0
Deluxe Garden Salad w/o Dressing	1 (9.5 oz)	110	6	1	0	7	9	3	180	350	—	36	—	6000
Eggs Hard Cooked	2 tbsp (0.9 oz)	40	3	1	110	3	0	0	20	30	—	0	—	200
Green Peas	2 tbsp (0.7 oz)	15	0	0	0	1	3	1	0	25	—	4	—	100
Green Peppers	2 pieces (0.3 oz)	0	0	0	0	0	1	0	0	0	—	6	—	0
Grilled Chicken Caesar Salad w/o Dressing	1 (9.2 oz)	260	9	3	60	26	17	2	70	1170	—	36	—	4000
Grilled Chicken Salad w/o Dressing	1 (11.9 oz)	200	8	2	50	25	9	3	190	720	—	36	—	6000
Lettuce Iceberg/ Romaine	1 cup (2.6 oz)	10	0	0	0	0	2	1	20	5	—	6	—	300
Mushrooms	¼ cup (0.5 oz)	0	0	0	0	0	1	0	0	0	—	0	—	0
Orange Sliced	2 slices (1.1 oz)	15	0	0	0	0	4	1	20	0	—	15	—	100
Parmesan Blend Grated	2 tbsp (0.5 oz)	70	4	2	10	4	5	0	0	290	—	0	—	100
Pasta Salad	2 tbsp (1.2 oz)	35	2	0	0	1	4	1	10	180	—	2	—	100
Peaches Sliced	1 piece (1 oz)	15	0	0	0	0	4	0	0	0	—	1	—	100
Pepperoni Sliced	6 slices (0.2 oz)	30	3	1	5	1	0	0	0	70	—	0	—	100
Potato Salad	2 tbsp (1.3 oz)	80	7	3	5	0	5	0	0	180	—	4	—	0
Pudding Chocolate	¼ cup (1.8 oz)	70	3	1	0	0	10	0	100	60	—	0	—	0
Red Onions	3 rings (0.5 oz)	0	0	0	0	0	1	0	0	0	—	1	—	0
Side Salad w/o Dressing	1 (5.4 oz)	60	3	0	0	4	5	2	100	180	—	18	—	3000
Soft Breadstick	1 (1.5 oz)	130	3	1	5	4	23	1	40	250	—	0	—	0
Sunflower Seeds & Raisins	2 tbsp (0.5 oz)	80	5	1	0	0	5	1	20	0	—	1	—	0
Taco Chips	15 (1.5 oz)	210	11	2	0	3	24	2	40	180	—	0	—	0
Taco Salad w/o Dressing	1 (16.4 oz)	380	19	10	65	26	28	7	370	1040	—	27	—	2250

FOOD	PORTION	CALORIES	FAT	SAT FAT	CHOL	PROTEIN	CARBO	FIBER	CALCIUM	SOD	POTAS	VIT C	FOLIC	VIT A
Tomatoes Wedged	1 piece (0.9 oz)	5	0	0	0	0	1	0	0	0	—	5	—	100
Turkey Ham Diced	2 tbsp (0.8 oz)	50	4	1	25	3	0	0	20	280	—	0	—	0
Watermelon Wedged	1 piece (2.2 oz)	20	0	0	0	0	4	0	0	0	—	6	—	100

WHATABURGER

BAKED SELECTIONS

FOOD	PORTION	CALORIES	FAT	SAT FAT	CHOL	PROTEIN	CARBO	FIBER	CALCIUM	SOD	POTAS	VIT C	FOLIC	VIT A
Biscuit	1	280	13	—	3	5	37	—	—	509	—	—	—	—
Blueberry Muffin	1	239	8	—	0	6	36	—	—	538	—	—	—	—
Cinnamon Roll	1	320	16	—	10	4	39	—	—	190	—	—	—	—
Cookie Chocolate Chunk	1	247	16	—	28	4	28	—	—	75	—	—	—	—
Cookie White Chocolate Macadamia Nut	1	269	16	—	34	3	31	—	—	80	—	—	—	—
Fried Apple Turnover	1	215	11	—	0	2	27	—	—	241	—	—	—	—

BREAKFAST SELECTIONS

FOOD	PORTION	CALORIES	FAT	SAT FAT	CHOL	PROTEIN	CARBO	FIBER	CALCIUM	SOD	POTAS	VIT C	FOLIC	VIT A
Biscuit w/ Bacon	1	359	20	—	15	10	37	—	—	730	—	—	—	—
Biscuit w/ Bacon Egg & Cheese	1	511	33	—	213	18	38	—	—	1010	—	—	—	—
Biscuit w/ Egg & Cheese	1	434	26	—	202	14	38	—	—	797	—	—	—	—
Biscuit w/ Sausage	1	446	29	—	37	12	37	—	—	794	—	—	—	—
Biscuit w/ Sausage Egg & Cheese	1	601	42	—	236	21	38	—	—	1081	—	—	—	—
Biscuit w/ Sausage Gravy	1	479	27	—	20	9	48	—	—	1253	—	—	—	—
Breakfast Platter w/ Bacon	1 serv	695	44	—	389	22	54	—	—	1162	—	—	—	—
Breakfast Platter w/ Sausage	1 serv	785	53	—	412	25	54	—	—	1234	—	—	—	—
Breakfast On A Bun w/ Bacon	1	365	19	—	210	18	29	—	—	815	—	—	—	—
Breakfast On A Bun w/ Sausage	1	455	28	—	232	20	30	—	—	886	—	—	—	—
Butter	1 pkg	36	4	—	11	0	0	—	—	42	—	—	—	—
Egg Omelette Sandwich	1	288	13	—	198	13	29	—	—	602	—	—	—	—
Grape Jelly	1 pkg	45	0	0	0	0	10	—	—	15	—	—	—	—
Hashbrown	1 serv	150	9	—	0	1	16	—	—	228	—	—	—	—
Honey	1 pkg	25	0	0	0	0	7	—	—	0	—	—	—	—
Margarine	1 pkg	25	3	—	0	0	0	—	—	40	—	—	—	—
Pancake Syrup	1 pkg	180	0	0	0	0	42	—	—	50	—	—	—	—
Pancakes	3	259	6	—	0	11	40	—	—	842	—	—	—	—
Pancakes w/ Bacon	1 serv	335	12	—	12	15	40	—	—	1074	—	—	—	—
Pancakes w/ Sausage	1 serv	426	21	—	34	18	40	—	—	1127	—	—	—	—

FOOD	PORTION	CALORIES	FAT	SAT FAT	CHOL	PROTEIN	CARBO	FIBER	CALCIUM	SOD	POTAS	VIT C	FOLIC	VIT A
Scrambled Eggs	2	189	15	—	374	11	2	—	—	211	—	—	—	—
Strawberry Jam	1 pkg	40	0	0	0	0	9	—	—	15	—	—	—	—
Taquito Bacon & Egg	1	335	16	—	286	15	32	—	—	761	—	—	—	—
MAIN MENU SELECTIONS														
Bacon	1 slice	38	3	—	6	2	0	—	—	106	—	—	—	—
Cheese Slice	1 lg	89	7	—	22	5	tr	—	—	338	—	—	—	—
Cheese Slice	1 sm	46	4	—	12	3	tr	—	—	176	—	—	—	—
Chicken Strips	2	120	5	—	14	7	10	—	—	420	—	—	—	—
Club Crackers	1 pkg	30	2	—	0	1	4	—	—	75	—	—	—	—
Croutons	1 pkg	30	1	—	0	1	5	—	—	90	—	—	—	—
Fajita Beef	1	326	12	—	28	22	34	—	—	670	—	—	—	—
Fajita Grilled Chicken	1	272	7	—	33	18	35	—	—	691	—	—	—	—
French Fries	1 lg	442	24	—	0	7	49	—	—	227	—	—	—	—
French Fries	1 reg	332	18	—	0	5	37	—	—	208	—	—	—	—
French Fries	1 junior	221	12	—	0	4	25	—	—	139	—	—	—	—
Garden Salad	1	56	1	—	0	3	11	—	—	32	—	—	—	—
Grilled Chicken Salad	1 serv	150	1	—	49	23	14	—	—	434	—	—	—	—
Grilled Chicken Sandwich	1	442	14	—	66	34	48	—	—	1103	—	—	—	—
Grilled Chicken Sandwich w/o Bun Oil w/ Mustard	1	300	3	—	66	33	35	—	—	994	—	—	—	—
Grilled Chicken Sandwich w/o Bun Oil & Dressing	1	358	6	—	66	34	46	—	—	989	—	—	—	—
Grilled Chicken Sandwich w/o Dressing	1	385	9	—	66	34	46	—	—	989	—	—	—	—
Jalapeno Pepper	1	3	tr	—	0	tr	1	—	—	190	—	—	—	—
Justaburger	1	276	11	—	34	13	30	—	—	578	—	—	—	—
Ketchup	1 pkg	30	0	0	0	0	7	—	—	344	—	—	—	—
Onion Rings	1 reg	329	19	—	0	5	34	—	—	596	—	—	—	—
Onion Rings	1 lg	493	29	—	0	8	51	—	—	893	—	—	—	—
Peppered Gravy	1 serv (3 oz)	75	5	—	0	0	8	—	—	375	—	—	—	—
Picante Sauce	1 pkg	5	0	—	0	tr	1	—	—	130	—	—	—	—
Taquito Potato & Egg	1	446	22	—	281	14	48	—	—	883	—	—	—	—
Taquito Sausage & Egg	1	443	26	—	315	20	32	—	—	790	—	—	—	—
Texas Toast	1 slice	147	5	—	0	4	22	—	—	250	—	—	—	—
Whataburger	1	598	26	—	84	30	61	—	—	1096	—	—	—	—
Whataburger Double Meat	1	823	42	—	168	49	62	—	—	1298	—	—	—	—
Whataburger Jr.	1	300	12	—	34	14	35	—	—	583	—	—	—	—

FOOD	PORTION	CALORIES	FAT	SAT FAT	CHOL	PROTEIN	CARBO	FIBER	CALCIUM	SOD	POTAS	VIT C	FOLIC	VIT A
Whataburger w/o bun oil	1	407	19	—	84	25	34	—	—	839	—	—	—	—
Whatacatch Sandwich	1	467	25	—	33	18	43	—	—	636	—	—	—	—
Whatachick'n Sandwich	1	501	23	—	40	27	51	—	—	1122	—	—	—	—
SALAD DRESSINGS														
Low Fat Ranch	1 pkg	66	3	—	15	1	9	—	—	607	—	—	—	—
Low Fat Vinaigrette	1 pkg	37	2	—	0	0	6	—	—	896	—	—	—	—
Ranch	1 pkg	320	33	—	50	0	4	—	—	750	—	—	—	—
Thousand Island	1 pkg	160	12	—	15	0	12	—	—	470	—	—	—	—

WHITE CASTLE

FOOD	PORTION	CALORIES	FAT	SAT FAT	CHOL	PROTEIN	CARBO	FIBER	CALCIUM	SOD	POTAS	VIT C	FOLIC	VIT A
Cheeseburger	2 (3.6 oz)	310	17	9	30	15	23	6	80	480	—	0	—	100
Grilled Chicken Sandwich	2 (4 oz)	250	9	3	20	17	24	5	40	490	—	0	—	0
Grilled Chicken Sandwich w/ Sauce	2 (4.8 oz)	290	9	3	20	17	24	5	40	600	—	0	—	0
Hamburger	2 (3.2 oz)	270	14	6	20	12	23	5	20	270	—	0	—	0

WINCHELL'S DONUTS

FOOD	PORTION	CALORIES	FAT	SAT FAT	CHOL	PROTEIN	CARBO	FIBER	CALCIUM	SOD	POTAS	VIT C	FOLIC	VIT A
Apple Fritter	1 (4.25 oz)	580	37	—	—	4	59	—	—	201	—	—	—	—
Cinnamon Crumb	1 (2 oz)	240	11	—	—	2	34	—	—	208	—	—	—	—
Cinnamon Roll	1 (3 oz)	360	21	—	—	5	39	—	—	179	—	—	—	—
Glazed Jelly	1 (3 oz)	300	13	—	—	5	43	—	—	172	—	—	—	—
Glazed Round	1 (1.75 oz)	210	12	—	—	1	24	—	—	100	—	—	—	—
Glazed Twist	1 (1.75 oz)	210	11	—	—	1	26	—	—	100	—	—	—	—
Iced Chocolate Bar	1 (2 oz)	220	11	—	—	3	28	—	—	125	—	—	—	—
Iced Chocolate Cake	1 (2 oz)	230	10	—	—	2	31	—	—	218	—	—	—	—
Iced Chocolate Devil's Food	1 (2 oz)	240	12	—	—	3	31	—	—	221	—	—	—	—
Iced Chocolate French	1 (1.89 oz)	220	13	—	—	3	23	—	—	217	—	—	—	—
Iced Chocolate Raised	1 (1.75 oz)	210	10	—	—	3	26	—	—	96	—	—	—	—
Plain	1 (1.58 oz)	200	11	—	—	1	24	—	—	211	—	—	—	—
Plain Donut Hole	1 (0.4 oz)	50	3	—	—	tr	5	—	—	13	—	—	—	—

ZUZU

FOOD	PORTION	CALORIES	FAT	SAT FAT	CHOL	PROTEIN	CARBO	FIBER	CALCIUM	SOD	POTAS	VIT C	FOLIC	VIT A
Bean & Cheese Burrito Platter	1 serv	475	15	—	15	—	—	—	—	—	—	—	—	—
Beans	1 cup	210	6	—	0	—	—	—	—	—	—	—	—	—
Cheese Enchilada Platter	1 serv	395	13	—	15	—	—	—	—	—	—	—	—	—
Chicken Burrito Platter	1 serv	580	19	—	60	—	—	—	—	—	—	—	—	—
Chicken Taco Platter	1 serv	440	13	—	70	—	—	—	—	—	—	—	—	—

FOOD	PORTION	CALORIES	FAT	SAT FAT	CHOL	PROTEIN	CARBO	FIBER	CALCIUM	SOD	POTAS	VIT C	FOLIC	VIT A
Chicken Taco w/o Mexican Cream	1	125	4	—	35	—	—	—	—	—	—	—	—	—
Frozen Yogurt	1 serv	200	0	0	0	—	—	—	—	—	—	—	—	—
Green Salad w/o Dressing or Avocado	1	20	0	0	0	—	—	—	—	—	—	—	—	—
Grilled Chicken Salad w/o Dressing	1 serv	305	10	—	70	—	—	—	—	—	—	—	—	—
Rice	1 cup	150	2	—	0	—	—	—	—	—	—	—	—	—
Salsa Roja Epazote	¼ cup	8	0	0	0	—	—	—	—	—	—	—	—	—
Tortilla Corn	1	35	0	0	0	—	—	—	—	—	—	—	—	—
Tortilla Flour	1	60	2	—	0	—	—	—	—	—	—	—	—	—

PART THREE

ALL THE FACTS—A TO Z

ACESULFAME-K—Sold as Sweet One and Sunett, this calorie-free sugar substitute is almost 200 times sweeter than sugar. It is used in desserts, confections, and beverages and retains its sweetness when heated.

ALCOHOL—Ethyl alcohol (ethanol) is the alcohol in beverages. Liquors such as vodka, gin, and rye are about 40 to 50 percent alcohol; wine is 10 to 14 percent alcohol, and beer is 2 to 4 percent. There are lower-alcohol and nonalcoholic versions of some of these beverages. Many over-the-counter drugs and herbal extracts contain alcohol. Alcohol doesn't need to be digested; it's simply absorbed from the stomach and small intestines. It is a central nervous system depressant that first impairs walking, coordination, judgment, and speech. Emotions, memory, and reflexes are affected next. Drunkenness and stupor will follow if drinking is continued. Excessive alcohol intake contributes to three leading causes of death—cirrhosis of the liver, accidents, and suicide. "Moderate" drinking for normal, healthy people is one drink a day for women, two drinks for men. Twelve ounces of regular beer, 5 ounces of wine, or 1½ ounces of liquor equal one drink. Studies show that moderate alcohol drinking increases the level of HIGH-DENSITY LIPOPROTEINS (HDLs), the good form of CHOLESTEROL, which appears to protect against heart attack. A survey of the research on alcohol use found that wine, beer, and liquor in moderation all reduce death rate from heart disease.

AMERICAN DIETETIC ASSOCIATION (ADA)—The world's largest organization of food and nutrition professionals. With nearly 70,000 members, ADA serves the public by promoting nutrition, health, and well-being. The ADA's Consumer Nutrition Hotline offers recorded food and nutrition messages and referrals to registered dietitians who give individual and group nutrition counseling services. The number is 1-800-366-1655.

AMINO ACIDS—Building blocks that make up the different proteins in foods and in your body. Nine of these amino acids come from food and cannot be made in the body. They are: histidine, isoleucine, leucine, lysine, methionine, phenylalanine, threonine, tryptophan, and valine. All other needed amino acids can be produced in the body. Some amino acids are said to have special benefits when taken as supplements. There is little solid evidence to back up these claims. Many athletes take amino acid powders and pills in the hope that they will help build extra muscle. In fact, extra amino acids do not turn into muscle; they are simply a source of extra calories that are used as fuel or turned into fat. Taking large amounts of single amino acids may be harmful. In 1990, the amino acid L-tryptophan, which was used by millions of Americans as a remedy for depression, insomnia, and premenstrual syndrome, was taken off the market after a contaminated form of the supplement was believed responsible for death and serious illness in some users. Recently, a similar contaminant was found in a new version of tryptophan, 5-hydroxy-L-tryptophan (5HTP), which is widely available and recommended in self-help books.

ANTIOXIDANTS—Help protect the body somewhat like a police force from potentially harmful substances called free radicals that can damage nearby healthy cells. Free radicals result from smoking, air pollution, and sun exposure and are also by-products of normal body functions. VITAMINS C and E, the mineral SELENIUM, and PHYTOCHEMICALS are some antioxidants. Some foods—fruits, vegetables, nuts, tea—are rich sources of antioxidants. Some food additives, such as BHA (butylated hydroxyanisole), sodium citrate, and EDTA (ethylenediamenetetraacetic acid) act as antioxidants by keeping processed foods fresh longer.

APHRODISIACS—Why did Casanova eat fifty raw oysters every day? The famous lover thought they would increase his libido. The list of supposed aphrodisiacs is long—asparagus, ginseng, yohimbe, mushrooms, vitamin E, chocolate, licorice root, truffles, garlic, foods that look like sex organs, and, of course, oysters. Most reports of foods acting as aphrodisiacs have no scientific basis.

ASPARTAME—See EQUAL.

BEANS—Legumes, sold canned, dried, fresh, and frozen. They are rich sources of carbohydrate, protein, and fiber. Studies show that substituting vegetable protein, such as beans, for animal protein lowers the risk for heart disease by reducing cholesterol and triglyceride levels.

BETA-CAROTENE—One of a group of over 500 deep-yellow, orange, and red pigments that color fruits and vegetables. Some of these are changed into vitamin A in the body, and beta-carotene is the most active carotenoid in this conversion. Carotenoids supply most of the world's vitamin A.

BIOTECHNOLOGY—Biotechnology, or genetic engineering, is a way of speeding up genetic change by taking DNA (made up of genes) from one organism and inserting it into another. This process passes on certain characteristics to plants and animals that are used for food. These foods may be more resistant to pests, be more nutritious, have a longer shelf life, need less water to grow, or produce larger crops. Although many gene-altered foods are already in the food supply, people may not be aware that they are eating them because the U.S. does not currently require that they be labeled. Some consumer advocate groups are raising health and environmental concerns about genetically engineered products.

BIOTIN—One of the B vitamin family. It is a part of the enzymes that help the body process carbohydrates, fat, and protein. Biotin is found in many foods. The best sources are egg yolks, liver, whole grains, and yeast. Some biotin is made by bacteria in the lower intestines. The Adequate Intake (AI) of biotin is 5 milligrams a day for adults.

BODY MASS INDEX (BMI)—BMI is often used to determine if a person is overweight. Weight and height are calculated together to estimate body fat. To figure your BMI:

1. Multiply your weight in pounds by 700.
2. Divide that number by height in inches.
3. Then divide that result by height in inches again.

Under new government guidelines, people with a BMI of 25 to 29.9 are considered overweight. Those with a BMI of 30 or more are considered obese. Waistline measurement is also considered a factor because fat deposited around the belly is a greater risk. For those with a BMI of 25 to 35, in men who have waists of more than 40 inches and in women who have waists greater than 35 inches, there is an increased risk for serious health problems.

BULGUR—Chewy wheat kernels that are steamed and dried before being crushed into granules, bulgar is used to make the popular Middle Eastern salad tabbouleh. Bulgur is low in fat, a moderate source of protein, and high in carbohydrate.

CAFFEINE—A stimulant found in coffee, tea, soft drinks, cocoa, chocolate, and many over-the-counter medications. Although it is not addictive, it is habit-forming and the body comes to depend on it. Many people can't get going without their "wake-up" coffee or cola. Caffeine is absorbed quickly and its effects can be felt within 30 minutes. The brain and heart are stimulated, increasing work capacity, urination, and stomach acid secretion. Some people have disturbed sleep, heartburn, and stomach upset from caffeine. Getting rid of caffeine in the body can take several hours. The caffeine in 5 ounces of drip coffee averages about 130 milligrams. Decaffeinated coffee has only 3 milligrams in a cup and a can of cola has about 40 milligrams.

CALCIUM—A major mineral in the body. Besides building bones and teeth, it is needed for blood clotting, muscle contraction, nerve function, and activating ENZYMES. Good food sources are milk, yogurt, and cheese; greens such as broccoli, collards, and kale; small fish—like sardines—eaten with the bones; beans; and calcium-fortified juice. All adults lose bone mass as they age, beginning at about age 40. When enough is lost, bones become fragile and can break. High calcium intake during the growing years can help build up more bone mass so that even though bone is lost, enough is left to protect against bone fractures. Some studies suggest that calcium can help lower blood pressure in older people and can also lower the risk for colon cancer. A study of 497 women found that daily doses of 1,200 milligrams of calcium reduced symptoms of premenstrual syndrome (PMS) by 54 percent. The Adequate Intake (AI) for calcium is 1,000 milligrams a day for adults age 19 to 50 years and 1,200 milligrams for those age 51 and over. The average daily calcium intake of women ranges between 400 and 600 milligrams.

CALORIES—A measure of the energy in food. We get calories whenever we eat CARBOHYDRATE, FAT, or PROTEIN. One gram of carbohydrate or protein has 4 calories while 1 gram of fat has a whopping 9.

CARBOHYDRATES—Sugars and starches—both those that can be digested, and cellulose and other fibers, which cannot. Over 50 percent of the calories (energy) in the average American diet comes from carbohydrates. A healthy intake is considered to be between 50 and 60 percent of total calories eaten. It's best to limit the amount of sugars you eat as sweets because they usually come without other useful nutrients. Eat more of the sugars in fruits and fruit juices instead. These come with vitamins, minerals, and other healthy plant substances. The Daily Value (DV) for carbohydrates for a 2,000 calorie diet is 300 grams.

CARCINOGEN—A cancer-causing substance that may be man-made, such as nitrites, or natural, like sassafras. Food often carries carcinogens into the body.

CARDIOVASCULAR DISEASES—Diseases affecting the heart and blood vessels, such as heart disease and stroke. These diseases are the leading causes of death and disability in the U.S. In 1996 nearly a million people died of heart disease and stroke, and an estimated $150 billion was spent to treat them. Major risk factors for these diseases are overweight, high blood pressure, and high CHOLESTEROL.

CAROB—Also known as St. John's Bread, carob is a long, edible, sweet pod. When the pod is ground it looks like cocoa (but doesn't taste like it). Some people use it in place of cocoa because it contains no stimulants while cocoa does.

CHERIMOYA—Also known as a custard apple because of its custardy texture, its flavor is a combination of many fruits—papaya, pineapple, and banana. Different varieties of cherimoya have slightly different flavors. The sweet and juicy flesh contains many inedible black seeds that must be removed before eating. Cherimoyas are a good source of vitamin C.

CHOLESTEROL—A white, waxy, fatlike substance that is part of every cell in the body. Hormones (including sex hormones), nerve coverings, vitamin D, bile (used in digestion), and the sebum that keeps your skin soft are all made from cholesterol. Cholesterol also makes up a major part of your brain. The body needs it to function normally. But when the level of cholesterol in your blood gets too high, it's not healthy. Some of the extra cholesterol can be deposited on the artery wall, narrowing it and interfering with normal blood flow. Every 1 percent rise in blood cho-

lesterol increases the risk of heart disease by 2 percent. We make some cholesterol in our body and we get some added cholesterol every time we eat any animal foods like meat, fish, poultry, milk, cheese, and eggs. Egg yolks, caviar, and organ meats, such as liver and brains, are very high in cholesterol. Most experts suggest that people limit cholesterol in food to 300 milligrams or less a day. The average cholesterol intake of Americans is over 400 milligrams a day.

CHOLINE—Sometimes classified as one of the B vitamin family, choline doesn't really fit the description of a vitamin because it can be made in the body. It is found in many foods, including beans, eggs, liver, nuts, wheat germ, wheat bran, and cabbage. Choline is part of the neurotransmitters, substances that carry messages from nerve cell to nerve cell—which is the basis for the belief that choline and lecithin, which contains choline, might help improve memory. Unfortunately, studies of choline and lecithin supplements did not seem to bear this out. In 1998, the Food and Nutrition Board issued recommended levels for choline intake. The AI (Adequate Intake), the amount believed to cover the need for a nutrient, for choline is 550 milligrams a day for men and 425 milligrams for women. Some of this requirement is met by the choline that is made in the body. If you still want to try choline supplements, be aware that taking large amounts can make you smell like a fish.

CHROMIUM—An essential mineral needed in tiny amounts in the body. It works along with insulin to move glucose (blood sugar) into the cells where the energy is released. It also plays a role in the body's use of fat and protein. A chromium deficiency may be a factor in some cases of diabetes that develop in older people. Chromium picolinate is a popular supplement advertised as an aid to weight loss, a muscle builder, and body fat reducer. None of these claims has been supported by research. Experts have warned against long-term use of high doses of chromium supplements because studies in animals suggest that it can cause gene damage. Good food sources of chromium are whole-grain breads and cereals, beans, meat, peanut butter, potatoes, brewer's yeast, broccoli, and mushrooms. The Estimated Safe and Adequate Daily Dietary Intake for chromium for adults is 50 to 200 micrograms. Intake of average Americans is only 25 micrograms for women and 33 for men.

COPPER—An essential mineral needed in tiny amounts in the body. It helps maintain a strong immune system, and is part of several enzymes involved in energy release, skin pigment production, and iron absorption. Excess zinc intake interferes with copper absorption and can cause a copper deficiency. Good food sources of copper are grains, nuts, liver, and beans. The Estimated Safe and Adequate Daily Dietary Intake of copper for adults is 1.5 to 3 milligrams, but most people get less, only 1 milligram a day. An FDA diet study found that estimated intakes of copper were below recommendations for all age groups.

CREATINE—An AMINO ACID that plays an essential part in the release of energy when muscles contract. The daily requirement for a normally active man is about 2 grams. Creatine is made in the body and is also found in meats, milk, and some fish. It is also available as a supplement. When creatine supplements are taken in large amounts, it is an effective muscle builder and can enhance performance. Because it is considered a nutritional supple-

ment, it is available without a prescription and is widely used by professional athletes. It is estimated that 50 percent of college and high school athletes are using it. Creatine is available as a powder, pill, gel, liquid, or candy and in 1997 racked up $200 million in sales in the U.S. There are no long-term studies of the effects of using creatine, but there are reports of diarrhea, dizziness, nausea, and muscle cramping in users. Creatine supplements also increase the risk of dehydration and gouty arthritis. Questions have been raised about the safety of creatine because of the deaths of three college wrestlers who had used it, but creatine was found not to be responsible for these deaths. There also was a report of a soccer player developing reduced kidney function while taking creatine. People with kidney problems are advised not to take the supplement. The FDA recommended that consumers get medical advice before taking a creatine supplement, as they would with any other dietary supplements.

DAIKON—A white Asian radish that can be eaten raw but is commonly eaten dried and pickled.

DAILY VALUE (DV)—DVs are used on NUTRITION LABELS as reference numbers. These numbers are set by the USDA and are based on current nutrition recommendations. The percent daily values (DV) are based on a 2,000 calorie diet; values are also calculated for an optional 2,500 calorie diet. These calorie levels cover the average intakes of most people, but they do not cover everyone. The DVs for total fat, saturated fat, cholesterol, and sodium set upper limits for the amount to eat each day to stay healthy. For total carbohydrate, fiber, vitamins, and minerals, DVs show the best levels to aim for each day.

DIABETES—A disease in which there is a high level of sugar (glucose) in the blood caused by either a lack of insulin or insulin that does not work normally. (Insulin is the hormone that controls blood sugar.) There are two main types of diabetes: Type 1, or insulin-dependent diabetes, and Type 2, noninsulin-dependent diabetes (the name is misleading because about one-third of people with this kind of diabetes do use insulin). Type 2 is more common, affecting about 14 million Americans (90 percent of all diabetics). The best defense against Type 2 is to stay slim. Other risk factors are age, lack of exercise, and family history of diabetes. For both types, the goal is to keep the blood sugar as close to normal as possible. That is accomplished for most people with Type 2 by weight loss, exercise, and diet; some people will also require oral medication or insulin at some point. People with Type 1 diabetes usually need to take insulin and to eat regular meals and snacks in prescribed amounts to control blood sugar levels.

DIARRHEA—Frequent, loose, watery stools caused by a virus, bacteria, food intolerance, food poisoning, or infection are both common and uncomfortable. There are many home remedies for the treatment of diarrhea. The BRAT diet—bananas, rice, applesauce, and tea or toast—offered in frequent, small, feedings is often helpful.

DIET—The usual foods and drinks eaten by an individual or group. But the term diet often means having certain foods and drinks in specified amounts at certain times to achieve weight loss or for some other healing effect.

DIETARY GUIDELINES FOR AMERICANS—The Guidelines are the federal government's advice about diets for healthy Americans ages 2 years and over. The fourth edition was released in 1995:

- Eat a variety of foods.
- Balance the food you eat with physical activity—maintain or improve your weight.
- Choose a diet with plenty of grain products, vegetables, and fruits.
- Choose a diet low in fat, saturated fat, and cholesterol.
- Choose a diet moderate in sugars.
- Choose a diet moderate in salt and sodium.
- If you drink alcoholic beverages, do so in moderation.

DIURETICS—Commonly referred to as "water pills," diuretics remove fluids from the body by increasing the flow of urine. Alcohol, caffeine, and water also act as diuretics and increase urine flow.

DOUBLE BLIND EXPERIMENT—In this type of experiment neither the test subjects nor the researchers performing the test know which subjects are being given the real treatment and which are receiving a PLACEBO. This keeps researchers from making biased interpretations as the results are being gathered.

ECHINACEA—An herb that reduces symptoms of colds. Studies suggest that this herb may help keep the immune system healthy and let the body fight off disease-causing bacteria and viruses. Although echinacea is not considered toxic, it's best not to take it daily. Check with your health care provider before you begin taking any herbs.

EDIBLE FLOWERS—Flowers that can safely be used in salads and for edible decoration include roses, pansies, nasturtiums, day lilies, sesbania, marigolds, hibiscus, jasmine, and squash blossoms—fun to eat and delicious. Some flowers are pretty to look at but dangerous to eat—lilies of the valley, sweet peas, and delphiniums, to name a few. That also goes for all flowers that have been sprayed with pesticide.

E. COLI—The *Eschericia* group of bacteria is normally found in the intestines of animals and people. It is a health problem when it appears in water, through contamination by animal or human feces, and in foods. One strain of this bacteria, *E. coli* 015:H, can cause serious symptoms, including severe stomach cramps and watery diarrhea, and in a small percentage of the cases, it progresses to serious kidney disease. Recently these deadly strains of bacteria were found in ground beef, fruits, vegetables, and unpasteurized apple cider and milk. Fruits and vegetables can be contaminated from fertilization with raw manure and irrigation with contaminated water. *E. coli* can be passed along by accidental contact of animal products with fecal matter during processing or by infected food handlers who have not properly washed their hands before touching food. Thorough cooking of all meats; avoiding unpasteurized fruit and vegetable juices, milk, and milk products; carefully washing fruits and vegetables in clean water; and washing hands thoroughly after using the bathroom and before preparing or eating food will reduce the risk of *E. coli* contamination.

ENZYME—Proteins that speed up chemical reactions in the body. They help break down substances, build up substances, and change some substances into others. Enzymes are not used up in these activities. Many enzymes are simply protein, while others need to have a vitamin or mineral attached (coenzyme) to the protein part. The names of many enzymes begin with the name of the substance they act on and end in *ase*. For example, lactase is an enzyme that digests lactose, or milk sugar.

EQUAL (ASPARTAME)—Also known as Nutrasweet, this sugar substitute is made of two AMINO ACIDS. It is 200 times sweeter than sugar and contains only 2 calories in the amount equal in sweetness to 1 teaspoon of sugar. It is a general, all-purpose sweetener. People with the inherited disorder PKU (phenylketonuria) are cautioned to limit sources of phenylalanine, an amino acid, including Equal or aspartame. The FDA requires foods containing aspartame to have a label stating that it contains phenylalanine.

ESTIMATED SAFE AND ADEQUATE DAILY DIETARY INTAKE (ESADDI)—These are ranges of values used for nutrients when there is less information on which to base recommendations. Because the toxic level for many of these nutrients may be only a few times the usual intake, upper levels of the range should not be exceeded regularly.

FAT—A concentrated source of calories (energy). It has 9 calories in a gram. A teaspoon of olive oil (about 5 grams) has more than 40 calories. Fat also supplies essential fatty acids, which the body cannot make but which are needed to make hormones. Fat insulates the body, keeping it warm as well as cushioning and protecting vital organs. It is also part of every cell and carries fat-soluble vitamins into the body where they are stored in fat. Fat makes food taste and smell good. Fats in foods slow down digestion so that, after eating, you feel full longer. Eating too much fat is not healthy. Americans, on the average, get about 33 percent of their calories from fat. The Daily Value (DV) for a 2,000 calorie diet is 65 grams or less of total fat. The average American eats almost 90 grams of fat a day. See also LIPOPROTEINS; TRIGLYCERIDES.

FIBER—CARBOHYDRATE that cannot be digested. It is found in plant foods like whole grains, fruits, and vegetables. Adequate fiber keeps your bowels regular, helps regulate weight, helps to control DIABETES, lowers CHOLESTEROL, and protects against some cancers. The average fiber intake in the U.S. is about 15 grams; experts recommend 25 to 30 grams.

FLAVONOIDS—Antioxidants found in fruits, vegetables, TEA, and red WINE. Studies show that people who eat large amounts of flavonoids lower their risk for heart attacks. It is thought that flavonoids may help reduce the formation of artery-clogging plaque.

FLUORIDE—An essential mineral found in tiny amounts in the body, mainly in the bones, teeth, thyroid gland, and skin. Fluoride protects against cavities and helps to stimulate new bone formation. Fluoride is added to the water supply in many areas of the U.S. at levels of 0.7 to 1.2 parts per million, and there is no evidence of harm in people who drink this water over long periods of time. Tea— herbal, green, or regular—is a good source of fluoride as is fluoridated water and fish. Bottled water and home-filtered water may not contain fluoride. The Adequate Intake (AI) is 4 milligrams a day for adult men and 3 for women.

FOLIC ACID—One of the B vitamins, found in green, leafy vegetables and orange juice, folic acid protects against some birth defects and also is becoming recognized as a preventive factor for heart disease. In 1998, the Food and Nutrition Board increased the recommended intake of folic acid to 400 micrograms

for those age 14 and over, with higher levels during pregnancy (600 micrograms) and breast-feeding (500 micrograms). As of January 1998, folic acid was added to flour, cereals, and grains at a level of 140 micrograms for each 100 grams.

FOOD AND DRUG ADMINISTRATION (FDA)—Federal government agency responsible for the wholesomeness and safety of foods sold in interstate commerce, except for meat, poultry, and eggs, which are monitored by the USDA. The FDA also inspects food plants and foods that are imported into the U.S.

FOOD AND DRUG INTERACTION—Drugs and food can each affect your body's reaction to the other. Drugs can change your sense of taste and smell, change appetite, cause nausea and vomiting, decrease nutrient absorption, or replace nutrients in body reactions. Food can change the effectiveness of a drug. Researchers have known for years that when some common blood pressure drugs were taken with grapefruit juice instead of water, much more of the drug got into the blood. Grapefruit juice can increase the effect of other drugs, too. The reaction can be so dangerous that some scientists are now asking that warning labels about the effects of grapefruit juice be put on pill bottles to prevent accidental drug overdoses.

FOOD GUIDE PYRAMID—The Food Guide Pyramid, published by the USDA in 1992, is the first visual guide to eating showing that all foods can fit into a healthy diet. It consists of six sections arranged to show the importance of each section in the diet. The base of the pyramid, its largest section, is bread, cereals, grains, and pasta. The message is that they are the foundation of healthy eating. Resting on this are the vegetable and fruit groups. On top of these and slightly smaller are the milk and meat groups. Last is the small tip of the pyramid representing the small contribution of fat and sweets to a healthy diet. Here is a rundown of each section of the pyramid:

- Bread, Cereal, Rice, and Pasta Group: 6 to 11 servings a day. A serving is 1 slice of bread, 3 to 4 crackers, 1 ounce of ready-to-eat cereal, ½ cup of cooked cereal, pasta, rice, or other grains.

- Vegetable Group: 3 to 5 servings a day. A serving is 1 cup of raw, leafy vegetables, ¾ cup of vegetable juice, ½ cup of other vegetables, cooked or raw.

- Fruit Group: 2 to 4 servings a day. A serving is one medium orange, apple, or banana, ¾ cup of fruit juice, ½ cup of cooked or canned fruit.

- Milk, Yogurt, and Cheese Group: 2 to 3 servings a day. A serving is 1 cup of milk or yogurt, 1½ ounces of natural cheese or 2 ounces of processed cheese.

- Meat, Poultry, Fish, Dry Beans, Eggs, and Nuts Group: 2 to 3 servings a day. A serving is 2 to 3 ounces of cooked lean meat, poultry, and fish; ½ cup of cooked dry beans, 1 egg, ⅓ cup nuts, or 2 tablespoons peanut butter count as 1 ounce of lean meat.

- Fat, Oils, and Sweets: Use sparingly.

FOOD POISONING—Illness caused by foods contaminated with harmful bacteria and other microorganisms. Although you can't see them and most times you cannot smell or taste them, bacteria can get into food during preparation, cooking, serving, or storage. Usual symptoms of food poisoning are DIARRHEA, cramps, fever, headache, and VOMITING.

Symptoms may start as early as half an hour after eating the contaminated food or as long as two weeks later. In healthy people, food poisoning may be uncomfortable but it is usually brief. In the very young, very old, and those with weakened immune systems, it may be more serious, requiring hospitalization, and may even lead to death. The Partnership for Food Safety Education sponsored by the USDA and FDA has put out guidelines under the logo FIGHT BAC on how to keep food safe from bacteria in four steps:

- Clean—Wash hands, utensils, and surfaces with hot soapy water before and after food preparation, and especially after preparing meat, poultry, eggs, or seafood to protect against bacteria. Using a disinfectant cleaner or a mixture of bleach and water on surfaces and antibacterial soap on hands can provide some added protection.
- Separate—Keep raw meat, poultry, eggs, seafood, and their juices away from ready-to-eat foods, and never place cooked food on an unwashed plate that previously held raw meat, poultry, eggs, or seafood.
- Cook—Cook foods to the proper internal temperatures (this varies for different cuts and types of meat and poultry) and check for doneness with a food thermometer. Cook eggs until both the yolk and white are firm.
- Chill—Refrigerate or freeze perishables, prepared food, and leftovers within two hours and make sure the refrigerator is set no higher than 40° F and that the freezer unit is set at 0° F.

GARLIC—Garlic has been used as a folk remedy since ancient times. Throughout history, garlic was used on wounds and parasites and to treat deafness and other ills. Garlic was also considered useful in warding off "the evil eye" and keeping vampires away. To this day, garlic has a reputation as a health food. Some studies suggest that eating large amounts of garlic (up to 20 cloves daily) can kill bacteria, reduce cancer risk, and lower high blood pressure and CHOLESTEROL levels. Experts have criticized the way some of these studies were carried out. A recent well-controlled study failed to show that garlic could lower cholesterol levels.

GAS (FLATULENCE)—We all produce gas—some more, some less. Lucky people expel it as it is produced so it does not make them uncomfortable. Swallowed air contributes to the gas load. Everyone swallows some air when they eat and drink. Mouth breathers swallow more. Eating slowly with a closed mouth and drinking through a straw reduces the amount of air swallowed; chewing gum and drinking soda increases it. You expel swallowed air by burping; so do babies. Bacteria in the intestines ferment undigested food, producing gas. Some foods, like beans, have a well-deserved reputation for causing gas. Other foods—onions, celery, broccoli, cabbage, radishes—are gas producers for some people. If you are bothered by gas, keep a record of what you eat so you'll find out which foods to eat less of.

GINGER—Relieves motion sickness, and a pinch of it in your tea may relieve a stuffy nose and intestinal gas. Researchers have shown that ginger is an ANTIOXIDANT that may help lower cholesterol when used in combination with other spices in Indian dishes. One-half teaspoon of ground ginger equals 2 teaspoons fresh or preserved.

GINKGO BILOBA—Widely used in Europe (as are many other herbs), it has been used to treat short-term memory loss, Alzheimer's Disease, and ringing in the ears. Ginkgo improves blood circulation by dilating blood vessels and so increases blood supply to the brain. Ginkgo also reduces blood clotting. This could cause problems when anticoagulants (blood thinners) are taken along with ginkgo. Be sure to check with your health care provider before taking any herbs.

GINSENG—Used in China for thousands of years as a health tonic, stimulant, and APHRODISIAC, ginseng is called an "adaptogen;" it is believed to improve the body's ability to adapt to stress. However, there is no proof of its effectiveness. Potency of ginseng products varies widely, with some containing mostly fillers. Some ginseng sold in small vials, about 1/3 ounce, can contain up to 34 percent alcohol (that's the equivalent of 68 proof) though most don't show that on the label. Large amounts of ginseng can cause insomnia, diarrhea, and skin eruptions in some users.

GLUCOSE—The sugar circulating in the blood, it provides the body's major source of energy. It comes from the digestion and absorption of CARBOHYDRATES from food and is also made in the liver. Fruits, sweet corn, corn syrup, and honey contain glucose.

GRAM—The basic unit of weight in the metric system. A teaspoon of sugar is equal to 4 grams. A small paper clip weighs 1 gram.

HEALTHY EATING INDEX—The Healthy Eating Index (HEI) was developed by the USDA's Center for Nutrition Policy and Promotion to provide a single measurement of how well a person's diet meets the recommendations in the Dietary Guidelines and the FOOD GUIDE PYRAMID. According to HEI, women generally have healthier diets than men. Those who have completed higher education or who have high incomes tend to have better diets. Smokers have poorer diets than nonsmokers. On a scale of 1 to 100, Americans scored an average of about 60 on the Healthy Eating Index.

HEARTBURN—Also known as acid indigestion, heartburn is a burning sensation felt in the area of the throat and heart. It actually has nothing to do with the heart, but the pain can be so strong that it is often mistaken for a heart attack. It is caused by a backflow of food and acid from the stomach that irritates the food pipe (esophagus). Overeating, alcohol, smoking, fatty or spicy foods, exercising, and lying down after a large meal all increase the risk of heartburn.

HIGH-DENSITY LIPOPROTEINS (HDL)— One kind of lipoprotein (the form in which cholesterol is ferried around in the blood). HDL cholesterol is called "good" cholesterol because it has small amounts of cholesterol and takes the cholesterol away from cells in the artery walls and carries it to the liver, where it is removed from the body. People with higher levels of HDL cholesterol (over 60) have less heart disease. Levels of HDL cholesterol under 35 are considered too low. Every 1 percent increase in HDLs reduces the risk of heart disease by 3 percent. See also LOW-DENSITY LIPOPROTEINS.

HIGH-FRUCTOSE CORN SYRUP (HFCS)— This sweetener, made from corn, is a mixture of glucose and fructose (fruit sugar). It is commonly used to sweeten fruit drinks and soft drinks. Some people experience a laxative effect when they eat more than a tablespoon of HFCS.

HOMOCYSTEINE—High levels of this protein are believed to be a major risk factor for heart disease. High blood levels of homocysteine are reduced with adequate amounts of the B vitamins FOLIC ACID, B_6, and B_{12}.

HOT PEPPERS—The Scoville heat unit is a commonly used method of rating the heat in hot peppers. It was first used in 1912 when Wilbur Scoville invented a test that analyzed the amount of *capsaicin*, the "heating element" in chili peppers. The heat in jalapeño peppers measures from 2,500 to 5,000 units, more or less acceptable for most people. The greater heat of cayenne or Tabasco falls between 30,000 to 50,000 units. A habañero pepper with 100,000 to 300,000 units has more heat than most people would enjoy. Most brand-name salsas have around 400 units.

IODINE—An essential mineral found in the body in tiny amounts. One teaspoon of iodine is all a person needs in a lifetime. But because iodine is not stored in the body, very small amounts are needed regularly. It is used to make thyroid hormones, which help regulate growth and development and also help control METABOLISM. When there is an iodine deficiency, the thyroid gland gets bigger in an attempt to compensate. An enlarged thyroid gland is called a goiter. The iodine level in foods depends on the amount of iodine in the environment where they are grown or produced. Seafood and seaweed are rich sources of iodine, as is iodized salt. Iodine was added to salt in the 1930s to cure the deficiency that was common in some parts of the U.S. The situation is different today because people eat foods grown in all parts of the country, so they usually get enough iodine from food. Additional iodine is obtained from iodine-containing food additives used in food processing and production and from the widespread use of iodized salt. The Recommended Dietary Allowance (RDA) for iodine is 150 micrograms daily for adults—the amount in less than half a teaspoon of iodized salt.

IRON—An essential mineral needed in tiny amounts in the body. Iron is part of the red blood cells, which carry oxygen in the blood. Some enzymes also contain iron, and others need iron to help them build new cells. Iron deficiency can cause anemia. This type of anemia is still fairly common in the U.S. in toddlers, adolescent girls, and women of childbearing age. Iron overload may occur when iron supplements are taken along with a lot of red meat and the body is not iron deficient. Research suggests that excess iron in the body can promote heart disease and increase the risk for cancer. Iron supplements should be taken only when iron deficiency has been established by blood tests. Good food sources of iron are meat, eggs, liver, seafood, vegetables, and whole grain or enriched cereals. Cooking in iron or stainless steel pans increases the amount of iron in the food. The Recommended Dietary Allowance (RDA) is 10 milligrams for adult men, 15 milligrams for adult women up to age 51, and 10 for women over 51. Iron has been added to all breads and grains labeled "enriched." Iron supplements and iron-containing drugs must carry warning labels advising parents to keep iron supplements in their original containers and out of the reach of children if the iron content is 30 milligrams or higher per dose. A high number of serious iron poisonings and some deaths from accidental overdoses in children under 6 prompted this regulation.

IRRADIATION—Irradiation of red meat, approved by the FDA in 1997, has many positive features. It reduces or eliminates common bacteria in meat that can make you sick. It also controls insects and parasites in foods and lengthens the shelf life of some foods by delaying ripening and reducing spoilage. Irradiation has been endorsed by the World Health Organization, the American Medical Association, and the American Dietetic Association. It has been approved for use on dry spices, poultry, fresh fruits, and vegetables. When it is done properly, it does not make food radioactive, affect nutrients, or change taste, appearance, or texture.

JUNK FOOD—An inaccurate term used to describe foods that are high in sugar and/or fat and low in vitamins and minerals. There really is no food that is junk food. All kind of foods can be enjoyed and be part of a healthy diet for most people. Foods that are less nutritious should be eaten in small quantities.

KIWI—What's green, fuzzy, and provides more vitamin C than a glass of orange juice, with 125 percent of your daily requirement for vitamin C? Kiwi, believe it or not, and you can eat the fiber-full skin, too.

LACTOSE INTOLERANCE—An inability to digest milk sugar (lactose) due to decreased amounts of the enzyme lactase. When more milk (and the milk sugar in it) is taken in than the body can digest, GAS, bloating, cramps, and DIARRHEA can result. As infants, most people produce enough lactase, but in many people the amount produced goes down after infancy. In the U.S., the percent of whites with low lactase levels is about 15 percent, 53 percent in Mexican-Americans, 62 percent to 100 percent in Native Americans, 80 percent in African-Americans, and 90 percent in Asian-Americans. Research shows that the majority of people with low lactase levels can tolerate 1 cup of milk with a meal and even 2 cups a day if it is taken in divided portions. Chocolate milk, ice cream, yogurt with live cultures, and most cheeses are better tolerated than plain, lowfat milk. Milk and milk products treated with Lact-Aid are more easily digested.

LICORICE—Used as a flavoring since ancient times and often used in medicines in China, where it is believed to have anti-inflammatory, antibacterial, and anticancer properties. The licorice candy sold in the U.S. usually is flavored with anise oil, not licorice. Anise oil tastes like licorice but does not have the same properties. Licorice that contains real licorice flavoring should not be eaten by people who have high blood pressure, heart trouble, or kidney problems. There are reports of toxic effects—headache, sodium and water retention, heart failure—in people who have eaten large amounts of licorice candy. These effects are caused by glycyrrhiza, a substance found in licorice.

LIPOPROTEINS—Because fat and water don't mix, cholesterol, a fat, is coated with protein so it can travel in the blood, which is mainly water. These packages of protein, cholesterol, and other fats are called lipoproteins.

LITER—A liter is 33.8 fluid ounces, 1.8 fluid ounces more than a quart, which is 32 ounces. Soft drinks and other beverages are often sold in liters.

LOW-DENSITY LIPOPROTEINS (LDL)—LDL CHOLESTEROL is called "bad" cholesterol because it has large amounts of cholesterol that can be deposited in the artery walls. Levels of LDL cholesterol above 130 are considered unhealthy. See also HIGH-DENSITY LIPOPROTEINS.

LYCOPENE—A pigment found in tomatoes, ketchup, tomato sauce, watermelon, and red grapefruit. Recent research suggests that high intake of lycopene, a strong ANTIOXIDANT, may reduce the risk for heart attack and cancers of the prostate, colon, and rectum. Surprisingly, the lycopene is absorbed more easily from cooked tomato products than from raw tomatoes. Absorption is increased even more if some fat is eaten along with the cooked tomatoes.

MAGNESIUM—An essential mineral. The body has less than 1 ounce of it, mainly in the bones. It functions in more than 300 enzymes, in muscle contraction, in blood clotting, and in passing messages from nerve to nerve. Magnesium is part of the green-colored pigment in vegetables (chlorophyll). In addition to green vegetables, magnesium is found in whole grains, beans, nuts, chocolate, and cocoa. In areas where the water is "hard," meaning that it contains the minerals magnesium and calcium, drinking water adds to the intake of these minerals. The Recommended Dietary Allowance (RDA) for magnesium is 350 milligrams a day for adult men and 280 milligrams for women. High intakes of magnesium in supplements can cause DIARRHEA.

MANGANESE—An essential mineral found in the body in very tiny amounts. It functions as part of many enzymes and as an activator for others. Manganese also is needed for bone growth and skin health. Good food sources of manganese are TEA, nuts, legumes, leafy vegetables, and fruit. The Estimated Safe and Adequate Daily Dietary Intake for adults is 2 to 5 milligrams.

MAPLE SYRUP—This sweetener is graded according to color and flavor. Lighter syrups, those graded U.S. Grade A, have a sweet, mild maple flavor. The color of dark syrups, grades

B and C, comes from the minerals in them. They have a stronger flavor.

MEDITERRANEAN DIET PYRAMID—Its full name is the Traditional Healthy Mediterranean Diet Pyramid and it was developed by the Oldways Preservation & Exchange Trust, the Harvard School of Public Health, and the World Health Organization (WHO) Regional Office of Europe. Developers say these guidelines are not intended to be an official recommendation by WHO or Harvard but rather a new way of thinking about WINE, FAT, and healthy diets. It reflects the traditional way of eating in the Mediterranean—the way people of Greece, Crete, and southern Italy were eating in the 1960s. At that time they had the lowest recorded rates of chronic diseases and the highest adult life expectancy. The Mediterranean diet is high in fruits, vegetables, and grains; limited in red meat (eaten no more than a few times a month or not more than 1 ounce a day); 4 to 6 ounces of poultry (3 or 4 times a week); 4 to 6 ounces of fish (3 to 7 times a week); and 1 cup of yogurt and ½ ounce or less of cheese (unless it is low-fat) daily. Beans are put in a separate category with other legumes and nuts, and it is recommended that foods from this category be eaten daily. The Mediterranean diet also includes an optional recommendation for some wine each day. Daily physical activity is also recommended. Olive oil is specified as the major source of fat. Suggested fat intake is between 25 and 40 percent of the calories eaten daily. Critics have disagreed with the recommendations for liberal use of fat, and some question the optional recommendation for wine.

METABOLISM—The sum total of all the chemical reactions that go on in cells.

MG/DL—Abbreviation for milligrams in a deciliter. Blood cholesterol is measured in milligrams. A milligram (mg) is one-thousandth of a gram. The number of milligrams of cholesterol in a deciliter (dl), a little less than ½ cup, is the ratio used to measure cholesterol level in the blood. When describing the cholesterol level of the blood, usually just the number is given.

MICROGRAMS (MCG)—One one-thousandth (.001) of a milligram.

MINERALS—There are 20 to 30 different minerals important in nutrition, which you get by eating a wide variety of foods. Minerals are not a source of energy in the body. They retain their identity and cannot be converted into another form. This indestructibility helps to protect minerals in food; they need no special handling to preserve them. Long soaking or cooking can draw minerals from food into the cooking water, but if the water is used in some other way, such as for gravy, the minerals are not lost. Minerals have many important functions in the body. Some become part of the body, like calcium and phosphorus in bones and teeth and iron in red blood cells; others float in body fluids, giving them certain characteristics that help the body stay in balance.

MISO—A thick, high-protein paste made from soybeans, salt, and a fermenting agent. Sometimes grain, such as rice or barley, is added for flavor. Miso is used to make soup and as a substitute for salt or soy sauce to flavor other foods. It is very high in sodium.

MOLYBDENUM—An essential mineral found in the body in tiny amounts. It functions as part of several enzymes. The amount of molybdenum in food varies depending on where it is grown. Milk, beans, cereals, and whole grains are the best sources. The Estimated Safe and Adequate Daily Dietary Intake for adults is 75 to 250 micrograms.

MONOUNSATURATED FAT—Monounsaturated fat, such olive oil, stays liquid at room temperature but gets cloudy in the refrigerator as it becomes partly solid. Monounsaturated fat has been getting lots of good press lately; it is part of the MEDITERRANEAN DIET. Research suggests that it lowers cholesterol. Foods that are high in monounsaturated fat include oils like olive, canola, peanut, and soybean, and nuts like peanuts, hazelnuts, pistachios, cashews, and pine nuts. Experts recommend that 10 percent or more of the calories eaten each day be monounsaturated fat.

NATIONAL CHOLESTEROL EDUCATION PROGRAM (NCEP)—An educational campaign to help teach Americans how to modify their lifestyles to reduce high CHOLESTEROL levels.

NATIONAL HEALTH AND NUTRITION EXAMINATION SURVEY (NHANES) I, II, and III—A continuing national program to obtain information on the health and nutrition of Americans. During the first nutritional survey, from 1971 to 1974, clinical examinations, biochemical tests, body measurements, and dietary intake were used to evaluate nutrition status. The second survey, from 1976 to 1980, used the same methods as the first. The Hispanic Health and Nutrition Examination Survey (HHANES), from 1982 to 1984, used the same methods as the earlier ones. The third survey, begun in 1988, will continue to survey the participants throughout their lives.

NIACIN—A member of the B vitamin family. It acts as a coenzyme (helper), often along with other B vitamins, in the release of energy from carbohydrate, protein, and fat. Niacin can be made in the body from the amino acid tryptophan. That is why high-protein foods are good sources of the vitamin. High doses of niacin are used to reduce CHOLESTEROL levels. Large doses of the acid form of niacin (not the nicotinamide form) may cause a sensation of burning, flushing, and tingling of the skin. This is called a "niacin flush." Taking large amounts of niacin of any type should be done under the direction of a physician; it is not a do-it-yourself treatment. Good food sources of niacin are meats, fish, poultry, and enriched breads and cereals. The Recommended Dietary Allowance (RDA) for niacin is 16 milligrams a day for males 14 and over and 14 milligrams for females 14 and over. A niacin equivalent is equal to 1 milligram of niacin or 60 milligrams of tryptophan.

NORI—A dark-green sea vegetable, a seaweed, that is dried and formed into sheets, and which is available as nori, which is untoasted, or as sushi nori, which is toasted to bring out the flavor and aroma.

NUTRACEUTICAL (FUNCTIONAL FOODS)—A term originated by Steven L. DeFelice, M.D., who defines it as a food or food-related substance that has a medical or health benefit. A nutraceutical could be a candy bar, soup, a vitamin or mineral supplement, or a diet plan. Examples are calcium-fortified orange juice, fortified high-fiber cereals, sports drinks, and gelatin fortified with vitamin C and calcium. Another example is Benecol margarine, which contains added sitostanol, a natural product made from pine trees. Popular in Finland, just three pats daily have been shown to lower cholesterol by 10 percent.

NUTRITION—The science of food and its nutrients and their relation to health. It is the study of how the contents of food affect our bodies and our health. While many things contribute to health—genetics, sleep, fresh air, exercise, housing, and medical care—the foremost consideration is food. We truly are what we eat.

NUTRITION LABEL—Found on almost all packaged foods, the "Nutrition Facts" label shows how the food fits into the daily diet and also makes it easier to compare one food with another. It lists the amount of calories in a typical serving along with the calories from fat. Total fat, cholesterol, sodium, total carbohydrate, and fiber are given both as numbers and as percentages of the DAILY VALUE (DV). DVs are set by the government and are based on current nutrition recommendations for a typical 2,000-calorie diet. The DV for total fat, saturated fat, cholesterol, and sodium set upper limits on the amount to eat to stay healthy. For total carbohydrate, fiber, vitamins, and minerals, DVs show the best levels to aim for. Foods in small packages and snack-size candies don't need nutrition labels. Neither do foods like coffee, tea, and most spices that do not have significant amounts of any nutrient.

OBESITY—Excess fat accumulation in the body. Under the new government standards, one-third of the U.S. population is considered obese. Recently, the American Heart Association Nutrition Committee named obesity as a major risk factor for coronary heart disease and noted that a modest weight loss of 5 to 10 percent of body weight can decrease blood pressure and total blood CHOLESTEROL, improve DIABETES symptoms, and reduce sleep apnea (breathing interruptions while sleeping).

OLEAN (OLESTRA)—It looks like fat, it tastes like fat, it can be used in frying, yet it has no calories. With olean, you can have fat-free snacks like potato chips that taste like the real thing. Olean is made from sugar and vegetable oil and was approved by the FDA in 1996 for use in snack foods like chips and crackers. Unlike ordinary fat, the olean molecule is so large that it cannot be digested. Without digestion, no calories are absorbed. Olean binds with fat-soluble vitamins A, D, E, K, and carotenoids so they are not absorbed either. The four vitamins are added back to compensate for this, but the carotene is not. Because it isn't digested, olean can have a laxative effect especially if eaten in large amounts. Products made with olean must have a label stating that they may cause cramping and loose stools.

OMEGA-3 FATTY ACIDS—Polyunsaturated fatty acids found in fish that function as hormone-like substances in the body. They are involved in many body functions, such as blood pressure, reproduction, and muscle contractions. Eicosapentaenoic acid (EPA) and docosahexaenoic acid (DHA) are two omega-3 fatty acids found in fish oils; they have been used to lower high TRIGLYCERIDES in the blood. Another omega-3 fatty acid, alpha-linolenic acid, is found in walnuts, Brazil nuts, soybeans, soy and canola oil, and the common weed purslane.

ONIONS—One of the most widely used vegetables in the U.S. They improve the flavor of many dishes and, as a bonus, they contain the antioxidant allicin. Have you ever wondered what it is in onions that makes your eyes tear? It's proanethial S-oxide. This chemical evaporates quickly as the onion is sliced. When it comes in contact with the water surrounding the eyes, it undergoes a chemical change into sulfuric acid, which stings the eyes and causes them to tear. Frequent onion slicers become more tolerant and produce less tears.

ORGANIC—Crops grown using only natural fertilizers or composts—but no chemical pesticides, fertilizers, or synthetic additives. Some states have established standards for foods that are advertised or labeled organic. Late in 1997, the USDA released its proposed rule for national standards for organic foods. The Department of Agriculture's organic seal may be used only on raw products that are 100 percent organic—grown and manufactured without the use of added hormones, pesticides, or synthetic fertilizers. Processed foods must contain at least 95 percent organic ingredients. Products containing 50 to 95 percent organic ingredients may be labeled "made with certain organic ingredients." Products with less than 50 percent organic ingredients can use the word "organic" only in the list of ingredients. Land on which organic products are grown cannot have pesticides applied for at least three years before harvesting an organic crop. Organically raised animals cannot be given hormones or antibiotics to stimulate growth and must be fed organic feeds. Sales of organic food have been increasing more than 20 percent a year since 1990; organic food is a $3.5 billion-a-year industry.

OSTEOPOROSIS—Osteoporosis affects 28 million Americans, 80 percent of them women. It is the contributing factor in more than 1.5 million bone fractures a year with an annual health care cost of $18 billion. Osteoporosis is usually painless, and often the first sign of the disease is a fracture. Bone loss can start as early as age 40 or younger, but during the first few years after menopause the loss is accelerated and women can lose 2 to 4 percent of total bone mass each year. Although osteoporosis mainly affects women, particularly slender white or Asian women, by age 75, one-third of all men will have it, too. Other risk factors include a family history of osteoporosis, early menopause, alcohol abuse, high caffeine intake, cigarette smoking, inactivity, and low intake of calcium. The best way to avoid osteoporosis is by prevention. You can maximize bone mass by getting enough CALCIUM, VITAMIN D, and exercise early in life. This can help bones stay strong throughout life.

PANTOTHENIC ACID—One of the family of B VITAMINS, pantothenic acid is part of coenzyme A, which is involved in processing carbohydrate, protein, and fat. At one time, pantothenic acid was tried as a way to restore gray hair to its previous color. This was believed possible because research animals that were made deficient in pantothenic acid turned gray. Unfortunately, it didn't work. Pantothenic acid is found in many foods; good sources include meat, fish, poultry, whole grains, and beans. The Adequate Intake (AI) for adults is 5 milligrams a day.

PHOSPHORUS—Found in bones and teeth, phosphorus plays a part in almost all body reactions and is part of every cell. Foods rich in phosphorus include milk, cheese, meats, whole grain cereals, beans, phosphate food additives, colas, and other sodas. For adults, the Recommended Dietary Allowance (RDA) is 700 milligrams a day.

PHYTOCHEMICALS—"Phyto" is the Greek word for plant. Fruits, vegetables, and other plants such as tea are rich sources of phytochemicals that seem to reduce the risk of chronic diseases like cancer and heart disease.

Current research trials are using phytochemicals as a treatment for existing cancers.

PLACEBO—When people are given sugar pills (an inactive substance) to relieve a symptom and they get results, this is known as a placebo effect—a result of the expectation that they would be helped by the "pill" even though no real treatment was given. A placebo is often used in research on one group of people to compare its results with that of a second group who were given an active substance.

POLYUNSATURATED FAT—Polyunsaturated fats are liquid at room temperature. These fats help lower CHOLESTEROL levels in the blood, but too much of these fats may not be good. High intake may cause gallbladder disease, depress the immune system, and put you at greater risk for some cancers. Foods high in polyunsaturated fats include corn, salmon, bluefish, soft margarine, mayonnaise, wheat germ, and soybean, walnut, and sesame oils. The recommended intake of polyunsaturated fat is 10 percent or less of daily total calories.

POTASSIUM—A mineral found in many foods such as meat, bananas, potatoes, tomatoes, and oranges, potassium helps maintain balance in the body and is part of enzyme reactions. Some high blood pressure medications increase the need for potassium; using laxatives for a long time also causes potassium loss. Adequate potassium may lower blood pressure and reduce the risk of strokes. The Daily Value (DV) for potassium is 3,500 milligrams.

PROTEIN—Protein is made up of chains of AMINO ACIDS. It is found in every cell of the body and almost all body substances. Protein is used in the growth, repair, and replacing of cells lost in wear and tear on the body. We get all the protein we need to build and maintain our bodies from food. The Recommended Dietary Allowances (RDA) for protein is 63 grams for adult men and 50 grams for women. Many people eat more than that. Good sources of protein are milk, cheese, yogurt, meat, fish, poultry, beans, and nuts.

QUINOA—This nutritious grain is native to South America, where it is ground into flour for tortillas and cereal. Quinoa has a light taste and pleasing texture and, unlike other grains, contains all the necessary amino acids so that it can substitute for meat. It takes only about 12 minutes to cook, but must always be rinsed before cooking.

RECOMMENDED DIETARY ALLOWANCES (RDAs)— RDAs have been published periodically since 1941 by the National Academy of Sciences. They are estimates, based on available scientific knowledge, designed to meet the needs of groups of healthy people over a period of time. The 1989 RDAs are the latest complete revision; these are currently being revised and will be published in a series of reports as DRIs (Dietary Reference Intakes), which will replace the RDAs. Instead of only a single reference, there are now several reference values included in the DRIs:

- Recommended Dietary Allowance (RDA) is the average daily intake that is enough to meet the needs of nearly all healthy individuals in a group.
- Adequate Intake (AI) is used when there is not enough information to set an RDA.
- Tolerable Upper Intake Levels (UL) is the maximum safe level.
- Estimated Average Requirement (EAR) is the nutrient value that meets the es-

timated nutrient need of 50 percent of a group of individuals with similar characteristics.

The current RDAs will remain in use until they are gradually replaced by the new DRIs.

RIBOFLAVIN—Also known as vitamin B_2, riboflavin is one of the B vitamin family. Riboflavin helps release energy from food and is needed for the health of skin, eyes, lips, and tongue. Good food sources are milk, yogurt, cottage cheese, meat, leafy green vegetables, and yeast. The Recommended Dietary Allowance (RDA) for riboflavin is 1.1 milligrams a day for adult women 19 and older, and 1.3 for adult men 19 and older.

SACCHARIN—Sold under the brand name Sweet 'n Low, this artificial sweetener is about 400 times sweeter than sugar. It provides no calories because it isn't broken down in the body. Saccharin is often combined with other low-calorie sweeteners to mask its bitter aftertaste. It is possibly a carcinogen, but because of the small amounts used, the risk is very minor. The FDA requires foods containing saccharin to have the following label: "Use of this product may be hazardous to your health. This product contains saccharin which has been determined to cause cancer in laboratory animals."

SALMONELLA—Salmonella bacteria is the most common cause of food poisoning. These bacteria are found in some raw or undercooked foods, including poultry, eggs, meat, and unpasteurized milk and other dairy products. Symptoms of salmonella food poisoning are headache, stomach ache, DIARRHEA, fever, and nausea, which usually begin 8 to 48 hours after eating contaminated food. The symptoms last from one to eight days. To avoid food poisoning from salmonella, thaw poultry and meat in the refrigerator or microwave and cook right after thawing. Watch out for cross-contamination of raw and cooked foods and the utensils and surfaces that have contact with foods. Never eat unpasteurized, raw, or undercooked animal foods. Reheat leftovers until steaming hot. Eggs should be fully cooked and never eaten raw. Always wash hands in warm, soapy water after going to the bathroom and before preparing or eating food.

SALSA—This spicy condiment, usually made with tomatoes, peppers, and onions, is outselling ketchup. The USDA recently announced that commercially made salsas can qualify as a vegetable in school lunch programs. It was explained that, unlike ketchup, which is high in sugar and did not qualify, salsa is essentially a vegetable salad. You can make salsa more like a salad at home by adding chopped raw vegetables.

SATURATED FAT—Saturated fat is solid at room temperature. If you leave a stick of butter (high in saturated fat) on the kitchen counter all day, it will soften but it won't melt. Research shows that eating saturated fat raises blood CHOLESTEROL levels. People with high cholesterol levels are at greater risk for a heart attack. There are different types of saturated fats. Not all saturated fats raise cholesterol; foods can contain some saturated fat that raises cholesterol and some that does not. The Daily Value (DV) for a 2,000 calorie diet is 20 grams or less of saturated fat.

SELENIUM—Tiny amounts of the essential mineral selenium are found in the body, where it acts as an ANTIOXIDANT along with vitamin E to protect body substances from oxidation. A study using selenium supplements in people who had a history of skin cancer suggested that, while the supplements did not prevent the development of new skin cancers, they did lower the risk of developing lung, colon, and prostate cancers. A recent Harvard study suggested that eating foods rich in selenium may keep men from getting advanced prostate cancer. Another study showed that people with low levels of selenium in their blood were 3 times as likely to die of a heart attack. Selenium supplements of about 200 micrograms a day have been shown to make subjects feel better, less anxious, more confident and energetic. Seafood, liver, Brazil nuts, dairy products, and meats are good sources of selenium. The amount of selenium in grains depends on the soil in which they are grown. The Recommended Dietary Allowance (RDA) for selenium is 70 micrograms for adult men and 55 for women. Americans get about 100 micrograms of selenium a day. Intakes of 750 to 850 micrograms a day can be toxic.

SELL BY OR PULL DATE—The sell by or pull date shows the last day a product should be offered for sale. This allows time for home use when stored properly. The label may read "January 9" or "sell by January 9". If a food has a long shelf life, the sell by or pull date may also include a year. For some foods, like bread, only the day of the week is given. These sell by dates are usually used on foods such as dairy products, baked goods, and meats that are more or less perishable. Other foods can be labeled "Best if used by January 9, 2000." Cereals and snacks often have this kind of label. Packaged yeast and refrigerated dough may be labeled "Use by January 9, 2000." This is the last day the item should be used.

SOBA—Tan-colored Japanese buckwheat noodles. These are delicious and a great source of protein and fiber. Often served cold with a peanut butter–based sauce, they are also used for dipping and in hot soups.

SODIUM—A major mineral essential to life. It keeps the body in balance, helps muscles contract, and carries signals from one nerve to another. Almost all foods contain sodium, either naturally or as added salt. Table salt is simply the mineral sodium combined with chloride, another mineral. Americans eat 2 to 3 teaspoons of salt a day. That's the equivalent of 4,000 to 6,000 milligrams of sodium. Most of this comes from the salt added to processed foods. We could get along with much less. High sodium intake makes it harder to treat high blood pressure and also causes more calcium to be lost in the urine. Eating less salt may help reduce high blood pressure and may also reduce the risk for osteoporosis. The Daily Value (DV) sodium intake is less than 2,400 milligrams.

SOY—Soy foods have been studied for their health benefits. Research has shown that eating a cup of soybeans a day will lower CHOLESTEROL. Soybeans contain a group of PHYTOCHEMICALS called isoflavones or phytoestrogens (genistein and daidzein). These are weak estrogens that may block the activity of other estrogens in the body. In that way, soy isoflavones may help reduce the risk of breast cancer.

ST. JOHN'S WORT—St. John's wort, an herbal remedy used to treat mild to moderate depression, has been in use for hundreds of years in Germany. It has become very popular in the U.S., with sales increasing by 1,900 percent between 1995 and 1997. A review of a number of studies concluded that extracts of St. John's wort were better than a PLACEBO for treating mild to moderate depression and that the herb may work as well as some standard drugs used for depression. St. John's wort has also been reported to have on antiviral effect, to relieve anxiety, to improve immune function, and to help insomnia. Be sure to check with your health care provider before taking any herbs.

SUCRALOSE—Sold as Splenda, this artificial sweetener was approved by the Food and Drug Administration in April 1998. Six hundred times sweeter than sugar and with no calories, sucralose will be used in soda, gum, baked goods, frozen desserts, and other foods.

SULFITES—Sulfites like sodium and potassium bisulfite, sulfur dioxide, and sodium sulfite are used to eliminate bacteria, preserve freshness and brightness, prevent browning, and increase the storage life of foods. They have been used as food preservatives for centuries. Sulfites are used on dried fruits, processed potatoes, fresh shrimp, imported peppers, and in wines. They are not removed by washing. Foods containing more than ten parts per million of added sulfites must have a warning label because some people may react to them.

SURIMI—A shellfish substitute made from Alaskan pollack, a whitefish of the cod family, Surimi is shaped and dyed to resemble crab, lobster, shrimp, and scallops. It sells at half the price of real shellfish and is very convenient to use but is high in sodium.

TEA—The most popular beverage in the world, second only to water. A cup of tea (black or green) has only half as much caffeine as a cup of coffee, only a few calories (before sugar and/or cream are added), and is a source of antioxidants and the mineral fluoride. In fact, studies show that one cup of green or black tea a day can keep the dentist at bay by actually strengthening tooth enamel and reducing plaque formation.

TOFU—Also called bean curd. A bland, cheeselike cake formed from soy milk with a coagulant added. When it is coagulated with calcium sulfate, the resulting curd is a good source of CALCIUM. Ounce for ounce, tofu has as much PROTEIN as meat. Firm tofu is often used as a meat substitute, while soft or silken (custard) tofu is good in recipes that call for blending it with other ingredients. It is a good substitute for cottage cheese. An added bonus is that tofu is easily digested and, though made from beans, is not likely to cause gas.

TRANS FATTY ACIDS—When liquid oils are hardened to make margarine and solid shortenings, some of the unsaturated fats become trans fatty acids, which, like saturated fat, can raise CHOLESTEROL. They are listed in the ingredients as "partially hydrogenated" or "hydrogenated vegetable oils." Besides margarine and shortening, trans fatty acids are found in cookies, crackers, chips, and other processed foods. Research suggests that trans fatty acids increase the risk of heart disease in the same way that saturated fat does. Trans fat is not listed separately on food labels; it is included in total fat. Americans get about one-fourth of their trans fatty acids from margarine.

TRIGLYCERIDES—Almost all the fats and oil in food and the fat in our bodies is in the form of triglycerides. Research suggests that high levels of triglycerides in the blood may be a risk factor for heart disease. Overweight is a major cause of high triglycerides and, in some people, sugar and/or large amounts of alcohol may have the same effect. Levels of triglycerides above 200 milligrams are considered too high. Some studies show that fish oil supplements can reduce triglyceride levels in the blood.

UNITED STATES DEPARTMENT OF AGRICULTURE (USDA)—A government agency responsible for monitoring the wholesomeness and quality of meat, poultry, and eggs produced in the U.S. The USDA hotline number for consumer questions is 1-800-535-4555. Other activities of the USDA include conducting nutrition research and public education programs and administering the Women, Infants, and Children Supplemental Food Program (WIC), and the School Lunch and Breakfast Programs on the national level.

U.S. RECOMMENDED DAILY VALUES—U.S. Recommended Daily Values for nutrition labeling refer to two sets of standards: RDIs (Reference Daily Intakes) are standards used for nutrition labeling that were formerly known as the USRDA. They use the 1968 RDA values for vitamins, minerals, and protein; and the DRV (Daily Reference Values) are values for other nutrients not included in the RDA.

VEGETARIANS—It's hard to define what vegetarianism is because there are many kinds of vegetarians with different eating habits. Some have no animal foods at all (vegan), eating only plant foods—fruits, vegetables, nuts, seeds, and grains. Others may eat these foods plus milk (lacto-vegetarian), or all plant foods with the addition of eggs (ovo-vegetarian). People who eat plant foods plus eggs and milk (lacto-ovo-vegetarians) make up the largest group of traditional vegetarians. Vegetarian eating is healthy. Studies (mostly done with lacto-ovo-vegetarians) show they are leaner and less likely to have heart disease, cancer, and diabetes. A lacto-ovo-vegetarian diet provides all the nutrients needed for good health; this is the kind of vegetarian diet recommended for growing children. Vegans, with more limited diets, need to be sure to get enough vitamins B_{12} and D and the minerals calcium, iron, and zinc. Fortified foods and supplements can be used. Today, many people eat what has been called a semi-vegetarian diet in which they eat some animal products like fish, eggs, and milk but do not eat "red meat." Vegetarian eating has become so popular that almost all restaurants offer at least one vegetarian entree.

VITAMIN A—Found in both animal and plant foods. In plant foods, it is BETA-CAROTENE, one of the pigments that color plants; all deep-yellow and orange vegetables and fruits have the plant form of vitamin A. Green vegetables are also rich in beta-carotene, but the color is masked by the green pigment chlorophyll. Taking large amounts of vitamin A supplements may not be safe. When added to the vitamin A in foods you eat, they can raise your intake to dangerous levels. Adults can be poisoned when they take doses equal to 10 times the Recommended Dietary Allowance (RDA). In children and in pregnant women, vitamin A can be harmful in even much smaller amounts. Retinol, one form of vitamin A used in antiwrinkle creams, is safe to use. A highly toxic form of vitamin A, Accutane, is used to treat severe acne. Because it can cause serious birth defects, Accutane cannot be used by women when they are pregnant or have a chance of becoming pregnant. Some people who overdose on supplements containing too much vitamin A can develop serious symptoms, including hair loss, headache, loss of menstruation, and other problems. Excess beta-carotene is not harmful, but it can turn the skin yellow. Vitamin A is currently measured in retinol equivalents (RE), a measure of the vitamin A activity that the body will get from food, but the amount of vitamin A in foods and supplements is sometimes still measured in international units (IU). The RDA for vitamin A is 1,000 RE a day for men and 800 for women. One RE is equal to 5 IUs, so the RDA for vitamin A in men can be expressed as 5,000 IUs and for women as 4,000.

VITAMIN B COMPLEX—A family of B vitamins including thiamin (B₁), RIBOFLAVIN (B₂), pyridoxine (B₆), cobalamin (B₁₂), biotin, CHOLINE, FOLIC ACID and niacin. These vitamins are usually found together in foods and have some similar roles in the body.

VITAMIN B₁₂—Vitamin B₁₂ has important functions in the body. It is needed for conversion of FOLIC ACID (another B vitamin) to its active form, for energy release, and for the normal functioning of all cells. A deficiency of either folic acid or B₁₂ can cause anemia, and either vitamin can cure it. But if folic acid is given when there is a B₁₂ deficiency (called pernicious anemia), the anemia is cured, but other serious nerve symptoms persist and can lead to permanent damage. B₁₂ is found only in animal foods such as liver, eggs, milk, fish, and meat. To avoid a deficiency, strict vegetarians (vegans) can use vitamin B₁₂-fortified soy milk or a supplement. The Recommended Dietary Allowance (RDA) for vitamin B₁₂ is 2.4 micrograms a day for adults. Because older people may have trouble absorbing B₁₂ from food, those over age 51 are advised to meet their RDA by eating fortified foods or supplements containing it. In years past, B₁₂ shots were often used as a tonic for older people who may or may not have had anemia. It fell out of favor, but a recent study showed that the shots did reduce anemia and also increased bone mineral density in people with pernicious anemia and osteoporosis.

VITAMIN C (Ascorbic acid)—Vitamin C performs a variety of important functions: helping cells cement together, building bones, teeth, and new red blood cells, helping the body resist infection, increasing iron absorption, and helping wounds heal. It works as an ANTIOXIDANT, protecting body cells and substances from damage. Good sources of vitamin C include oranges, grapefruit, strawberries, peppers, and potatoes. A Finnish study concluded that vitamin C deficiency, as shown by low plasma levels, is a risk factor for heart disease. Vitamin C is the second most commonly purchased supplement in the U.S. Large doses (over 2 grams a day) can cause nausea and DIARRHEA and may not be safe for people with diabetes. Excess vitamin C can also interfere with some lab tests such as those for sugar in the urine and blood in the stool. The Recommended Dietary Allowance (RDA) for vitamin C is 60 milligrams a day for people 15 and over. Smokers are advised to take 100 milligrams a day because they use up the vitamin more quickly.

VITAMIN D—Vitamin D aids in the absorption of CALCIUM and maintains normal blood levels of calcium. Vitamin D is different from other vitamins because it can be made in the skin when skin is exposed to sunlight. In fact, about 90 percent of the vitamin D most people get is from casual sun exposure, but the use of sunscreens (with an SPF of 8 or higher) to protect against skin cancer prevents the formation of vitamin D in the skin. People who live in the North or are confined to the home may not have enough sun exposure, and some experts believe that they should take a supplement of 800 IUs a day. Recent studies suggest that many Americans do not get enough vitamin D to protect their bones. A study showed that elderly women taking supplements of calcium and 800 units of vitamin D decreased their risk of hip fracture by 43 percent in two years. Only a few foods are good sources of vitamin D—egg yolk, liver, butter, fortified milk, and margarine. The Recommended Dietary Allowance (RDA) is 200 IUs for adults up to age 50, 400 IUs for ages 51 to 70, and 600 for those over 70.

VITAMIN E (TOCOPHEROL)—A strong ANTIOXIDANT that seems to protect body cells from damage. Earlier claims for this vitamin, when it was referred to as a fertility vitamin and was believed to cure fibrocystic breast disease, are no longer accepted. But more recent studies suggest that vitamin E supplements of at least 100 IUs may protect against heart disease, cancer, cataracts, and other diseases. The Recommended Dietary Allowance (RDA) for vitamin E is small and only a fraction of the 200 to 400 IUs found in many supplements. Natural and synthetic vitamin E are not the same, and a recent study shows that pregnant women should be using the natural form because natural vitamin E can be transferred to the developing baby in greater amounts than the synthetic form. In the ingredient panel on vitamin supplements, natural vitamin E begins with a "d," as in "d-alpha-tocopherol." The synthetic version begins with "dl" as in dl-alpha-tocopherol. Vitamin E is the most commonly purchased single nutrient supplement in the U.S. Food sources of the vitamin are soybeans, sunflower and wheat germ oils, milk, and avocados.

VITAMIN K—Needed for normal blood clotting and bone growth. The daily need is small and can easily be met because many foods contain the vitamin. Good sources are cabbage, lettuce, broccoli, spinach, turnip greens, and liver. In addition, "friendly" bacteria in the digestive tract make a small supply (though not enough to meet the body's need). Babies are born with a sterile digestive tract so they do not make any vitamin K until bacteria take up residence. To protect against bleeding, a single dose of vitamin K is given at birth. The Recommended Dietary Allowance (RDA) for vitamin K is 80 micrograms for adult men and 65 for women.

VITAMINS—Chemicals that help regulate your body's activities. You can think of them as the body's spark plugs. They are vital to your life and health. Although they do not give you energy, they help turn the food you eat into energy you can use. They also help your body grow and your nerves, muscles, and organs work normally. You get vitamins from the foods you eat, and many people get them from supplements, too. A vitamin is something we either cannot make in our bodies or, if we do make it, we don't make as much as we need.

VOMITING—"Throwing up" or forced expulsion of stomach contents out of the mouth can be caused by too much alcohol, an infection, or food poisoning. Vomiting is the way the body gets rid of something irritating. Do not eat anything right after vomiting. After half an hour or so, try a little water. If it stays down, move on to other drinks or try a good home remedy—the thick syrup in canned fruit. It works! For teens and adults, take 2 tablespoons every 10 to 15 minutes. For young children, offer 2 to 3 teaspoons every 10 to 15 minutes.

WASABI (Japanese horseradish)—Used to make a spicy, hot, pale-green condiment that is part of the sushi presentation, wasabi is also used to give a punch of heat to snack foods.

WATER—The average person can go for long periods without food but only for a few days without water. Water is needed in every body process to control body temperature and to maintain normal performance levels. You lose water through sweat even when sitting quietly, when breathing, and through normal elimination. Exercise and hot weather increase water loss. Experts recommend 8 to 12 glasses of water a day, but this does not all have to be plain water. Water from food and beverages plus 6 to 8 glasses of plain water will meet the water need for the average adult. The color of your urine shows you if you are getting enough. It should be pale yellow or clear, and you should make a trip to the bathroom at least every 4 hours.

WELLNESS—A lifestyle that is balanced with appropriate nutrition, exercise, work, and rest so that a person has the best experience from life.

WINE—Drinking wine has been shown to have health benefits. All kinds of wine can be heart healthy, but red wine may be especially beneficial in protecting against heart disease. Substances called phenolic FLAVONOIDS that are extracted from red wine may prevent the buildup of fat that can block arteries. The fats that form these buildups become a problem when they are oxidized. Research suggests that phenolic flavonoids from wine act as ANTIOXIDANTS, preventing fat from oxidizing and accumulating in the arteries. Research in France showed that a daily glass or two of red wine can reduce the risk of heart disease by at least 40 percent. French researchers did the studies to find out why the French people enjoyed a high-fat diet and still had fewer deaths from heart disease. The good news is that the same protective flavonoids in red wine are also found in smaller amounts in purple grape juice. But you'll have to drink three times as much grape juice as wine to get the same amount of flavonoids.

YEAST—A fungus available as baker's yeast, brewer's yeast, and nutritional yeast. Baker's yeast, sold in dry and cake form, ferments sugar to produce alcohol, carbon dioxide, and heat; the carbon dioxide gas bubbles make bread rise and the alcohol evaporate. Nutritional yeast, a concentrated source of B vitamins and protein, is used as a supplement, especially by vegetarians.

ZINC—An essential mineral in the body needed in tiny amounts. It is needed for the function of over 200 different enzymes, helps make protein, and is needed for normal taste and immune function. Correcting a zinc deficiency improves immune function. The Recommended Dietary Allowance (RDA) is 15 milligrams a day for men and 12 for women. An American's average daily intake is between 10 and 15 milligrams of zinc but VEGETARIANS and people on low-protein diets may get less. Meat, fish, poultry, milk and foods made with milk, are the best sources of zinc. Large amounts can interfere with the absorption of other minerals, interfere with immune function, and even be toxic. Zinc supplements of 50 milligrams a day can decrease HDL (good) CHOLESTEROL. Too much zinc (over 100 milligrams a day) is not healthy.

ZINC LOZENGES—Zinc lozenges have become popular as a treatment for the common cold and many people take them at the first sign of one. Ten studies evaluating the use of zinc for colds in adults had mixed results; only half showed a benefit. A recent study in children and adolescents found that the zinc lozenges were not effective in relieving cold symptoms. If you are using zinc lozenges, it's not wise to take additional zinc supplements.